SEIDEL'S GUIDE TO

Physical Examination

AN INTERPROFESSIONAL APPROACH

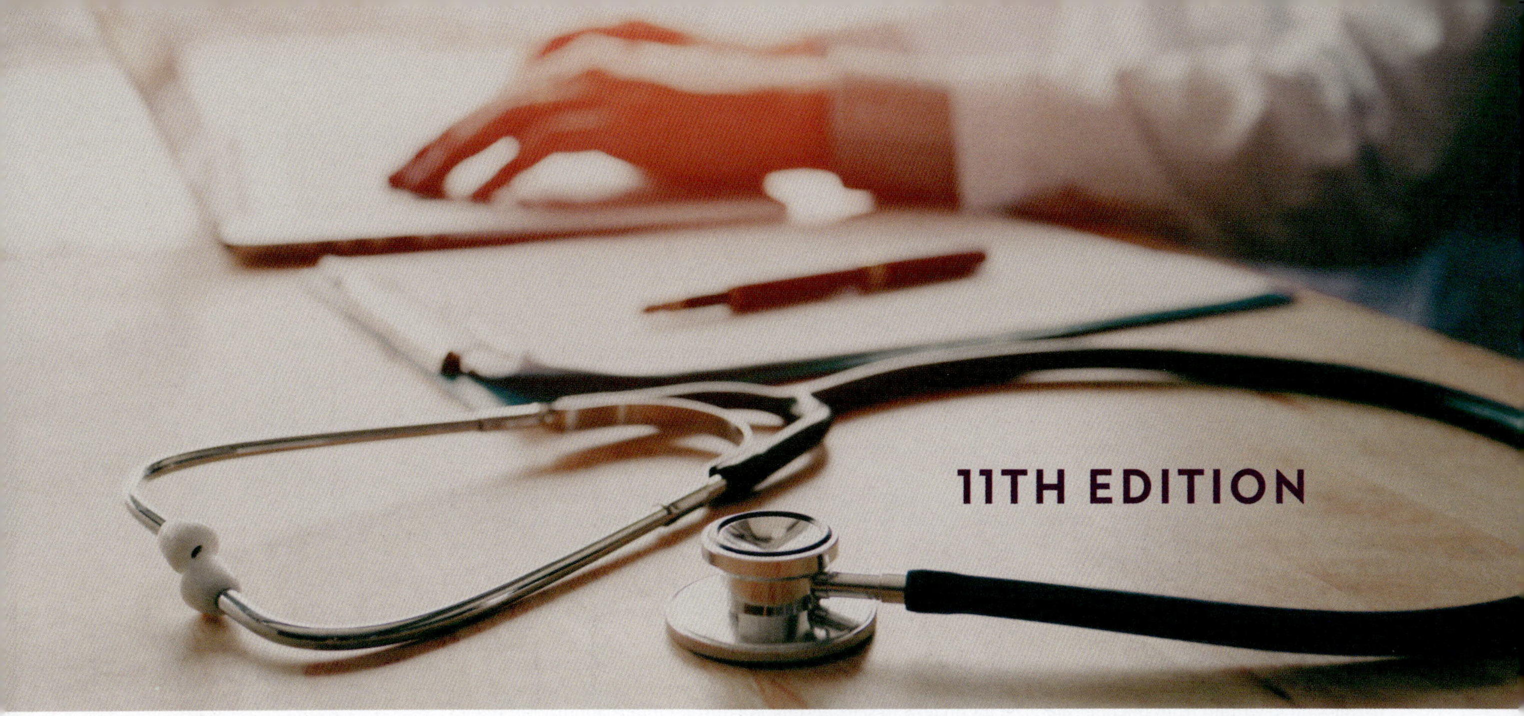

11TH EDITION

SEIDEL'S GUIDE TO

Physical Examination

AN INTERPROFESSIONAL APPROACH

Joyce E. Dains,
DrPH, JD, APRN, FNP-BC, FNAP, FAANP, FAAN
Professor
The University of Texas MD Anderson Cancer Center
Houston, Texas

John A. Flynn,
MD, MBA, MEd
Professor of Medicine
Baylor College of Medicine
Houston, Texas

Joanne Silbert-Flagg,
DNP, CPNP-PC, IBCLC, CNE, FAAN, FAANP
Associate Dean for Clinical Practice
Johns Hopkins University
Baltimore, Maryland
Pediatric Nurse Practitioner
Columbia Medical Practice
Columbia, Maryland

Barry S. Solomon,
MD, MPH
Professor of Pediatrics
Assistant Dean for Medical Student Affairs
The Johns Hopkins University School of Medicine
Baltimore, Maryland

Rosalyn W. Stewart,
MD, MS, MBA
Associate Professor of Internal Medicine and Pediatrics
Johns Hopkins University
Baltimore, Maryland

ELSEVIER

ELSEVIER
3251 Riverport Lane
St. Louis, Missouri 63043

SEIDEL'S GUIDE TO PHYSICAL EXAMINATION:
AN INTERPROFESSIONAL APPROACH, ELEVENTH EDITION ISBN: 978-0-443-34813-6

Content Strategist: Sonya Seigafuse
Content Development Specialist: Elizabeth McCormac
Senior Publishing Services Manager: Deepthi Unni
Project Manager: Prasanna Kalyanaraman
Design Direction: Brian Salisbury

Printed in India

Last digit is the print number: 9 8 7 6 5 4 3 2 1

About the Authors

Joyce E. Dains, DrPH, JD, APRN, FNP-BC, FNAP, FAANP, FAAN

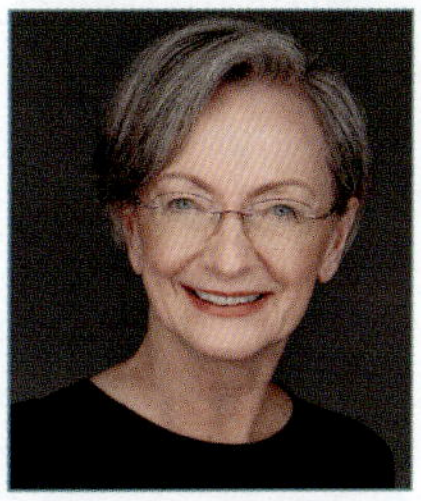

As a board-certified family nurse practitioner with doctorates in both public health and law, Joyce E. Dains has had a rich and productive career in education and clinical practice. She graduated as valedictorian from the New England Baptist Hospital School of Nursing in Boston and subsequently earned a baccalaureate degree in nursing from Boston College, graduating magna cum laude; a master's degree in nursing from Case Western Reserve University; and a doctorate in public health from the University of Texas–Houston. She also completed a postgraduate nurse practitioner program at the Texas Woman's University. She earned her law degree at the University of Houston and practiced law for a brief period. In addition to her current position and affiliation, Dr. Dains has been in clinical practice, teaching, and leadership positions at major universities and medical institutions including the Ohio State University, the University of Texas–Houston, the Texas Woman's University, and Baylor College of Medicine. She has been instrumental in the education of nursing students, nurse practitioners, medical students, and other health care professionals. As a family nurse practitioner, she has maintained a clinical practice in a variety of primary care settings. She is currently at the University of Texas MD Anderson Cancer Center where she is Executive Director for Advanced Practice and a family nurse practitioner in the Cancer Prevention Center. Dr. Dains is a fellow of the American Association of Nurse Practitioners and a fellow of the American Academy of Nursing and is the recipient of other distinguished honors, including election to the National Academies of Practice. Dr. Dains is also the author of Elsevier's *Advanced Health Assessment and Clinical Diagnosis in Primary Care.*

John A. Flynn, MD, MBA, MEd

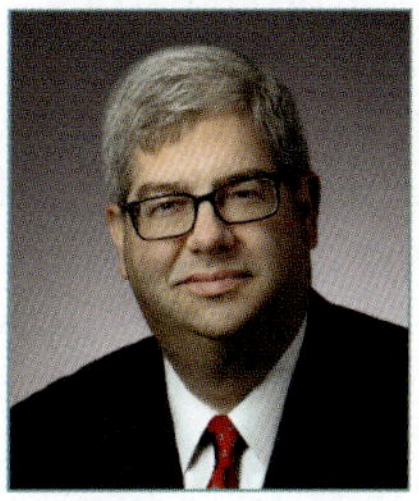

John A. Flynn graduated with a degree in mathematics from Boston College, received his medical degree from the University of Missouri–Columbia, and completed his residency and rheumatology fellowship both at the Johns Hopkins University School of Medicine. He later earned an MBA from Hopkins and a Master of Medical Education from the University of Cincinnati. Board certified in internal medicine and rheumatology, for over 30 years Dr. Flynn held several joint appointments at Johns Hopkins in the Schools of Nursing, Education, and Public Health and has been recognized as a fellow of the American College of Rheumatology and the American College of Physicians. His clinical research focuses on the advancement of care for patients with spondyloarthritis, as well as innovations in ambulatory medical education and clinical practice. At Hopkins, he achieved the rank of Professor of Medicine and served as Vice President of the Office of Johns Hopkins Physicians. Dr. Flynn earned numerous honors at Hopkins where he received the Osler Housestaff Teaching Award, the Chairman's Award for Excellence in Teaching, the Alumni Association Excellence in Teaching Award, and the David M. Levine Award for Excellence in Mentoring. He also won the National Award for Scholarship in Medical Education from the Society of General Internal Medicine, the Young Alumni Award from the University of Missouri–Columbia, and the Clinician Scholar Educator Award from the American College of Rheumatology. At Hopkins, his grateful patients recognized his clinical excellence through the establishment of an endowed professorship in his name. Dr. Flynn then served as Chief Physician and Dean for Clinical Affairs and as President of the University of Chicago Medicine Care Network. Currently he is Professor of Medicine at the Baylor College of Medicine in Houston, Texas. Dr. Flynn has published over 100 book chapters and articles. He has served as an editor of *Cutaneous Medicine: Cutaneous Manifestations of Systemic Disease* and the first and second editions of the *Oxford American Handbook of Clinical Medicine.*

JoAnne Silbert-Flagg, DNP, CPNP-PC, IBCLC, CNE, FAAN, FAANP

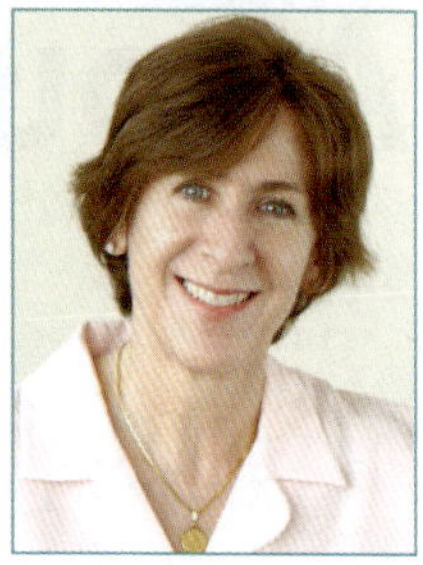

JoAnne Silbert-Flagg graduated from the University of Maryland where she earned her BSN and MSN as a pediatric nurse practitioner. She received her DNP from Columbia University in New York. She is an Associate Professor and the Associate Dean for Clinical Practice at the Johns Hopkins University School of Nursing. She has previously served as Director of the MSN Program and Track Director of the Pediatric Nurse Practitioner Program. She provides primary care to pediatric patients at Columbia Medical Practice. As an International Board of Lactation Consultant (IBCLC), she provides lactation support to parents of infants in the practice. She has provided lactation education to nursing students and teaches the Breastfeeding: Practice and Research course to graduate nursing students. She is coauthor of the National Association of Pediatric Nurse Practitioners (NAPANP) Position Paper Statement on Breastfeeding published in the *Journal of Pediatric Health Care*. She is past chair of the Breastfeeding Expert Panel for the American Academy of Nursing. She is a member of the affiliate staff at Johns Hopkins Howard County Medical Center where she provides care for newborns for admission and discharge. She is also a member of the Center for Equity in Child and Youth Health and Wellbeing. The mission of the Center for Equity in Child and Youth Health and Wellbeing is to advance the health and well-being of infants, children, adolescents, young adults, and their families, particularly those in underserved, under-resourced, and systematically disadvantaged communities locally and globally. She was a coinvestigator with a team from the Bloomberg School of Public Health, through a Health Resources and Services Administration (HRSA) grant, to study the impact of the Baby-Friendly Hospital Initiative in Maryland on selected WIC agency breastfeeding rates and maternal experiences of breastfeeding support.

Barry S. Solomon, MD, MPH

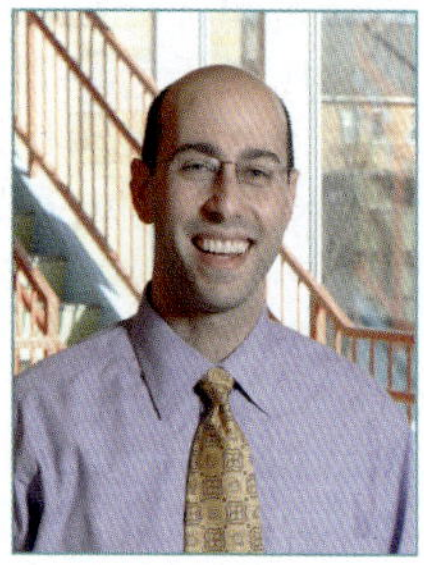

Barry S. Solomon graduated from the University of Pennsylvania School of Medicine and completed his residency at the Children's Hospital of Pittsburgh. He then completed a fellowship in general academic pediatrics at The Johns Hopkins University School of Medicine, during which time he received a master of public health degree from The Johns Hopkins University Bloomberg School of Public Health. Dr. Solomon is currently the Catherine DeAngelis, MD, MPH, and Jackie Julio Endowed Professor of Pediatrics; director of the Division of General Pediatrics; and Assistant Dean for Medical Student Affairs in the School of Medicine. With institutional and community partners, he works to improve health equity by addressing social drivers of health for children and families through innovations in pediatric primary care. Dr. Solomon holds a joint appointment in the Department of Health, Behavior and Society in the Bloomberg School of Public Health, where he conducts research with faculty in the Center for Injury Research and Policy to reduce disparities in childhood injury. For 10 years, as medical director of The Johns Hopkins Children's Center Harriet Lane Clinic, Dr. Solomon developed a nationally recognized model for delivering family-centered care in an urban pediatric primary care setting. Many of the clinic's patients and families experience significant social and financial challenges. Dr. Solomon helped bring a variety of services to the clinic, including a social needs screening and case management program staffed by undergraduates and community health workers. Dr. Solomon is also an active clinical teacher and research mentor to medical students, residents, fellows, and junior faculty. He is a member of the American Academy of Pediatrics, the Society of Pediatric Research, the American Pediatric Society, and past leader of the Academic Pediatric Association. Dr. Solomon's academic career and personal mission have been centered on providing high-quality, family-centered primary care while training new generations of child health professionals to become advocates for vulnerable populations.

Rosalyn W. Stewart, MD, MS, MBA

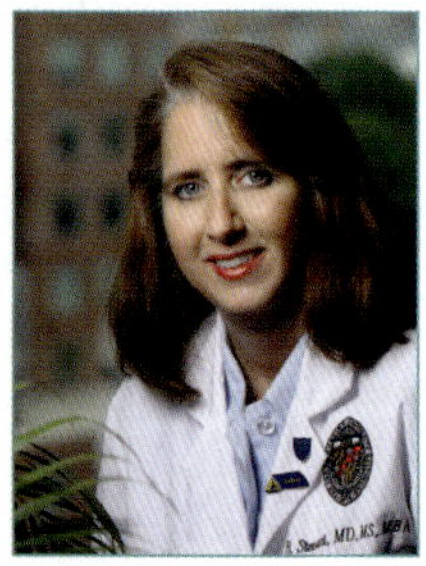

Rosalyn Stewart began her career at the University of Texas Medical Branch where she earned her medical degree and subsequently completed her combined internal medicine–pediatrics residency and a master of science degree in preventive medicine. She is currently a professor of Internal Medicine and Pediatrics at Johns Hopkins University School of Medicine. She completed a master of business administration degree with an emphasis on health care at the Johns Hopkins Carey Business School. She practices general internal medicine, general pediatrics, pediatric hospital medicine, and addiction medicine. Her academic focus is on improving systems of health care delivery for the medically underserved, medical education, the patient care continuum, and health equity. She holds many positions centered on these interests and has been recognized for her ability to carry forth the Osler philosophy, discipline, and practice of medicine. She has been recognized for her teaching acumen, clinical excellence, and clinical innovation by induction into the Miller Coulson Academy of Clinical Excellence and serves as core faculty in the Armstrong Institute of Quality Improvement and Patient Safety. As a clinical program builder, educator, and mentor, the culmination of her efforts is to create medical providers who are leaders and systems-level change agents while providing high-quality, safe, effective, equitable, comprehensive, well-coordinated, person-focused care.

Reviewers and Contributors

Yong Choi, MD
Assistant Professor
Department of Surgery
Baylor College of Medicine
Houston, Texas

Sunjay Devarajan, MD
Assistant Professor
Pulmonary/Critical Care
Department of Medicine
Baylor College of Medicine
Houston, Texas

Christopher LaVergne, MD
Assistant Professor
Cardiology
Department of Medicine
Baylor College of Medicine
Houston, Texas

Oyetewa Oyerinde, MD
Assistant Professor of Dermatology
Specialist in Hair and Scalp Disorders
Director, Skin of Color Clinic
Baylor Medicine Department of Dermatology
Houston, Texas

Joel Ward, DO
System VP of Medical Informatics
CommonSpirit Health

Preface

Seidel's Guide to Physical Examination: An Interprofessional Approach was a landmark text when first published, in part because of the interprofessional team of nurse practitioner and physician authors. The use of interprofessional authors has continued through all editions, and the current team of nurse practitioner and physician authors brings the strengths of their respective disciplines to help students of all health disciplines learn to conduct a patient-centered interview and perform a physical examination. This text is written primarily for students beginning their careers as health care professionals.

The core message of the book is that patients are our central focus and it is an honor to care for them. Learning how to take a history and perform a physical examination is necessary, but it does not provide a full understanding of your patients' lives and health needs. A trusting relationship with your patients most often begins with conversation. Patients will more comfortably share personal and sensitive information when you develop a rapport grounded in respect and curiosity. Such a relationship helps you obtain reliable information and develop a strong therapeutic alliance with the patient and family. You are learning the stories of individuals with unique experiences and cultural heritage, and our interaction with them involves far more than the sum of body parts, systems, and maladies. The art and skills involved in history taking and the physical examination are common to all of us, regardless of our particular health profession or specialty.

Organization

The achievement of a constructive relationship with a patient begins with your mastery of sound history taking and physical examination. Chapter 1 stresses that "knowing" is incomplete without the mutual understanding of cultural backgrounds and differences. Chapter 2 offers vital "getting to know you" guidelines to help you learn about the patient as the patient learns about you. Chapter 3 gives an overview of examination processes and the equipment you will need.

Chapter 4 assists with the process of analyzing the information collected during the history and physical examination and using clinical reasoning to support decision making and problem solving. Chapter 5 provides guidance on recording the information collected into the patient's health record with particular emphasis on the Problem-Oriented Medical Record (POMR) and the use of SOAP (**S**ubjective findings, **O**bjective findings, **A**ssessment, and **P**lan).

Chapters 6 through 8 introduce important elements of assessment: vital signs and pain; mental status; and growth, development, and nutrition. Chapters 9 through 23 discuss specific body systems and body parts, with each chapter divided into four major sections:

- Anatomy and Physiology
- Review of Related History
- Examination and Findings
- Abnormalities

Each of these sections begins with consideration of the adult patient and ends, when appropriate, with variations for infants, children, and adolescents; pregnant persons; older adults; and individuals with disabilities. We have also updated language and content to reflect gender-diverse considerations. Language throughout the book supports the inclusive nature of a physical examination, including physical examination changes related to transgendered persons.

To help you get organized, each chapter starts with a preview of physical examination components discussed. The Anatomy and Physiology sections begin with the physiologic basis for the interpretation of findings as well as the key anatomic landmarks to guide physical examination. The Review of Related History sections detail a specific method of inquiry when a system- or organ-related health issue is discovered during the interview or examination. The Examination and Findings sections list needed equipment and then describe in detail the procedures for the examination and the expected findings. These sections encourage you to develop an approach and sequence that is comfortable for you and also for the patient. In some chapters advanced examination procedures are described for use in specific circumstances or when specific conditions exist. You will note that the terms *normal* and *abnormal* are avoided whenever possible to describe findings because, in our view, these terms suggest a value judgment that may or may not prove valid with experience and additional information. The Abnormalities sections provide an overview of diseases and associated problems relevant to the particular system or body part. The Abnormalities sections include tables clearly listing pathophysiology in one column and patient subjective and objective data in another column for selected conditions. Full-color photos and illustrations are often included.

Chapter 24 details the issues relevant to the sports participation evaluation. Chapter 25 provides guidance for integrating examination of all body systems into an organized sequence and process. Chapter 26 provides guidelines for the change in standard examination approaches in emergency and life-threatening situations. This information is only a beginning and is intended to be useful in your clinical decision making. You will need to access other resources to enhance your knowledge base.

The companion Evolve website content (at http://evolve.elsevier.com/Seidel/) provides clinical tools and resources to document observations or problems and complete the physical examination, preserving a continuous record.

Special Features

The basic structure of the book—with its consistent chapter organization and the inclusion of special considerations sections for infants, children, adolescents, pregnant persons, and older adults—facilitates learning.

- Differential Diagnosis tables—a hallmark of this text—appear throughout the text.
- Evidence-Based Practice in Physical Examination boxes are reminders that our clinical assessment—as much as possible—should be empirically supported.
- Risk Factors boxes highlight modifiable and nonmodifiable risk factors for a variety of conditions.
- Functional Assessment boxes help students to consider specific physical problems and to evaluate their effect on patient function.
- Patient Safety boxes offer guidance about ways to promote patient safety during the physical examination or about patient education that supports safe practices at home.
- Think About It boxes help guide students to the next steps when a particular cluster of findings is noted.

New to This Edition

The entire book has been thoroughly updated for this edition. This includes the replacement of illustrations of abnormal findings with updated photos and the use of new full-color photos and drawings. There are approximately 1200 illustrations in addition to the numerous tables and boxes that have traditionally given readers easy access to information. Among the many changes:

- Evidence-Based Practice in Physical Examination boxes have been thoroughly updated. These boxes focus on the ongoing need to incorporate recent research into clinical practice and decision making.
- Clinical Pearls boxes have been updated and revised.
- The Examination Techniques and Equipment chapter includes updated recommendations for Standard Precautions.
- Updated cancer screening controversies and summary evidence are included in the abdomen, breast, and prostate chapters.
- Information about sensitive and respectful approaches to history taking and physical examination of lesbian, gay, bisexual, and gender-diverse patients has been integrated throughout the book.
- The Emergency or Life-Threatening Situations chapter has been updated.
- The Sports Participation Evaluation chapter includes updated recommendations for assessing and managing patients with sports-related concussions.

Our Ancillary Package

Seidel's Physical Examination Handbook is a concise, pocket-sized companion for clinical experiences. It summarizes, reinforces, and serves as a quick reference to the core content of the textbook.

Student Laboratory Manual for Seidel's Guide to Physical Examination is a practical printed workbook that helps readers integrate the content of the textbook and ensure content mastery through a variety of engaging exercises.

Instructor Resources on the companion Evolve website (http://evolve.elsevier.com/Seidel/) include an extensive electronic image collection and a PowerPoint lecture slide collection that includes integrated animations, case studies, and a series of audience response questions. In addition, *TEACH* provides learning objectives, key terms, nursing curriculum standards, content highlights, teaching strategies, and case studies. Also available on the Evolve website is a thoroughly revised Test Bank in ExamView format, which faculty can use to create customized examinations for medical, allied health, or nursing programs. Together these resources provide the complete building blocks needed for course preparation.

Student Resources on the companion Evolve website include a wide variety of activities, including animations depicting content and processes, review questions that promote clinical reasoning, and downloadable student checklists.

This edition is also available on Elsevier eBooks on VitalSource. Easy-to-use, interactive features let you make highlights, share notes, run instant searches, and much more. You can access your eBook online through Evolve or with apps for PC, Mac, iOS, and Android.

Our Core Values

In the 11th edition of *Seidel's Guide to Physical Examination: An Interprofessional Approach*, we have made every attempt to consider patients in all of their variety and to preserve the fundamental messages explicit in earlier editions. These include the following:

- Respect the patient.
- Achieve the complementary forces of competence and compassion.
- The art and skill essential to history taking and physical examination are the foundation of care; technologic resources complement these processes.

- The history and physical examination are inseparable; they are one.
- The use of technology should not serve as a distraction. Your care and skills are what build a trusting, meaningful relationship with the patient.
- That relationship can be indescribably rewarding.

We hope that you will find this a useful text and that it will continue to serve as a resource as your career evolves.

Acknowledgments

The 11th edition of our textbook is possible only because of the professionalism and skills of so many others who really know how to fashion a book and its ancillaries so that it is maximally useful to you. First, there are those instructors and students who have so thoughtfully and constructively offered comments over the years. Improvements in content and style are often the results of their suggestions. Furthermore, we are very grateful to Paula M. Neira, JD, MSN, RN, CEN, FAAN, clinical program director of the Johns Hopkins Center for Transgender Health, for her previous contributions to providing care to transgender and gender-diverse patients that continue to guide us.

While the authors have provided the content, it must be accessible to the reader. A textbook needs a style that ensures readability, and our partners at Elsevier have made that happen. Sonya Seigafuse, our executive content strategist, provided oversight and guidance with the eye of an experienced editor along with strategies to meet the changing environment of print and electronic publishing. The whole textbook revision is a demanding project requiring effective teamwork. Betsy McCormac, our senior content development manager, maintained professional skill and calm while moving the project forward. Brian Salisbury's design is visually appealing and showcases the content.

We also want to recognize the indispensable efforts of the entire marketing team led by Kristen Oyirifi as well as the sales representatives, who make certain that our message is honestly portrayed and that comments and suggestions from the field are candidly reported. Indeed, there are so very many people who are essential to the creation and potential success of our 11th edition, and we are indebted to each of them.

The remarkable teaching tools we call the ancillaries need special attention. They demand an expertise—if they are to be useful—that goes beyond that of the authors. Frances Donovan Monahan offers hers for the laboratory manual, and Matthew J. Zdilla offers his for the test bank. The careful attention to all Evolve asset development is overseen by Joy C. Neumarin.

We want to acknowledge Henry M. Seidel, MD; William Benedict, MD; and Jane Ball, DrPH, RN, CPNP, three of our original four authors, who served on the sixth, seventh, and tenth editions, respectively. Their commitment to the relationship with the patient and their appreciation of the importance of interprofessional collaboration helped shape this text.

And finally—our families! They are patient with our necessary absences, support what we do, and are unstinting in their love. They have our love and our special thanks.

Joyce E. Dains, DrPH, JD, APRN, FNP-BC, FNAP, FAANP, FAAN
John A. Flynn, MD, MBA, MEd
JoAnne Silbert-Flagg, DNP, CPNP-PC, IBCLC, CNE, FAAN, FAANP
Barry S. Solomon, MD, MPH
Rosalyn W. Stewart, MD, MS, MBA

Contents

CHAPTER 1

Cultural Competency

Achieving cultural competence is an ongoing process that requires self-awareness, reflective practice, knowledge of core cultural issues, and the use of effective patient-centered communication. It is important to recognize one's own culture, values, and biases. Culturally competent clinicians adapt to the unique needs of patients with backgrounds and cultures that differ from their own. This adaptability, coupled with a genuine curiosity about a patient's beliefs, values, and lived experience, lay the foundation for a trusting patient-provider relationship.

AN OVERVIEW OF CULTURE

A Definition of Culture and Cultural Values

Culture is a system of shared beliefs and values that are not defined by ethnicity or race. A culture may form around religion, language, gender, sexual orientation, disability, or socioeconomic status. *Cultural values* are beliefs, behaviors, and ideas that a group of people share and expect to be observed in their interactions with others (Hagan et al., 2017).

Distinguishing Physical Characteristics

A cultural group or subgroup should not be distinguished by physical characteristics (e.g., anatomy or skin color) of its members. To assume homogeneity in the beliefs, attitudes, and behaviors of all individuals in a particular group leads to misunderstandings about an individual. A *stereotype* is a fixed image of any group that denies the potential of originality or individuality within the group. People can and do respond differently to the same environment or situation. Stereotyping occurs through two cognitive phases. In the first phase, a stereotype becomes activated when an individual is categorized into a social group. When this occurs, beliefs and feelings (prejudices) come to mind about what members of that particular group are like. Over time, this first phase occurs without effort or awareness. In the second phase, people use these activated beliefs and feelings when they interact with the individual, even when they explicitly deny these stereotypes. Multiple studies have shown that clinicians activate these implicit stereotypes, or unconscious biases, when communicating with and providing care to patients from minoritized and marginalized backgrounds (FitzGerald and Hurst, 2017). With this in mind, you can begin learning cultural competence by acknowledging your implicit, or unconscious, biases toward patients based on physical characteristics and understanding the negative impact they may have on patients and their families.

At the same time, this does not minimize the value of understanding the cultural characteristics of groups, nor does this deny the interdependence of the physical with the cultural. Genotype, for example, precedes the development of the intellect, sensitivity, and imagination that leads to unique cultural achievements, such as the creation of classical or jazz music. Similarly, a person's phenotype, such as skin color, precedes most of the experience of life and the subsequent interweaving of that phenotype with cultural experience. Although traditionally used in clinical practice, the use of phenotypic traits to classify an individual's race is unacceptable. The term *race* has been used to categorize individuals based on their continent or subcontinent of origin (e.g., Asian, Southeast Asian). However, there is ongoing debate about the usefulness of race, considering the degree of phenotypic and genetic variation of individuals from the same geographic region (Duello et al., 2021). In addition, the origins of race date back to the 17th century, long before scientists identified genetic similarities. Over time, beliefs about particular racial groups were shaped by economic and political factors, and most believe race is a social construct (Richeson and Sommers, 2016). *Racism*, defined as discrimination directed against a person or people of a particular racial or ethnic group, has been shown to negatively affect health over the life course. This occurs through inequitable access to resources and opportunities, such as education and health care, and stressful experiences that result in altered physiologic responses and changes in health behavior (Williams et al., 2019). Historically, the American health care system has discriminated against racial and ethnic minorities in education, research, and direct patient care. Structural racism remains an ongoing problem within the health care system and is reflected in well-documented health disparities and inequities. As clinicians, you will encounter patients affected by racism on a daily basis. After identifying and examining your own biases, you can strive to create a safe space for dialogue with patients, provide support, and refer to resources when appropriate (Trent et al., 2019).

Genomics and Precision Medicine

A growing body of research examines genomics, the study of multiple genes and their interactions with environmental determinants, in predicting disease susceptibility and response to medical treatment. An explosion of genome-wide association studies (GWASs) has linked genomic loci, or single-nucleotide polymorphisms (SNPs), with common diseases such as rheumatoid arthritis, type 1 and type 2 diabetes mellitus, Crohn disease, and schizophrenia (Visscher et al., 2017). *Personalized medicine* is a term used to describe patient care that considers an individual's genetic susceptibility in preventing and treating disease. In 2015, the Precision Medicine Initiative was launched by the U.S. Department of Health and Human Services to bring researchers, policymakers, and technology innovators together with the goal of developing individualized care. *Precision medicine* is defined as "an emerging approach for disease treatment and prevention that takes into account individual variability in genes, environment, and lifestyle for each person" (Garrido et al., 2018). Many believe precision medicine will transform health care delivery by leveraging genomics and other molecular technologies with data sharing, advanced data analytics, and digital health platforms (Ginsburg and Phillips, 2018). As clinicians learn to integrate precision medicine into their practice, direct-to-consumer genetic testing continues to evolve and has become more affordable and accessible to their patients. Clinicians in all disciplines will need to become fluent in the language of genomics and learn how to discuss risks and benefits of genetic testing with their patients and families (Calzone et al., 2013; Demmer and Waggoner, 2014). With this new emphasis, it may be even more important to acknowledge unconscious biases and seek to understand the patient's unique cultural and personal health beliefs and expectations.

CULTURE IN HEALTH CARE

Cultural Competence

Cultural competency requires that clinicians be aware of and responsive to patients' backgrounds and cultural experiences, including their preferences, values, languages, and traditions, among other things (Stubbe, 2020). Many models have been proposed to teach cultural competence. Most include the domains of acquiring knowledge (e.g., understanding the meaning of culture), shaping attitudes (e.g., respecting differences of individuals from other cultures), and developing skills (e.g., eliciting a patient's cultural beliefs about health and illness) (Saha et al., 2008). Some of these domains overlap with core aspects of the patient-centered care model (Fig. 1.1). Seeleman et al. (2009) have proposed a framework for teaching cultural competence that emphasizes an awareness of the social context in which specific ethnic groups live. Assessing the social context includes inquiring about stressors and support networks, sense of life control, and literacy. A clinician needs to be flexible and creative in working with

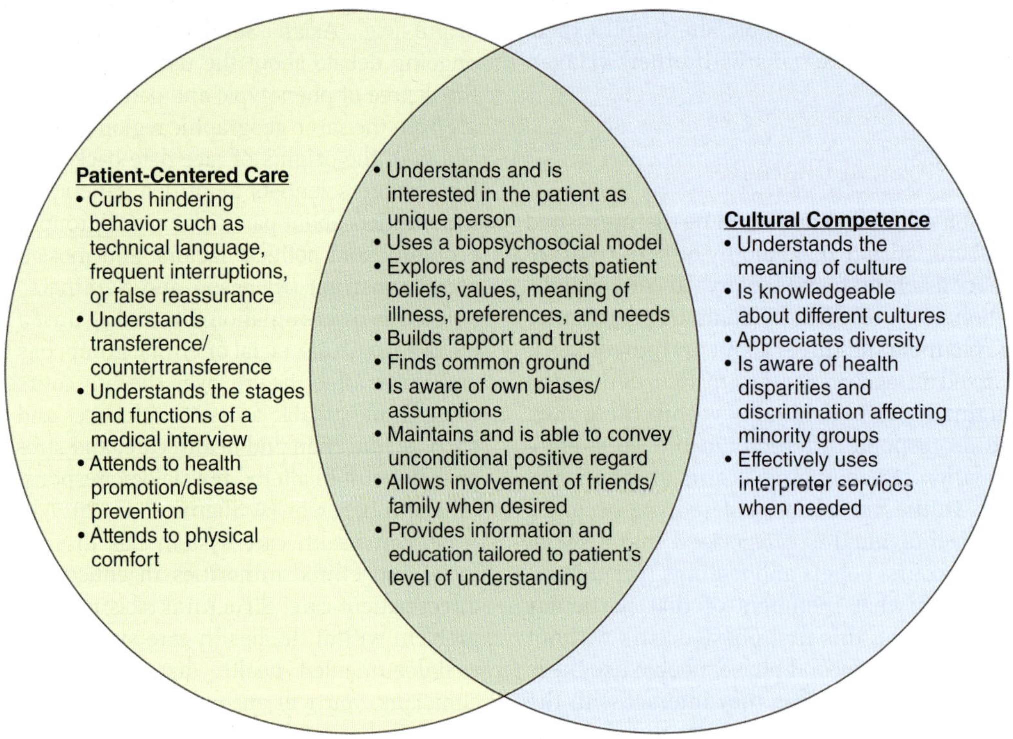

FIG. 1.1 Overlapping concepts of patient-centered care and cultural competence. (From Saha, S., Beach, M. C., & Cooper, L. A. (2008). Patient centeredness, cultural competence and healthcare quality. *Journal of the National Medical Association, 100*(11), 1275–1285.)

BOX 1.1 Dimensions of Cultural Competence

- **Cultural Encounters**—The continuous process of interacting with patients from culturally diverse backgrounds to validate, refine, or modify existing values, beliefs, and practices about a cultural group and to develop cultural desire, cultural awareness, cultural skill, and cultural knowledge.
- **Cultural Desire**—The motivation of the clinician to "want to" engage in the process of becoming culturally competent, not "have to."
- **Cultural Awareness**—The deliberate self-examination and in-depth exploration of one's biases, stereotypes, prejudices, assumptions, and "isms" that one holds about individuals and groups who are different from them.
- **Cultural Knowledge**—The process of seeking and obtaining a sound educational base about culturally and ethnically diverse groups.
- **Cultural Skill**—The ability to collect culturally relevant data regarding the patient's presenting problem, in addition to accurately performing a culturally based physical assessment in a culturally sensitive manner.

From Campinha-Bacote, J. (2011). Delivering patient-centered care in the midst of a cultural conflict: The role of cultural competence. *Online Journal of Issues in Nursing, 16*(2), 5.

patients. Campinha-Bacote's (2011) Process of Cultural Competence Model is another approach and includes five cultural constructs: encounters, desire, awareness, knowledge, and skill. Box 1.1 defines these five constructs.

Cultural Humility

Cultural humility involves the ability to recognize one's limitations in knowledge and cultural perspective and be open to new perspectives. Rather than assuming all patients of a particular culture fit a certain stereotype, clinicians should view patients as individuals. In doing so, cultural humility helps to equalize the imbalance in the patient-provider relationship (Borkan et al., 2008). A clinician may know many specific details about a patient's particular cultures, yet not show cultural humility. Cultural humility involves self-reflection and self-critique, with the goal of having a more balanced, mutually beneficial relationship. It involves meeting patients "where they are" without judgment to avoid the development of stereotypes. Attaining cultural humility is an ongoing process shaped by every patient encounter that involves openness, partnership, and genuine interest in understanding our patients' belief systems and lives (Fahlberg et al., 2016).

The Impact of Culture

The information in Box 1.2 suggests that racial and ethnic differences, in addition to social and economic conditions, may affect the provision of specific health care services to certain groups and subgroups in the United States. Although death rates have declined overall in the United States over the past 50 years, individuals with less

BOX 1.2 The Influence of Age, Race, Ethnicity, Socioeconomic Status, and Culture

Age, gender, race, ethnic group, and, with these variables, cultural attitudes, regional differences, and socioeconomic status influence the way patients seek medical care and the way clinicians provide care. For example, consider the ethnic and racial differences in the treatment of depression in the United States. The prevalence of major depressive disorders is similar across groups; however, compared with White Americans, Black and Latino patients are less likely to receive treatment. Although some of the disparity is related to differing patient attitudes and perceptions of counseling and medication, there is growing evidence suggesting clinician communication style and treatment recommendations differ on the basis of patient race and ethnicity (Shao et al., 2016). Similarly, in the pediatric population, Black and Latino children in the United States also experience health disparities, including lower overall health status and lower receipt of routine medical care and dental care compared with White children. Flores and colleagues (2010), in a systematic literature review, demonstrated that, compared with White children, Black children have lower rates of preventive and population health care (e.g., breastfeeding and immunization coverage), higher adolescent health risk behaviors (e.g., sexually transmitted infections), higher rates of asthma emergency visits, and lower mental health service use. There is a clear need to better understand why these differences exist more globally, but removing cultural blindness at the individual patient level is an important first step.

Furthermore, the possible beneficial and harmful effects of many culturally important herbal medicines, which are used but not always acknowledged, must be understood and, in trusting relationships, reported to us if we are to guide their appropriate use. Crossing the cultural divide helps, but skepticism is a barrier. For example, many allopathic medical providers question the notion that complementary and alternative medicine might be a helpful adjuvant therapy for the prevention and treatment of acute otitis media. However, in several randomized controlled studies, xylitol, probiotics, herbal ear drops, and homeopathic treatments have been shown, compared with placebo, to have a greater effect in reducing pain duration and decreasing the use of antibiotics. Although skepticism can be put aside, evidence-driven guidance is still essential. Cultural competence is entirely consistent with that.

Data from Bukutu, C., Deol, J., & Vohra, S. (2008). Complementary, holistic, and integrative medicine: Therapies for acute otitis media. *Pediatrics in Review, 29*(6), 193–199; Flores, G. (2010). Committee on Pediatric Research: Technical report—racial and ethnic disparities in the health and health care of children. *Pediatrics, 125*, e979–e1020; and Shao, Z., Richie, W. D., & Bailey, R. K. (2016). Racial and ethnic disparity in major depressive disorder. *Journal of Racial and Ethnic Health Disparities, 3*(4), 692–705.

education and those living in poverty still die at higher mortality rates from the same conditions than those who are better educated and economically advantaged. Morbidity, too, is greater among the poor. A variety of health care disparities are reported in the 2023 Centers for Disease Control and Prevention (CDC) Health Disparities and Inequalities Report. Hispanic and non-Hispanic Blacks were uninsured at a significantly higher rate compared with Asians and Pacific Islanders and non-Hispanic Whites. The infant mortality rate among infants born to non-Hispanic Black females is more than double the rate for infants born to non-Hispanic White females. Compared with White females, a much higher percentage of Black females die from coronary heart disease before age 75 (37.9% vs. 19.4%). This same difference was observed between Black and White males (61.5% vs. 41.5%) (CDC, 2023). From 2017 to 2020, the rate of obesity was higher among Black (50%) and Hispanic (48%) adults than White adults (41%). This was true for diabetes prevalence (21% among Hispanic adults, 19% among Black adults, 19% among Asian adults, and 12% among White adults) (CDC, 2023). Because of societal stigmatization and discrimination, when compared with cisgender populations, transgender and gender-diverse individuals are at greater risk for suicidality, being victims of violence, mental health comorbidities, human immunodeficiency virus (HIV)/sexually transmitted infection (STI) exposure, homelessness, and lower rates of insurance coverage (Kota et al., 2020; Office of Disease Prevention and Health Promotion [ODPHP], 2010).

Health equity is achieved when everyone has the opportunity to attain their full health potential (CDC, 2023). Three major modifiable health risk behaviors are responsible for many early deaths related to chronic disease: tobacco use, poor nutrition, and lack of physical activity (CDC, 2023). Health disparities related to chronic conditions may be seen in the following groups: people of color; people with disabilities; people living in rural communities; older adults; people with mental health or substance use disorders; people with less than a high school education; people with low income or those experiencing poverty; and people who identify as lesbian, gay, bisexual, or transgender (LGBTQ+) (CDC, 2023). Improving health equity includes a focus on the following: food service and nutrition guidelines; fruit and vegetable voucher incentives and/or produce prescription programs; safe and accessible physical activity; continuity of care in breastfeeding support; early care and education settings; family healthy weight programs; tobacco prevention and control policies; and COVID-19, flu, and other routine vaccines (CDC, 2023). Nutrition and exercise behaviors begin in childhood, where the availability of nutritious foods and the opportunity for outdoor play have an impact on these behaviors. Cultural and practice differences exist among clinicians as well. Allopathic clinicians often demonstrate skepticism regarding the use of complementary and alternative medicine (CAM) without considering the possibility of potential benefit to patients.

The Blurring of Cultural Distinctions

Some cultural differences may be malleable in a way that physical characteristics are not. For example, one group of people can be distinguished from another by language (see Clinical Pearl, "Language Is Not All"). However, globalization, the growing diversity of the U.S. population, and evidence of health care disparities mandate more and more that we learn one another's languages. Although modern technology and economics may eventually lead to universality in language, we can begin by acknowledging and overcoming our individual biases and cultural stereotypes. Because it is impossible to learn the native languages of all of our patients, when language barriers arise, we must become aware of our resources and know how to effectively use interpreters. Use of medical interpreters has a positive impact on health care quality, but some continue to use suboptimal methods of communication (e.g., family members). Although greater adoption of medical interpreter use involves policy and system-level changes, clinician training and encouragement remain critically important (DeCamp et al., 2013).

CLINICAL PEARL

Language Is Not All

A patient who knows the English language, however well, cannot be assumed to know the culture. Consider the diversity of the populations in Britain, India, American Samoa, and South Africa who are English speaking. The absence of a language barrier does not preclude a cultural barrier. You will likely still need to achieve a "cultural translation."

The Primacy of the Individual in Health Care

The individual patient may be visualized at the center of an indefinite number of concentric circles. The outermost circles represent constraining universal experiences (e.g., death). The circles closest to the center represent the various cultural groups or subgroups to which anyone must, of necessity, belong. The constancy of change forces adaptation and acculturation. The circles are constantly interweaving and overlapping. For example, a common experience in the United States has been the economic gain at the root of the assimilation of many ethnic groups. Although this results in greater homogeneity among the population, an individual's ethnic behaviors or sexual orientation and gender identity will likely be unique. Predicting the individual's character merely on the basis of the common cultural behavior, or stereotype, can cause harm. Based on The Joint Commission 2010 report, "Checklist to Improve Effective Communication, Cultural Competence, and Patient- and Family-Centered Care Across the Care Continuum," White and Stubblefield-Tave (2016) remind us that unconscious bias, stereotyping, racism, gender bias, and limited English proficiency underlie healthcare inequalities. They offer their own checklist of recommendations for clinicians to address these issues, with the goal of reducing disparities in care (Box 1.3).

Ethical issues often arise when the care of an individual comes into conflict with the utilitarian needs of the larger community, particularly with the recognition of limited resources and, in the United States, rising health care costs. Cultural attitudes of our patients, at times vague and poorly understood, may constrain our professional behavior and confuse the context in which we serve the individual. Box 1.4 offers a guide to help understand

BOX 1.3 Provider Role in Reducing Disparities in Health Care

This modified "culturally competent checklist" is provided as a guide to help providers partner with patients and families to provide high-quality care. Although some items are simple, others are quite complicated and difficult to achieve. On our path to achieving cultural humility, we should strive to incorporate as many of these recommendations as possible into our routine clinical practice.

1. Humanize your patient.
2. Identify and monitor conscious and unconscious biases.
3. Do a teach-back.
4. Help the patient to learn about their disease or condition.
5. Welcome a patient's friend, partner, and/or family members.
6. Learn a few key words and phrases in the most common languages in your area.
7. Use a qualified medical interpreter as appropriate.
8. Be aware of the potential for "false fluency" (clinician language skill should be tested and certified).
9. Seek training in working with an interpreter.
10. Consider the health literacy of one's patients.
11. Respond thoughtfully to patient complaints.
12. Hold one's institutions accountable for providing culturally and linguistically competent care.
13. Advocate that the affiliated institution's analyses of patient satisfaction and outcome include cultural group data and that the results lead to concrete action.
14. Encourage patients to complete patient satisfaction and demographics forms.

Modified from White, A. A., & Stubblefield-Tave, B. (2017). Some advice for physicians and other clinicians treating minorities, women, and other patients at risk of receiving health care disparities. *Journal of Racial and Ethnic Health Disparities*, *4*(3), 472–479.

the patient's beliefs and practices that can lead to individualized, culturally competent care. Particular attention should be paid to caring for patients who are sexual or gender minorities (SGMs): those who self-identify as lesbian, gay, bisexual, transgender, queer, or questioning. Unfortunately, these individuals often face discrimination and disrespect in the health care setting. Thus it is imperative that clinicians invest time in becoming culturally competent and develop cultural humility to work effectively with SGM patients. Specific responsibilities include providing a welcoming and safe environment, gathering a history with sensitivity and compassion, and performing a physical examination using a "gender-affirming" approach (e.g., using the patient's correct name and preferred pronouns). Box 1.5 provides useful terminology (Center for Excellence for Transgender Health, 2016), and Box 1.6 reviews the social, legal, and medical dimensions of transition for transgender and gender-diverse people.

Interprofessional Care: A Culture Shift in the Health Professions

There is a harmony—a unity—in the care of patients that is not constricted by the cultural and administrative boundaries of individual health professions. To the extent that we stake out territories of care by allowing individual professional cultures and needs to take precedence over patient needs, we may impede the achievement of harmony. In 2010, the World Health Organization (WHO) published "The Framework for Action on Interprofessional Education and Collaborative Practice." In this publication, interprofessional education is described as training in which "students from two or more professions learn about, from, and with each other to enable effective collaboration and improve health outcomes." The WHO believes this type of training can lead to "interprofessional collaborative practice," in which health team members from different professional backgrounds work together to deliver high-quality care. A surge in published curricula on interprofessional education and team-based training for students and faculty has occurred. Although most curricula for nursing and medical students focus on improving communication skills, training programs need to evolve to address cultural humility and valuing diversity in patient populations (Foronda et al., 2016).

The Impact of Culture on Illness

Disease is shaped by illness, and illness—the full expression of the impact of disease on the patient—is shaped by the totality of the patient's experience. Cancer is a disease. The patient dealing with, reacting to, and trying to live with cancer is having an illness—is "ill" or "sick." The definition of "ill" or "sick" is based on the individual's belief system and is determined in large part by their enculturation. This is so for a brief, essentially mild episode or for a chronic, debilitating, life-altering condition. If we do not consider the substance of illness—the biologic, emotional, and cultural aspects—we will too often fail to offer appropriate care. To make the point, imagine that while taking a shower you have conducted a self-examination and, still young, still looking ahead to your career, you have discovered an unexpected mass in a breast or a testicle. How will you respond? How might other individuals respond?

Evidence-Based Practice in Physical Examination

Cultural Adaptations for Screening

We often use a variety of screening tools to identify health concerns and help our patients stay well. These screening tools are based on norms that may not be consistent across cultures. Screening tools may contain cultural biases and result in misleading information. Whenever possible, we should use instruments that have been adapted for and tested with individuals from our patients' specific cultural groups. Fortunately, a variety of instruments have been validated in racial and ethnic subgroups (Manuel et al., 2015). Before implementing a screening tool, it is our responsibility to ensure the instrument is valid and at an appropriate literacy level for our specific patient populations.

BOX 1.4 Cultural Assessment Guide: The Many Aspects of Understanding

Health Beliefs and Practices
- How does the patient define health and illness? How are feelings concerning pain, illness in general, or death expressed?
- Are particular methods used to help maintain health, such as hygiene and self-care practices?
- Are particular methods being used for treatment of illness?
- What is the attitude toward preventive health measures such as immunizations?
- Are there health topics that the patient may be particularly sensitive to or consider taboo?
- Are there restrictions imposed by modesty that must be respected; for example, are there constraints related to exposure of parts of the body, discussion of sexual health, and attitudes toward various procedures such as termination of pregnancy or vasectomy?
- What are the attitudes toward mental illness, pain, chronic disease, death, and dying? Are there constraints in the way these issues are discussed with the patient or with reference to relatives and friends?
- Is a person in the family responsible for various health-related decisions such as where to go, whom to see, and what advice to follow?
- Does the patient prefer a health professional of the same gender, age, and ethnic and racial background?

Faith-Based Influences and Special Rituals
- Is there a religion or faith to which the patient adheres?
- Is there a significant person to whom the patient looks for guidance and support?
- Are there any faith-based special practices or beliefs that may affect health care when the patient is ill or dying?

Language and Communication
- What language is spoken in the home?
- How well does the patient understand English, both spoken and written?
- Are there special signs of demonstrating respect or disrespect?
- Is touch involved in communication?
- Is an interpreter needed? (If so, this person ideally should be a trained professional and not a family member.)

Parenting Styles and Role of Family
- Who makes the decisions in the family?
- What is the composition of the family? How many generations are considered to be a single family, and which relatives compose the family unit?
- What is the role of and attitude toward children in the family?
- Do family members demonstrate physical affection toward their children and each other?
- Are there special beliefs and practices surrounding conception, pregnancy, childbirth, lactation, and childrearing? Is co-sleeping practiced? (If so, further inquiry is necessary regarding safe sleep practices for infants 12 months and younger.)

Sources of Support Beyond the Family
- Are there ethnic or cultural organizations that may have an influence on the patient's approach to health care?
- Are there individuals in the patient's social network that can influence perception of health and illness?
- Is there a particular cultural group with which the patient identifies? Can this be clarified by where the patient was born and has lived?

Dietary Practices
- Who is responsible for food preparation?
- Are any foods forbidden by the culture, or are some foods a cultural requirement in observance of a rite or ceremony?
- How is food prepared and consumed?
- Are there specific beliefs or preferences concerning food, such as those believed to cause or to cure an illness?
- Are there periods of required fasting? What are they?

Modified from Stulc, D. M. (1991). The family as a bearer of culture. In J. M. Cookfair (Ed.), *Nursing process and practice in the community.* St. Louis: Mosby.

BOX 1.5 Gender, Transgender, and Sexuality Terminology

Gender/gender identity: Term used to describe a person's internal sense of self and how they fit into the world from the perspective of gender.

Sex: Refers to the sex assigned at birth, historically based on a cursory visualization of external genitalia. Sex is often used interchangeably with gender, although the terms are not synonymous.

Transgender: Person whose gender identity differs from sex assigned at birth; a transgender man is someone with a male gender identity and a female birth-assigned sex, while a transgender woman is someone with a female gender identity and a male birth-assigned sex.

Gender-diverse: Person whose gender identity differs from that sex assigned at birth but may be more complex or fluid. It can encompass individuals who identify as nonbinary, genderqueer, gender fluid, and a host of other descriptors.

They/them/their: Gender-neutral pronouns used by some who identify as nonbinary (meaning that they do not identify as exclusively male or female within the traditional gender binary of Western European–based culture).

Sexual orientation: Term describing a person's sexual, romantic, emotional, or physical attraction toward other people.

From Center of Excellence for Transgender Health. (2016). *Department of Family and Community Medicine, University of California, San Francisco: Guidelines for the primary and gender-affirming care of transgender and gender nonbinary people* (2nd ed.). www.transhealth.ucsf.edu/guidelines

THE COMPONENTS OF A CULTURAL RESPONSE

When cultural differences exist, seek to fully understand what the patient means and know exactly what they think you mean in words and actions. Asking the patient if you are unsure demonstrates curiosity and is far better than making an assumption, which could result in a damaging mistake. Avoid assumptions about cultural beliefs and behaviors made without validation from the patient.

Beliefs and behaviors that will have an impact on patient assessment include the following:
- Modes of communication: the use of speech, body language, and space
- Health beliefs and practices that may vary from your own or those of other patients you care for
- Diet and nutritional practices
- The nature of relationships within a family and community

Attitudes toward autonomy may be based on a patient's cultural background and belief system. The patient-centered

BOX 1.6 Health Care Delivery for Transgender and Gender-Diverse People

In the 21st century, a trend in medicine is to move away from a psychopathological approach to transgender and gender-diverse (TGD) care. This former historical approach was found to be unsupported by scientific evidence, and it served to foster continued stigma and discrimination faced by TGD people. Being transgender or gender diverse is not a mental disease or disorder—gender identity disorder was removed from the *Diagnostic and Statistics Manual of Mental Health Disorders* (DSM) in 2013. In the *International Classification of Diseases,* 11th edition (ICD-11), gender incongruence will be removed from mental health and will be listed in sexual health. As our knowledge about TGD people evolves, the understanding of clinicians must also evolve. Within the framework of discussing physical examinations, it is beneficial to change from a perspective that ascribes anatomy to a binary gender or legal sex. Rather, view patients as individuals and "meet them where they are at" holistically.

Transition is a term used by many to describe the process of going from living aligned with one's sex assigned at birth to living aligned with one's gender identity. Transition is a multidimensional process affected by social, legal, and medical influences.

Social Transition

The process of modifying how one is seen by and interacts with society in a gendered way. A person may modify their gender expression (e.g., appearance or mannerisms), come out to others (e.g., family, friends, coworkers, community members), or use prosthetics (e.g., wigs, breast forms, or packers) (UCSF, 2019). Of note for practitioners, a person may also bind the chest for a more masculine appearance or tuck (placing the testes into the inguinal canal) to appear more feminine. Either practice may have clinical implications.

Legal Transition

The process of updating one's government-issued identity documents such as a birth certificate, driver's license, or passport. The requirements to update these documents vary by jurisdiction, including any medically related requirements. Many jurisdictions no longer require genital surgery as a requirement, and more are recognizing nonbinary as a legal sex. Of note for practitioners, this means a practitioner should not assume a patient's legal sex simply based on anatomy.

Medical Transition

Many TGD people will not seek any medical care related to their transition or in living as their authentic self. For those who do seek medical care or treatment, the interventions are also highly individual. What may be medically necessary for one person may not be necessary for another person. In general, medical transition may involve mental health care and support, hormone therapy, and gender-affirming surgical procedures, in addition to hair removal, speech therapy, and fertility preservation, among other specialties (UCSF, 2019). The World Professional Association for Transgender Health (WPATH) Standards of Care provide a person-centered, flexible approach to care. The UCSF Center of Excellence for Transgender Health has created guidelines for primary care providers. The Endocrine Society has established a standard of care for gender-affirming hormone therapy. As of 2020, the use of hormones for gender affirmation remains a U.S. Food and Drug Administration (FDA) off-label use.

Commonly used feminizing hormones include:
- Estrogen
- Spironolactone
- Progesterone
- Leuprolide

Commonly used masculinizing hormone:
- Testosterone

Note: Leuprolide or other gonadotropin-releasing hormone (GnRH) agonists are often used for puberty blocking for TGD adolescents.

Common gender-affirming surgical procedures include:
- Facial surgery (jaw, forehead, nose, cheeks)
- Chest ("top") surgery (breast augmentation or chest masculinization/bilateral mastectomy)
- Genital ("bottom") surgery (orchiectomy, vaginoplasty, hysterectomy, metoidioplasty, phalloplasty)

From University of California, San Francisco (UCSF). (2019). Transition roadmap. https://transcare.ucsf.edu/transition-roadmap

care model, firmly respected in the United States, could be at odds with a more family-centered model that is more likely dominant elsewhere. In Japan, for example, the family is generally considered the legitimate decision-making authority for patients who have capacity and for those patients who lack capacity. Persons of some cultures (e.g., Middle Eastern and Navajo Native American) believe that a patient should not be told of a diagnosis of a metastatic cancer or a terminal prognosis for any reason, but this attitude is not likely to be shared by Americans with European or African traditions. Traditionally, the members of the Navajo culture believe that thought and language have the power to shape reality. Talking about a possible outcome is thought to ensure the outcome. It is important, then, to avoid thinking or speaking in a negative way. The situation can be dealt with by talking in terms of a third person or an abstract possibility. You might even refer to an experience you have had in your own family. Obviously, the conflicts that may arise from differing views of autonomy, religion, and information sharing require an effort that is dominated by a clear understanding of the patient's goals. However, it is also important to remember that a patient may not typify the attitudes of the group of origin.

Modes of Communication

Communication and culture are interrelated, particularly in the way feelings are expressed verbally and nonverbally. The same word may have different meanings for different people. For example, in the United States, a "practicing physician" is an experienced, trained person. However, "practicing" suggests inexperience and the status of a student to an Alaskan Native or to some Western Europeans. Similarly, touch, facial expressions, eye movement, and body posture all have varying significance.

In the United States, for example, people may tend to talk more loudly and to worry less about being overheard than others do. The English, on the other hand, may worry more about being overheard and speak in modulated voices. In the United States, people may be direct in conversation and logical, preferring to avoid the subjective and to come to the point quickly. The Japanese may do the opposite, using indirection, talking around points, and emphasizing attitudes and feelings. Silence, although sometimes uncomfortable for many of us, affords patients who are Native American time to think; the response should not be forced and the quiet time should be allowed.

Many groups use firm eye contact. Spanish individuals often meet one another's eyes and look for the impact of what is being said. The French, too, may have a firm gaze and often stare openly at others. However, this might be thought rude or immodest in some Asian or Middle Eastern cultures. Americans are more apt to let the eyes wander and to grunt, nod their head, or say, "I see" or "Uh huh," to indicate understanding. The British may avoid touch and may be less apt to pat you on the arm in a reassuring way than are, for example, Italians.

These are but a few examples of cultural variation in communication. They do, however, suggest a variety of behaviors within groups. As with any example we might use, they are not to be thought of as rigidly characteristic of the indicated groups. Still, the questions suggested in Box 1.4 can at times provide insight to particular situations and can help avoid misunderstanding and miscommunication.

The cultural and physical characteristics of both patient and clinician may significantly influence communication (Fig. 1.2). Social class, race, age, and gender are variables that characterize everyone; they can intrude on successful communication if there is no effort for mutual knowledge and understanding. The young student or clinician and the older adult patient may have to work harder to develop a meaningful relationship. Recognizing these differences and talking about them, evoking feelings sooner rather than later, can result in a more positive encounter for both patient and provider. It is permissible to ask whether the patient is uncomfortable with you or your background and whether they are willing to talk about it.

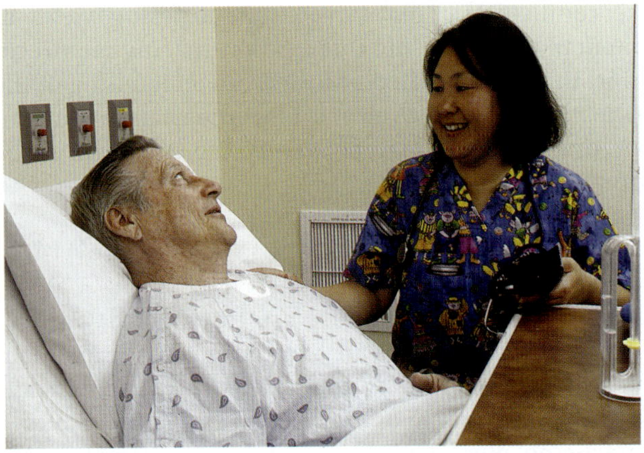

FIG. 1.2 Being sensitive to cultural differences that may exist between you and the patient can help to avoid miscommunication.

Health Beliefs and Practices

The patient may have a view of health and illness and an approach to a cure that are shaped by a particular cultural and/or faith belief or paradigm. If that view is "scientific," in the sense that a cause can be determined for every problem in a very precise way, the patient is more apt to be comfortable with Western approaches to health and medical care. However, the scientific view is reductionist and looks to a very narrow, specific cause and effect. A more naturalistic or "holistic" approach broadens the context. It views our lives as part of a much greater whole (the entire cosmos) that must be in harmony. If the balance is disturbed, illness can result. The goal, then, is to achieve balance and harmony. Aspects of this concept are evident among the beliefs of many Hispanics, Native Americans, Asians, and Middle Eastern groups, and they are increasingly evident in people of all ethnic groups in the United States nowadays (Box 1.7). Other groups believe in the supernatural or forces of good and evil that determine individual fate. In such a context, illness may be thought of as a punishment for wrongdoing.

Clearly, there can be a confusing ambivalence in many of us, patient and clinician alike, because our genuine faith-based or naturalistic beliefs may conflict with the options available for the treatment of illness. For example, consider a child with a broken bone, the result of an unintentional injury that occurred while the child was under the supervision of a babysitter. The first need is to tend to the fracture. That done, there is a need to talk with the parents about the guilt they may feel because they were away working. They might think this injury must be God's punishment. It is important to be aware of, to respect, and to discuss without belittlement a belief that may vary from yours in a manner that may still allow you to offer your point of view. This can apply to the guilt of a parent and to the use of herbs, rituals, and religious artifacts. After all, the pharmacopeia of Western medicine is replete with plants and herbs that we now call drugs (see Clinical Pearl, "Complementary and Alternative Treatments for the Common Cold"). Our difficulty in understanding the belief of another does not invalidate its substance, nor does a patient's adherence to a particular belief preclude concurrent reliance on allopathic or osteopathic health practitioners.

BOX 1.7 The Balance of Life: The "Hot" and the "Cold"

A naturalistic or holistic approach often assumes that there are external factors—some good, some bad—that must be kept in balance if we are to remain well. The balance of "hot" and "cold" is a part of the belief system in many cultural groups (e.g., Middle Eastern, Asian, Southeast Asian, and Hispanic). To restore a disturbed balance (i.e., to treat) requires the use of opposites (e.g., a "hot" remedy for a "cold" problem and vice versa). Different cultures may define "hot" and "cold" differently. It is not a matter of temperature, and the words used might vary: for example, the Chinese have named the forces yin (cold) and yang (hot). The bottom line: we cannot ignore the naturalistic view if many of our patients are to have appropriate care.

Hot and Cold Conditions and Their Corresponding Treatments

COLD CONDITIONS	HOT TREATMENTS	HOT CONDITIONS	COLD TREATMENTS
CONDITIONS	**FOODS**	**CONDITIONS**	**FOODS**
Cancer	Beef	Constipation	Barley water
Cold	Cereals	Diarrhea	Chicken
Earaches	Chili peppers	Fever	Dairy products
Headaches	Chocolate	Infection	Fresh vegetables
Joint pain	Eggs	Kidney problems	Fruits
Malaria	Goat's milk	Rash	Honey
Menses	Liquor	Sore throat	Goat meat
Pneumonia	Onions		Raisins
Stomach cramps	Peas		
Teething	Ginger		
Tuberculosis	Herbs		
	MEDICINES AND HERBS		**MEDICINES AND HERBS**
	Anise		Bicarbonate of soda
	Aspirin		Milk of magnesia
	Castor oil		Orange flower water
	Cinnamon		Sage
	Cod liver oil		
	Garlic		
	Ginger root		
	Iron		
	Tobacco		
	Penicillin		
	Vitamins		

Modified from Purnell, L. D. (Ed.). (2013). *Transcultural health care: A culturally competent approach* (4th ed.). Philadelphia: F. A. Davis.

CLINICAL PEARL

Complementary and Alternative Treatments for the Common Cold

Home-based remedies for common colds are widely used. In children, the following therapies may be effective: buckwheat honey, vapor rub, geranium, and zinc sulfate. In adults, *Echinacea purpurea,* geranium extract, and zinc gluconate may be effective. When asking about medications, always remember to ask about use of complementary and alternative therapies. Using a nonjudgmental approach, you may wish to start with the question, "What else have you tried?"

From Fashner, J., Ericson, K., & Werner, S. (2012). Treatment of the common cold in children and adults. *American Family Physician, 86,* 153–159.

Family Relationships

Family structure and the social organizations to which a patient belongs (e.g., faith-based organizations, clubs, social media, and schools) are among the many imprinting and constraining cultural forces. The expectations of children and how they grow and develop are key in this regard and often culturally distinct. Determining these family and social structures needs emphasis in the United States today, with its shift toward dual-income families, single-parent families, and a significant number of teenage parents. The prevalence of divorce (nearly one for every two marriages) and the increasing involvement of both parents in childcare in two-parent families suggest cultural shifts that need to be recognized.

One type of already-known behavior may predict another type of behavior. For example, mothers who are low-income living in an urban setting who attend prenatal care visits generally bring their infants for routine care, regardless of educational level (Van Berckelaer et al., 2011). Adolescents who are not monitored by their parents are more likely to smoke, use alcohol and cannabis, be depressed, and initiate sexual activity compared with are those who are monitored (Dittus et al., 2015; Pesola et al., 2015). Being aware of this sequence of related behaviors is especially important because it may be unrelated to the integrity of the family structure, gender, or background. Parenting style and childrearing practices such as setting boundaries and expectations may be culturally driven. Many adolescents and young adults find comfort in their families' cultural traditions and practices and benefit from their connectedness. In a large study of U.S. college students from immigrant families, compared with their peers, students who retained their heritage practices reported fewer health risk behaviors such as substance use, unsafe sex, and impaired driving (Schwartz et al., 2011). These examples remind us that one individual may belong to many subgroups and that the behaviors and attitudes of a subgroup (e.g., a young person who remains connected to their cultural heritage) can override the impact of the cultural values of the larger group (e.g., youth whose peers are engaged in risk-taking behaviors).

Diet and Nutritional Practices

Beliefs and practices related to food, along with the social significance of food, play an obvious vital role in everyday life. Some of these beliefs of cultural and/or faith-based significance may have an impact on the care you provide to patients. An Orthodox Jewish patient will not take some medicines, particularly during a holiday period such as Passover, because the preparation of a drug does not meet the religious rules for food during that time. A patient who is Muslim may respect *halal* (a prescribed diet), even throughout pregnancy. A Chinese person with hypertension and a salt-restricted diet may need to consider a limited use of monosodium glutamate (MSG) and soy sauce. Attitudes toward vitamins vary greatly, with or without scientific proof, in many of the subgroups in the United States. It is possible to work out a mutually agreed-on management plan if the issues are recognized and freely discussed. This is also possible with attitudes toward home, herbal, and natural—complementary or alternative—therapies. Many have benefits; others may be dangerous. For example, some herbal medications containing cassia senna may cause liver damage, and other herbal preparations interact with prescribed medications (Posadzki et al., 2013).

SUMMING UP

As clinicians, we face a compelling need to meet each patient on their own terms and to resist forming a sense of the patient based on prior knowledge of the race, religion, gender, ethnicity, gender identity and sexual orientation, or cultures from which that patient comes. That knowledge should not be formative in arriving at conclusions; rather, we must draw on it to help make the questions we ask more constructively probing to avoid viewing the patient as a stereotype (Box 1.8). You need to understand yourself well. Your involvement with any patient gives that interaction a unique quality, and your contribution to that interaction, to some extent, makes it different from what it might have been with anyone else. Remember that your attitudes and prejudices, which are largely culturally derived, may interfere with your understanding of the patient and increase the probability of unconscious bias and stereotypic judgment. When you're able to adapt to the unique needs of your patients and display genuine curiosity

BOX 1.8 Communication

This list of questions, derived over the years from our experience and multiple resources, illustrates the variation in human responses. Try not to be intimidated by the mass of "need to know" cultural issues, but begin reflecting on them as you work with patients to raise your cultural awareness and develop a greater sense of cultural humility.

- How important are nonverbal clues?
- Are moments of silence valued?
- Is touching to be avoided?
- Are handshakes, or even embracing, avoided or desired at meeting and parting?
- What is the attitude toward eye contact?
- Is there a greater-than-expected need for "personal space"?
- What is the verbal or nonverbal response if your suggestions are not understood?
- Is there candor in admitting lack of understanding?
- What are the attitudes concerning respect for self and for authority figures?
- What are the attitudes toward persons in other groups, such as minorities and majorities?
- What are the language preferences?
- What is the need for "chit-chat" before getting down to the primary concern?
- Is there a relaxed or rigid sense of time?
- What is the degree of trust of clinicians?
- How easily are personal matters discussed?
- Is there, even with you, a wish to avoid discussing income and other family affairs?

Health Customs/Health Practices

- What is the degree of dependence on the healthcare system, both for illness alone and for preventive and health maintenance needs?
- What is generally expected of a health professional, and what defines a "good one"?
- What defines health?
- Are there particularly common folk practices?
- Is there a greater (or lesser) inclination to invoke self-care and use home remedies?
- Is there a particular suspicion or fear of hospitals?
- What is the tendency to use alternative care approaches and/or herbal remedies exclusively or as a complement?
- What are the tendencies to invoke the magical or metaphysical?
- Who is ultimately responsible for outcomes: you or the patient?
- Who is ultimately responsible for maintaining health: you or the patient?
- Is there a particular fear of painful or intrusive testing?
- Is there a tendency toward stoicism?
- What is the dependence on prayer?
- Is illness thought of as punishment and a means of penance?
- Is "shame" attached to illness?
- What is the belief about the origins of illness?
- Is illness thought to be preventable and, if so, how?
- What is the attitude toward autopsy?
- Does a belief in reincarnation mandate that the body be left intact?
- Are there particular cultural cooking habits that can influence diagnosis or management?
- Is the degree of modesty in both males and females more than you would generally expect?
- Do females, considering modesty, need a much more cautious and protected approach than usual (e.g., during the examination)?

Family, Friends, and the Workplace

- How tightly organized (and multigenerational) is the family hierarchy?
- How tight is the family?
- Is social life extended beyond the family and, if so, to what degree?
- Does the family tend to be matriarchal or patriarchal?
- What are the relative roles of females and males?
- Are particular tasks assigned to individual genders (e.g., who does the laundry, family finances, grocery shopping)?
- To what extent are older adults and other authority figures given deference and how?
- Who makes decisions for the family?
- To what extent is power shared?
- Who makes decisions for the children and adolescents?
- How strongly are children valued?
- Is a greater value placed on one specific gender?
- How much are self-reliance and personal discipline valued?
- What is the work ethic?
- What is the sense of obligation to the community?
- How is education sought, that is, from school, reading, and/or experience?
- What is the emphasis on tradition and ritual practice?

The RESPECT Model

What is most important in considering the effectiveness of your cross-cultural communication, whether it is verbal, nonverbal, or written, is that you remain open and maintain a sense of respect for your patients. The RESPECT Model can help you remain effective and patient-centered in all of your communication with patients.

Rapport
- Connect on a social level
- See the patient's point of view
- Consciously suspend judgment
  Recognize and avoid making assumptions

Empathy
- Remember the patient has come to you for help
- Seek out and understand the patient's rationale for their behaviors and illness
- Verbally acknowledge and legitimize the patient's feelings

Support
- Ask about and understand the barriers to care and compliance
- Help the patient overcome barriers; involve family members if appropriate
- Reassure the patient you are and will be available to help

Partnership
- Be flexible
- Negotiate roles when necessary
- Stress that you are working together to address health problems

Explanations
- Check often for understanding
- Use verbal clarification techniques

Cultural competence
- Respect the patient's cultural beliefs
- Understand that the patient's views of you may be defined by ethnic and cultural stereotypes
- Be aware of your own cultural biases and preconceptions
- Know your limitations in addressing health issues across cultures
- Understand your personal style and recognize when it may not be working with a given patient

Trust
- Recognize that self-disclosure may be difficult for some patients; consciously work to establish trust

Guide to Providing Effective Communication and Language Assistance Services
www.ThinkCulturalHealth.hhs.gov

OMH U.S. Department of Health and Human Services Office of Minority Health

THINK CULTURAL HEALTH

FIG. 1.3 The RESPECT Model.

about their beliefs and values, you will be making strides toward cultural competence. The RESPECT Model is one useful tool to bridge the cultural divide between patients and clinicians (Fig. 1.3).

It is not unusual to find tables of information about health care–related cultural attitudes for a variety of religious and ethnic groups in reference materials. Although this provides quick access to information about various population groups, our experience suggests that the rigid superficiality in this information often does not adequately describe the beliefs and attitudes of a particular individual. Our purpose in this chapter is to review many of the questions and frameworks that might be relevant as you prepare to meet and care for your patients. Patient by patient, your insights will develop as you examine your own biases, avoid stereotypes, consider the individual, and become increasingly culturally competent. View cultural competence as a lifelong journey and not a destination or end point in and of itself.

CHAPTER

2

The History and Interviewing Process

This chapter discusses the development of relationships with patients and the building of histories or health care narratives. We write of it as "building" a history rather than "taking" one because you and your patient are involved in a partnership that should have, among other outcomes, a history that reflects the patient's perspectives and unique status. In essence, you are capturing the patient's story. This chapter discusses the context of the relationship in emotional, physical, and ethical terms and offers suggestions in verbal and nonverbal behavior that you may adapt to your individual comfort and style. Finally, we offer widely accepted approaches to history building with suggested adaptations for children, adolescents, pregnant persons, older adults, and patients with disabilities. The history is vital to building relationships with patients, guiding the physical examination, and interpreting physical examination findings.

Developing a Relationship With the Patient

In this chapter we offer instruction in learning about well and sick patients as they seek care. History and physical examination are at the heart of this effort. It is not easy to get the sense of another person or to fully appreciate someone else's orientation in the world. You and the patient may seem to have a similar experience but may, in all likelihood, interpret it differently (see Clinical Pearl, "'Unique,' Originally Derived From Latin 'Unus,' Meaning 'One'"). On the other hand, you and your patient may come from very different backgrounds without any shared experiences. To prevent misunderstandings, misinterpretations, and misperceptions, you must make every effort to sense the world of the individual patient as that patient senses it. (See Chapter 1 for additional discussion.)

CLINICAL PEARL

"Unique," Originally Derived From Latin "Unus," Meaning "One"

We use "unique" in that sense of being the only one. Each of us is unique, incomparably different from anyone in the past, present, or future. No relationship, then, has an exact counterpart. Each moment is unique, different from the time before with the same patient.

The first meeting with the patient sets the tone for a successful partnership, indicating that you want to know all that is needed and you will be open, flexible, and eager to answer questions and provide explanations. You can also explain the boundaries of your practice and the degree of your availability in any situation. Trust evolves from honesty, integrity, candor, and demonstrating dignity and respect toward the patient.

A primary objective is to discover the details about a patient's concern; explore expectations for the encounter; and display genuine interest, curiosity, and partnership. Identifying underlying worries, believing them, and trying to address them optimizes your ability to help. You need to understand what is expected of you.

CLINICAL PEARL

The Patient Relationship

You will, in the course of your career, have numerous relationships with patients. Never forget that each time a patient has an experience with you, it is important to them and a privilege for you.

Much has been written about technology and artificial intelligence (AI) replacing the history and physical examination in some part (e.g., pre-encounter electronic surveys), but personalized care of patients goes far beyond any scientific or technical advances. Appropriate care satisfies a need that can be met by human touch, intimate conversation, providing education, and respect for privacy. Personal interactions and physical examination play an integral role in developing meaningful and therapeutic relationships with patients (Artandi and Stewart, 2018; Goroll, 2015). The relationship with patients, particularly when illness compounds vulnerability, cannot be replaced (see Clinical Pearl, "The Patient Relationship").

Because cost containment is also essential, the well-performed history and physical examination can justify the appropriate and cost-effective use of resources. This underscores the need for judgment and the use of resources in a balance appropriate for the individual patient.

At a first meeting, you are in a position of authority and your patients are vulnerable. You may not have similar perspectives, lifestyles, religious backgrounds, sexual orientation, or gender identity, but you need to understand the patient's if you are to establish a meaningful partnership. This partnership has been conceptualized as patient-centered care, identified by the Institute of Medicine (IOM) as an important element of high-quality care. The IOM report defined patient-centered care as "respecting and responding to patients' wants, needs and preferences, so that they can make choices in their care that best fit their individual circumstances" (IOM, 2001). Box 2.1 identifies questions that represent a patient-centered approach in building a history. Your own beliefs, attitudes, and values cannot be discarded, but you do have to discipline them. Be aware of your cultural beliefs, faith, and conscience so that they do not inappropriately intrude as you discuss with patients a variety of issues. That means knowing yourself and leading with curiosity (Curlin et al., 2007; Gold, 2010) (see also Chapter 1).

You react differently to different people. Why? How? Do you want to be liked too much? Does thinking about how you are doing get in the way of your effort? Why does a patient make you angry? Is there some frustration in your life? Which of your prejudices may influence your response to a patient? Bias is an example of mental associations that can influence behavior or feelings toward an individual and encompasses attitudes, stereotypes, and prejudices. Possible sources of bias include race, ethnicity, religion, sexual orientation, gender identification, socioeconomic status, and disabilities. In medicine, these constructs can affect how we care for a patient. If providers are unaware of these biases, then the biases are considered implicit. Implicit biases can be further confounded by stigmatizing diagnoses such as physical handicap, HIV, obesity, psychiatric illness, and substance use disorders. In total, implicit bias is an attribution of certain qualities (prejudices and stigma) by an individual to a person. Implicit bias can be shaped by experience (Greenwald and Banaji, 1995). Implicit bias, if not taken into consideration with each encounter, can lead to discriminatory care without conscious intent (Narayan et al., 2019; Pritlove et al., 2019) (see Risk Factors box "Bias in Health Care"). Implicit bias can be overcome; learn about people, have a basic understanding of the culture from which your patient comes, avoid stigmatizing language and stereotypes, explore awkwardness and discomfort with your conversations, respect the magnitude of unconscious bias and situations that may magnify it, and assiduously practice evidence-based medicine (Williams & Wyatt, 2015).

Establishing a positive patient relationship depends on communication built on courtesy, comfort, connection, and confirmation (Box 2.2).

Be courteous, ensure physical and emotional comfort, be sure that you have connected with the patient with trust and candor, and confirm that all that has happened during the interaction is clearly understood by all parties and your patient is able teach back the agreed-on plan. That is communication.

BOX 2.1 Patient-Centered Questions

The following questions represent a patient-centered approach in building a history:

- How would you like to be addressed?
- How are you feeling today?
- What would you like for us to do today?
- What do you think is causing your symptoms?
- What is your understanding of your diagnosis? Its importance? Its need for management?
- How do you feel about your illness? Frightened? Threatened? Angry? As a wage earner? As a family member? (Be sure, however, to allow a response without putting words in the patient's mouth.)
- Do you believe treatment will help?
- How are you coping with your illness? Crying? Drinking more? Tranquilizers? Talking more? Less? Changing lifestyles?
- Do you want to know all the details about your diagnosis and its effect on your future?
- How important to you is "doing everything possible"?
- How important to you is "quality of life"?
- Have you prepared advance directives?
- Do you have people you can talk with about your illness? Where do you get your strength?
- Is there anyone else we should contact about your illness or hospitalization? Family members? Friends? Employer? Religious advisor? Attorney?
- Do you want or expect emotional support from the health care team?
- Are you troubled by financial questions about your medical care? Insurance coverage? Tests or treatment you may not be able to afford? Timing of payments required from you?
- If you have had previous hospitalizations, does it bother you to be seen by teams of physicians, nurses, and students on rounds?
- How private of a person are you?
- Are you concerned about the confidentiality of your medical records?
- Would you prefer to talk to an older/younger, male/female health care provider?
- Are there medical matters you do not wish to have disclosed to others?

We suggest that use of these questions should be determined by the particular situation. For example, talking about a living will might alarm a patient seeking a routine checkup but may relieve a patient hospitalized with a life-threatening disease. Cognitive impairment, anxiety, depression, fear, or related feelings in addition to racial, gender, ethnic, or other differences should modify your approach.

Seeking Connection

Examine your habits and modify them when necessary so that you are not a barrier to effective communication. Stiff formality may inhibit the patient; a too-casual attitude may fail to instill confidence. Do not be careless with words—what you think is innocuous may seem vitally important to a patient who may be anxious and searching for meaning in everything you say. Consider intellectual and emotional constraints related to how you ask

BOX 2.2 Communication
Courtesy, Comfort, Connection, Confirmation

Courtesy
- Knock before entering a room.
- Address the patient first formally (e.g., Miss, Ms., Mrs., Mr., Mx., or the manner of address preferred by the patient). It is all right to shake hands.
- Meet and acknowledge others in the room and establish their roles and degree of participation. Learn their names.
- Ensure confidentiality.
- Be in the room, sitting, with no effort to reach too soon for the doorknob.
- If taking notes, do so sparingly; note key words as reminders, but do not let note-taking distract from your observing and listening.
- If typing in the electronic health record, type briefly and maintain eye contact with the patient, if possible.
- Respect the need for modesty.
- Allow the patient time to be dressed and comfortably settled after the examination. Follow-up discussion with the patient still "on the table" is often discomfiting.

Comfort
- Ensure physical comfort for all, including yourself.
- Try to have a minimum of furniture separating you and the patient.
- Maintain privacy, using available curtains and shades.
- Ensure a comfortable room temperature or provide a blanket—a cold room will make a patient want to cover up.
- Ensure good lighting.
- Ensure necessary quiet. Turn off the television set.
- Try not to overtire the patient. It is not always necessary to do it all at one visit.

Connection
- Look at the patient; maintain good eye contact if cultural practices allow.
- Watch your language. Avoid professional jargon. Do not patronize with what you say.
- Do not dominate the discussion. Listen alertly. Let the patient order priorities if several issues are raised.
- Do not accept a previous diagnosis as a chief concern. Do not too readily follow a predetermined path.
- Find out whether the patient has turned from other health care providers to come to you.
- Take the history and conduct the physical examination before you look at previous studies or tests. Consider first what the patient has to say.
- Avoid leading or direct questions at first. Open-ended questions are better for starters. Let specifics evolve from these.
- Avoid being judgmental.
- Respect silence. Pauses can be productive.
- Be flexible. Rigidity limits the potential of an interview.
- Assess the patient's potential as a partner.
- Seek clues to problems from the patient's verbal behaviors and body language (e.g., talking too fast or too little).
- Look for the hidden concerns underlying chief complaints.
- Never trivialize any finding or clue.
- Problems can have multiple causes. Do not leap to one cause too quickly.
- Define any concern completely: Where? How severe? How long? In what context? What soothes or aggravates the problem?

Confirmation
- Ask the patient to summarize the discussion. There should be clear understanding, and uncertainty should be eased.
- Allow the possibility of more discussion with another open-ended question: "Anything else you want to bring up?"
- If there is a question that you cannot immediately answer, say so. Be sure to follow up later if at all possible.
- If you seem to have made a mistake, make every effort to repair it. Candor is important for development of a trusting partnership. Most patients respect it.

questions and offer information, how fast you talk, and how often you punctuate speech with verbal utterances like "uh-huh." The interaction requires the active encouragement of patient participation, with questions and responses addressed to social and emotional issues as much as the physical nature of health problems.

This introduction (for use with every patient) forms the foundation of the rest of the interaction. By stating how you want to be addressed and your pronouns, you invite the patient to share this information about themselves and avoid assumptions on your part. For patients who are transgender and gender diverse, this helps create a welcoming and supportive environment. Welcome others and ask how they are connected to the patient. Begin by asking open-ended questions ("How have you been feeling since we last met?" "What are your expectations for today's visit?" "What would you like to discuss?" "What do you want to make sure we cover?"). Resist the urge to interrupt. You will be amazed how many times a complete history is provided without prompting. Later, as information accumulates, you will need to be more specific. However, early on, it is entirely appropriate to check the patient's agenda and concerns and let the information flow. It is important not to interrupt the patient at the start of the interview. By initially remaining silent and then asking whether there is "anything else" a few times, you will be amazed how the patient's primary concerns are identified early in the visit. Thus you and the patient can collaboratively set the agenda for the visit.

Having clear and agreed-upon goals for each interaction leads to successful communication. You should strive to be a skilled listener and observer with a polished sense of timing and a kind of repose that is at once alert and reassuring. Your nonverbal behavior complements your listening. In the absence of infectious control issues, your face should not be masked. Be expressive and nod in agreement. It is better to avoid the extremes of reaction (e.g., startle, surprise, or grimacing). Eye contact should be assured and comfortable, and your body language should show that you are emotionally present and open to and engaged with the patient. You should be comfortably seated close to the patient and, if using an electronic health record, should position the computer screen so both you and the patient can visualize it. Do not stand and do not reach for the doorknob (see Clinical Pearl, "Professional Dress and Grooming").

Remember that patients also communicate nonverbally, and understanding this is advantageous to both you and the patient (Henry et al., 2012).

CLINICAL PEARL

Professional Dress and Grooming

Appropriate dress and grooming go a long way toward establishing a good first impression with the patient. Although clean fingernails, modest clothing, and neat hair are imperative, you need not be formal to be neat. You should avoid extremes so that appearance does not become an obstacle in the patient's response to care.

Confidentiality, which is important in all aspects of care, is another essential element. The patient should provide the information. It is important to identify everyone in the room to be sure the patient is comfortable and wants others to participate in the visit. You may want to ask the parent, spouse, or other person to step out of the room so you can have a confidential discussion with the patient. If language is a barrier, a professional interpreter, rather than a family member, should be used (Fig. 2.1).

Gentle guidance and polite redirection are sometimes necessary to keep the visit focused and moving forward (e.g., "Now let's also talk about . . ." or "Thank you for sharing this, but let me make sure I understand . . ."). Be prepared with questions you think are important to address based on the patient's history and main concerns.

If the patient touches on something that does not seem immediately relevant to your purposes (e.g., introducing a possible problem not previously mentioned), be flexible enough to clarify at least the nature of the concern. Some apparent irrelevancies may contain clues to the care-seeking behaviors or concerns that may be hidden beneath the primary concern or concerns and may be held until a certain level of trust has developed between you and the patient. The patient's body language will also suggest the intensity of an underlying feeling. Although too many digressions can lead to misspent time, paying attention may save a lot of time later, and information learned may be important to the future plan of care.

Enhancing Patient Responses

Carefully phrased questions can lead to more accurate responses. Ask one question at a time, avoiding a barrage that discourages the patient from being complete or that limits answers to a simple yes or no:

- The open-ended question gives the patient discretion about the extent of an answer: "Tell me about . . ." "And then what happened?" "What are your feelings about this?" "What else would you like to talk about?"
- The direct question seeks specific information: "How long ago did that happen?" "Where does it hurt?" "Please put a finger where it hurts." "How many pills did you take each time?" and "How many times a day did you take them?"
- The leading question is the riskiest because it may limit the information provided to what the patient thinks you want to know: "It seems to me that this bothered you a lot. Is that true?" "That wasn't very difficult to do, was it?" "That's a horrible-tasting medicine, isn't it?" When asking how often something happened, allow the patient to define "often," rather than asking, "It didn't happen too often, did it?"

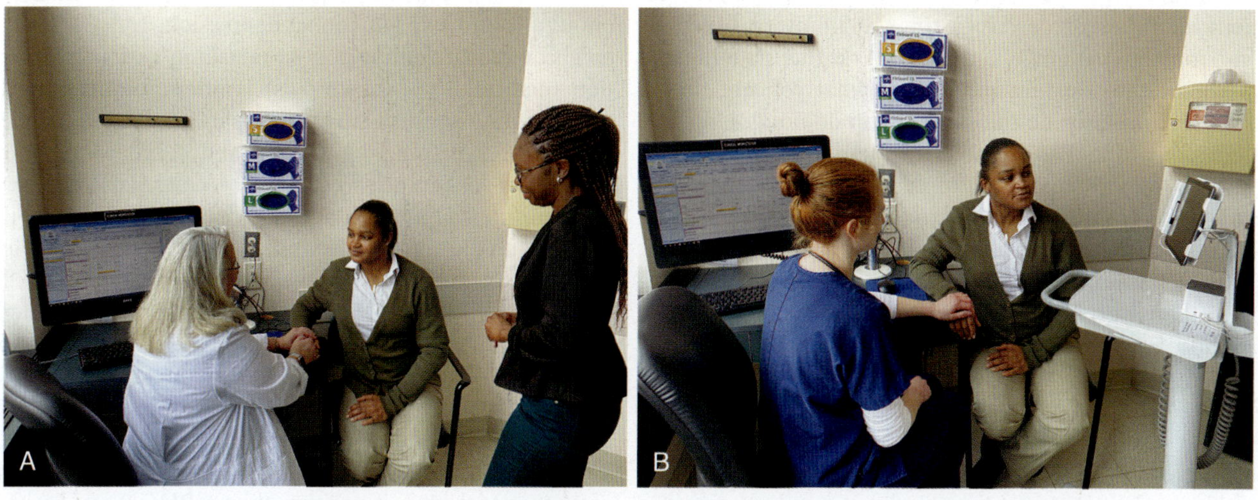

FIG. 2.1 (A) Interviewing a patient with the help of a live interpreter. (B) Interviewing a patient with the help of a video interpreter. Someone other than a family member should act as interpreter to bridge the language difference between the health care provider and the patient. An interpreter can be live, on video, or available telephonically.

Sometimes the patient does not quite understand what you are asking and says so. Recognize the need when it is appropriate to:

- Facilitate—encourage your patient to say more, either with your words or with a silence that the patient may break when given the opportunity for reflection.
- Reflect—repeat what you have heard to encourage more detail.
- Clarify—ask, "What do you mean?"
- Empathize—show your understanding and acceptance. Do not hesitate to say "I understand" or "I'm sorry" if the moment calls for it.
- Confront—do not hesitate to discuss a patient's disturbing behavior.
- Interpret—repeat what you have heard to confirm the patient's meaning.

What you ask is complemented by how you ask it. Take the following actions, if necessary, to clarify the patient's point of view. Do not assume you know what a patient is thinking:

- Ask what the patient thinks and feels about an issue.
- Make sure you know their chief concern.
- Ask about the patient's life situation, so that nothing seemingly extraneous to the chief concern and present illness has gone unnoticed.
- Suggest at appropriate times that you have the "feeling" that the patient could say more or that things may not be as well as they are reported.
- Suggest at appropriate times that it is all right to be angry, sad, or nervous, and it is all right to talk about it, ensuring confidentiality when appropriate.
- Make sure that the patient's expectations in the visit are met and that there are no further questions.

Make sure your questions are clearly understood. Define words when necessary and choose them carefully. Avoid technical terms if possible. Adapt your language when necessary to the patient's education level. Adapt your terminology, particularly in reference to how a patient identifies or describes their anatomy or illness, to mirror the patient's language. Ask the patient to stop you if they do not understand what you are talking about. Similarly, do the same if you do not grasp the patient's meaning. For example, a patient may report that he had "low blood" (anemia), "high blood" (hypertension), "bad blood" (syphilis), or "thin blood" (they are taking anticoagulants). It can take a bit of exploring to sort it all out. Do not assume every question needs a complex and technical answer. Avoid medical jargon with all patients, even those who are in the health care field.

Moments of Tension: Potential Barriers to Communication

Curiosity About You. Patients will sometimes ask about you. Although you are not the point, you may be comfortable revealing some relevant aspects of your experience ("I have trouble remembering to take medicines too" or "I remember when my children had tantrums"). A direct answer will usually do. Often, simply informing your patients that you have experienced similar life events (e.g., illness, pregnancy, and childbirth) can help alleviate fears and, with further exploration, can help in the identification of the patient's concerns. The message that you are a "real" person can lead to a trust-enhancing or even therapeutic exchange. At the same time, it is wise to exercise caution and remain professional in what and how much you disclose.

Anxiety. Anxiety has multiple sources, such as an impending procedure, risk exposure, or anticipated diagnosis. Some disorders will be more likely to cause an intense response, such as those associated with crushing chest pain or difficulty in breathing; with other disorders, just seeing a health care professional can cause anxiety. You can help by avoiding an overload of information, pacing the conversation, and presenting a calm demeanor.

Silence. Sometimes intimidated by silence, many clinicians feel the urge to break it. Be patient. Do not force the conversation. You may have to move the moment along with an open-ended question ("What seems to worry you?") or a mild nudge ("And after that?"). Remember, though, that silence allows the patient a moment of reflection or time to summon courage, especially when sharing traumatic and other emotional experiences. Some issues can be so painful and sensitive that silence becomes necessary and should be allowed. Most people will talk when they are ready. The patient's demeanor, use of hands, facial expressions, or teary eyes will help you interpret the moment. For teary eyes, be prepared to offer a tissue. Silence may also be cultural; for example, some cultural groups take their time, ponder their responses to questions, and answer when they feel ready. Do not push too hard. Be comfortable with silence and give it reasonable bounds.

Depression. Being sick or thinking that you are sick can be enough to provoke situational depression. Indeed, serious or chronic, unrelenting illness or taking certain prescription medications (e.g., steroids) is often accompanied by depression. A sense of sluggishness in the daily experience; disturbances in sleeping, eating, and social contact; and feelings of loss of self-worth can be clues. In addition to screening for depression at every visit, pay attention. First ask, "When did you start feeling this way?" Then ask, "How do you feel about it?" "Have you stopped enjoying the things you like to do?" "Do you have trouble sleeping?" "Have you had thoughts about hurting yourself?" "Are you depressed?" The Patient Health Questionnaires (a two-item screening tool, PHQ-2, or nine-item screening tool, PHQ-9) are validated tools used to screen for depression. The PHQ-2, the first two questions of the PHQ-9, is a preliminary screening tool, and, if positive, then a PHQ-9 can be used to help aid in diagnosis, determine severity, and follow response to treatment. See Box 2.3, "The Patient Health Questionnaire for Depression Screening." A patient in this

BOX 2.3 The Patient Health Questionnaire for Depression Screening

Depression can be screened for using a variety of tools. Adolescents aged 12–18 and adults, including pregnant and postpartum persons, should be screened for depression. The Patient Health Questionnaire (PHQ) is one of these tools. The PHQ-2 is made up of the first two questions from the PHQ-9. It asks about the frequency of depressed mood and anhedonia over the past 2 weeks. Each question is scored from 0 ("not at all") to 3 ("nearly every day"). The numeric values of each response is summed. PHQ-9 scores of 5, 10, 15, and 20 represent mild, moderate, moderately severe, and severe depression, respectively. The PHQ is as follows:

Over the last 2 weeks, how often have you been bothered by any of the following problems:

	NOT AT ALL	SEVERAL DAYS	MORE THAN HALF OF THE DAYS	NEARLY EVERY DAY
1. Little interest or pleasure in doing things	0	1	2	3
2. Feeling down, depressed, or hopeless	0	1	2	3
3. Trouble falling or staying asleep or sleeping too much	0	1	2	3
4. Feeling tired or having little energy	0	1	2	3
5. Poor appetite or overeating	0	1	2	3
6. Feeling bad about yourself or that you are a failure or have let yourself or your family down	0	1	2	3
7. Trouble concentrating on things such as reading the newspaper or watching television	0	1	2	3
8. Moving or speaking so slowly that other people could have noticed. Or the opposite—being so fidgety or restless that you have been moving around a lot more than usual	0	1	2	3
9. Thoughts that you would be better off dead or of hurting yourself in some way	0	1	2	3

Kroenke, K., Spitzer, R. L., & Williams, J. B. (2001). The PHQ-9: Validity of a brief depression severity measure. *Journal of General Internal Medicine, 16*(9), 606–613.

circumstance cannot be hurried and certainly cannot be relieved by superficial assurance. You need not worry about introducing the idea of suicide (see Clinical Pearl, "Adolescent Suicide"). It has most often been considered, if only briefly (see Chapter 7 Risk Factors box, "Suicide").

CLINICAL PEARL

Adolescent Suicide

Suicide is a major cause of mortality in the preteen and teen years, more often in young males. If the thought of it occurs to you, you can be quite sure that it has to the patient too. You can mention it and thus give permission to talk about it. You will not be suggesting anything new. You may actually help prevent it. The Ask Suicide-Screening Questions (ASQ) is a suicide risk screening tool approved for all ages. It consists of four questions:

1. In the past few weeks, have you wished you were dead?
2. In the past few weeks, have you felt that you or your family would be better off if you were dead?
3. In the past week, have you been having thoughts about killing yourself?
4. Have you ever tried to kill yourself?

If a patient answers yes to any of the four questions, the screen is considered positive.

Adapted from https://www.nimh.nih.gov/research/research-conducted-at-nimh/asq-toolkit-material

Crying and Compassionate Moments. People will cry. Let the emotion proceed at the patient's pace. Resume your questioning only when the patient is ready. If you suspect a patient is holding back, give permission. Offer a tissue or simply say, "It seems like you're feeling sad. It's OK to cry." Name the emotion. Be direct about such a tender circumstance, but gently, not too aggressively or insistently. Do not hesitate to say that you feel for the patient, that you are sorry for something that happened, and that you can tell it was painful. At times, the touch of a hand or even a hug is in order. (See Clinical Pearl, "Appropriate Touch in Medical Encounters.") Sometimes, a concern—a difficult family relationship, for example—must be confronted. You may have to check an assumption and hope that you have guessed correctly in bringing the patient's feelings to the surface. If uncertain, ask without presupposing what the response might be.

Physical and Emotional Intimacy. It is not easy to be intimate with the emotions and the bodies of others. Cultural norms and behaviors are at once protective of and barriers to trusting relationships. The patient is in a dependent status as well. You cannot be sure of the degree to which a given patient has been "desensitized" to the issues of

CLINICAL PEARL

Appropriate Touch in Medical Encounters

Touch during the history and physical examination process should be brief and purposeful by the clinician to perform an examination maneuver, provide comfort, or establish a connection with the patient. It should always have explicit consent and respect for the patient's boundaries.

Things to remember regarding physical contact during medical encounters:

- Consent is necessary: Seek permission before touching a patient, even for routine examinations
- Professionalism is paramount: Maintain a professional demeanor and avoid unnecessary or overly intimate touch
- Cultural sensitivity: Consider cultural differences and patient preferences regarding touch (see Box 2.4 "Trauma-Informed Care")
- Context counts: Appropriate touch depends on the clinical situation (e.g., sensitive conversation, painful procedure, or physical examination)

EXAMPLES OF APPROPRIATE TOUCH	THINGS TO AVOID
Gentle hand on the shoulder	Touching sensitive area like chest or groin without a clear medical indication and explicit consent.
Light touch on the back	Hugging is generally not considered appropriate unless the patient initiates it and there has been an existing strong therapeutic relationship.
Palpation during the examination	Touching beyond what is needed for the examination.
Hand holding in certain situations while providing emotional support	Ignoring patient cues or discomfort. If a patient expresses discomfort with any touch, immediately stop.

BOX 2.4 Trauma-Informed Care

It is common for people to experience trauma or adverse childhood experiences (ACEs) and for this trauma to have a lasting impact on their lives. Trauma comes from an individual's experiences and can be the result of an event or series of events or from circumstances. These events are perceived as emotionally harmful or threating and have lasting adverse effects on a person's functioning and/or physical, social, emotional, or spiritual well-being. Screening for trauma or an ACE is not for diagnostic purposes, but rather to help identify risks for trauma. Trauma-informed care (TIC) helps improve the care provided, health care experiences, and health outcomes for patients who have experienced trauma. Remembering the 5 R's can help prevent further harm when talking with patients.

Realize that trauma, ACEs, and adversity are common
  Screening and trauma recognition

Recognize different ways that trauma can affect people
  Understanding the health effects of trauma

Respond by considering how people can be affected by trauma to support recovery and recognize and support resilience
  Practice patient-centered communication and care

Resist retraumatization and offer opportunities for choice, control, empowerment, collaboration, and safety
  Emphasis on emotional safety and avoiding triggers

Recognize the importance of relationships
  Relationships provide a foundation of trust and safety

TIC requires changing interactions, policies, and environments to prevent retraumatization. For example, a trauma-informed clinician will:

- Explain why they need to perform a physical examination
- Let a patient bring a trusted friend or family member into the room
- Respond with compassion if a patient refuses an examination or test

Adapted from Substance Abuse and Mental Health Services Administration, Trauma-informed care in behavioral health services. Treatment improvement protocol (TIP) Series 57. HHS Publication No. (SMA) 13-4801, Substance Abuse and Mental Health Services Administration, Rockville, MD (2014) and Roberts, S. J., Chandler, G. E., & Kalmakis, K. (2019). A model for trauma-informed primary care. *Journal of the American Association of Nurse Practitioners, 31*(2), 139–144. http://dx.doi.org/10.1097/JXX.0000000000000116

intimacy. You also cannot be sure of the patient's trauma history. You can acknowledge this while explaining clearly and without apology what you must do for the patient's benefit while ensuring your care is patient centered and allows for the patient to maintain control. Be careful about the ways in which you use words or frame questions. Box 2.4 discusses trauma-informed care. Mirror the patient's language about their anatomy, and respect modesty, using covers appropriately without hampering a complete examination. By being calm and asking questions with professional poise and by being empathetic yet straightforward, explaining the consequences of not performing an examination, such as skipping examination of the genitals, because of modesty or past-trauma concerns may help keep the necessary from becoming an issue.

Inappropriate Attraction. Some patients can be excessively flattering and manipulative and even seductive. Their illness and insecurity beg for extra-special attention. Do not be taken in by this. There are limits to warmth and cordiality. Certainly not all touch is sexually motivated; a heartfelt hug is sometimes just right. Nevertheless, beware of that trap. Avert it courteously and firmly, delivering the immediate message that the relationship is and will remain professional. It takes skill to do this while maintaining the patient's dignity, but there is no room for sexual misconduct in the relationship, and there can be no tolerance for exploitation of the patient in this regard.

Anger. Sometimes patients who express anger (or persons with them) are the ones who may need you the most. Of course, it can be intimidating. Confront it. It is all right to say, "It seems like you're angry. Can you tell me why? I want to hear." Speak softly and try not to argue the point. You may not know if or why you made someone angry. Most often, you have done nothing wrong, and the patient's emotion is unrelated to you or the visit. Still, the stress of time, heavy workload, and tension of caring for the acutely—even terminally—ill can generate your own impatience and potential for anger. Avoid being defensive but acknowledge the problem. Only when appropriate, apologize and ask how to make things better.

Explore the feelings. Often, you can continue on a better footing after anger is vented. On occasion, nothing will seem to help. It is then all right to defer to another time or even to suggest a different professional.

Afterward, do not hesitate to talk about the episode with a trusted colleague. It helps. Discussing the incident later may lend insight into behaviors and help prevent the occurrence again. Better ways of responding can be explored.

Avoiding the Full Story. Patients may not always tell the whole story, or even the truth, either purposely or unconsciously. Dementia, illness, substance abuse, past experience of or fear of discrimination because of sexual orientation or gender identity in health care settings, intimate partner violence (IPV), and child abuse are among some of the reasons. Do not push too hard when you think this is happening. Allow the interview to go on and then come back to a topic with gentle questioning. You might say, "I think that you may be more concerned than you are saying" or "I think you're worried about what we might find out." Unless there is concern about the safety of the patient or another individual, learning all that is necessary may not come in one sitting. You may have to pursue the topic at a later visit or perhaps with other members of the family or friends or your professional colleagues.

Financial Considerations. The cost of care and the resulting drain on resources (and the potential impact on employment or insurance coverage) are often sources of stress for the patient. Talk about them with candor and accurate knowledge. Provide resources (social worker or financial counselor). Otherwise, an appropriate care plan acceptable to the patient cannot be devised or implemented. Pressing circumstances and obligations may still present barriers to appropriate care. (See Clinical Pearl, "Social Determinants of Health.")

The Patient History

A first objective in building the history is to identify those matters the patient defines as problems, the subtle and the obvious. You need to establish a sense of the patient's reliability as an interpreter of events. Consider the potential for intentional or unintentional suppression or underreporting of certain experiences that may give context to a problem that is at odds with your expectations. Constantly evaluate the patient's words and behavior. The history is built on the patient's perspective and story, not yours. Make modifications as required for the patient's age and their physical and emotional disabilities. There are times when collateral information is needed to fully appreciate the patient's narrative.

Setting for the Interview

Regardless of the setting, make everyone as comfortable as possible. Position yourself so that there are no bulky desks, tables, computer screens, or other electronic equipment between you and the patient (Fig. 2.2). If possible, have a clock placed where you can see it without obviously looking at your watch (preferably behind the patient's chair). Sit comfortably and at ease, maintaining eye contact and a conversational tone of voice. Your manner can assure the patient that you care and that the patient is your primary focus. You can do this only by concentrating on the matter at hand, giving the encounter primacy in your life, and putting aside both personal and professional distractions.

Structure of the History

You build the history to establish a relationship with the patient, so that you jointly discover the issues and problems that need attention and priority. A widely accepted

CLINICAL PEARL

Social Determinants of Health

Social determinants of health (SDOH) are conditions and environments where people live, learn, worship, work, play, and age. SDOH have a major impact on health, functioning, well-being, and quality of life. SDOH contribute to health disparities and inequities. For example, people without access to healthy foods or grocery stores are less likely to have good nutrition and are more likely to have heart disease, diabetes, and obesity. As a result, these individuals have a shorter life expectancy. SDOH can be divided into five domains:

1. Economic stability
2. Education access and quality
3. Health care access and quality
4. Neighborhood and working environment
5. Social and community context

Modified from https://health.gov/healthypeople/objectives-and-data/social-determinants-health, https://www.who.int/gender-equity-rights/understanding/sdh-definition/en/, and https://www.cdc.gov/socialdeterminants/index.htm

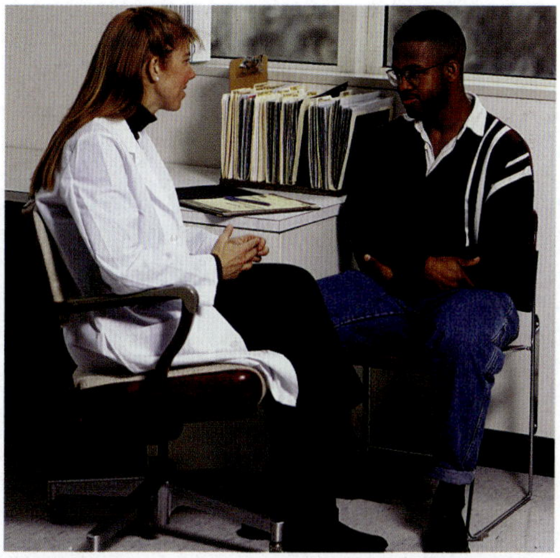

FIG. 2.2 Interviewing a young adult. Note the absence of an intervening desk or table.

approach is provided that can and should be modified to fit individual circumstances:

- First, the identifiers: name, date, time, age, sex assigned at birth, sexual orientation, gender identity, preferred language, identified race/ethnicity, source of information, and referral source
- Chief concern (CC)
- History of present illness or problem (HPI)
- Past medical history (PMH)
- Family history (FH)
- Personal and social history (SH)
- Review of systems (ROS)

The chief concern is a brief statement about why the patient is seeking care. Direct quotes are helpful. It is important, however, to go beyond the given reason and to probe for underlying concerns that cause the patient to seek care. If the patient has a sore throat, why is help sought? Is it the pain and fever, or is it concern caused by past experience with a relative who developed rheumatic heart disease? Many interviewers include the duration of the problem as part of the chief concern.

Understanding the present illness or problem requires a step-by-step evaluation of the circumstances that surround the primary reason for the patient's visit. A complete history includes an exploration of the patient's overall health before the chief concern, in addition to past medical and surgical experiences. The spiritual, psychosocial, and cultural contexts of the patient's life are essential to an understanding of these events. The patient's family also requires attention—their health; PMH; illnesses; deaths; and the genetic, social, and environmental influences. Careful inquiry about the personal and social experiences of the patient should include work habits and the variety of relationships in the family, school, and workplace. Finally, the ROS includes a detailed inquiry of possible concerns in each of the body's systems, looking for complementary or seemingly unrelated symptoms that may not have surfaced during the rest of the history. Flexibility, the appreciation of subtlety, lack of judgment, and the opportunity for the patient to ask questions and to explore feelings are explicit needs in the process.

Think About It

One question should underlie all of your inquiry: Why is this happening to this particular patient at this particular time? In other words, if many people are exposed to a potential problem and only some of them become ill after the exposure, what are the unique factors in this individual that led to that outcome? For example, if 100 people wake up with a bad headache and 97 go to work while 3 seek care, what underlying dimension prompted those decisions?

Building the History

Introduce yourself to the patient and accompanying persons if you have not already met, clearly stating your name and your role. If you are a student, say so. Be certain that you know the patient's full name and that you pronounce it correctly. Ask if you are not certain.

Ask the patient how they would like to be addressed and then address the patient properly (e.g., as Mr., Miss, Mrs., Ms., Mx., or the manner of address preferred by the patient) and repeat the patient's name at appropriate times. Avoid the familiarity of using a first name for an adult when you do not expect familiarity in return. Do not use a surrogate term for a person's name; for example, when the patient is a child, do not address the parent as "Mother" or "Father." It is respectful and courteous to take the time to learn each name.

It is respectful to look at the patient and not at the electronic health record. Use it if you must but position it so that it does not distract you from the patient. More and more electronic devices for documentation and educational purposes (e.g., capturing a picture of a lesion to follow over time, demonstrating the findings on an imaging study, showing the trend of a laboratory result over time, or reviewing a website together) are being used. Unless you already know the patient and know that there is urgency, proceed at a reasonable pace, asking for the reason for the visit with the intent of learning what their specific expectations of the visit are. Listen, and do not be too directive. You will often be surprised at how much of the story and how many details you will hear without pushing. Let the patient share their full story and reasons for seeking care.

You have begun to give structure to the present illness or problem, giving it a chronological and sequential framework. Unless there is urgency, go slowly, hear the full story, and refrain from interrupting with what seems the obvious course of questioning. The patient will take cues from you on the leisure you will allow. You must walk a fine line between permitting this leisure and meeting the many time constraints you are sure to have. Fix your attention on the patient, avoid interjecting as much as possible, and do not ask the next question before you have heard the complete answer to the prior one.

The patient's responses may at times be unclear. Seek certainty:

- "Of what you've told me, what concerns you the most?"
- "What do you want to make sure we pay attention to today?"
- "Do you have any ideas about what we ought to do?"
- Or a leading question sometimes: "I think _________ worries you the most. Am I right? Shall we talk about that first?"
- As the interview proceeds, thoroughly explore each positive response with the following questions:
  - Where? Where are symptoms located, as precisely as possible? If they seem to move, what is the range of their movement? Where is the patient when the symptom occurs—at work or play, active or resting?
  - When? Everything happens in a chronological sequence. When did it begin? Does it come and go? If so, how often and for how long? What time of day? What day of the week?

- What? What does it mean to the patient? What is its impact? What does it feel like? What is its quality and intensity? Has it been bad enough to interrupt the flow of the patient's life, or has it been dealt with rather casually? What else happened during this time that might be related? What makes it feel better? Worse?
- How? The background of the symptoms becomes important in answering the "how" question. How did they come about? Are other things going on at the same time, such as work, play, mealtime, or sleep? Is there illness in the family? Have there been similar episodes in the past? If so, how were they treated or were they resolved without treatment? Is there concern about similar symptoms in friends or relatives? Are there spouse concerns? How is the patient coping? Are there social supports? Nothing ever happens in isolation.
- Why? Of course, the answer to "why" is the solution to the problem. All other questions lead to this one.

Once you have understood the patient's chief concern and present problem and you have a sense of underlying issues, you may go on to other segments of the history: the family and past medical histories; emotional, spiritual, and cultural concerns; and social and workplace accompaniments to the present concerns. Remember that nothing in the patient's experience is isolated. Aspects of the present illness or problem require careful integration with the medical and family history. The life of the patient is not constructed according to your outline, with many factors giving shape to the present illness and with one chief concern possibly involving more than one illness.

A visit should conclude with a review:

- Ask the patient to try to satisfy gaps in your understanding.
- Ask for questions.
- Interpret and summarize what you have heard.
- Ask the patient to summarize for you to ensure complete understanding.
- Repeat instructions and ask to hear them back.
- Explain the next steps: needed examinations and/or studies, appointment times, keeping in touch.

Sensitive Issues

Sensitive issues, which may be difficult to discuss (e.g., sex, sexual orientation, gender identity, drug or alcohol use, concerns about death) are important to address. The following guidelines, keys to any successful interview, are essential in an approach to sensitive issues:

- Provide privacy.
- Do not waffle. Be direct and firm. Avoid asking leading questions.
- Do not apologize for asking a question. But ensure you are asking an appropriate question, in an appropriate manner, for an appropriate reason, at an appropriate time.
- Do not preach. Avoid confrontation. You are not there to pass judgment or proselytize.
- Use language that is understandable to the patient, yet not patronizing (see Clinical Pearl, "Watch the Use of Jargon").
- Do not push too hard.

Afterward, document carefully, using the patient's words (and those of others with the patient) whenever possible. It is all right to take notes, but try to do this sparingly, especially when discussing sensitive issues.

> **CLINICAL PEARL**
>
> **Watch the Use of Jargon**
>
> Unfortunately, many of us may too often lapse into the use of jargon, the language of our profession that is not accessible to the patient. Patient-demeaning words are worse. Stress, frustration, fatigue, and anger are common underlying causes for these lapses. Know yourself. Understand why you might fall into the habit, and do your best to avoid it.

You must always be ready to explain again why you examine sensitive areas. A successful approach will have incorporated four steps:

1. An introduction, the moment when you bring up the issue, alluding to the need to understand its context in the patient's life.
2. Open-ended questions that are free of assumptions and that first explore the patient's feelings about the issue—whether, for example, it is alcohol, drugs, sex, cigarettes, education, or problems at home—and then the direct exploration of what is actually happening.
3. A period in which you thoughtfully attend to what the patient is saying and then repeat the patient's words or offer other forms of feedback. This permits the patient to agree that your interpretation is appropriate, thus confirming what you have heard.
4. Finally, an opportunity for the patient to ask any questions that might be relevant.

Alcohol and Drugs. TAPS (Tobacco, Alcohol, Prescription medication, and other Substance use Tool) (https://www.drugabuse.gov/taps/#/) is a two-component screening tool. The first is TAPS-1, and if this is positive, it is followed by TAPS-2. TAPS-2 screens for risk level for the substance that was identified in TAPS-1. This tool can be self-administered by an adult patient or given as part of an interview. TAPS is one of several tools on the NIDAMED portal (https://www.drugabuse.gov/nidamed-medical-health-professionals) that can help providers choose brief, evidence-based substance use screening tools. The CAGE-AID questionnaire (Brown and Rounds, 1995) is one model for discussing the use of alcohol (see Box 2.5). **CAGE** is an acronym for **C**utting down, **A**nnoyance by criticism, **G**uilty feeling, **E**ye-openers. **CAGE-AID** is the CAGE questionnaire **A**dapted to **I**nclude **D**rugs. Its use does not ensure absolute sensitivity in the detection of a problem. Another common screening tool is the AUDIT-C (Bush et al., 1998; Box 2.6). It can be used to screen for

BOX 2.5 CAGE and CAGE-AID Questionnaire

The CAGE questionnaire was developed in 1984 by Dr. John Ewing, and it includes four interview questions designed to help screen for alcoholism. The questions were adapted by Dr. Richard Brown in 1991 to include illicit drugs. It is a screening questionnaire to help determine if a more complete assessment is needed.

The CAGE acronym helps practitioners quickly recall the main concepts of the four questions (**C**utting down, **A**nnoyance by criticism, **G**uilty feeling, **E**ye-openers). The CAGE-AID questionnaire is publicly available and can be downloaded at http://www.integration.samhsa.gov/clinical-practice/screening-tools.

BOX 2.6 AUDIT-C Questionnaire

The three-question AUDIT-C questionnaire is scored on a scale of 0 to 12 (0 = no alcohol use). In males, a score of 4 or more is considered positive, and in females, a score of 3 or more is considered positive (Bradley et al., 2003). The greater the score, the more likely it is that drinking is affecting the patient's health. The AUDIT-C is a modified version of the 10-item Alcohol Use Disorders Identification Test (AUDIT) developed by the World Health Organization and published in 1998. The AUDIT is available at: https://www.who.int/publications/i/item/WHO-MSD-MSB-01.6a. The AUDIT-C is available at: https://www.hepatitis.va.gov/alcohol/treatment/audit-c.asp.

hazardous drinking or for alcohol use disorders (see Clinical Pearl, "Alcohol Consumption Definitions"). These screens can be complemented or supplemented by the T-ACE model (Box 2.7), particularly in the identification of alcoholism in a pregnant patient (because of the potential for damage to the fetus), or by CRAFFT for identification of an alcohol problem in adolescents (Box 2.8). There is similarity in all of these questionnaires. You can adapt them to your style and to the particular patient. You can also adapt them to concerns about drugs or substances other than alcohol (see Clinical Pearl, "Screening," and Risk Factors box for developing a substance use disorder).

BOX 2.7 T-ACE Model

The following questions are included in the T-ACE model:

T How many drinks does it **T**ake to make you feel high? How many when you first started drinking? When was that? What do you prefer: beer, wine, or liquor? (More than two drinks suggests a tolerance to alcohol, which is a red flag.)

A Have people **A**nnoyed you by criticizing your drinking?

C Have you felt you ought to **C**ut down on your drinking?

E Have you ever had an **E**ye-opener drink first thing in the morning to steady your nerves or get rid of a hangover?

An answer to T alone (more than two drinks) or a positive response to two of A, C, or E may signal a problem with a high degree of probability. Positive answers to all four signal a problem with great certainty.

From Sokol, R. J., Martier, S. S., & Ager, J. W. (1989). The T-ACE questions: Practical prenatal detection of risk-drinking. *American Journal of Obstetrics and Gynecology, 160*, 863–870.

BOX 2.8 CRAFFT Questionnaire

The CRAFFT questionnaire was developed in 2002 as a screening tool for alcohol and substance abuse in adolescents.

The CRAFFT acronym helps clinicians remember the main concepts of the six questions: **C**ar, **R**elax, **A**lone, **F**orget, **F**riends, **T**rouble.

The exact wording of the CRAFFT questions is available at: http://archpedi.jamanetwork.com/article.aspx?articleid=203511.

Knight, J. R., Sherritt, L., Shrier, L. A., Harris, S. K., & Chang, G. (2002). Validity of the CRAFFT substance abuse screening test among adolescent clinic patients. *Archives of Pediatrics & Adolescent Medicine*, 156(6), 607–614.

CLINICAL PEARL

- Alcohol consumption definitions: One standard drink is equal to any one of the following:
  - 12 oz. regular beer, usually about 5% alcohol
  - 8–9 oz. malt liquor (7% alcohol)
  - 5 oz. table wine (12% alcohol)
  - 1.5 oz. 80-proof hard liquor (40% alcohol)
- Drinking in moderation: Two standard drinks or less daily for males and one standard drink or less for females
- Binge drinking: Five or more alcoholic drinks on at least 1 day in the past month for males or four or more alcohol drinks for females on the same occasion
- Heavy alcohol use: Five or more drinks on any day or 15 or more per week for males and 4 or more or 8 or more drinks per week for females

CLINICAL PEARL

Screening

There is a difference between a screening and an assessment interview. The goal of screening is to find out if a problem exists. It is effective, but it is only the start, and assessment continues after a positive screen. Discovering a problem early may lead to a better outcome.

Intimate Partner Violence. We frequently underestimate the incidence of IPV in the experience of our patients of any age, sexual orientation, or gender identity. IPV includes a range of abusive behaviors perpetrated by someone who is or was involved in an intimate relationship with the victim. It affects primarily females, children, and dependent older adults as victims and, in lesser frequency, males. Intimate partners are usually the perpetrators. Same-sex partners probably have the same prevalence, although underreporting may be more of a problem in this population. Alcohol use is a common facilitator. Children exposed to IPV are at increased risk for social and emotional problems. There is significant overlap between IPV and child abuse, so when IPV is detected, child abuse should be considered.

Reluctance to screen for fear of offending patients and families is a misplaced concern. This is occasionally compounded by an inappropriate response to an abused person, such as making too little of their experience or even laying the blame on them. They are twice a victim. Although IPV affects both males and females as victims and perpetrators, more females experience IPV (Nelson et al., 2012), and transgender women are at higher risk of physical and psychological IPV than are cisgender adults (Pitts et al., 2006). Likewise, lesbian, gay, bisexual, and transgender (LGBT) youth are at high risk for being victims of IPV (Whitton et al., 2016; Whitton et al., 2019). Few victims will discuss IPV willingly with a clinician, and the patient is usually the initiator of the discussion. We recommend that all individuals be screened. A validated brief Partner Violence Screen (PVS) uses three questions to detect partner violence (MacMillan et al., 2006):

1. Have you been hit, kicked, punched, or otherwise hurt by someone within the past year?
2. Do you feel safe in your current relationship?
3. Is there a partner from a previous relationship who is making you feel unsafe now?

These cover two dimensions of partner violence, and a positive response to any one of them constitutes a positive screen. The first question addresses physical violence. The latter two questions evaluate the individual's perception of safety and estimate their short-term risk of further violence and need for counseling.

Additionally, you may see something suggestive on the physical examination and ask the following: "The bruises I see. Can you tell me how you got them?"

Positive answers require accurate documentation, using words, drawings, and, if possible, photographs and the preservation of any tangible evidence. Positive answers require that the patient's safety be ensured. Ask the following:

- Are you afraid to go home?
- Are there guns or knives at home?
- Is alcohol (or other drugs) part of the problem?
- Has it gotten worse lately?
- Are children involved?

A "yes" answer mandates an intervention that requires utilization of other health care professionals such as social workers and mental health providers, who may be able to provide more in-depth assessment and linkage to resources. Get the patient's viewpoint. Let them speak; assure them that they are not alone and that you will do your best to help.

A "no" answer may still leave you uncomfortable. Get permission from the patient to document your concern and your suspicion of injury. Be unafraid to ask direct questions about your suspicion ("Where did that bruise come from?"). Ask them to come back to see you again.

Evidence-Based Practice in Physical Examination

Screening for Abuse and Intimate Partner Violence

Data from a systematic review indicate that screening practices by health care professionals are inconsistent for several reasons, including the existence of a variety of screening instruments, a lack of consensus on which instrument to use, lack of specificity of risk factors, lack of training, lack of effectiveness studies about what to do if violence is identified, discomfort with screening, and time constraints. Several instruments have been developed for IPV screening, and their diagnostic accuracy has been evaluated in studies of different populations using various reference standards. Six instruments with one to eight items demonstrated sensitivity and specificity greater than 80% in clinical populations of asymptomatic females; results varied between studies and across instruments. The PVS three-item screening instrument had a higher sensitivity and specificity compared with two longer instruments and can identify females at high risk for subsequent IPV (Houry et al., 2004). The HITS (Hurt-Insult-Threaten-Scream) four-item screening instrument for abuse (Box 2.9) demonstrated 86% sensitivity and 99% specificity (English version) and 100% sensitivity and 86% specificity (Spanish version).

Studies to develop and evaluate tools are generally lacking to assess screening older and vulnerable adults for abuse. Existing instruments to detect child abuse are not designed for direct administration to the child, thus missing opportunities to screen older children in the context of usual health care.

Data from Chen, P. H., Rovi, S., Vega, M., Jacobs, A., & Johnson, M. S. (2005). Screening for domestic violence in a predominantly Hispanic clinical setting. *Family Practice, 22*(6), 617–623. http://dx.doi.org/10.1093/fampra/cmi075; Kliegman, R., Stanton, B., St. Geme, J. W., et al. (Eds.). (2016). *Nelson textbook of pediatrics* (20th ed.). Philadelphia: Elsevier; and Nelson, H. D., Nygren, P., McInerney, Y., & Klein, J. (2004). Screening women and elderly adults for family and intimate partner violence: A review of the evidence for the U.S. Preventive Services Task Force. *Annals of Internal Medicine, 140*, 387–396.

BOX 2.9 Brief Screening Tool for Domestic Violence: HITS

Verbal abuse is as intense a problem as physical violence. HITS stands for **H**urt, **I**nsult, **T**hreaten, or **S**cream. The wording of the question is: In the past year, how often did your partner:

Hurt you physically?
Insult or talk down to you?
Threaten you with physical harm?
Scream or curse at you?

This approach works for all persons. Infants and children have the protection of the legal mandate for you to report your suspicions. Questioning a child about abuse suffered or witnessed at home can be problematic because you want to avoid suggestion. In general, open-ended questions are comfortably asked of the young child or of a parent in their presence:

- "Why did you come to see me today?" (Do not mention the concern directly.)
- "Tell me everything that happened to you, please." (No leading questions.)
- With infants, a bruise or burn with an odd shape or unexpected location is very concerning for child abuse.

It is difficult for an infant who is not yet crawling or toddling to break a femur or to have fingerprint-size bruises on the arms, for example.

- Adolescents may endure violence, particularly sexual, at home or away. The clue may be changes in behavior (such as dress and makeup), school effort, sleeping, and eating. Routinely screen adolescents for partner violence. Alcohol or drug use can become an issue. Former friends may be avoided. Most important, take your time and ask the following questions:
  - "What sexual experiences have you had?"
  - "When did you start?"
  - "Did you want to, or were you forced or talked into it?"
  - "Do the people you are with ever scare you?"
  - "Did anyone ever touch you in a sexual way?"

Always be available for more conversation. The questions are just a start. Note that young patients may also witness and endure violence at home, with a profound effect on their lives and behavior (see Risk Factors box for developing a substance use disorder). These problems should be dealt with as if the patient were the direct victim. Additionally, adolescents may be victims of human trafficking (see next section).

The risk of abuse of older adults, often underreported, is greater if the older adult has had a history of mental illness, is physically or cognitively impaired, or is living in a dependent situation with inadequate financial resources. The abusers may have similar risks, perhaps alcohol or drug related. Both groups may have a past history of domestic violence.

Human Trafficking. "Human trafficking involves the use of force, fraud, or coercion to obtain some type of labor or commercial sex act" (https://www.dhs.gov/blue-campaign/what-human-trafficking). It is a significant problem that is often not considered, and adolescents and adult patients should be screened to help identify trafficking victims or people at risk for trafficking victimization. There are guides to help providers use trauma-informed and survivor-informed practices with their screening (https://www.ncjrs.gov/pdffiles1/nij/grants/246713.pdf and https://www.acf.hhs.gov/sites/default/files/otip/adult_human_trafficking_screening_tool_and_guide.pdf). Examples of the screening tools and associated provider guides are the Trafficking Victim Identification Tool (TVIT), Adult Human Trafficking Screening Tool (AHTST), and Human Trafficking Screening Tool (HTST) (Dank et al., 2017) for youth (between the ages of 12 and 24 years). Before using these screening tools with persons who may be victims of human trafficking, the victim's personal safety and comfort should be assured; try not to be judgmental or shocked by details they may reveal and to be understanding when victims do not wish to repeat the details. Trafficking victims have often endured profound physical and psychological injuries.

Spirituality. The basic condition that life imposes is death. It often stirs in us a spiritual or "sacred" feeling—always with us, frequently sublimated, sometimes not. Illness, however mild, may stir that feeling and may carry with it a sense of dread. Faith may be an intimate contributor to one's perspective. An understanding of "spirituality" is, then, integral to the care we offer, but it is complicated by the fact that there is no universally agreed-on definition; each of us brings our own understanding to the care provided.

Many patients want attention paid to spirituality, and faith can be a key factor in the success of a management plan. Others may prefer that you not broach the subject. This requires the same degree of sensitivity and caution as talking about drugs, cigarettes, sex, and alcohol. The questions suggested by Puchalski and Romer (2000) with the acronym FICA and adapted by us suggest an approach:

- Faith, belief, and meaning
  - What is your spiritual or religious heritage? Is the Bible, the Quran, or a similar writing important to you?
  - Do these beliefs help you cope with stress?
- Importance and influence
  - How have these beliefs influenced how you handle stress? To what extent?
- Community
  - Do you belong to a formal spiritual or religious community? Does this community support you? In what way? Is there anyone there with whom you would like to talk?
- Address/action in care
  - How do your religious beliefs affect your health care decisions (e.g., choice of birth control)? How would you like me to support you in this regard when your health is involved?

Answers to these questions may guide you to involve clergy or other spiritual care providers or to become more deeply involved. There is some evidence that prayer can aid in healing. You may, if you are asked and are inclined, pray with a patient, although it is best that you not lead the prayer. You may even suggest it if the patient is sorely troubled and you understand the need. There are, however, boundaries. Except for very few of us, we are not theologians, and it is inappropriate to go beyond the limits of our professional expertise.

Auster (2004) suggests sensitivity on our part when patients ask about our personal beliefs and express their wish to talk only with someone of their own faith. You might say, "I want to help you as best I can, so please tell me why you ask about my faith" or, more directly, "I understand your feeling. Would it help if I found another person for you?" Let your sense of the situation guide you (Fosarelli, 2003; Puchalski and Romer, 2000).

Sexuality and Gender Identity

Patients should be told that discussion is routine and confidential. Questions about the patient's sexual history may first be indirect, addressing feelings rather than facts: "Are you satisfied with your sexual life, or do you have worries or concerns? Many people do." Although this is a leading question, it does not suggest what the patient's feelings should be. Rather, if there are concerns about sex, it may be comforting to know that one is not alone. The age of the patient should not deter discussion. Do not assume sexual practices or concerns for anybody, particularly older adults. It is also important to ask questions about a patient's sexual orientation and gender identity.

Identity. You should directly ask about your patient's sexual orientation and gender identity. In general, patients support health care providers asking questions related to sexual orientation and gender identity and understand the importance of health care providers' knowing their patients (Cahill et al., 2014).

The sexual orientation and gender identity of a patient must be known if appropriate continuity of care is to be offered. Working with sexual and gender minorities (SGM) demands knowing yourself regarding any potential feelings about cisgender-heteronormativity, homophobia, biphobia, and transphobia that you may have. Apprehension these patients may feel in revealing their information should be respected. Reassuring, nonjudgmental words help: "I'm glad you trust me. Thank you for telling me." It is also supportive if the health care setting offers some recognition of the patients involved (e.g., by making relevant informational pamphlets available in waiting areas).

- Trust can be better achieved if questions are "gender neutral":
  - Tell me about your living situation.
  - Are you sexually active?
  - In what way?
- Rather than:
  - Are you married?
  - Do you have a boyfriend/girlfriend?

If you use a nonjudgmental approach and a variety of questions applicable to any patient, understanding the patient's situation becomes possible. The patient's vernacular may be necessary. Once the barrier is broken, you can be more direct, asking, for example, about frequency of sexual intercourse, problems in achieving orgasm, variety and numbers of "partners" (a nongender-linked term), masturbation, and particular likes and dislikes. Identifying risk factors for unintentional pregnancy and sexually transmitted infections (STIs) is an important part of the sexual history. See Risk Factor box on unintentional pregnancy and STIs.

Outline of the History

The outline offered is a guide derived from multiple sources. It is not rigid, and you can decide what meets the needs of your patient and your style. Take advantage of the patient's photographs and videos that complement what you learn in the history.

Chief Concern or the Reason for Seeking Care. This answers the question, "Why are you here?" (see Clinical Pearl, "Chief Complaint or Chief Concern?"). Follow-up questions ask about duration (e.g., "How long has this been going on?" or "When did these symptoms begin?"). The patient's age, gender identity, sexual orientation, marital status, previous hospitalizations, military/veteran status, and occupation should be noted for the record. Other concerns may surface. A seemingly secondary issue may have greater significance than the original concern because the driving force for the chief concern may be found in it. What really made the patient seek care? Was it a possibly unexpressed fear or concern? Each hint of a care-seeking reason should be thoroughly explored (Box 2.10).

BOX 2.10 The Basis of Understanding

The following are vital questions that probe the unique experience of each patient:

Why is this happening with this particular person at this time?

How is this patient different from other patients?

Can I assume that what is generally true for others is true for this patient?

How does this bear on my interpretation of possible problems and solutions?

CLINICAL PEARL

Chief Complaint or Chief Concern?

Many of us do not view patients as "complainers" and prefer to express the "chief complaint" differently, adopting "chief concern," "presenting problem," or "reason for seeking care" as a more appropriate term. Feel free to use the words that suit you best or are most appropriate in your health care setting.

History of Present Illness or Problem. You will often find that it is easiest to question the patient on the details of the current problem immediately after hearing the chief concern. Sometimes it may be of value to take the patient's past and family history before returning to the present. The specific order in which you obtain the patient's story is not critical. You want the patient's version without the use of leading questions. Box 2.11 suggests many of the variables that can influence the patient's version.

A complete HPI will include the following:

- Chronological ordering of events.
- State of health just before the onset of the present problem.
- Complete description of the first symptoms: The question "When did you last feel well?" may help define the time of onset and provide a date on which it might have been necessary to stop work or school, miss a planned event, or be confined to bed.

BOX 2.11 Factors That Affect the Patient's Expression of Illness

Disease is a real condition that prevents the body or mind from working normally (Merriam-Webster.com). Illness is the unique way in which a disease is expressed by the afflicted individual. An infinite number of variables come into play and may even cause illness without disease:

- Recent termination of a significant relationship because of death, divorce, or other stressors such as moving to a new city
- Physical or emotional illness or disability in family members or other significant individuals
- Inharmonious spousal or family relationships
- School problems and stresses
- Poor self-image
- Drug and alcohol misuse
- Poor understanding of the facts of a physical problem and its treatment
- Influence from social media
- Peer pressure (among adults in addition to adolescents and children)
- Secondary gains from the expression of symptoms (e.g., indulgent family response to symptoms, providing extra comforts or gifts, solicitous attention from others, distraction from other intimidating problems)

At any age, such circumstances can contribute to the intensity and persistence of symptoms or, quite the opposite, the denial of an insistent, objective concern. The patient may then be led to seek help or, at other times, to avoid it.

- Symptom analysis: Questions in the following categories assist the patient in specifying characteristics of the presenting symptom(s): location, duration, intensity, description/character, aggravating factors, alleviating factors.
- Description of a typical attack, including its persistence: If the present problem involves intermittent attacks separated by an illness-free interval, ask the patient to describe a typical attack (e.g., onset; duration; variation in intensity; and associated symptoms, such as pain, chills, fever, jaundice, hematuria, or seizures). Then ask the patient to define inciting, exacerbating, or relieving factors such as specific activities, positions, diet, or medications.
- Possible exposure to infection, toxic agents, or other environmental hazards.
- Impact of the illness on the patient's usual lifestyle (e.g., sexual experience, leisure activity, ability to perform tasks or cope with stress) and an assessment of the ability to function in the expected way, with an indication of the limitations imposed by illness.
- Immediate reason that prompted the patient to seek care, particularly if the problem has been long standing.
- Appropriate relevant system review.
- Medications: current and recent, including dosages of prescriptions, home remedies, and nonprescription medications.
- Use of complementary or alternative therapies and medications.
- A review, at the end of the interview, of the chronology of events, seeking the patient's confirmations and corrections (if there appears to be more than one problem, the process should be repeated for each one).

Past Medical History. The PMH is the baseline for assessing the present concern.

- General health
- Gender identity: as described by the patient (e.g., male, female, nonbinary, queer, among many other terms); the sex they were assigned at birth; pronouns; history of gender-affirming care (e.g., hormones and/or gender-affirming surgeries)
- Childhood illnesses: measles, mumps, pertussis, chickenpox, scarlet fever, acute rheumatic fever, diphtheria, poliomyelitis, asthma
- Major adult illnesses or chronic diseases: tuberculosis, hepatitis, diabetes, hypertension, myocardial infarction, heart disease, stroke, respiratory disease, tropical or parasitic infections, other infections; any nonsurgical hospital admissions
- Immunizations: polio; diphtheria, pertussis, and tetanus toxoid; COVID-19; hepatitis A and hepatitis B; rotavirus; respiratory syncytial virus; measles, mumps, and rubella; varicella; herpes zoster vaccine; pneumococcus; meningococcus; human papillomavirus (HPV); bacille Calmette-Guérin; last tuberculosis or other skin tests; annual influenza; unusual reactions to immunizations or travel-related immunizations (e.g., typhoid, yellow fever)
- Surgery: dates, hospital, diagnosis/indication, complications
- Serious injuries and resulting disability; obtain complete details if the present problem has potential medicolegal relation to an injury
- Limitation of ability to function as a result of past events
- Medications: past, current, and recent medications, including dosages of prescription and over-the-counter medications and complementary, alternative, and integrative therapies (when not mentioned in present problem); ask the patient why they take each medication; this allows for an opportunity to identify education gaps if the patient does not understand why the medication is prescribed or recommended
- Allergies and the nature of reactions, especially to medications, but also to environmental allergens and foods
- Transfusions: reactions and the nature of reactions, date, and number of units transfused
- Recent screening tests (e.g., cholesterol, Pap smear/HPV testing, colonoscopy, mammogram)
- Emotional status: mood disorders, psychiatric problems

Evidence-Based Practice in Physical Examination

History Taking

There is evidence that the risk for type 2 diabetes or cardiovascular disease is detectable in childhood and that the diseases share risk factors, including obesity and dyslipidemia. Other studies suggest that these risks can be reduced in childhood. The pathway to detecting risk is the family history. Adults with one or more second-degree relatives with diabetes or cardiovascular disease are at high risk. So, too, are children with similar histories. The family history provides insight into the genetic effects on health and disease and offers clues that can lead to prevention strategies.

From Yang, Q., Liu, T., Valdez, R., et al. (2010). Improvements in ability to detect undiagnosed diabetes by using information on family history among adults in the United States. *American Journal of Epidemiology, 171*(10), 1079–1089. http://dx.doi.org/10.1093/aje/kwq026

Family History. Blood relatives in the immediate or extended family with illnesses with features similar to the patient's are an immediate concern. If a disease "runs in the family," such as sickle cell disease, ask about everyone from grandparents to cousins and children. A pedigree diagram helps illustrate the family members with the disorder (see Chapter 5). Determine the health and, if applicable, the cause of death of first-degree relatives (parents, children, and siblings), including age at death; after that, second-degree relatives (grandparents, grandchildren, aunts, nieces, uncles, and nephews); and then third-degree relatives (first cousins). There should be at least three generations in the pedigree.

- Include the following in your list of illnesses: heart disease, high blood pressure, cancer (including the type), tuberculosis, stroke, sickle cell disease, cystic fibrosis, epilepsy, diabetes, gout, kidney disease, thyroid disease, asthma or other allergic conditions, forms of arthritis, blood diseases, STIs, familial hearing, and visual or other sensory problems.
- In particular, determine whether cancers have been multiple or bilateral and occurring more than once in the family and at a young age (<50 years).
- Note the age and outcome of any illness.
- Note the ethnic and racial background of the family.
- Note the age and health of the patient's spouse/partner or the child's parents.

Personal and Social History

- Personal status: birthplace, where raised, home environment when young (e.g., parental divorce or separation, socioeconomic class, cultural and ethnic background), education, position in family, marital status, general life satisfaction, hobbies and interests, occupation, activities, and sources of stress or strain (see Clinical Pearl, "Who Are You?").

CLINICAL PEARL

Who Are You?

We cannot assume how patients define themselves (e.g., gender, ethnic or cultural affiliation) without asking them. "Male," "female," "cisgender," "transgender," "Hispanic," "non-Hispanic," "Black," "White," "Latino," and "Asian," among many other designations, are subject to a variety of interpretations. Just ask, "How do you see yourself?" "How do you define yourself?" "I respect your values and beliefs; what do I need to know to provide care for you?" Remember not to stereotype just because a patient is a member of a culture. Each person has their own unique culture.

- Habits: nutrition and diet; regularity and patterns of eating and sleeping; quantity of coffee, tea, tobacco, alcohol; use of substances (e.g., frequency, type, and amount); ability to perform activities of daily living (ADLs; see "Functional Assessment for All Patients"). The extent of cigarette use can be reported in "pack-years": the number of packs a day multiplied by the number of years (e.g., 1.5 packs per day × 10 years = 15 pack-years; see Evidence-Based Practice in Physical Examination, "Smoking Cessation").
- Self-care: exercise (quantity and type) and use of home, herbal, natural, complementary, or alternative therapies.
- Sexual history: concerns with sexual feelings and performance, frequency of intercourse, ability to achieve orgasm, number and variety of partners, specific sexual practices, modes of birth control, protection against STIs and past STIs. ("Partner" is a gender-free term appropriate in the early stages of discussion; see Clinical Pearl, "The Five P's of a Sexual History.")

CLINICAL PEARL

The Five P's of a Sexual History

The five P's stand for:

- Partners
- Practices
- Protection from STIs
- Past history of STIs
- Prevention of pregnancy (if necessary)

These are the areas that you should openly discuss with your patients. You will need to ask additional questions that are appropriate to each patient's special situation or circumstances.

From Centers for Disease Control and Prevention. *Guide to taking a sexual history.* https://www.cdc.gov/sti/hcp/clinical-guidance/taking-a-sexual-history.html

- Home conditions: housing, economic condition, types of furnishings (e.g., carpeting and drapes), pets and their health.
- Occupation: description of usual work (and present work if different); list of job changes; work conditions

and hours; physical or mental strain; duration of employment; present and past exposure to heat and cold or industrial toxins (especially lead, arsenic, chromium, asbestos, beryllium, poisonous gases, benzene, and polyvinyl chloride or other carcinogens and teratogens); any protective devices required (e.g., ear plugs, goggles, or masks); excessive screen time.

- Environment: travel and other exposure to contagious infections, residence in tropics, water and milk supply, other sources of infection if applicable.
- Military service: branch of service, military occupational specialty/job in the military, dates and geographic area of assignments/deployments, current status (active duty, reserves, retired, veteran). Box 2.12 highlights veteran-specific histories to assess for common problems and unique risks for people who have served in the military.

BOX 2.12 Have You Ever Served?

"Have you ever served?" is an initiative to address special health needs of military veterans. It provides specific histories to assess veterans for both common health concerns and unique health care risks encountered by them.

Initial Intake Questions

Have you or has someone close to you ever served in the military?

- When did you serve?
- Which branch?
- What did you do while you were in the military?
- Were you assigned to a hostile or combative area?
- Did you experience enemy fire, see combat, or witness casualties?
- Were you wounded, injured, or hospitalized?
- Did you participate in any experimental projects or tests?
- Were you exposed to noise, chemicals, gases, demolition of munitions, pesticides, or other hazardous substances?
- Have you ever used Veterans Affairs (VA) for health care?
- When was your last visit to the VA?
- Do you have a service-connected disability or condition? Do you have a claim pending? If so, what is the nature of the claim?
- Do you have a VA primary care provider?
- Do you have a safe place to go when you leave today?
- Do you need assistance in caring for yourself or members of your household?

General Areas of Concern for All Veterans

- Posttraumatic stress
- Military sexual trauma
- Blast concussions/traumatic brain injury
- Suicide risk

Unique Health Risks

These relate to exposures experienced by veterans at specific times or locations, which increase their risk for development of cancers, hepatitis C, respiratory illnesses, and other health conditions.

Modified from American Academy of Nursing. For further information, specific history questions, and additional resources, visit https://www.haveyoueverserved.com/.

- Religious and cultural preferences: any religious proscriptions concerning food, medical care, and spiritual needs.
- Access to care: transportation and other resources available to patient, type of health insurance coverage (if any), worries in this regard, primary care provider, customary pattern of seeking care.
- Social needs: insurance/medication coverage, food insecurity, housing instability, employment assistance needs.

It is important to have a candid discussion of issues.

Evidence-Based Practice in Physical Examination

Smoking Cessation

Abundant evidence indicates that patients in a trusting relationship with nurses, physicians, or other health professionals will respond positively to even brief, simple advice about smoking cessation.

Pooled data from 17 trials of brief advice versus no advice (or usual care) detected a significant increase in the rate of quitting (relative risk [RR] 1.66). Among 11 trials where the intervention was more intensive, the estimated effect was higher (RR 1.84), but there was no statistical difference between the intensive and minimal subgroups. Direct comparison of intensive versus minimal advice showed a small advantage of intensive advice (RR 1.37). The bottom line is that it pays to offer even minimal advice if given respectfully and earnestly. Simple advice has an effect on cessation rates. The challenge is to incorporate smoking cessation interventions as part of standard practice.

From Stead, L. F., Buitrago, D., Preciado, N., et al. (2013). Physician advice for smoking cessation. *Cochrane Database of Systematic Reviews, 5*, CD000165 http://dx.doi.org/10.1002/14651858.CD000165.pub4

Review of Systems. Identify the presence or absence of health-related issues in each body system. You may not ask all of the questions relevant to each system each time you take a given patient's history. Nevertheless, many should be asked, particularly at the first interview. A targeted ROS is appropriate in some circumstances. More comprehensive questions for particular circumstances in each system are detailed in subsequent chapters. Negative responses to ROS questions are as important as positive responses.

- General constitutional symptoms: pain, fever, chills, malaise, fatigue, night sweats, sleep patterns, weight (i.e., average, preferred, present, change)
- Skin, hair, and nails: rash or eruption, itching, pigmentation or texture change, excessive sweating, abnormal nail or hair growth
- Head and neck
- General: frequent or unusual headaches and their location, dizziness, syncope, severe head injuries, concussions, periods of loss of consciousness (momentary or prolonged)
- Eyes: visual acuity, blurring, diplopia, photophobia, pain, recent change in appearance or vision, glaucoma,

use of eye drops or other eye medications, history of trauma

- Ears: hearing loss, pain, discharge, tinnitus, vertigo, infections
- Nose: sense of smell, frequency of colds, obstruction, epistaxis, postnasal discharge, sinus pain
- Throat and mouth: hoarseness or change in voice, frequent sore throats, bleeding or swelling of gums, recent tooth abscesses or extractions, soreness of tongue or buccal mucosa, ulcers, disturbance of taste, dental care
- Lymph nodes: enlargement, tenderness, suppuration
- Chest and lungs: pain related to respiration; dyspnea; cyanosis; wheezing; cough; sputum (character and quantity); hemoptysis; night sweats; exposure to tuberculosis; indication, date, and result of last chest x-ray
- Breasts: development, pain, tenderness, discharge, lumps, galactorrhea, presence of implants, mammogram results
- Heart and blood vessels: chest pain or distress, precipitating causes, timing and duration, relieving factors, palpitations, dyspnea, orthopnea (number of pillows needed), edema, hypertension, previous myocardial infarction, estimate of exercise tolerance, past electrocardiogram or other cardiac tests and their results
- Peripheral vasculature: claudication (frequency and severity), tendency to bruise or bleed, thromboses, thrombophlebitis
- Hematologic: anemia, bruising, any known abnormality of blood cells
- Gastrointestinal: appetite; digestion; intolerance for any class of foods; dysphagia; heartburn; nausea; vomiting; hematemesis; regularity of bowels; constipation; diarrhea; change in stool color or contents (e.g., clay-colored, tarry, fresh blood, mucus, undigested food); flatulence; hemorrhoids; jaundice, history of ulcers, gallstones, polyps, or tumors; previous diagnostic imaging (indication, where, when, results)
- Diet: appetite, likes and dislikes, restrictions (e.g., preferential, religious, allergy, or other disease), vitamins and other supplements, use of caffeine-containing beverages (e.g., coffee, tea, and cola), an hour-by-hour detailing of food and fluid intake (sometimes a written diary covering several days of intake may be necessary)
- Endocrine: thyroid enlargement or tenderness, heat or cold intolerance, unexplained weight change, diabetes, polydipsia, polyuria, distribution and changes in facial or body hair, increased hat and ring size, skin striae
- Genitourinary: dysuria, flank or suprapubic pain, urgency, frequency, nocturia, hematuria, polyuria, dark or discolored urine, hesitancy, dribbling, loss in force of stream, passage of stone, edema of face, stress incontinence, hernias, STIs (type and treatment), presence of implants/implant functionality
- Musculoskeletal: joint stiffness, pain, restriction of motion, swelling, redness, heat, bony deformity
- Neurologic: syncope, seizures, weakness or paralysis, abnormalities of sensation or coordination, tremors, loss of memory
- Psychiatric: depression, mood changes, difficulty concentrating, anxiety, agitation, tension, suicidal thoughts, irritability, sleep disturbances

People Assigned Female at Birth

- Menses: age at menarche, regularity, duration and amount of flow, dysmenorrhea, last menstrual period (LMP), intermenstrual discharge or bleeding, itching, date of last Pap smear and/or HPV test and result, age at menopause, libido, frequency of intercourse, pain during intercourse, sexual difficulties, infertility
- Pregnancies: number, living children, multiple births, miscarriages, abortions, duration of pregnancy, each type of delivery, any complications during any pregnancy or postpartum period or with neonate, use of oral or other contraceptives

People Assigned Male at Birth

- Puberty onset, difficulty with erections, emissions, testicular pain, libido, infertility

Concluding Questions. Give the patient further opportunity: "Is there anything else that you want me to know?" If there are several issues, ask, "What problem concerns you most?" When situations are vague, complicated, or contradictory, it may be helpful to ask, "What do you think is the matter with you?" or "What worries you the most about how you are feeling?"

Adaptations for Age, Pregnancy, and Possible Disabilities

Some concerns are pervasive and universally shared among patients, others are specific to particular subgroups, and certain concerns are uniquely individual, serving to distinguish one patient from another.

Infants and Children

Many young children love it when you get down on the floor to play with them. They often have anxieties and fears that must be eased (Fig. 2.3). Use language that they

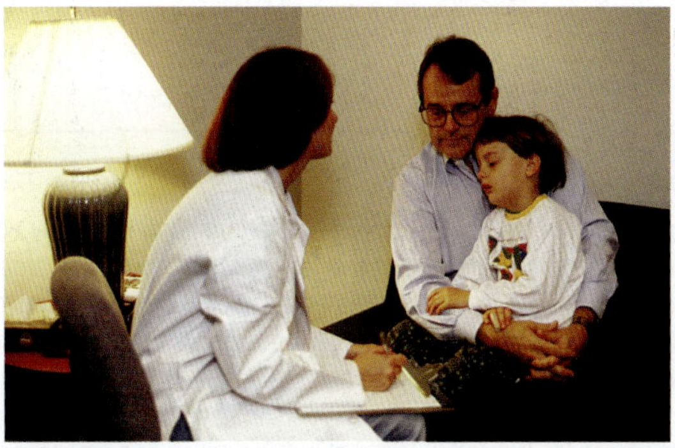

FIG. 2.3 Interviewing a child with his parent. Note that the interviewer is sitting close to the patient and that the child is secure on his parent's lap.

understand. When they are old enough, allow them to participate in the interview. Starting at age 7 years, children can be dependable reporters on some aspects of their health (Olson et al., 2007). The older the child, the more productive it becomes to ask questions and to give information directly. The older child and the adolescent may seem passive and sometimes appear resistant to some degree. This may suggest a wish to be alone with you, which may help to get a more accurate history. Be proactive and arrange for this routinely (see Clinical Pearl, "Twins or More").

> **CLINICAL PEARL**
>
> **Twins or More**
>
> Your patients may be twins, triplets, or more! Each is an individual entitled to separate consideration. Ensure that each has confidential and separate time with you.

Family dynamics become evident during history taking and may even lead to clues that a parent is in need of help. For example, an excessively tearful parent who does not seem to be having much pleasure in a child or seems self-absorbed, unresponsive, and uncommunicative—or even hostile—may be depressed. Your responsibility goes beyond the child. It is appropriate to screen the mother for depression (Weiss-Laxer et al., 2016) and suggest ways to help (see Chapter 7). Respect parental concerns about their children and do what is needed to ease worry.

There are aspects of the history concerning the young that may complement the approach suggested for adults or vary from it. They are as follows.

Chief Concern. A parent or other responsible adult (Box 2.13) often makes a threesome. The relationship of that person should be recorded. However, the child should be included as much as possible and as is age appropriate. The latent fears underlying any chief concerns of the adults and children should be explored.

> **BOX 2.13 Consent by Proxy**
>
> Infants, children, and many adolescents are minors. They may come to you accompanied by someone other than their custodial parent or guardian, often a grandparent or other member of their extended family. Sometimes your informant might be a babysitter; an au pair or nanny; or, in the event of divorce and remarriage, a noncustodial parent, stepparent, or friend. Does that person have the right to consent to your care for the child? Learn about the policy and procedure for consent in your health care setting.

History of Present Illness. The degree and character of the reaction to the problem on the part of parent/guardian and child should be noted.

Past Medical History

- Note general health: the age of the child and/or the nature of the problem determine the approach to questioning
- Health during pregnancy:
  - General health as related by the patient, if possible; extent of prenatal care; gravidity; parity
  - Specific diseases or conditions: infectious disease (approximate gestational month), weight gain, edema, hypertension, proteinuria, bleeding (approximate gestational month), preeclampsia
  - Medications, hormones, vitamins, special or unusual diet, general nutritional status
  - Quality of fetal movements and time of onset
  - Emotional and behavioral status (e.g., attitudes toward pregnancy and children)
  - Radiation exposure
  - Substance use
- Birth
  - Gestational age
  - Place of delivery
  - Labor: spontaneous or induced, duration, analgesia or anesthesia, complications
  - Delivery: presentation; forceps, vacuum extraction, spontaneous, or cesarean section; complications
  - Condition of infant, time of onset of cry, Apgar scores if available
  - Birth weight

> **Patient Safety**
>
> **Putting Prevention Into Practice**
>
> Take time to consider prevention. Consider how you can include prevention-related advice when talking with your patient or surrogate. For example, infants should sleep alone on their backs in a crib or bassinet to decrease the risk of sleep-related infant death. Additionally, child safety seats are frequently used incorrectly. Their correct use should be reviewed.

- Neonatal period
  - Congenital anomalies; baby's condition in hospital, oxygen requirements, color, feeding characteristics, vigor, cry; duration of baby's stay in hospital and whether infant was discharged with the patient who gave birth; bilirubin phototherapy; prescriptions (e.g., antibiotics)
  - First month of life: jaundice, color, strength of cry, bleeding, convulsions, or other evidence of illness
  - Degree of early bonding: opportunities at birth and during the first days of life for the parents to hold,

talk to, and caress the infant (i.e., opportunities for both parents to relate to and develop a bond with the baby)
  - The feelings of the patient after giving birth: loss of laughter, unreasonable anxiety or sense of panic, excessive crying and sadness, sleeplessness, feelings of guilt, suicidal ideation, clues singly but most often in combination may be related to postpartum depression
- Feeding
  - Formula or breast milk, reason for changes, if any; type of formula and how it is prepared, amounts offered and consumed; frequency of feeding and weight gain
  - Present diet and appetite; age of introduction of solids; age when child achieved three feedings per day; present feeding patterns, elaboration of any feeding problems; age weaned from bottle or breast; type of milk and daily intake; food preference; ability to feed self; cultural variations
- Development: Obtain the age when the child achieved common developmental milestones:
  - Holds head erect while in sitting position
  - Rolls over from front to back and back to front
  - Sits alone and unsupported
  - Stands with support and alone
  - Walks with support and alone
  - Uses words
  - Talks in sentences
  - Dresses self

Expand the list when indicated. Parents may have baby books, which can stimulate recall, or photographs may be helpful. Additional developmental information to inquire about includes the following:
- Age when toilet trained: approaches to and attitudes regarding toilet training
- School: grade, performance, problems
- Dentition: age of first teeth, loss of deciduous teeth, eruption of first permanent teeth; last dental visit
- Growth: height and weight in a sequence of ages; changes in rates of growth or weight gain
- Pubertal development: present status; in females, development of breasts, nipples, sexual hair, menstruation (onset, cycle, regularity, pain, description of menses), acne; in males, development of sexual hair, voice changes, acne, nocturnal emissions
- Puberty suspension/suppression in gender-diverse or transgender minors
- Illnesses: immunizations, communicable diseases, injuries, hospitalizations

Family History
- Pregnant patient's gestational history listing all pregnancies, together with the health status of living children. For deceased children, include date, age, cause of death, and dates and duration of pregnancies in the case of miscarriages.
- Patient's health during pregnancies and the ages of parents at the birth of this child.
- Are the parents consanguineous? Again, a pedigree diagram helps (see Chapter 5).

Personal and Social History
- Family structure: who lives in the home, their relationship to the child, who cares for the child, are biologic parents involved, additional adults involved with the child.
- Behavioral status: childcare or school adjustment; masturbation, nail biting, thumb sucking, breath holding, temper tantrums, pica, tics, rituals; bed wetting, constipation or fecal soiling of pants; playing with fire; reactions to prior illnesses, injuries, or hospitalization.
- An account of a day in the life of the patient (from parent, child, or both) is often helpful in providing insights. Box 2.14 emphasizes the particular needs of children who are adopted or are in foster care.
- Family circumstances: parents' occupations, the principal caretakers of the child, whether parents are divorced or separated, educational attainment of parents; spiritual orientation; cultural heritage; food preparation and by whom; adequacy of clothing; dependence on relief or social agency.
- Setting of the home: number of rooms in house and number of persons in household; sleep habits, sleeping arrangements available for the child, possible environmental hazards.

Review of Systems. In addition to the usual concerns, inquire about any past medical or psychological or education testing of the child (Box 2.15). Ask about the following:
- Skin: eczema, seborrhea, "cradle cap"
- Ears: otitis media (frequency, laterality)
- Nose: snoring, mouth breathing, allergic reaction
- Teeth: dental care
- Genitourinary: bedwetting

BOX 2.14 Adoption and Foster Care

Patients who are adopted or in foster care may not have a sufficient history available. Learn as much as you can. Our outline for history taking is a starter and should be filled out by an exploration of the circumstances that led to adoption or foster care. Do this with care. Some adoptive parents may not yet have shared the knowledge with their children. The trials of the adoptive parents as they sought a child, the process of adoption, the country of origin of the adoptee, and the particular concerns of all involved must be explored.

The needs of foster children vary considerably from those who are adopted. The history may be offered by a social worker, and the issues you encounter will differ in variety and intensity. Foster parents have varying experience, and foster children have often lived in more than one home. Invariably, difficult social circumstances underlie the separation from their parents. The probable lack of stability and security and incomplete knowledge of past illnesses or other conditions make it more difficult to understand the full range of the child's complex and urgent needs.

BOX 2.15 Adverse Childhood Experiences

Witnessing or experiencing violence or injury is a fact of life for many children and is a barrier to appropriate growth and development. Talk about the event in a straightforward, simple, and direct fashion:

- Can you tell me what happened?
- What did you see? What did you hear?
- What scared you the most?
- What were you doing when it happened?
- Do you ever dream about it?
- Do you think about it during the day?
- Do you worry it will happen again?
- Whom do you talk to when you feel worried or scared?
- Why do you think it happened?
- For the older child and adolescent:
- How do you think it changed your life (for the older child and adolescent)?

These questions are not value laden and are not too constraining. The child is free to talk if you can be comfortable with the silences that may often ensue. Parents can also respond to the same questions to fill out the story, and you can then learn how they dealt with the circumstance and what they observed in their child's behavior.

Modified from Augustyn, M., Parker, S., Groves, B. M., & Zuckerman, B. (1995). Silent victims: Children who witness violence. *Contemporary pediatrics, 12*, 35. Reprinted with permission from *Contemporary pediatrics*, Vol. 12, 1995. *Contemporary pediatrics* is a copyrighted publication of Advanstar Communications, Inc. All rights reserved.

Adolescents

Adolescence, the time from puberty to maturity, is different from childhood and adulthood both physically and psychosocially. It is a time made vulnerable by a tendency to experiment with risky behaviors. Adolescents may be reluctant to talk and have a clear need for confidentiality. All adolescent patients should be given the opportunity to discuss their concerns with you privately. At the start of the visit, it is wise to let the parent or other caregiver know you will be asking them to step out of the room to provide this important opportunity for the adolescent. The visit can be an opportunity to provide a safe space for teens to talk with their caregivers about sensitive issues with your support. Every effort should be made to maintain confidentiality. The limits regarding confidentiality should be clearly discussed. Information that suggests the adolescent's safety or the safety of another is at risk may be reasons to "break" confidentiality.

If a parent/guardian is present, acknowledge the patient first. In the beginning it is helpful to talk about what is happening in the patient's day-to-day experiences. Do not force conversation because adolescents do not respond readily to confrontation. On the other hand, you will often sense a need to talk and an inability to get the words out. Silences can be long, sometimes sheepish, occasionally angry, and not always constructive.

The peer group and the desire to be like peers take on a dominant role during middle adolescence. Experimentation with risky behaviors begins, and frequent arguments with parents are common. Immature decision making can lead to destructive, life-changing experiences and lifelong bad habits. During late adolescence with approaching adulthood, a more thoughtful consideration of consequences ordinarily occurs, along with a more secure sense of self and an ability to establish intimate relationships and to start planning a career.

The adoption of risky behaviors depends on a number of factors:

- Peer pressure
- Loosening attachment to parents
- Poor school performance
- Nonparticipation in school extracurricular activities
- Poor self-esteem
- Need to act older
- Susceptibility to advertising, the internet, or social media

These issues may make it difficult to transcend the barrier imposed by age in caring for the adolescent (see Clinical Pearl, "Identification of Concerns by Adolescents"). Make generous use of open-ended questions, and do not force an adolescent to talk.

CLINICAL PEARL

Identification of Concerns by Adolescents

Previsit screeners or questionnaires allow the adolescent to identify their concerns prior to the start of the visit. Sometimes allowing an opportunity to write a concern or allowing a choice of concerns presented in written, silent fashion may help (Box 2.16). Then you can phrase the appropriate questions and make the transition to a verbal discussion reasonably comfortable. Take an open-ended approach, always indicating a sense of alliance and partnership.

BOX 2.16 Adolescents' Concerns

The following subjects may be of concern to adolescents. These are highly charged issues, mandating the effort for discussion but requiring sensitivity, knowledge of adolescent language, and an unforced approach.

- Bed-wetting
- Menstrual pain
- Concern with height or weight: too short, too tall, underweight, overweight
- Concern with breast size: too big, too small
- Concern with penis size: too small
- Worry about pregnancy
- Questions about sexual orientation
- Questions about gender identity
- Interpersonal violence
- Sex? Ready or not?
- HIV, AIDS
- Gambling
- Smoking
- Substance use
- Parents' attitudes and demands
- Friends and their pressures
- Bullying
- School: not doing well, excessive work
- What am I going to do in life?
- Thoughts about dying

Flexibility, respect, and confidentiality are key; otherwise, little productive discussion will result. On occasion, the patient may ask to talk with someone of the same gender, and this should be facilitated if possible. Box 2.17 provides useful screening tools for adolescent issues. You can use them as a guide for an exploratory interview. Some questions that you can ask to structure the interview include the following:

- "How are things at home?" "Tell me about your living situation." Do not assume the family structure. Do not ask directly about who else lives in the house. The open-ended question at the start can lead to greater specifics later on.
- "How is school?" "Are you working?" "What is it about school that appeals to you?" "What is it about school that doesn't appeal to you?" You may expect to hear somewhat more about jobs outside of school and ideas about the future when the patient approaches 20 years of age.

BOX 2.17 Screening Tools for Adolescent Issues

SSHADESS

- **S**trengths
- **S**chool
- **H**ome
- **A**ctivities
- **D**rugs and substance use
- **E**motions, eating, and depression
- **S**exuality
- **S**afety

PACES

- **P**arents, peers
- **A**ccidents, alcohol/drugs
- **C**igarettes
- **E**motional issues
- **S**chool, sexuality

CRAFFT

- Have you ridden in a CAR driven by someone who was high or had been using drugs and alcohol?
- Do you ever use alcohol or drugs to RELAX, feel better about yourself, or fit in?
- Do you ever use drugs or alcohol when you are ALONE?
- Do you FORGET things you did while using drugs or alcohol?
- Do your family and FRIENDS ever tell you that you should cut down your drinking or drug use?
- Have you ever gotten into TROUBLE while using drugs or alcohol?

From Goldenring, J. M., & Rosen, D. (2004). Reprinted with permission from *Contemporary pediatrics*, Vol. 12, 2004, pp. 64–90. *Contemporary pediatrics* is a copyrighted publication of Advanstar Communications, Inc. All rights reserved.

From Ginsburg, K. R. (2020). Chapter 32: The SSHADESS screening: A strength-based psychosocial assessment. In K. R. Ginsburg & Z. B. Ramirez McClain, Z. B. (Eds.), *Reaching teens: strength-based, trauma-sensitive, resilience-building communication strategies rooted in positive youth development*, 2nd ed. Itasca: American Academy of Pediatrics, pp. 225–228.

From Knight, J. R., Sherritt, L., Shrier, L. A., Harris, S. K., & Chang G. (2002). Validity of the CRAFFT substance abuse screening test among adolescent clinic patients. *Archives of Pediatrics & Adolescent Medicine, 156*, 607–614.

- "Tell me about your friends." "Where do you go with them?" "What do you do with them?" "To what groups do you belong?" "How would a friend describe you?"
- "What types of computer and electronic games do you play?"
- "What are you good at doing?"

Open-ended conversations about home, school, jobs, activities, and friends can suggest the areas that may trouble the adolescent (e.g., sex, drugs, bullying, suicidal ideation). Talk does not always flow easily as the adolescent transitions from dependency to independency, from parent/guardian to peer group, and ultimately to self, but you can help.

Pregnant Persons

Care during the prenatal period depends on the commitment of the patient to both patient and fetal health in partnership with the health care provider. The patient's approach to pregnancy is influenced by many factors, including previous experiences with childbearing and child-rearing, the relationship with the patient's parent and other individuals significant to the patient's life, the patient's desire for children, and the patient's present life circumstances. The interaction of the patient with the fetus increases the complexity of care. The initial interview includes past history; assessment of health practices; identification of potential risk factors; and assessment of the patient's knowledge, expectations, and perceptions as they affect pregnancy.

If you use an electronic device or preprinted history form to gather the history, bridge the distance by talking comfortably and at some length with the patient, particularly about the patient's expectations and concerns. There will, of course, be much "laying on of hands" as the pregnancy matures.

Basic Information

- Patient's age and ethnicity
- Marital status, partner, or relationship and involvement in the pregnancy
- LMP
- Previous usual/normal menstrual period (PUMP or PNMP)
- Expected date of confinement/delivery (EDC)
- Occupation
- Parent(s) of the baby and occupation(s) (if applicable)

History of Present Illness or Problem. Obtain a description of the current pregnancy and identify previous medical care. Identify specific problems (e.g., bleeding or spotting, nausea, vomiting, fatigue, or edema). Include information about illness, injuries, surgeries, or accidents or other injuries since conception.

Obstetric History. Information on each previous pregnancy (gravidity and parity) includes the date of delivery; length of pregnancy; weight and gender of infant(s); type of delivery (e.g., spontaneous vaginal; cesarean delivery and type of scar [an evaluation of the competency of the scar is needed for females attempting vaginal birth after cesarean delivery]); or spontaneous, therapeutic, or elective abortion and the type of procedure; length of labor; and complications in pregnancy or labor, postpartum, or with the infant. It is also important to determine whether any previous children have been removed from the home (e.g., because of abuse or neglect or inability to care for the children).

Menstrual History. In addition to previous information, include age at menarche, characteristics of the cycle, unusual bleeding, and associated symptoms. If known, include dates of ovulation and conception and the use of contraceptives before or during conception.

Gynecologic History. Record the date of the most recent Pap smear and HPV test along with any history of abnormalities, treatments, or gynecologic surgery. A sexual history includes age of first intercourse and whether it was consensual, number of sex partners, safe-sex methods, partner orientation, and, if a minor, age of partner. Information regarding the types of contraceptives used and reason for discontinuing them, along with plans for use postpartum, is obtained. Any history of infertility should be explored. If any STIs are reported, discuss the type, dates, treatments, and complications. Give full attention to any history of sexual assault.

Past Medical History. The same information identified previously for adults is obtained, with the addition of risk factors for HIV, hepatitis, herpes, tuberculosis, and exposure to environmental and occupational hazards.

Family History. Obtain a family history of genetic conditions, multiple births, gestational diabetes, preeclampsia/eclampsia or pregnancy-induced hypertension (PIH), and/or congenital anomalies.

Personal and Social History. Other children and pets (cats can carry toxoplasmosis, which can be teratogenic to the fetus). In addition, obtain information about feelings toward the pregnancy, whether it was planned, consideration of adoption or abortion, gender preference, social and spiritual resources, experiences with parenting, experience with and plans for labor and breastfeeding, and history of past or present abuse in relationships (IPV).

Review of Systems. Perform a complete ROS because the effects of pregnancy are seen in all systems. Give special attention to the reproductive system (including breasts) and cardiovascular systems (documentation of pre-pregnancy blood pressure if possible). Assess the endocrine system for signs of diabetes and thyroid dysfunction. Assess the urinary tract for infection, and review kidney function. Assess respiratory function because it may be compromised later in pregnancy or with tocolytic therapy for preterm labor. Evaluate dental care needs because treatment of periodontitis can prevent preterm birth and/or low birth weight (George et al., 2011).

Risk Assessment. Identify conditions from the history and physical examination or circumstances that threaten the well-being of the patient and/or fetus. These include gestational diabetes, preterm labor, preeclampsia/eclampsia, pregnant patient malnutrition and vitamin deficiency, and use of potentially teratogenic agents such as lithium valproic acid or angiotensin-converting enzyme inhibitors.

Postpartum. Postpartum depression is a significant mental health problem, and universal screening for this problem is recommended (see Chapter 7). The clues are similar to those of depression in other circumstances—feeling down, depressed, or hopeless; sleep disturbance; loss of energy; eating disturbance; trouble concentrating; restlessness; sad mood; anxiety; fatigue; feelings of worthlessness and inappropriate guilt; and suicidal ideation. A cluster of these symptoms should strongly suggest postpartum depression (O'Connor et al., 2016; O'Hara & McCabe, 2013).

Older Adults

A change in knowledge, experience, cognitive abilities, and personality may occur with aging (Box 2.18). It is important to anticipate the effect these changes may have on the interview. However, physiologic age and chronologic age may not match. It is equally important to recognize that not all adults experience the same changes, they do not occur at the same rate, and some abilities may not decline with age.

Some older adults have sensory losses, such as hearing, that make communication more difficult. Position yourself so that the patient can see your face. Speak clearly and slowly, taking care to always face the patient while you are talking. Shouting magnifies the problem by distorting consonants and vowels. In some instances, a written interview may be necessary. Impaired vision and light-dark adaptation are a problem with written interview forms. Ensure large print and ample lighting with a source that does not glare or reflect in the eyes.

Some older adults may be confused or experience memory loss, particularly for recent events. Take whatever extra time is needed. Ask short (but not leading) questions, and keep your language uncomplicated and free of double negatives. Consult other family members to clarify discrepancies, provide collateral information, or fill in the gaps. On the other hand, older patients have a lifetime of experience that may be a rich source of wisdom and perspective. Listen for it.

BOX 2.18 Competency to Make Medical Decisions

Patients or their surrogates have the right to decide the extent of care they will accept under your guidance. Many may have lost the ability to make relevant competent decisions. To give informed consent, patients must be well informed about what is proposed, and they must be able to voluntarily give consent. Competency to make medical decisions is used interchangeably with the word *capacity*. In a report from the President's Commission for the Study of Ethical Problems in Medicine, clinical decision-making capacity includes three specific elements: the patient has a set of values and goals, the patient is able to understand and communicate information, and the patient is able to reason and deliberate about the choice being made by the patient. Competency may fluctuate from hour to hour or day to day, depending on the age and the physical/emotional circumstance. It is often necessary to seek consultative help in deciding a patient's status. The law in your state may require this, and it may ultimately be left to a judge to decide on legal competence. It is important to recognize that the patient who disagrees with you is not necessarily incompetent and the patient who agrees with you is not necessarily competent.

From Appelbaum, P. S. (2007). Assessment of patients' competence to consent to treatment. *New England Journal of Medicine, 357*, 1834–1840; Magauran, Jr., B. G. (2009). Risk management for the emergency physician: Competency and decision-making capacity, informed consent, and refusal of care against medical advice. *Emergency Medicine Clinics of North America, 27*(4), 605–614; President's *Commission for the Study of Ethical Problems in Medicine and Biomedical and Behavioral Research, 1982*, US Code Annot US, 1982. Title 42 Sect. 300v.

The history is more complex and increasingly intricate with the chronic, progressive, and debilitating problems that occur with aging. Symptoms may be less dramatic, vague, or nonspecific. Confusion may be the only indication of a major problem. Pain may be unreliably reported because, with age, its perception varies. The excruciating pain usually associated with pancreatitis, for example, may be perceived as a dull ache, and myocardial infarction can occur without any pain. Some patients may not report symptoms because they attribute them to old age or because they believe that nothing can be done. They may have lived with a chronic condition for so long that it has been part of their expectation of daily living.

Patient Safety

Multiple problems needing multiple medications increase risk for iatrogenic disorders. A medication history with attention to interactions of drugs, diseases, and aging is needed for prescribed and over-the-counter medications and herbal preparations. It is particularly helpful to have patients of all ages bring in their medications.

Routinely include functional assessment as part of the older adult's history (see "Functional Assessment for All Patients" and individual chapters with functional assessment specific to systems). Questions concerning the ability to take care of one's daily needs are part of the ROS. The personal and social history should include other dimensions of functional capacity such as social, spiritual, and economic resources; recreational activity; sleep patterns; environmental control; and use of the health care system. Maintaining function is a compelling concern of older adults.

For all ages, a cognitive impairment that deprives the patient of the ability to join in the decision-making process emphasizes the need for a designated health care agent (guardianship or medical power of attorney for health care) and/or advance directives (a document outlining the patient's wishes regarding life support). Be aware of the specific rules governing these issues in your state. Encourage the patient and family to pursue these documents if steps have not yet been taken.

FUNCTIONAL ASSESSMENT

Functional Assessment for All Patients

Quite simply, functional assessment is an attempt to understand a patient's ability to achieve the basic ADLs. This assessment should be made for all older adults and for any person limited by disease or disability, acute or chronic. A well-taken history and a meticulous physical examination can bring out subtle influences, such as tobacco and alcohol use, sedentary habits, poor food selection, overuse of medications (prescribed and nonprescribed), and less-than-obvious emotional distress. Even some physical limitations may not be readily apparent (e.g., limitations of cognitive ability or of the senses). Keep in mind that patients tend to overstate their abilities and, quite often, to obscure reality.

When performing a functional assessment, consider a variety of disabilities: physical, cognitive, psychological, social, and sexual. An individual's social and spiritual support system must be as clearly understood as the physical disabilities. There are a variety of physical disabilities, including the following:

- Mobility
  - Difficulty walking standard distances: ½ mile, 2–3 blocks, ½ block, across a room
  - Difficulty climbing stairs, up and down
  - Problems with balance
- Upper extremity function
  - Difficulty grasping small objects, opening jars
  - Difficulty reaching out or up overhead, such as taking something off a shelf
- Household chores
  - Heavy (vacuuming, scrubbing floors)
  - Light (dusting)
  - Meal preparation

Continued

FUNCTIONAL ASSESSMENT—cont'd

- ADLs
  - Eating
  - Toileting
  - Selecting proper attire and putting on clothes
  - Grooming and bathing
  - Maintaining continence
  - Walking and transferring (moving from bed to [wheel] chair, chair to standing)
- Instrumental ADLs
  - Shopping
  - Medication management
  - Money management
  - Transportation (driving or navigating public transit)
  - Preparing meals
  - Using telephone and other communication devices
  - Housework and basic home maintenance

Any limitations, even mild, in any of these areas will affect a patient's independence and autonomy and, to the extent of the limitation, increase reliance on other people and on assistive devices. These limitations indicate the loss of physical reserve and the potential loss of physical function and independence that indicate the onset of frailty. The patient's social support system and material resources are then integral to the development of reasonable management plans. (See Clinical Pearl, "Activities of Daily Living and Instrumental Activities of Daily Living.")

CLINICAL PEARL

Activities of Daily Living and Instrumental Activities of Daily Living

Activities of daily living (ADLs) and instrumental activities of daily living (IADLs) represent key life tasks that people need to perform in order to live at home and be fully independent. Following is a mnemonic to aid in remembering examples of ADLs and IADLs.

DEaTTH SHAFT (DEaTTH = ADLs, SHAFT = IADLs)

Dressing
Eating
Tabulating
Toileting
Hygiene
Shopping
Housekeeping
Accounting
Food preparation
Transportation

The Frail. Frailty has its onset with the loss of physical reserve and the increased risk for loss of physical function and independence. Its prevalence increases with age, particularly past 80 years. Frailty is characterized by weakness, weight loss, low activity, and diminished ability to respond to stress and is associated with adverse health outcomes. It is considered an at-risk state caused by the age-associated accumulation of deficits. With multisystem dysregulation, decreased physiologic reserves, and increased vulnerability to stressors, frailty shares features of normal aging (Bandeen-Roche et al., 2015). Nonetheless, age and frailty are not necessarily synonymous.

Patients With Disabilities

You must adapt to the needs of all patients of any age with disabling physical or emotional states (e.g., deafness, blindness, depression, psychosis, developmental delays, or neurologic impairments). They may or may not be effective historians but respect them regardless. Their perspectives and attitudes matter. Involve each fully to the limit of emotional and mental capacity or physical ability (Fig. 2.4). Still, when necessary, use the family, other health professionals involved in care, and the patient's record for collateral information. Some of the most common communication barriers can be overcome by keeping the following in mind:

- Family members are often available to make the patient more comfortable and to provide information.
- Persons with impaired hearing often read, write, sign, wear hearing aids, and/or read lips. You should speak slowly and clearly enunciate each word. A translator who signs may be necessary.
- Persons with visual impairment usually can hear, and talking louder to make a point does not help. Remember that you must always vocalize what you are trying to communicate; gestures may not be seen.
- Aging, debilitating illness, and frailty increase dependency on others, worry about tomorrow, and grieving for what has been lost. Recognize these concerns and the sense of loss in both the patient and the caregivers. You can acknowledge this and offer to talk about it.

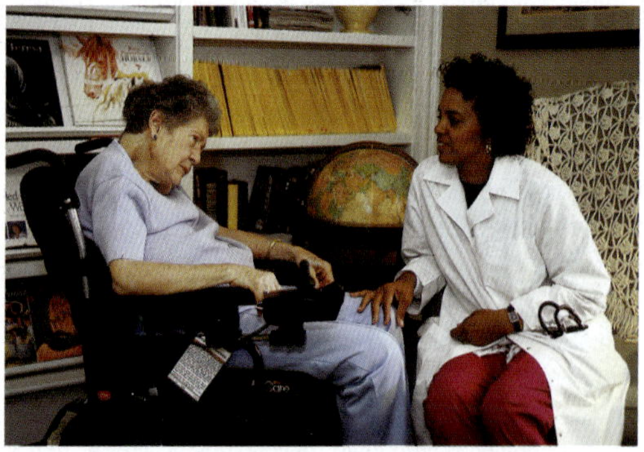

FIG. 2.4 Interviewing a patient with a physical disability. Note the uncluttered surroundings; be sure the patient in a wheelchair has room to maneuver.

The Next Step

Once the history (Box 2.19) has been built, move on to the physical examination, the laying on of hands, which is discussed in subsequent chapters. These chapters are segmented and are not meant to reflect the natural flow that you will develop with experience. Do not be intimidated because your patients expect you to be perfect. Just be disciplined and alert and recognize that your value judgments are not necessarily imbued with wisdom.

BOX 2.19 Types of Histories

A "complete" history is not always necessary. You may already know the patient well and may be considering the same problem over time. Therefore adjust your approach to the need at the moment. There are variations:

- The **complete history** makes you as thoroughly familiar with the patient as possible. Most often, this history is recorded the first time you see the patient.
- The **inventory history** is related to but does not replace the complete history. It touches on the major points without going into detail. This is useful when it is necessary to get a "feel" for the situation and the entire history taking will be completed in more than one session.
- The **problem (or focused) history** is taken when the problem is acute, possibly life threatening, and requiring immediate attention so that only the need of the moment is given full attention.
- The **interim history** is designed to chronicle events that have occurred since your last meeting with the patient. Its substance is determined by the nature of the problem and the need of the moment. The interim history should always be complemented by the patient's previous record.
- Key information to gather regardless of the type of history includes current medications and allergies.

Risk Factors

Bias in Health Care

Implicit Bias

Unconscious bias that is outside of someone's awareness. It can be activated by various identities we perceive in others such as race/ethnicity, gender, weight, height, age, language, (dis)ability, income, and insurance status.

- Stressful situations
- Uncertainty
- Time pressures
- Actions or words of others
- Situations that have promoted stereotyping

Explicit Bias

Attitudes and beliefs we have about a person or group on a conscious level; positive or negative preferences for a particular group, which are conscious.

- Personal background or prejudices
- Learned associations between particular qualities or social categories
- Stereotyping of patients
- Personal experiences
- Lack of cultural awareness
- Exposure to images and messages about certain groups of people

Risk Factors

Risk Factors for Developing a Substance Use Disorder

- Environmental stressors
- Exposure to the substance
- Genetic vulnerability
- Individual personality characteristics
- Psychiatric problems
- Social pressures
- Trauma

Risk Factors

Risk Factors for Unintentional Pregnancy or Sexually Transmitted Infection

Unintentional Pregnancy

- Age (<20 or >35 years)
- Being single
- Binge drinking
- Having more sexual partners
- History of unplanned pregnancies or abortions
- Inadequate family planning services or access to family planning services
- Low socioeconomic status
- Lower educational level
- Not using contraception
- Psychiatric problems
- Smoking
- Substance use
- Unawareness of family planning methods
- Younger age at sexual debut

Sexually Transmitted Infection

- Anal, vaginal, or oral sex without a barrier contraception
- Anonymous sex partners
- Having sex while under the influence of substances
- Multiple sex partners
- Sexual acts that tear or break the skin

Adapted from https://www.cdc.gov/sti/prevention/index.html

CHAPTER

3 Examination Techniques and Equipment

This chapter provides an overview of the techniques of inspection, palpation, percussion, and auscultation that are used throughout the physical examination. In addition, general use of the equipment for performing the physical examination is discussed (Box 3.1). Details regarding techniques and equipment as they relate to specific parts of the examination can be found in the relevant chapters. This chapter also addresses special issues related to the physical examination process.

Precautions

Infection Prevention

Because persons of all ages and backgrounds may be sources of infection, it is important to take proper precautions when examining patients. Standard Precautions are to be used for the care of all patients in any setting in which health care is delivered. These precautions are designed to prevent the transmission of HIV, hepatitis B, and other blood-borne pathogens based on the principle that all blood, body fluids, secretions, excretions except sweat, nonintact skin, and mucous membranes may contain transmissible infectious agents. Standard Precautions include the following:

- Hand hygiene
- Personal protective equipment (PPE): use of gloves, gown, mask, eye protection, or face shield, depending on the anticipated exposure
- Respiratory hygiene/cough etiquette
- Safe injection practices
- Safe handling of potentially contaminated equipment or surfaces in the patient's environment. Guidelines for Standard Precautions are summarized in Table 3.1. Use precautions to protect yourself and your patients.

A second tier of precautions, Transmission-Based Precautions, are designed to supplement Standard Precautions in the care of patients who are known or suspected to be infected by epidemiologically important pathogens that are spread by airborne or droplet transmission or by contact with dry skin or contaminated surfaces. The emergence of novel viral infections underscores the need to always exercise hand hygiene, follow appropriate respiratory precautions, and use designated PPE.

Guidelines and recommendations for the prevention of health care–associated infections are available from the Centers for Disease Control and Prevention (https://www.cdc.gov/infection-control/hcp/basics/index.html).

Latex Allergy

Allergic reactions to latex can be potentially serious, although rarely fatal with anaphylaxis. Latex allergy occurs when the body's immune system reacts to proteins found in natural rubber latex. Latex products also contain added chemicals, such as antioxidants, that can cause irritant or delayed hypersensitivity reactions. Box 3.2 describes the various types of latex reactions.

Clinicians are at risk of developing latex allergy because of exposure to latex in the form of gloves and other equipment and supplies. Sensitization to the latex proteins occurs by direct skin or mucous membrane contact or through airborne exposure. Box 3.3 contains a summary of recommendations to protect you from latex exposure in the workplace. Be aware that some patients who have had multiple procedures or surgeries performed are at higher risk of developing latex allergy. Those patients with latex allergies are at risk when exposed to latex gloves if worn by the clinician. Direct contact is not necessary; inhalation of latex airborne molecules from powder-filled latex gloves can trigger an allergic reaction.

> **Patient Safety**
>
> ***The Vulnerability of the Health Professional***
>
> Clinicians do not have better immune systems than other people, although we sometimes behave as though we do. Nor are we invincible against everyday work-related injuries. We stand a much better chance of staying well if we are scrupulous in protecting ourselves:
>
> - Follow Standard Precautions.
> - Use personal protective equipment (PPE) when appropriate.
> - Minimize latex exposure.
> - Use good body mechanics or lift devices in transferring or assisting patients into various positions. NO EXCEPTIONS!

Examination Technique

Patient Positions and Draping

Most of the physical examination is conducted with the patient in seated and supine positions. Other positions

BOX 3.1 What Equipment Do You Need to Purchase?

Students are confronted by a large number and variety of pieces of equipment for physical examination. A commonly asked question is "What do I really need to buy?" The answer depends somewhat on the expectations from your educational program and where you will be practicing. If you are in a clinic setting, for example, wall-mounted ophthalmoscopes and otoscopes are typically provided. This is not necessarily true in a hospital setting.

The following list is intended only as a guideline to the equipment that you will use most often and should personally own. The price of stethoscopes, otoscopes, ophthalmoscopes, and blood pressure equipment can vary markedly. Different models, many with optional features, can affect the price. Because these pieces of equipment represent a significant monetary investment, evaluate the quality of the instrument, consider the manufacturer's warranty and support, and decide on the features that you will need.

- Stethoscope
- Ophthalmoscope
- Otoscope
- Blood pressure cuff and manometer
- Centimeter ruler
- Tape measure
- Reflex hammer
- Tuning forks: 500–1000 Hz for auditory screening; 100–400 Hz for vibratory sensation
- Penlight
- Near-vision screening chart

TABLE 3.1 Recommendations for Application of Standard Precautions for the Care of All Patients in All Health Care Settings

COMPONENT	RECOMMENDATIONS
Hand hygiene	The preferred method of hand hygiene in most clinical situations is with an alcohol-based hand sanitizer. Use soap and water when hands are visibly soiled (e.g., blood, body fluids) or after caring for patients with known or suspected *Clostridium difficile* or norovirus during an outbreak. Use hand hygiene: • Immediately before touching a patient. • Before performing an aseptic task (e.g., insertion of IV, preparing an injection). • Before moving from work on a soiled body site to a clean body site on the same patient. • After touching a patient or patient's surroundings. • After contact with blood, body fluids, or contaminated surfaces. • Immediately after glove removal. • After removal of PPE.
Use of personal protective equipment (PPE)	PPE, other than respirators, should be removed and discarded before leaving the patient's room or care area. If a respirator is used, it should be removed and discarded (or reprocessed if reusable) after leaving the patient's room or care area and closing the door. Perform hand hygiene immediately after removal of PPE.
Gloves	Wear gloves for potential contact with blood, body fluids, mucous membranes, nonintact skin, or contaminated equipment. Do not wear the same pair of gloves for the care of more than one patient. Do not wash gloves for the purpose of reuse. Perform hand hygiene after glove removal.
Gown	Wear a gown that is appropriate to the task to protect skin and clothing during procedures or activities where contact with blood or body fluids is anticipated. Do not wear the same gown for the care of more than one patient. Perform hand hygiene before leaving the patient's environment.
Mouth, nose, eye protection*	Wear mouth, nose, and eye protection during procedures that are likely to generate splashes or sprays of blood or other body fluids, secretions, and excretions, especially during suctioning, endotracheal intubation, or lumbar puncture.
Safe injection practices	Wear a surgical mask when performing lumbar puncture. Properly handle needles. Dispose of used sharps at the point of use in a sharps container that is closable, puncture resistant, and leak proof.
Safe handling of potentially contaminated equipment or surfaces in the patient's environment	• Follow policies and procedures for routine cleaning and disinfection of environmental surfaces in the facility and for appropriate cleaning and decontamination of spills of blood or other potentially infectious materials. • Remove organic material from critical and semicritical instruments/devices using recommended cleaning agents before high-level disinfection and sterilization. • Wear PPE according to the level of anticipated contamination when handling patient-care equipment and instruments that are visibly soiled or may have been in contact with blood or body fluids.
Respiratory hygiene/ cough etiquette	Instruct symptomatic persons to cover their mouth/nose when sneezing/coughing, use tissues and dispose in a no-touch receptacle, and perform hand hygiene after hands have been in contact with respiratory secretions. Wear a surgical mask and maintain spatial separation, >3 feet if possible, from others.

*During aerosol-generating procedures on patients with suspected or proven infections transmitted by respiratory aerosols, wear a fit-tested N95 or higher respirator in addition to gloves, gown, and face/eye protection.

From Siegel, J. D., et al. (2024). *Centers for Disease Control and Prevention: The guide to infection prevention for outpatient settings.* https://www.cdc.gov/infection-control/hcp/basics/standard-precautions.html (Accessed April 24, 2025).

BOX 3.2 Types of Latex Reactions

Irritant contact dermatitis—Chemical irritation that does not involve the immune system. Symptoms are usually dry, itching, irritated areas on the skin, typically the hands.

Type IV dermatitis (delayed hypersensitivity)—Allergic contact dermatitis that involves the immune system and is caused by the chemicals used in latex products. The skin reaction usually begins 24–48 hours after contact and resembles that caused by poison ivy. The reaction may progress to oozing skin blisters.

Type I systemic reactions—True allergic reactions caused by protein antibodies (immunoglobulin E antibodies) that form as a result of interaction between a foreign protein and the body's immune system. The antigen-antibody reaction causes release of histamine, leukotrienes, prostaglandins, and kinins. These chemicals cause the symptoms of allergic reactions. Type I reactions include the following symptoms: local urticaria (skin wheals), generalized urticaria with angioedema (tissue swelling), asthma, eye/nose itching, gastrointestinal symptoms, anaphylaxis (cardiovascular collapse), chronic asthma, and permanent lung damage.

BOX 3.3 Summary of Recommendations for Workers to Prevent Latex Allergy

- Use NONLATEX gloves for activities not likely to involve infectious materials. Hypoallergenic gloves are not necessarily latex free, but they may reduce reactions to chemical additives in the latex.
- For barrier protection when handling infectious materials, use powder-free latex gloves with reduced protein content.
- Use vinyl, nitrile, or polymer gloves appropriate for infectious materials.
- When wearing latex gloves, do not use oil-based hand creams or lotions because they may cause glove deterioration.
- After removing gloves, wash hands with mild soap and dry thoroughly.
- Use good housekeeping practices to remove latex-containing dust from the workplace.
- Take advantage of latex allergy education and training provided.
- If you develop symptoms of latex allergy, avoid direct contact with latex gloves and products.

From National Institute for Occupational Safety and Health. (2023). https://www.cdc.gov/niosh/docs/98-113/ (Accessed April 24, 2025).

are used for specific aspects of the examination. Special positioning requirements are discussed in the relevant chapters.

Seated. When seated, position the drape to cover the patient's lap and legs. You can move it to uncover parts of the body as they are examined.

Supine. In the supine position, the patient lies on their back, with arms at the sides and legs extended. The drape should cover the patient from chest to knees or toes. Again, you can move or reposition the drape to give appropriate exposure.

Prone. The patient lies on the stomach. This position may be used for special maneuvers as part of the musculoskeletal examination. Drape the patient to cover the torso.

Dorsal Recumbent. This position may be used for examination of the genital or rectal areas. The patient lies supine with knees bent and feet flat on the table. Place the drape in a diamond position from chest to toes. Wrap each leg with the corresponding lateral corner of the "diamond." Turn back the distal corner of the drape to perform the examination.

Lateral Recumbent. This is a side-lying position, with legs extended or flexed. The left lateral recumbent position (patient's left side is down) may be used in listening to heart sounds or palpating the spleen. This position can also be used for examination of the rectum or obtaining a rectal temperature. The patient starts in a lateral recumbent position. The torso is rolled toward a prone position; the top leg is flexed sharply at the hips and knee, and the bottom leg is flexed slightly. Drape the patient from shoulders to toes.

Lithotomy. The lithotomy position is generally used for the pelvic examination. Variations of positioning are discussed in Chapter 19. Begin with the patient in the dorsal recumbent position, with the feet at the corners of the table. Help the patient to stabilize the feet in the stirrups and slide the buttocks down to the edge of the table. Drape in the diamond position as with the dorsal recumbent position.

Inspection

Inspection is the process of observation. Your eyes and nose are sensitive tools for gathering data throughout the examination (Box 3.4). Take time to practice and develop this skill. Challenge yourself to see how much information you can collect through inspection alone. As the patient enters the room, observe the gait and stance and the ease or difficulty with which getting onto the examining table is accomplished. These observations alone will reveal a great deal about the patient's neurologic and musculoskeletal integrity. Is eye contact made? Is the demeanor appropriate for the situation? Is the clothing appropriate for the weather? The answers to these questions provide clues to the patient's emotional and mental status. Color and moisture of the skin or an unusual odor can alert you to the possibility of underlying disease. These preliminary observations require only a few seconds yet provide basic information that can influence the rest of the examination.

Inspection—unlike palpation, percussion, and auscultation—can continue throughout the history-taking process and during the physical examination. With this

BOX 3.4 The Sense of Smell: The Nose as an Aid to Physical Examination

The first observation when entering an examining room may be an odor, obvious and pervasive. Distinctive odors provide clues leading to the diagnosis of certain conditions, some of which need early detection if life-threatening sequelae are to be avoided. However, do not rush to premature diagnosis. A foreign body that has been present in a child's nose may cause this. Appreciate these odors for what they are—clues that must be followed up with additional investigation. Examples of odor clues follow.

CONDITION	SOURCE OF ODOR	TYPE OF ODOR
Inborn errors of metabolism	Phenylketonuria	Mousy
	Tyrosinemia	Fishy
Infectious diseases	Tuberculosis	Stale beer
	Diphtheria	Sweetish
Ingestions of poison or intoxication	Cyanide	Bitter almond
	Chloroform and salicylates	Fruity
Physiologic nondisease states	Sweaty feet	Cheesy
Foreign bodies (e.g., in the nose or vagina)	Organic material (e.g., bead in a child's nose)	Foul-smelling discharge

The odors may range from objectionable, to bland, to rather pleasant. The examiner often is the one to determine the characterization of the odor.

From Kippenberger, S., Havlíček, J., Bernd, A., et al. (2012). 'Nosing around' the human skin: What information is concealed in skin odour? *Experimental Dermatology, 21*(9), 655–659. https://doi.org/10.1111/j.1600-0625.2012.01545.x

kind of continuity, observations about the patient can constantly be modified until a complete picture is created. Be aware of both the patient's verbal statements and body language right up to the end of the encounter. The stance, stride, and body position can tell you a great deal about the patient's perception of the encounter (see Clinical Pearl, "Greeting the Patient").

CLINICAL PEARL

Greeting the Patient

Although a handshake is a nice gesture (coupled with appropriate hand washing), consider that in addition to infection prevention, cultural differences may preclude a handshake. If you do shake hands, be careful not to harm your patients by squeezing too tightly, especially those patients with conditions that may involve their hands—rheumatoid arthritis or osteoarthritis, for example. A good rule of thumb is to reciprocate the pressure applied by the patient but not exceed it.

Some general guidelines will be helpful as you proceed through the examination and inspect each area of the body. Adequate lighting is essential. The primary lighting should be direct enough to reveal color, texture, and mobility without distortion from shadowing. Secondary, tangential lighting from a lamp that casts shadows is also important for observing contour and variations in the body surface. Inspection should be unhurried. Give yourself time to carefully observe what you are inspecting. Pay attention to detail and note your findings. An important rule to remember is that you must expose what you want to inspect. Unwarranted concession to modesty, convenience, or haste comes at the cost of important information. Part of your job is to look and observe (and document) critically.

Knowing what to look for is essential to the process of focused attention. Be willing to validate inspection findings with your patient. The ability to narrow or widen your perceptual field selectively will come with time, experience, and practice.

Palpation

Palpation involves the use of the hands and fingers to gather information through the sense of touch. Certain parts of your hands and fingers are better than others for specific types of palpation (Table 3.2). The palmar surface of the fingers and finger pads is more sensitive than the fingertips. Use this surface whenever discriminatory touch is needed for determining position, texture, size, consistency, masses, fluid, and crepitus. The ulnar surface of the hand and fingers is the most sensitive area for distinguishing vibration. The dorsal surface of the hands is best for estimating temperature. Of course, this estimate provides only a crude measure—use it to compare temperature differences among parts of the body.

Specific techniques of palpation are discussed in more detail as they occur in each part of the examination (see Clinical Pearl, "Right-Sided Examination?"). Palpation may be either light or deep and is controlled by the amount of pressure applied with the fingers or hand. Short fingernails are essential to avoid discomfort or injury to the patient.

CLINICAL PEARL

Right-Sided Examination?

It is the convention, at least in the United States, to examine patients from the right side and to palpate and percuss with the right hand. We continue with this convention, if only to simplify description of a procedure or technique. We feel no obligation to adhere strictly to the right-sided approach. Our suggestion is that students learn to use both hands for examination and that they be allowed to stand on either side of the patient, depending on both the patient's and clinician's convenience and comfort. The important issue is to develop an approach that is useful and practical and yields the desired results.

TABLE 3.2 Areas of the Hand to Use in Palpation

TO DETERMINE	USE
Position, texture, size, consistency, fluid, crepitus, form of a mass, or structure	Palmar surface of the fingers and finger pads
Vibration	Ulnar surfaces of hand and fingers
Temperature	Dorsal surface of hand

TABLE 3.3 Percussion Tones

TONE	INTENSITY	PITCH	DURATION	QUALITY	EXAMPLE WHERE HEARD
Tympanic	Loud	High	Moderate	Drumlike	Gastric bubble
Hyperresonant	Very loud	Low	Long	Boomlike	Emphysematous lungs
Resonant	Loud	Low	Long	Hollow	Healthy lung tissue
Dull	Soft to moderate	Moderate to high	Moderate	Thudlike	Over liver
Flat	Soft	High	Short	Very dull	Over muscle

Touch is in many ways therapeutic, and palpation is the actuality of the "laying on of hands." Our advice for a gentle approach with warm hands is not only practical but also symbolic of your respect for the patient and for the privilege the patient gives you.

Percussion

Percussion involves striking one object against another to produce vibration and subsequent sound waves. In the physical examination, your finger functions as a hammer, and the impact of the finger against underlying tissue produces the vibration. Sound waves are heard as percussion tones (called *resonance*) that arise from vibrations 4 to 6 cm deep in the body tissue. The density of the medium through which the sound waves travel determines the degree of percussion tone. The more dense the medium, the quieter the percussion tone. The percussion tone over air is loud, over fluid less loud, and over solid areas soft. The degree of percussion tone is classified and ordered as listed in Table 3.3 and as follows:

- Tympany
- Hyperresonance
- Resonance
- Dullness
- Flatness

Tympany is the loudest, and flatness is the quietest. Quantification of the percussion tone is difficult, especially for the beginner. For points of reference, as noted in Table 3.3, the gastric bubble is considered to be tympanic, air-filled lungs (as in emphysema) to be hyperresonant, healthy lungs to be resonant, the liver to be dull, and muscle to be flat. Degree of resonance is more easily distinguished by listening to the sound change as you move from one area to another. Because it is easier to hear the change from resonance to dullness (rather than from dullness to resonance), proceed with percussion from areas of resonance to areas of dullness. A partially full milk carton is a good tool for practicing percussion skills. Begin with percussion over the air-filled space of the carton, appreciating its resonant quality. Work your way downward and listen for the change in sound as you encounter the milk. This principle applies in percussion of body tissues and cavities.

The techniques of percussion are the same regardless of the structure you are percussing. Immediate (direct) percussion involves striking the finger or hand directly against the body. Indirect or mediate percussion is a technique in which the finger of one hand acts as the hammer (plexor) and a finger of the other hand acts as the striking surface. To perform indirect percussion, place your nondominant hand on the surface of the body with the fingers slightly spread. Place the distal phalanx of the middle finger firmly on the body surface with the other fingers slightly elevated off the surface. Snap the wrist of your other hand downward, and with the tip of the middle finger, sharply tap the interphalangeal joint of the finger that is on the body surface (Fig. 3.1). You may tap just distal to the interphalangeal joint if you choose, but decide on one and be consistent because the sound varies from one to the other. Percussion must be performed against bare skin. If you are not able to hear the percussion tone, try pressing harder against the patient's skin with your finger that lies on the body surface. Failing to press firmly enough is a common error. On the other hand, pressing too hard on an infant or very young chest can obscure the sound.

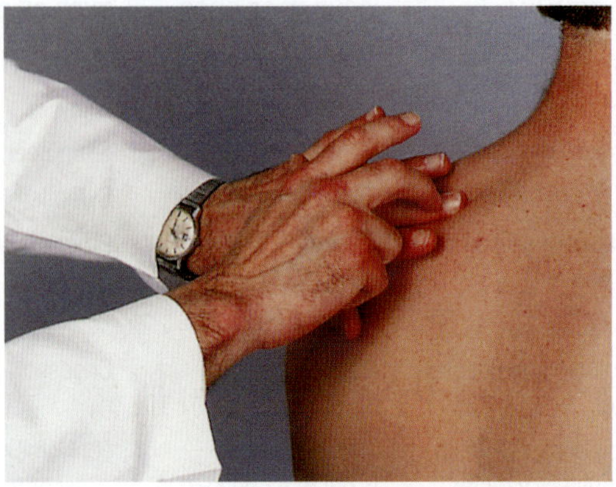

FIG. 3.1 Percussion technique: tapping the interphalangeal joint. Only the middle finger of the examiner's nondominant hand should be in contact with the patient's skin surface.

Several points are essential in developing the technique of percussion. The downward snap of the striking finger originates from the wrist and not the forearm or shoulder. Tap sharply and rapidly; once the finger has struck, snap the wrist back, quickly lifting the finger to prevent dampening the sound. Use the tip and not the pad of the plexor finger (short fingernails are a necessity). Percuss one location several times to facilitate interpretation of the tone. Like other techniques, percussion requires practice to

BOX 3.5 Common Percussion Errors

Percussion requires practice. In learning percussion, beginning clinicians often make the following errors:

- Failing to exert firm pressure with the finger placed on the skin surface
- Failing to separate the hammer finger from other fingers
- Snapping downward from the elbow or shoulder rather than from the wrist
- Tapping by moving just the hammer finger rather than the whole hand
- Striking with the finger pad rather than the fingertip of the hammer finger
- Failing to trim the fingernail of the hammer finger

obtain the skill needed to produce the desired result. Box 3.5 describes common percussion errors. In learning to distinguish between the tones, it may be helpful to close your eyes to block out other sensory stimuli, concentrating exclusively on the tone you are hearing.

You can also use your fist for percussion. Fist percussion is most commonly used to elicit tenderness arising from the liver, gallbladder, or kidneys. In this technique, use the ulnar aspect of the fist to deliver a firm blow to the flank and back areas. Too gentle a blow will not produce enough force to stimulate the tenderness, but too much force can cause unnecessary discomfort, even in a well patient. The force of a direct blow can be mediated by use of a second hand placed over the area. Practice on yourself or a colleague until you achieve the desired middle ground.

Auscultation

Auscultation involves listening to sounds produced by the body. Some sounds, such as speech, are audible to the unassisted ear. Most others require a stethoscope to augment the sound. Specific types of stethoscopes, their use, and their desired characteristics are discussed later in the section on stethoscopes.

Some general principles apply to all auscultatory procedures. The environment should be quiet and free from distracting noises. Place the stethoscope on the naked skin because clothing obscures the sound. Listen not only for the presence of sound but also for its characteristics: intensity, pitch, duration, and quality. The sounds are often subtle or transitory, and you must listen intently to hear the nuances. Closing your eyes may prevent distraction by visual stimuli and narrow your perceptual field to help you focus on the sound. Try to target and isolate each sound, concentrating on one sound at a time. Take enough time to identify all the characteristics of each sound. Auscultation should be carried out last, except with the abdominal examination, after other techniques have provided information that will assist in interpreting what you hear (see Clinical Pearl, "Unexpected Findings").

CLINICAL PEARL

Unexpected Findings

Respect your judgment and your instinct when you identify a physical examination finding you had not expected to find. Pay attention when this occurs, even if it does not seem to make sense or you cannot explain it easily. The flip side—not finding a previously documented "abnormal" finding—may simply be a learning opportunity, or it may reflect a change in the patient's condition. It is OK if you say, "I couldn't hear that" or "I'm not sure I felt that." If in doubt, have someone with more experience check it with you.

One of the most difficult achievements in auscultation is learning to isolate sounds. You cannot hear everything all at once. Whether it is a breath sound, a heartbeat, or the sequence of respirations and heartbeats, each segment of the cycle must be isolated and listened to specifically. After the individual sounds are identified, they are put together. Do not anticipate the next sound; concentrate on the one at hand. Auscultation of the lungs is discussed in Chapter 14, of the heart in Chapter 15, and of the abdomen in Chapter 18.

Modifications for Patients With Disabilities

Each disability affects each person differently; therefore it is important for clinicians to educate themselves about relevant aspects of a patient's disability. Sensitivity in asking only pertinent questions about the disability will increase the patient's comfort and cooperation.

Keep some considerations in mind about the environment and the encounter. Speak directly to the patient if they have capacity. Often people will address a disabled person's spouse, friend, attendant, or an interpreter instead of speaking directly to the person. Remove or rearrange the furnishings in the examination room to provide needed space, such as for a wheelchair. Take the paper covering off the examination table if it is a bother during transfers and positioning. Equipment such as a high-low examination table, a particularly wide examination table, or a slide board can be obtained to facilitate safer, easier transfers and positioning. Obstetric or foot stirrups can be padded or equipped with a strap to increase the patient's comfort and safety during a pelvic examination. For the pelvic examination, a patient can wear an easily removable skirt or pair of pants. A button-up or zippered shirt will facilitate the breast examination. Musculoskeletal examinations of the lower extremities can be accomplished with the patient wearing shorts.

Patients With Mobility Impairments

The patient is the expert in transferring from the wheelchair or in using assistants to transfer to the examination table. Transfers are relatively simple if the patient, assistant, and clinician all understand the method that will best suit the patient's disability, the room space, and the

BOX 3.6 Transfer Guidelines

Guidelines for the Assistant

- The patient/parent/caregiver should direct the transfer and positioning process.
- Assistants should not overestimate their ability to lift.
- Keep in mind that not all nonambulatory patients need assistance.
- Assistants should keep their backs straight, bend their knees, and lift with their legs.
- It may be helpful to perform a test lift or to practice the transfer by lifting the patient just over the wheelchair before attempting a complete transfer.
- Assistants who feel that they may drop a patient during a transfer should not panic. It is important, whenever possible, to explain what is happening to reassure the patient throughout the situation. Assistants will usually have time to lower the patient safely to the floor until they can get additional help.

Guidelines for the Patient

- Explain clearly the preferred transfer method and direct the clinician and assistants during the process.
- Assistants can help by preparing equipment. Because many people are not familiar with wheelchairs or supportive devices, the patient may need to explain to the health care clinicians and assistants how they can handle belongings. Patients who use wheelchairs should explain how to apply the brakes, detach the footrests and armrests, or turn off the motor of an electric wheelchair. Have the patient who wears adaptive devices (e.g., leg braces or supportive undergarments) explain how to remove them, if necessary, and where to put them if the patient cannot do so.
- Patients who use urinary equipment should direct assistants in the moving or straightening of catheter tubing. The patient may wish to unstrap the leg bag and place it on the table beside or across the abdomen for proper drainage while supine. Assistants should be reminded not to pull on the tubing or allow kinks to develop.
- Have the patient inform the clinician and assistants when they are comfortable and balanced after the transfer is completed.
- All parties should be aware of jewelry, clothing, tubing, or equipment that might catch or otherwise interfere with the transfer.

examination table (Box 3.6). You need to know your own physical limits for lifting or moving a patient—always seek assistance if uncertain. This will avoid falls and injuries to both you and the patient.

Pivot Transfer. Stand in front of the patient, take the patient's knees between your own knees, grasp the patient around the back and under the arms, raise the patient to a vertical position, and then pivot from the wheelchair to the table. The examination table must be low enough for the patient to sit on; therefore a hydraulic high-low table may be needed when using this transfer method.

Cradle Transfer. While bending or squatting beside the patient, put one arm under the patient's knees and the other arm around the back and under the armpits. Stand and carry the patient to the table.

Two-Person Transfer. In all two-person transfers, the assistants must be careful to work together to lift the patient over the arms of the wheelchair from a sitting position onto the examination table. The stronger, taller person should always lift the upper half of the patient's body.

- *Method 1* requires the patient to fold the arms across the chest. The assistant standing behind the patient kneels, putting their elbows under the patient's armpits, and grasps the patient's opposite wrists. The second assistant lifts and supports the patient under the knees.
- *Method 2* can be used if the patient cannot fold the arms. The assistant standing behind the patient puts their own hands together around the patient, if possible, so that there is less likelihood of losing hold of the patient. The second assistant lifts and supports the patient under the knees.
- *Cradle transfer* is a variation of the one-person cradle transfer. Two assistants grasp each other's arms behind the patient's back and under the knees and then stand and carry the patient to the table.

Equipment. Some persons with mobility impairments use a slide board, which forms a bridge to slide across from the wheelchair to the examination table. For this method to work, the table and chair must be approximately the same height. Most examination tables, however, are quite a bit higher than wheelchairs. Some examining rooms have high-low examination tables that can be adjusted to a height that will facilitate the safest and easiest transfer. A wider table, even if it is not adjustable in height, can also make transfers and positioning easier.

Patients With Sensory Impairment

At the beginning of the visit with a patient with a hearing or speech impairment, discuss the communication system that will be used (e.g., a sign language interpreter, word board, talk box, or typing questions on a tablet or computer). Specialized educational materials (e.g., Braille or audiotaped information or three-dimensional anatomic models) can be acquired to make information accessible to sensory-impaired patients.

Impaired Vision. Remember to identify yourself upon entering the examination room and inform the patient when you are leaving the room. A red-tipped white cane and guide animal are mobility aids used by many persons with visual impairments. If a patient is accompanied by a guide animal, do not pet or distract the animal, which is trained to respond only to its owner. A patient may prefer to keep the guide animal or white cane nearby in the examination room. Do not move either of these without the patient's permission. Before the examination, ask whether the patient would like to examine any equipment or instruments that will be used during the examination. If three-dimensional models are available, they can be used to acquaint the patient with the examination process (e.g., with the genital examination). During the examination, the patient may feel more at ease if you maintain continuous tactile or verbal contact (e.g., by keeping a hand on the arm or by narrating what is taking place during the examination).

Some patients with visual impairments will want to be oriented to their surroundings, whereas others may not. Each should be encouraged to specify the kind of orientation and assistance needed. Verbally describe and assist the patient in locating where to put the clothes, where the various furnishings are positioned, how to approach the examination table, and how to get positioned on the table.

Impaired Hearing or Speech. Federal regulations require clinicians to provide effective communication, using auxiliary aids and services that ensure communication with patients who have a hearing loss is as effective as communication with others. The patient should choose which form of communication to use during the examination (e.g., qualified interpreters, assistive listening devices, written materials, telecommunications devices for the deaf). Although a patient may use an interpreter throughout most of the visit, they may decide not to use the interpreter during parts of the actual examination. If an interpreter is used, you and the patient should decide where the interpreter should stand or sit. When working with an interpreter, speak at a regular speed and directly to the patient instead of to the interpreter. Qualified interpreters may be live or virtual. As with language interpreters, family members are not appropriate.

Special Concerns for Patients With Spinal Cord Injury or Lesion

Bowel and bladder concerns and other conditions such as autonomic dysreflexia (hyperreflexia), hypersensitivity, and spasticity should be given special attention during the examination process.

Bowel and Bladder Concerns. Some patients do not have voluntary bladder or bowel movements. A bladder or bowel routine could affect the pelvic or rectal examination. The physical stimulation of a speculum, bimanual, or rectal examination can mimic the stimulation for the bowel routine and cause a bowel movement during the examination. An indwelling catheter need not be removed during the examination unless it is not working; if it is removed, another catheter should be available for insertion. Likewise, it is not necessary to remove the catheter during a pelvic examination, as it will not interfere.

If a patient uses intermittent catheterization to manually open the bladder sphincter at regular intervals during the day, tactile stimulation in the pelvic area during the examination could cause the bladder sphincter to open and produce incontinence.

Autonomic Dysreflexia. Autonomic dysreflexia, also called *hyperreflexia,* is a potentially life-threatening condition associated with high-level spinal cord injury (T6 or higher), which can occur even after the acute injury phase. Symptoms include severe high blood pressure, sweating, blotchy skin, nausea, or goosebumps caused by stimulation of the bowel, bladder, or skin below the spinal lesion. Some causes of dysreflexia that may occur during the physical examination include reactions to a cold, hard examination table or cold stirrups; insertion and manipulation of a vaginal speculum; pressure during the bimanual or rectal examination; or tactile contact with hypersensitive areas. If the patient experiences high blood pressure, identify and remove the source of the stimulation. Sit the patient upright with legs dangling. Remove tight or constrictive clothing. Once the dysreflexia ceases, you and the patient should mutually decide whether to continue the examination. If the examination is continued and dysreflexia recurs, stop the examination and reschedule for another time. If the blood pressure does not decrease with removal of the stimulus or if the dysreflexia symptoms persist and lead to a throbbing headache or nasal obstruction, treat the situation as a medical emergency. Do not leave unaccompanied a patient experiencing any degree of dysreflexia.

Think About It

Autonomic Dysreflexia

Autonomic dysreflexia occurs because of dysregulation of the autonomic nervous system. Cutaneous or visceral stimulation below the level of the spinal cord injury initiates afferent impulses that elicit reflex sympathetic nervous system activity. The sympathetic response leads to diffuse vasoconstriction, typically to the lower two-thirds of the body, causing a rise in blood pressure. In the compromised autonomic nervous system, the normal compensatory parasympathetic response cannot travel below the level of the spinal cord injury. Sitting the patient upright and removing any tight clothing or constrictive devices orthotactically helps lower blood pressure by inducing pooling of blood in the abdominal and lower extremity vessels.

Hypersensitivity. To help prevent possible discomfort or spasms, ask the patient about hypersensitive areas of the body before the examination. Some patients may experience variable responses (e.g., spasms or pain) to ordinary tactile stimulation. Often, you can avoid sensitive areas or use an extra amount of lubricant jelly to decrease friction or pressure.

Spasticity. Spasms may range from slight tremors to quick, violent contractions. Spasms may occur during a transfer, while assuming an awkward or uncomfortable position, or from stimulation of the skin with an instrument. If spasm occurs during the examination, gently support the area (usually a leg, an arm, or the abdominal region) to avoid any injury to the patient. Allow the spasms to resolve before continuing the examination. A feeling of physical security can decrease spasm intensity or frequency. A patient who experiences spasms should never be left alone on the examination table. Have an assistant stand near the examination table and maintain physical contact with the patient to provide a feeling of safety.

Equipment

Weight Scales and Height Measurement Devices

Height and weight of adults are measured on a standing platform scale with a height attachment. Scales can be manual or electronic. Note what the patient is wearing: adults and older children should wear lightweight clothing for more accurate measurement.

The manual scale uses a system of adding and subtracting weight in increments as small as 0.1 kg to counterbalance the weight placed on the scale platform. Calibrate the scale to zero before the patient mounts the platform by moving both the large and small weights to zero. Level and steady the balance beam by adjusting the calibrating knob. Pull up the height attachment before the patient steps on the scale and then position the headpiece at the patient's crown. Place a paper towel on the platform before the patient steps on it to avoid the potential transmission of organisms from bare feet.

With electronic scales, weight is calculated electronically and provided as a digital readout (Fig. 3.2). These scales are automatically calibrated each time they are used.

The infant platform scale is used for measuring weights of infants and small children (Fig. 3.3). It works the same as the adult scale but measures in grams. Scales can be manual or electronic. The scale has a platform with curved sides in which the child may sit or lie. Place paper under the child, and never leave the child unattended on the scale. Weigh the infant either nude or with only a diaper for accuracy of weight.

Infant lengths can be measured by using an infant measuring device that comes with a rigid headboard and movable footboard (Fig. 3.4A). An alternative to the rigid measuring device is a commercially available measure mat, consisting of a soft rubber graduated mat attached to a plastic headboard and footboard (see Fig. 3.4B). Place the measuring board on the table so that the headboard and footboard are perpendicular to the table. Position the infant supine on the measuring board with the head against the headboard and knees held straight. Move the footboard until it touches the bottom of the infant's feet. The infant's length can be read in either inches or centimeters. Be sure to clean the mat between uses.

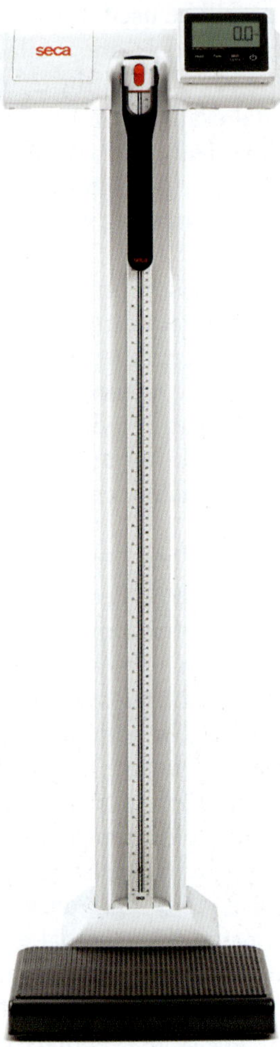

FIG. 3.2 Platform scale with height attachment.

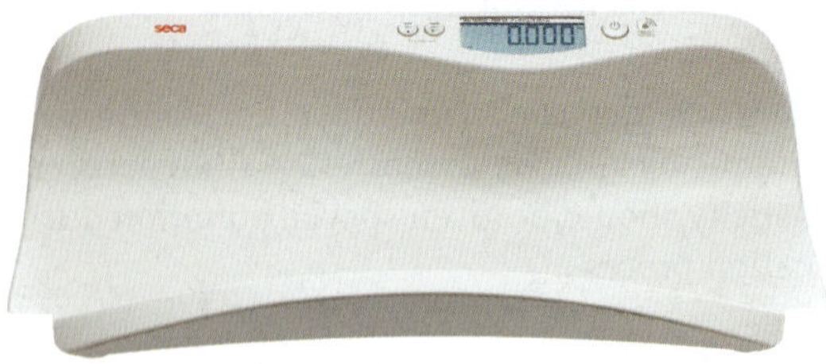

FIG. 3.3 Infant platform scale.

Infants can also be measured by placing them on a pad or disposable paper sheet and making a mark at the top of the head and another at the heel of the extended leg. Then measure the length from marking to marking.

Once a child can stand erect without support, use a stadiometer, a stature-measuring device, to measure height. The device consists of a movable headpiece attached to a rigid measurement bar and platform. Standing height is measured barefoot. With the child standing with the shoulders, buttocks, and heels in alignment, lower the head piece to the crown of the child's head (Fig. 3.5).

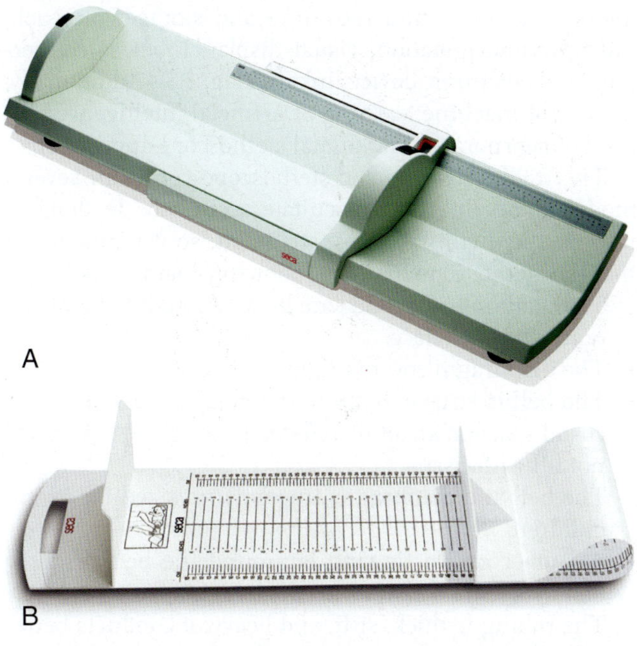

FIG. 3.4 **Devices used to measure the length of an infant.** (A) Infant length board. (B) Measure mat. (A, Courtesy Perspective Enterprises, Inc., Portage, MI. B, Courtesy Seca North America, Medical Scales and Measuring Systems, Seca Corp., Chino, CA.)

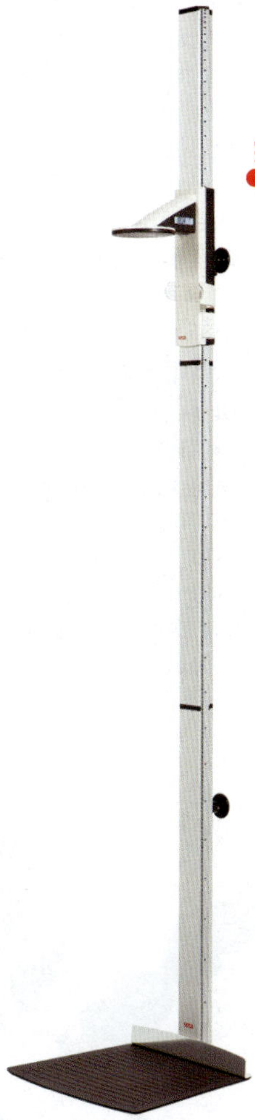

FIG. 3.5 Device used to measure height of a child. (Courtesy Perspective Enterprises, Portage, MI.)

Devices can be mobile or attached to the wall. Height is calibrated either manually or digitally. Digital touchless models use sonar technology to triangulate the top of the head and provide a digital readout.

Thermometer

Electronic temperature measurement has decreased the time required for accurate temperature readings. One piece of equipment that contains an electronic sensing probe can be used for measurement of rectal, oral, and axillary temperatures (Fig. 3.6A). The probe, covered by a disposable sheath, is placed under the tongue with the mouth tightly closed, in the rectum, or in the axillary space with the arm held close to the torso. A temperature reading (in either Fahrenheit or Celsius) is revealed on a digital display within 15 to 60 seconds, depending on the model used.

Professional-grade infrared thermometers are also available, which infer temperature from the thermal radiation from the patient source such as the temporal artery or the tympanic membrane, which shares its blood supply with the hypothalamus in the brain. The measurements obtained vary somewhat from those obtained by oral or rectal routes (see Fig. 3.6B). In some situations, as with very young infants or with the critically ill, traditional routes of measurement may be more accurate; in other situations, such as with children in an outpatient setting, an infrared thermometer, with its ease of use and no-contact feature, is preferred. For tympanic membrane temperature measurement, a specially designed probe similar in shape to an otoscope is required. Gently place the covered probe tip at the external opening of the ear canal. Do not try to force the probe into the canal or to occlude it. The temperature is displayed in a few seconds.

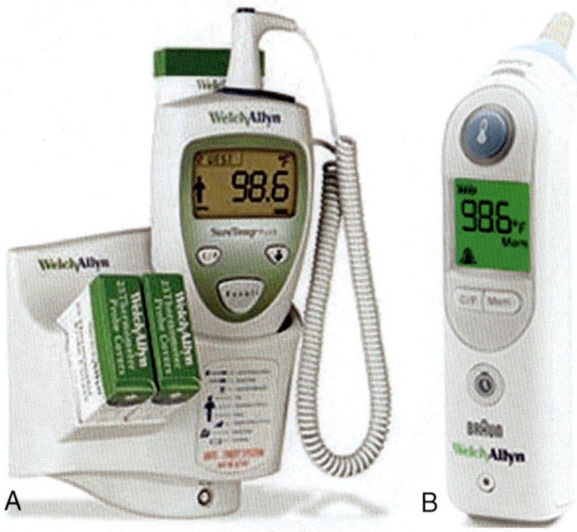

FIG. 3.6 **Devices for electronic temperature measurement.** (A) Rectal, oral, or axillary thermometer. (B) Tympanic membrane thermometer. (Courtesy Welch Allyn, Inc., Skaneateles Falls, NY.)

Stethoscope

Auscultation of most sounds requires a stethoscope. Several types are available: acoustic, magnetic, electronic, and digital.

The acoustic stethoscope is a closed cylinder that transmits sound waves from their source and along its column to the ear (Fig. 3.7). Its rigid diaphragm has a natural frequency of around 300 Hz. It screens out low-pitched sounds and best transmits high-pitched sounds such as the second heart sound. The bell end piece has a natural frequency that varies with the amount of pressure exerted. It transmits low-pitched sounds when very light pressure is used. With firm pressure, the skin converts it to a diaphragm end piece. The chest piece contains a closure valve so that only one end piece, either the diaphragm or bell, is operational at any one time (thus preventing inadvertent dissipation of sound waves).

The stereophonic stethoscope, a type of acoustic stethoscope, is used to differentiate between the right and left auscultatory sounds using a two-channel design. With a single tube, diaphragm, and bell, it looks and functions like an acoustic stethoscope. However, the right and left ear tubes are independently connected to right and left semicircular microphones in the chest piece.

The magnetic stethoscope has a single end piece that is a diaphragm. It contains an iron disk on the interior surface; behind this is a permanent magnet. A strong spring keeps the diaphragm bowed outward when it is not compressed against a body surface. Compression of the diaphragm activates the air column as magnetic attraction is established between the iron disk and the magnet. Rotation of a dial adjusts for high-, low-, and full-frequency sounds.

The electronic stethoscope picks up vibrations transmitted to the surface of the body and converts them into electrical impulses. The impulses are amplified and transmitted to a speaker, where they are reconverted to sound. Digital versions of the electronic stethoscope can also provide additional features such as extended listening ranges, digital readout, sound recording and storage, playback, murmur interpretation, visual display, tubeless connection, and electronic device linkage (Fig. 3.8). Additionally, the use of machine learning or artificial intelligence (AI) can be incorporated into digital stethoscope applications.

The traditional acoustic stethoscope comes in several models. The ability to auscultate accurately depends in part on the quality of the instrument, so it is important that the stethoscope have the following characteristics:

- The diaphragm and bell are heavy enough to lie firmly on the body surface.
- The diaphragm cover is rigid.
- The bell is large enough in diameter to span an intercostal space in an adult and deep enough so that it will not fill with tissue.
- The bell and diaphragm are pediatric sized for use in children.
- A rubber or plastic ring is around the bell edges to ensure secure contact with the body surface.
- The tubing is thick, stiff, and heavy; it conducts better than thin, elastic, or very flexible tubing.
- The length of the tubing is between 30.5 and 40 cm (12 and 18 inches) to minimize distortion.
- The earpieces fit snugly and comfortably. Some instruments have several sizes of earpieces, and some have hard and soft earpieces. The determining factors are how they fit and feel to the examiner. The earpieces should be large enough to occlude the auditory canal, thus blocking outside sound. If they are too small, they will slip into the ear canal and be painful.
- The angled binaural earpieces are pointed toward the nose so that sound is projected toward the tympanic membrane.

To stabilize the stethoscope when it is in place, hold the end piece between the fingers, pressing the diaphragm firmly against the skin (Fig. 3.9). The diaphragm piece should never be used without the diaphragm. Because the bell functions by picking up vibrations, it must be positioned so that the vibrations are not dampened. Place the bell evenly and lightly on the skin, making sure there is skin contact around the entire edge. To prevent extraneous noise, do not touch the tubing with your hands or allow the tubing to rub against any surfaces. Be sure to appropriately disinfect your stethoscope after each use.

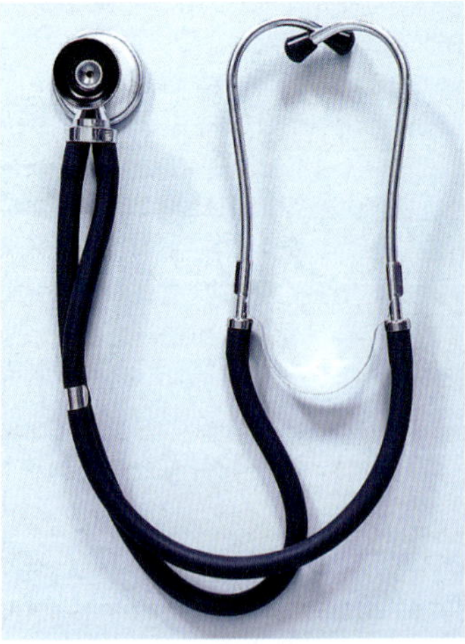

FIG. 3.7 Acoustic stethoscope.

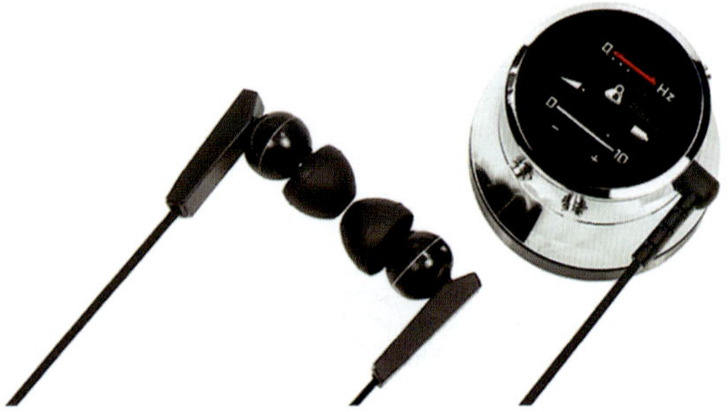

FIG. 3.8 Electronic stethoscope. (Courtesy Thinklabs One, Centennial, CO.)

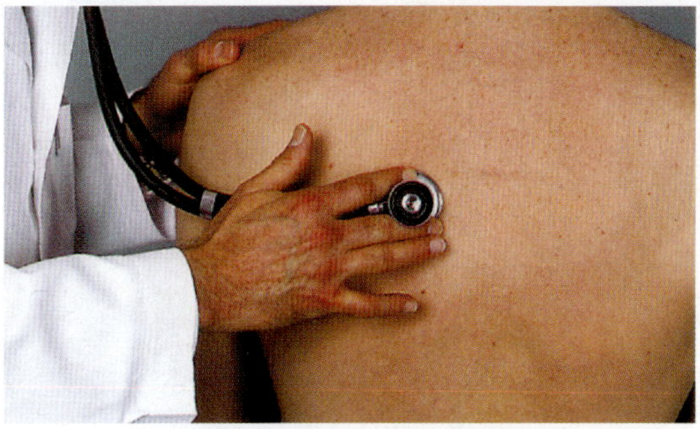

FIG. 3.9 Position the stethoscope between the index and middle fingers against the patient's bare skin.

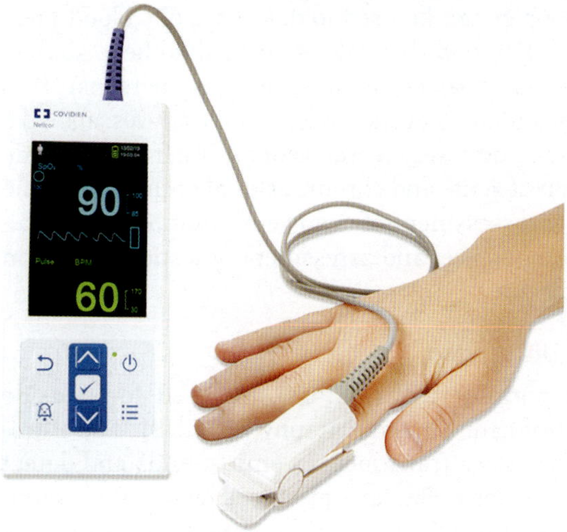

FIG. 3.10 Pulse oximeter monitor and sensor. (©2017 Medtronic. All rights reserved. Used with the permission of Medtronic, Minneapolis, MN.)

Sphygmomanometer

Blood pressure is measured indirectly with a stethoscope and an aneroid sphygmomanometer or with an electronic sphygmomanometer, which does not require the use of a stethoscope. Each sphygmomanometer is composed of a cuff with an inflatable bladder, a pressure manometer, and a rubber hand bulb with a pressure control valve to inflate and deflate the bladder. The electronic sphygmomanometer senses vibrations and converts them into electric impulses. The impulses are transmitted to a device that translates them into a digital readout. The instrument is relatively sensitive and is also capable of simultaneously measuring the pulse rate. It does not, however, indicate the quality, rhythm, and other characteristics of a pulse and should not be used in place of your touch in assessing pulse. An elevated blood pressure detected by an electronic sphygmomanometer should be repeated using a manual approach. Particularly in children, electronic blood pressure readings may be falsely elevated.

Pulse Oximeter

Pulse oximetry measures the percentage of hemoglobin saturated with oxygen (oxyhemoglobin). Oxygen saturation is a measure of how much oxygen the blood is carrying as a percentage of the maximum it could carry. A sensor attached to a digit or an ear has two light-emitting diodes: one that sends out invisible infrared light and one that sends out red light. Oxygenated hemoglobin absorbs more infrared light and allows more red light to pass through. Deoxygenated hemoglobin absorbs more red light and allows more infrared light to pass through. The ratio of the absorption is used to calculate the oxy/deoxyhemoglobin ratio. The difference between the two gives a measure of the fraction of the oxyhemoglobin in the blood. The readout displays the result as a percentage.

Pulse oximetry requires a reasonably translucent site with good blood flow. Typical adult/pediatric sites are the finger, toe, or pinna (top) or lobe of the ear (Fig. 3.10). Infant sites are the foot or palm of the hand and the big toe or thumb. The oximeter detects the slight change in color of the arterial blood caused by the beat of the heart when blood is pushed into the finger (or earlobe or toe). Because the change in color is so minute, it is imperative to ensure a strong pulse during testing. When the pulse is weak, the results may be inaccurate.

Doppler

Some sounds are so difficult to auscultate that a regular stethoscope will not suffice. Dopplers are useful at these times (Fig. 3.11). Dopplers are ultrasonic stethoscopes that detect blood flow rather than amplify sounds, and they vary in frequency from 2 to 10 MHz. The use of a Doppler requires that you first place transmission gel over the skin area where you will be listening. Then place the tip of the instrument directly over the area being examined. Tilt the tip at an angle along the axis of blood flow to obtain the best signal. Arterial flow is heard as a pulsatile pumping sound, and venous flow resembles the sound of rushing wind. When using a Doppler, do not press so hard as to impede blood flow.

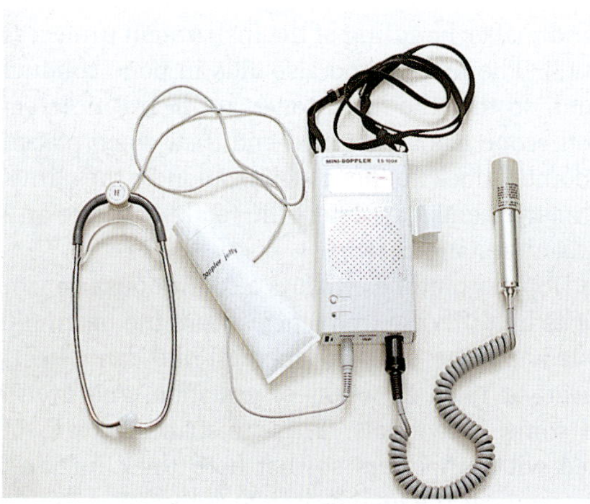

FIG. 3.11 Doppler.

The Doppler can be used to detect systolic blood pressures in patients with weak or difficult-to-hear sounds (e.g., patients in shock, infants, or obese persons). It is used to auscultate fetal heart activity, locate vessels, take weak pulses, and assess vessel patency. Other uses include localization of acute and chronic arterial occlusions in the extremities, assessment of deep vein thrombosis and valvular incompetence, and assessment of testicular torsion and varicoceles.

Portable Ultrasound

Compact portable units (CPUs) are used for bedside and point-of-care ultrasonography (POCUS). The ultrasound unit uses a transducer to emit sounds and detect returning echoes that are produced when the sound wave strikes an object. The returning echoes identify the distance, size, and shape of the object. A CPU analyzes the echoes and transforms them into a two- or three-dimensional image of the organs or tissues being examined. Ultrasound waves pass easily through fluids and soft tissues, making the procedure especially useful for assessing fluid-filled organs, such as the urinary bladder for fullness, distention, and incomplete emptying, and soft organs, such as the gallbladder and liver. Because ultrasound produces dynamic moving images, it can show the structure and movement of the body's internal organs, in addition to blood flowing through blood vessels. Abnormalities that can be detected by ultrasound include cysts, tumors, fluid collection, infections, structural abnormalities of organs, and blockages in major blood vessels. Ultrasound provides a visual aid to improving targeted clinical procedures such as aspiration and drainage of pleural effusions, abscesses, and biopsies. Use of the ultrasound device requires training and skilled operation.

Fetal Monitoring Equipment

The fetal heart rate is determined using specially designed instruments called the *fetoscope* and *Leff scope;* by use of the clinical stethoscope, addressed previously; or with an electronic instrument that uses the Doppler effect. The fetoscope has a band that fits against the head of the listener and makes handling of the instrument unnecessary (Fig. 3.12). The metal band also aids in bone conduction of sound, so that the heart tones are heard more easily. The Leff scope has a weighted end that, when placed on the abdomen, does not need stabilization by the clinician. These instruments can detect the fetal heart rate at 17 to 19 weeks of gestation.

The Doppler method employs a continuous ultrasound that picks up differing frequencies from the beating fetal heart. It is a more sensitive method and can detect the fetal heart at 10 to 12 weeks of gestation, and even earlier in some individuals. These instruments are often supplied with amplifiers so that both the clinician and parents can hear the fetal heartbeat at the same time.

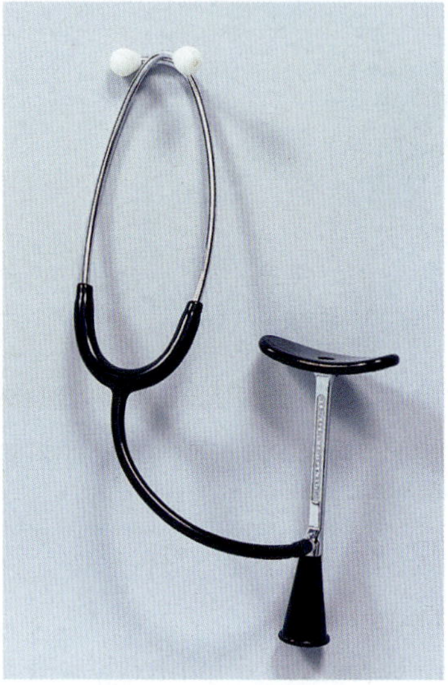

FIG. 3.12 Fetoscope.

Ophthalmoscope

The traditional handheld ophthalmoscope has a system of lenses and mirrors that enables visualization of the interior structures of the eye (Fig. 3.13). The instrument has a light source that projects through various apertures while you focus on the inner eye. The large aperture, the one used most often, produces a large round beam. The various apertures (described in Table 3.4) are selected by rotating the aperture selection dial.

The lenses in varying powers of magnification are used to bring the structure under examination into focus by

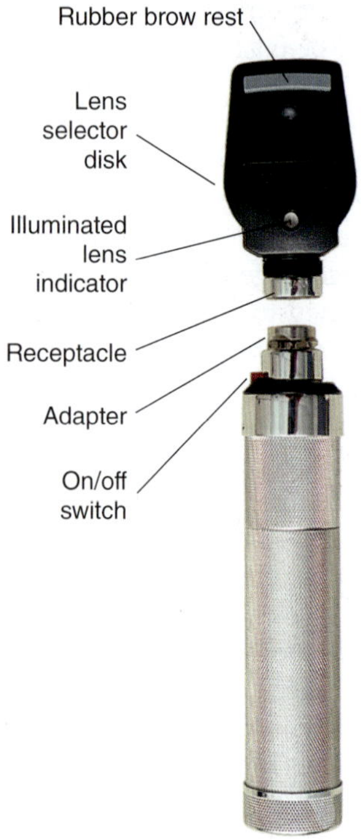

FIG. 3.13 Ophthalmoscope.

TABLE 3.4 Apertures of the Ophthalmoscope

APERTURE	EXAMINATION USE
Small aperture	Small pupils
Red-free filter	Produces a green beam for examination of the optic disc for pallor and minute vessel changes; also permits recognition of retinal hemorrhages, with blood appearing black
Slit	Examination of the anterior eye and determination of the elevation of lesions on the retina
Grid	Estimation of the size of fundal lesions

converging or diverging light. An illuminating lens indicator displays the lens number positioned in the viewing aperture. The number, ranging from about ±20 to ±140, corresponds to the magnification power (diopter) of the lens. The positive numbers (plus lenses) are shown in black, and the negative numbers (minus lenses) are shown in red. A way to remember this is that when you are using a minus lens, you are in the red. Clockwise rotation of the lens selector brings the plus sphere lenses into place. Counterclockwise rotation brings the minus sphere lenses into place. Fig. 3.14 shows the expected lens diopters to focus on eye structures. The system of plus and minus lenses can compensate for myopia or hyperopia in both the examiner and the patient. There is no compensation for astigmatism.

Seat the ophthalmoscope head in the handle by fitting the adapter of the handle into the head receptacle and pushing downward while turning the head in a clockwise direction. The two pieces lock into place.

Turn on the ophthalmoscope by depressing the on/off switch and turning the rheostat control clockwise to the desired intensity of light. Turn the instrument off when you have finished using it to preserve the life of the bulb.

The ophthalmoscopic examination is discussed in more detail in Chapter 12.

PanOptic Ophthalmoscope

The "panoramic" ophthalmoscope head uses an optical design that allows a larger field of view (25 degrees versus the standard 5 degrees) and increases magnification. As a result, the view of the fundus is five times larger than the view achieved with the standard ophthalmoscope in an undilated eye. The PanOptic head connects to a standard handle (Fig. 3.15). Both the PanOptic and other models come with a smartphone adapter that can be used to photograph and video the fundus.

StrabismoScope

The StrabismoScope is used for detecting strabismus (eye misalignment) and can be used as part of eye testing in children (Fig. 3.16). Instruct the child to focus on an accommodative target, such as the wall poster that comes with the instrument. Turn on the StrabismoScope and place it over the patient's eye. Because of a one-way mirror, you are able to see in but the patient is not able to see out. As a result, subtle eye movements associated with strabismus are more easily detected. With the StrabismoScope in place, watch for movement in both the covered and the uncovered eye. Repeat with the other eye. The instrument,

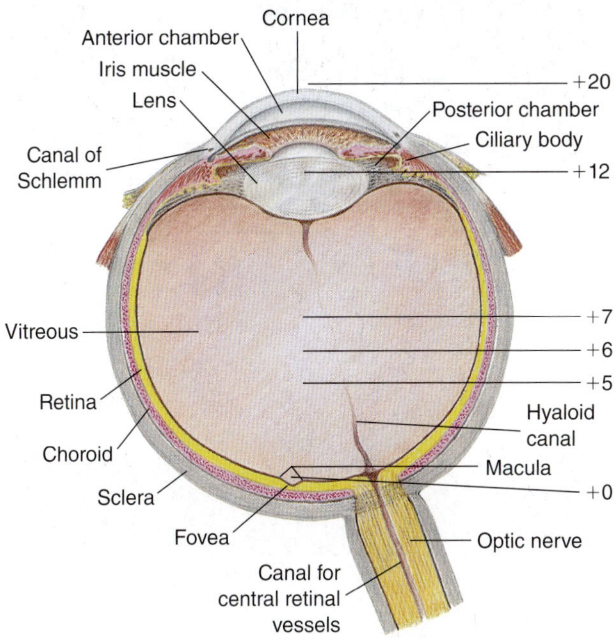

FIG. 3.14 Longitudinal cross section of eye showing lens diopters to focus on eye structures.

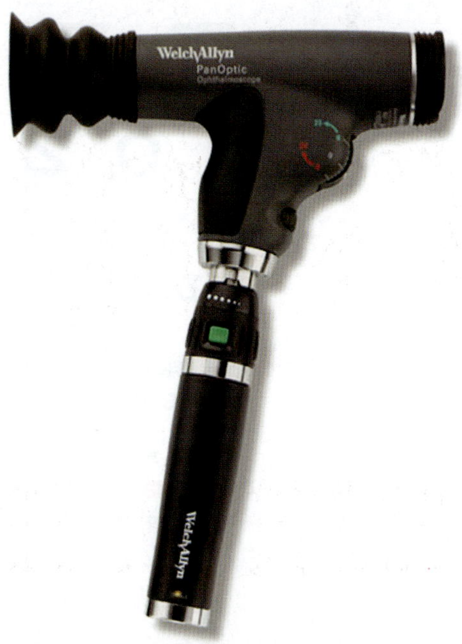

FIG. 3.15 PanOptic ophthalmoscope. (Courtesy Welch Allyn, Skaneateles Falls, NY.)

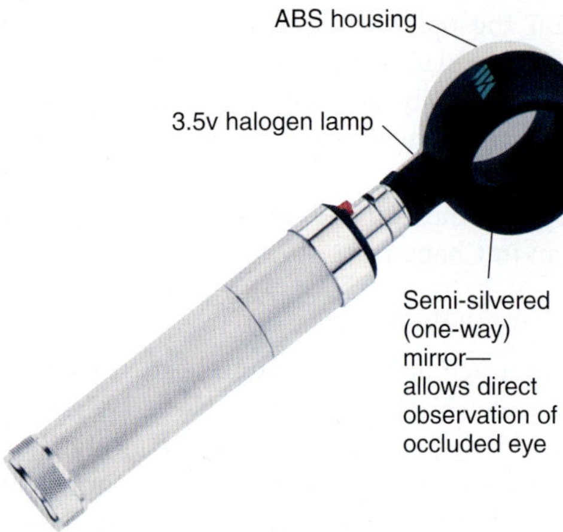

FIG. 3.16 StrabismoScope. (Courtesy Welch Allyn, Skaneateles Falls, NY.)

typically used by specialists, comes with test instructions and a guide to interpretation of test results.

Photoscreening

Photoscreening is used to detect amblyopia (lazy eye) and strabismus in children using an appropriately equipped camera or video system to obtain images of pupillary reflexes and red reflexes. Various optical systems can be used for photoscreening. The child need only visually fixate on the appropriate target long enough for the photoscreening to occur. Data are then analyzed by the evaluator, by the reviewing center, or electronically.

Visual Acuity Charts

While traditionally designed as stand-alone charts positioned at a distance on a wall or as a handheld card, digital systems that incorporate the various individual acuity charts are also available.

Snellen Alphabet and Sloan Letters Charts. The Snellen alphabet and Sloan letters charts are used for a screening examination of far vision (Fig. 3.17) for literate, verbal, and English-speaking adults and school-age children. The Snellen chart contains letters of graduated sizes; the Sloan letters chart presents letters that are almost equal in legibility (C, D, H, K, N, O, R, S, V, Z). There are five proportionally spaced letters on each line with geometric progression up and down the chart. Both types of charts come with standardized numbers at the end of each line of letters. These numbers indicate the degree of visual acuity when read from a distance of 20 feet. Some charts are standardized for use at 10 feet.

Test visual acuity for each eye using the standardized numbers on the chart. Visual acuity is recorded as

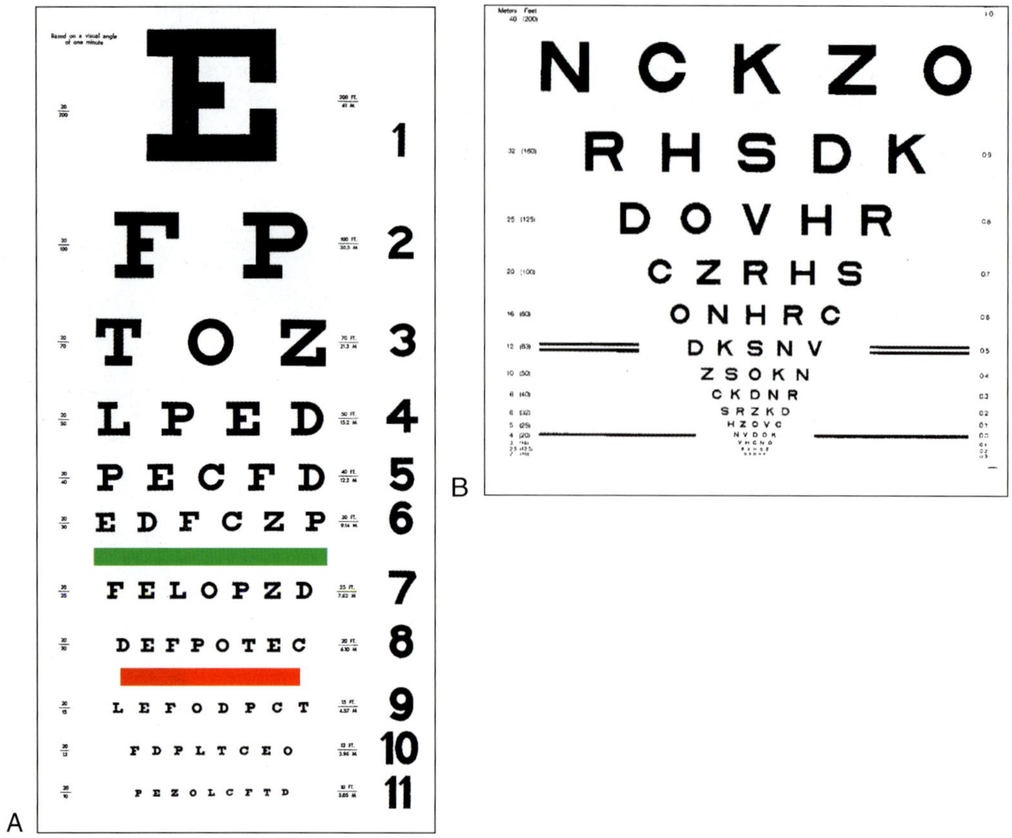

FIG. 3.17 Charts for testing distant vision (not to scale). (A) Snellen chart. (B) Sloan chart. (B, From Drum, B., Calogero, D., Rorer, E. [2007]. Assessment of visual performance in the evaluation of new medical products. *Drug Discoveries Today Technologies, 4*[2], 55–61.)

a fraction, with the numerator of 20 (the distance in feet between the patient and the chart) and the denominator as the distance from which a person with normal vision could read the lettering. The larger the denominator, the poorer the vision. The standard used for normal vision is 20/20. Measurement other than 20/20 indicates either a refractive error or an optic disorder. Record the smallest complete line that the patient can read accurately without missing any letters. If the patient is able to read some but not all letters of the next smaller line, indicate this by adding the number of letters read correctly on that next line (e.g., 20/25 + 2). This would indicate that the patient read all the letters in the 20/25 line correctly and two of the letters of the 20/20 line correctly.

For young children or adults not able to use the Snellen or Sloan chart, other options are available. The highest difficulty of test that the child is capable of performing should be used. In general, the HOTV characters or LEA symbols should be used for children 3 to 5 years of age and Sloan letters or Snellen letters or numbers for children 6 years and older (American Academy of Pediatrics, 2015). For children, cover the nontested eye with an occluder held by the examiner or with an adhesive occluder patch applied to the eye. Ensure that it is not possible to peek with the nontested eye. Children usually stand 10 feet (3 m) away from the visual chart to minimize distraction (one standardized for that distance). Young children require training before testing.

HOTV. This test consists of a wall chart composed only of H's, O's, T's, and V's. The child is given a testing board containing a large H, O, T, and V. Point to a letter on the wall chart and ask the child to point to (match) the correct letter on the testing board.

LH Symbols (LEA Symbols). The LEA Symbols chart consists of four optotypes (circle, square, apple, house) that blur equally. The child must find a matching block or point to the shape that matches the target presented. The visual acuity is determined by the smallest symbols that the child is able to identify accurately at 10 feet. For example, if the child is able to identify the 10/15 symbols at 10 feet, then the child's visual acuity is 10/15 or 20/30. If it is not possible to perform testing at 10 feet, move closer to the child until they correctly identify the largest symbol. Proceed down in size to the smallest symbols that the child is consistently able to correctly identify. Record the acuity as the smallest symbol identified (bottom number) at the testing distance (top number). For example, correctly identifying the 10/15 symbols at 5 feet is recorded as 5/15 or 20/60.

Near-Vision Charts

To assess near vision, a specially designed chart such as the Rosenbaum or Jaeger chart can be used, or simply use standard-sized printed material such as newsprint. The Rosenbaum chart contains a series of numbers, E's, X's, and O's in graduated sizes. Test and record vision for each eye separately. Acuity is recorded as either distance equivalents, such as 20/20, or Jaeger equivalents, such as J-2. Both these measures are indicated on the chart. If printed material is used, the patient should be able to read it without difficulty.

Amsler Grid

A screening test for use with individuals at risk of macular degeneration is provided with the Amsler grid. The grid monitors about 10 degrees of central vision and is used when retinal drusen bodies are seen during an ophthalmologic examination or when there is a strong family history of macular degeneration. The grid consists of straight lines that resemble graph paper. At the center of the grid is a black dot that acts as a fixation point. The patient views the grid with one eye at a time and notes the occurrence of line distortion or actual scotoma (see Chapter 12).

Otoscope

The otoscope provides illumination for examining the external auditory canal and the tympanic membrane. The traditional otoscope head is seated in the handle in the same manner as the ophthalmoscope and is turned on the same way. Newer models can provide a macroview and operate slightly differently (Fig. 3.18). Some allow adjustment of focus. Digital models contain a camera that allows images to be visually shared and recorded on an accompanying screen or with a smartphone. Select the

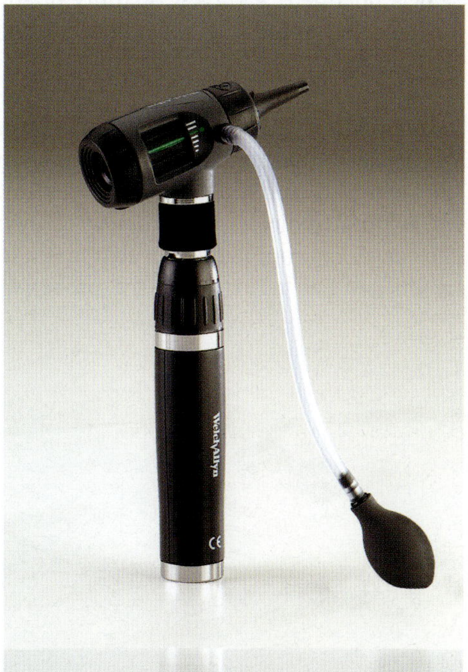

FIG. 3.18 Digital macroview otoscope with pneumatic attachment. (Courtesy Welch Allyn, Skaneateles Falls, NY.)

largest size speculum that will fit comfortably into the patient's ear canal. Chapter 13 discusses the specific techniques of examination.

You can also use the otoscope for the nasal examination if a nasal speculum is not available. Use the shortest, widest otoscope speculum and insert it gently into the patient's naris.

The pneumatic attachment for the otoscope is used to evaluate the fluctuating capacity of the tympanic membrane. A short piece of rubber tubing is attached to the head of the otoscope. A hand bulb attached to the other end of the tubing, when squeezed, produces puffs of air that cause the tympanic membrane to move.

Nasal Speculum

Use the nasal speculum with a penlight to visualize the lower and middle turbinates of the nose (Fig. 3.19). Be sure that the patient is in a comfortable position. You may need to support the patient's head, or you can have the patient lie down. You will need to tilt the patient's head at various angles for a complete nasal examination. Stabilize the speculum with your index finger to avoid contact of the blades with the nasal septum, which can cause discomfort. Squeezing the handles of the instrument opens the blades.

Tympanometer

Various instruments are used to perform screening tympanometry. Tympanometry is a simple, reliable, and objective means of assessing the functions of the ossicular chain, eustachian tube, and tympanic membrane, in addition to the interrelation of these parts (Fig. 3.20).

Position the probe at the opening of the ear canal. When a tight seal is obtained, a known quantity of sound energy is introduced into the ear. The amount of the sound energy transmitted is the amount of sound energy introduced minus the amount of sound energy that returns to the probe microphone. The amount of energy transmitted is directly related to the compliance of the system. Compliance (measured in milliliters or cubic centimeters of equivalent volume) indicates the amount of mobility in the middle ear. A low compliance measurement indicates that more energy has returned to the probe, with less energy admitted to the middle ear. A high compliance reading indicates a flaccid or highly mobile system.

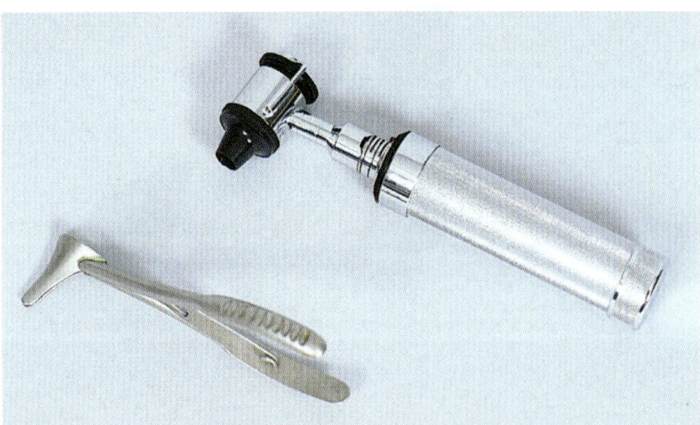

FIG. 3.19 Nasal specula.

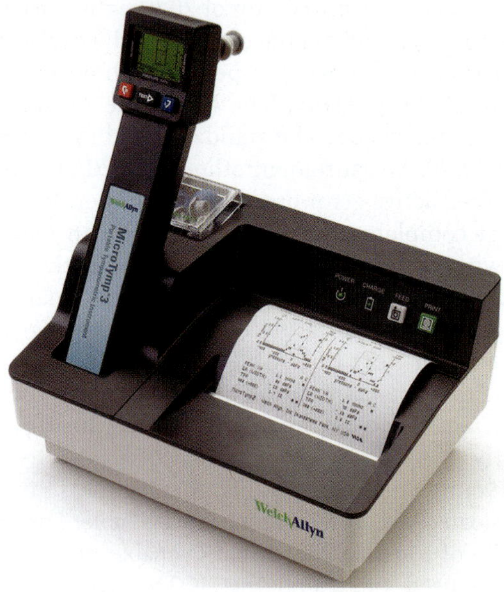

FIG. 3.20 Tympanometer. (Courtesy Welch Allyn, Skaneateles Falls, NY.)

At this point, the probe introduces a pressure of 200 daPa (decapascals; a measurement of air pressure) to the middle ear canal. This positive pressure forces the tympanic membrane inward, and the approximate ear canal volume is recorded. This volume gives a baseline from which the compliance curve is drawn. The pressure is then varied in the negative direction, constantly monitoring the compliance of the system. The pressure continues toward the negative direction until a pressure peak has been detected or until a pressure of 2400 daPa is present in the ear canal, whichever comes first. The point of peak compliance occurs once the pressure is equalized on both sides of the tympanic membrane.

A tympanogram is a graphic representation of the change in compliance of the middle ear system as air pressure is varied. The tympanogram results are displayed on the probe monitor or can be printed out for a hard copy.

Tuning Fork

Tuning forks are used in screening tests for auditory function and for vibratory sensation as part of the neurologic examination (Fig. 3.21). As tuning forks are activated, vibrations are created that produce a particular frequency of sound wave, expressed as cycles per second (cps) or Hertz (Hz). Thus a fork of 512 Hz vibrates at 512 cps.

For auditory evaluation, use a fork with a frequency of 500 to 1000 Hz because it estimates hearing loss in the range of normal speech, approximately 300 to 3000 Hz. Forks of lower frequency can cause you to overestimate bone conduction and can be felt as vibration and heard. Activate the fork by gently squeezing and stroking the

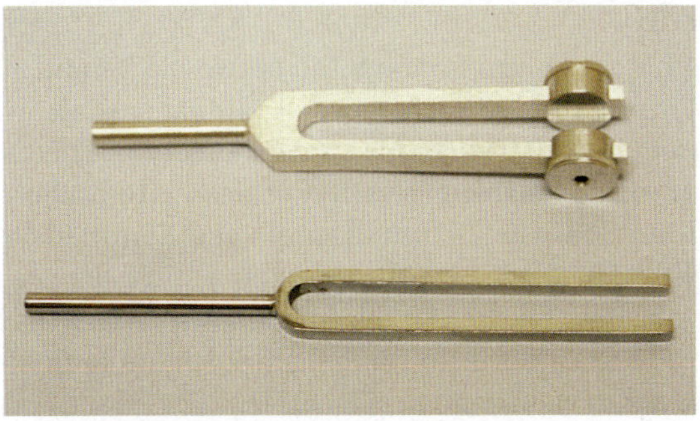

FIG. 3.21 Tuning forks for testing vibratory sensation *(top)* and auditory screening *(bottom)*.

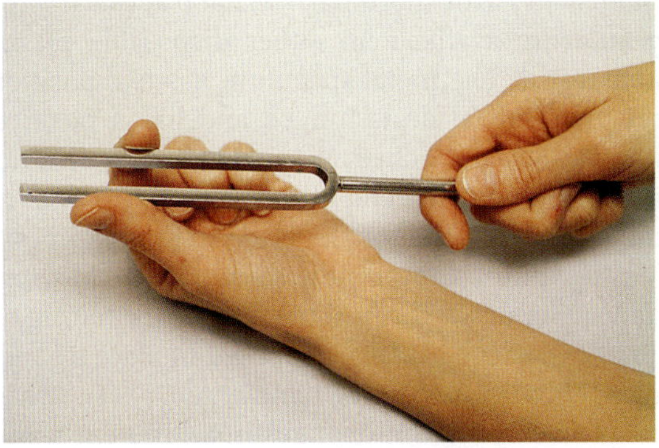

FIG. 3.22 Squeezing and stroking the tuning fork to activate it. Hold the fork only by the handle so as not to dampen the sound.

prongs or by tapping them against the knuckles of your hand so that they ring softly (Fig. 3.22). Because touching the tines will dampen the sound, hold the fork by the handle. Hearing is tested at near-threshold level; this is the lowest intensity of sound at which an auditory stimulus can be heard. Striking the prongs too vigorously results in a loud tone that is above the threshold level and requires time to quiet to a tone appropriate for auditory testing. The specific tuning fork tests for hearing are described in Chapter 13.

For vibratory sensation, use a fork of lower frequency. The greatest sensitivity to vibration occurs when the fork is vibrating between 100 and 400 Hz. Activate the tuning fork by tapping it against the heel of your hand, then apply the base of the fork to a bony prominence. The patient feels the vibration as a buzzing or tingling sensation. The specific areas of testing are described in Chapter 23.

Percussion (Reflex) Hammer

The percussion hammer is used to test deep tendon reflexes. Hold the hammer loosely between the thumb and index finger so that it moves in a swift arc and in a controlled direction. As you tap the tendon, use a rapid downward snap of the wrist, tap quickly and firmly, and then snap your wrist back so that the hammer does not linger on the tendon (Fig. 3.23). The tap should be brisk and direct. Practice this action to achieve smooth, rapid, and controlled motion. You can use either the pointed or flat end of the hammer. The flat end is more comfortable when striking the patient directly; the pointed end is useful in small areas, such as on your finger placed over the patient's bicep tendon. Chapter 23 contains a detailed discussion of evaluation of deep tendon reflexes.

Your finger can also act as a reflex hammer; this can be particularly useful when you are examining very young patients. Certainly, it is less threatening to a child than a hammer. Many pediatric specialists let the child hold the hammer while they use their fingers.

Neurologic Hammer

A variant of the percussion hammer is the neurologic hammer, which is also used for testing deep tendon reflexes. Available in a variety of models, the hammer has two additional features that make it a multipurpose neurologic instrument: a soft brush (usually concealed in the handle) and a tapered tip. These additional implements were designed to determine sensory perception as part of the neurologic examination. Some models come with a rotating

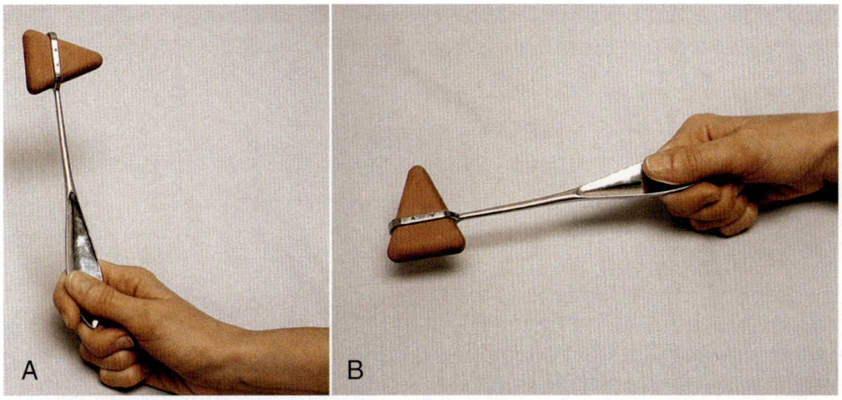

FIG. 3.23 (A) Reflex hammer. (B) Use a rapid downward snap of the wrist.

wheel to test sharp sensation. The procedure for testing sensory perception is described in detail in Chapter 23.

Tape Measure

Use a tape measure 7 to 12 mm wide for determining circumference, length, and diameter. It may be helpful to have one that measures in both inches and metric units. Tape measures are available in a variety of materials, including paper (disposable), plastic or vinyl, and cloth. The tape measure should not be able to be stretched to assure accuracy and pliable for circumference measurement. Because it is placed against the skin, beware of edges that are sharp and can cut.

When measuring, make sure that the tape is not caught or wrinkled beneath the patient. Pull the tape closely but not tightly enough to cause depression of the skin when measuring circumference.

When monitoring serial measures, such as head circumferences or abdominal girth, it is important to place the tape measure in the same position each time. If serial measures are made over a period of days, an easy way to ensure accurate placement is to use a pen to mark the borders of the tape at several intervals on the skin. Subsequently, the tape can be placed within the markings. Accurate placement of the tape for specific measurements is described in Chapter 8 and related chapters.

Transilluminator

A transilluminator consists of a strong light source with a narrow beam. The beam is directed to a particular body cavity and is used to differentiate between various media present in that cavity. Air, fluid, and tissue differentially transmit light; this allows you to detect the presence of fluid in sinuses or the presence of blood or masses in the scrotum (see Clinical Pearl, "Transillumination").

Specific transilluminating instruments are available, or a flashlight with a rubber adapter can be used. It is fine, when situations demand, to use a plain flashlight or penlight. Do not use a light source with a halogen bulb because this can burn the patient's skin. Perform transillumination in a darkened room. Place the beam of light directly against the area to be observed, shielding the beam with your hand if necessary. Watch for the red glow of light through the body cavity. Note the presence or absence of illumination and any irregularities.

> **CLINICAL PEARL**
>
> **Transillumination**
>
> Compared with imaging technology, transillumination may seem archaic and imprecise. Imaging is used, when necessary, but transillumination maintains its value as a clinical tool and is far less expensive. Transillumination is effective, for example, in assessing for a hydrocele in the scrotum of an infant.

Vaginal Speculum

A vaginal speculum is composed of two blades and a handle. There are three basic types of vaginal specula, which are used to view the vaginal canal and cervix. The Graves speculum is available in a variety of sizes with blades ranging from 76 mm to 170 mm in length and 22 mm to 36 mm in width. The blades are curved, with a space between the closed blades. The bottom blade is slightly longer than the top blade to conform to the longer posterior vaginal wall and to aid in visualization (Fig. 3.24A). The Pederson speculum has blades that are the same lengths as those of the Graves speculum but are both narrower (16 to 25 mm) and flatter. It is used for females with small vaginal openings (see Fig. 3.24B). Pediatric or virginal specula are smaller in all dimensions, with short, narrow, flat blades.

Specula are available in either disposable plastic or reusable metal. The metal speculum has two positioning devices. The top blade is hinged and has a positioning thumb piece lever attached. When you press down on the thumb piece, the distal end of the blade rises, thus opening the speculum. To lock the blade in an open position, tighten the thumbscrew on the thumb piece. Moving the top blade up or down controls the degree of opening of the proximal end of the blades; it is locked in place by another thumbscrew, which is on the handle.

The plastic speculum operates in a different way. The bottom blade is fixed to a posterior handle, and an anterior lever handle controls the top blade. As you press on the lever, the distal end of the top blade elevates. At the same time, the base of the speculum also widens. Lock the speculum into position with a catch on the lever handle that snaps into place in a positioning groove. Some models come with an integrated light source.

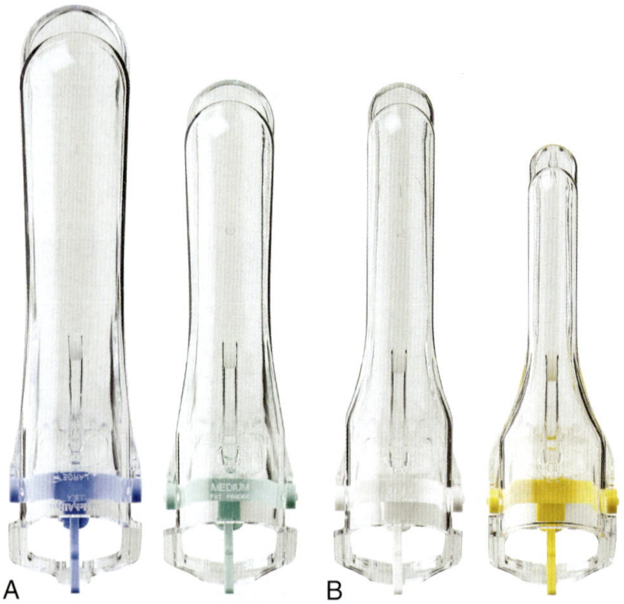

FIG. 3.24 Vaginal specula. (A) Graves, large and small. (B) Pederson, large and small. (From Welch Allyn, Skaneateles Falls, NY.)

Become familiar and practice with both types of specula to feel comfortable with them. Do not wait until you are in the process of doing your first examination, or you are likely to be embarrassed and cause discomfort to the patient because of your initial clumsiness in handling the instrument. The procedure for performing the speculum examination is described in detail in Chapter 19.

Goniometer

The goniometer is used to determine the degree of joint flexion and extension. The instrument consists of two straight arms that intersect and can be angled and rotated around a protractor marked with degrees. Place the center of the protractor over the joint and align the straight arms with the long axes of the extremities. The degree of angle flexion or extension is indicated on the protractor. Electronic models provide a digital angle measurer (Fig. 3.25). The specific joint examinations are discussed in Chapter 22.

Wood's Lamp

The Wood's lamp contains a light source with a wavelength of 360 nm (Fig. 3.26). This is the black light that causes certain substances to fluoresce. It is used primarily to determine the presence of fungi on skin lesions. Darken the room, turn on the Wood's lamp, and shine it on the area or lesion you are evaluating. A yellow-green fluorescence indicates the presence of fungi.

Darkening the room can sometimes be intimidating, particularly to children. Children and their parents react positively when they know what to expect. You can accomplish this by shining the lamp on something fluorescent (e.g., a nondigital watch) to give them the sense of what you are looking for.

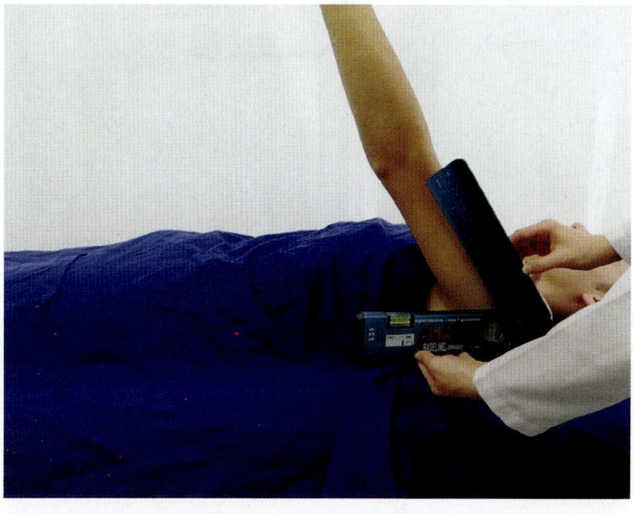

FIG. 3.25 Electronic goniometer. (From Çubukçu, B., Yüzgeç, U., Zileli, R., & Zileli, A. [2020]. Reliability and validity analyzes of Kinect V2 based on measurement system for shoulder motions. *Medical Engineering and Physics, 76*, 20–31.)

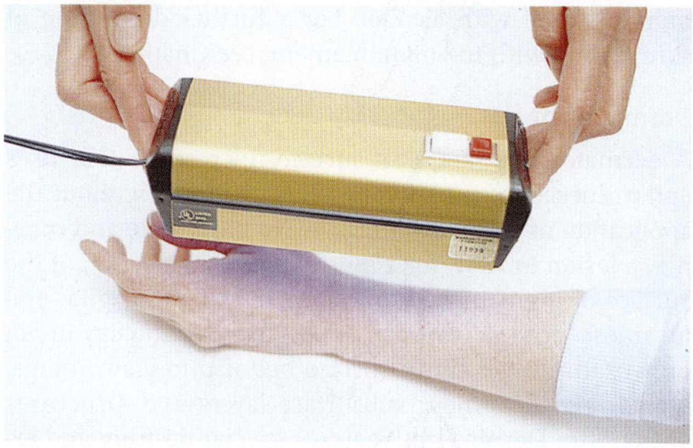

FIG. 3.26 Wood's lamp. The purple color on the skin indicates no fungal infection is present. (From Wilson, S. F., & Giddens, J. (2013). *Health assessment for nursing practice* (5th ed.). St Louis: Mosby.)

Monofilament

The monofilament is a device designed to test for loss of protective sensation, particularly on the plantar surface of the foot (Fig. 3.27A) such as in diabetic or other peripheral neuropathy and nerve damage. It bends at 10 g of linear pressure. Patients who cannot feel the application of the monofilament at the point that it bends have lost their protective sense and are at increased risk for injury.

Test intact skin on the plantar surface of the foot at multiple areas, including the great toe, and the first, third, and fifth metatarsal heads (see Fig. 3.27B). Lock the monofilament in its handle at a 90-degree angle. With the patient's eyes closed, apply the monofilament perpendicular to the surface of the skin. Press hard enough to allow the monofilament to bend, holding pressure for approximately 1 to 2 seconds, then slowly release the pressure. Test at various locations in random order. Ask the patient to indicate when the monofilament is felt. Vary the interval between applications. Note the response at each location in the patient's medical record. Dispose of or clean the

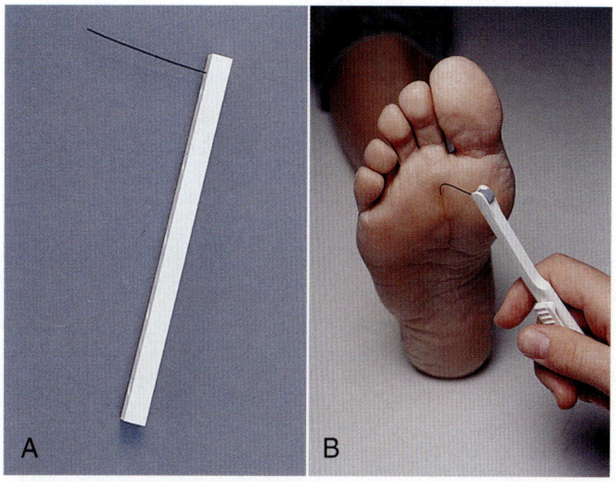

FIG. 3.27 (A) Monofilament. (B) Press the monofilament against the skin hard enough to allow it to bend.

monofilament with alcohol. For a further discussion of skin testing with the monofilament, see Chapter 23.

Dermatoscope

A dermatoscope is a skin surface microscope that uses epiluminescence microscopy (ELM), with or without the application of oil on a skin lesion, to illuminate and magnify a lesion to allow for a more detailed inspection of the surface of pigmented skin lesions (Fig. 3.28). Digital epiluminescence microscopy (DELM) uses technology to not only examine the skin's surface but also to view, image, record, and document subsurface layers and structures of the skin. Dermoscopy requires special training and expertise and is used to confirm a diagnosis or determine which skin lesions require biopsy or removal.

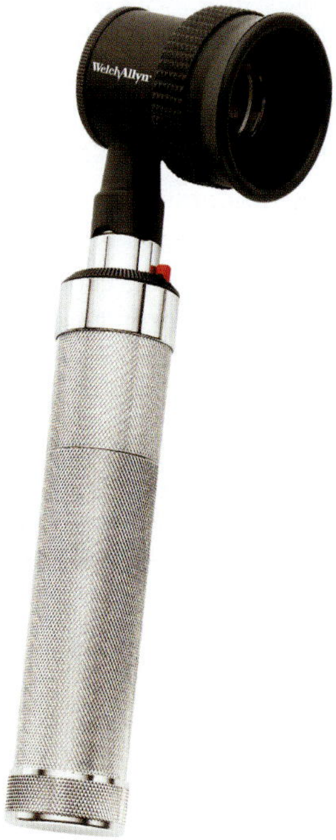

FIG. 3.28 EpiScope. (From Welch Allyn, Skaneateles Falls, NY.)

Scoliometer

A scoliometer measures the degree of rotation of the spine to screen for scoliosis. Ask the patient to bend forward slowly, stopping when the shoulders are level with the hips. View from the back. Note any rib elevation and/or asymmetry in the low back area. Before measuring with the scoliometer, adjust the height of the patient's bending position to the level at which the deformity of the spine is most pronounced. This position will vary depending on the location of the curvature. Lay the scoliometer across the deformity at right angles to the body, with the "0" mark over the top of the spinous process (Fig. 3.29). Let the scoliometer rest gently on the skin. Do not push down. Read the number of degrees of rotation. The screening examination is considered positive if the reading on the scoliometer is 7 degrees or more at any level of the spine. Lesser degrees of rotation may or may not indicate a mild degree of scoliosis.

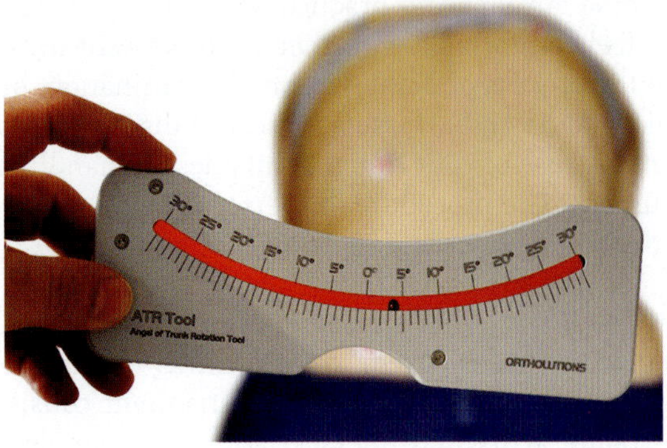

FIG. 3.29 The scoliometer. (Courtesy Ortholutions GmbH & Co. KG, Rosenheim, Germany.)

Orchidometer

An orchidometer measures testicular volume and is used to assess testicular size and inform Tanner staging. The orchidometer consists of testicle-shaped numbered beads ranging in size generally from 1 mL to 25 mL (Fig. 3.30). The beads are compared with the testicles of the patient, and the volume is determined by the bead that matches most closely in size. Charts to track testicular volume over time are available.

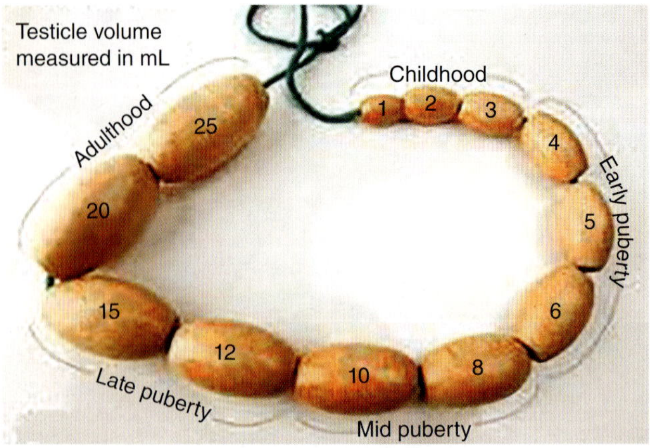

FIG. 3.30 Prader orchidometer. (From Mathews, K. G., & Aggarwal, P. [2023] *Medicine: Prep manual for undergraduates* (7th ed.). St. Louis: Elsevier.)

CHAPTER 4

Taking the Next Steps: Clinical Reasoning

Clinical reasoning is the process by which the information gathered from the history and physical examination is merged with clinical knowledge, experience, and the current best evidence to formulate the next steps in patient care—development of the diagnostic and management plans. Critical reflection involves thinking through the reasoning for these decisions. This reflection can help you progress from rote decision making to clinical reasoning.

Thus far, we have been concerned with the initial patient interaction, establishment of respectful rapport, and information-gathering processes (i.e., history and physical examination). Organizing, integrating, and analyzing information comprise the next step in caring for patients. This process, called *clinical reasoning,* leads to the development of potential diagnoses, diagnostic evaluation priorities, and management plans (Box 4.1). Formulating management plans should occur in partnership with patients and their families. Working with the patient to determine the best course of action is often called *shared decision making* or *patient-centered care.*

Clinical Reasoning

When you document your clinical reasoning, other people involved in the patient's care can follow your logic as you move from recording the subjective and objective parts of an evaluation to the management phase.

Assessment, Judgment, and Evidence

Clinical reasoning involves bringing knowledge of the patient, clinical experience, and decision-making skills together with the current evidence and expert recommendations. The best available evidence must be carefully obtained from the latest research and provisional society guidelines. Use of evidence in decision making is called *evidence-based practice* (Box 4.2).

The first step in clinical reasoning is to assess what has been learned from the patient and to determine its value and significance. Priorities are then assigned to information that might influence clinical judgment as management plans and clinical impressions are created.

Further assessment depends on clinician, patient, and family preferences, which may be influenced by feelings, attitudes, and values. By using clinical reasoning, you can think through your own beliefs, values, cultural practices, and attitudes for potential bias affecting the decision-making process (see Chapter 1). Clinical impressions help direct further assessment, which must be balanced by benefits and risks to the patient, cost considerations, and available resources. Determining the leading diagnoses and potential diagnostic and management plans can be formulated using shared decision making.

Problem Identification

A problem may be defined as any concern that may need further evaluation and/or attention. It may be related to one or more of the following:

- An uncertain diagnosis
- New symptoms or physical examination findings related to a previous diagnosis
- New symptoms or findings of unknown etiology
- Unusual findings from the physical examination or by diagnostic tests
- Personal, social, or emotional difficulties

Formulate problems as specifically as possible. Identify and list the signs and symptoms associated with each of the patient's concerns in addition to abnormalities discovered during the physical examination. This listing of findings—the problem list—is key to developing a complete understanding of a patient's concern. The problem list is the foundation for clinical reasoning and is used to form hypotheses based on the available information (Box 4.3). Review the problem list and note the absence of findings that you might expect in support of your hypotheses. Think through the patient's verbal and nonverbal communication and determine whether there are questions you may have neglected to ask or information you did not fully understand. Gather additional information from the patient or family members to fill in these gaps. Beware of "red herrings"—the bits of information that are distracting and draw your thinking away from central issues (Box 4.4). Critically evaluate unexpected or unusual findings, but do not let them distract from your consideration of what you have learned.

After a match between the data (both subjective and objective) and a presumed diagnosis is made, consider the appropriate laboratory studies, imaging studies, or specialty consultation needed to confirm the diagnosis. When determining next steps, it is important to consider the

BOX 4.1 Steps for Clinical Reasoning

The clinical examination (information gathering)
↓
Organization and integration of information
↓
Assessment of organized information
↓
Assignment of priorities (the need for clinical judgment)
↓
Clinical opinions
↓
Integration of preferences; the patient's and the professional's
- Consideration of feelings, attitudes, and values
- Consideration of probabilities and risks

↓
Further assessment; balancing advantages with risks in the light of feelings, attitudes, and values
↓
Identification of problems (be as specific as possible)
↓
Hypothesis formation and determination of the next steps

BOX 4.2 Evidence-Based Practice

Evidence-based practice (EBP) incorporates best evidence, along with individual experience and patient preference, into making medical decisions. EBP involves questioning physical examination findings, the effects of therapy, the utility of diagnostic tests, disease prognosis, and/or the etiology of disorders (see https://www.cancer.gov/publications/dictionaries/cancer-terms/def/evidence-based-medicine).

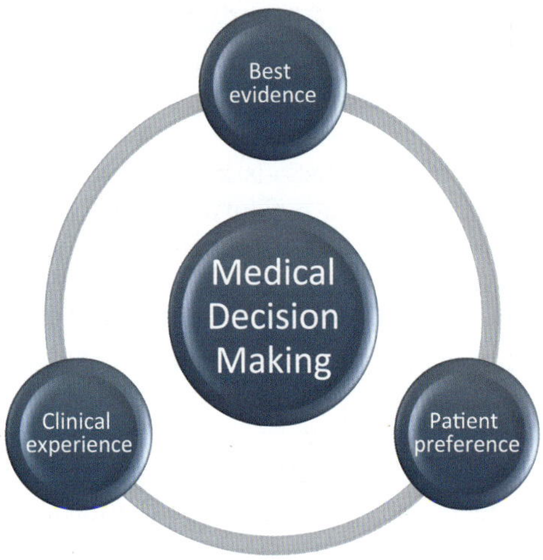

primacy of patient welfare, patient autonomy, and need for resource allocation.

We are strong advocates for our patients and, at times, their only voice. As such, we are responsible for appropriate resources; we should make judicious choices with testing and evaluation. See Risk Factor box "Health Care Waste and Unnecessary Testing."

BOX 4.3 Decision Making

There are several ways to make a diagnosis:
- Pattern recognition (e.g., "If it walks like a duck, swims like a duck, and quacks like a duck—it is most likely a duck.")
- Sampling the universe (including everything precludes missing anything)
- Using algorithms (a rigidly defined thought process precludes error)

Although each of these may have limited use in specific situations, consideration of all your findings should most often result in the development of one or more hypotheses needing an evidence-based approach to solutions.

Guidelines to a sound decision-making process include the following:
- Always derive possibilities that are consistent with the chief concern, your findings, and known psychosocial and pathophysiologic mechanisms.
- Remember that common problems occur commonly and rare ones do not.
- Common problems can have unusual presentations, and rare ones may have a seemingly common concern.
- Rare problems that have an available treatment should be considered.
- Do not rush to a diagnosis with no available treatment, and do not pursue a line of reasoning that will not alter your course of action. For example, if a patient cannot tolerate cancer treatment, do not pursue the screening and diagnostic evaluation.
- Do not undertake procedures that are not related to your hypotheses.
- Always consider potential harm and cost in addition to benefit when determining the need for a test or action.
- Consider whether the risk is worth the potential gain in information, invoking the ethical principle of nonmaleficence: *Primum non nocere*—"First, do no harm."
- Remain open in your thinking, and be ready to discard or modify your hypotheses when necessary. Recognize that your leading hypotheses may not be valid, and avoid the tendency to discount information that may invalidate your favorite ideas.
- Try to have a single process explain all or most of your data, but do not be rigid in this regard. After all, a patient with many concerns and problems may have more than one disease; two common diseases may occur simultaneously more often than one rare disease alone.

Probability and utility should always be your guides to sequencing your actions unless a life-threatening situation exists. A conscientious estimate of probability is the best way to define the limits of uncertainty and the best way to establish priorities.

BOX 4.4 Red Herrings

A patient with swollen cervical nodes and fever owns a cat, which had claws, but the patient did not have cat scratch disease. The too obvious apparent source of the problem, a "red herring," delayed the ultimate diagnosis of non-Hodgkin lymphoma.

Valid Hypotheses

Clinical reasoning allows you to consider the variety of possible diagnoses—from the common to the rare—before settling on the best match between the patient's signs and symptoms and a specific disorder. Many experts feel we should consider three to five diagnoses for every disease: the one that unifies what you have learned, the one you cannot afford to miss, and the one that it is. Sometimes they are the same one, but usually not. Avoid tunnel vision and letting your initial thoughts or bias narrow the focus of questions during the interview. In other words, do not jump to conclusions.

One of the clichés of clinical practice is that all findings should be unified into one diagnosis—Occam's razor, or *lex parsimoniae* ("law of parsimony" or "law of succinctness") (Thorburn, 1918). Although you should strive to look for the fewest possible causes that will account for all the symptoms, this may not always be possible. More than one disease process can exist at one time in the same person, an acute illness can occur in the context of a chronic one, and a chronic disease can cycle through remission and relapse. Carefully chosen laboratory or imaging studies can often help validate your observations and confirm your clinical impressions (Box 4.5).

BOX 4.5 "A Patient Can Have as Many Diagnoses as He Darn Well Pleases"

Common problems happen commonly and can occur at the same time (Hilliard et al., 2004). As Hilliard and colleagues note, C. F. M. Saint stated several decades ago that more than one disease may be responsible for a patient's signs and symptoms when he could find no pathophysiologic explanation for the coexistence of hiatal hernia, gallbladder disease, and diverticulosis in one of his patients. That, they added, was the same point made by Hickam's dictum: "A patient can have as many diagnoses as he darn well pleases." It was William Osler, however, who invoked the competing 14th-century philosophy of William of Occam: "Plurality must not be posited without necessity." In other words, do not consider more than one diagnosis unless you really have to and "among competing hypotheses, favor the simplest one." Thus we are given the term *Occam's razor* to signify this.

But suppose Occam's razor doesn't always work. Hilliard and coworkers write, "As the population continues to age—and as diagnostic studies increase in number and sophistication—the dulling of Occam's razor is certain to continue." Thus we suggest that you think critically about Saint and Occam and use their hypotheses for appropriate balance as you make your clinical judgments.

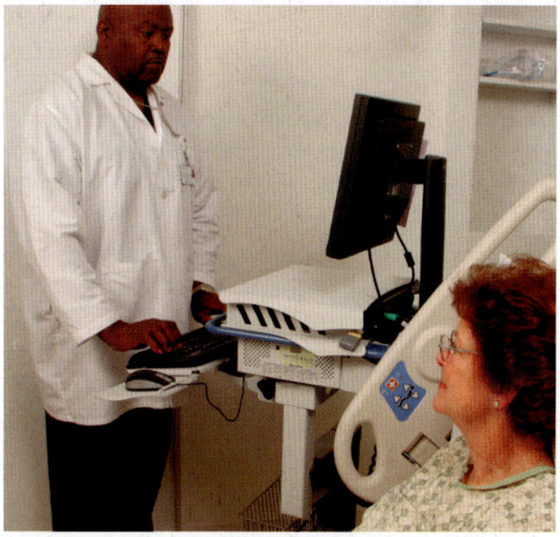

Think About It

- Occam's razor states that the single simplest cause is the most likely to be the diagnosis.
- Hickam's dictum implies that there can be several simultaneous diagnoses.

These two competing principles of medicine must be balanced.

Possible Barriers to Clinical Reasoning

Illness evolves from disease and is usually multifaceted. Not all of the findings can be explained on a pathophysiologic level because physical symptoms are frequently inseparable from emotional symptoms. Therefore avoid being misled into believing that, given a pathophysiologic conclusion, management targeted to that finding will necessarily solve the problem. You must consider the full range of issues—from the physical to the emotional, psychological, social, and economic—that might affect the expected outcomes. The pitfall is that in allowing yourself to be lost in physical details, you lose the context of the broader view.

Feelings, Attitudes, and Values. Clinical reasoning becomes complex because of emotions in both the patient and the clinician. Feelings, attitudes, bias, and values can be strong enough that our decision making may be impaired. If these feelings are to be given a proper context, you must know yourself and take time for personal reflection (see Chapter 1 for a discussion of self-awareness). Critical reflection involves thinking through the reasoning for these decisions. The questioning of yourself must be relentless:

- "What is really happening?"
- "Do I have preconceived ideas?"
- "Has my bias overtaken logic?"
- "Have ethical concepts been ignored?"
- "What are the issues that matter?"
- "What should take precedence?"
- "Do I understand my contribution to the interaction?"
- "Do I understand the patient?"
- "How does the patient feel about it?"

The Ethical Context. Ethics does not provide answers. Consideration of ethical principles provides the framework for respectful, flexible discussion and a disciplined approach to decision making. For example, for a given problem, several concepts must be considered.

- Autonomy: The patient's need for self-determination. Autonomy suggests that choices exist, and a patient may choose between alternatives. Patients may choose something you would not choose; patients have a right to make a seemingly poor decision even when you share (and the patient/family understands) the risks of doing so. Uncertainty exists when the patient is a child or is cognitively impaired. Parents, guardians, family, or other significant persons should then be included, and the boundaries of that participation must be clearly set. In some cases, the boundaries are established by an advance directive from the patient. Competency is not always easily determined, and there may be disagreement. Both the mental status examination (see Chapter 7) and consultation with individuals who know the person well can assist.

- Beneficence: Do good for the patient. This may be too eagerly pursued and may result in a paternalism that might preclude autonomy of the patient. However, paternalism can have some benefit when used with constraint and respect for autonomy.
- Nonmaleficence: Do no harm to the patient.
- Utilitarianism: Consider appropriate use of resources with concern for the greater good of the larger community. Choose wisely.
- Fairness and justice: Recognize the balance between autonomy and competing interests of the family and community.
- Deontological imperatives: Our dutiful responsibilities for offering care are established by tradition and in cultural contexts. Because cultures vary, your culture may be different from your patient's; these will not be universally binding for all patients. Ethical principles can come into conflict in any given circumstance. If it is difficult to make a decision, consider the following:
  - Is the problem one of ethics and not of poor communication, internal family conflict, financial strain, legal confusion, or cultural or personality conflict?
  - Are the facts clearly stated and the attitudes of patients and/or their representatives clearly communicated?
  - Is there a reasonable chance for a satisfactory health or medical care outcome?

In the end, the competent and autonomous patient's point of view should prevail without a compelling argument to do otherwise.

Mechanism and Probabilism. Mechanistic (deterministic) thinking is governed by a sense that knowledge must be certain and not subject to attributes of the observer. Knowledge is to be free of bias, personal beliefs, attitudes, and values. Our decision making must have a balance between mechanism and probabilism (certainty in knowledge is impossible). There are variables in the decision-making process such as the individual patient, our age and experience, and fatigue. Accepting the inevitability of probability simply recognizes that the certainty of truth, whatever that may be, is hard to achieve. Why is this so?

- Causes may act or interact differently at different times.
- The same effect may not always have the same cause.
- The effect of a given cause cannot be isolated with certainty.

Causes, effects, and our interpretations of them change probabilistically with time. They involve uncertainty, conjecture, and chance. Dependence on the purely scientific and technical offers an unrealistic comfort (Box 4.6). Acknowledging this may be viewed as gambling. A high probability diminishes uncertainty; a low probability does not.

Do not be dominated by the mechanistic assumption that there is a precise and discoverable cause for every event. Make judgments based on well-informed probabilities and recognize the complexity of the decision-making process. Clinical reasoning does not require a compulsive listing of all the possible options in diagnosis and management. Rather, it is dominated by hypothesis development, asking whether a particular diagnosis should be made depending on its probability, and whether a test may

BOX 4.6 The Ubiquity of Information

Patients now present to clinicians with a wealth of data, including myths that need to be discredited and other false information. The internet can be a terrific source of patient education information, but knowing which websites have accurate and valid information is challenging. Use caution when using nonscientific resources and be leery of medical advice from social media sources. It can remind you about unrecognized diagnostic possibilities and place the patient's health record at your fingertips. Still, it can also be considered a threat. There is at times an unacceptable temptation to substitute electronic support for clinical reasoning and judgment. As sophisticated and accessible as internet resources have become, the most advanced software coupled with the sleekest hardware still has no sense of the subtleties of the human dimension. It is your responsibility to artfully merge subjective and objective data with best evidence and your knowledge and experience to make a clinical judgment.

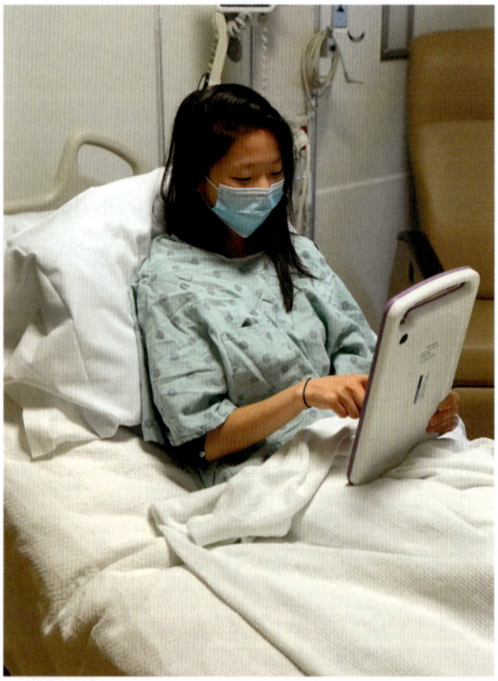

	Has disease	Does not have disease	
Test positive	True positive (TP)	False positive (FP)	Positive predictive value (people with positive test who have disease) (TP/(TP + FP)
Test negative	False negative (FN)	True negative (TN)	Negative predictive value (people with negative test who do NOT have disease) (TN/(TN + FN)
	Sensitivity: people with disease who test positive (true positive rate) TP/(TP = FN)	Specificity: people without disease who test negative (true negative rate) TN/(FP + TN)	

FIG. 4.1 Sensitivity and specificity, true positive/negative, and positive/negative predictive values.

be indicated, depending on the likelihood suggested by its sensitivity and specificity.

Validity of the Clinical Examination

We practice in a time when there is considerable effort to reduce health care costs. Recognize that the majority of diagnoses can be achieved with information from a comprehensive history and physical examination and then limit indiscriminate use of unnecessary technology.

Keep the following definitions in mind (Fig. 4.1):

- Sensitivity: the ability of an observation to identify correctly those who have a disease
- Specificity: the ability of an observation to identify correctly those who do not have a disease
- True positive: an expected observation that is found when the disease characterized by that observation is present
- True negative: an expected observation that is not found when the disease characterized by that observation is not present
- False positive: an observation made that suggests a disease when that disease is not present
- False negative: an observation that suggests a disease is not present when in fact it is (e.g., absence of cough or respiratory findings when lung cancer is present)
- Positive predictive value: the proportion of persons with an observation characteristic of a disease who have it (e.g., when an observation is made 100 times and on 95 of those occasions that observation proves to be consistent with the ultimate diagnosis, the positive predictive value of the observation is 95%)
- Negative predictive value: the proportion of persons with an expected observation who ultimately prove not to have the expected condition (e.g., if 100 observations are made expecting a disease and 95 times that observation is not found and the condition proves not to have been the diagnosis, the negative predictive value of the observation is 95%)

Bayes' Theorem

As a critical thinker, you will discover that the likelihood of your diagnosis being related to your findings depends on:

1. The probability of those findings being associated with that diagnosis
2. The prevalence of both that particular diagnosis and that combination of findings in the community where you practice

These considerations have been formalized as Bayes' theorem. Bayes' theorem considers a test result and relates it to the conditional probability of that test result given other factors. (See Box 4.7.) This juggling of probabilities is implicit during diagnostic decision making. We do not think consciously of Bayes' theorem most of the time, but we are using it at some level all the time.

We have stressed that diagnostic decision making is generally best served by the development of hypotheses that will provide a disciplined approach to solutions. If you are uncertain about an observation, never hesitate to confirm its validity. That is vital to clinical reasoning. As much as you strive to be scientific and base what you do on the disciplined principles of science, at times you will make undeniable intuitive judgments. Intuition, however, must be as fully subject to clinical reasoning as any other aspect of your effort.

Evidence-Based Practice

Evidence-based practice (EBP) is a system that incorporates the best available scientific evidence to clinical decision making in the care of the individual patient. EBP balances the strength of the evidence, the risks and benefits of treatment (or lack of treatment), and diagnostic tests while integrating clinical expertise. Evidence-based decision making is the intersection of your clinical observations from the history and physical examination, clinical expertise, patient values and preferences, and the best evidence (Fig. 4.2).

BOX 4.7 Bayes' Theorem

Bayes' theorem was created by the mathematician Thomas Bayes and is mathematically the following equation:

$$P(A|B) = \frac{P(B|A)P(A)}{P(B)}$$

A, B	=	events
P(A|B)	=	a conditional probability: the probability of *A* given *B* is true
P(B|A)	=	probability of *B* given *A* is true
P(A), *P(B)*	=	prior or marginal probability: the probabilities of observing *A* and *B*, respectively, without any given conditions

Risk Factor Box

Health Care Waste and Unnecessary Testing

- **Defensive medicine:** ordering unnecessary tests to avoid malpractice or litigation
- **Fear of uncertainty:** ordering unnecessary tests to reduce uncertainty or "to be safe"
- **Lack of knowledge:** ordering unnecessary tests because the clinician does not understand the evolution of a disease or its management
- **Cognitive bias:** ordering unnecessary tests because of personal beliefs or previous experiences
- **Profit motive:** ordering unnecessary tests for the reimbursement
- **Medical culture:** prioritizing more tests, leading to unnecessary testing
- **Patient pressure:** patient requesting particular tests or imaging
- **Protocol-based testing:** ordering tests based on protocols without consideration
- **Failure to follow up:** not following up on test results or obtaining other records leading to repeated testing

Negative Consequences of Unnecessary Testing

- Misdiagnosis
- False-positive or false-negative results
- Overdiagnosis
- Wasted health care resources
- Increased cost of medical care
- Decreased clinician productivity
- Disruption to the therapeutic alliance between clinician and patient

Evaluation and Management Plan and Setting Priorities

You decide what you think is going on (the diagnosis) and what you are going to do about it (the management plan). You may need to investigate further, deciding on which of the available laboratory and imaging techniques you might use and who might help you with them. Having thought critically (using shared decision making), you and the patient can jointly arrive at an approach that may include the following:

- Laboratory and imaging studies
- Subspecialty consultation
- Medications, equipment (e.g., walker or wheelchair), or assistive technology (e.g., telemetry monitor, ventilator)
- Special care (e.g., home nursing, physical therapy, respiratory therapy)
- Diet modification
- Activity or lifestyle modification
- Patient education
- Follow-up visit

In addition, you need to decide the degree of urgency, the next step, and what underlies the issues in terms of the social, economic, and pathophysiologic considerations. Priorities must be set. The following is only a partial guide:

- What is the patient's physical condition?
- Is something going on that overrides every other consideration (e.g., a problem with the central nervous system, heart, kidneys, pain, a change in mental status) and needs immediate attention?
- Are there abnormal laboratory values or imaging findings (e.g., mass identified on mammogram) that need immediate attention?
- What are the patient's social circumstances?
- Will a job be threatened if there is an absence from work?
- Are there small children at home for whom no other caretaker is available?
- Is there available and convenient transportation to and from services and care?

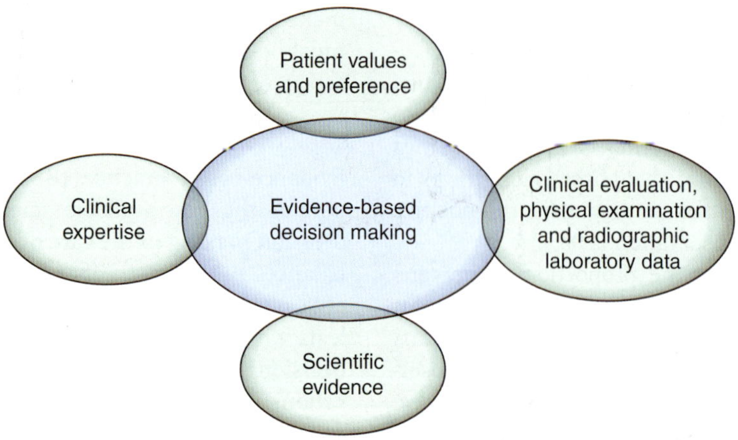

FIG. 4.2 Evidence-based decision making.

- What are the patient's economic circumstances?
- Does the patient have adequate health insurance coverage?
- Is the cost of care or medication going to compromise other areas of the patient's life?

These considerations suggest the kind of critical judgment that helps to set priorities and develop a management plan in collaboration with the patient. Perhaps in some cases, tests, treatments, or therapies can be delayed without risk. Alternatively, there might be a sequence of steps that meets priority needs, some that need to be done now, and some that might await the information gleaned from an earlier step or the result of a first therapeutic attempt.

Certainly, the patient's subsequent behavior is a major variable in their health status (e.g., smoking cessation) or therapy (e.g., medication adherence). The patient must be actively and positively involved for an optimal outcome. Does the patient want to take the necessary steps? Behavior change is a process involving progress through a series of stages. The transtheoretical model of behavior change assesses an individual's readiness to change (Table 4.1). What is the extent of the patient's commitment and recognition that the benefits of action outweigh any possible disadvantages? What is the patient's ability to sustain the effort?

Developing a sequence for your clinical reasoning can be facilitated by careful attention to your documentation in the health record (see Chapter 5) and its consideration of the problem-oriented health record. Careful attention to recording the findings in the history and physical examination will aid in organizing your thoughts and lead to clinical reasoning.

TABLE 4.1 Stages of Change

STAGE OF CHANGE	DESCRIPTION
Precontemplation	Not yet admitting there is a problem behavior that needs to be changed or not intending to take action
Contemplation	Admitting that there is a problem but not yet ready or sure of wanting to make a change; starting to think about pros and cons for continued action
Preparation	Intending to take action in the immediate future; beginning to take small steps toward change
Action	Changing behavior, overt modification in behavior
Maintenance	Being able to sustain action and working to prevent relapse
Termination	No temptation and confidence in not returning to old behavior
Relapse	Not considered a stage in itself, but rather the shift from action or maintenance to an earlier stage (precontemplation or contemplation)

From DiClemente, C., & Prochaska, J. (1998). Toward a comprehensive transtheoretical model of change. In W. R. Miller & N. Healther (Eds.), *Treating addictive behaviors*. New York: Plenum Press.

CHAPTER

5 The Health Record

After performing the history and physical examination, the clinician must organize, synthesize, and record the data along with the health and social concerns identified and the rationale for the diagnostic evaluation and plan of care. This cognitive effort goes well beyond simply transcribing or importing data that may exist from other sources or completing prescribed templates. The information in the patient's health record must enable you and your colleagues to know and care for the patient by identifying health problems, making diagnoses and judgments regarding the diagnostic testing needed, planning appropriate care, and monitoring the patient's responses to treatment. The patient's health record is only as good as the accuracy, pertinent depth and detail, and thoughtful synthesis provided by the documenting caregivers. With the transition to the electronic health record (EHR), it is even more critical to maintain standards of documentation excellence, especially as EHRs can consume data from multiple sources, including patient-entered data Within the EHR environment, there is great risk in overwhelming the reader with volumes of insignificant or inaccurate data through importing preexisting and unverified information from other sources within the record. This phenomenon, sometimes referred to as *note bloat,* must be guarded against.

Multiple beneficial functions can now be achieved with the EHR beyond documentation and communication among the team of the patient's caregivers and with the patient directly through patient portals. These functions include, among others, order entry, risk stratification, population health reporting, provision of care pathways, and the exchange of health information among different health care systems through health information exchanges (HIEs).

Increasingly, technology is being developed to allow additional methods for capturing the information exchanged during the visit. This includes having live scribes accompany the clinician during the visit or recording the visit for subsequent transcription or natural language processing. Regardless of the method of production, the patient's health record is a legal document. Any information contained in it may be used in court and in other legal proceedings as well as to determine health care payment. Your documentation will be read by many individuals; increasingly, and appropriately, this includes the patient and their family members through the use of patient portals. It is your responsibility to document the facts of the history and your physical examination findings accurately.

General Guidelines

When using an in-person scribe, they should be introduced to the patient, explaining their purpose and seeking approval from the patient. If the visit is being recorded for subsequent documentation, that too should be explained to the patient. It is quite acceptable to take brief written or typed notes regarding the patient's concerns and history along with your findings during the course of the interview and physical examination. Similarly, it is important and respectful to request permission and inform the patient you will be taking these notes during the visit. It is not necessary to record all the details during the visit, as this may distract your attention from the patient. Documenting simple notes should be sufficient in preparation for the subsequent complete note. This allows you to gather, reflect, and organize all the data appropriately before making the record final. Certain data should be recorded as you obtain it, specifically the vital signs and any measurements. It is essential to complete the essence of the patient's story and key findings as soon as possible after the examination while your memory for detail is fresh. Resist going on to other patients before doing so. Although this is sometimes unavoidable, you can easily become confused about which patient had a particular finding and even forget to record an important finding.

In the EHR all entries will be dated and timed when signed and cannot be subsequently erased. If using a paper chart, recorded information should not be erased. Instead, make necessary changes by lining out data and leaving this crossed-out information legible while initialing and dating the changes. When using an EHR, include an addendum to correct or update your documentation. Any portion of the examination that has been deferred or omitted should be so noted, rather than neglecting to mention particular findings. It is appropriate in some circumstances to defer a portion of an examination, stating the reason for deferral. For example, if doing a virtual visit through video transmission, your ability to do a complete examination will be limited. A clear and exact record of your assessment, an analysis of the problem, and your rationale for the management plan are vital for communicating with other health care providers and for your protection in case a question is ever raised relevant to your care of the patient.

It is unacceptable to copy other health care providers' documented work (e.g., history taken, examination performed, or thought processes outlined) and enter it into your own documentation as if you did the work. Text copied from another person's note must always be attributed to the source. *Information integrity* refers to the dependability of information and is further defined as the accuracy, consistency, and reliability of information content. This is not only an important concept in a legal proceeding; it is also critical for safe patient care. Hospital care is often fragmented, and handoffs and cross-coverage prevail. Health care providers need to be able to trust the documentation on which they will base clinical decisions at the point of care.

Be concise, yet avoid the use of abbreviations and symbols as much as possible, as meanings may differ among health professionals (Box 5.1 and Table 5.1; Garbutt et al., 2008). Similarly, avoid the use of words such as "normal," "good," "poor," and "negative" because these words are open to various interpretations by other examiners.

Document what you observe and what the patient tells you, rather than the conclusions you interpret or infer. Use direct quotes from the patient when a description is particularly vivid, especially when documenting the patient's chief concern. This is an effective way to capture the patient's perspective of their health situation. Keep subjective and symptomatic data in the history, making sure these aspects are not woven into the physical findings. Physical examination findings should be the result of your direct observation. For example, when a patient reports pain (a symptom) during palpation, you should note tenderness (a sign) in the record and report the patient's reaction to pain, such as crying, withdrawal, rigid posturing, or facial expression. Record both what the patient tells you and what you observe. Detectable changes can then be better compared and documented in the future. Clues about health changes and trends over time are lost if such details are not recorded in the patient's record.

BOX 5.1 Abbreviations and Acronyms: The Initial Challenge to Reliability

There was a time when recorded histories and physical examinations contained few, if any, acronyms. After World War II, the use of initials began to proliferate. Today it is a compulsive problem leading to misunderstanding that is at times inconvenient and at times dangerous.

When our interprofessional languages are obscured by acronyms, communication suffers and the safety of patients may be compromised. For example, ROM has many meanings. The obstetrician uses ROM for "rupture of membranes." The pediatrician uses ROM for "right otitis media." The physiatrist uses ROM for "range of motion." The following statement taken from a hospital chart demonstrates how abbreviations can cause confusion.

67yo CM who CVA, CABG×2, GERD, CRI on HD, POD #5 - Ex Lap for MVC with OA, s for WO & RFCOAW.

TABLE 5.1 Prohibited Abbreviations

The Joint Commission has identified "improving communications among caregivers" as a patient safety goal (Joint Commission, 2020). Certain abbreviations have been placed on a "do not use" list when an error in misreading the abbreviation could cause harm.

When considering the use of initials, abbreviations, and acronyms to work quickly, resist the temptation.

OFFICIAL "DO NOT USE" LIST[a]

DO NOT USE	POTENTIAL PROBLEM	USE INSTEAD
U (unit)	Mistaken for "0" (zero), the number "4" (four), or "cc"	Write "unit"
IU (International Unit)	Mistaken for "IV" (intravenous) or the number "10" (ten)	Write "International Unit"
Q.D., QD, q.d., qd (daily)	Mistaken for each other	Write "daily"
Q.O.D., QOD, q.o.d., qod (every other day)	Period after the "Q" mistaken for "I" and the "O" mistaken for "I"	Write "every other day"
Trailing zero (X.0 mg)[b]	Decimal point is missed	Write X mg
Lack of leading zero (.X mg)		Write 0.X mg
MS	Can mean "morphine sulfate" or "magnesium sulfate"	Write "morphine sulfate"
MSO_4 and $MgSO_4$	Confused for one another	Write "magnesium sulfate"

[a]Applies to all orders and all medication-related documentation that is handwritten (including free-text computer entry) or on preprinted forms.

[b]Exception: A "trailing zero" may be used only where required to demonstrate the level of precision of the value being reported, such as for laboratory results, imaging studies that report the size of lesions, or catheter/tube sizes. It may not be used in medication orders or other medication-related documentation.

From The Joint Commission. Reprinted with permission.

Electronic Health Record Functions

Multiple functions can now be achieved within the EHR, well beyond the documentation and communication purposes that were achieved through traditional paper-based charting. These activities include, among others, order entry, risk stratification, population health reporting, provision of care pathways, and the exchange of health information among different healthc are systems and direct communication between patients and their health care teams through patient portals. By combining the clinical and administrative data that exist within a single EHR and among other data sources, additional benefit can be attained to enhance patient care.

Order Entry. Computerized provider order entry (CPOE) has been a major emphasis in achieving meaningful use of the EHR. By using CPOE for medications and laboratory and radiology studies, a health system can reduce errors and enhance patient safety through several mechanisms. These orders are legible and congruent with the standardized inventory of pharmaceutical therapies and diagnostic studies performed. Clinical decision algorithms can be applied to alert the clinician to such risks as medication allergies, drug interactions, and dosage inaccuracies. This can also expand into condition-specific care plans to facilitate team-based care goals.

Risk Stratification. Risk stratification can facilitate clinicians in assigning risks of specific clinical outcomes to subgroups of patients. By using data that exist within the EHR, this information can then be used to direct specific interventions to those patient cohorts that carry the highest risk. Although a specific risk score may be generated by the particular algorithm, it is generally translated into a "low," "medium," or "high" risk category. This allows high-intensity interventions to be focused on patients who carry the greatest risk of developing an adverse outcome, with the aim of achieving a greater benefit. Examples of such stratification algorithms include the evaluation of the risk of a cardiac event as a result of noncardiac surgery or the risk of progression of a patient's prostate cancer. With the advent of artificial intelligence and enhanced computational capabilities, there are greater opportunities to develop strategies to advance the care of patients with chronic diseases, improve clinical trial enrollment. and offer precision therapies for complex medical conditions.

Population Health Reporting. *Population health* is a term used to signify the synergistic activity of various organizations to improve the health outcomes of the communities that they serve. Such participating organizations within a community can be drawn from local businesses, health systems, government agencies, service organizations, or public policy entities. This represents the intersection of clinical outcomes, determinants of health, and public policy. By leveraging the capacity of the EHR to analyze and report clinical and demographic data regarding the community health status, population health interventions can be designed and implemented. One such example is through the analysis of gaps in care within a specific population. This can lead to targeted interventions to enhance community wellness and prevention programs.

Care Pathways. Care pathways, also referred to as *critical* or *clinical pathways,* are standardized evidence-based health care plans and processes designed for patients within a specific clinical setting to enhance their care (Hipp et al., 2016). By drawing upon each member of the interprofessional team caring for the patient, the designed pathway reduces the unnecessary variation in care to achieve improved patient outcomes. Through incorporating these established pathways into the EHR, each member of an interdisciplinary team can clearly understand the team goals for the care of the patient and the specific role of each team member in achieving those goals. One area where this has been found to be successful is with the enhanced recovery of patients after surgery.

Health Information Exchange. The electronic HIE allows clinicians and patients and, when designated, their family members to secure access to pertinent and appropriate portions of the patient's health record. By facilitating the timely sharing of vital health information that has been generated across multiple health systems, clinicians can potentially avoid duplicate testing, unnecessary admissions, and medication errors and can improve diagnostic and therapeutic plans.

Replication and Templates. Although potentially an effective tool, the ability to easily copy and paste or carry forward text from one note to another has become the latest hazard in medical documentation and presents a patient safety, legal, and regulatory challenge (Box 5.2). When used inappropriately, it can render meaningless an essential communication tool relied on at the point of care (Box 5.3). All copied information must be verified and

BOX 5.2 Use and Misuse of Copy and Paste or Carry Forward

Although text replication is generally discouraged, it can improve efficiency, decrease information drop-off, and decrease typing errors; therefore some uses are potentially acceptable.

Potentially Acceptable Uses of Copy and Paste or Carry Forward

1. The author's previously documented assessment and plan on a given patient that has carried forward to subsequent notes, subject to editing for relevance and accuracy
2. Auto-populated, presumably static information (e.g., past medical history and family history) entered by other health care providers and carried forward into new documents, subject to confirmation and editing if needed
3. Cumulative dated information that carries forward to create a running log of daily hospital events
4. Copying and pasting important lists or information (e.g., medication lists), which can prevent potential clinically relevant retyping errors

Unacceptable Uses of Copy and Paste or Carry Forward

1. Copying previous health care providers' documented work (e.g., history, examination, or thought processes) and entering it into a new note unedited (or minimally edited) as if the new author did the work
2. Unedited text carried forward from other notes (including the author's) that results in conflicting or inaccurate information
3. Unedited or minimally edited notes carried forward from day to day that do not allow readers to determine changes in clinical course

BOX 5.3 Implications of Misuse of Copy and Paste or Carry Forward

1. Copying subjective information obtained by other health care providers without appropriate editing degrades patient narratives, which form the basis for complex decision making.
2. Perpetuation of inaccurate data or diagnoses cloned from previous notes can result in poor patient care decisions.
3. Incorporating (or not removing) redundant or irrelevant information lengthens the document, dwarfs the information that is most important at the time, and makes it difficult to determine what is old and new. When urgent information is needed at the point of care, patient safety can suffer.
4. Unless edited and reorganized daily, copied assessments and plans may not reflect changes in a patient's status or clinical course (e.g., "pulmonary" is always on top though it may not be currently relevant); in handwritten notes, health care providers usually filter and organize pieces of information that are most relevant to the patient's care at the time.
5. When health care providers authenticate their notes containing large amounts of text from previous health care providers, it can appear as though they did not do the work (e.g., take the history, formulate the plan) themselves. Taking credit for parts of a note that one did not create not only is unethical, but can also result in mistrust of the entire document by the legal system and be considered fraud by payers and regulators such as The Joint Commission.
6. When copied text is not edited appropriately, conflicting information or improper time representation can call into question the reliability of the entire note.

subsequently edited or removed as necessary to ensure that it is not erroneous or out of date. Text copied from another health care professional's note must always be attributed to the source.

Organization of the Note

Most health care providers use a customary organization of information from the interview and physical examination. Health care facilities often incorporate the information in standardized forms or templates within the health record. Following this customary outline of information enables all health care providers in an integrated system to find and use the patient information more efficiently. The problem-oriented health record (POHR) with SOAP (**S**ubjective, **O**bjective, **A**ssessment, and **P**lan) notes is one such system. The POHR can also be created in the APSO (**A**ssessment, **P**lan, **S**ubjective, and **O**bjective) format.

Organizing the Patient's Health Record With SOAP Notes

S Subjective data—the information, including the absence or presence of pertinent symptoms, that the patient tells you

O Objective data—your direct observations from what you see, hear, smell, and touch and from diagnostic test results

A Assessment—your interpretations and conclusions, your rationale, the diagnostic possibilities, and present and anticipated problems

P Plan—diagnostic testing, therapeutic modalities, need for consultants, and rationale for these decisions

Subjective Data

Subjective data are the information that patients offer about their condition.

Describe the patient's concerns or unexpected findings by their quality or character. For example, indicating the presence of pain without providing characteristics (e.g., timing, location, severity, and quality) is not useful either for determining the extent of the present problem or for future comparison. Record the severity of pain using the patient's response or score on a pain scale. Be sure to name the pain scale in the record. The severity of pain may also be described by its interference with activity or disruption of sleep. Note whether the patient is able to continue regular activity despite pain or whether it is necessary to decrease or stop all activity until pain subsides (see Chapter 6). Similar detail should be provided for other signs.

Objective Data

Objective data are the findings resulting from direct observation—what you see, hear, and touch.

Relate physical findings to the processes of inspection, palpation, auscultation, and percussion, making clear the process of detection so confusion does not occur. For example, "no masses on palpation" may be stated when recording abdominal findings. Include details about expected objective findings, such as "tympanic membranes pearly gray, translucent, light reflex and bony landmarks present, mobility to positive and negative pressure bilaterally." Also, provide an accurate description of unexpected objective findings. Suggestions for recording the character and quality of objective findings follow.

Location of Findings. Use topographic and anatomic landmarks to add precision to your description of findings. Indicating the liver span measurement at the midclavicular line enables future comparison because measurement at this location can be replicated. The location of the apical impulse is commonly described by both a topographic landmark (the midsternal line) and an anatomic landmark (a specific intercostal space); for example, "the apical impulse is 4 cm from the midsternal line at the fifth intercostal space."

In some cases, location of a finding on or near a specific structure (e.g., tympanic membrane, rectum, vaginal vestibule) may be described by its position on a clock. It is important that others recognize the same landmarks for the 12 o'clock reference point. For rectal findings, use the anterior midline, and for vaginal vestibule findings (e.g., Bartholin glands, episiotomy scar), use the clitoris.

Incremental Grading. Findings that vary by degrees are customarily graded or recorded in an incremental scale format. Pulse amplitude, heart murmur intensity, muscle strength, and deep tendon reflexes are findings often recorded in this manner. In addition, retinal vessel changes and prostate size are sometimes graded similarly. See the chapters in which these examination techniques are discussed for the grading system used to describe the findings.

Organs, Masses, and Lesions. For organs, any type of mass (e.g., an enlarged lymph node), or skin lesions, describe the following characteristics noted during inspection and palpation:

- Texture or consistency: smooth, soft, firm, nodular, granular, fibrous, matted
- Size: recorded in centimeters on two dimensions, plus height if the lesion is elevated. Future changes in the lesion size can then be accurately detected. (This is more precise than comparing the lesion's size to fruit or nuts, which have different dimensions.)
- Shape or configuration: annular, linear, tubular, elliptical
- Mobility: moves freely under skin or is fixed to overlying skin or underlying tissue
- Tenderness
- Induration
- Heat
- Color: hyperpigmentation or hypopigmentation, redness or erythema, or the specific color of the lesion
- Location
- Other characteristics; for example, oozing, bleeding, discharge, scab formation, scarring, excoriation

Discharge. Regardless of the site, describe discharge by color and consistency (e.g., clear, serous, mucoid, white, green, yellow, purulent, bloody, or sanguineous); odor; and amount (e.g., minimal, moderate, copious).

Illustrations and Photographs

Illustrations and photographs can sometimes provide a better description than words and should be used when appropriate. Illustrations with labeling are particularly useful in describing the origin of pain; where it radiates; and the size, shape, and location of a lesion (Fig. 5.1). Photographs included in the EHR can provide useful information, although you need to be aware of any institutional consent policies that apply to this practice.

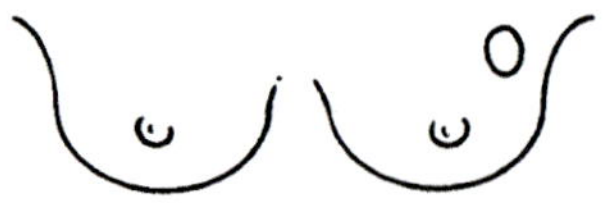

FIG. 5.1 Illustration of the location of a breast mass. Illustration shows an oval mass above the areola on the right breast. The left breast is normal in appearance.

Problem-Oriented Health Record

The POHR is a commonly used process to organize patient data gained during the history and physical examination. After the history and physical examination are completed, the POHR provides a format for collecting and recording your thoughts that assists with critical thinking and clinical decision making—determining the patient's problems as well as the possible and probable diagnoses.

After the subjective and objective data are documented, along with the problems identified, the diagnostic and therapeutic plan is made with the patient as a full participant. The health record describes plans made and the rationale for actions taken to address these problems, lists the information and education provided to the patient, and describes the patient's response to care provided.

The record must be well organized, precise, and concise to facilitate your thinking and the thinking of your colleagues who may need to care for the patient. The consistent recording format enables more effective communication and coordination among professionals caring for the patient.

There are six components of the POHR:

1. Comprehensive health history
2. Complete physical examination
3. Problem list
4. Assessment and plan
5. Baseline and problem-directed laboratory and radiologic imaging studies
6. Progress notes

Comprehensive Health History and Complete Physical Examination

All relevant data regarding the comprehensive health history should be documented, including both absence and presence of pertinent findings that contribute directly to your assessment. Arrange the history in chronological order, starting with the current episode and then filling in relevant background information. Arrange the physical examination findings in a consistent order and style. This allows future readers, and you, to find specific points of information. It also enables you to quickly remember key components for assessment on each encounter.

Make your headings clear, using indentations and spacing to accentuate the organization of your documentation. Be concise yet complete! Avoid abbreviations as much as possible.

Problem List

The problem list is created after the subjective and objective information has been organized. All pertinent data and examination findings, illustrations or pictures, laboratory data, imaging studies, and prior diagnoses are reviewed to develop a problem list in the form of a running log with the following information: problem number, date of onset, description of problem, and date problem was resolved or became an inactive concern.

A problem may be defined as anything that will require further evaluation or attention. Problems arise in many varieties, for example, the questions regarding diagnosis, the availability of diagnostic and therapeutic resources, ethical issues, and factors in the patient's life—social, emotional, financial, work related, school related, family related, and even the availability of caretakers. A problem may be related to any of the following:

- A firmly established diagnosis (e.g., diabetes mellitus, hypertension)
- A new symptom or physical finding of unknown etiology or significance (e.g., right knee effusion)
- New findings revealed by laboratory tests (e.g., microcytic anemia)
- Personal or social difficulties (e.g., unemployment, homelessness)
- Risk factors for serious conditions (e.g., smoking, family history of coronary artery disease)
- Factors crucial to remember long term (e.g., allergy to penicillin)

You may describe problems in separate lists (e.g., diagnostic issues, care and therapeutic issues, and long-range issues), or you may make one list. The needs of a particular patient and the resources available to you will influence your judgment and your ultimate approach. The nature of the patient's problems determines the sequence in which you list them. Problems may be listed in chronological order or listed according to the problems' severity. Some controlling variables with regard to the sequencing of listed problems include the following:

- Possibility that the diagnosis is life threatening and needs immediate attention; the relative gravity of the problem
- Probability/possibility ratio: priority given to the probable diagnoses or therapeutic actions
- Likelihood of the probabilities in a differential diagnosis—with the more probable taking precedence
- Availability and cost of the diagnostic, therapeutic, and caretaking resources; cost relative to need and availability
- Time sequence in which the problems arose and the time sequence dictated by their relative urgency

This list enables all health care providers to quickly assess the patient's history by the summary presented on this list. When a problem is resolved, the date of resolution should be entered, and this item can then be removed from the active problem list. Surgical correction of a condition and recovery from an acute infectious process are examples of resolved problems.

Assessment

The assessment section is composed of your interpretations and conclusions, their rationale, the diagnostic strategy, present and anticipated problems, and the needs of ongoing as well as future care—what you think (see Chapter 4).

Develop an assessment for each problem on the problem list. Begin the process of making a differential diagnosis by discussing and giving priority to possible causes and contributing factors for a problem or symptom. Present the rationale for the potential causes and validate the assessment from data contained in the comprehensive health history, physical examination, consultations, and any laboratory data available. When a serious potential cause is no longer under consideration, explain why.

Describe any pertinent absence of information when other portions of the history or physical examination suggest that an abnormality might exist or develop in an area (e.g., absence of wheezing in someone with dyspnea). Avoid the use of words such as "normal" or phrases such as "within normal limits" or, worse yet, "WNL," because they do not describe what is inspected, palpated, percussed, or auscultated. Be as objective as possible. Assessment may include anticipated potential problems such as complications or progression of the disease.

Plan

The plan describes the need to invoke diagnostic resources, therapeutic modalities, other professional resources, and the rationale for these decisions—what you intend to do.

Develop a plan for each problem on the problem list. The plan can be divided into three sections: diagnostics, therapeutics (if known), and patient education:

- **Diagnostics.** List the diagnostic tests and consultations to be performed or ordered.
- **Therapeutics.** Describe the therapeutic treatment plan. Provide a rationale for any change or addition to an established treatment plan. List any referrals initiated with their purpose and to whom the referral is made. State the target date for reevaluating the plan.
- **Patient education.** Describe health education provided or planned. This should address the role of new therapies initiated and plans for patient requirements upon discharge. Include materials dispensed and evidence of the patient's understanding or lack thereof.

SOAP Notes

The organization of the patient data within the POHR, especially for care beyond the initial evaluation, is often recorded in a series of SOAP notes. Each problem is recorded separately. Subjective and objective data relevant to each problem are clustered together, followed by the assessment and the plan (Box 5.4). Alternatively, all of the subjective and objective data can be recorded in totality. Then the list of problems with the assessment and plan for each are written.

APSO Notes

With widespread use of the EHR, one consequence that has occurred is an increased amount of data that can be incorporated into the note. Although we should be ever vigilant against inappropriate "note bloat," the busy health

BOX 5.4 Governing Principles for Using POHR, APSO, and SOAP

- Record legibly the information you judge is needed; you will write more early in your career, but as time goes by, you will learn to edit with experience and wisdom, especially under the time pressures you will face.
- Organize! Tell the unique story of your patient chronologically and precisely, including positive as well as relevant negative information.
- Use clear headings.
- Precision requires exact description; for example, use a tape measure to measure the size of swelling.
- Be terse. An "erythematous" throat may also be described as "red," and a bulge in an "eardrum" is as well understood as "tympanic membrane."

care provider may be challenged to quickly find the most clinically useful information: the assessment and plan. In the SOAP format one may be required to scroll or click through multiple screens before locating this. With the APSO format, the assessment and plan are moved to the beginning of the document, with all remaining data available in the remainder of the note.

Notes From Subsequent Evaluations

Whether it is during each of the hospital days after an inpatient admission (progress notes) or subsequent outpatient visits for episodic illness or preventive care (ambulatory care notes), the encounter is recorded within the health record. Because there exists in the record an established amount of baseline information, recording of the POHR can be focused primarily on updating information.

An interval history—including subjective status of the problem, current medications, and review of systems related to the problem—is presented in the subjective portion of the note. Medication reconciliation is a critical part of every visit in order to prevent adverse drug events. This is the process of determining an accurate list of all of the medications being taken by the patient. This includes the medication name along with the dosage, route, frequency, and any special instructions. It is not uncommon, especially when the patient is seeing multiple clinicians or has recently been hospitalized, that this list requires correction. The objective portion includes vital signs, a record of any physical examination performed at the time of the visit, and results of laboratory data or radiographic studies performed since the last visit.

The assessment section includes your evaluation of the problem status. If the problem was formerly a symptom, such as shortness of breath, you may have enough data to make a diagnosis. The rationale for the diagnosis is presented in this section, and the problems, allergies, and medications list is updated accordingly.

Similar to the comprehensive health history and examination documentation, plans are presented in three components: diagnostic, therapeutic, and patient education.

Problem-Oriented Health Record Format

The History

The patient's history, especially for an initial visit, provides a comprehensive database. The following organized sequence will guide you in creating a POHR.

Identifying Information. The patient's name, date of birth, and an assigned health record number are the first items of information recorded. Most health agencies have forms or EHR templates with headings for each category of information to be recorded. This information should be contained on every page of documentation.

Problems, Allergies, Medications, and Immunizations List. Although the problems, allergies, medications, and immunizations (PAMI) list itself is added to the record after the subjective and objective information has been organized, the POHR form can be reviewed at a glance by medical personnel. The PAMI list is an ongoing record of a patient's medical problems, allergies with associated reactions, medications with dosages and instructions of how these are administered, and past immunizations. This list should be reviewed, reconciled, and updated with the patient at each visit and when admitted to the hospital.

For each entry, the date of onset or initiation is recorded along with the date that the problem was resolved, the medication discontinued, or the date and route that an immunization was given.

General Patient Information. Additional identifying information for each patient includes address, home and/or cell phone number, employer, work address and telephone number, email address, marital status, health insurance status, and health plan name with the member identification number. Often this information now includes the patient's primary language, need for an interpreter, and preferred method of contact (phone, email, patient portal).

Source and Reliability of Information. Document the historian's identity—that is, the patient or the person's relationship to the patient. State your judgment about the reliability of the historian's information. Indicate when the history is taken from the patient's health record.

Chief Concern/Presenting Problem/Reason for Seeking Care. The chief concern or presenting problem is a brief description of the patient's main reason for seeking care. The information may be stated verbatim in quotation marks. Always include the duration of the chief concern or problem.

History of Present Illness. This section contains a detailed description of all symptoms that may be related to the chief concern, and it describes the concern or problem chronologically, dating events and symptoms. When describing the present illness, it is important for the examiner to record the absence of certain symptoms commonly associated with the particular area, or system, involved. Also inquire about anyone in the household with the same symptoms or possible exposure to infectious or toxic agents. If pertinent to the present illness, include relevant information from the review of systems, family history, and personal/social history. When more than one problem is identified, address each problem in a separate paragraph. Include the following details of each symptom's occurrence, described in narrative form by categories:

- Onset: when the problem or symptom first started; chronological order of events; setting and circumstances (e.g., while exercising, sleeping, working); manner of the onset (sudden versus gradual)
- Location: exact location of pain (localized, generalized, radiation patterns)
- Duration: length of problem or episode; if intermittent, duration of each episode
- Character: nature of pain (e.g., stabbing, burning, sharp, dull, gnawing)
- Aggravating and associated factors: food, activity, rest, certain movements; nausea, vomiting, diarrhea, fever, chills
- Relieving factors and effect on the problem: food, rest, activity, position, prescribed and/or home remedies, alternative or complementary therapies
- Temporal factors: frequency of occurrence (single attack, intermittent, chronic); describe typical attack; change in symptom intensity, improvement or worsening over time
- Severity of the symptoms: 0 to 10 scale, effect on lifestyle, work performance

Recording the History of the Present Illness: OLDCARTS. The OLDCARTS mnemonic helps make sure all characteristics of a problem are described in the history of present illness (HPI) to ensure a comprehensive presentation. The order of recording these characteristics does not need to be consistent.

Onset
Location
Duration
Character
Aggravating/associated factors
Relieving factors
Temporal factors
Severity of symptoms

Past Medical History. The past medical history (PMH) includes general health over the patient's lifetime and disabilities and functional limitations as the patient perceives them. List and describe each of the following with dates of occurrence and any specific information available:

- Hospitalizations and/or surgery (including outpatient surgery): dates, hospital, diagnosis, complications, injuries, disabilities
- Major childhood illnesses: congenital heart defects, previous cancer, inflammatory bowel disease, asthma
- Major adult illnesses: tuberculosis, hepatitis, diabetes mellitus, hypertension, myocardial infarction, tropical or parasitic diseases, other infections
- Serious injuries: traumatic brain injury, liver laceration, spinal injury, fractures
- Immunizations: polio, diphtheria, pertussis, tetanus toxoid, hepatitis B, measles, mumps, rubella, *Haemophilus influenzae,* varicella, influenza, hepatitis A, COVID-19, meningococcal, human papillomavirus (HPV), pneumococcal, zoster, cholera, typhus, typhoid, anthrax, smallpox, Bacille Calmette-Guérin (BCG), unusual reaction to immunizations
- Medications: past, current, and recent medications (dosage, nonprescription medications, vitamins); complementary and herbal therapies
- Allergies: drugs, foods, environmental allergens, along with the allergic reaction (e.g., rash, anaphylaxis)
- Transfusions: reason, date, and number of units transfused; reaction, if any
- Mental health: mood disorders, psychiatric therapy, or medications
- Recent laboratory tests: glucose, cholesterol, Pap smear/HPV, HIV, mammogram, colonoscopy

Family History. Include a pedigree (with at least three generations). An example is shown in Fig. 5.2. Many EHRs allow health care providers to create a pedigree. If it is not part of the pedigree, include a family history of major health or genetic disorders (e.g., hypertension, cancer, cardiac, respiratory, kidney disease, strokes, or thyroid disorders; asthma or other allergic manifestations; blood dyscrasias; psychiatric illness; tuberculosis; rheumatologic diseases; diabetes mellitus; hepatitis; or other familial disorders). Spontaneous abortions and stillbirths suggest genetic problems. Include the age and health of the spouse and children.

Personal and Social History. The information included in this section varies according to the concerns of the patient and the influence of the health problem on the patient's life.

- Cultural background and practices, birthplace, where raised, home environment as youth, education, position in family, marital status, general life satisfaction, hobbies, interests, sources of stress, religious preference (religious or cultural proscriptions concerning medical care)
- Home environment: number of individuals in household, pets, economic condition

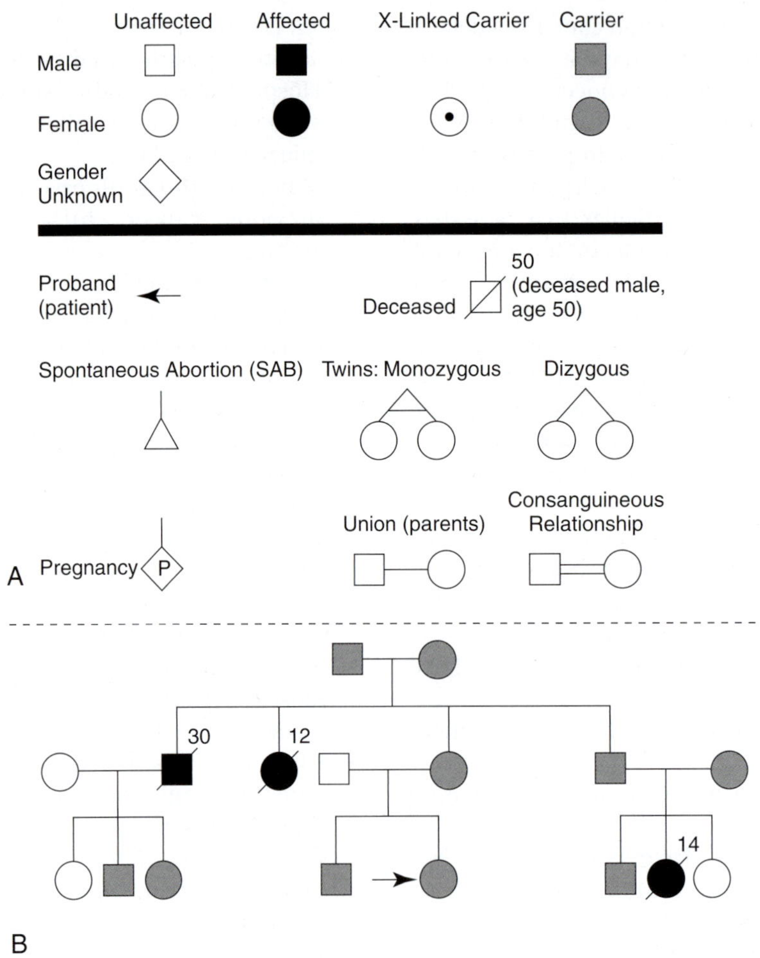

FIG. 5.2 (A) Common pedigree symbols. (B) Sample pedigree for autosomal recessive condition. (A) The different pedigree symbols are as follows: unaffected male: square, unaffected female: circle, gender unknown: diamond, affected male: black square, affected female: black circle, X-linked carrier: a circle with a dot at the center, male carrier: gray square, female carrier: gray circle, proband (patient): leftward arrow, spontaneous abortion (SAB): a triangle with a straight line at top, deceased male, age 50: a square with a diagonal line at the center and a straight line at the top, twins—monozygous: a triangle where its two vertices are each attached to a circle, dizygous: two circles each with a line connected at the top, pregnancy: diamond shape with a line, union (parents): a square attached to a circle through a single line, and consanguineous relationship: a square attached to a circle through a double line. (B) In the sample pedigree chart, the details for different generations are as follows: First generation: Carrier male marries carrier female. Second generation: Couple has one affected deceased boy labeled 30, one affected deceased girl labeled 12, one carrier girl, and one carrier boy. Affected boy marries unaffected girl, carrier girl marries unaffected boy, and carrier boy marries carrier girl. Third generation: Affected boy and unaffected girl have unaffected girl, carrier boy, and carrier female. Carrier girl and unaffected boy have carrier boy and carrier girl (proband patient). Carrier boy and carrier girl have carrier boy, affected deceased girl labeled 14, and unaffected girl.

- Occupation: usual work and present work if different, list of job changes, work conditions and hours, physical or mental strain, duration of employment; present and past exposure to heat and cold, industrial toxins; protective devices required or used; military service
- Environment: home, school, work, structural barriers if physically disabled, community services used; travel and other exposure to contagious diseases, residence in tropics; water and milk supply, other sources of infection when applicable
- Current health habits and/or risk factors: exercise; smoking (packs per day times duration); salt intake; obesity/weight control; diet; alcohol intake: beer, wine, hard liquor (amount/day), duration; CAGE (see Box 2.5) or TACE (see Box 2.7) question responses; blackouts, seizures, or delirium tremens; drug or alcohol treatment program or support group; illicit drugs used (e.g., marijuana, cocaine, heroin, LSD, PCP, methamphetamine) and methods (e.g., injection, ingestion, sniffing, smoking, or use of shared needles)

- Exposure to chemicals, toxins, poisons, asbestos, or radioactive material at home or work and duration; caffeine use (cups or glasses/day)
- Military service record: branch of service, military occupational specialty/job in the military, dates and geographic area of assignments/deployments, current status (active duty, reserves, retired, veteran)
- Sexual activity: contraceptive or barrier protection method used; past sexually transmitted infections (e.g., syphilis, gonorrhea, chlamydia, herpes, warts); treatment
- Concerns about cost of care, health care coverage

Review of Systems

- General constitutional symptoms: fever, chills, malaise, easily fatigued, night sweats, weight (average, preferred, present, change over a specified period and whether this change was intentional)
- Skin, hair, and nails: rash or eruption, itching, pigmentation or texture change; excessive sweating, unusual nail or hair growth
- Head and neck: frequent or unusual headaches, their location, dizziness, syncope; brain injuries, concussions, loss of consciousness (momentary or prolonged)
- Eyes: visual acuity, blurring, double vision, light sensitivity, pain, change in appearance or vision; use of glasses/contacts, eye drops, other medication; history of trauma, glaucoma, cataracts, familial eye disease
- Ears: hearing loss, pain, discharge, tinnitus, vertigo
- Nose: sense of smell, frequency of colds, obstruction, nosebleeds, postnasal discharge, sinus pain
- Throat and mouth: hoarseness or change in voice; frequent sore throats, bleeding or swelling of gums; recent tooth abscesses or extraction; soreness of tongue or buccal mucosa, ulcers; disturbance of taste
- Lymphatic: enlargement, tenderness, suppuration
- Chest and lungs: pain related to respiration, dyspnea, cyanosis, wheezing, cough, sputum (character and quantity), hemoptysis, night sweats, exposure to tuberculosis; last chest radiograph
- Breasts: development, pain, tenderness, discharge, lumps, galactorrhea, mammograms (screening or diagnostic)
- Heart and blood vessels: chest pain or distress, precipitating causes, timing and duration, relieving factors, palpitations, dyspnea, orthopnea (number of pillows), edema, hypertension, previous myocardial infarction, exercise tolerance (flights of steps, distance walking), past electrocardiogram and cardiac tests
- Peripheral vasculature: claudication (frequency, severity), tendency to bruise or bleed, thromboses, thrombophlebitis
- Hematologic: anemia, any known blood cell disorder
- Gastrointestinal: appetite, digestion, intolerance of any foods, dysphagia, heartburn, nausea, vomiting, hematemesis, bowel regularity, constipation, diarrhea, change in stool color or contents (clay, tarry, fresh blood, mucus, undigested food), flatulence, hemorrhoids, hepatitis, jaundice, dark urine; history of ulcer, gallstones, polyps, tumor; previous radiographic studies, sigmoidoscopy, colonoscopy (where, when, findings)
- Diet: appetite, likes and dislikes, restrictions (because of religion, allergy, or other disease), vitamins and other supplements, caffeine-containing beverages (coffee, tea, cola); food diary or daily listing of food and liquid intake as needed
- Endocrine: thyroid enlargement or tenderness, heat or cold intolerance, unexplained weight change, polydipsia, polyuria, changes in facial or body hair, increased hat and glove size, skin striae
- Assigned male at birth: puberty onset, erections, emissions, testicular pain, libido, infertility
- Assigned female at birth: menses onset, regularity, duration, amount of flow; dysmenorrhea; last period; intermenstrual discharge or bleeding; itching; date of last Pap smear/HPV test; age at menopause; libido; frequency of intercourse; sexual difficulties
- Pregnancy: infertility; gravidity and parity (G = number of pregnancies, P = number of childbirths, A = number of abortions/miscarriages, L = number of living children); number and duration of each pregnancy, delivery method; complications during any pregnancy or postpartum period; use of oral or other contraceptives
- Genitourinary: dysuria, flank or suprapubic pain, urgency, frequency, nocturia, hematuria, polyuria, hesitancy, dribbling, loss in force of stream, passage of stone, edema of face, stress incontinence, hernias, sexually transmitted infection
- Musculoskeletal: joint stiffness, pain, restriction of motion, swelling, redness, heat, bony deformity, number and pattern of joint involvement
- Neurologic: syncope, seizures, weakness or paralysis, problems with sensation or coordination, tremors
- Mental health: depression, mania, mood changes, difficulty concentrating, nervousness, tension, suicidal thoughts, irritability, sleep disturbances

Physical Examination Findings

Record the objective data by body systems and anatomic location. Begin with a general statement about the overall health status of the patient. All observations of physical signs should be described in the appropriate body system or region, usually organized in sequence from head to toe. Take care to describe findings in detail rather than make diagnostic statements. The findings generally included in each category follow.

General Statement

- Age, general appearance
- Weight, height, body mass index

- Vital signs: pain score and location of pain if present, temperature, pulse rate, respiratory rate, and blood pressure
- When appropriate you should include pulse oximetry reading and orthostatic (lying, sitting, and standing) pulse and blood pressure

Mental Status

- Physical appearance and behavior
- Cognitive: consciousness level, response to questions, reasoning or judgment, arithmetic ability, memory, attention span, specific mental test scores
- Emotional stability: depression, anxiety, disturbance in thought content, hallucinations
- Speech and language: voice quality, articulation, coherence, comprehension

Skin

- Color, uniformity, integrity, texture, temperature, turgor, hygiene, tattoos, scars
- Presence of edema, moisture, excessive perspiration, unusual odor
- Presence and description of lesions (size, shape, location, color, configuration, blanching, inflammation, tenderness, induration, discharge), trauma
- Hair texture, distribution, color, quality
- Nail configuration, color, texture, condition, nail base angle for clubbing, ridging, beading, pitting, peeling, nail plate firmness, adherence to nail bed

Head

- Size and contour of head, scalp appearance, head position
- Symmetry and spacing of facial features, tics, characteristic facies
- Presence of edema or puffiness
- Temporal arteries: pulsations, thickening, hardness, tenderness, bruits

Eyes

- Visual acuity (near, distant), visual fields
- Appearance of orbits (edema, sagging tissue, puffiness), color of conjunctivae and sclerae, eyelids (redness, flakiness, fasciculations, ptosis), eyebrows
- Extraocular movements, corneal light reflex, cover-uncover test, nystagmus
- Pupillary shape, size, consensual response to light and accommodation, depth of anterior chamber
- Ophthalmoscopic findings of cornea, lens, retina, red reflex, optic disc and macular characteristics, retinal vessel size, caliber, and arteriovenous (AV) crossings, arteriole-venule ratio, exudates, hemorrhages

Ears

- Configuration, position, and alignment of auricles; nodules; tenderness of auricles or in mastoid area
- Otoscopic findings of canals (cerumen, lesions, discharge, foreign body) and tympanic membranes (integrity, color, bony landmarks, light reflex, mobility, bulging, retraction), fluid, air bubbles
- Hearing: Weber and Rinne tests, whispered voice, conversation

Nose

- Appearance of external nose, nasal patency
- Presence of discharge, crusting, flaring, polyp
- Appearance of turbinates, alignment of septum
- Presence of sinus tenderness, swelling
- Discrimination of odors

Throat and Mouth

- Number, occlusion, and condition of teeth; missing teeth; presence of dental appliances
- Characteristics of lips, tongue, buccal and oral mucosa, and floor of mouth (color, moisture, surface characteristics, symmetry, induration)
- Appearance of oropharynx, palate, and tonsils; tonsil size
- Symmetry and movement of tongue, soft palate, and uvula; gag reflex
- Voice quality
- Discrimination of taste

Neck

- Fullness, mobility, suppleness, and strength
- Position of trachea, tracheal tug, movement of hyoid bone and cartilages with swallowing
- Thyroid size, shape, nodules, tenderness, bruits
- Presence of masses, webbing, skin folds

Chest

- Size and shape of chest, anteroposterior versus transverse diameter, symmetry of movement with respiration, superficial venous patterns
- Tenderness over ribs, bony prominences
- Presence of retractions, use of accessory muscles
- Diaphragmatic excursion

Lungs

- Respiratory rate, depth, regularity, quietness or ease of respiration
- Palpation findings: symmetry and quality of tactile fremitus
- Percussion findings: quality and symmetry of percussion notes
- Auscultation findings: characteristics of breath sounds (intensity, pitch, duration, quality), phase and location where audible
- Characteristics of cough, stridor
- Presence of friction rub, egophony, bronchophony, whispered pectoriloquy, vocal resonance

Breasts
- Size, contour, symmetry, supernumerary nipples, venous patterns, lesions
- Tissue consistency, presence of masses, scars, tenderness, thickening, retractions or dimpling
- Characteristics of nipples and areolae (inversion, eversion, retraction), discharge

Heart
- Anatomic location of apical impulse, pulsations
- Heart rate, rhythm
- Palpation findings: thrills, heaves, or lifts
- Auscultation findings: characteristics of S_1 and S_2 (location, intensity, pitch, timing, splitting, systole, diastole)
- Presence of murmurs, clicks, snaps, S_3 or S_4; description by timing, location, radiation, intensity, pitch, quality, variation with respiration

Blood Vessels
- Amplitude, symmetry of pulses in extremities
- Jugular vein pulsations and distention, pressure measurement; jugular vein and carotid artery pulse waves
- Presence of bruits over abdominal aorta and carotid, temporal, renal, iliac, and femoral arteries
- Temperature, color, hair distribution, skin texture, muscle atrophy, nail beds of lower extremities
- Presence of edema, swelling, vein distention, varicosities, circumference of extremities
- Tenderness of lower extremities or along superficial vein

Abdomen
- Shape, contour, visible aorta pulsations, surface motion, venous patterns, scars, hernia or separation of muscles, peristalsis
- Auscultation findings: presence and character of bowel sounds, friction rub over liver or spleen
- Palpation findings: aorta, organs, feces, masses; location, size, contour, consistency, tenderness, muscle resistance
- Percussion findings: tone in each quadrant, areas of different percussion notes, costovertebral angle (CVA) tenderness, liver span

Male Genitalia
- Appearance of external genitalia, penis (symmetry, circumcision status, unusual thickening, color, texture, location and size of urethral opening, discharge), urethral discharge with stripping, lesions, distribution of pubic hair
- Palpation findings: penis, testes, epididymides, vas deferens contour, consistency, tenderness
- Presence of hernia or scrotal swelling, transillumination findings

Female Genitalia
- Appearance of external genitalia and perineum, distribution of pubic hair, tenderness, scarring, discharge, inflammation, irritation, lesions, caruncle, polyps
- Internal examination findings: appearance of vaginal mucosa, cervix (color, position, surface characteristics, shape of os), discharge, odor
- Bimanual examination findings: size, contour, and position of uterus; tenderness and mobility of cervix, uterus, adnexa, and ovaries (size, shape, consistency, tenderness)
- Rectovaginal examination findings
- Urinary incontinence when patient bears down

Anus and Rectum
- Perianal area: appearance, presence of hemorrhoids, fissures, skin tags, pilonidal dimpling, hair tufts, inflammation, excoriation
- Rectal wall contour, tenderness, sphincter tone and control
- Prostate size, contour, consistency, mobility
- Color and consistency of stool

Lymphatic System
- Presence of lymph nodes in head, neck, submandibular, supraclavicular, infraclavicular, epitrochlear, axillary, or inguinal areas
- Size, shape, warmth, tenderness, mobility, consistency (matted or discreteness of nodes)
- Redness or streaks in localized area

Musculoskeletal System
- Posture: alignment of extremities and spine, symmetry of body parts
- Symmetry of muscle mass, tone, fasciculation, spasms
- Range of motion (active and passive)
- Appearance of joints: presence of deformities, tenderness, crepitus, swelling
- Muscle strength

Neurologic System
- Cranial nerves: specific findings for each or specify those tested if findings are recorded in head and neck sections
- Gait (posture, rhythm, sequence of stride and arm movements)
- Balance, coordination with rapid alternating motions
- Sensory function: presence and symmetry of response to pain, touch, vibration, temperature stimuli; monofilament test
- Superficial and deep tendon reflexes: symmetry, grade, plantar reflex, ankle clonus

Assessment (for Each Problem on Problem List)

The diagnosis with rationale, derived from the subjective and objective data, is stated. If a diagnosis cannot yet be made, differential diagnoses are prioritized. Assessment includes anticipated potential problems, if appropriate (e.g., complications, progression of disease, sequelae).

Plan (for Each Problem on Problem List)

- Diagnostic tests performed or ordered
- Therapeutic treatment plan, including changes or additions to the established treatment plan, with rationale
- Patient education: health education provided or planned; materials such as websites provided, handouts/pamphlets dispensed; evidence of patient's understanding (or lack of understanding); counseling
- Referrals initiated (including to whom the patient is referred and the purpose)
- Target dates for reevaluating the results of the plan

Infants

The organizational structure for recording the history and physical examination of newborns and infants is the same as for adults. The recorded information varies from the adult's primarily because of the developmental status of the infant. With newborns, the focus is on their transition to extrauterine life and the detection of any congenital anomalies. Specific additions to the history and physical examination follow.

History

Present Problem. For older infants, record information as for adults; however, for newborns, include the details of the pregnancy and any untoward events occurring since birth.

Details of Pregnancy

- Patient's health during pregnancy, age, specific conditions (e.g., hypertension, diabetes, lupus, seizures, bleeding, proteinuria, preeclampsia); infectious illnesses (gestational month of infection); radiation exposure; medications taken; use of tobacco, alcohol, or illicit drugs
- Prenatal care: weight gained, planned pregnancy, attitude toward pregnancy, duration of pregnancy, support from partner and family members
- Labor and delivery: spontaneous, induced, duration, analgesia or anesthesia, complications, presentation, forceps, vacuum extraction, vaginal or cesarean delivery

Infant's Status at Birth

- Birth weight, gestational age, respiratory status, color, Apgar scores at 1 and 5 minutes if known; newborn's condition and duration of hospital stay, nutrition; congenital anomalies, meconium staining, bilirubin phototherapy, bleeding, seizures, prescriptions (e.g., antibiotics)

First Month of Life

- Jaundice, bleeding, seizures, other evidence of illness

Past Medical History. Birth history represents the newborn's PMH. Older infants should have general health as well as prenatal and neonatal events added to this category unless this information is directly related to the present problem.

Family History. Focus on the number of miscarriages, number of deceased children, congenital anomalies, and hereditary disorders in the family.

Personal and Social History. Focus on the newborn's and infant's family and household structure, number of siblings, other children in the home, presence of both parents in the home, other adult caregivers in and outside of the home, financial stressors, housing situation, arrangements for child care, and parents' plans to return to work.

Growth and Development. Placement of this information is according to the purpose of the examination. For the infant with no growth or development problems, it may be recorded as either history or review of systems, or it may be a separate category. When a problem with growth or development is apparent, the information will be recorded in the section for the present problem. Passing or failing of a developmental screening tool would be recorded with objective data.

Developmental Milestones. List developmental milestones with the age at which they are attained (e.g., holds head erect while in sitting position, rolls over front to back and back to front, sits unsupported, stands and walks without support, first words and sentences, dresses self).

Injury Prevention. List parents' efforts to consistently prevent injuries based on infant's chronological and developmental age (e.g., use of a car seat, stair gates).

Diet. Placement of this information varies by healt hcare facility; it may appear in the present illness or review of systems, or it may be a separate category.

Breastfed Infants. Note the frequency; use of supplemental formula and vitamin D supplementation; patient's diet, fluid intake, concern with milk supply, any problems with nipple soreness, cracking, or infections; and age weaned.

Formula-Fed Infants. Note the specific formula and preparation method; concentration or powder and amount of water added; frequency of feeding; amount per feeding; total ounces per day; and whether juice, water, or vitamins are given.

Solid Foods. Note the age at which cereal and other foods were introduced; specifics about feeding methods, amount, food preparation; and the response of infant to foods.

Physical Examination Findings

General

- Age in hours, days, weeks, or months; sex assigned at birth
- Gestational age
- Length, weight, and head circumference with percentiles; for newborns, percentiles for gestational age

Mental Status
- Infant state during examination (irritable, crying, sleeping, alert, quiet)

Skin
- Color, texture, presence of lanugo or vernix, hyperpigmented macule, nails
- Presence of hemangiomas, nevi, telangiectasia, milia

Lymphatics
- Visible or palpable lymph nodes

Head
- Shape, molding, forceps or electrode marks
- Fontanel size, dysmorphic facial features, swelling

Eyes
- Red reflex, corneal light reflex, follows object with eyes
- Swelling of lids, discharge

Ears
- Shape and alignment of auricles, presence of skin tags or pits
- Startle to noise or response to voice

Nose
- Patency of nares, nasal flaring, discharge

Mouth
- Palate and lip integrity
- Presence and number of teeth
- Strength of sucking, coordinated sucking, and swallowing

Neck
- Head position, neck control
- Presence of masses, webbing, excess skinfolds

Chest and Lungs
- Symmetry of shape, circumference
- Breast swelling or discharge
- Abdominal or thoracic breathing
- Presence of retractions (intercostal, supraclavicular, substernal), presence of grunting or stridor
- Quality of cry

Heart and Blood Vessels
- Recording as for adults but with peripheral vascular findings integrated in this section

Abdomen
- Number of umbilical arteries and veins, stump dryness, color, odor
- Any bulging or separation of abdominal wall
- Apparent peristaltic waves

Male Genitalia
- Appearance of penis, scrotum; position of urethra
- Location of testes: descended, descendible, not descended, not palpable
- Urinary stream
- Presence of hernia or hydrocele

Female Genitalia
- Appearance of labia, presence of discharge

Anus and Rectum
- Perforate, sphincter control
- Character of meconium or stool, if observed
- Presence of sacral dimple, skin pigmentation, or hair tuft

Musculoskeletal System
- Alignment of limbs and spine
- Presence of joint deformity, fixed or flexible; integrity of clavicles
- Symmetry of movement in all extremities, hip abduction
- Number of fingers and toes, webbing or extra digits, palmar creases

Neurologic System
- Presence and symmetry of primitive reflexes
- Consolability, presence of tremors or jitteriness
- Gross and fine motor development

Children and Adolescents

As during infancy, some adaptations in the recorded history reflect the developmental progress of the child. Such modifications in recording the child's history are discussed next.

History

Past Medical History. Prenatal and neonatal history are less important as the child gets older. Birth weight and major neonatal problems are generally included in the history of an initial examination until the child reaches school age. If a health problem can be related to birth events, more detail is recorded, often summarized from previous records because the parent's recall may not be as accurate as time elapses.

Personal and Social History. Record how the child interacts with parents and other adult caregivers, siblings, and other children; their temperament and behavior in group situations; and any evidence of family problems. Include the principal caretaker; parents' relationship (e.g., married, divorced, separated, single parent, foster parent); education attainment of parents; and involvement with social service agencies. Describe injury prevention strategies used by family.

For older children, record school performance: grade level, progress, adjustment to school, and parents' attitude toward education. Note any habits of the child, such as nail biting or thumb sucking; note hobbies, sports participation, and clubs.

For adolescents, add peer group activities, conflicts, relationships, sexual activity, alcohol or illicit drug use, concerns with gender identity and independence, self-esteem, favorite activities, type of job, and potential hazards. This may be summarized with the HEEADSSS tool (see Box 1.13).

Growth and Development. For toddlers and young children, list motor skills and language milestones attained, age toilet trained, and age weaned from bottle.

Physical Examination Findings. The physical findings are recorded in the same format used for adults and infants.

Some additional notations related to development include the following:

Mental Status. Record mental status and cognitive development status.

Breasts. For females, record the Tanner stage of breast development.

Genitalia. Record the Tanner stage of pubic hair and genital development as appropriate.

Neurologic System. Findings should indicate developmental expectations of cerebellar function, cranial nerves, and deep tendon reflexes.

Pregnant Patients

The organizational structure of the record does not vary from that of other adults; however, information about the pregnancy is added, and some aspects of the examination are modified.

History

History of Present Illness. List the gravidity and parity, last menstrual period, and expected delivery date. Is it a planned pregnancy? Describe details about specific problems such as bleeding or spotting, nausea, vomiting, fatigue, edema, illness, injury, surgery, or exposure to drugs, chemicals, radiation, or infections since conception.

Obstetric History. This additional category should provide information on previous pregnancies, type of delivery, length of labor; complications in pregnancy, labor, postpartum; weight and gender of newborn; and previous abortions.

Menstrual and Gynecologic History. Age at menarche, characteristics of cycle, unusual bleeding, use of contraceptives, sexual history, most recent Pap smear/HPV test, infertility.

Personal and Social History. In addition to the information usually obtained, include the adjustment to the pregnancy by the patient and the patient's significant other, information about whether pregnancy was planned, acceptance by the other parent and family, any history of partner violence, and the other parent's role or other support available to the parent who gave birth and to the child after delivery.

Physical Examination Findings

Abdomen

- Status of the pregnancy, fundal height in relation to dates
- Fetal heart rate, position, well-being, movement
- Contractions

Pelvic Region

- Pelvic measurements
- Uterine size
- During late pregnancy and labor: centimeters of dilation and effacement, station of the fetus, position of the fetal head or presenting part
- Leaking of fluid or rupture of membranes

Older Adults

The organizational structure, again, does not vary from that recorded for other adults. A few modifications in aspects of the history and physical examination are made as described in the following.

History

Personal and Social History. Describe the community and family support systems. Add the functional assessment of ability to prepare meals, manage personal affairs, and engage in social and other meaningful activities. Identify plans for advance directives and power of attorney for health care decisions.

Physical Examination Findings

General Assessment

- Extra time to assume positions for physical examination
- Position modifications needed for specific systems
- Mental status
- Functional assessment of cognitive function, memory, and reasoning and calculation
- Skin
- Presence of common lesions of older age
- Turgor, resilience of skin
- Condition and thickness of nails, especially toenails
- Character and color of hair, baldness patterns

Chest and Lungs

- Change in chest shape and percussion tones
- Effect of chest shape on respiratory status

Heart and Blood Vessels

- Location of the apical pulse
- Characteristics of superficial vessels and distal pulses

Musculoskeletal System

- Posture and muscle mass changes
- Functional assessment of mobility and muscle strength

Neurologic System

- Functional assessment of fine motor movements
- Gait and balance, sensation

Sample Records

Information must be recorded as precisely as possible. Select words for the patient's history carefully because some words may have different implications. Health care providers have commonly used the term *denies* when a patient reports that no symptom has occurred. The term *denies* may imply a confrontational or unproductive relationship. It is better to write either "reports no" or "indicates no" symptoms, statements that more positively record the patient's cooperation in providing needed information. It is safe to assume that your note will be carefully read by many people.

Inpatient Admission Note

Box 5.5 shows an example of a written admission note.

BOX 5.5 Admission Note

Identifying Information: R.S. is a 68-year-old male admitted to the hospital on July 3, 2024. The history is obtained from the patient, and he is considered to be a reliable historian. His preferred pronouns are he/him/his.

Chief Concern: "Having a hard time catching my breath."

History of Present Illness

The patient is a 68-year-old male with type 2 diabetes mellitus and hypertension who presented to the emergency department on 7/2/24 with 5 days of increasing difficulty in breathing. He began to notice the difficulty when he walked up the steps in his home. This became progressively worse over the next several days to the point where he was feeling uncomfortable breathing even at rest. He also had been having increasing difficulty sleeping at night, having to prop himself up on four pillows and waking up short of breath over the past 3 nights. He had to spend the entire night before his admission sitting up in a chair because he couldn't lie down without becoming short of breath. Finally, when he "couldn't talk without losing [his] breath," he called 911 and was transported to the hospital.

R.S. has no prior history of these episodes and reports no prior history of cardiac or pulmonary disease. He reports no chest pain. Before the onset of these symptoms 5 days ago, he went for daily walks up to 1 mile with his golden retriever ("Millie") and had no dyspnea or chest pain. He does report swelling developing in his ankles and feet over the past several days. He has also noticed a weight gain over the past several days of about 8 pounds, despite having a poor appetite. As far as he knows, his diabetes and hypertension have been well controlled, and he last saw his physician 4 months ago. He has had no cough, sputum production, hemoptysis, wheezing, fever, or chills. He does not report a history of hyperlipidemia or smoking but does report a family history of coronary artery disease in his mother and older brother.

Past Medical History

Childhood Illnesses: Reports having all "usual childhood illnesses"; unable to recall specific ones.

Adult Illnesses

1. Hypertension—diagnosed in 2011, on medication since 2012 and reportedly well controlled
2. Diabetes mellitus (type 2)—diagnosed in 2006, on oral medicine since time of diagnosis. Last hemoglobin A1c 7.2% 4 months ago. No history of retinopathy, nephropathy, or peripheral neuropathy.
3. Hypothyroidism—diagnosed in 2010, last thyroid-stimulating hormone (TSH) was 1.05 in 2023

Prior Surgery

1. Appendectomy—1962
2. Inguinal hernia repair, left side—1970
3. Sigmoid colectomy for sessile villous adenoma, 2003; last colonoscopy was 2023 and was without pathology

Medications on Admission

Hydrochlorothiazide 25 mg by mouth each day (hypertension)
Lisinopril 20 mg by mouth each day (hypertension)
Metformin 1000 mg by mouth twice daily (diabetes)
L-Thyroxine 100 mcg by mouth each day (hypothyroidism)
Acetaminophen as needed (used rarely for knee pain)
Multivitamin (Centrum Silver) one by mouth each day
No herbal medicines or other over-the-counter medicines

Allergies

Penicillin: causes hives, no history of anaphylaxis
No known environmental or food allergies

Family History

The patient's parents are deceased. His father died at age 61 of complications of colon cancer and also had type 2 diabetes mellitus. His mother died at age 72 of a myocardial infarction. She also had an ischemic stroke at age 68. She was a smoker and had hypertension and hypothyroidism. The patient has one living brother at age 70 who has coronary artery disease and had a coronary artery bypass graft last year. He also has type 2 diabetes, is a smoker, and has mild chronic obstructive pulmonary disease (COPD). One brother died in a motor vehicle accident at age 20. He had no prior medical problems. One sister died at age 54 of breast cancer without other medical problems. The patient has three children (two sons aged 46 and 44 and a daughter aged 41), two of whom are in good health. One of his sons was diagnosed with hypertension at age 37. There is no other family history of heart disease, diabetes, or cancer. He has no history of anyone in his family having a similar presentation to his current illness.

Social History

R.S. was born in St. Louis, Missouri, and completed school through the 10th grade, then joined the military for 5 years, serving as a supply technician in San Diego. After his military service, he moved to Baltimore and worked at Marine Terminal as a dock supervisor for his entire career. He retired at age 60. He has had no exposure to asbestos or chemical agents through his career. He is now retired and spends time with his grandchildren and working on his house.

He was married at age 20. He and his wife were together for 44 years until her death 4 years ago due to lung cancer. He has three children, all of whom live in the area, and five grandchildren; he reports a good relationship with them. He is still grieving his wife's death but feels that things are getting easier. He has a good social network of friends through his neighborhood. He lives independently in the same house in which he and his wife raised their children.

He is not currently sexually active and has not been since his wife's death. He has no prior history of sexually transmitted infections. He has never smoked, and he drinks one to two beers a month. He reports that he used to drink heavily during his military service but has not since that time. He reports no illicit drug use.

The patient does not get regular exercise other than walking his dog for about 30 to 40 min each morning. He does not watch his diet as closely as he thinks he should but does try to avoid sweets because of his diabetes.

Review of Systems

Constitutional: weight as per history of present illness (HPI); no weakness, fatigue, fever, or night sweats
Eyes: He does wear glasses for reading only. He has no blurred vision, eye pain, redness, tearing, diplopia, or flashing lights.
Ears: no hearing loss, tinnitus, discharge
Nose: no nasal congestion, epistaxis
Mouth and throat: wears upper dentures; last saw dentist 4 months ago; no mouth dryness, throat pain, hoarseness
Neck: no lumps or swollen glands, pain, or neck stiffness
Respiratory: as per HPI
Cardiac: as per HPI
Gastrointestinal: No dysphagia, heartburn, dyspepsia, nausea, vomiting. He does report constipation over the last 5 to 6 years, no change

Continued

BOX 5.5 Admission Note—cont'd

recently. No blood in stool or black tarry stool. No abdominal pain or diarrhea.

Genitourinary: Urinary frequency and nocturia over the past year, 2 times per night. No hesitancy, urgency, dysuria, or hematuria. No penile discharge or pain, no testicular pain. He has not been able to have an erection for the past 3 years.

Peripheral vascular: no intermittent claudication, no leg cramps

Musculoskeletal: mild bilateral knee pain with extended ambulation, stable over the last 1 to 2 years; no other joint pain, stiffness, swelling, or muscle pain

Hematologic: no easy bruising, bleeding, or history of blood clots; no prior blood transfusions

Endocrine: as per HPI and PMH

Skin: no rashes, dryness, color change, or abnormalities of hair or nails

Neurologic: no headaches, head injuries, lightheadedness, vertigo, syncope, seizures, focal weakness, numbness, paresthesias, tremor, gait instability or falls, or declining memory

Mental health: Despite experiencing grief over his wife's death at times, he expresses no pervasive sadness or worry and feels optimistic about the future. Before this current illness, he had good energy and reports good memory, concentration, and interest in activities.

Physical Examination

General appearance: This is a well-developed male appearing his stated age, in no respiratory distress sitting up in bed. He is alert and cooperative with the examination.

Vital signs: heart rate 68 beats/min, blood pressure (left arm, regular adult cuff) 135/70, temperature (oral) 37°C, respiratory rate 18/min, pain 0/10, weight 65 kg

HEENT: Head is normocephalic without scalp or facial tenderness. Eyes: Conjunctivae are pink and sclerae are without injection or jaundice. Bilateral arcus senilis is present. Pupils are equal in size and react equally (4 to 2 mm) to light. Fundi showed sharp disc margins, and arteriole/venous nicking was present. No hemorrhages or exudates seen. Ears: External auditory canals had moderate cerumen (left greater than right). Tympanic membranes were intact and without erythema. Hearing was grossly intact. Nasopharynx mucosa was pink with slight septal deviation from left to right. The oropharynx had no lesions or exudates, and the mucus membranes were moist. Upper dentures were present, lower teeth were in good repair.

Neck: Trachea was midline, the thyroid was not palpable. Jugular venous distention was present (approximately 9 cm). Hepatojugular reflux was present. Carotid upstrokes were strong without bruits. No meningismus.

Lymph nodes: No cervical or axillary lymph nodes were palpable. Small, shoddy, rubbery, mobile, nontender inguinal nodes were present bilaterally, all approximately 5 mm in size.

Chest: Thoracic expansion was symmetric. There was dullness to percussion at both bases. Diaphragmatic excursion was difficult to assess due to dullness to percussion at the bases. Breath sounds were remarkable for crackles up to the angle of the scapula bilaterally. No rhonchi, wheezes, or stridor. No egophony, bronchophony, or tactile fremitus.

Cardiac: Point of maximal impulse is noted in the fifth intercostal space 4 cm laterally from the midclavicular line. Regular rate and rhythm. S_1 normal, S_2 physiologically split. S_3 is present, no S_4. A II/VI blowing, holosystolic murmur was present at the apex radiating into the axilla.

Abdomen: Nondistended, no tenderness to palpation. Bowel sounds were present but hypoactive. No masses were palpable. The liver span percussed to 8 cm and the edge was smooth and palpable 2 cm below the right costal margin. The spleen was not palpable.

Genitourinary (GU): Penis and testicles are without lesions. No inguinal hernias are present. Rectal examination had intact tone. Moderately enlarged, firm, symmetric, nontender prostate without nodules.

Extremities: No cyanosis or clubbing. 2+ pitting edema was present in the lower extremities up to the midcalf and was symmetric. Peripheral pulses at the dorsalis pedis and posterior tibial positions were palpable and strong bilaterally.

Musculoskeletal: Hands were without joint deformities with good finger curl and wrist movement. Bilateral knees showed mild hypertrophic joint deformity with reduced range of motion in extension bilaterally (to about 170 degrees). No erythema, warmth, tenderness, or effusion. Bulge sign negative. Other joints unremarkable.

Skin: Warm and dry, no rashes. Tattoo present on right shoulder. Well-healed incisions over abdomen in the left inguinal region and right lower quadrant. Hair with male-pattern baldness. No skin or nail lesions.

Neurologic

1. Mental status—Awake, alert, and attentive. Oriented in all spheres. Speech fluent and repetition intact, able to point way out of room. Mood is euthymic and affect is appropriate to situation with full range. Thoughts are appropriate; no evidence of disordered thinking.
2. Cranial nerves—II to XII are intact: visual acuity 20/20 with correction, visual fields intact, extraocular movements intact, facial sensation and movement intact, hearing intact, soft palate elevates well, tongue protrudes in midline, intact shoulder shrug.
3. Motor—Intact and symmetric; no pronator drift; strength 5/5 in deltoids, finger extensors, hip flexors, and foot dorsiflexion bilaterally.
4. Sensory—Intact to monofilament and fine touch, fingers, midthighs, toes bilaterally. Vibratory sense intact of great toes bilaterally. Proprioception in toes intact.
5. Reflexes—2+ and symmetric in biceps and patella. Babinski reflex negative.
6. Coordination/gait—Intact finger to nose bilaterally. Intact rapid alternating movement. Stands and walks 10 feet without difficulty. Romberg negative; tandem walk, heel walk, toe walk intact.

Assessment

R.S. is a 68-year-old male who presents with new-onset dyspnea on exertion, orthopnea, and paroxysmal nocturnal dyspnea of 5 days' duration. His physical examination is significant for the presence of jugular venous distention, hepatojugular reflux, a displaced point of maximal impulse with an S_3 and a holosystolic murmur, and peripheral edema. The most likely etiology for his illness is congestive heart failure. Other etiologies for the progressive dyspnea include pneumonia, pulmonary embolus, pneumothorax, pleural effusion, and pericardial effusion. However, the history and findings are most consistent with congestive heart failure, and the absence of fever and constitutional symptoms argues against pneumonia. His physical examination is not consistent with a pneumothorax or pulmonary embolus. He likely does have pleural

BOX 5.5 Admission Note—cont'd

effusions present based on his examination, but this is most likely secondary to congestive heart failure.

In this patient the most likely explanation for congestive heart failure is coronary artery disease given his multiple risk factors, with the possibility of a silent myocardial infarction in the setting of diabetes. Other etiologies to consider would be primary valvular disease given a murmur consistent with mitral regurgitation, but the rapidity with which his symptoms developed argues against this being the sole answer. He could have a primary cardiomyopathy either from long-standing hypertension, hypothyroidism, or alcohol (although his use is limited, unless he is underreporting his current use). Much less likely would be an occupational exposure such as to heavy metals given his work in the shipyard.

Plan

1. Cardiac:
   - Obtain chest radiograph, metabolic panel, complete blood count, and an electrocardiogram.
   - Perform serial cardiac enzyme screening to evaluate for myocardial infarction.
   - Obtain echocardiogram to assess chamber size and valvular and left ventricular function.
   - Give oxygen 2 L/min and begin diuresis with furosemide 20 mg IV every 12 h.
   - Monitor intake/urine output, daily weight, and electrolytes.
   - Consider further assessment for coronary artery disease pending results of previous data.
2. Endocrine: Hold metformin while in the hospital if contrast studies needed. Monitor finger sticks with sliding-scale insulin for glucose control. Obtain hemoglobin A1c and thyroid-stimulating hormone.
3. Musculoskeletal: As-needed acetaminophen for likely bilateral osteoarthritis of his knees.
4. Health maintenance: Recommend pneumococcal vaccine given diabetes. Recommend influenza and zoster vaccine. Up to date with cancer screening.

Thepedigreechartisshownasfollows:Firstgeneration:Deceasedmale (61) suffering from colon cancer and diabetes was married to deceased female (72), who was suffering from myocardial infarction, ischemic strokes, hypertension, tobacco abuse, and hypothyroidism. Second generation: Two boys and two girls are born. Male (68) is married to deceased female (65) who suffered from lung cancer. Deceased boy (20) met with motor vehicle accident. Deceased female (54) was affected with breast cancer. The other male (70) has coronary artery disease, heart bypass, diabetes, tobacco abuse, and COPD. Third generation: Male and deceased female have two girls, 41 (A plus W) and 46 (hypertension). Third child is a male, 44 (A plus W). Proband: leftward arrow.

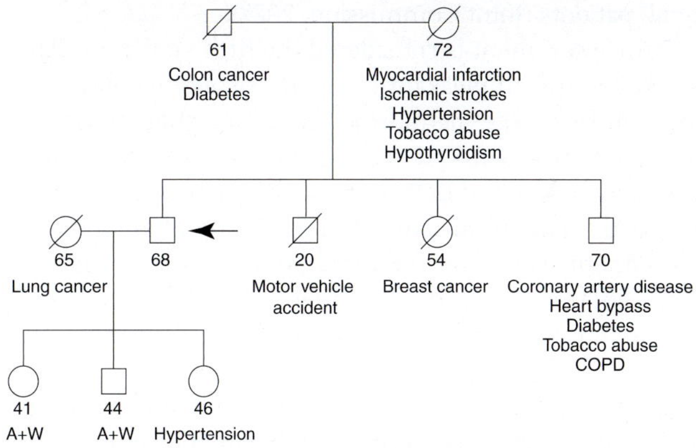

Summary

As you begin to examine patients, it is often difficult to determine how to cluster information that will lead to a diagnosis. As a result, all collected information is initially part of the puzzle. With experience, you will be able to identify appropriate groupings of information, enabling you to better organize and synthesize the raw data. Your first attempts to write a complete history and physical examination will be lengthy and perhaps disorganized, but clinical experience will eventually lead to a more concise and organized record.

CHAPTER

6 Vital Signs and Pain Assessment

The vital signs include assessment of temperature, pulse, respiration, and blood pressure. They are considered the baseline indicators of a patient's health status. Pulse oximetry is often included as a vital sign, but should be obtained based on clinical judgement and is not required for all patients (Joint Commission, 2022).

Pain assessment is considered the fifth vital sign. Pain is a subjective unpleasant symptom of many conditions and injuries. The pain experience, its characteristics, and intensity are unique for each person. A pain "screening" may be used to determine if the patient has pain or not. If the patient answers "yes," a comprehensive pain assessment would be indicated. If the patient answers "no," no further pain assessment would be expected, unless required by organizational policy. Organizations are responsible for ensuring that appropriate screening and assessment tools are readily available and used appropriately. The tools required to adequately assess pain may differ depending on a patient's age, condition, and ability to understand and should be evidence based. The Joint Commission (2022) requires health care facilities to make pain assessment and pain management a priority. Repeat assessment of pain is performed to evaluate the treatment response and to identify the presence of new or recurring pain.

Physical Examination Components

Temperature
Pulse rate
Respiratory rate
Blood pressure
Self-report pain rating scales
Assessing pain behaviors
Pain scales for children

ANATOMY AND PHYSIOLOGY

Vital Signs

Temperature

Body temperature is regulated and maintained by the hypothalamus. When pathogens invade the body, exogenous pyrogens—endotoxins produced by the pathogens—are released and travel to the hypothalamus. Pyrogenic cytokines are produced when phagocytic cells destroy microorganisms, leading to production of prostaglandin E_2. The hypothalamus raises the body's temperature set point, stimulating heat production and a fever (pyrexia). Release of epinephrine and norepinephrine increases heat production by raising the basal metabolic rate (Huether and Rodway, 2019; Osilla et al., 2024). Increased muscle tone and shivering—a rapid contraction and relaxation of the skeletal muscles—also produce heat. The body conserves heat by vasoconstriction, which reduces heat loss through the skin. Body cooling occurs through the skin by radiation, vasodilation, conduction, convection, evaporation, decreased muscle tone, and an increased respiratory rate.

Pulse Rate

The arterial pulse results when the ventricular heart contraction pushes a pressure wave of blood throughout the arterial system.

Respiratory Rate

The primary muscles of respiration are the diaphragm and the intercostal muscles. The diaphragm is the dominant muscle. It contracts and moves downward during inspiration to increase the intrathoracic space. The external intercostal muscles increase the anteroposterior chest diameter during inspiration, and the internal intercostal muscles decrease the lateral diameter during expiration. Air is drawn into the lungs during inspiration and expelled during expiration when the intercostal muscles and diaphragm relax, allowing the chest wall to recoil.

Blood Pressure

The arterial blood pressure is the force of the blood against the wall of an artery as the ventricles of the heart contract and relax. Systolic pressure—the force exerted when the ventricles contract—is largely the result of cardiac output, blood volume, and compliance of the arteries. Diastolic pressure is the force exerted by peripheral vascular resistance when the heart is in the filling or relaxed state. Blood pressure is highest during systole and falls to the lowest point during diastole. The pulse pressure is the difference between the systolic and diastolic pressures.

Pain

Pain is an uncomfortable sensation and emotional experience associated with actual or potential tissue damage. Acute pain is of short duration and has a sudden onset in association with injury, surgery, or an acute illness episode. Inflammation helps sustain the pain response. Persistent (chronic) pain lasts several months or longer and is often sustained by a pathophysiologic process (e.g., joint disease, chronic inflammation, headache, or cancer). Neuropathic pain is long-term pain associated with damage or dysfunction of the central or peripheral nervous system (e.g., amputation, complex regional pain syndrome, diabetic neuropathy).

Nociceptors are free nerve endings in the peripheral nervous system activated by tissue damage from injury or inflammation. Biochemical mediators such as bradykinin, prostaglandins, serotonin, glutamate, and substance P facilitate the transmission of pain impulses from the nerve endings along nerve pathways. Pain impulses travel from the site of tissue damage to the dorsal horn of the spinal cord through the ascending spinal tracts to the thalamus and cerebral cortex. Two specialized nerve fibers transmit pain impulses (nociception) to the dorsal horn of the spinal cord. Sharp, well-localized pain is quickly transmitted by the large, myelinated A-delta fibers. Dull, burning, diffuse, and chronic pain is slowly transmitted by the small, unmyelinated C fibers (Fig. 6.1). Specific spinal tracts transmit the pain signals to the brain where perception occurs.

After the pain impulses reach the spinal cord's dorsal horn, the pain signal may be modified when other stimuli are present from either the brain or the periphery. Substances such as endorphins (endogenous opioids) and gamma-aminobutyric acid (GABA) can change or inhibit the pain perceived. Pain impulse transmission may be reduced when nonpain impulses (e.g., ice, massage) compete to transmit sensations along the same spinal pathways to the brain.

Response to pain is individualized because it is a physiologic, behavioral, and emotional phenomenon. Individuals have different thresholds at which pain is perceived and different pain tolerance levels. Emotions, cultural background, sleep deprivation, previous pain experience, and age are some factors that have an impact on a person's perception and interpretation of pain.

Infants

Infants are more susceptible to hypothermia—low body temperature—because of their large body surface area for weight ratio, thinner skin, inability to shiver, and limited ability to cope with cold stress. Infants have a higher pulse rate and respiratory rate than adults, and the rates decrease as children age. Infants have a lower blood pressure than adults, and blood pressure increases as children age.

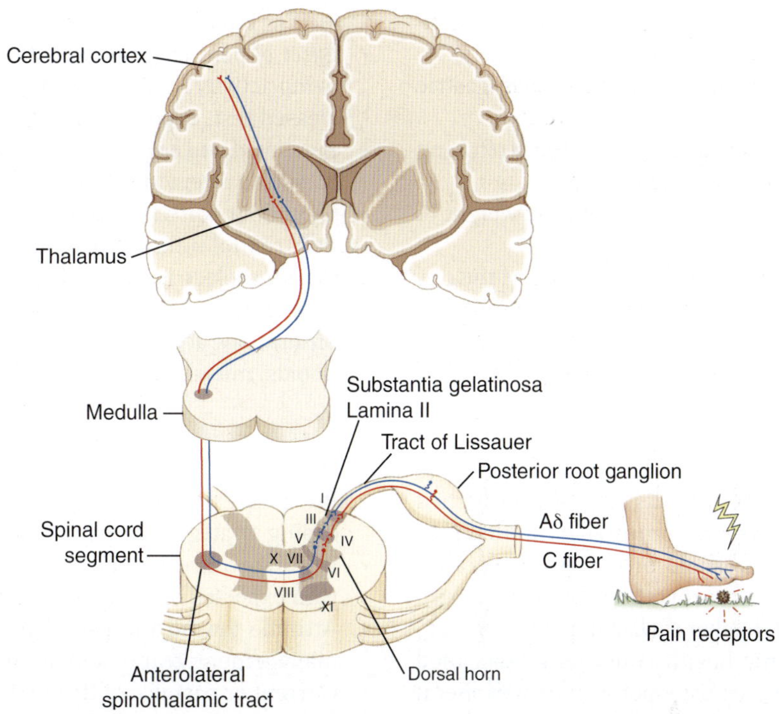

FIG. 6.1 Transmission of pain impulses from pain receptors to the central nervous system. Nociceptors transmit pain impulses from the periphery along A-delta (Aδ) and C fibers to the dorsal horn of the spinal cord. Pain impulses from pain receptors pass through the A-delta fiber, C fiber, posterior root ganglion, and tract of Lissauer and reach the substantia gelatinosa lamina II, anterolateral spinothalamic tract, and dorsal horn in the spinal cord segment. The pain impulses then pass through the medulla, thalamus, and cerebral cortex in the brain.

The nociceptor system for pain processing develops early in fetal life, enabling preterm and full-term newborns to feel pain. The immaturity of the neurologic system results in some differences in pain transmission and processing. Most pain impulses are transmitted along the unmyelinated slower C fibers because myelination of the A-delta fibers continues to develop after birth. The transmission distance to the brain is short. Infants are less able to modify pain impulses because of immaturity of their dorsal horn synaptic connection and inhibition circuits in the descending spinal cord pathways. This results in greater sensitivity of the central nervous system to repeated painful stimuli (American Academy of Pediatrics, Committee on Fetus and Newborn and Section on Anesthesiology and Pain Medicine, 2016).

Pregnant Patients

Blood pressure commonly decreases because of lowered systemic vascular resistance beginning at about 8 weeks' gestation, gradually falling until a low point is reached at mid-pregnancy. The diastolic value decreases more than the systolic value, and it gradually rises to prepregnant levels by term (Antony et al., 2017; Shen et al., 2017).

During pregnancy, some patients may experience pain because of several physiologic processes:

- Back pain may be related to lax ligaments, weight gain, hyperlordosis, and anterior tilt of the pelvis.
- Cramping or pressure may be signs of premature labor or Braxton-Hicks contractions (sporadic uterine contractions that start at around 6 weeks of pregnancy).
- Pressure from the gravid uterus may cause epigastric pain.
- Round ligament pain may be caused by the stretching of the ligaments by the enlarging uterus.
- Pressure on the bladder may occur from the weight of the enlarging uterus.

During labor, pain may be related to dilation of the cervix, stretching of the lower uterine segment, and pressure on adjacent structures. During delivery, additional pain is caused by pressure of the fetal head against the pelvic floor, vagina, and perineum.

Older Adults

No evidence exists that older adults have a diminished perception of pain. However, some older adults may have an increased pain threshold or less pain tolerance associated with peripheral neuropathies, thickened skin, or cognitive impairment (Huether et al., 2019; Mullins et al., 2022). Many have chronic health conditions associated with pain, such as arthritis, osteoporosis, or peripheral neuropathy.

REVIEW OF RELATED HISTORY

For each of the conditions discussed in this section, topics to include in the history of the present illness are listed. Responses to questions about these topics help to assess the patient's condition and provide clues for focusing the physical examination.

Present Problem

Fever

- *Onset:* date of onset, duration, cyclic nature, variability; related to injury or illness exposure
- *Associated symptoms:* sweating, chills, irritability, nausea, vomiting, fatigue
- *Medications:* acetaminophen or nonsteroidal antiinflammatory drugs (NSAIDs)

Pain

- *Onset:* date of onset, sudden or gradual onset, time of day, duration, precipitating factors, variation, rhythm (constant or intermittent)
- *Quality:* throbbing, shooting, stabbing, sharp, cramping, gnawing, hot or burning, aching, heavy, tender, splitting, tiring or exhausting, sickening, fear producing, punishing or cruel
- *Intensity:* ranges from slight to severe using a pain scale from 1 to 10 or from little to worst pain ever felt
- *Location:* identify all sites (Can the patient point a finger to it? Does it travel or radiate?)
- *Associated symptoms:* nausea, fatigue, behavior change, irritability, disturbed sleep, distress caused by pain
- *What the patient thinks is causing the pain or what was the inciting event*
- *Effect of pain on daily activities:* recreational and daily living activity limitations, sleep disruption, need for increased rest, appetite change
- *Emotional and behavioral effects of pain:* change in mood or social interactions, poor concentration, can think only about pain; irritability
- *Pain control measures:* distraction, relaxation, ice, heat, massage, electrical stimulation, acupuncture, mindfulness exercises, meditation
- *Medications:* acetaminophen, NSAIDs, opioids, gabapentinoids, muscle relaxants, anxiolytics, antidepressants

Personal and Social History

- Previous experiences with pain and its effect; typical coping strategies for pain control
- Family's concerns and cultural beliefs about pain: Is pain expected or tolerated in certain situations?
- Attitude toward the use of pain medications for pain management; fear of addiction
- Current or past use of drugs that affect pain sensation

Children

- Word(s) the child uses for pain, such as "owie," "ouch," "ache," or "hurt"
- What do you tell your parent when you hurt? What do you want them to do for the hurt?

- What kinds of things caused hurt in the past? What made the hurt feel better?
- Pain behaviors (facial expressions, grimacing, protective posture) the parent identifies in the infant or child

Pregnant Patients

- Discomforts associated with increasing fetal size; description of discomfort, location, and when it occurs
- Investigate all known medical conditions and physical limitations to identify sources for persistent or acute pain.

Older Adults

- Investigate all known medical conditions and physical limitations to identify potential sources for persistent or acute pain.
- Word(s) used by the older adult for pain, such as "achy," "sore," or "discomfort": Use this word consistently during the pain assessment.
- When the older adult is cognitively impaired, have a family member describe cues to the patient's expression of pain.

EXAMINATION AND FINDINGS

Temperature

The assessment of body temperature may provide an important clue to the severity of a patient's illness. Temperature measurement is most commonly performed by oral, rectal, axillary, tympanic, and forehead routes. The temperature is read in either Fahrenheit or Celsius. The expected temperature range is 97.2°F to 99.9°F (36.2°C to 37.7°C) with an average of 98.6°F or 37.0°C. Core body (rectal) temperature is 0.9°F (0.5°C) higher than oral temperature (Huether et al., 2019). The body temperature fluctuates over a 24-hour period and in response to activity.

Pulse Rate

The pulse rate is best palpated over an artery close to the surface of the body that lies over bones, such as the carotid, brachial, radial, femoral, popliteal, dorsalis pedis, and posterior tibial arteries (Fig. 6.2). The radial pulse is most often used to assess the heart rate. With a thumb or finger pad, palpate the radial pulse on the flexor surface of the wrist laterally. If you have difficulty finding a pulse, vary your pressure, feeling carefully throughout the area (see Fig. 16.8C). Count the pulsations for 60 seconds or count for 30 seconds and multiply by 2.

The average resting pulse rate in adults is 70 beats/min and ranges between 60 and 100 beats/min. Well-conditioned athletes or individuals taking beta-blockers may have a resting pulse rate of 50 to 60 beats/min. In adults, tachycardia is a pulse rate that exceeds 100 beats/min, and bradycardia is a pulse rate less than 60 beats/min.

Determine the steadiness of the heart rhythm; it should be regular. If an irregular rhythm is detected, count for a full 60 seconds. See Chapter 15 for more information about heart rhythm assessment. While counting the heart rate, also note the contour (waveform) and amplitude (force) of each pulsation. See Chapter 16 for a more detailed discussion of arterial pulse evaluation.

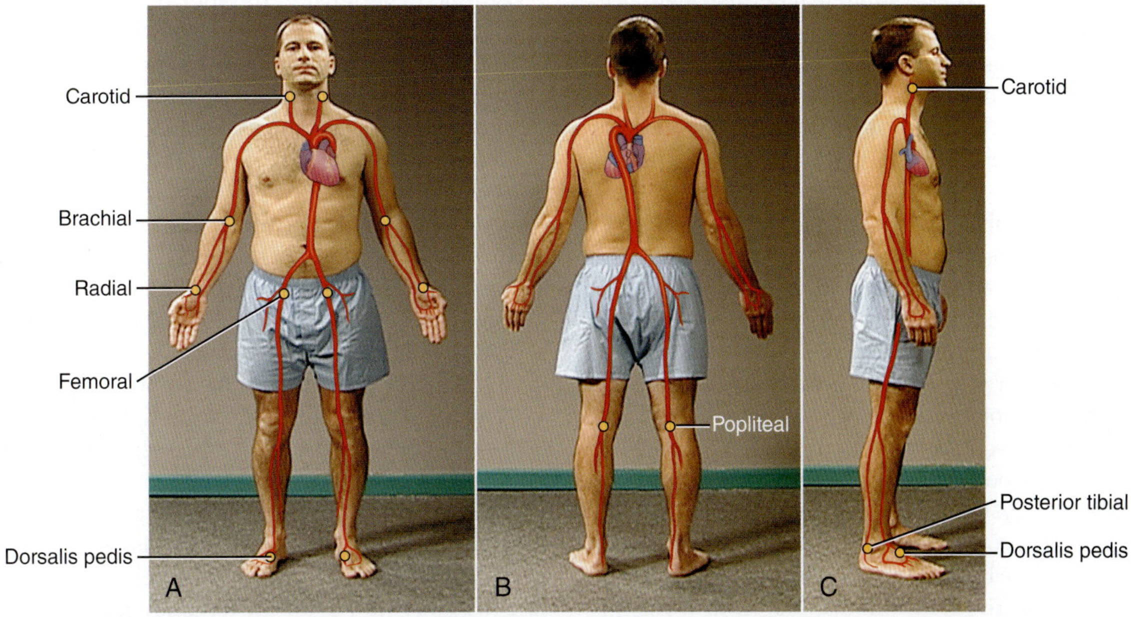

FIG. 6.2 Location of the sites to palpate the pulse. (A) Anterior view of man shows labels as follows: carotid, brachial, radial, femoral, and dorsalis pedis. (B) Posterior view of man shows popliteal at the back side of knee. (C) Lateral view of man shows carotid below the right ear and posterior tibial and dorsalis pedis on the foot.

Respiratory Rate

Assess the respiratory rate (number of breaths per minute) by inspecting the rise and fall of the chest. Count the number of breaths (inspiration and expiration) that occur in 1 minute or count the number of breaths for 30 seconds and multiply by 2. Avoid telling the patient that you are counting the respiratory rate so the patient will not vary the rate or pattern of breathing. A good way to do this is to count the respirations just after counting the pulse, while you are still palpating the radial artery.

The expected adult resting respiratory rate is 12 to 20 breaths/min. The ratio of the respiratory rate to the heart rate is approximately 1:4. Respiratory rates can vary between waking and sleep states. The normal rate of respirations (breaths per minute) depends on a number of factors, including the age of the individual and the amount of activity. Tachypnea is a faster-than-normal respiratory rate. Bradypnea is a slower-than-normal respiratory rate. See Chapter 14 to further evaluate respiratory patterns.

Blood Pressure

The blood pressure is most often measured in the arm when the patient is seated with both feet on the ground and the back supported. Blood pressure readings taken in supine position tend to be lower than those taken in sitting position. Standards for blood pressure readings are based upon the seated position using the right arm.

Free the arm of clothing and apply a cuff of appropriate size around the upper arm (Box 6.1). Center the deflated bladder over the brachial artery, just medial to the bicep tendon, with the lower edge 2 to 3 cm above the antecubital crease. Make sure the cuff is snug and secure because a loose cuff will give an inaccurate diastolic reading. Flex the patient's arm to be at the level of the heart and support it comfortably on a table, a pillow, or your arm.

Check the palpable systolic blood pressure first to avoid being misled by an auscultatory gap when using the stethoscope. Place the fingers of one hand over the brachial or radial artery and palpate the pulse. Rapidly inflate the cuff with the hand bulb 20 to 30 mm Hg above the point at which you no longer feel the peripheral pulse. Deflate the cuff slowly at a rate of 2 to 3 mm Hg per second until you again feel at least two beats of the pulse. This point is the palpable systolic blood pressure. Immediately deflate the cuff completely (Fig. 6.3A).

Pause for 30 seconds, and then place the bell of the stethoscope over the brachial artery. The bell of the stethoscope is more effective than the diaphragm in transmitting the low-pitched sound produced by the turbulence of blood flow in the artery (Korotkoff sounds). Inflate the cuff until it is 20 to 30 mm Hg above the palpable systolic blood pressure (see Fig. 6.3B). Deflate the cuff slowly 2 to 3 mm Hg per second, listening for the following sounds (see Fig. 6.4):

- Two consecutive beats indicate the systolic pressure reading and the beginning of the Korotkoff sounds, phase 1.
- Sometimes the Korotkoff sounds will be heard, then disappear, and then reappear 10 to 15 mm Hg below the systolic pressure reading (Korotkoff sounds, phase 2). The period of silence is the auscultatory gap. Be aware of the possibility of this gap to avoid underestimation of the systolic pressure or overestimation of the diastolic pressure. The auscultatory gap widens with systolic hypertension in older persons because of the loss of arterial pliability. It also widens with a drop in diastolic pressure when chronic severe aortic regurgitation is present. The auscultatory gap narrows in the case of pulsus paradoxus because of asthma exacerbation, cardiac tamponade, or other constrictive cardiac events.
- Note the point at which the initial crisp sounds (Korotkoff sounds, phase 3) become muffled (Korotkoff sounds, phase 4). The muffled sound is the first diastolic sound, and it is considered to be the closest approximation of direct diastolic arterial pressure. It signals disappearance of the Korotkoff sounds.
- Note the point at which the sounds disappear (Korotkoff sounds, phase 5). This is the second diastolic sound. Now deflate the cuff completely.

The two blood pressure readings recorded are the first systolic and second diastolic sounds (e.g., 110/68). The systolic pressure is expected to be below 120 mm Hg and less than 80 mm Hg for the (second) diastolic sound. The difference between the systolic and diastolic pressures is the pulse pressure. The pulse pressure should range from 30 to 40 mm Hg, even to as much as 50 mm Hg. Some studies suggest that the pulse pressure may be a more

BOX 6.1 Selecting the Correct Cuff Size

Cuffs are available in several sizes to match the size of the patient's limb. The correct cuff size ensures that equal pressure will be exerted around the artery, resulting in an accurate measurement. If the cuff is too wide, the blood pressure will be underestimated. If the cuff is too narrow, an artificially high blood pressure reading will result. The size of the cuff is measured by the width and length of the bladder, not the material covering the bladder.

- For adults, choose a width that is one-third to one-half the circumference of the limb.
- The length of the bladder should be twice the width or about 80% of the limb circumference. The bladder should not completely encircle the limb.
- If the patient has an obese arm, attempt to find a cuff size appropriate for the size of the arm. If a sufficiently large cuff is not available, wrap a standard-size cuff around the forearm and auscultate over the radial artery.
- If the adult patient is very thin, a pediatric cuff may be necessary.

Record the size of the cuff used and the site of auscultation.

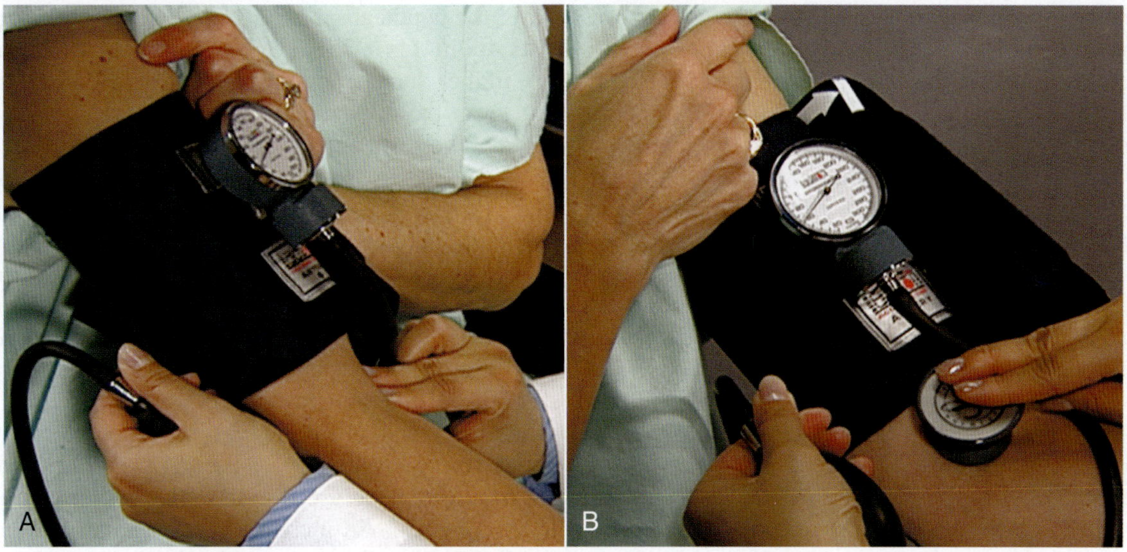

FIG. 6.3 Blood pressure measurement. (A) Checking the systolic blood pressure by palpation. (B) Using bell of the stethoscope to auscultate the blood pressure. (A) Close-up of a patient's arm tied with a blood pressure cuff. A health care professional measures the blood pressure of the patient by pressing inflation bulb with left hand and touching the skin surface with index and middle finger of right hand. (B) Close-up of hands of a health care professional measuring the blood pressure of patient by placing fingers on bell. The diaphragm of bell touches the skin surface of patient.

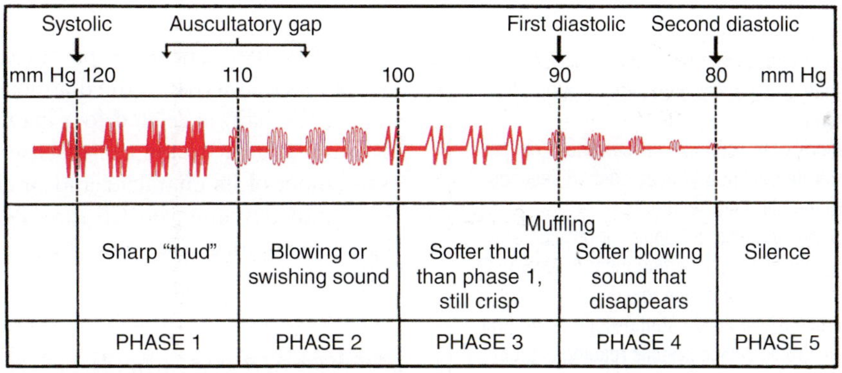

FIG. 6.4 Phases of Korotkoff sounds, including an example of auscultatory gap. A spectrum shows five phases of Korotkoff sounds. Phase 1: Systolic 120 to 110 millimeters of mercury: sharp "thud." Phase 2: Systolic 110 to 100 millimeters of mercury: blowing or swishing sound. The auscultatory gap is marked from 115 to 105 millimeters of mercury. Phase 3: 100 to 90 millimeters of mercury: softer thud than phase 1, still crisp. Text at 90 millimeters of mercury reads muffling. Phase 4: First diastolic 90 to 80 millimeters of mercury: softer blowing sound that disappears. Phase 5: After second diastolic at 80 millimeters of mercury: silence.

important predictor of heart disease than either the systolic or diastolic pressure alone.

Blood pressure levels for adults are classified into healthy, elevated, and two stages of hypertension (Table 6.1). Two well-established clinical practice guidelines on hypertension include the 2017 American College of Cardiology/American Heart Association (ACC/AHA) Guideline for the Prevention, Detection, Evaluation, and Management of High Blood Pressure in Adults and the 2023 European Society of Hypertension (ESH) Guidelines for the Management of Arterial Hypertension (Vemu et al., 2024). Because the systolic pressure is labile and responsive to a wide range of physical, emotional, and pharmacologic (e.g., caffeine) stimuli,

TABLE 6.1 Categories for Blood Pressure Levels for Adults

CATEGORY	SYSTOLIC (MM HG)		DIASTOLIC (MM HG)
Normal	Less than 120	*and*	Less than 80
Elevated	120–129	*and*	Less than 80
Hypertension			
Stage 1	130–139	*or*	80–89
Stage 2	140 or higher	*or*	90 or higher

From Whelton, P. K., Carey, R. M., Aronow, W. S., et al. (2018). 2017 ACC/AHA/AAPA/ABC/ACPM/AGS/APhA/ASH/ASPC/NMA/PCNA guideline for the prevention, detection, evaluation, and management of high blood pressure in adults: A report of the American College of Cardiology/American Heart Association Task Force on Clinical Practice Guidelines. *Journal of the American College of Cardiology, 71*, e127–e248.

high blood pressure or hypertension is usually diagnosed on the basis of several measurements taken over time.

Repeat the process in the other arm. Readings between the arms may vary by as much as 5 to 10 mm Hg. Record both sets of measurements. The higher reading should be used as the patient's blood pressure. Measure the blood pressure in both arms at least once annually and during a hospitalization (Box 6.2).

Most cases of hypertension in adults have no discoverable cause, and the condition is referred to as *essential* or *primary hypertension.* An elevated blood pressure may be the only significant clinical finding, and persons with hypertension are often asymptomatic. Some individuals with severe hypertension may have frequent nosebleeds (epistaxis) or recurrent severe headaches.

If the diastolic pressure reading in the arm is greater than 80 mm Hg or if you suspect coarctation of the aorta, measure the blood pressure in the legs. Place the patient in a prone position (if the patient is in supine position, flex the leg as little as possible). Center the thigh cuff bladder over the popliteal artery and wrap the cuff securely on the distal third of the femur. Auscultate the blood pressure over the popliteal artery. A Doppler measurement may be helpful in this regard. Leg blood pressures are expected to be higher than arm pressures. The leg blood pressure will be lower than the arm blood pressure in cases of coarctation of the aorta or aortic stenosis.

If the patient is taking antihypertensive medications, has a depleted blood volume, or complains of fainting or postural lightheadedness, measure the blood pressure in the arm one minute after the patient stands (Ringer and Lappin, 2024). Compare this reading to the sitting blood pressure. As a patient changes position from sitting to standing, a slight drop or no drop in systolic pressure and a slight rise in diastolic pressure occurs. If orthostatic (postural) hypotension is present, expect to see a significant drop in systolic pressure (greater than 20 mm Hg) and a 10 mm Hg drop in diastolic pressure (Ringer and Lappin, 2024). An increase in heart rate often occurs as well. Mild blood loss (e.g., blood donation), drugs, autonomic nervous system disease, or prolonged time in a recumbent position can contribute to orthostatic hypotension. Patients with active gastrointestinal bleeding will often have dramatic changes in blood pressure with postural change.

BOX 6.2 Pointers for Taking the Blood Pressure

- Position the dial of the aneroid sphygmomanometer so it faces you directly, no more than 3 feet away. An aneroid manometer needs periodic calibration.
- Slow or repeated inflations of the cuff can cause venous congestion and result in inaccurate readings. Wait at least 15 seconds between readings, with the cuff fully deflated.
- Electronic sphygmomanometers with a Doppler or oscillometric device work by sensing vibrations, converting them to electrical impulses, and transmitting the information to a digital readout. These devices are more sensitive than a stethoscope to the first Korotkoff sound. The electronic device systolic reading is thus somewhat higher than the auscultatory systolic reading. The two techniques are not interchangeable. If the electronic reading and clinical impression are not consistent, take a manual blood pressure to validate the electronic reading.
- When documenting a patient's blood pressure measurements over time, use the same position and the same arm.
- The accuracy of the blood pressure reading may be undermined by some conditions, even when using impeccable technique:
  - *Cardiac dysrhythmias.* If heart rate irregularity is sustained, take the average of several blood pressure readings and document the problem.
  - *Aortic regurgitation.* If the sounds of aortic regurgitation do not disappear, the diastolic pressure reading will be obscured.
  - *Venous congestion.* If sluggish venous flow occurs because of a pathologic event or repeated slow inflations of the cuff, the systolic pressure will be heard lower than it actually is, and the diastolic pressure will be higher.
  - *Cardiac valve replacement.* If the sounds are heard all the way down to a zero-gauge reading, listen carefully for the first muffling of the sound (Korotkoff phase 4) to determine the diastolic pressure. More modern valves do not cause this discrepancy.

Pain Assessment

When the chief concern is pain, the location and related symptoms may assist in the diagnosis of a patient's condition. If the pain is related to a diagnosed condition (e.g., trauma, surgery, sickle cell disease, cancer, or arthritis), assessment of its character and intensity is necessary for pain management (see Clinical Pearl, "The Fifth Vital Sign"). Remember that more than one cause of pain may exist.

CLINICAL PEARL

The Fifth Vital Sign

Pain is often referred to as the fifth vital sign because of its association with tissue damage, the pathophysiologic effect of pain on body systems, and the patient's emotional response, which may worsen the pain perceived.

Self-Report Pain Rating Scales

Because of the subjective nature of pain, assessment is often based on history and patient responses to various tools that evaluate pain intensity and quality. The patient's report of pain is the most reliable indicator of pain and should be believed, even when observed behaviors do not seem to correspond. Encourage patients to report the presence, intensity, and character of discomfort.

Several pain-rating scales have been developed for patients to report their pain intensity and quality; only a sample is presented here (Figs. 6.5–6.8). The patient's rating of

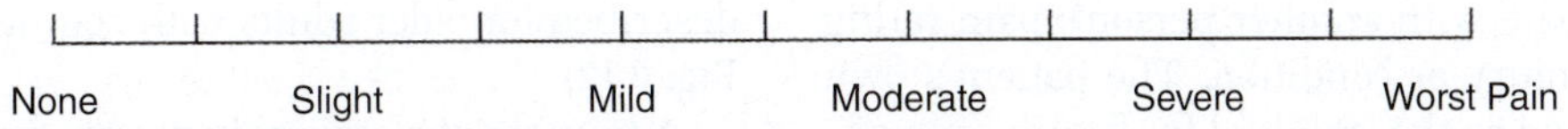

FIG. 6.5 Descriptive pain intensity scale. Pain intensity scale shows 11 divisions indicating "None," "Slight," "Mild," "Moderate," "Severe," and "Worst Pain" from left to right.

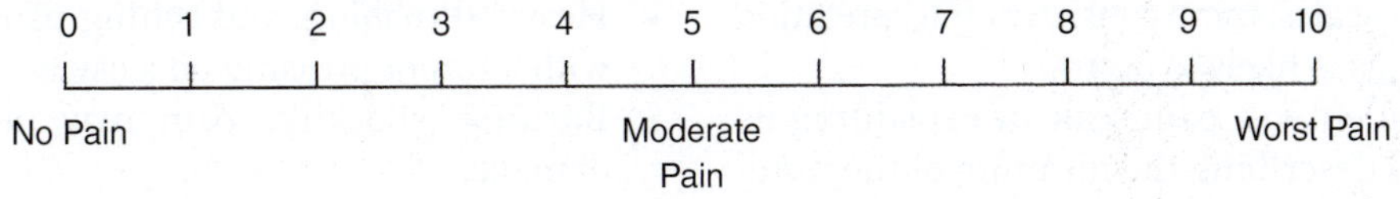

FIG. 6.6 Numeric pain intensity scale. Pain intensity scale shows 11 divisions, numbered from 0 through 10. The divisions at 0, 5, and 10 are marked "No Pain," "Moderate pain," and "Worst pain," respectively.

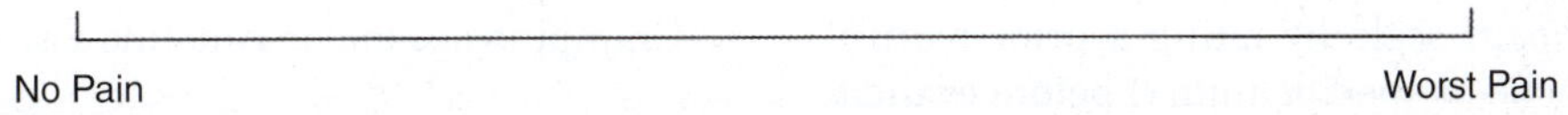

FIG. 6.7 Visual analog scale. Use a 10-cm line with word anchors ("No Pain" and "Worst Pain") on each end. Ask the patient to mark the level of pain felt on the line. A centimeter ruler is then used to identify a numeric pain rating for future comparison. Visual analog scale is marked "No Pain" on the left and "Worst Pain" on the right.

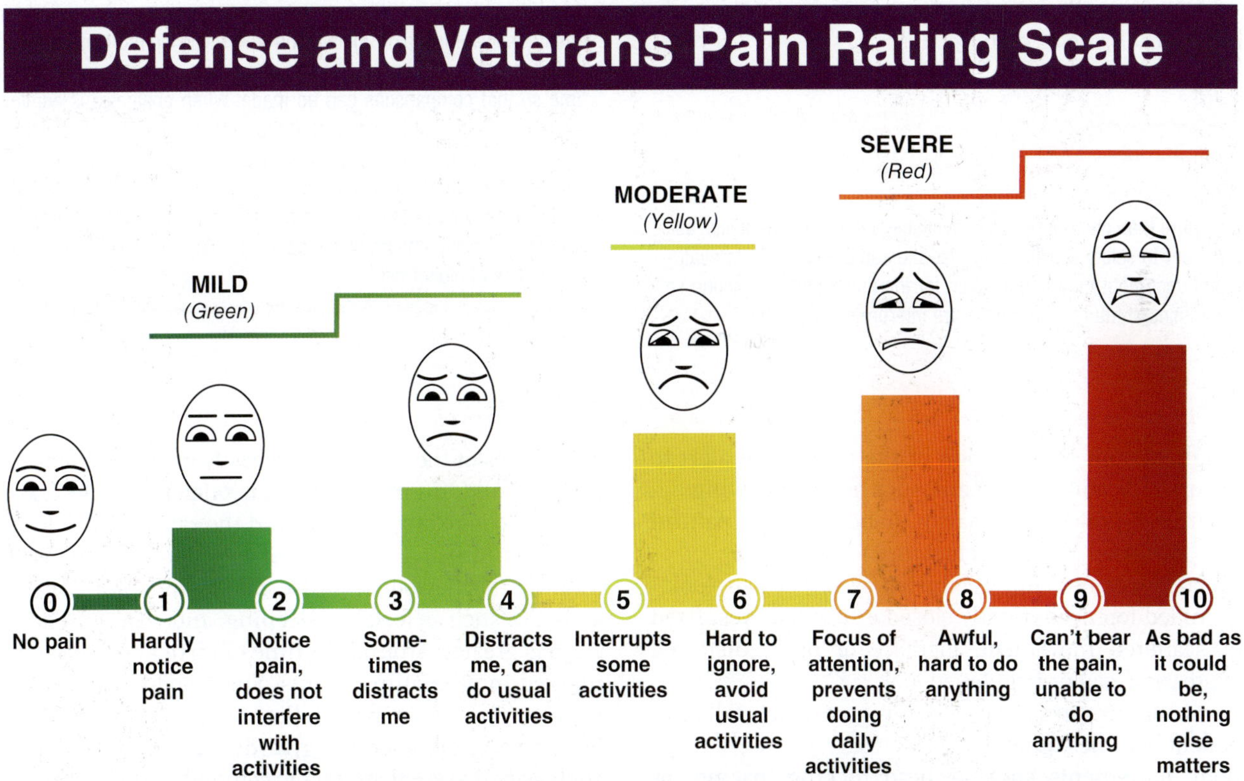

FIG. 6.8 Defense and Veterans Pain Rating Scale. This recently developed and validated tool for military personnel, which is useful for all adults, includes a numerical rating scale, facial expressions, word descriptions, and color coding matched to different pain levels (Steven et al., 2024). Ask the patient to review the facial expressions and pain descriptors when selecting a pain level. Pain rating scale shows facial expressions, color codes, and description corresponding to different ratings. The description of different ratings is as follows: 0: No pain; 1: Hardly notice pain; 2: Notice pain, does not interfere with activities; 3: Sometimes distracts me; 4: Distracts me, can do usual activities; 5: Interrupts some activities; 6: Hard to ignore, avoid usual activities; 7: Focus of attention, prevents doing daily activities; 8: Awful, hard to do anything; 9: Can't bear the pain, unable to do anything; 10: As bad as it could be, nothing else matters. The color coding corresponding to different levels, 0 through 4, 5 through 7, and 7 through 10 is mild (green), moderate (yellow), and severe (red). From https://www.dvcipm.org/clinical-resources/defense-veterans-pain-rating-scale-dvprs/

pain may not compare with another person's pain rating for an equivalent injury or condition. The patient's own rating should be used as the standard for future comparison after pain treatment. It is often helpful for a facility or group of health care providers to select a few self-report pain scales to use routinely. If all health care providers use the same set of pain scales, more consistent interpretation of patient pain ratings is likely to occur.

Introduce the patient to a pain scale by explaining its purpose and clearly describing the meaning of the numbers or figures on the scale (see Clinical Pearl, "Selecting a Pain Scale"). Ask about the patient's usual terms for different kinds of pain (e.g., "aching," "burning," "stabbing," "sharp," or "dull"). Encourage the patient to practice using the pain scale by rating a prior painful episode (e.g., headache or specific injury) before evaluating the current pain level. Ask the patient to rate the pain level in all painful sites, as each site may have different pain characteristics. The pain rating may also vary with procedures performed and activities such as moving, coughing, and deep breathing. Body drawings may help patients to identify painful sites. Document the pain rating for each site of pain.

CLINICAL PEARL

Selecting a Pain Scale

When more than one pain scale is available and used in a facility, ask the patient to select a pain scale. Use the same pain scale to evaluate and document the patient's pain for the entire painful episode so comparisons of future pain ratings are interpreted accurately.

Assessing Pain Behaviors

Throughout your examination of the patient, be alert to behaviors indicating acute pain, such as the following:

- Guarding, protective behavior, hands over the painful area, distorted posture, reluctance to move
- Facial mask of pain: lackluster eyes, "beaten look," wrinkled forehead, tightly closed or opened eyes, fixed or scattered movement, grimace or other distorted expression, sad or frightened look
- Vocalizations: grunting, groaning, crying; talkative patient becomes quiet
- Body movements such as head rocking, pacing, or rubbing; an inability to keep the hands still
- Changes in vital signs: blood pressure, pulse, or respiratory rate and depth with acute onset of pain. Fewer changes in vital signs are found in patients with persistent pain or after they adapt to acute pain.
- Pallor and diaphoresis
- Pupil dilation
- Dry mouth
- Decreased attention span, greater confusion, irritability

Cognitively impaired adults who are unable to use a self-rating pain scale should have pain evaluated as described for older adults with cognitive impairment (see Fig. 6.12).

A number of classic pain patterns may provide valuable clues to underlying conditions, such as the following:

- Bone and soft tissue pain may be tender, deep, and aching.
- Heavy, throbbing, and aching pain may be associated with a tumor pressing on a cavity.
- Burning, shocklike pain may indicate nerve tissue damage.
- A clenched fist over the chest with diaphoresis and grimacing is the classic picture of myocardial infarction. Even a mild pain can require immediate attention in this regard.
- Cramping spasms may define visceral or colic pain.

Patient Safety

Pain Assessment

Assess a patient's pain during every health care visit and frequently during hospitalization. When pain is reported, repeat the assessment after administering pain medication and using comfort measures or complementary therapies. Use the same pain assessment tool each time so that comparisons can be made. When analgesia is administered, reassessment is essential at the expected time of the analgesic peak action to determine its effectiveness and to be assured that acute complications (e.g., respiratory depression) or an acute problem that analgesia may mask (e.g., compartment syndrome) have not occurred. This is especially important for patients with chronic conditions that place them at higher risk.

Newborns and Infants

The pulses of the newborn are easily palpable. Rates close to 200 beats/min may occur in neonates. The decrease in pulse rate is relatively rapid, and the rate may be closer to 120 beats/min at a few hours of age. Compared with older infants, the newborn's pulse rate is more variable with activities such as feeding, sleeping, and waking. The variation is greatest around the time of birth and is even more marked in premature infants. Sustained tachycardia in a neonate may be the first indication of infection, or it may be a clue to an underlying cardiac rhythm disturbance, such as paroxysmal atrial contractions. See Chapter 15 for more information.

Count the respiratory rate for 1 minute. The expected rate for neonates varies from 40 to 60 breaths/min, but a rate of up to 80 may be noted. Infants delivered by cesarean section may have a more rapid respiratory rate than babies delivered vaginally.

The blood pressure of infants is often determined using an electronic sphygmomanometer with a Doppler or other oscillometric technique. The expected newborn blood pressure ranges from 60 to 96 mm Hg systolic and 30 to 62 mm Hg diastolic. A sustained increase in blood pressure is almost always significant (see Clinical Pearl, "Blood Pressure in Infants"). Hypertension in the newborn may be the result of many conditions, such as thrombosis after the use of an umbilical artery catheter, coarctation of the aorta, renal disorders (e.g., renal artery stenosis, cystic disease, or hydronephrosis), congenital adrenal hyperplasia, or central nervous system disease.

CLINICAL PEARL

Blood Pressure in Infants

A very ill baby can maintain a "normal blood pressure" as hemodynamic instability develops. Check the capillary refill, which is usually less than 2 seconds (see Chapter 16). Capillary refill time prolonged 4 or more seconds is an indication of poor perfusion, even when the blood pressure seems normal. The lesson: both measurements are needed to fully evaluate the infant.

Pain Assessment

Valid and reliable pain behavior scales have been developed for the assessment of pain in neonates and infants. Physiologic measures and behaviors are combined for development of these scales. A pain behavior score helps identify the presence of pain and can be used to evaluate pain management efforts. These scales are not designed to measure pain intensity.

- The Premature Infant Pain Profile (PIPP) is used to assess procedural pain in preterm and full-term neonates between 28 and 40 weeks' gestation. It measures physiologic signs (heart rate and oxygen saturation), pain behaviors (brow bulge, eye squeeze, and nasolabial furrow), gestational age, and behavioral state (Llerena et al., 2023).
- The Neonatal Infant Pain Scale is used to assess procedure pain in preterm and full-term infants up to 6 weeks of age. The infant's facial expression, cry, breathing pattern, arm and leg movements, and state of arousal are observed and scored (Llerena et al., 2023).
- The Neonatal Pain, Agitation and Sedation Scale (N-PASS) is used to assess acute pain, ongoing pain, agitation, and sedation of critically ill newborns. The pain portion of the scale involves observation of crying/irritability, behavioral state, facial expression, extremity tone, and vital signs for scoring (Llerena et al., 2023).
- The CRIES Scale (**C**rying, **R**equires oxygen to keep saturation greater than 95, **I**ncreased vital signs, **E**xpression, and **S**leeplessness) is designed to evaluate postoperative pain in newborns and infants. The infant's behaviors (crying, expression, and sleeplessness) as well as physiologic signs (oxygen saturation, heart rate, and blood pressure) are scored (Sansone et al., 2023).

Children

The heart rates of children are more variable than those of adults and react with wider swings related to exercise, fever, or stress. A child's heart rate increases with fever. The mean resting heart rate ranges gradually decrease as the child ages (Sansone et al., 2023).

AGE	MEAN RESTING HEART RATE (BEATS PER MINUTE)
Less than 1 year	128–130
1 year	116–119
2–3 years	106–108
4–5 years	94–97
6–11 years	77–88
12–19 years	72–80

The usual range of respiratory rates for children of different ages is listed in the following table. Rates decrease with age, with a greater variation in the first 2 years of life and without significant gender difference. If the respiratory rate is sustained at a level higher or lower than the expected range, further evaluation is needed (see Chapter 14).

AGE	RESPIRATIONS PER MINUTE
Newborn	24–50
1 year	20–40
3 years	20–30
6 years	16–22
10 years	16–20
17 years	12–20

Select the correct cuff size to obtain an accurate blood pressure reading (Box 6.3). Children become more cooperative for the blood pressure measurement at 2 to 3 years of age. Allow the child to explore the sphygmomanometer. Explain that the cuff is a balloon that will

BOX 6.3 Selecting a Blood Pressure Cuff for the Child

Consider the child's age and body build when choosing the blood pressure cuff size. Use the following guidelines to select an appropriately sized cuff to obtain the most accurate blood pressure reading:

- The cuff width should cover approximately 70% of the distance between the acromion and the olecranon (tip of the elbow).
- The bladder length should be 80% to 100% of the upper arm circumference, and the bladder width should be at least 40% of the arm circumference at the midpoint of the acromion-olecranon distance.

From Flynn, J. T., Kaelber, D. C., Baker-Smith, C. M., Blowey, D., & Carroll, A. E. (2017). Subcommittee on screening and management of high blood pressure in children: Clinical practice guideline for screening and management of high blood pressure in children and adolescents. *Pediatrics, 140*(3), e20171904. http://dx.doi.org/10.1542/peds.2017-1904.

squeeze the arm and then slowly stop squeezing. Take time to allow the child to play with the equipment and squeeze the bulb to gain better cooperation. Use the bell of the stethoscope to auscultate. Korotkoff phase 5 (disappearance of sound) is the diastolic reading unless the sounds are heard down to zero or very low, in which case Korotkoff phase 4 sound (muffling) is the diastolic reading (Bonita et al., 2023).

Blood pressure standards for children aged 1 to 13 years are based on gender, age, and height percentiles. Measure the child's height and determine the child's height percentile using the standard length or height growth curve. Refer to blood pressure tables and compare the child's systolic and diastolic blood pressure reading to that expected for gender, age, and height percentile (nhlbi.nih.gov/files/docs/guidelines/child_tbl.pdf). Expect the child's systolic and diastolic blood pressure values to be below the 90th percentile for age and height. An elevated blood pressure is a reading between the 90th and 94th percentile. Stage I hypertension is the 95th percentile up to the 95th percentile + 12 mm Hg. Stage II hypertension is a blood pressure greater than the 95th percentile + 12 mm Hg. Use the adult ranges for adolescents older than 13 years for expected blood pressure, elevated blood pressure, and stage I and stage II hypertension (Bonita et al., 2023).

Take at least three readings over several visits to diagnose hypertension. If the systolic pressure is elevated and the diastolic is not, anxiety may be the cause. Take time to reassure the child and reduce anxiety. If the blood pressure is in the 90th to 95th percentile range, repeat the blood pressure later during the same visit and average the two systolic and diastolic readings. If the pressure is more than the 95th percentile, have the child return soon for additional blood pressure measurements. Many young children with a diagnosis of hypertension have an identifiable cause (secondary hypertension), such as renal disease, but the incidence of primary hypertension is increasing with the rise in obesity in children in the United States (see Clinical Pearl, "Obesity in Children and Adolescents").

CLINICAL PEARL

Obesity in Children and Adolescents

The overall prevalence of hypertension in childhood is 2%, most commonly primary hypertension, especially in adolescence (Bonita et al., 2023). As in adults, the leading risk factors for children with primary hypertension are excess adipose tissue and suboptimal lifestyles; however, environmental stress, low birth weight, and genetic factors may play a role (Bonita et al., 2023).

Pain Assessment

Some children as young as 3 years of age have adequate communication skills to self-report their pain perception. Assess the child's ability to use a self-report pain scale by determining whether the child understands concepts of higher–lower and more–less. Give the child a chance to practice using the chosen pain scale by describing a previous painful episode (e.g., immunization, earache, or skinned knee).

Valid and reliable self-rating pain scales for young children include the Wong-Baker Faces Rating Scale (Fig. 6.9) and the Oucher Scale (Fig. 6.10). Give the child clear instructions about the amount of pain each face means, beginning with the face with no pain/hurt and ending with the last face that is the most pain/hurt ever felt. Ask the child to select the face that is the best match for the amount of pain felt. Do not compare the child's facial expression to that on the pain scale to evaluate the child's pain. Older children and adolescents may use these pain scales or those listed for adults.

For nonverbal children, the FLACC Behavioral Pain Assessment Scale can be used (Fig. 6.11). FLACC is an acronym for the five assessment categories: *f*ace, *l*egs, *a*ctivity, *c*ry, and *c*onsolability. This scale is used most commonly to assess acute pain associated with surgery in children between 2 months and 7 years of age.

The Revised FLACC, with additional score descriptors for children with cognitive disabilities, can also be used to develop a customized pain behavioral scale. The parent identifies pain behaviors (e.g., specific facial expressions,

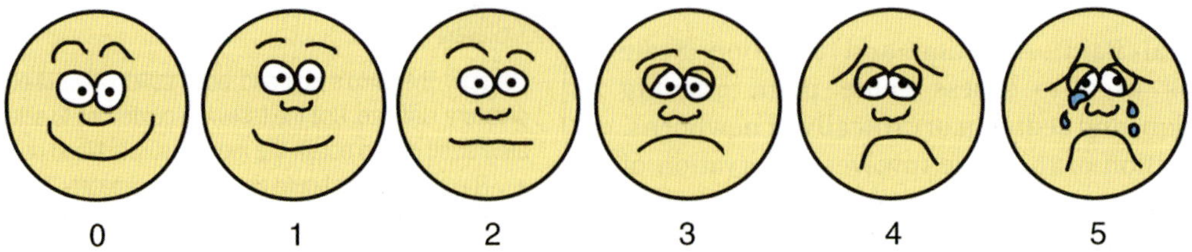

FIG. 6.9 The Wong/Baker Faces Rating Scale. Six facial expressions from mild to severe pain are numbered 0 through 5. Explain to the patient that each face is for a person who feels happy because he has no pain (hurt) or sad because he has some or a lot of pain. Face 0 is very happy because the person does not hurt at all. Face 1 hurts just a little bit. Face 2 hurts a little more. Face 3 hurts a little more. Face 4 hurts a whole lot. Face 5 hurts as much as you can imagine, although you do not have to be crying to feel this bad. Ask the patient to choose the face that best describes how they are feeling. Recommended for persons 3 years of age and older. (From Hockenberry, M. J., Wilson, D., & Rodgers, C. C. (2017). *Wong's essentials of pediatric nursing* (10th ed.). St Louis" Elsevier.)

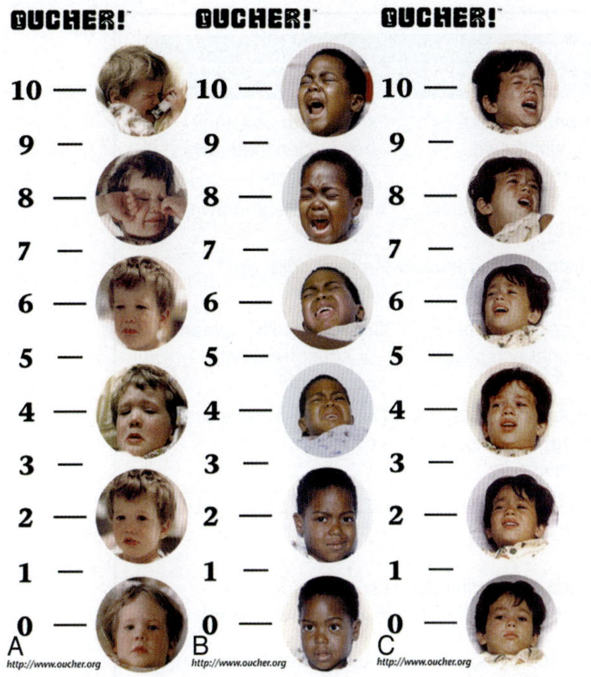

FIG. 6.10 (A) Version of the Oucher for White children. (B) Version of the Oucher for Black children. (C) Version of the Oucher for Hispanic children. (A, Developed and copyrighted in 1983 by Judith E. Beyer, PhD, RN [University of Missouri–Kansas City School of Nursing. B, Developed and copyrighted in 1990 by Mary J. Denyes, PhD, RN [Wayne State University], and Antonia M. Villarruel, PhD, RN [University of Michigan]. Cornelia P. Porter, PhD, RN, and Charlotta Marshall, RN, MSN, contributed to the development of this scale. C, Developed and copyrighted in 1990 by Antonia M. Villarruel, PhD, RN [University of Michigan], and Mary J. Denyes, PhD, RN [Wayne State University]. The scale shows three series of faces marked A through C, each series ranging from "no pain" at 0 to "crying face" at 10.

body movements, emotional behaviors, self-injurious behaviors). These behaviors can be added to the category descriptors and used during pain assessments (Sansone et al., 2023).

Pregnant Patients

Vital Signs

The heart rate gradually increases throughout pregnancy until it is 10% to 30% higher at term.

To identify the onset of hypertension during pregnancy, measure the blood pressure consistently in the right arm in the sitting position in the ambulatory setting. Alternatively, measure the blood pressure consistently in the supine position. The left lateral recumbent position blood pressure reading is lower than supine (Luger and Kight, 2024). Document both Korotkoff phase 1 (muffling) and Korotkoff phase 5 (disappearance of sounds) at each visit (Luger and Kight, 2024). A gradual increase in blood pressure is common from the second to the third trimester. Gestational hypertension, or pregnancy-induced hypertension (blood pressure reading greater than or equal to 140 mm Hg systolic or 90 mm Hg diastolic), develops in 5% to 10% of pregnant patients (Foo et al., 2015). A blood pressure reading greater than or equal to 160 mm Hg systolic or 110 mm Hg diastolic is one sign of preeclampsia; see Chapter 15 for more information.

Pain Assessment

The majority of patients have some degree of pain during labor. It is challenging to assess a patient's pain during labor, as a pain assessment should match individual preferences for mode and timing during labor to provide accurate results (Rantala et al., 2022). Pain assessment scales such as the Visual Analogue Scale (VAS), Numeric Rating Scale (NRS), Verbal Rating Scale (VRS), or McGill pain questionnaire can be used to measure pain during labor (Rantala et al., 2022).

Older Adults

Vital Signs

The heart rate may be slower because of increased vagal tone or more rapid, with a wide range that may vary from the low 40s to more than 100 beats/min.

Because of stiffness of the blood vessels and increased vascular resistance during the process of aging, the systolic blood pressure often increases. Hypertension in older adults is defined as a blood pressure greater than 140/90. Recent studies suggest that individuals who are normotensive at 55 years of age will have a 90% lifetime risk of developing hypertension. Vital sign changes in older patients may be subtle because of reduced physiologic ranges and inability to respond appropriately to stressors (Su et al., 2022). The prevalence of orthostatic hypotension increases with aging.

Pain Assessment

Use self-report pain scales with older adults, but make sure the patient can see, hear, and understand the instructions for use of the scale. Repeat the instructions if necessary. If the patient has vision problems, use a scale with large print and give verbal descriptors for the self-report pain scale. As with children, consider alternate words for pain, such as "ache" or "hurt." Provide adequate time for the older adult to respond. For cases where pain may be localized, help the older adult focus by touching or pointing to the body area when asking about the patient's current pain and chronic pain.

Many patients with mild or moderate cognitive impairment can use a simple pain rating scale (e.g., the NRS, faces scale, verbal descriptor scale, and pain thermometer) to report pain reliably. When a self-report pain rating scale cannot be used, ask family members or observe for pain behaviors (e.g., vocalizing, facial grimacing, guarding a body area, resisting care, or a change in

		SCORING	
CATEGORIES	**0**	**1**	**2**
Face	No particular expression or smile	Occasional grimace or frown; withdrawn, disinterested	Frequent to constant frown, clenched jaw, quivering chin
Legs	Normal position or relaxed	Uneasy, restless, tense	Kicking or legs drawn up
Activity	Lying quietly, normal position, moves easily	Squirming, shifting back and forth, tense	Arched, rigid, or jerking
Cry	No cry (awake or asleep)	Moans or whimpers, occasional complaint	Crying steadily, screams or sobs; frequent complaints
Consolability	Content, relaxed	Reassured by occasional touching, hugging, or being talked to; distractable	Difficult to console or comfort

Guidelines for Scoring the FLACC

Face

Score 0 if the patient has a relaxed face, makes eye contact, shows interest in surroundings.

Score 1 if the patient has a worried facial expression, with eyebrows lowered, eyes partially closed, cheeks raised, mouth pursed.

Score 2 if the patient has deep furrows in the forehead, closed eyes, an open mouth, deep lines around nose and lips.

Legs

Score 0 if the muscle tone and motion in the limbs are normal.

Score 1 if patient has increased tone, rigidity, or tension; if there is intermittent flexion or extension of the limbs.

Score 2 if patient has hypertonicity, the legs are pulled tight, there is exaggerated flexion or extension of the limbs, tremors.

Activity

Score 0 if the patient moves easily and freely, normal activity or restrictions.

Score 1 if the patient shifts positions, appears hesitant to move, demonstrates guarding, a tense torso, pressure on a body part.

Score 2 if the patient is in a fixed position, rocking; demonstrates side-to-side head movement or rubbing of a body part.

Cry

Score 0 if the patient has no cry or moan, awake or asleep.

Score 1 if the patient has occasional moans, cries, whimpers, sighs.

Score 2 if the patient has frequent or continuous moans, cries, grunts.

Consolability

Score 0 if the patient is calm and does not require consoling.

Score 1 if the patient responds to comfort by touching or talking in 30 seconds to 1 minute.

Score 2 if the patient requires constant comforting or is inconsolable.

Interpreting the Behavioral Score

Each category is scored on the 0–2 scale, which results in a total score of 0–10.

0 = Relaxed and comfortable

1–3 = Mild discomfort

4–6 = Moderate pain

7–10 = Severe discomfort or pain or both

FIG. 6.11 **FLACC Behavioral Pain Assessment Scale for nonverbal children.** A chart at the top shows scoring for different categories, face, legs, activity, cry, and consolability, as follows: Face: 0: no particular expression or smile; 1: occasional grimace or frown; 2: frequent to constant frown. Legs: 0: normal position or relaxed; 1: uneasy, restless, tense; 2: kicking or legs drawn up. Activity: 0: lying quietly; 1: squirming; 2: arched, rigid, or jerking. Cry: 0: no cry; 1: moans or whimpers; 2: crying steadily. Consolability: 0: content, relaxed; 1: reassured by occasional touching; 2: difficult to console or comfort. Below the chart, the guidelines for scoring the FLACC and range for behavioral score are given. From Merkel, S., Voepel-Lewis, T., Shayevitz, J. R., et al. (1997). The FLACC: A behavioral scale for scoring postoperative pain in young children. *Pediatric Nursing, 23*(2), 293–297.

mental status [increased confusion, agitation, or withdrawal]) when a painful condition is present (Su et al., 2022). The PAINAD tool has good validity and reliability for scoring pain behaviors in older adults with dementia and the inability to communicate (Fig. 6.12). Perform the assessment when some activity is occurring, such as turning, walking, or transferring to the bed or chair. If pain behaviors are observed, an analgesia trial may confirm that the observed behaviors are caused by pain.

PAIN ASSESSMENT IN ADVANCED DEMENTIA (PAINAD) SCALE

Items	Score = 0	Score = 1	Score = 2	Score
Breathing (independent of vocalization)	Normal	• Occasional labored breathing • Short period of hyperventilation	• Noisy, labored breathing • Long period of hyperventilation • Cheyne-Stokes respirations	
Negative vocalization	None	• Occasional moan or groan • Low level of speech with a negative or disapproving quality	• Repeated trouble calling out • Loud moaning or groaning • Crying	
Facial expression	Smiling or inexpressive	• Sad • Frightened • Frown	• Facial grimacing	
Body language	Relaxed	• Tense • Distressed pacing • Fidgeting	• Rigid • Fists clenched • Knees pulled up • Pulling or pushing away • Striking out	
Consolability	No need to console	• Distracted or reassured by voice or touch	• Unable to console, distract, or reassure	
Total				

Note. Total scores range from 0 to 10 (based on a scale of 0 to 2 for each of five items), with a higher score indicating more behaviors indicating pain (0-10 = no observable pain to highest observable pain).
Adapted from Warden, V., Hurley, A.C., & Volicer, L. (2003). Development and psychometric evaluation of the Pain Assessment in Advanced Dementia (PAINAD) scale. Journal of the American Medical Directors Association, *4, 9-15.*

FIG. 6.12 Pain Assessment in Advanced Dementia (PAINAD) Scale. A chart titled Pain Assessment in Advanced Dementia (PAINAD) scale shows the details of scores from 0 through 2 for different items as follows: Item: Breathing; 0: normal; 1: occasional labored breathing; 2: noisy labored breathing, long period of hyperventilation. Item: Negative vocalization; 0: none; 1: occasional moan, low level of speech; 2: repeated trouble calling out. Item: Facial expression; 0: smiling; 1: sad, frightened, frown; 2: facial grimacing. Item: Body language; 0: relaxed; 1: tense, distressed pacing; 2: rigid, fists clenched, knees pulled up. Item: consolability; 0: no need to console; 1: distracted by voice; 2: unable to console, distract, or reassure. In the last column, score column is blank.From Warden, V., Hurley, A. C., & Volicer, L. (2003). Development and psychometric evaluation of the pain assessment in advanced dementia (PAINAD) scale. *Journal of the American Medical Directors Association, 4*(1), 9–15.

ABNORMALITIES

Hypertension

Hypertension is one of the most common diseases in the world; it is often responsible for stroke, renal failure, and congestive heart failure.

PATHOPHYSIOLOGY

- In adults, defined as blood pressure consistently at 130/80 mm Hg or higher. See Table 6.1.
- For essential hypertension, its pathologic origin is poorly understood.
- For secondary hypertension, potential causes include renal disease, renal artery stenosis, primary aldosteronism, thyroid disorders, coarctation of the aorta, or pheochromocytoma.

PATIENT DATA

Subjective Data

- Essential hypertension is asymptomatic.
- In malignant (severe) hypertension, headache, blurred vision, dyspnea, or encephalopathy may be present.

Objective Data

- Multiple confirmed blood pressure readings at or above 130/80 or in children greater than 94th percentile for age, gender, and height percentile.
- End-organ damage (e.g., papilledema and evidence of heart failure) may be present with long-standing hypertension.

Neuropathic Pain

A form of chronic pain caused by a primary lesion or dysfunction of the central nervous system that persists beyond expected after healing.

PATHOPHYSIOLOGY

- Potential causes include postherpetic neuralgia, diabetic peripheral neuropathy, trigeminal neuralgia, or radiculopathy.
- Damaged peripheral nerves fire repeatedly. Dorsal horn neurons are hyperexcited and transmit enhanced pain to the brain. This causes sustained pain.

PATIENT DATA

Subjective Data

- Burning, intense tightness, shooting, stabbing, electric shock–like sensations
- Pain sensations may worsen at night
- Exaggerated pain response to pain stimuli (hyperalgesia)
- Pain response to stimuli that are not typically painful (allodynia)
- Sleep disturbance
- Interference with activities of daily living, work, or social activities

Objective Data

- Confirmed self-report of pain for all painful body regions
- Distribution of pain sensations (e.g., glove or stocking, leg)
- Pain response to nonpainful stimulus (e.g., stroking skin)
- Sensory loss (light touch, pin prick, vibration sense, proprioception, numbness) may be present in painful areas (Steven et al., 2024).

Complex Regional Pain Syndrome

Chronic condition (greater than 6 months) in which regional pain extends beyond a specific peripheral nerve injury in an extremity with motor, sensory, and autonomic changes.

PATHOPHYSIOLOGY

- No relationship between the original trauma severity and the severity and cause of the symptoms.
- Cause is unknown, but the sympathetic nervous system helps maintain symptoms.

PATIENT DATA

Subjective Data

- Burning, shooting, or pain with aching character
- Exaggerated sensitivity to cold or sweating changes
- Pain increases or persists after light pressure
- Allodynia
- Numbness may be present

Objective Data

- Edema
- Changes in skin blood flow: abnormal skin color; red and hot, cyanotic, temperature difference of up to 1°C between the affected and unaffected extremity
- Increased sweating may be seen

CHAPTER

7

Mental Status

Mental status is the total expression of a person's emotional responses, mood, cognitive functioning (ability to think, reason, and make judgments), and personality. A major focus of the mental status evaluation is to identify an individual's strengths and capabilities. This chapter focuses on the mental status evaluation, which occurs through the full patient encounter with some specific components during the neurologic examination. See Chapter 23 for the assessment of neurologic lesions that cause alterations in mental status.

Physical Examination Components

1. Observe physical appearance and behavior.
2. Investigate cognitive abilities:
   - State of consciousness
   - Response to analogies
   - Abstract reasoning
   - Arithmetic calculation
   - Memory
   - Attention span
3. Observe speech and language for voice quality, articulation, coherence, and comprehension.
4. Evaluate emotional stability for signs of depression, anxiety, thought content disturbance, and hallucinations.

ANATOMY AND PHYSIOLOGY

Two cerebral hemispheres of the brain, each divided into lobes, comprise the cerebrum, which is primarily responsible for a person's mental status. The gray outer layer—the cerebral cortex—houses the higher mental functions and is responsible for perception and behavior (Fig. 7.1).

The frontal lobe, containing the motor cortex, is associated with speech formation (in the Broca area). This lobe is responsible for decision making, problem solving, the ability to concentrate, and short-term memory. Associated areas—related to emotions, affect, drive, and awareness of self and the autonomic responses related to emotional states—also originate in the frontal lobe.

The parietal lobe is primarily responsible for receiving and processing sensory data.

The temporal lobe is responsible for the perception and interpretation of sounds as well as localizing their source. It contains the Wernicke speech area, which allows a person to understand spoken and written language. The temporal lobe is also involved in the integration of behavior, emotion, and personality as well as long-term memory.

The limbic system, located beneath the temporal lobe, mediates certain patterns of behavior that determine survival (e.g., mating, aggression, fear, and affection). Reactions to emotions such as anger, love, hostility, and envy originate here, but the expression of emotion and behavior is mediated by connections between the limbic system and the frontal lobe. The limbic system also interacts with the hippocampus, which plays a major role in converting short-term memories into long-term memories.

The reticular activating system, a collection of nuclei in the brainstem, regulates vital reflexes such as heart and respiratory functioning. It also maintains wakefulness, which is important for consciousness and for awareness and arousal functions. Disruption of the reticular activating system can lead to altered mental status (e.g., confusion and delirium).

Infants and Children

All brain neurons are present at birth in a full-term infant, but brain development continues with the myelination of nerve cells over years. Brain insults, such as infection (e.g., meningitis or encephalitis), trauma, or metabolic imbalance, can damage brain cells, which may result in serious permanent dysfunction in mental status. Genetic, metabolic, and chromosomal disorders may also affect cognitive development and mental status.

Adolescents

Brain maturation continues, with greater capacity for attaining and processing new information, building vocabulary, and growth in social-emotional development. Abstract thinking (i.e., the ability to develop theories, use logical reasoning, make future plans, use generalizations, and consider risks and possibilities) develops during this period. Judgment and decision-making skills continue to develop with education and experience.

Older Adults

Cognitive function should be intact in healthy adults, but with advancing age cognitive abilities may decline.

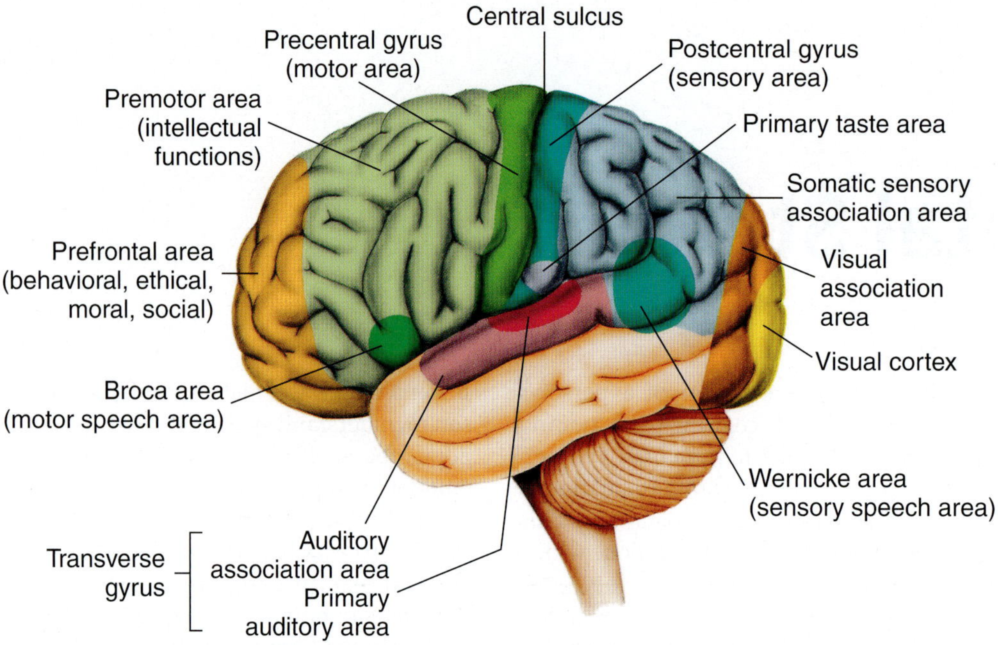

FIG. 7.1 Functional subdivisions of the cerebral cortex. Patton, K. T., & Thibodeau, G. (2016). Anatomy & physiology (9th ed.). St. Louis: Elsevier.

Variations in genetics, environment, diet, exercise, and chronic disease have an impact on the cognitive function of older adults. Decreases in the speed of information processing and psychomotor speed accompanied by less cognitive flexibility are expected with healthy aging. However, cognitive declines in executive functioning (the ability to plan and develop strategies, organize, concentrate and remember details, and manage activities) and memory are associated with cognitive impairment (Wischenka et al., 2016). An estimated 6.2 million persons in the United States have dementia, with increasing prevalence by age (Hudomiet et al., 2022).

REVIEW OF RELATED HISTORY

For each of the symptoms or conditions discussed in this section, targeted topics to include in the history of the present illness are listed. Responses to questions about these topics provide clues for focusing the physical examination and the development of an appropriate diagnostic evaluation. Questions regarding medication use (prescription and over-the-counter preparations) as well as complementary, alternative, and integrative therapies are relevant for each area.

History of Present Illness

Disorientation and Confusion

- Abrupt or insidious onset: intermittent, fluctuating, or persistent; association with time of day or emotional crisis
- Associated health problems: new hearing or vision impairment; neurologic disorder, vascular occlusion, or brain injury; systemic infection; withdrawal from alcohol; metabolic or electrolyte disorder
- Associated symptoms: delusions, hallucinations (imaginary perceptions), mood swings, anxiety, sadness, lethargy or agitation, insomnia, change in appetite, drug toxicity
- Medications: anticholinergics, benzodiazepines, opioid analgesics, tricyclic antidepressants, levodopa or amantadine, diuretics, digoxin, antiarrhythmics, sedatives, hypnotics, or therapies such as ginkgo biloba and St. John's wort

Depression

- Troubling thoughts or feelings, constant worry; change in outlook on life; feelings of hopelessness; inability to control feelings
- Low energy level, awakens feeling fatigued, agitation, feels best in the morning or at night
- Recent changes in living situation, death or relocation of friends or family members, changes in physical health
- Thoughts or plans for hurting self and/or others, thoughts about dying, hopelessness, no plans for the future
- Medications: antidepressants; medications that may cause or worsen depression (e.g., antihypertensive agents, corticosteroids, beta-blockers, calcium channel blockers, barbiturates, phenytoin, anabolic steroids)

Anxiety

- Sudden, unexplained episodes of intense fear, worry, anxiousness, or panic; afraid will be unable to escape or get help in certain situations; cannot control worrying;

spends excessive time repeatedly doing or checking things
- Feels uncomfortable in or avoids situations or events that involve being with people
- Exposure to frightening or traumatic events
- Associated symptoms: panic attacks, obsessive thoughts, or compulsive behaviors
- Medications: antidepressants, steroids, benzodiazepines

Past Medical History

- Neurologic disorder, brain surgery, brain injury, residual effects, chronic disease, intellectual delay, or debilitating condition
- Psychiatric disorder or hospitalization

Family History

- Psychiatric disorders, mental illness, alcoholism
- Alzheimer disease or other dementia
- Learning disorders, intellectual disability, autism

Personal and Social History

- Emotional status: feelings about self; anxious, restless, or irritable; discouraged or frustrated; problems with finances, job, legal system, spouse, partner, children, or other family member; trauma history, ability to cope with current life stressors
- Life goals, attitudes
- Relationships with family members and friends
- Intellectual level: education history, access to information, mental stimulation
- Communication pattern, able to understand questions, coherent and appropriate speech, change in memory or cognitive thought processes
- Changes in sleeping or eating patterns; change in appetite or diet, weight loss or gain; decreased interest in sexual activity
- Use of alcohol or recreational drugs, especially mood-altering drugs

Children

- Speech and language development: timing of first words, words understood, progression to phrases and sentences
- Behavior: temper tantrums, ease in separating from family or adjusting to new situations
- Performance of self-care activities: dressing, toileting, feeding
- Personality and behavior patterns: changes related to any specific event, illness, or trauma
- Learning or school difficulties: associated with interest, hyperactivity, or ability to concentrate

Adolescents

- Risk-taking behaviors
- School performance and peer interactions
- Family interactions
- Reluctance to talk about attitudes, behaviors, and experience

Older Adults

- Changes in cognitive functioning, thought processes, memory; association with prescribed medications (e.g., opioids, benzodiazepines, antidepressants, corticosteroids, muscle relaxants)
- Changes in activities of daily living (ADLs; e.g., finance management, food preparation)
- Depression: somatic complaints, hopelessness, helplessness, lack of interest in personal care

EXAMINATION AND FINDINGS

Mental status is assessed continuously during the entire patient interaction by evaluating their alertness, orientation, cognitive abilities, and mood (Box 7.1). Observe the patient's physical appearance, behavior, and responses to questions asked during the history (Fig. 7.2). Note any reliance on an accompanying adult to answer questions. If another adult is present, make a point of asking the patient to provide responses. Note any variations in response to questions of differing complexity. Speech should be clear and at an appropriate volume. Questions should be answered appropriately, with ideas expressed logically, relating current and past events.

BOX 7.1 Procedures of the Mental Status Screening Examination

The shorter screening examination is commonly used for health visits when no known mental status problem is apparent. Information is generally obtained during the history by observation of behavior and responses to questions in the following areas.

Appearance and Behavior
- Grooming
- Emotional status
- Body language

Emotional Stability
- Mood and feelings
- Thought processes

Cognitive Abilities
- State of consciousness
- Memory
- Attention span
- Judgment

Speech and Language
- Voice quality
- Articulation
- Comprehension
- Coherence
- Aphasia

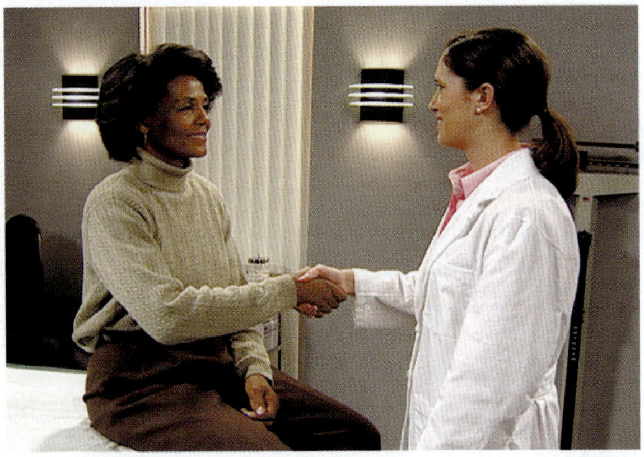

FIG. 7.2 During the initial greeting, observe the patient for behavior, emotional status, grooming, and body language. Note the patient's body posture and ability to make eye contact.

TABLE 7.1 Common Causes of Unresponsiveness

TYPE OF DISORDER	CAUSE
Focal lesions of the brain	Hemorrhage, hematoma, infarction, tumor, abscess, trauma
Diffuse brain dysfunction	Drug intoxications Disturbances of glucose, sodium, or calcium metabolism; renal failure; myxedema; pulmonary insufficiency Hypothermia, hyperthermia Hypoxic or anoxic event such as strangulation, drowning, cardiac arrest, pulmonary embolism Encephalitis, meningitis Seizures
Psychogenic unresponsiveness	Catatonia, severe depression, conversion disorder

Physical Appearance and Behavior

Grooming

Assess the patient's hygiene, grooming, and appropriateness of dress for age and season. Poor hygiene, lack of concern with appearance, or inappropriate dress for season or occasion may occur in individuals with depression, another psychiatric disorder, or dementia.

Emotional Status

Note the patient's overall behavior and demeanor. The patient's manner should demonstrate concern appropriate for the topics discussed. Consider cultural variations when assessing emotional responses. Note patient behavior that conveys carelessness, apathy, loss of sympathetic reactions, unusual docility, hostility, rage reactions, or excessive irritability.

Nonverbal Communication (Body Language)

Note the patient's posture, eye contact, and facial expression. Some cultural groups will not maintain eye contact with others. Slumped posture and a lack of facial expression may indicate depression or a neurologic condition such as Parkinson disease. Excessively energetic movements or constantly watchful eyes suggest tension, mania, anxiety, a metabolic disorder, or the effects of recreational or prescription drug use (e.g., methamphetamine, amphetamine salts, opioids, cocaine, and steroids).

State of Consciousness

Assess the patient's orientation to person, place, and time with responses to questions as well as to physical and environmental stimuli. Person disorientation may result from cerebral trauma, seizures, or amnesia. Place disorientation occurs with psychiatric disorders, delirium, and cognitive impairment. Time disorientation is associated with anxiety, delirium, depression, and cognitive impairment.

See Table 7.1 for potential causes of unresponsiveness. The Glasgow Coma Scale is used to quantify the level of consciousness after an acute brain injury or medical condition (see Chapter 26).

Cognitive Abilities

Evaluate cognitive functions from the patient's responses to questions during the history. Specific questions and tasks can provide a detailed assessment of cognition, the execution of complex mental processes (e.g., learning, perceiving, decision making, and memory). See tools (e.g., Montreal Cognitive Assessment and Mini-Cog) later in the chapter to assess cognitive function in older adults if quantification is needed.

Signs of possible cognitive impairment include the following: significant memory loss; confusion (impaired cognitive function with disorientation, attention and memory deficits, and difficulty answering questions or following multiple-step directions); impaired communication; inappropriate affect; personal care difficulties; aggressive behavior; agitation; and suspiciousness (see Clinical Pearl, "The Importance of Collateral Information").

CLINICAL PEARL

The Importance of Collateral Information

Talk with a family member or friend of the patient if you have any concerns about a patient's responses or behavior. Ask whether the patient has any problems remembering appointments or important events; paying bills; shopping independently for food, clothing, or other goods; preparing meals; taking medication; getting lost while walking or driving; making decisions about daily life; or asking the same question again and again.

Analogies

Ask the patient to describe simple analogies first and then more complex analogies:

- What is similar about these objects: Peaches and lemons? Ocean and lake? Trumpet and flute?
- Complete this comparison: An engine is to an airplane as an oar is to a _____.
- What is different about these two objects: A magazine and a cookbook? A bush and a tree?

Correct responses should be given when the patient has average intelligence. An inability to describe similarities or differences may indicate a lesion of the left or dominant cerebral hemisphere.

Abstract Reasoning

Ask the patient to tell you the meaning of a fable, proverb, or metaphor, such as the following:

- A stitch in time saves nine.
- A bird in the hand is worth two in the bush.
- A rolling stone gathers no moss.

When the patient has average intelligence, an adequate interpretation should be given. Inability to explain a phrase may indicate poor cognition, dementia, brain trauma, or psychiatric illness like schizophrenia.

Arithmetic Calculation

Ask the patient to do simple arithmetic, without use of an electronic device or paper and pen, such as the following:

- Subtract 7 from 50, subtract 7 from that answer, and so on, until the answer is 8.
- Add 8 to 50, add 8 to that total, and so on, until the answer is 98.

The calculations should be completed with few errors and within 1 minute when the patient has average intelligence. Impairment of arithmetic skills may be associated with depression, cognitive impairment, and diffuse brain dysfunction.

Writing Ability

For a comprehensive mental status examination, ask the patient to write their name and address or a dictated phrase. Omission or addition of letters, syllables, words, or mirror writing may indicate aphasia (impairment of comprehension or language formulation). Alternatively, if low literacy is a concern, ask the patient to draw simple geometric figures (e.g., a triangle, circle, or square) and then more complex figures such as a clock face, house, or flower. Uncoordinated writing or drawing may indicate dementia, parietal lobe damage, a cerebellar lesion, or peripheral neuropathy.

Execution of Motor Skills

Ask the patient to unbutton a shirt button or tie a shoelace. Apraxia (the inability to translate an intention into action that is unrelated to paralysis or lack of comprehension) may indicate a cerebral disorder.

Memory

Immediate recall or new learning: Ask the patient to listen and then repeat a sentence or a series of numbers. Five to eight numbers or words forward or four to six numbers or words backward can usually be repeated.

Recent memory: Give the patient a short time to view four or five test objects, telling them that you will ask about the objects in a few minutes. Ten minutes later, ask the patient to list the objects. All objects should be remembered. (See Clinical Pearl, "Testing Memory in a Patient With Visual Impairment.")

Remote memory: Ask the patient about verifiable past events or information such as their city of birth, high school attended, or a subject of common knowledge.

Memory loss may result from chronic disease, acute infection, or temporal lobe trauma. Impaired memory occurs with various neurologic or psychiatric disorders, such as anxiety and depression. Loss of immediate and recent memory with retention of remote memory suggests dementia.

CLINICAL PEARL

Testing Memory in a Patient With Visual Impairment

When a patient is visually impaired, test recent memory with unrelated words rather than observed objects. Pick four unrelated words that sound distinctly different, such as "green," "daffodil," "hero," and "sofa" or "bird," "carpet," "treasure," and "orange." Tell the patient to remember these words. After 5 minutes, ask the patient to list the four words.

Attention Span

Ask the patient to follow a short set of commands. Alternatively, ask the patient to say either the days of the week or to spell the word "world" forward or backward. The ability to perform arithmetic calculations is another test of attention span. Appropriate response to directions is expected. Easy distraction, confusion, negativism, and impairment of recent and remote memory may all indicate a decreased attention span. This may be related to fatigue, depression, delirium, or toxic or metabolic causes that result in confusion.

Judgment

Determine the patient's judgment and reasoning skills by exploring the following topics:

- How is the patient meeting personal, social, and family obligations?
- What are the patient's plans for the future? Do they seem appropriate?
- Ask the patient to provide solutions to hypothetical situations, such as: "What would you do if you found someone's wallet?" or "What would you do if a police officer gave you a ticket after you drove through a red light?"

If the patient is meeting personal, social, and family obligations and adequately dealing with financial obligations, judgment is generally considered intact. The patient should be able to evaluate the situations presented and

DIFFERENTIAL DIAGNOSIS

Distinguishing Characteristics of Aphasias

CHARACTERISTICS	BROCA APHASIA (EXPRESSIVE)	WERNICKE APHASIA (RECEPTIVE)	GLOBAL APHASIA (EXPRESSIVE AND RECEPTIVE)
Word comprehension	Fair to good	Can hear words but cannot relate them to previous experiences	Absent or reduced to a person's own name, few select words
Spontaneous speech	Impaired speech flow; laborious effort to speak; know what they want to say but cannot articulate properly; telegraphic speech (mostly nouns and verbs)	Fluent speech but uses words inappropriately, such as neologisms or word substitutions; may be totally incomprehensible	Absent or reduced to only a few words or sounds
Reading comprehension	Intact	Impaired	Severely impaired
Writing	Impaired	Impaired	Severely impaired

recognize the consequences of action. Impaired judgment may indicate intellectual disability, emotional disturbance, frontal lobe injury, dementia, or psychosis.

Speech and Language Skills

An in-depth evaluation of the patient's language skills, both receptive and expressive, should be performed if they have difficulty communicating during the history. The patient's voice should have inflections, be clear and strong, and be able to increase in volume. Determine whether the patient's rate of speech is excessively fast or slow, normal, or has hesitations. Speech should be fluent with a clear expression of thoughts.

Voice Quality

Determine whether there is any difficulty or discomfort in phonation or if abnormal speech sounds are present. Dysphonia, a disorder of voice volume, quality (e.g., harsh, nasal, or breathy), or pitch (e.g., monotony of pitch or loudness), suggests a problem with laryngeal innervation or disease of the larynx.

Articulation

Evaluate spontaneous speech for pronunciation and ease of expression. Abnormal articulation includes imprecise pronunciation of consonants, slurring, difficulty articulating a single speech sound, hesitations, repetitions, and stuttering. Dysarthria, a motor speech disorder, is associated with many conditions of the nervous system such as stroke, alcohol intoxication, cerebral palsy, and Parkinson disease.

Comprehension

Ask the patient to follow simple one- and two-step directions as you perform the examination, such as during the attention span assessment. The patient should be able to follow simple instructions.

Coherence

The patient's intentions or perceptions should be clearly conveyed to you. Communication characteristics that may be associated with a psychiatric disorder include the following:

- Circumlocution—use of an unnecessarily large number of words to avoid revealing a word was forgotten
- Perseveration—repetition of a word, phrase, or gesture
- Flight of ideas or use of loose associations—disordered words or sentences
- Word salad—meaningless, disconnected word choices
- Neologisms—made-up words that have meaning only to the patient
- Clang association—word choice based on sound so that words rhyme in a nonsensical way (e.g., the far car mar to the star)
- Echolalia—Repetition of another person's words
- Utterances of unusual sounds

Aphasia, a speech disorder that can be receptive (understanding language) or expressive (speaking language), may be indicated by hesitations and other speech rhythm disturbances, omission of syllables or words, word transposition, circumlocutions, and neologisms. Aphasia can result from facial muscle or tongue weakness or from neurologic damage to brain regions controlling speech and language. Characteristics of different types of aphasia are listed in the Differential Diagnosis box following this section.

Emotional Stability

Emotional stability should be evaluated when a patient does not seem to be coping well or does not have the resources to meet their personal needs.

Mood and Feelings

During the history and physical examination, observe the mood and emotional expression from the patient's verbal and nonverbal behaviors. Note any mood swings or behaviors indicating anxiety, depression, anger, hostility, or hypervigilance.

Ask the patient how they feel right now, whether feelings are a problem in daily life, and whether any time or experience is particularly difficult for the patient. The U.S. Preventive Services Task Force recommends depression screening of all adults using the self-administered Patient Health Questionnaire (PHQ) (U.S. Preventive Services Task Force, 2023). Two- and nine-item versions of the PHQ exist. The PHQ-2 questions are:

- Over the past 2 weeks, have you felt down, depressed, or hopeless?
- Over the past 2 weeks, have you felt little interest or pleasure in doing things?

If the response is positive to both questions, perform the PHQ-9 or explore depressive symptoms with additional questions, such as trouble sleeping or sleeping too much, moving too slow or restlessness, poor appetite or overeating, poor concentration, feeling like a failure, or thoughts of hurting oneself. The PHQ-9 is a valid and sensitive tool for identifying a major depressive disorder in adults (Nandakumar et al., 2019). This tool has been translated into several languages and is publicly available.

Be concerned if the patient's behaviors do not correspond to a situation being discussed. For example, does the patient laugh when talking about a seriously ill family member? Hopelessness, agitation, aggression, anger, euphoria, irritability, or wide mood swings indicate disturbances in mood, affect, and feelings.

Suicide is a leading cause of death in the United States, with over 40,000 fatalities in persons 10 years and older in 2021 (Nguyen et al., 2024). Although universal suicide risk screening is strongly encouraged, assessing suicide risk is particularly important when a patient exhibits signs or symptoms of depression. See "Risk Factors: Suicide." Two questions on the Columbia-Suicide Severity Risk Screener (C-SSRS) help identify the patient at higher risk for suicide ideation and behavior:

- Have you wished you were dead or wished you could go to sleep and not wake up?
- Have you actually had any thoughts of killing yourself?

A positive response to the second item places the patient at higher risk, especially if the patient made any recent preparations for how to end their life. Implement a patient safety monitoring plan with the patient and family, and obtain an immediate psychiatry referral if preparations have occurred within the past two to three weeks. Arrange a more thorough suicide risk assessment for other patients with a positive response (Posner et al., 2016). Full access to the C-SSRS is available at https://cssrs.columbia.edu/wp-content/uploads/C-SSRS_Pediatric-SLC_11.14.16.pdf. Patients, family members, and clinicians can call the 988 Suicide & Crisis Lifeline or chat 988lifeline.org 24 hours per day, 7 days per week for confidential support in the United States.

Risk Factors

Suicide

- Personal history of suicide attempts
- Depression or other psychiatric disorder
- Substance use disorder
- Chronic pain
- Family history of psychiatric disorder or substance use
- Exposure to family violence, including physical or sexual abuse
- Presence of guns or other firearms in the home
- Having recently been released from prison or jail
- Exposure, either directly or indirectly, to suicidal behavior of others (e.g., family, peers, celebrities)
- Stressful life events (legal or financial difficulty, loss of a loved one, relationship challenges, bullying)

From Suicide Prevention—National Institute of Mental Health (NIMH) at https://www.nimh.nih.gov/health/topics/suicide-prevention#part_2474

Thought Process and Content

Observe the patient's thought patterns, especially the appropriateness of sequence, logic, coherence, and relevance to the topics discussed. The patient's thought process should be easy to follow with logical and goal-directed ideas expressed. Illogical, disorganized, or unrealistic thought processes, flight of ideas (rapid disconnected thoughts), blocking (i.e., an inappropriate pause in the middle of a thought, phrase, or sentence), or an impaired stream of thinking (e.g., repetition of a word, phrase, or behavior) indicates an emotional disturbance or a psychiatric disorder.

Evaluate disturbance in thought content by asking about obsessive thoughts related to fears, guilt, or making decisions. Does the patient ever feel like they are being watched or followed, controlled or manipulated, or losing touch with reality? Does the patient compulsively repeat actions or check and recheck to make sure something is done? Obsessive thoughts, compulsive behaviors, phobias, or anxieties that interfere with daily life should be further evaluated by a mental health professional.

Does the patient have delusions (false personal beliefs not shared by others in the same culture), such as delusions of grandeur or of being controlled by an outside force? Does the patient feel unrealistic persecution, jealousy, or paranoia? Delusions are often associated with psychiatric disorders, delirium, and alcohol or drug intoxication. (See Clinical Pearl, "Cognitive Distortions.")

CLINICAL PEARL

Cognitive Distortions

A patient who demonstrates an unrealistic sense of persecution, jealousy, grandiose ideas, irrational thought or belief, or ideas of reference (e.g., neutral things in the environment have a special meaning to the person) may be experiencing cognitive distortions.

MENTAL STATUS

Perceptual Distortions and Hallucinations

Determine whether the patient perceives any sensations that are not caused by external stimuli (e.g., hears voices, sees vivid images or shadowy figures, smells offensive odors, tastes offensive flavors, feels worms crawling on the skin). Find out when these experiences occur. Auditory and visual hallucinations are associated with psychiatric disorders, severe depression, acute intoxication, withdrawal, delirium, and dementia. Tactile hallucinations are most commonly associated with alcohol withdrawal.

Infants and Children

Evaluate an infant's general behavior and level of consciousness by observing their activity and responsiveness to caregivers and environmental stimuli. Note whether the baby is lethargic, drowsy, stuporous, alert, active, or irritable (Fig. 7.3A). By 2 months of age, the infant should appear alert, quiet, and content and should recognize the face of a primary caregiver (see Fig. 7.3B). The examiner who devotes time to developing a relationship with a 2- to 3-month old infant should be able to coax a smile. When it is difficult or impossible to elicit a social smile in an infant who appears ill, be concerned about a neurologic condition or infection, such as meningitis. Be concerned if the parent or primary caregiver seems detached or depressed. An infant's social and emotional development is heavily influenced by interaction with the primary caregiver.

Crying and other vocal sounds are evaluated when language has not yet developed. The infant's cry should be loud and angry. A shrill or whiny, high-pitched cry or catlike screeching cry suggests a central nervous system disorder. Cooing and babbling are expected after 3 and 4 months of age, respectively.

Evaluate the types of words and speech patterns used by the child. For example, does the child pronounce most words correctly as expected for age, do persons outside the immediate family understand the child's speech, and does the child stutter? What is the child's voice quality? Does the child's voice have intonation (e.g., excitement)? Table 7.2 describes expected expressive language milestones for infants, toddlers, and preschoolers. Language development should be adjusted for prematurity, and speech should become more clearly understandable as the child ages.

Questionnaires completed by parents (e.g., Ages and Stages Questionnaire, see www.agesandstages.com; and Parent's Evaluation of Developmental Status, see www.pedstest.com) are two commonly used screening tools recommended for developmental assessment during routine well-child visits. These questionnaires have good sensitivity and specificity for detecting developmental concerns. Ask children 5 years and older to draw a picture of a person, doing the best job possible. Scores for the detail in 14 body part attributes are available to assess cognitive development (Kwan, 2018) (Fig. 7.4).

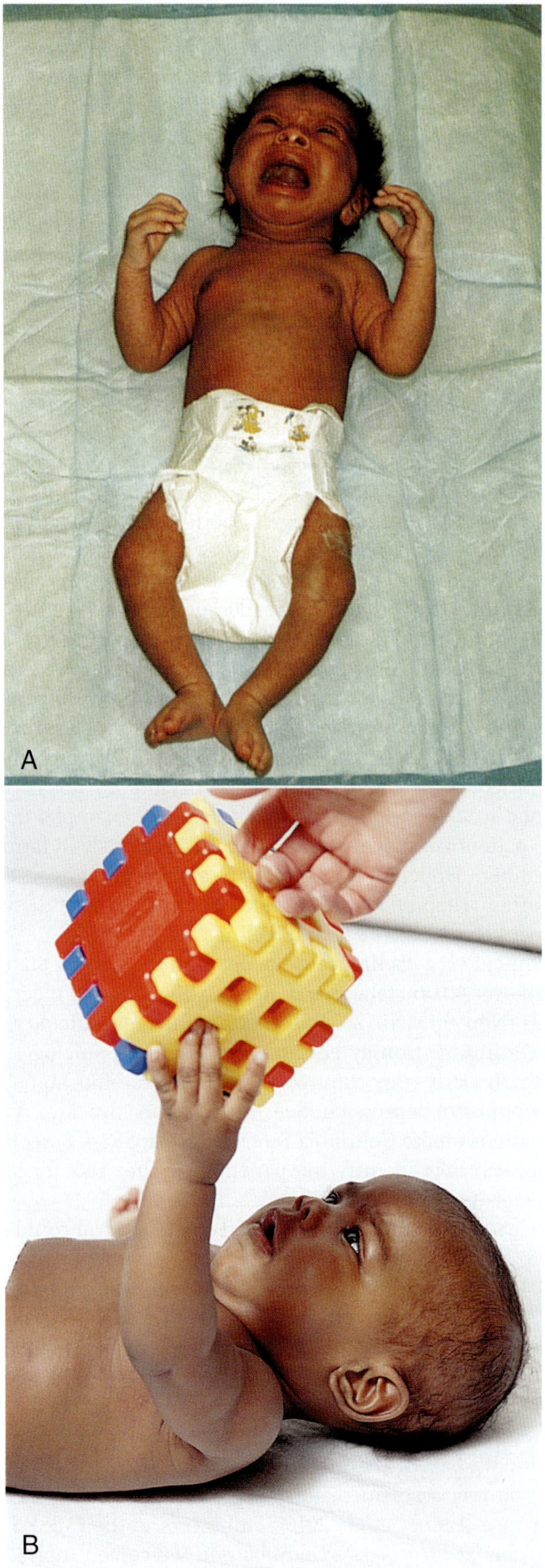

A

B

FIG. 7.3 (A) Note this newborn's irritability and posturing associated with neonatal abstinence syndrome. (B) Note this infant's level of alertness and interest in various objects and people.

TABLE 7.2 Expressive Language Milestones for Toddlers and Preschoolers

AGE (MONTHS)	EXPRESSIVE LANGUAGE MILESTONES
4–6	Babbles speechlike sounds, including p, b, and m
10–12	Imitates different speech sounds, has 1 or 2 words, such as "mama," "dada," "bye-bye," but sounds may not be clear
12–24	Increases words each month, two-word questions or phrases (e.g., "Where baby?" and "Want cookie")
24–36	Uses two- to three-word sentences to ask for things Large vocabulary, speech understood by family members most of the time
36–48	Answers simple questions, talks about activities Sentences have four or more words, speech understood by most people
48–60	Says most sounds correctly, except l, s, r, v, z, ch, sh, and th Uses sentences, gives many details Tells stories and stays on topic

Data from National Institutes of Health, National Institute on Deafness and Other Communication Disorders (2017).

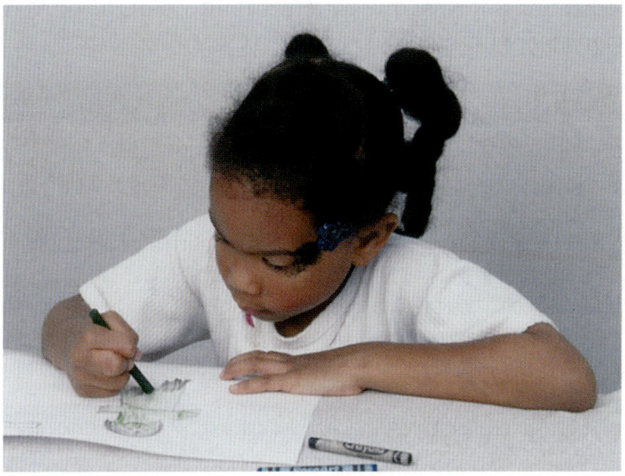

FIG. 7.4 Ask the child to draw a picture of a person. The presence and form of body parts provide a clue about the child's development when following the scoring criteria of the Goodenough-Harris Drawing Test.

Observe the child's behaviors while obtaining the history to identify mood, activity level, communication pattern, preferences, responsiveness to the parent or caregiver, and ability to separate. Does the child have self-comforting measures? Does the child play and have fun?

Attempt memory testing at about 4 years of age if the child pays attention and is not too anxious. Expected memory skills vary with the age of the child. When testing immediate recall, a 4-year-old can typically repeat three digits or words, a 5-year-old can repeat four digits or words, and a 6-year-old can repeat five digits or words. Test recent memory in a child starting at 5 to 6 years by showing the child familiar objects and waiting no longer than 5 minutes to ask the child to recall the objects (Fig. 7.5).

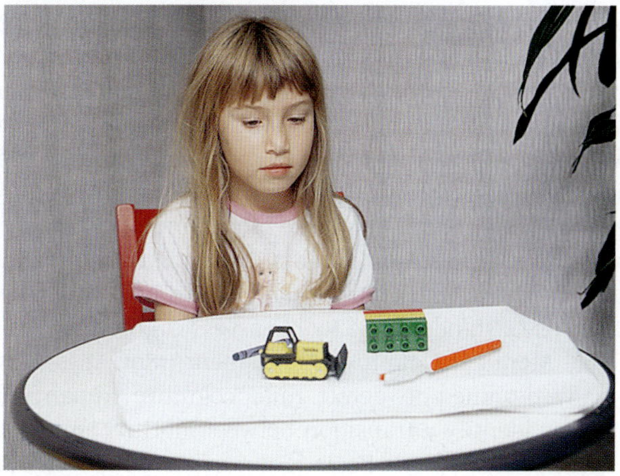

FIG. 7.5 Test a child's memory recall by using familiar objects.

Remote memory is tested by asking the child to recite a nursery rhyme, say what they had for dinner last night, or tell you the name of their school.

Concerns about behaviors and mood disorders may be assessed in children 4 to 18 years of age with validated tools like the Pediatric Symptom Checklist (https://www.massgeneral.org/psychiatry/treatments-and-services/pediatric-symptom-checklist). An adolescent version of the PHQ-9 is also available to screen for depression. Positive responses should prompt questions about school, family, friends, moods, and activities.

Pregnant Patients

An estimated 39% of patients who have depression during pregnancy will experience postpartum depression. Overall, about 13% of patients have postpartum depression, and postpartum psychosis occurs in up to 3% of postpartum patients (Wilkinson et al., 2017). Risk factors for postpartum depression include a history of depression, postpartum depression after a previous birth, and poor social support. Because depression may interfere with the patient's health, ability to work, personal relationships, attachment to the newborn, and the infant's subsequent development, all pregnant patients should be screened for depressive symptoms during and after pregnancy, including during routine well-child visits.

The PHQ-2 described in the section on "Mood and Feelings" can be used for screening. When a screening is positive for depressive symptoms, explore with additional questions. The Edinburgh Postnatal Depression Scale is a 10-item self-administered screening tool that may be used during pregnancy and in the postpartum period. Patients are asked to identify the frequency of feelings (e.g., happy, anxious or worried, scared or panicky, and sad or miserable) over the past 7 days. See https://psychology-tools.com/epds/for access to this tool.

Older Adults

Assess cognitive function to identify mild impairment that may indicate the onset of dementia or cognitive changes associated with normal aging. As with all adults, assess the patient's response to questions and directions throughout the history and physical examination. Recent memory for important events and conversations is usually not impaired. An older adult may complain about episodic memory loss, but this is not predictive of cognitive decline. The concern of a close family member or friend about the patient's memory loss or a patient's report that memory loss interfered with daily activities is an indication to use a standardized tool to assess cognition.

The Montreal Cognitive Assessment (MoCA) is a tool initially designed to detect mild cognitive impairment that may identify a transition between normal aging and dementia. The MoCA-Basic is a version for low-literacy adults. This tool also helps identify patients needing a more comprehensive cognitive assessment. See "Evidence-Based Practice in Physical Examination: Montreal Cognitive Assessment Battery."

Evidence-Based Practice in Physical Examination

Montreal Cognitive Assessment Battery

The Montreal Cognitive Assessment tools (MoCA and low-literacy MoCA-Basic) include items in the following domains, providing a broader assessment of cognitive status than the Mini-Mental State Examination (MMSE):

- Immediate and delayed memory recall
- Visuospatial abilities with clock drawing and copying a three-dimensional cube
- Executive functioning with trailmaking, phonemic fluency, and verbal abstraction tasks
- Attention, concentration, working memory, sustained attention, serial subtraction, and digits forward and backward tasks
- Language with identification of low-familiarity animals, repetition of two complex sentences
- Orientation to time and place

It has more cognitively demanding tasks related to memory recall and executive functioning than the MMSE and takes approximately 10 to 15 minutes to administer. With a cutoff score of 24 in a 30-point test, the MoCA-Basic has a sensitivity of 79.5% and specificity of 83.7% in the identification of mild cognitive impairment in a general practice population (Islam et al., 2023). The MoCA was found to better discriminate between patients with mild cognitive impairment and no cognitive impairment than the MMSE, though both screening tools can accurately detect patients with Alzheimer disease (Pinto et al., 2019). For access to the screening tool, visit www.mocatest.org.

The Mini-Cog is another screening tool for measuring cognitive function that takes up to 5 minutes to administer. It involves immediate and delayed recall of three unrelated words and a clock-drawing test (see Fig. 7.6 for test administration and scoring guidelines). A score of 0 to 5 points is possible, and a score of 2 or less may be associated with dementia. In a systematic review, the Mini-Cog had a sensitivity of 76% and specificity of 83% for detecting dementia across adult health care settings (Abayomi et al., 2024). It has been used successfully in non–English-speaking and culturally diverse populations as well as those with varying educational levels.

The MMSE is a standardized tool to assess cognitive function changes over time. The 11 items—measuring orientation, registration, attention and calculation, recall, ability to follow commands, and language—take approximately 5 to 10 minutes to administer. Fig. 7.7 shows testing of the copying skill under the language portion of the MMSE. The maximum score is 30. A score of 20 or less may be associated with dementia, and a score of 26 or higher is not associated with dementia. The MMSE has been translated into multiple languages and adapted for many cultures; however, age, ethnicity, and education have an impact on scoring (Hwang et al., 2019). MMSE Version 2 was developed to replace problematic items and to improve item translation (Folstein and Folstein, 2020).

Determine whether any changes in cerebral function could be the result of cardiovascular, hepatic, renal, or metabolic disease. Medications can also impair central nervous system function, causing slowed reaction time, disorientation, confusion, loss of memory, tremors, and anxiety. Problems may develop because of the dosage, number, or interaction of prescribed and over-the-counter medications. Review the patient's ability to perform ADLs associated with mental status.

FUNCTIONAL ASSESSMENT

Activities of Daily Living Related to Mental Status

The ability to perform basic and instrumental activities of daily living (ADLs), or the ability to live independently, is an important assessment. When assessing the patient's mental status, attempt to determine the patient's ability to perform the following ADLs:

- Shop, cook, and prepare meals
- Personal hygiene (includes bathing and dental, nail, and hair care)
- Manage medications (includes obtaining medications and taking them as directed)
- Manage personal finances (includes paying bills and managing assets)
- Cleaning and home maintenance
- Communicating with others (includes ability to seek help when needed)
- Remember appointments, family occasions, holidays, and household tasks

Edemekong, P. F., Bomgaars, D. L., Sukumaran, S., et al. (2024). Activities of daily living. [Updated June 26, 2023]. In StatPearls [Internet]. Treasure Island, FL: StatPearls Publishing. https://www.ncbi.nlm.nih.gov/books/NBK470404/

Older adults are expected to maintain the same level of interpersonal skills and have no personality changes. Depression, one of the most common conditions in older adults, may contribute to cognitive impairment. Depression can be identified with the Geriatric Depression Scale (Fig. 7.8). Paranoid thought may be a striking alteration in personality. Attempt to determine whether the thought process is accurate or a paranoid ideation, keeping in mind the incidence of elder abuse. Facial expressions that are masklike or overly dramatic or a stance that is stooped and fearful may indicate a progressive disease in an older adult.

The Mini-Cog Assessment Instrument for Dementia

The Mini-Cog assessment instrument combines an uncued three-item recall test with a clock-drawing test (CDT). The Mini-Cog can be administered in about three minutes, requires no special equipment, and is relatively uninfluenced by level of education or language variations.

Administration

The test is administered as follows:

1. Instruct the patient to listen carefully to and remember three unrelated words and then to repeat the words.

2. Instruct the patient to draw the face of a clock, either on a blank sheet of paper or on a sheet with the clock circle already drawn on the page. After the patient puts the numbers on the clock face, ask their to draw the hands of the clock to read a specific time, such as 11:20. These instructions can be repeated, but no additional instructions should be given. Give the patient as much time as needed to complete the task. The CDT serves as the recall distractor.

3. Ask the patient to repeat the three previously presented words.

Scoring

Give 1 point for each recalled word after the CDT distractor. Score 1 to 3.

A score of O indicates positive screen for dementia.

A score of 1 or 2 with an abnormal CDT indicates positive screen for dementia.

A score of 1 or 2 with a normal CDT indicates negative screen for dementia.

A score of 3 indicates negative screen for dementia.

The CDT is considered normal if all numbers are present in the correct sequence and position, and the hands readably display the requested time.

FIG. 7.6 The Mini-Cog is a brief screening tool for measuring cognitive function. Borson S, et al: The Mini-Cog: a cognitive 'vital signs' measure for dementia screening in multi-lingual elderly. *Int J Geriatr Psychiatry* 15 (11):1021-1027, 2000.

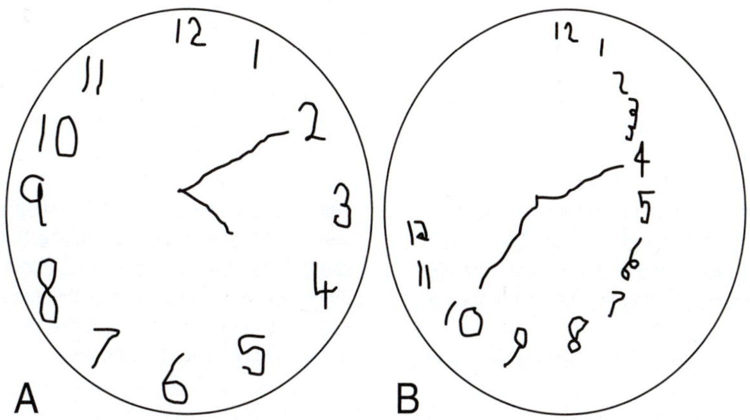

FIG. 7.7 (A) Acceptable drawing of a clock with numbers appropriately spaced around the face and the requested time of 10 minutes after 4 o'clock noted correctly by the long and short hands. (B) Unacceptable drawing that shows poor planning regarding number placement around the clock face and hands pointing to the 10 and 4, for 10 minutes after 4 o'clock. Stern, T. A., Fricchione, G. L., et al. (2010). *Massachusetts general hospital handbook of general hospital psychiatry* (6th ed.). Philadelphia: Elsevier.

Ask the patient to choose the best answer for how their felt over the preceding week.

1. Are you basically satisfied with your life?	Yes/No
2. Have you dropped many of your activities and interests?	Yes/No
3. Do you feel that your life is empty?	Yes/No
4. Do you often get bored?	Yes/No
5. Are you in good spirits most of the time?	Yes/No
6. Are you afraid that something bad is going to happen to you?	Yes/No
7. Do you feel happy most of the time?	Yes/No
8. Do you feel helpless?	Yes/No
9. Do you prefer to stay at home rather than going out and doing new things?	Yes/No
10. Do you feel you have more problems with memory than most people?	Yes/No
11. Do you think it is wonderful to be alive now?	Yes/No
12. Do you feel pretty worthless the way you are now?	Yes/No
13. Do you feel full of energy?	Yes/No
14. Do you feel that your situation is hopeless?	Yes/No
15. Do you think most people are better off than you are?	Yes/No

Correct responses are the following:
Yes for questions 2, 3, 4, 6, 8, 9, 10, 12, 14, and 15.
No for questions 1, 5, 7, 11, and 13.
Give 1 point for each correct answer. A score greater than 5 suggests depression.

FIG. 7.8 Geriatric Depression Scale (short form). Sheikh J.I., Yesavage J.A.: Geriatric depression scale: recent evidence and development of a shorter version, *Clin Gerontol* 5:165-172, 1986.

Patient Safety

Living Arrangements for Older Adults

When impairment in the ability to perform ADLs is identified, determine safety in an older adult's living arrangements. Is a caregiver present in the home, or does someone check in each day? Is food delivered to the home, or are meals provided? Are medication dosages provided or monitored? Has the older adult stopped driving a car? How well can they safely move around the home? If safety is a concern, have a discussion with the older adult's family member or friend to encourage changes that will improve safety.

Think About It

Mental Status

An older adult expresses concern about forgetfulness, such as not remembering her last appointment to see you. She lives alone, her closest family members live an hour away, and she worries about being a burden to her family. During the history, she responded to all questions indicating good recall, an ability to shop for and prepare healthy meals, and take her prescribed medications. During the physical examination, she followed two-step directions correctly. Findings indicate appropriate cognitive functioning at this time. If concerns about cognitive function were revealed, a validated tool such as the MoCA could help reveal mild cognitive impairment.

ABNORMALITIES

MENTAL STATUS

Disorders of Altered Mental Status

Traumatic Brain Injury. Brain injury resulting from an outside force like a blow, forceful bump, or jolt to the head or body or an object penetrating the brain

PATHOPHYSIOLOGY	PATIENT DATA
Concussion (Mild TBI) A direct blow to the head or rapid movement of the brain within and against the skull; often caused by a sports injury, motor vehicle crash, or fall	**Subjective Data** • Headache • Dazed or dizzy, may have a brief loss of consciousness • Nausea and vomiting • Blurred vision • Ringing in ears • Restless or irritable **Objective Data** • Dazed expression • Slow motor and verbal responses, slurred speech • Emotional lability • Hypersensitivity to stimuli • Deficits in coordination, cognition, memory, and attention • Symptoms may disappear within 15 min or persist for several weeks to months • See the Sports Concussion Assessment Tool in Chapter 25
Chronic Traumatic Encephalopathy Progressive neurologic disorder from repetitive head injuries over many years, including repeated concussions in individuals playing contact sports or in military service	**Subjective Data** • Difficulty thinking, communicating, and memory loss • Impaired judgment • Sleep disturbance **Objective Data** • Depression • Confusion and irritability • Emotional lability • Impulsive behavior • Aggression
Moderate to Severe Brain Injury Higher forces cause acceleration-deceleration and rotational movement of the brain in the skull. Nerve fibers are stretched, compressed, or torn. Brain chemicals responsible for brain functioning are disrupted, and inflammation leads to brain swelling (see Chapter 23).	**Subjective Data** • May be in a minimally conscious state with some awareness of environment and ability to respond to simple commands **Objective Data** • Unresponsive wakefulness syndrome (unconscious with periods of alertness) • Coma (unconscious, unaware, and unable to respond to stimuli) • Glasgow Coma Score <13 (see Chapter 26) • Increased intracranial pressure • Seizures

Disorders of Mood

Depression. A mood disorder in which feelings of sadness, loss, anger, or frustration interfere with everyday life for an extended period (weeks or longer).

PATHOPHYSIOLOGY

Although the cause is unknown, likely involves disturbance in serotonin and other neurotransmitter activity.

Multifactorial with genetic and environmental influences.

Higher rates occur in patients with neurodegenerative diseases, stroke, cancer, seizure disorders, chronic pain, and other illnesses.

Traumatic and stressful life events, grief, interpersonal difficulties, caregiver burden, and lack of social support can trigger depression.

PATIENT DATA

Subjective Data

- Feelings of sadness, emptiness, hopelessness, worthlessness, guilt
- Loss of interest or pleasure in what was previously of interest or pleasurable
- Irritable mood
- Fatigue or loss of energy
- Insomnia or excessive sleeping
- Increased or decreased appetite; weight gain or loss (>5%) in a month

Objective Data

- Poor concentration
- Slowed thought processes and speech
- Agitation, irritability, or restlessness
- See the Differential Diagnosis table later in the chapter

Mania. A persistently elevated, expansive, euphoric, or irritable and agitated mood lasting longer than a week; one phase of bipolar I disorder usually followed by depressive episodes.

PATHOPHYSIOLOGY

Although the cause is unknown, likely the result of a combination of genetic, psychological, and social factors.

30%–50% of patients with bipolar disorder have a co-occurring substance use disorder (Substance Abuse and Mental Health Services Administration, 2016).

PATIENT DATA

Subjective Data

- Hyperactivity
- Overconfidence, exaggerated view of own abilities
- Impaired occupational, social, and interpersonal functioning
- Excessive involvement in pleasurable activities with high potential for serious or painful consequences
- Decreased need for sleep
- Racing thoughts
- Lack of impulse control

Objective Data

- Grandiose or persecutory delusions, euphoria
- Increased talkativeness or pressure to keep talking, may involve excessive rhyming or puns; flight of ideas
- Impaired attention, easily distracted
- Impaired judgment
- Hypersexual behavior

Anxiety Disorder. A group of disorders with such marked anxiety or fear that it causes significant interference with personal, social, and occupational functioning.

PATHOPHYSIOLOGY

- Norepinephrine, serotonin, dopamine, and gamma-aminobutyric acid (GABA) are thought to be mediators of anxiety; activation of the amygdala and limbic system play a role.
- Genetic and environmental factors may underlie risk for anxiety.

Specific disorders include the following:

Panic attacks
Generalized anxiety disorder
Specific phobias
Obsessive-compulsive disorder (OCD)
Posttraumatic stress disorder (PTSD)

PATIENT DATA

Subjective Data

- *Panic attacks:* palpitations, sweating, shaking, dizziness, faintness, chest pain, nausea, abdominal distress, chills or hot flashes, chronic social avoidance, fear of losing control and dying

Objective Data

- *Panic attacks:* tachycardia, diaphoresis, tremors

Subjective Data

- *Generalized anxiety disorder:* chronic worry, restlessness, irritability, tension, fatigue, poor concentration, sleep disturbance

Objective Data

- *Generalized anxiety disorder:* impaired attention, motor tension, tremors, restlessness

Subjective Data

- *OCD:* preoccupation with contamination or religious or sexual themes; belief that failure to perform a specific act will lead to a bad outcome

Objective Data

- *OCD:* Ritualized acts performed compulsively (washing, cleaning, hoarding, organizing, counting)

Subjective Data

- *PTSD:* recurrent intrusive flashbacks (e.g., images, odors, sounds, and negative emotions), dreams, thoughts; avoidance behavior; sleeping difficulty; hypervigilance; poor concentration

Objective Data

- *PTSD:* anger or rage reactions, impulsive behavior, hyperarousal, emotional numbing, detachment from others

Schizophrenia. A severe, persistent, psychotic syndrome with impaired reality that relapses throughout life.

PATHOPHYSIOLOGY

Complex genetic disorder that involves many genes on different chromosomes in patients who are vulnerable because of factors such as intrauterine infection, maternal nutritional deficiencies, perinatal complications, and neonatal hypoxia. Structural brain abnormalities exist such as enlarged lateral and third ventricles, reduced size of the temporal lobe and thalamus, and abnormal amygdala connectivity, which has a role in social and emotional processing networks (Takahashi, 2019).

PATIENT DATA

Subjective Data

- Hears voices
- Unpleasant tastes or odors
- Sees images
- Paranoid thoughts
- Unable to experience emotions, blunted affect, apathy, detached from environment
- Poor personal hygiene

Objective Data

- Incoherent speech, loose associations, illogical answers to questions
- Hallucinations (tactile, auditory, visual, somatic, gustatory, or olfactory)
- Delusions
- Repetitive or aimless behavior
- Inappropriate affect in response to a situation

Infants and Children

Intellectual Disability

A neurodevelopmental condition that impairs cognitive and adaptive function and typically begins before 18 years of age.

PATHOPHYSIOLOGY

May be associated with structural brain defects, genetic disorders (e.g., Down syndrome, fragile X syndrome), environmental exposures (e.g., fetal alcohol syndrome), inborn error of metabolism (e.g., phenylketonuria), or serious brain insult (infection or injury) during neonatal period or childhood

Genetic link (e.g., parents have intellectual disability)

Cause may not be identified

PATIENT DATA

Subjective Data

- Delayed motor development
- Delayed speech and language skills

Objective Data

- Delayed developmental milestones
- Impaired cognitive function and short-term memory
- Poor academic performance
- Lack of motivation

Attention-Deficit/Hyperactivity Disorder

A neurobehavioral disorder characterized by three core symptoms of inattention, hyperactivity, and impulsivity that affects 11% of children aged 3 to 17 years in the United States (Centers for Disease Control and Prevention, 2024).

PATHOPHYSIOLOGY

High heritability (70%–80%) likely from genetic and environmental influences

Associated with prenatal and perinatal risk factors (e.g., prematurity, low birth weight)

Associated with intrauterine tobacco exposure, maternal stress, and obesity, though may in part be explained by confounding genetic factors (Posner et al., 2020)

Boys more than twice as likely to be diagnosed, possibly because they display more externalizing symptoms (e.g., hyperactivity and impulsiveness) compared with girls, who show more inattentiveness

Co-occurrence with other behavioral conditions (e.g., anxiety, oppositional defiant disorder, depression)

PATIENT DATA

Subjective Data

- Short attention span, easily distracted, fails to complete school assignments or follow instructions
- Forgetful, loses things necessary for tasks
- Fidgets and squirms, often moving, running, climbing
- Disruptive behavior, talks excessively, difficulty with quiet play activities, "on the go," poor impulse control

Objective Data

- Symptoms often present before 6 years of age
- Increased motor activity
- Difficulty organizing tasks
- Difficulty sustaining attention
- Poor school performance
- Low self-esteem
- Has problems in more than one setting

Autism Spectrum Disorder

A neurodevelopmental disorder with deficits in social communication, restricted interests, and repetitive behaviors.

PATHOPHYSIOLOGY

- No single causal pathway has been identified; genetic and environmental factors influence the developing brain and have been associated with autism spectrum disorder (ASD).
- Siblings of affected individuals have an increased risk of diagnosis compared with the general population.
- Advanced maternal and paternal age increase risk.
- Prevalence is 1 in 59 children in the United States (Hodges et al., 2020).

PATIENT DATA

Subjective Data

- Avoids or does not make eye contact
- Does not respond to name or show facial expressions (e.g., happy, sad) by 9 months of age
- Uses few or no gestures by 12 months of age
- Does not share interests with others by 15 months of age
- Does not point to objects by 18 months of age
- Does not notice or join other children in play by 3 years of age
- Lines up toys or other objects, becomes upset when order is changed
- Must follow certain routines

Objective Data

- Delayed language skills
- May have delay in motor skills
- May have cognitive delay
- Poor eye contact
- May become upset with certain smells, sounds, and tastes
- Repeats words or phrases (echolalia)
- Lack of interest in peers
- Repetitive movements (e.g., flaps hands, rocks body)

Older Adults

Delirium

Impaired cognition, arousal, consciousness, mood, and behavioral dysfunction of acute onset.

PATHOPHYSIOLOGY

Disorder that may arise from disturbances in neurotransmitters, inflammatory pathways, stress responses, and anatomic changes in the brain, but causes are usually multifactorial (Bennett, 2019). Advanced age is a predisposing factor. Other potential risk factors include inadequate pain management, neurovascular insult, metabolic disturbance, and medication induced.

PATIENT DATA

Subjective Data

- Suspicious, fearful
- Mood swings
- See Differential Diagnosis later in the chapter

Objective Data

- Altered consciousness, staring, unawareness, apathy, or combativeness
- Incoherence, illogical flow of ideas
- Illusions, hallucinations, delusions
- Poor memory

Dementia

A chronic progressive disorder of failing memory, cognitive impairment, behavioral abnormalities, and personality changes that often begins after age 60 years.

PATHOPHYSIOLOGY

Usually related to structural diseases of the brain. Incidence increases with advancing age.

Dementia of Alzheimer Type

Most common; accumulation of amyloid plaques and neurofibrillary tangles, deteriorating synapses, and neuron death. Presence of e4 allele gene for apolipoprotein E is present in 60% of affected persons (Ulep et al., 2019).

Vascular Dementia

About 10%–15% of cases; associated with reduced blood flow to the brain from multiple emboli and hemorrhages in different parts of the brain, stroke, or small blood vessel narrowing (Boss and Huether, 2019).

Other Dementias

Associated with diffuse Lewy bodies in the brain, Parkinson disease, and frontal lobe degeneration (Boss and Huether, 2019).

PATIENT DATA

Subjective Data

- Impaired memory, forgets appointments
- Gets lost in familiar areas, wanders
- Unable to manage shopping, food preparation, medication, finances, and driving
- Behavioral changes, such as socially inappropriate dress or conduct, impaired grooming, impulsiveness, disinhibition
- Aphasia, agnosia, apraxia
- Apathy, withdrawal
- Anxiety, irritability
- Changes in mood (depression, uncharacteristic anger, anxiety, agitation)
- See Differential Diagnosis later in this chapter

Objective Data

- Memory impairment
- Disturbance in executive functioning
- Impairment in social and occupational functioning
- Impaired use of language
- Impaired functioning in activities of daily living (ADLs)
- Eventual profound disintegration of personality and complete disorientation
- Stepwise deterioration of cognitive function with plateaus and occasional episodes of improvement characteristic of vascular dementia

DIFFERENTIAL DIAGNOSIS

Distinguishing Characteristics of Delirium, Dementia, and Depression

CHARACTERISTIC	DELIRIUM	DEMENTIA	DEPRESSION
Onset	Acute	Insidious, relentless	Acute or insidious
Duration	Hours, days	Persistent	For longer than 2 weeks
Time of day	Fluctuates during the day	Stable, no change	Throughout most of the day
Consciousness	Altered	Not impaired except in severe cases	Not impaired
Cognition	Impairment of memory, attentiveness, numerous errors in assessment tasks	Minimal cognitive impairment initially, progresses to impaired abstract thinking, judgment, memory, thought patterns, calculations, agnosia	Impaired concentration, reduced attention span, indecisiveness, slower thought processes, impaired short-term and long-term memory
Activity	Increased or decreased activity, may fluctuate	Unchanged from usual behavior	Insomnia or excessive sleeping, fatigue, restlessness, anxiety, increased or decreased appetite
Speech/language	Rambling and irrelevant conversation, illogical flow of ideas, incoherent	Disordered, rambling, incoherent; struggles to find words	Slower speech or possibly rapid speech
Mood and affect	Rapid mood swings; fearful, suspicious	Depressed, apathetic, uninterested	Sad, hopeless, feels worthless, loss of interest or pleasure
Delusions/hallucinations	Misperceptions, illusions, hallucinations, and delusions	Misperceptions usually absent, delusions, no hallucinations	Usually no delusions or hallucinations
Reversibility	Potential	No, progressive	Can be treated, may recur
Pathophysiology	Acute onset may be associated with inflammation, inadequate pain management, metabolic derangements, and medications in an older adult	Usually related to structural diseases of the brain	Associated with grief, a stressful life event, reaction to medical or neurologic diseases or a change in lifestyle

CHAPTER

8

Growth and Nutrition

An individual's weight and body composition (proportion of fat and fat distribution) offer information about current and future health status. Nutrition is considered the science of food as it relates to promoting optimal health and preventing chronic disease. A nutritional assessment is an analysis of an individual's approximate nutrient intake and relates it to the history, physical examination findings, body size measurements, and biochemical measures. This chapter focuses on the assessment of an individual's body size and nutritional status and the examination for growth, gestational age, and pubertal development.

Physical Examination Components

Nutritional Assessment

From the history and physical examination, assess the patient's nutritional status, including:

- Changes in height and weight
- Chronic illnesses affecting nutritional status or intake
- Medication and supplement use
- Assessment of nutrient intake

Growth Assessment

Obtain the following body size measurements and compare them to standardized tables:

- Standing height (ages 2 and older) or lying length (under age 2)
- Weight
- BMI (BMI percentile ages 2 to 19)
- Waist circumference (generally ages 6 and older)
- Calculate waist-height ratio (generally ages 6 and older)
- Head circumference and chest circumference (ages 2 and under)

ANATOMY AND PHYSIOLOGY

In this chapter, the terms *female* and *male* are used in order to differentiate between the body composition, physical and sexual development, and growth measurements in patients assigned as female or male at birth, respectively. This becomes important to the examination and health assessment of patients who are transgender male, transgender female, and nonbinary.

Food provides essential nutrients and calories to function in one or more of the following:

- To provide energy for activities
- To build and maintain body tissues
- To regulate body processes

The nutrients necessary to the body are classified as macronutrients (carbohydrates, protein, and fat); micronutrients (vitamins, minerals, and electrolytes); and water. Energy requirements are based on the balance of energy expenditure associated with body size, composition, and the level of physical activity. Adequate intake provides for optimal growth, development, and physical activity. Inadequate or excessive intake may negatively affect overall current or long-term health status. Adequate nutrition, from a well-balanced diet, supports growth—the increase in size of an individual or of a single organ. Growth is also dependent on a sequence of endocrine, genetic, environmental, and nutritional influences.

Hormones influence the progression and maintenance of growth and development (Fig. 8.1). Two hypothalamic hormones control growth hormone synthesis and secretion in the anterior pituitary gland. Growth hormone–releasing hormone (GHRH) stimulates the pituitary to release growth hormone. Somatostatin, or growth hormone–inhibiting hormone (GHIH), inhibits the secretion of both GHRH and thyroid-stimulating hormone (TSH). Growth hormone is secreted in pulses, with most secretion occurring during deep sleep. (Growth hormone promotes growth and increases in organ size, and it regulates carbohydrate, protein, and lipid metabolism.)

Thyroid hormone stimulates growth hormone secretion and the production of insulin-like growth factor 1 (IGF-1) and interleukins 6 and 8 (IL-6 and IL-8), which have important roles in bone formation and resorption. The thyroid hormone also affects the growth and maturation of other body tissues.

IGF-1 is a growth hormone produced by the liver and in peripheral tissues, like bone. Through activation of IGF-1 receptors throughout the body, IGF-1 exerts a negative feedback effect on growth hormone secretion and mediates the effect of growth hormone on bone, muscle, the nervous system, and immune system cells (Bioletto et al., 2024; Werner et al., 2008). Ghrelin, a peptide, known as the *hunger hormone,* helps control growth hormone

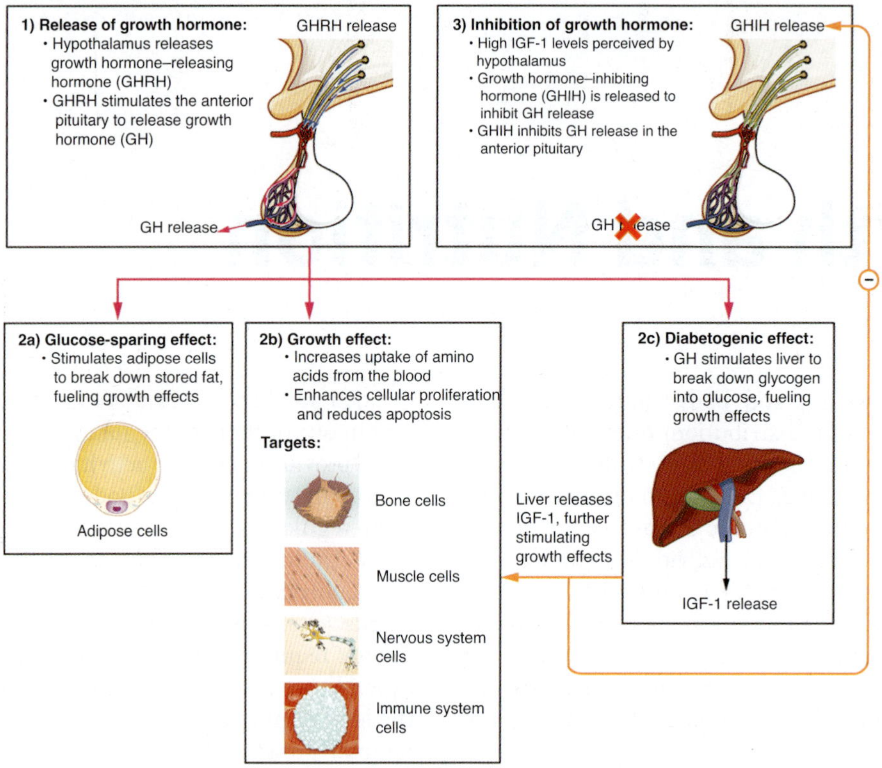

FIG. 8.1 Growth hormone (GH) directly accelerates the rate of protein synthesis in skeletal muscle and bones. Insulin-like growth factor 1 (IGF-1) is activated by growth hormone and indirectly supports the formation of new proteins in muscle cells and bone. (From Telleen, S. (2015, July 3). *The hypothalamus and pituitary gland.* OpenStax CNX. http://cnx.org/contents/ec7736ed-8658-4b58-9977-fa963a12caa8@1.)

release and influences food intake and obesity development (Bioletto et al., 2024; Sakata & Sakai, 2010).

Leptin has a key role in regulating body fat mass, and its concentration is thought to be a trigger for puberty by informing the central nervous system that adequate nutritional status and body fat mass are present to support pubertal changes and growth (Low, 2011; Roddick et al., 2024). Before puberty, body composition does not differ much between males and females. During puberty, with an increase in leptin, a relative decrease in fat percentage develops in males and an increase occurs in females (Roddick et al., 2024; Rogol, 2010). During puberty, the gonads begin to secrete testosterone and estrogen. Rising levels of these hormones trigger the release of gonadotropins (luteinizing hormone [LH] and follicle-stimulating hormone [FSH]) from the hypothalamus that stimulates the gonads to release more sex hormones. The genitalia begin growing to adult proportions. Testosterone enhances muscular development and sexual maturation and promotes bone maturation and epiphyseal closure. Estrogen stimulates the development of female secondary sexual characteristics, regulating the timing of the growth spurt and the acceleration of skeletal maturation and epiphyseal fusion. Androgens, secreted by the adrenal glands, promote masculinization manifested by secondary sex characteristics and skeletal maturation.

Growth at puberty is dependent on the interaction of growth hormone, IGF-1, leptin, and sex steroids (androgens). The sex steroids stimulate an increased secretion of growth hormone, which in turn mediates the dramatic increase in IGF-1. This leads to the adolescent growth spurt.

Differences in Growth by Organ System

Each organ or organ system has its particular period of rapid growth marked by rapid cell differentiation. Each individual has a unique growth timetable and final growth outcome, but the sequential growth patterns are consistent. An external environmental or abnormal pathophysiologic process may intervene and influence the expected growth pattern (Fig. 8.2).

The growth of the musculoskeletal system and most organs such as the liver and kidneys follows the growth curves described for stature. Skeletal growth is considered complete when the epiphyses of long bones have completely fused during late puberty. More than 90% of the skeletal mass is present by 18 years of age (Nguyen et al., 2024; Reiter & Rosenfield, 2008).

Weight is closely related to growth in stature and organ development. Growth and development are influenced by nutritional adequacy, which contributes to the number and size of adipose cells. The number of adipose cells increases throughout childhood. Gender-related differences in fat deposition appear in infancy and continue through adolescence.

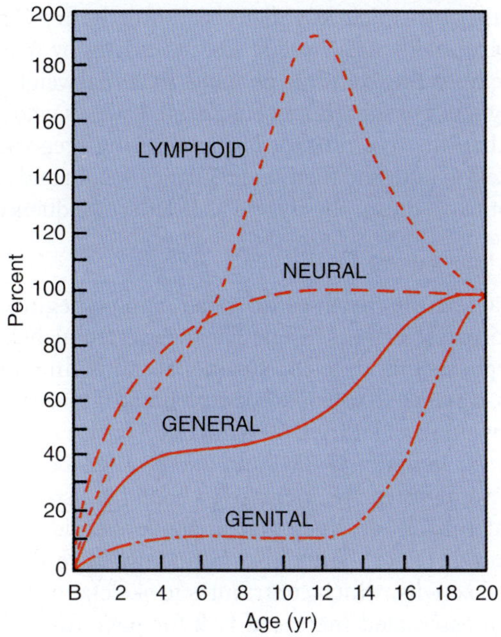

FIG. 8.2 Growth rates for the body as a whole and three types of tissues. Lymphoid type: thymus, lymph nodes, and intestinal lymph masses. Neural type: brain, dura, spinal cord, optic apparatus, and head dimensions. General type: body as a whole; external dimensions; and respiratory, digestive, renal, circulatory, and musculoskeletal systems. Genital type: includes the reproductive organ system. (Modified from Harris, J. A., Jackson, C. M., Paterson, D. J., et al. (1930). *The measurement of man.* Minneapolis: University of Minnesota Press.)

Lymphatic tissues (i.e., lymph nodes, spleen, tonsils, adenoids, and blood lymphocytes) are small in relation to total body size but are well developed at birth. These tissues grow rapidly to reach adult size by 6 years of age. By age 10 to 12 years, the lymphatic tissues are at their peak—about double adult size. During adolescence, they decrease to adult size.

The internal and external reproductive organs grow slowly before puberty. The reproductive organs double in size during adolescence, achieving maturation and function.

The brain, along with the skull, eyes, and ears, completes physical development more quickly than any other body part. The most rapid and critical period of brain growth occurs between conception and 3 years of age. By 34 weeks' gestation, 65% of the weight of a newborn's brain is present. Gray matter and myelinated white matter increase dramatically between the 34th and 40th weeks of gestation. By 37 weeks' gestation, the brain's structure is complete and an estimated 1 billion neurons are present. Glial cells, dendrites, and myelin continue to develop after birth, and by 3 years of age, most brain growth is completed (Fiegelman, 2011; Zonuzirad, 2024). The head circumference increases in infants and toddlers as brain growth occurs. During adolescence, the size of the head further increases because of the development of air sinuses and the thickening of the scalp and skull.

Infants and Children

As infants and children grow, the change in body proportion is related to the pattern of skeletal growth (Fig. 8.3).

Growth of the head predominates during the fetal period. Fetal weight gain follows growth in length, but weight reaches its peak during the third trimester with the increase in organ size. An infant's birth weight is influenced by genetic predisposition, gestational age, the mother's prepregnancy weight, weight gain during pregnancy, environmental exposures like secondhand smoke, overall maternal health, and intercurrent disease or complications in pregnancy such as gestational diabetes.

During infancy, the growth of the trunk predominates. Weight gain is initially rapid, but the speed with which weight is gained decreases over the first year of life. The fat content of the body increases slowly during early fetal development and then increases during infancy.

The legs are the fastest-growing body part during childhood, and weight is gained at a steady rate. Fat tissue increases slowly until 7 years of age, at which time a prepubertal fat spurt occurs before the true growth spurt.

The trunk and the legs lengthen during adolescence, and lean body mass averages 80% in males and females

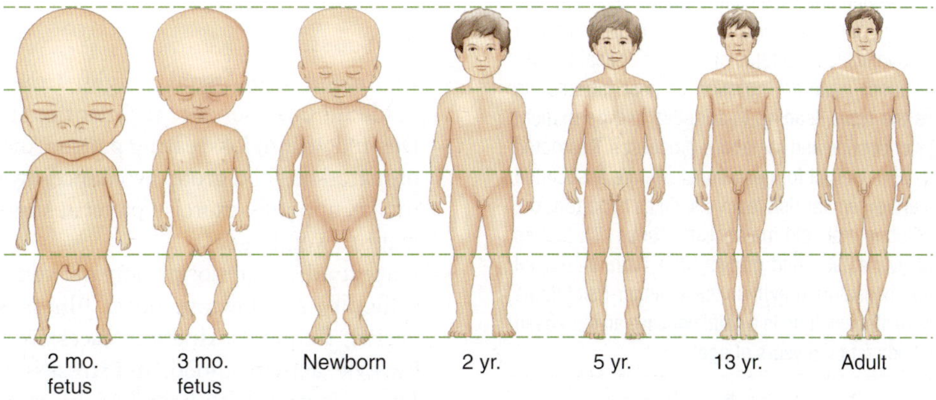

FIG. 8.3 Changes in body proportions from 8 weeks of gestation through adulthood.

(Bennett et al., 2024; Cromer, 2011). During adolescence, about 50% of the individual's ideal weight is gained and the skeletal mass and organ systems double in size.

During adolescence, males develop broader shoulders and greater musculature; females develop a wider pelvic outlet. Males have a slight increase in body fat during early adolescence and then have an average gain in lean body mass to 90%. Females accumulate subcutaneous fat and have a slight decrease in lean body mass to an average of 75% (Bennett et al., 2024; Cromer, 2011).

Pregnant Persons

Progressive weight gain is expected during pregnancy, but the amount varies among patients. The growing fetus accounts for 6 to 8 pounds of the total weight gained. The remainder results from an increase in maternal tissues:

- Fluid volume—2 to 3 pounds
- Blood volume—3 to 4 pounds
- Breast enlargement—1 to 2 pounds
- Uterine enlargement—2 pounds
- Amniotic fluid—2 pounds
- Maternal fat and protein stores—4 to 6 pounds

The rate of desirable weight gain follows a curve through the trimesters of pregnancy, slowly during the first trimester and more rapidly during the second and third trimesters. Maternal tissue growth accounts for most of the weight gained in the first and second trimesters. Fetal growth accounts for most weight gained during the third trimester.

Maternal nutrition before and during pregnancy and during lactation may have subtle effects on the developing brain of the infant and on the outcome of the pregnancy. Patients who have inadequate weight gain are at greater risk for delivering a low-birth-weight infant. Epigenetic research is revealing the potential consequences of inadequate maternal nutrition on the adult health of the fetus (Box 8.1).

BOX 8.1 Epigenetic Research and Nutrition

Epigenetic research is revealing an association between an individual's genome and environmental exposures during fetal life and adult health. Undernutrition during the second and third trimesters of pregnancy is believed to influence the fetus during the critical growth stages. Undernutrition (poor maternal nutrition or poor intrauterine environment) stresses the fetus, leading to adaptive and permanent changes in the infant's endocrine and metabolic processes. Restricted fetal growth and a low birth weight for gestational age are associated with increased adult cardiovascular risk factors such as hypertension, insulin resistance, and abnormal lipid metabolism. These risk factors are further influenced by nutrition and growth after birth. Increased nutrition can lead to compensatory growth in these higher-risk infants during the first 2 years of life, resulting in a child who has an increased body mass index and body fat by 5 years of age.

From Cota, B. M., & Allen, P. J. (2010). The developmental origins of health and disease hypothesis. *Pediatric Nursing, 36*(3), 157–167.

Postpartum weight loss often occurs over the first 6 months after birth, with most weight loss occurring by 3 months after delivery. Breastfeeding promotes maternal weight loss to prepregnancy weight (Boyd et al., 2024). Patients who gained more than the recommended weight during pregnancy are less likely to return to their prepregnancy weight and may be susceptible to future obesity and its health consequences.

Older Adults

Physical stature declines in older adults beginning at approximately 50 years of age. The intervertebral disks thin, and kyphosis may develop. Nutritional status, among other factors, can lead to osteoporotic vertebral compression.

Individuals older than 60 years often have a decrease in weight for height and BMI and a loss of 5% body weight over several years. An increase in body fat also occurs as skeletal muscle declines and anabolic steroid secretion is reduced. Older adults also frequently have decreased physical activity, which contributes to skeletal muscle loss with an associated increased risk for poor function and disability (Kalyani et al., 2014; Pabla et al., 2024). Physical activity recommendations vary by age. See Table 8.1 for guidelines for physical activity by age group from the U.S. Department of Health and Human Services (HHS).

Along with a decline in physical activity, an increase in overweight and obese older adults has been documented over the past 15 to 20 years. An age-associated reduction in size and weight of various organs has been identified, especially of the liver, lungs, and kidneys (McCance et al., 2015; Wen et al., 2024).

REVIEW OF RELATED HISTORY

For each of the symptoms or conditions discussed in this section, topics to include in the history of the present illness are listed. Responses to questions about these topics provide clues for focusing the physical examination and developing an appropriate diagnostic evaluation. Questions regarding medication use (prescriptions and over-the-counter preparations) as well as complementary, alternative, and integrative therapies are relevant for each area.

History of Present Illness

Weight Loss

- Compared with usual weight: time period (sudden, gradual); intentional or unintentional
- Desired weight loss: eating pattern, diet plan used, food preparation, food group avoidance, average daily calorie intake, appetite, exercise pattern, support group participation, weight goal
- Undesired weight loss: anorexia; vomiting or diarrhea, difficulty swallowing, other illness symptoms, time period; frequent urination, excessive thirst; change in lifestyle, activity, mood, and stress level
- Preoccupation with body weight or body shape: never feeling thin enough, fasting, unusually strict caloric

TABLE 8.1 Physical Activity Guidelines for Americans Recommendations

AGE	RECOMMENDATIONS
3–5 years	Preschool-aged children should be physically active throughout the day (ideally 3 hours per day of active play and structured activities).
6–17 years	Children and adolescents should do 60 minutes or more of physical activity daily. • Aerobic (e.g., running, swimming, dancing, bicycling): Most of the 60 or more minutes a day should be either moderate-[a] or vigorous-intensity[b] aerobic physical activity and should include vigorous-intensity physical activity at least 3 days a week. • Muscle strengthening[c]: As part of their 60 or more minutes of daily physical activity, children and adolescents should include muscle-strengthening physical activity on at least 3 days of the week. • Bone strengthening[d]: As part of their 60 or more minutes of daily physical activity, children and adolescents should include bone-strengthening physical activity on at least 3 days of the week. • It is important to encourage young people to participate in physical activities that are appropriate for their age, are enjoyable, and offer variety.
18–64 years	• All adults should move more and sit less throughout the day. Some physical activity is better than none, and adults who participate in any amount of physical activity gain some health benefits. • For substantial health benefits, adults should do at least 150 minutes (2 hours and 30 minutes) a week of moderate-intensity or 75 minutes (1 hour and 15 minutes) a week of vigorous-intensity aerobic physical activity or an equivalent combination of moderate- and vigorous-intensity aerobic activity. Aerobic activity should be performed in episodes of at least 10 minutes, preferably spread throughout the week. • For additional and more extensive health benefits, adults should increase their aerobic physical activity to 300 minutes (5 hours) a week of moderate-intensity activity. • Adults should also include muscle-strengthening activities that involve all major muscle groups on 2 or more days a week.
65 years and older	• Older adults should follow the adult guidelines. When older adults cannot meet the adult guidelines, they should be as physically active as their abilities and conditions will allow. • Older adults should do exercises that maintain or improve balance as well as aerobic and muscle-strengthening activities. • Older adults should determine their level of effort for physical activity relative to their level of fitness. • Older adults with chronic conditions should understand whether and how their conditions affect their ability to do regular physical activity safely.

[a]Moderate-intensity physical activity: Aerobic activity that increases a person's heart rate and breathing to some extent. On a scale relative to a person's capacity, moderate-intensity activity is usually a 5 or 6 on a 0–10 scale. Brisk walking, dancing, swimming, or bicycling on a level terrain are examples.

[b]Vigorous-intensity physical activity: Aerobic activity that greatly increases a person's heart rate and breathing. On a scale relative to a person's capacity, vigorous-intensity activity is usually a 7 or 8 on a 0–10 scale. Jogging, singles tennis, swimming continuous laps, or bicycling uphill are examples.

[c]Muscle-strengthening activity: Physical activity, including exercise that increases skeletal muscle strength, power, endurance, and mass. It includes strength training, resistance training, and muscular strength and endurance exercises.

[d]Bone-strengthening activity: Physical activity that produces an impact or tension force on bones, which promotes bone growth and strength. Running, jumping rope, and lifting weights are examples.

Adapted from US Department of Health and Human Services. (2018). *Physical activity guidelines for Americans* (2nd ed.). US Department of Health and Human Services.

intake; unusual food restrictions or cravings; laxative abuse, induced vomiting; amenorrhea; excessive exercise; mood, stress level; alcohol intake

- Medications: chemotherapy, diuretics, insulin, fluoxetine, glucagon-like peptide 1 (GLP-1) agonist drugs, prescription and nonprescription appetite suppressants, laxatives, oral hypoglycemics, steroids, herbal supplements
- Substance use

Weight Gain

- Total weight gained: time period, sudden or gradual, desired or undesired, possibility of pregnancy
- Change in lifestyle: change in social aspects of eating; more meals eaten out of the home; meals eaten quickly and "on the go"; change in meal preparation patterns; change in exercise patterns, mood, stress level, or alcohol intake
- Medications: steroids, oral contraceptives, antidepressants, insulin

Changes in Body Proportions

- Coarsening of facial features, enlargement of hands and feet, moon facies
- Change in fat distribution: trunk versus generalized

Increased Metabolic Requirements

- Infancy, prematurity, congenital heart disease, chronic obstructive lung disease
- Fever, infection, burns, trauma, pregnancy, hyperthyroidism, cancer, athlete
- External losses (e.g., fistulas, wounds, abscesses, chronic blood loss, chronic dialysis)

Past Medical History

- Chronic illness: liver disease, celiac disease, inflammatory bowel disease, surgical resection of the gastrointestinal tract, diabetes, congestive heart failure, hypothyroidism, hyperthyroidism, pancreatic insufficiency, chronic infection (e.g., human immunodeficiency virus [HIV] and tuberculosis), or allergies
- Previous weight loss or gain efforts: maximum body weight, minimum weight as an adult
- Previously diagnosed eating disorder, hypoglycemia

Family History

- Obesity (Box 8.2)
- Dyslipidemia
- Constitutionally short or tall stature, precocious or delayed puberty

BOX 8.2 Statistics on Obesity and Diet-Related Chronic Diseases in the United States

Nutrition-related chronic health conditions continue to be a major public health issue in the United States. Thirty-eight percent of adolescents ages 12 through 19 years have prediabetes, a particularly concerning finding as it may contribute to an increased risk of developing cardiovascular and metabolic diseases later in life. Chronic disease rates are especially high among adults and older adults. Variation in prevalence, incidence, and mortality rates indicate health disparities for some chronic health conditions, such as higher prevalence of obesity and diabetes among individuals of lower socioeconomic position. Some chronic health conditions—including obesity, diabetes, and (for females only) osteoporosis—have become more prevalent compared with 10 to 20 years ago.

- Seventeen percent of children and adolescents ages 2 through 19 years are overweight. Among adults and older adults ages 20 years and older, the prevalence of overweight is 43%. Obesity and severe obesity among adolescents and adults ages 20 years and older are 41% and 9%, respectively.
- The total prevalence of coronary heart disease (CHD) among adults and older adults ages 18 years and older is 5% and varies by sex, age, and educational attainment. The prevalence of CHD is 4% in adult females and 6% in adult males. By age, prevalence of CHD ranges from 1% among adults ages 18 through 44 years to 20% among older adults ages 75 years and older.
- Cancers linked to poor diet include breast (postmenopausal), endometrial, colon, kidney, gallbladder, and liver.
- The Division of Nutrition, Physical Activity, and Obesity at the Centers for Disease Control and Prevention has a wealth of information and useful resources for patients and health care professionals (www.cdc.gov/nccdphp/dnpao/index.html).

From the Centers for Disease Control and Prevention, & 2025 Dietary Guidelines Advisory Committee (2024). *Scientific report of the 2025 Dietary Guidelines Advisory Committee: Advisory report to the Secretary of Health and Human Services and Secretary of Agriculture.* U.S. Department of Health and Human Services (https://doi.org/10.52570/DGAC2025); and the *2020–2025 Dietary guidelines for Americans.*

- Genetic or metabolic disorder: diabetes (see list of chronic illnesses under "Past Medical History")
- Eating disorder: anorexia, bulimia
- Alcohol use disorder, substance use disorders

Personal and Social History

- Nutrition: appetite; usual calorie intake; vegetarianism; medical nutrition therapy guidelines followed; religious/cultural food practices; proportion of fat, protein, carbohydrate in the diet; intake of major vitamins and minerals (e.g., vitamins A, B_{12}, C, and D; iron; calcium; folate)
- Use of vitamin, mineral, and herbal supplements
- Usual weight and height; current weight and height; ability to maintain weight, goal weight
- Use of alcohol
- Substance use
- Food insecurity (i.e., limited or uncertain availability of nutritionally adequate and safe foods); limited/fixed income; eligibility for the Supplemental Nutrition Assistance Program (SNAP); financial and psychosocial stressors
- Functional assessment (i.e., ability to shop and prepare foods); access to healthy foods in their neighborhood; access to food storage/preparation equipment (refrigerator, stove, oven)
- Typical mealtime situations, companions, living environment
- Use of oral supplements, tube feedings, parenteral nutrition
- Dentition: dentures, missing teeth, gum disease

Infants

- Estimated gestational age, birth weight, length, head circumference
- Following an established percentile growth curve
- Unexplained changes in length, weight, or head circumference
- Poor growth/failure to thrive: falling one or more standard deviations off growth curve pattern; below the fifth percentile for weight and height; infant small for gestational age; quality of parent-infant bond and interaction; psychosocial stressors and food insecurity
- Rapid weight gain: overfeeding
- Nutrition: breastfeeding frequency and duration; maternal nutritional intake or any health conditions of the mother that may affect nutritional adequacy of breast milk, such as B_{12} deficiency
- Type and amount of infant formula; method of formula preparation; time it takes to drink one feeding; intake of protein, calories, vitamins, and minerals adequate for growth; vegetarian or veganism, cow's milk protein and other food allergies; vitamin and mineral supplements; number of fast-food meals eaten per week; eligibility for Women, Infants, and Children (WIC) program or school breakfast and lunch programs
- Hours of screen time per day (i.e., television, computer use, video and electronic games); access to safe areas for physical activity
- Chronic illness: cystic fibrosis, phenylketonuria (PKU), celiac disease, inborn errors of carbohydrate metabolism, amino acid and fatty acid oxidation disorders, tyrosinemia, homocystinuria, Prader-Willi syndrome
- Development: achieving milestones at appropriate ages
- Congenital anomalies, prematurity, prolonged neonatal hospitalization, cleft palate, malformed palate, tongue thrust, feeding and swallowing disorders, prolonged enteral tube feeding (gastrostomy and gastrojejunostomy), gastroesophageal reflux, malabsorption syndrome or chronic diarrhea, formula intolerance, neurologic disorders, congenital heart disease, others

Adolescents

- Initiation of sexual maturation of females: early (before 7 years) or delayed (beyond 13 years); signs of breast development and pubic hair, age at menarche
- Initiation of sexual maturation of males: early (before 9 years) or delayed (beyond 14 years); signs of genital development and pubic hair
- Short stature: not growing as fast as peers, change in shoe and clothing sizes in the past year, extremities short or long for the size of the trunk, height of parents, size of head disproportionate to the body
- Tall stature: height of parents, growing faster than peers, signs of early sexual maturation
- Nutrition: intake of protein, calories, vitamins, and minerals adequate for growth; vegetarian or veganism, number of fast-food meals eaten per week; food allergies; vitamin and mineral supplements; herbal supplements; appetite suppressants; laxative use; alcohol use, substance use
- Preoccupation with weight; overly concerned with developing muscle mass, losing body fat; excessive exercise; weighs self daily, excessive boasting about weight loss, weight goals; omits perceived fattening foods and food groups from the diet
- Risk factors for eating disorders
  - Weight preoccupation
  - Poor self-esteem, perfectionist personality
  - Self-image perceptual disturbances
  - Chronic medical illness (insulin-dependent diabetes)
  - Family history of eating disorders, obesity, alcohol use disorder, or affective disorders
  - Cultural pressure for thinness or outstanding performance
  - Athlete driven to excel (e.g., gymnasts, ice skaters, dancers, boxers, and wrestlers)
  - Food cravings, restrictions
  - Compulsive/binge eating
  - Difficulties with communication and conflict resolution; separation from family
  - Use of appetite suppressants and/or laxatives
- Chronic disease, such as inflammatory bowel disease, cystic fibrosis, malignancy
- Medications: steroids, growth hormones, anabolic steroids

Pregnant Persons

- Prepregnancy weight and BMI, age, dietary intake
- Age at menarche
- Date of last menstrual period, weight gain pattern, following established weight gain curve for gestational course
- Eating disorders
- Weight gain during pregnancy; nutrient intake during pregnancy (particularly protein, calories, iron, folate, calcium); supplementation with vitamins, iron, folic acid; eligibility for WIC program

BOX 8.3 Food-Nutrient-Medication Interactions

Medications can affect nutritional intake and status just as some foods, and the nutrients contained in them can affect absorption, metabolism, and excretion of medications. For example, a consistently high intake of grapefruit juice while taking simvastatin increases the bioavailability of the medication, often resulting in an increased risk of myopathy. It is important to assess the medications that a patient is taking to determine appropriateness and whether there are any possible interactions. The term *medications* includes those prescribed as well as those purchased over the counter. Often patients do not remember to list vitamin, mineral, herbal, and protein supplements during the history unless specifically asked about them.

- Pica (cravings for and eating nonnutritive substances such as laundry starch, ice, clay, raw icing)
- Nausea and vomiting
- Lactation: nutrient intake during lactation (particularly protein, calories, calcium, vitamins A and C); fluid intake (water, juice, milk, caffeine)
- Chronic illness: diabetes, renal disease, others

Older Adults

- Nutrition: weight gain or loss, adequate income for food purchases, interest and capability in preparing meals, participant in older adult feeding programs, social interaction at mealtime, number of daily meals and snacks, nutritional supplements, transportation to grocery stores, food delivery and access to healthy foods, poorly fitting dentures, missing teeth
- Energy level, regular exercise/activities
- Chronic illness: diabetes, renal disease, cancer, depression, heart disease; difficulty feeding self, chewing, or swallowing; swallowing dysfunction after stroke; functional status
- Food/nutrient/medication interactions (Box 8.3)

Risk Factors

Possible Medication Effects on Nutritional Intake and Status

- Altered food intake resulting from altered taste/smell, gastric irritation, bezoars (food ball found in the stomach and/or intestines), appetite increase/decrease, nausea/vomiting
- Modified nutrient absorption resulting from altered gastrointestinal pH, increased/decreased bile acid activity, altered gastrointestinal motility, inhibited enzymes, damaged mucosal cell walls, insoluble nutrient-drug complexes
- Modified nutrient metabolism resulting from vitamin antagonism (e.g., warfarin is a vitamin K antagonist)
- Modified nutrient excretion resulting from urinary loss, fecal loss

Determination of Diet Adequacy

The history of an individual's food and beverage intake allows estimation of the adequacy of the diet.

Histories may be obtained through 24-hour diet recalls or with a 3- or 4-day food diary that includes 1 weekend day. Various methods for measuring nutrient intake are available.

Twenty-Four-Hour Recall Diet

The 24-hour recall is an often-used method for obtaining a food intake history. Ask the patient to list all foods, beverages, and snacks eaten during the past 24 hours. Ask specific questions about the method of food preparation, portion sizes, amount of sugar-sweetened beverages, and use of salt or other additives. Some believe the 24-hour recall method provides a limited view of an individual's actual intake over time and may be misleading. Individuals may be unable to accurately remember everything they ate the day before, causing further inaccuracies in interpreting the information. There are now a variety of web-based 24-hour recall tools, including the Automated Self-Administered 24-Hour (ASA24) Dietary Assessment Tool (https://epi.grants.cancer.gov/asa24/). Patients report minimal burden and high rates of satisfaction with these types of tools compared with a typical diet history assessment (Arab et al., 2010; Vasiloglou et al., 2023).

Food Diary and Nutrient Intake

The food diary can be an accurate but time-consuming method for the patient and health professional. It provides a retrospective view of an individual's eating habits and dietary intake, recorded as it happened. It can also collect relevant data that may aid in identifying problem areas. The U.S. Department of Agriculture (USDA) MyPlate.gov website and mobile device application are useful tools for tracking daily food and beverage intake by food groups (grains, vegetables, fruits, dairy, and protein foods; Box 8.4).

Patients may ask for recommendations on calorie intake to guide their food choices. An interactive Dietary Reference Intake (DRI) calculator on the USDA Food and Nutrition Information Center website (https://www.nal.usda.gov/fnic/dri-calculator/) uses patient age, gender, height, and activity level to generate a tailored report.

BOX 8.4 Calculating the Body Mass Index

The formula to calculate BMI using pounds (be sure to convert ounces to a decimal) and inches:

$$\left[\text{Weight [in pounds]} \div \text{Height [in inches]}^2\right] \times 70$$

The formula to calculate BMI using kilograms and centimeters:

$$\text{Weight [in kg]} \div \text{Height [in meters]}$$

From https://www.nhlbi.nih.gov/health/educational/lose_wt/BMI/bmicalc.htm.

Patient Safety

MyPlate.gov

MyPlate.gov provides practical information, tips, web-based tools, and mobile device applications to help individuals build healthier diets (Fig. 8.4). MyPlate.gov is based on the most up-to-date recommendations from the 2020 to 2025 Dietary Guidelines for Americans. The guidelines, published every 5 years by HHS and the USDA, provide evidence-based information and advice for choosing a healthy eating pattern that focuses on nutrient-dense foods and beverages and helps individuals achieve and maintain a healthy weight. The full guidelines are available at https://www.dietaryguidelines.gov/resources/2020-2025-dietary-guidelines-online-materials.

Individuals can use the MyPlate.gov website to calculate their daily caloric needs and create a food plan based on age, sex, weight, height, and physical activity level. Individuals can also download an app to their mobile device to analyze their diet habits, set goals, and track progress. Additional resources include printed materials (English and Spanish) and videos.

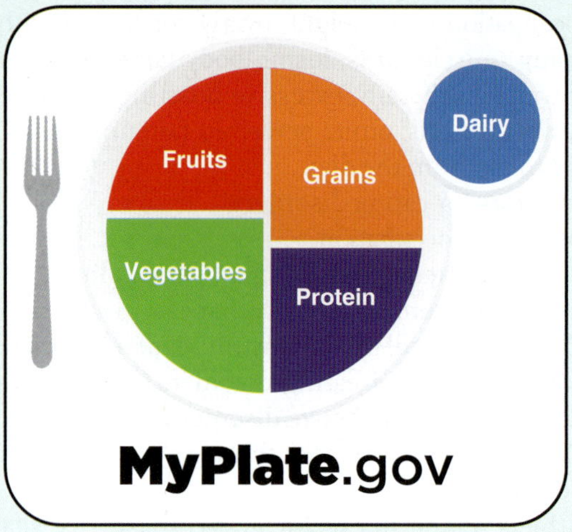

FIG. 8.4 My Plate. (From U.S. Department of Agriculture. MyPlate.gov.)

Limit foods and beverages high in added sugars, saturated fat, and sodium; limit alcoholic beverages.

CLINICAL PEARL

The 2020–2025 Dietary Guidelines for Americans emphasize the following key messages:

- Follow a healthy diet at every life stage.
- Customize nutrient-dense foods and beverages based on personal preferences, culture, and budget.
- Consume nutrient-dense foods and beverages (rich in vitamins and minerals with no or little added sugars, saturated fat, and sodium) and stay within calorie limits.

Vegetarian/Vegan Diets

Vegetarian/vegan diets can meet all the recommendations for nutrients. The key is to consume a variety and the appropriate amount of foods to meet an individual's caloric needs. Five nutrients may be deficient in a vegetarian diet if it is not carefully planned: protein, calcium (lacto-ovo and vegan), iron, vitamin B_{12} (vegan), and vitamin D. The Office of Dietary Supplements at the National Institutes of Health has a variety of useful educational materials for patients and health care providers about the effectiveness, safety, and quality of dietary supplements (https://ods.od.nih.gov).

Cultural and Ethnic Food Guide Pyramids

Food guide pyramids for ethnic populations are available (e.g., Mediterranean, Indian, Mexican, and Asian). To see examples of ethnic and cultural food guide pyramids, go to the USDA Food and Nutrition Information Center (www.nal.usda.gov/fnic/ethniccultural-food-pyramids). In addition, Oldways Preservation Trust (www.oldwayspt.org) is a useful resource.

EXAMINATION AND FINDINGS

Equipment

- Standing platform scale with height attachment
- Measuring tape with millimeter markings
- Infant scale
- Recumbent measuring device (for infants)
- Stature-measuring device (for children)
- Calculator

Weight and Standing Height

To measure the weight, ask the patient to remove excess clothing and shoes. Have the patient stand in the middle of the scale platform and note the digital reading. If using a balance scale, move the largest weight to the last 50-pound or 10-kg increment under the patient's weight. Adjust the smaller weight to balance the scale. Read the weight to the nearest 0.25 pound or 0.1 kg. Weight variations occur during the day and from day to day with changes in body fluid and intestinal contents. When monitoring a patient's weight daily or weekly, weigh the patient at the same time each day using the same scale.

To measure height, have the patient stand erect with their back to the stature-measuring device. Pull up the height attachment and position the headpiece on the top of the head. Make the reading at the nearest centimeter or 0.5 inch.

Body Mass Index

The BMI, an anthropometric index of weight and height, is the most common method used to assess nutritional status and total body fat. Although not a direct measure of body fat, BMI correlates to body fat measures using underwater body measuring and dual-energy x-ray absorptiometry. Although most electronic health records automatically calculate BMI, Box 8.4 presents the formula. For adults, the following are classifications of weight for height by BMI values (in kg/m^2):

- Underweight—under 18.5
- Healthy weight—18.5 to 24.9
- Overweight—25 to 29.9
- Obesity—30 or greater

Track the change of a patient's BMI over time (Emmerich et al., 2024; Hales et al., 2020).

CLINICAL PEARL

Controlling Weight

Exercise is a key factor in maintaining body weight or in reducing body weight. Vigorous-intensity aerobic exercise such as 25 minutes of brisk walking at least three times a week is recommended for adults 18 to 64 years of age. Look for ways to increase activity, such as using the stairs rather than an elevator or parking farther from the doors to businesses and workplaces. Limit the screen time for children and adolescents. Encourage children to walk, ride a bicycle (with a helmet), and participate in sports or recreational activities. The ability to participate in outdoor activity may vary depending on weather, time of year, and opportunities for safe outdoor play in the children's neighborhood.

Waist Circumference and Waist-Height Ratio

Waist circumference and waist-height ratio are indicators of visceral fat or abdominal obesity. Waist circumference should be measured at the high point of the iliac crest when the individual is standing and at minimal respiration. Persons of healthy weight who have increased waist circumferences often fall into a higher disease risk classification. A large waist circumference (>35 inches in females, >40 inches in males) is associated with an increased risk for type 2 diabetes, dyslipidemia, hypertension, and cardiovascular disease. Monitoring changes in a person's waist circumference over time, with or without changes in BMI, may aid in predicting relative disease risk in terms of cardiovascular risk factors and obesity-related diseases.

The waist-height ratio is calculated as a ratio of the waist circumference (cm) and height (cm). Like waist circumference, the waist-height ratio has been shown to be a strong predictor for diabetes and cardiovascular disease in adults (Ashwell & Gibson, 2016; Chan et al., 2024). A waist-height ratio greater than 0.5 is associated with increased risk.

See the Centers for Disease Control and Prevention (CDC) Waist Circumference tables at https://stacks.cdc.gov/view/cdc/40572.

Infants

The care of children is exciting because of the continuous change that accompanies growth and development. Give careful attention to measuring weight and length and the sequence of developmental achievements as you get to know a child over time.

The newborn with the best chance to be a healthy infant is born at term (at least 37 weeks' gestational age), is an appropriate size for gestational age, and has no history of prenatal or perinatal difficulty. Most babies born at term to the same parents weigh within 6 ounces of their siblings at birth. Pay close attention to an unexpected birth weight difference. If the baby has a lower birth weight than older siblings, carefully assess for congenital abnormality or factors that may have contributed to intrauterine growth restriction. Newborns with a greater birth weight than older siblings, at 10 pounds or greater, are at risk for hypoglycemia. A more rapid weight gain than expected during early infancy (e.g., the infant's weight percentile keeps increasing rather than following a specific growth curve) is associated with increased cardiovascular disease risk and hypertension as an adult (Amati et al., 2024; Howe et al., 2014).

Recumbent Length

Measure the length of infants between birth and 24 months of age in the supine position on a measuring device (Fig. 8.5). Have the parent hold the infant's head against the headboard. Hold the infant's legs straight at the knees and place the footboard against the bottom of the infant's feet. Read the length measurement to the nearest 0.5 cm or 0.25 inch. The infant's length should be plotted on the World Health Organization (WHO) growth curve for age and gender to identify the infant's percentile placement. Although most electronic health records include automated growth chart plotting, the WHO charts can be accessed at https://www.cdc.gov/growthcharts/who_charts.htm. Future length measurements should be plotted on the same chart to monitor the infant's growth over time (see Clinical Pearl, "Using the Correct Growth Chart").

At birth, healthy term newborns have length variations between 45 and 55 cm (18 and 22 inches). Length increases by 50% in the first year of life (see Clinical Pearl, "Reliability of Length Measurements").

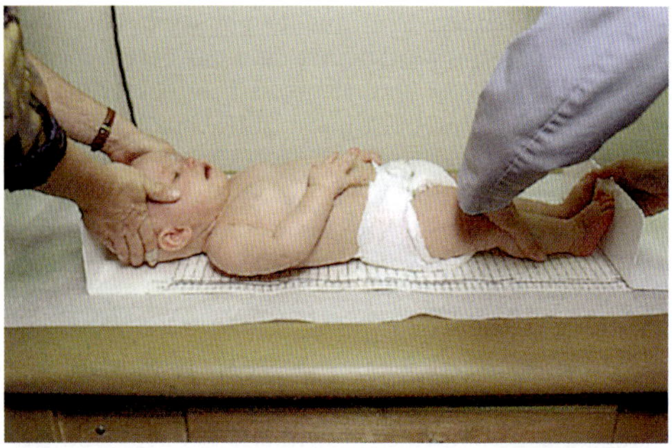

FIG. 8.5 Measurement of infant length. (From Hockenberry, M. H., & Wilson, D. (2017). *Wong's essentials of pediatric nursing* (10th ed.). St. Louis: Elsevier.)

CLINICAL PEARL

Using the Correct Growth Chart

Despite the toddler's ability to stand, continue measuring length until 24 months of age and continue plotting the length on the WHO growth curve. Measurements of length are 0.7 to 0.8 cm greater than height or stature (Grummer-Strawn et al., 2010). Using the child's height rather than length on the WHO growth curve will give an incorrect impression of poor growth. At 24 months of age, begin measuring the child's height and plotting the child's measurements on the Centers for Disease Control and Prevention growth curves for children ages 2 to 18 years (https://www.cdc.gov/growthcharts/clinical_charts.htm). Most electronic health record systems have embedded the WHO and CDC growth charts.

CLINICAL PEARL

Reliability of Length Measurements

Obtaining a reliable length measurement in newborns is difficult because of the natural flexion of the infant and the molding of the head. In infants, the reliability of the length measurement is difficult if the infant resists and moves. Use a consistent technique to increase reliability between examiners, and verify the length with a second measurement.

Weight

Use an infant scale, measuring weight in grams for infants and small children. Infants and children are weighed only in grams and kilograms to reduce medication errors because pediatric dosages are calculated per kilogram of body weight. Have the parent assist and use distraction to help keep the infant quiet and still until the digital reading appears or until the scale is balanced. Read the weight to the nearest 10 g when the infant is most still. Assess the infant's weight on the WHO growth curve for age and gender, comparing the infant's weight with the population standard. Identify the infant's percentile placement. As with length, monitor the child's weight by plotting future measurements on the same growth curve. Beginning at 2 years of age, convert to the CDC growth curve for the child's gender (https://www.cdc.gov/growthcharts/clinical_charts.htm). Use conversion tables available online to give parents the infant's weight in pounds and ounces (https://www.thecalculatorsite.com/conversions/common/kg-to-pounds-ounces.php).

Most term newborns vary in weight between 2500 and 4000 g (5 lb, 8 oz to 8 lb, 13 oz). Infants may lose up to 10% of their birth weight by day three, regain that weight within 2 weeks, and then gain weight at a rate of approximately 30 g (1 oz) per day. This rate of weight gain decreases starting at about 3 months of age (Fiegelman, 2011; Muth et al., 2024). In general, infants double their birth weight by 4 to 5 months of age and triple their birth weight by 12 months of age.

After obtaining the length and weight, plot the infant's weight for length on the WHO growth curve. This provides information about whether the infant's weight is proportional to length (see Clinical Pearl, "Uses of Growth Charts").

CLINICAL PEARL

Uses of Growth Charts

Growth charts are designed to plot and track anthropometric data to screen for atypical size and growth patterns and to make an overall clinical assessment. For example, growth charts for children between birth and 24 months of age make it possible to identify excessive weight gain for length. A separate growth curve for very low-birth-weight infants compares the growth of these infants with the growth of other low-birth-weight infants, although the WHO growth charts may also be used to evaluate the growth of these infants.

Head Circumference

Measure the infant's head circumference at every health visit until 2 to 3 years of age. Wrap a paper measuring tape snugly around the child's head at the occipital protuberance and the supraorbital prominence to find the point of the largest circumference (Fig. 8.6). Make the reading to the nearest 0.5 cm or 0.25 inch. Confirm the accuracy of the head circumference measurement at least once. Plot the measurement on the appropriate growth curve and identify the child's percentile in comparison with the population standard. Compare measurements over time to monitor the head circumference growth pattern using the WHO growth curve.

Expected head circumferences for term newborns range between 32.5 and 37.5 cm (12.5 to 14.5 inches) with a mean of 33 to 35 cm (13 to 14 inches). At 2 years of age, the child's head circumference is two-thirds its adult size. If the head circumference increases rapidly and plots in higher percentile curves, increased intracranial pressure may be present. If the head circumference does not grow as expected and plots in lower percentile curves, microcephaly may be present and further investigation may be warranted.

Chest Circumference

Although the chest circumference is not used routinely, it is a useful measurement for comparison with the head circumference when a problem is suspected with either the head size or chest size. Wrap the measuring tape around the infant's chest at the nipple line firmly but not tight enough to cause an indentation of the skin (Fig. 8.7). Read the chest circumference measurement midway between inspiration and expiration to the nearest 0.5 cm or 0.25 inch.

The newborn's head circumference may equal or exceed the chest circumference by 2 cm (0.75 inches) until 5 months of age. Between the ages of 5 months and 2 years, the infant's chest circumference and head circumference are close to the same size. If an infant's head circumference is smaller than the chest circumference, consider evaluating the infant for microcephaly. After 2 years of age, the chest circumference exceeds the head circumference because the chest grows faster than the head.

Gestational Age

Gestational age is an indicator of a newborn's maturity. One method of determining gestational age is to calculate the number of completed weeks between the first day of the mother's last menstrual period and the date of birth. An estimate of gestational age is used to evaluate an infant's developmental progress. It is also used to identify preterm newborns of appropriate size and term newborns who are small for gestational age.

The Ballard Gestational Age Assessment Tool evaluates six physical and six neuromuscular newborn characteristics within 36 hours of birth to establish or confirm the newborn's gestational age (https://perinatology.com/calculators/Ballard.htm). The assessment is accurate within 2 weeks of the assigned gestational age. Scores are more accurate for extremely preterm newborns when the assessment occurs within 12 hours of birth.

The gestational ages of 37 through 41 weeks are considered term and are associated with the best health outcomes. Infants born before 37 weeks of gestation are

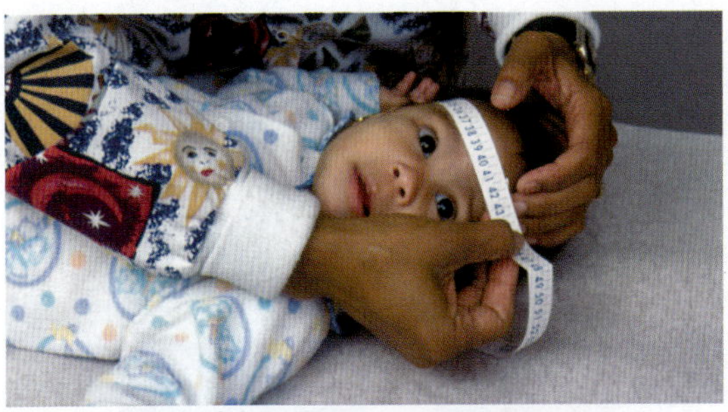

FIG. 8.6 Place the measuring tape around the largest circumference of the infant's head, across the occiput and the forehead.

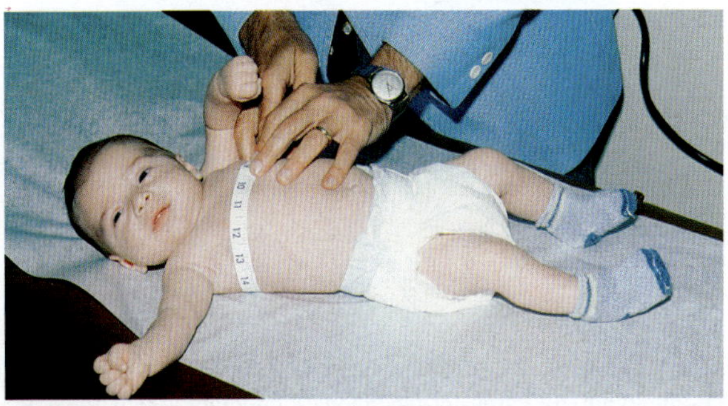

FIG. 8.7 Measurement of infant chest circumference with the measuring tape at the level of the nipple line.

preterm, and infants born after 41 completed weeks of gestation are postterm. The incidence of premature birth in the United States reached a peak in 2006 when 12.8% of all infants were born at gestational age less than 37 weeks The preterm birth rate declined 1% from 2021 to 2022, to 10.4%, following an increase of 4% from 2020 to 2021. However, racial and ethnic differences in preterm birth rates remain. In 2022, preterm birth among Black women (14.6%) was about 50% higher than White (9.4%) or Hispanic women (10.1%). https://www.cdc.gov/maternal-infanthealth/.

Size for Gestational Age

A newborn's fetal growth pattern and size for gestational age can be determined once gestational age is assigned. An intrauterine growth curve is used to plot the newborn's birth weight, length, and head circumference. The Fenton Growth Chart is recommended for tracking premature growth until 50 weeks postmenstrual age (https://live-ucalgary.ucalgary.ca/resource/preterm-growth-chart/preterm-growth-chart). The infant is classified as small, appropriate, or large for gestational age by percentile curve placement for weeks of gestation (Fig. 8.8). The classification system is as follows:

- Appropriate for gestational age: 10th to 90th weight percentile
- Small for gestational age: less than 10th weight percentile
- Large for gestational age: greater than 90th weight percentile

Infants who are small or large for gestational age have an increased risk for morbidity and mortality. Small-for-gestational-age infants who are full term have an increased risk for respiratory distress, hypoglycemia, and other health problems. For the year 2022, in the United States, the number of low-birth-weight infants born (less than 2500 grams) was 315,2288, or 8.60%. The percentage of very low-birth-weight infants (less than 1500 grams) was 1.26% (https://www.cdc.gov/nchs/fastats/birthweight.htm).

Large-for-gestational-age infants are at higher risk for birth injuries such as shoulder dystocia as well as health conditions such as respiratory distress syndrome, intraventricular hemorrhage, and bronchopulmonary dysplasia.

Children

Stature and Weight

Standing height (stature) is obtained beginning at 24 months when the child is walking well. Ask the parent to remove the child's shoes and heavy clothing. To get the most accurate measurement, use a stature-measuring device (stadiometer) mounted on the wall rather than the height measurement device on a scale. Have the child stand erect with heels, buttocks, and shoulders against the wall or freestanding stadiometer, looking straight ahead (Fig. 8.9). The outer canthus of the eye should be on the same horizontal plane as the external auditory canal while you position the headpiece at the top of the head. The stature reading is made to the nearest 0.5 cm or 0.25 inch (see Clinical Pearl, "Special Growth Charts").

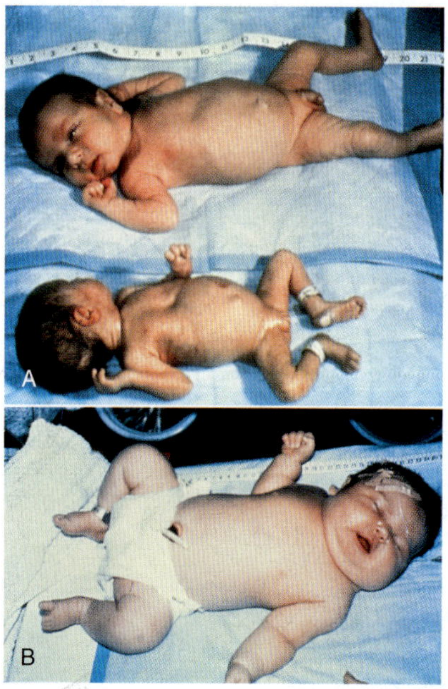

FIG. 8.8 (A) Small-for-gestational-age infant and appropriate-for-gestational-age infant. (B) Large-for-gestational-age infant. (From Zitelli, B. J., McIntire, S. C., & Nowalk, A. J. (2012). *Zitelli and Davis' atlas of pediatric physical diagnosis* (6th ed.). Philadelphia: Saunders.)

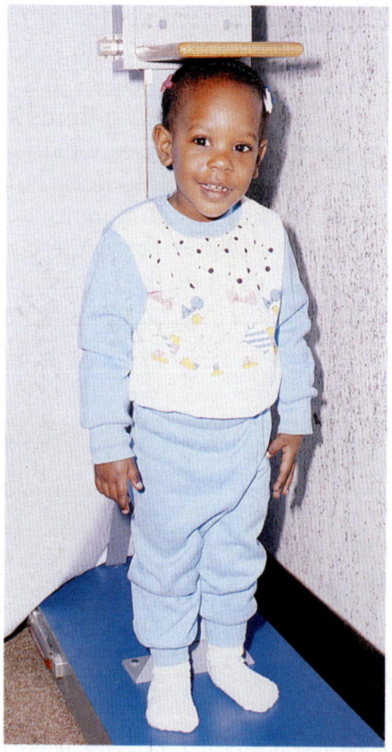

FIG. 8.9 Measuring the stature of a child.

CLINICAL PEARL

Special Growth Charts

Special growth charts exist for children with specific conditions such as Down syndrome and Turner syndrome, but use them in association with the WHO and Centers for Disease Control and Prevention standardized charts. These special growth charts may be obtained online at https://www.cdc.gov/birth-defects/hcp/down-syndrome-growth-charts/index.html https://pedsendo.org/wp-content/uploads/2020/07/Growth-Chart-Turner-syndrome.pdf

Height velocity represents the increase in height during a fixed period. It is often assessed when concerns arise about poor linear growth in childhood or adolescence. To calculate height velocity, determine the change in height over a time interval (e.g., 1 year). Shorter time intervals may reflect seasonal variations in growth. Make height measurements as close to 12 months apart as possible—no fewer than 10 months and no more than 14 months. Weigh young children older than 2 years of age on a standing scale in light garments. Read the weight to the nearest 0.1 kg. Plot the child's height and weight on the CDC growth curves for gender and age, comparing the child's growth with other children the same age.

The BMI is now standardized for use in children and adolescents, and it is calculated the same way as for adults. In children and adolescents, the amount of body fat changes with age, and the body fat values differ between males and females. As a result, the BMI is interpreted using age- and gender-specific percentiles. Once the BMI is calculated, plot the value on the appropriate growth chart for gender. Established cutoff points used to identify underweight and overweight children and adolescents are based on the following percentiles:

- Underweight—BMI for age under the 5th percentile
- Healthy weight—BMI for age 5th percentile to less than the 85th percentile
- Overweight—BMI for age 85th percentile to less than the 95th percentile
- Obese—BMI for age equal to or greater than the 95th percentile

For children, obesity is defined as having a BMI at or above the 95th percentile for age and sex. Approximately one in five U.S. children and adolescents is obese. Obesity affects some groups more than others, including adolescents, Hispanic and non-Hispanic Black children, and children in families with lower incomes. From 2017 to 2020, the prevalence of obesity among U.S. children and adolescents was 19.7%. This accounts for 14.7 million U.S. youths ages 2 to 19. The prevalence of obesity increased with age from 2017 to 2020. In U.S. children, obesity prevalence was 12.7% among children 2 to 5 years old, 20.7% among those 6 to 11, and 22.2% among adolescents. Overall, obesity prevalence was highest in Hispanic children (26.2%) and non-Hispanic Black children (24.8%), followed by non-Hispanic White (16.6%) and non-Hispanic Asian (9.0%) children. Among U.S. girls, obesity prevalence was highest among non-Hispanic Black girls (30.8%). Among U.S. boys, obesity prevalence was highest among Hispanic boys (29.3%). Obesity prevalence was 11.5% among U.S. children with family income more than 350% of the Federal Poverty Level (FPL), 21.2% among children with family income 130% to 350% of the FPL, and 25.8% among children with family income 130% or less of the FPL (https://www.cdc.gov/obesity/childhood-obesity-facts/childhood-obesity-facts.html#:~:text=Approximately%201%20in%205%20U.S.,percentile%20for%20age%20and%20sex).

Evaluate the child's growth pattern over time by placing all weight and height measurements on the growth curve. The child is expected to consistently follow a percentile curve on the growth curve. Children adopted from other countries may not fit the U.S. population standard, but they should have a consistent growth pattern (percentile), even if it is near or below the fifth percentile. Infants and children who suddenly fall below or rise above their established percentile growth curve should be examined more closely to determine the cause.

Upper-to-Lower Segment Ratio

The upper-to-lower segment ratio is calculated when a child's body may have inappropriate proportions between the head and trunk to the lower extremities. Measure the lower body segment (distance from the symphysis pubis to the floor when a child stands). Calculate the upper body segment by subtracting the lower body segment from the total height. Then divide the upper body segment by the lower body segment to calculate the ratio. Expected ratios by age are as follows (Hawkes et al., 2020; Keane, 2011):

- At birth—1.7
- At 3 years—1.3
- After 7 years—1.0

A higher upper-to-lower body segment ratio than expected may be associated with dwarfism or bone disorders.

Arm Span

The arm span measurement is not routinely obtained but may be useful when evaluating a child with tall stature. Have the child hold the arms fully extended from the sides of the body. Measure the distance from the middle fingertip of one hand to that of the other hand. The arm span should equal the child's height or stature. Arm span that exceeds height is associated with Marfan syndrome.

Sexual Maturation

Assessment of children and adolescents involves evaluation of secondary sexual characteristic development. In children assigned female at birth, breast and pubic hair development is evaluated; in children assigned male at birth, genital and pubic hair development is evaluated. The duration and tempo of each stage vary between individuals. Sexual maturation begins earlier in females with a higher BMI. On average, Black females enter puberty first, followed by Mexican American females and then White females. Sexual maturation, as measured by the onset of pubic hair development, begins earlier in Black males than in White males (Barton et al., 2024).

When assessing children and adolescents for pubertal development, ask a clinical team member to serve as a chaperone. Have the child sit while assessing the stage of breast development. Breast tissue may be seen and possibly palpated below a slightly enlarging areola (1 cm in diameter of palpable glandular tissue). Most females start puberty between 9 and 12 years of age with breast enlargement. A female's breasts often develop at different rates and appear asymmetric. Pubic hair begins lightly pigmented, sparse, and straight along the labia majora. See Figs. 8.10 and 8.11 for expected stages of female sexual maturation.

Ask the child to stand to assess pubertal development. Most males start puberty between 10 and 13 years of age with testicular enlargement. Pubic hair development, enlargement of the penis, and the growth spurt follow. See Figs. 8.12 and 8.13 for expected stages of male sexual maturation.

After the secondary sexual characteristics are assessed and staged, a sexual maturity rating (SMR), also known as the *Tanner stage,* may be assigned to determine the child's overall pubertal development. The height growth spurt and timing of other physiologic events occurring during puberty (e.g., menarche or nocturnal emissions) are associated with the stage of secondary sexual characteristic development. An SMR is calculated by averaging the female's stages of pubic hair and breast development or the male's stages of pubic hair and genital development.

The onset of puberty in females is the age at which breast stage 2 or pubic hair stage 2 is reached, whichever occurs first. Most females have breast development before pubic

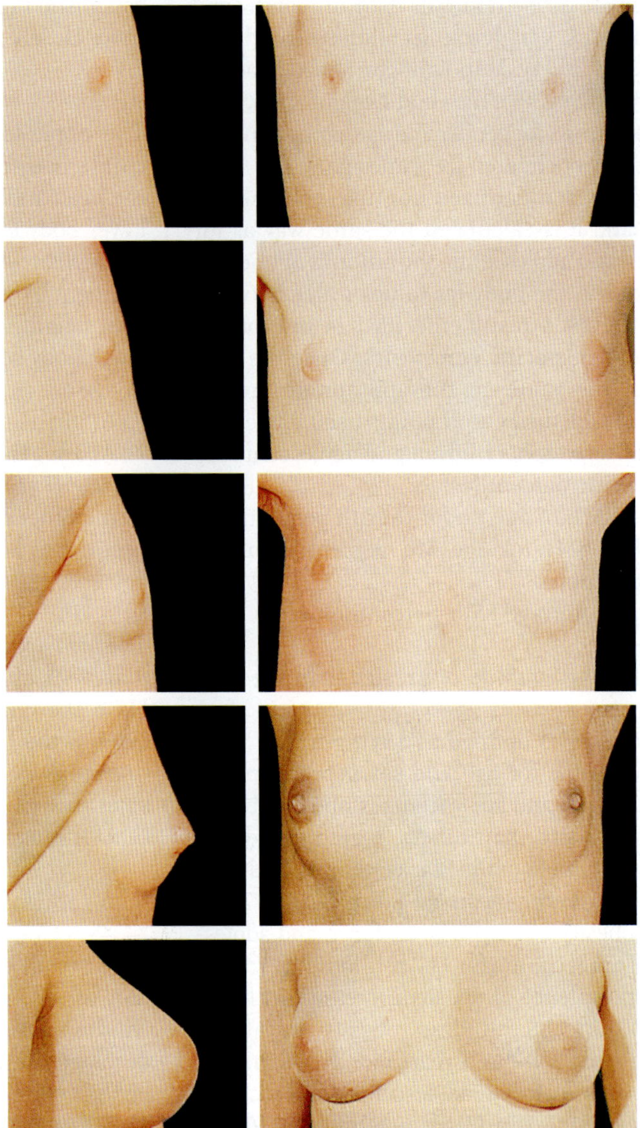

M_1—Tanner 1 (preadolescent). Only the nipple is raised above the level of the breast, as in the child.

M_2—Tanner 2. Budding stage; bud-shaped elevation of the areola; areola increased in diameter and surrounding area slightly elevated.

M_3—Tanner 3. Breast and areola enlarged. No contour separation.

M_4—Tanner 4. Increasing fat deposits. The areola forms a secondary elevation above that of the breast. This secondary mound occurs in approximately half of all girls and in some cases persists in adulthood.

M_5—Tanner 5 (adult stage). The areola is (usually) part of general breast contour and is strongly pigmented. Nipple projects.

FIG. 8.10 Five stages of breast development in females. (From Van Wieringen, J. C., Wafelbakker, F., Verbrugge, H. P., et al. (1971). *Growth diagrams 1965 Netherlands: Second national survey on 0–24-year-olds.* Groningen, Netherlands: Wolters-Noordhoff Publishing.)

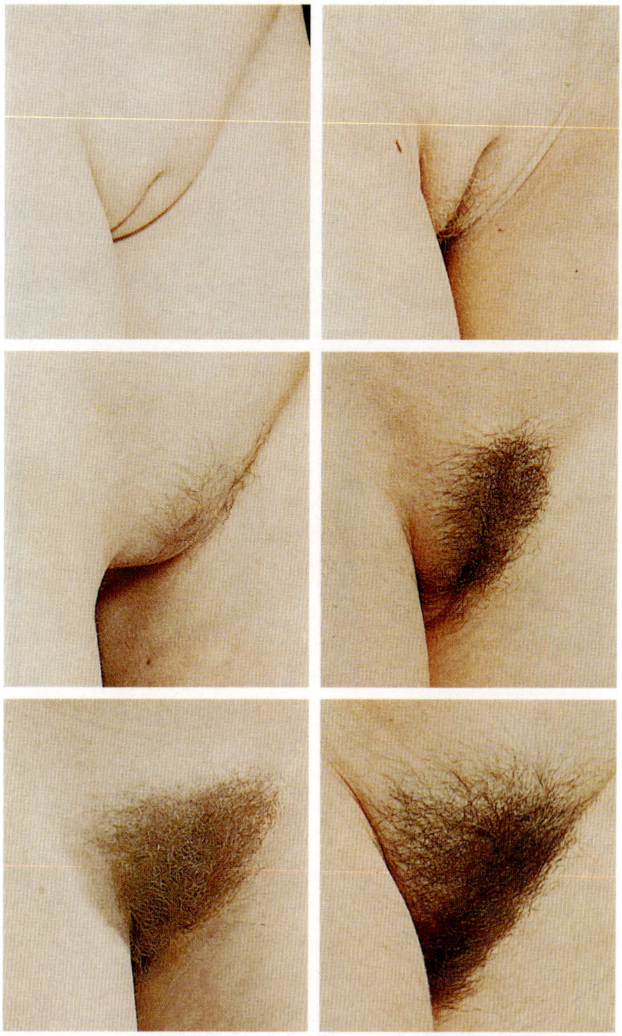

P_1—Tanner 1 (preadolescent). No growth of pubic hair.

P_2—Tanner 2. Initial, scarcely pigmented straight hair, especially along medial border of the labia.

P_3—Tanner 3. Sparse, dark, visibly pigmented, curly pubic hair on labia.

P_4—Tanner 4. Hair coarse and curly, abundant but less than adult.

P_5—Tanner 5. Lateral spreading; type and triangle spread of adult hair to medial surface of thighs.

P_6—Tanner 6. Further extension laterally, upward, or dispersed (occurs in only 10% of women).

FIG. 8.11 Six stages of pubic hair development in females. (From Van Wieringen, J. C., Wafelbakker, F., Verbrugge, H. P., et al. (1971). *Growth diagrams 1965 Netherlands: Second national survey on 0–24-year-olds.* Groningen, Netherlands: Wolters-Noordhoff Publishing.)

hair appears. Completion of puberty is when breast stage 4 or pubic hair stage 5 has been reached. Menarche generally occurs in SMR 4 or breast stage 3 to 4. Over the past few decades, the age of menarche and stage 2 breast development has become younger over time. In a national survey of females conducted between 2013 and 2017, one-half reported menarche before 11 years and 10 months of age (Martinez, 2020). The peak height velocity usually occurs before menarche. These events may be plotted on the standardized height growth chart for adolescents. Breast development may begin as early as 6 years in Black females and 7 years in White females. Breast development before these ages is abnormal and needs further evaluation (Leung et al., 2024).

The stage of genital and pubic hair development in males is related to age and the height spurt. External genital changes usually precede pubic hair development. Ejaculation generally occurs at SMR 3, with semen appearing between SMR 3 and 4. The peak height velocity occurs at a mean age of 13.5 years, usually in SMR 4 or genital development stage 4 to 5. These events may be plotted on the standardized height growth chart for adolescents. Development of genitals or pubic hair in prepubertal males younger than 9 years should be further investigated for the cause.

Delayed onset of puberty and secondary sexual characteristic development (at an age later than the average) may be a normal variant in both males and females or may be a deliberate consequence of the use of puberty blockers in transgender and gender-diverse youth. It is usually accompanied by a lag of stature growth. A parent or sibling often may have had a similar adolescent growth pattern. Once pubertal changes begin, the sequence of development is the same as for other adolescents, but it may occur over a different time span. Ultimate height may still be the same. Further evaluation is needed if no evidence of pubertal development is seen in a male by 14 years of age or a female by 13 years of age (Abaci & Besci, 2024).

Early development of sexual hair without signs of sexual maturation may be an indication of premature pubarche. In these children, pubescence usually occurs at the expected time, as with healthy children.

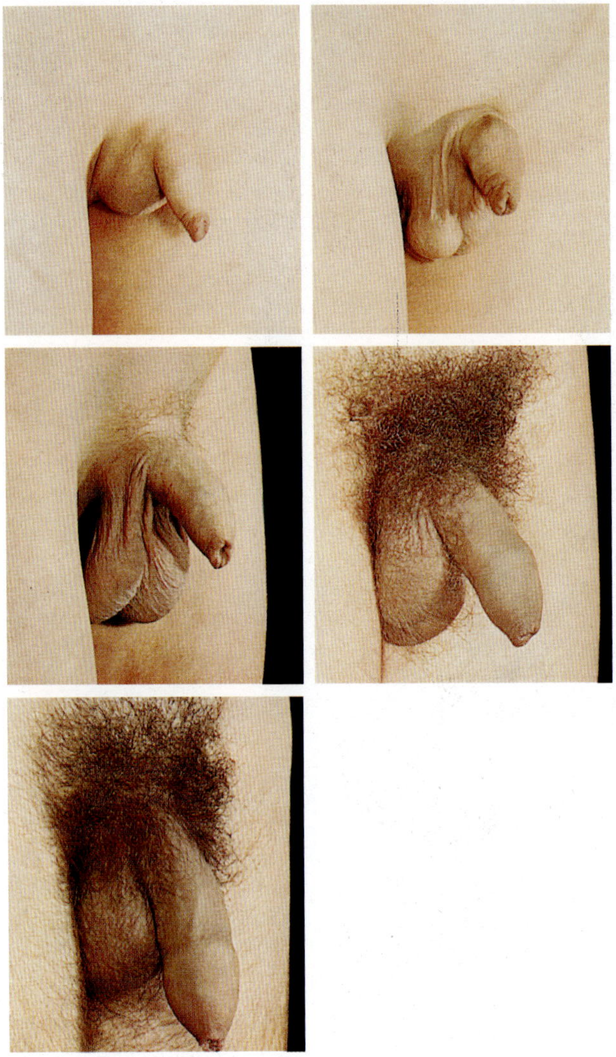

G_1—Tanner 1. Testes, scrotum, and penis are the same size and shape as in the young child.

G_2—Tanner 2. Enlargement of scrotum and testes. The skin of the scrotum becomes redder, thinner, and wrinkled. Penis no larger or scarcely so.

G_3—Tanner 3. Enlargement of the penis, especially in length; further enlargement of testes; descent of scrotum.

G_4—Tanner 4. Continued enlargement of the penis and sculpturing of the glans; increased pigmentation of scrotum. This stage is sometimes best described as "not quite adult."

G_5—Tanner 5 (adult stage). Scrotum ample, penis reaching nearly to bottom of scrotum.

FIG. 8.12 Five stages of penis and testes/scrotum development in males. (From Van Wieringen, J. C., Wafelbakker, F., Verbrugge, H. P., et al. (1971). *Growth diagrams 1965 Netherlands: Second national survey on 0–24-year-olds.* Groningen, Netherlands: Wolters-Noordhoff Publishing.)

Think About It

How Do Puberty Blockers Work?

Gonadotropin-releasing hormone (GnRH) analogs are a synthetic form of the human body's GnRH hormone. When taken regularly, GnRH analogs work by suppressing the secretion of luteinizing hormone (LH) and follicle-stimulating hormone (FSH), which ultimately suppresses the body's release of sex hormones, including testosterone and estrogen, during puberty. Blocking the release of these hormones delays changes in both the primary and secondary sex characteristics that can affect gender expression. In those identified as male at birth, GnRH analogs decrease the growth of facial and body hair, prevent voice deepening, and limit the growth of genitalia. In those identified as female at birth, GnRH analogs stop breast development and widening of the hips and delay or stop menstruation. Puberty blockers do not stop acne, body odor, or axillary and pubic hair development, as these changes are not controlled only by estrogen or testosterone. The use of GnRH analogs does not cause permanent changes in an adolescent's body. Instead, it pauses puberty, providing time to solidify gender identity, treat gender dysphoria, and promote mental well-being. If an adolescent stops taking GnRH analogs, puberty will resume.

Pregnant Persons

Calculate the weight gain during pregnancy from the patient's prepregnancy weight. To provide guidance in weight gain during pregnancy, first determine the prepregnancy BMI. Then, monitor the patient's weight throughout pregnancy using the BMI weight gain curve guidelines on the prenatal weight gain chart (Fig. 8.14).

Guidelines for recommended weight gain during pregnancy are based on the patient's prepregnancy BMI to improve reproductive outcomes. Patients with a prepregnancy BMI of 19.8 to 26.0 should gain 11.5 to 16 kg (25 to 35 lb) over the entire pregnancy. Underweight patients (BMI <19.8) should gain up to 12.2 to 18.2 kg (28 to 40 lb). Overweight patients (BMI 26.1 to 29) should gain 7 to 11.5 kg (15 to 25 lb). Those who are obese (BMI >29) should gain no more than 5 to 9.1 kg (11 to 20 lb) (Institute of Medicine and National Research Council, 2009). Adjust the recommended weight gain for patients with a twin or triplet pregnancy.

Obese patients are at increased risk of complications during pregnancy such as gestational hypertension, preeclampsia, gestational diabetes, cesarean delivery, and

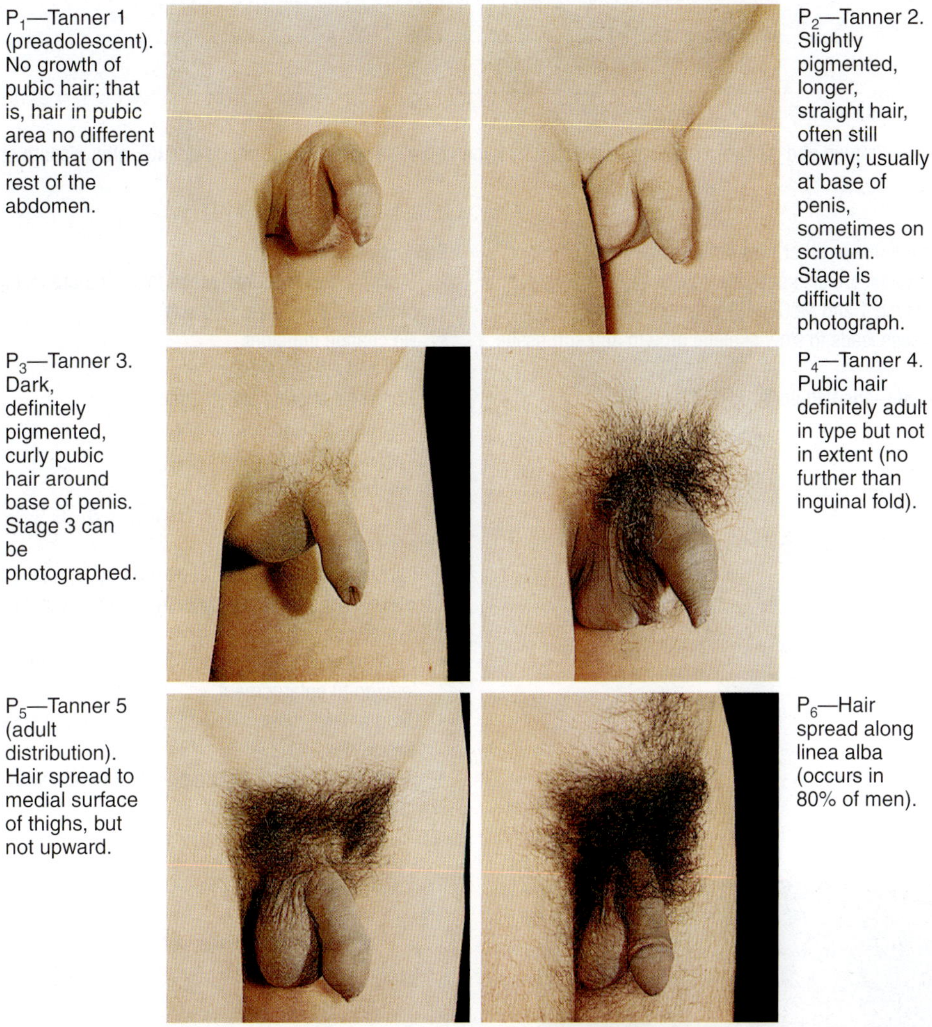

FIG. 8.13 Six stages of pubic hair development in males. (From Van Wieringen, J. C., Wafelbakker, F., Verbrugge, H. P., et al. (1971). *Growth diagrams 1965 Netherlands: Second national survey on 0–24-year-olds*. Groningen, Netherlands: Wolters-Noordhoff Publishing.)

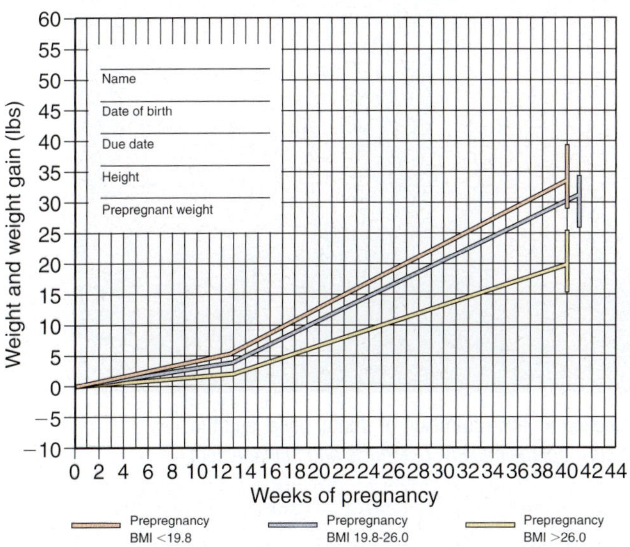

FIG. 8.14 Prenatal weight gain curve by weeks of gestation. (From Food and Nutrition Board. *Prenatal weight gain curve by weeks of gestation.* Washington, DC, 2003.)

failure to initiate breastfeeding (Alves et al., 2024). Pregnant adolescents younger than 16 years, or less than 2 years after menarche, may still be in their growth spurt. They may require higher weight gains during pregnancy to achieve an optimal infant birth weight (Marković et al., 2009).

Note any variation from the expected weight gain. First-trimester gain is variable, from 1.4 to 2.7 kg (3 to 6 lb). In the second and third trimesters, weekly weight gain should be approximately 0.23 to 0.45 kg (0.5 to 1 lb) per week. Patients who gain too little weight during pregnancy are at risk for having a low-birth-weight infant. Those who gain too much weight are at risk for having a high-birth-weight infant, which may lead to a difficult delivery (Teede et al., 2022).

Older Adults

Measurement procedures for the older adult are the same as those used for other adults. First, calculate the BMI. Second, identify any problems with underweight that could be associated with a health condition or food insecurity. From 2021 to 2023, the prevalence of obesity in adults age 60 and older was 38.9%.

ABNORMALITIES

GROWTH

Acromegaly

A rare disease of excessive growth and distorted proportions caused by hypersecretion of growth hormone and IGF after closure of the epiphyses.

PATHOPHYSIOLOGY

- A benign pituitary adenoma or other rare tumor is the most common cause; familial syndromes are also possible causes (e.g., multiple endocrine neoplasia type 1 and McCune-Albright syndrome).
- Growth hormone excess leads to slow skeletal growth and soft tissue enlargement.
- Most common in middle-aged adults.

PATIENT DATA

Subjective Data

- Slow progressive changes in facial feature exaggeration
- Increased shoe size, ring size
- No change in height
- Oily and sweaty skin
- Excessive snoring, sleep apnea
- Decreased exercise tolerance
- Pain in joints and hands
- See Fig. 8.15

Objective Data

- Face and skull—frontal skull bossing, cranial ridges, mandibular overgrowth, maxillary widening, teeth separation, malocclusion, overbite
- Skin thickening on the face (tongue, lips, and nose); hands; and feet leading to enlargement
- Joint enlargement, swelling, pain; vertebral enlargement, kyphoscoliosis
- Cardiac ventricular enlargement bilaterally with decreased exercise tolerance

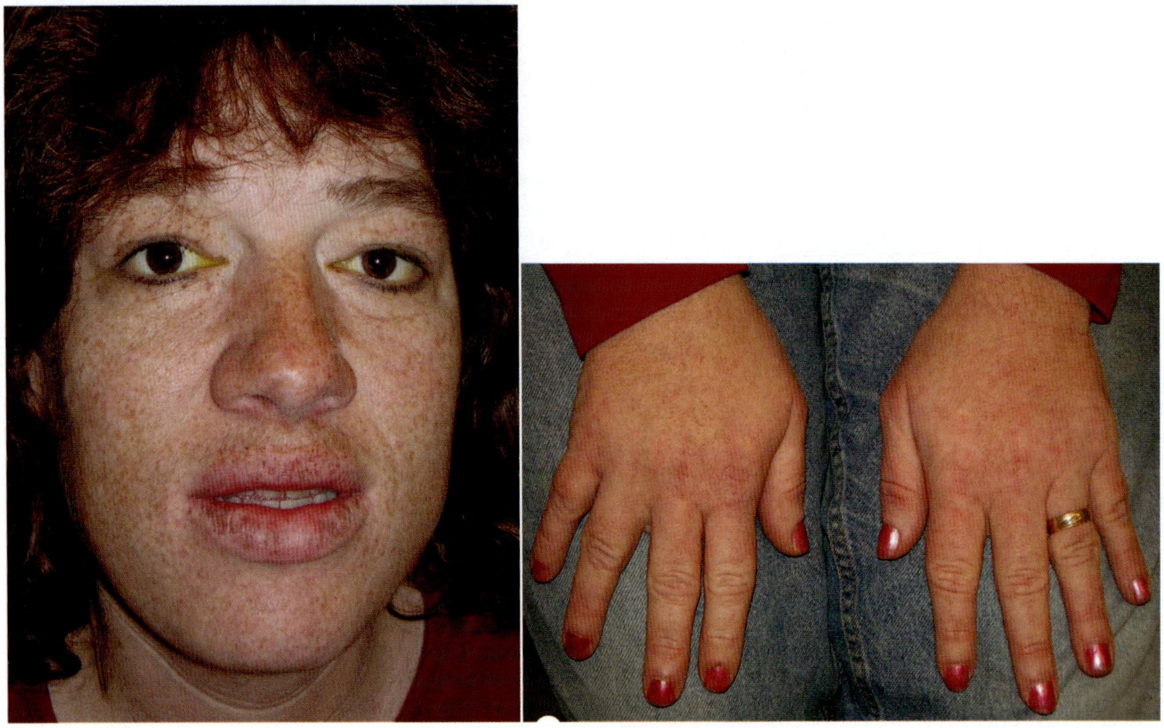

FIG. 8.15 Acromegaly. Note the large head, forward projection of jaw, protrusion of frontal bone, and the large hands. (From Liu, G. T., Volpe, N. J., & Galetta, S. L. *Neuro-ophthalmology: Diagnosis and management* (2nd ed.). London: Saunders; 2010.)

Cushing Syndrome

A disorder associated with a prolonged and excessively high exposure to glucocorticoids.

PATHOPHYSIOLOGY

- Most commonly caused by the use of medically prescribed corticosteroids.
- Other causes include adrenal gland oversecretion leading to excessive production of cortisol or a pituitary tumor leading to excessive secretion of adrenocorticotropic hormone (ACTH).
- Leads to conditions caused by the excess cortisol such as diabetes, hypertension, depression, and menstrual irregularities.

PATIENT DATA

Subjective Data

- Weight gain, changes in appetite
- Depression, irritability, decreased libido
- Decreased concentration, impaired short-term memory
- Easy bruising
- Menstrual abnormalities
- Weight gain but slow height velocity in children
- See Fig. 11.8

Objective Data

- Obesity, "buffalo hump" fat pad, supraclavicular and pendulous abdominal fat distribution
- Facial plethora or moon facies
- Thin skin, reddish-purple striae, poor skin healing
- Proximal muscle weakness
- Hirsutism or female balding
- Peripheral edema
- In children—short stature, abnormal genital virilization, delayed puberty, or pseudoprecocious puberty

Turner Syndrome

A genetic disorder in which there is partial or complete absence of a second X chromosome.

PATHOPHYSIOLOGY

- Phenotype results from a reduced complement of genes that are typically expressed from both X chromosomes in females.
- Turner syndrome incidence is 1 per 2500–3000 live births.

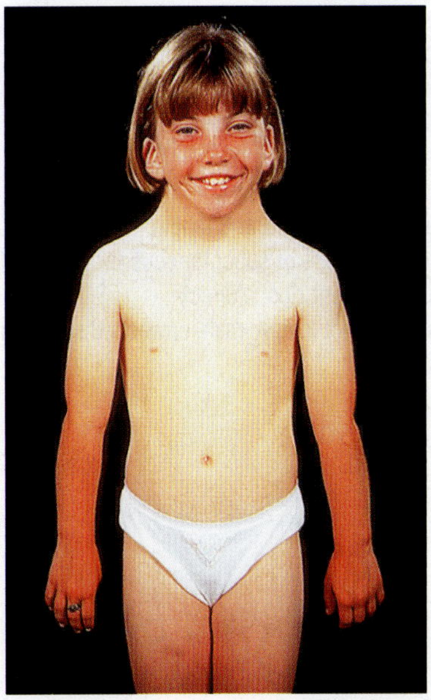

FIG. 8.16 Turner syndrome. (From Patton, K. T., & Thibodeau, G. *Anatomy & physiology* (9th ed.). St. Louis: Elsevier; 2016.)

PATIENT DATA

Subjective Data

- Poor height growth
- Lack of breast development and amenorrhea
- Normal intelligence

Objective Data

- Short stature
- Webbed neck
- Broad chest with widely spaced nipples
- Wide carrying angle of the elbow (cubitus valgus)
- Low posterior hairline, misshapen or rotated ears, narrow palate with crowded teeth
- Coarctation of the aorta, bicuspid aortic valve
- Sensorineural hearing loss
- Infertility
- May be diagnosed prenatally by amniocentesis or chorionic villous sampling
- Karyotype or chromosome analysis to confirm the diagnosis
- See Fig. 8.16

Hydrocephalus

An excess volume of cerebrospinal fluid (CSF) in the brain leading to an enlarged head circumference or increased intracranial pressure.

PATHOPHYSIOLOGY

- May be caused by an infection or obstruction in the subarachnoid space that interferes with the reabsorption of CSF or from an infection or injury that obstructs the flow of CSF to the subarachnoid space, where it can be reabsorbed.
- Often occurs in association with meningomyelocele.

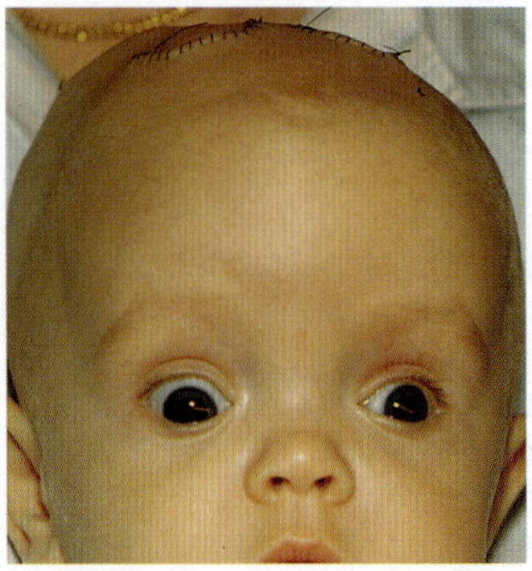

FIG. 8.17 Infantile hydrocephalus. Paralysis of the upward gaze is seen in an infant with hydrocephalus resulting from aqueductal stenosis. It appears more apparent on the right. This phenomenon is often termed the *sunsetting sign.* (Courtesy Dr. Albert Biglan, Children's Hospital of Pittsburgh.)

PATIENT DATA

Subjective Data

- Enlarged head
- Difficulty holding head up or inability to lift the head off the bed
- Irritable, lack of energy, poor feeding
- After sutures close: severe headache, diplopia or other vision problems, vomiting not associated with an illness

Objective Data

- Rapidly increasing head circumference
- Tense, full, or bulging fontanel; split sutures
- Bossing (protrusion) of frontal area, face disproportionate to the skull size
- Prominent, distended scalp veins, translucent scalp skin
- Increased tone or hyperreflexia, brisk deep tendon reflexes, positive Babinski sign
- Once skull sutures are closed, increased intracranial pressure, papilledema
- Paralysis of upward gaze (sixth cranial nerve palsy)
- See Fig. 8.17

Failure to Thrive

Growth in an infant or child below the 3rd to 5th percentiles on a growth chart or a slower-than-expected rate of growth or crossing down two percentile lines in a short period (e.g., from the 50th percentile to below the 10th percentile on the growth chart).

PATHOPHYSIOLOGY

- Psychosocial causes include poverty and inadequate food, errors in food preparation, or a poor parent-child interaction (e.g., maternal depression, child abuse or neglect, or family dysfunction).
- Organic causes include an underlying medical condition such as major infection or organ system disease.
- May result from a combination of organic disease and psychosocial stressors.

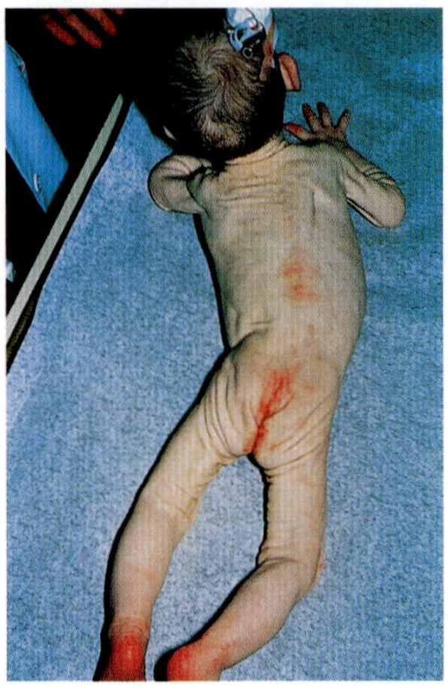

FIG. 8.18 Psychosocial failure to thrive as the result of neglect. This 4-month-old infant was brought to the emergency department because of congestion. She was found to be below weight expectations and suffering from severe developmental delay. Note the marked loss of subcutaneous tissue manifested by the wrinkled skinfolds over the buttocks, shoulders, and upper arms. (From Zitelli, B. J., & Davis, H. W. (2018). *Zitelli and Davis' atlas of pediatric physical diagnosis* (7th ed.). Philadelphia: Elsevier.)

PATIENT DATA

Subjective Data

- Insufficient food for infant or child, poor dietary intake
- Breastfeeding failure, tires or sweats when feeding, refuses food
- Smaller than infants or children of the same age

Objective Data

- Does not meet expected weight and length (height) norms for age
- Reduced muscle mass, loss of subcutaneous fat, wasted buttocks, thin extremities, prominent ribs, alopecia
- May show signs of neglect (diaper rash, unwashed skin, skin infections, unwashed clothing)
- Developmental delay
- See Fig. 8.18

Growth Hormone Deficiency

Failure of the anterior pituitary to secrete adequate growth hormone to support growth in stature.

PATHOPHYSIOLOGY

- May be congenital or develop from a pituitary tumor, radiation therapy for a tumor, or brain trauma.

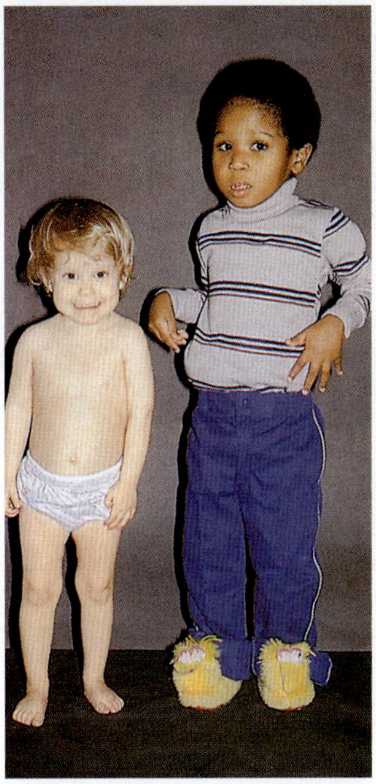

FIG. 8.19 The normal 3-year-old boy is in the 50th percentile for height. The short 3-year-old girl exhibits the characteristic "Kewpie doll" appearance, suggesting a diagnosis of growth hormone deficiency. (From Zitelli, B. J., McIntire, S. C., & Nowalk, A. J. (2012). *Zitelli and Davis' atlas of pediatric physical diagnosis* (6th ed.). Philadelphia: Saunders.)

PATIENT DATA

Subjective Data

- Normal birth weight and growth during the first year
- Smaller than a child of the same age

Objective Data

- Short stature; growth begins leveling off at 9–12 months
- Body proportions of younger-age child, cherubic or elfin appearance, child appears younger than chronologic age
- Excess subcutaneous fat
- High-pitched voice
- See Fig. 8.19

Precocious Puberty

The onset of secondary sexual characteristics before 7 years of age in White females, 6 years in Black females, and 9 years in males with progressive sexual maturation (Alonso, 2024).

PATHOPHYSIOLOGY

- A brain tumor or lesion (e.g., hypothalamic hamartoma) may activate the hypothalamic-pituitary-gonadal axis with gonadotropins, triggering the growth of the gonads, secretion of the sex hormones, and progressive sexual maturation.
- May also be related to McCune-Albright syndrome.

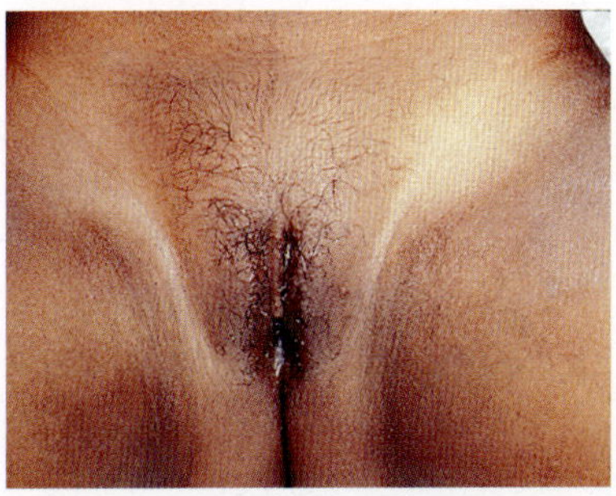

FIG. 8.20 Precocious puberty with pubic hair development in a young female. (From Zitelli, B. J., McIntire, S. C., & Nowalk, A. J. (2012). *Zitelli and Davis' atlas of pediatric physical diagnosis* (6th ed.). Philadelphia: Saunders.)

PATIENT DATA

Subjective Data

- Development of breast tissue or pubic hair at an earlier age than expected in females
- Enlargement of testes, then the penis, and appearance of pubic hair at an earlier age than expected in males

Objective Data

- In young females—breast development, pubic hair, maturation of external genitalia, axillary hair development, and the onset of menses
- In males—progressive signs of sexual maturation with testicular and penis enlargement, pubic hair, acne, erections, and nocturnal emissions
- Accelerated height growth at an early age
- Sex hormone concentrations are appropriate for the stage of puberty
- See Fig. 8.20

NUTRITION

Obesity

Excessive proportion of total body fat.

PATHOPHYSIOLOGY

- Genetic, behavioral, and environmental factors contribute to the development of obesity.
- Excess body fat develops as a result of energy imbalance of caloric intake and energy expenditure (physical activity).
- Disproportionately affects some racial groups (e.g., Blacks) and those of low socioeconomic status.
- Body fat, especially visceral fat, increases the risk for numerous health problems, including type 2 diabetes, cardiovascular disease, dyslipidemia, and cancer.
- Medications (e.g., steroids) and certain disease processes (e.g., Cushing disease and polycystic ovarian syndrome) may cause weight gain and contribute to obesity.

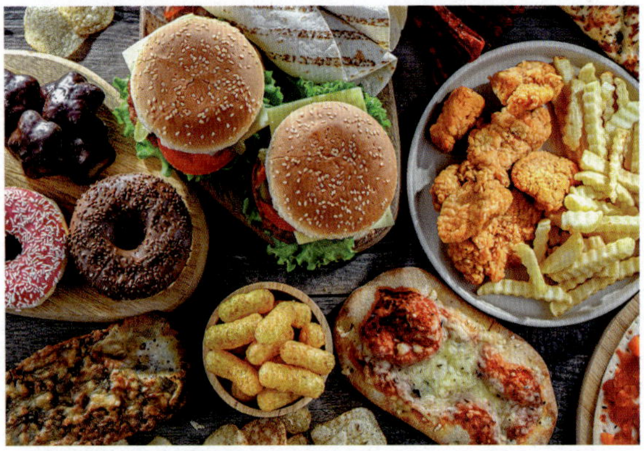

FIG. 8.21 **Poor food choices can lead to obesity, which is increasing in childhood.** (From iStock.com/monticelllo.)

PATIENT DATA

Subjective Data

- Weight gain; increase in daily caloric intake and high-fat foods
- Decrease in physical activity
- Medications
- Recent life change or stressors
- Obesity-related symptoms or conditions include snoring and sleep apnea, shortness of breath, headaches, musculoskeletal symptoms, depression, irregular menses, polyuria, and polydipsia

Objective Data

- Excess fat tissue generally located in breasts, buttocks, and thighs
- May have acanthosis nigricans (see Fig. 9.57) and pale striae
- Physical examination findings of obesity-related conditions can be found in Table 8.2
- Characteristic features of genetic disorders should be assessed (e.g., Prader-Willi syndrome)
- Adult classification of BMI: overweight 25–29.9; obesity $\geq$30
- Children and adolescents 2–18 years old: obesity is a BMI $\geq$95th percentile for age and gender or BMI $>$30; overweight is a BMI $\geq$85th percentile but $<$95th percentile for age and gender or BMI 25–29.9 (Fig. 8.21)

TABLE 8.2 Physical Examination Findings in Obesity Assessment and Possible Causes

SYSTEM	FINDINGS	POSSIBLE EXPLANATIONS
Anthropometric features	High BMI percentile	Overweight or obesity
	Short stature	Underlying endocrine or genetic condition
Vital signs	Elevated blood pressure	Hypertension if systolic blood pressure ≥140 or diastolic blood pressure ≥90 on ≥3 occasions; for children and adolescents systolic or diastolic blood pressure ≥95th percentile for age, gender, and height percentile on ≥3 occasions
Skin	Acanthosis nigricans	Common in obese children, especially when skin is dark; increased risk of insulin resistance
	Excessive acne, hirsutism	Polycystic ovary syndrome
	Irritation, inflammation	Consequence of severe obesity
	Violaceous striae	Cushing syndrome
Eyes	Papilledema, cranial nerve VI paralysis	Pseudotumor cerebri
Throat	Tonsillar hypertrophy	Obstructive sleep apnea
Neck	Goiter	Hypothyroidism
Chest	Wheezing	Asthma (may explain or contribute to exercise intolerance)
Abdomen	Tenderness	Gastroesophageal reflux disorder, gallbladder disease, NAFLD
	Hepatomegaly	NAFLD
Reproductive system	Tanner stage	Premature puberty in <7-yr-old White females, <6-yr-old Black females, and <9-yr-old males
	Apparent micropenis	May be normal penis that is buried in fat
	Undescended testes	Prader-Willi syndrome
Extremities	Abnormal gait, limited hip range of motion	Slipped capital femoral epiphysis
	Bowing of tibia	Blount disease
	Small hands and feet, polydactyly	Some genetic syndromes

NAFLD, Nonalcoholic fatty liver disease.

From Barlow, S. E. (2007). Expert committee recommendations regarding the prevention, assessment, and treatment of child and adolescent overweight and obesity: summary report. *Pediatrics, 120,* S164–S192.

Anorexia Nervosa

Eating disorder classified by the *Diagnostic and Statistical Manual of Mental Disorders,* Fifth Edition *(DSM-V)* as a psychiatric disease, characterized by low body weight and body image distortion.

PATHOPHYSIOLOGY

- Cause is unknown, but genetic, environmental, and sociocultural factors likely contribute to the development of anorexia.
- Adolescent and young adult women, usually from middle- and upper-class families, are most commonly affected; also occurs in adolescent and adult males.
- Two types: restricting (food intake is voluntarily limited) and purging (patients engage in purging after eating).

PATIENT DATA

Subjective Data

- May report preoccupation with weight, excessive exercise, and unusual eating habits including voluntary starvation, purging, vomiting, and weight control measures such as diet pills, use of laxatives, and diuretics
- May report being overweight as a child and unhappiness with current weight as well as poor body image
- Symptoms may include fatigue, dizziness, low energy, amenorrhea, weight loss or gain, constipation, bloating, abdominal discomfort, heartburn, intolerance to cold, palpitations, depression or irritability, decreased libido, and interrupted sleep

Objective Data

- Physical examination findings may include dry skin, lanugo hair, brittle nails, bradycardia, hypothermia, orthostatic hypotension, and loss of muscle mass and subcutaneous fat
- May have hypoglycemia, elevated liver enzymes, and thyroid hormone abnormalities
- *DSM-V* criteria for diagnosis include refusal to maintain body weight at or above a minimally normal weight for age and height (failure to maintain weight at 85% of ideal body weight); intense fear of gaining weight; disturbance in self-perception of body weight; and amenorrhea in females
- BMI ≤17.5 also characteristic

Bulimia Nervosa

Eating disorder classified by the *DSM-V* as a psychiatric disease.

PATHOPHYSIOLOGY

- Cause unknown, but genetic, environmental, and sociocultural factors likely contribute to the development of bulimia.
- Adolescent and young adult females most commonly affected.
- Two types are purging and nonpurging episodes followed by fasting or excessive exercising.

PATIENT DATA

Subjective Data

- Binge-eating episodes on average two times a week, usually high-calorie or high-carbohydrate foods in purging type, followed by purging behaviors (e.g., vomiting, laxatives, diuretics)
- Bloating, fullness, lethargy, abdominal pain, heartburn, and sore throat

Objective Data

- Body weight can be normal, underweight, or overweight
- Knuckle calluses, dental enamel erosion, salivary gland enlargement
- Metabolic alkalosis from vomiting, hypokalemia from laxative or diuretic use, and elevated salivary amylase
- *DSM-V* criteria for diagnosis include recurrent binge-eating episodes over a discrete period and lack of control over eating; recurrent compensatory behaviors to prevent weight gain (e.g., self-induced vomiting); behaviors occur on average twice per week for 3 months

CHAPTER 9

Skin, Hair, and Nails

Skin provides an elastic, self-regenerating, protective covering for the body. The skin and its appendages are an important means by which we are viewed in the world, and physical appearances are often critical to the well-being of patients. Examination of the skin, hair, and nails is performed as part of both the comprehensive and focused physical examination. The skin, hair, and nails can provide external visible clues to systemic disease that may not otherwise be apparent.

ANATOMY AND PHYSIOLOGY

The skin is a stratified organ composed of several functionally related layers. Fig. 9.1 shows the main structural components and their approximate spatial relationships. It is important to note that the anatomy of the skin varies from one part of the body to another.

Skin structure and its physiologic processes perform the following integral functions:

- Protect against microbial and foreign substance invasion and minor physical trauma
- Restrict body fluid loss by providing a restrictive barrier
- Regulate body temperature
- Provide sensory perception via free nerve endings and specialized receptors
- Produce vitamin D from precursors in the skin
- Contribute to blood pressure regulation through constriction of skin blood vessels
- Repair surface wounds by exaggerating the normal process of cell replacement
- Excrete sweat, urea, and lactic acid
- Express emotions

Components of Physical Examination

Skin

1. Systematically inspect the entire skin surface. During evaluation of each organ system, evaluate the overlying skin for:
   - Color
   - Uniformity
   - Thickness
   - Symmetry
   - Hygiene
   - Lesions
   - Odors
2. Palpate skin surfaces for:
   - Moisture
   - Temperature
   - Texture
   - Turgor (fullness or tension produced by the fluid content of the cells and tissue)
   - Elasticity

Hair

1. Inspect hair for:
   - Color
   - Distribution
   - Density
2. Palpate hair for texture and fragility.

Nails

1. Inspect for:
   - Pigmentation of nail plates and nail beds
   - Length
   - Symmetry
   - Surface changes (ridging, beading, pitting, peeling)
2. Inspect and palpate proximal and lateral nail folds for:
   - Redness
   - Swelling
   - Pain
   - Exudate
   - Growths (warts, cysts, tumors)
   - Shape of lunulae
3. Palpate nail plate for:
   - Texture
   - Firmness
   - Thickness
   - Uniformity
   - Adherence to nail bed
4. Measure nail base angle.
5. Observe the cuticles for:
   - Color
   - Vasculature
   - Integrity

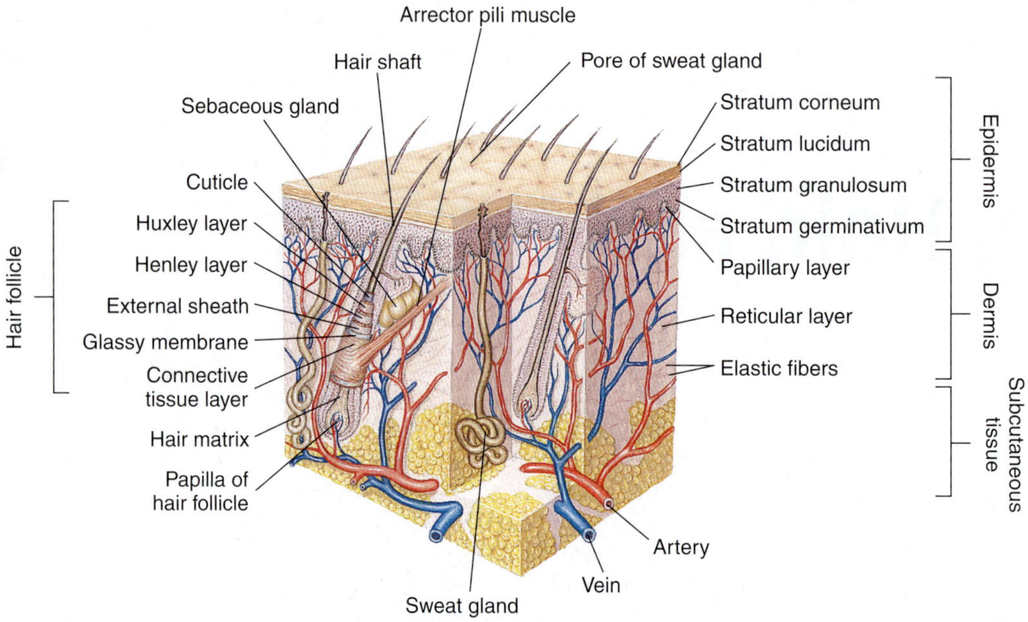

FIG. 9.1 Anatomic structures of the skin.

Epidermis

The epidermis is the outermost portion of the skin and is composed of several cellular layers. The topmost layer is the stratum corneum (cornified layer), which is composed of closely packed, dead, keratin-filled squamous cells; it is the chief mechanical barrier, protecting the body against environmental exposures and pathogens and restricting water loss. The keratins contained in the stratum corneum are synthesized in the lower layers of the skin, beginning at the stratum basale (basal layer). This lower layer contains stem cells, which allow for the regenerative properties of the skin to manifest. As keratinocytes mature, they pass from the basal layer through the granular layer to the cornified layer, a process that takes, on average, 28 days.

The thick skin of the palms and soles contains an additional layer compared with other parts of the body called the *stratum lucidum,* which lies just below the stratum corneum. Mucosal skin, on the other hand, lacks a stratum corneum, allowing for diffusion through the skin surface. The stratum basale also contains melanocytes, the cells that synthesize melanin, which gives the skin its color.

Dermis

The dermis is the richly vascular connective tissue layer of the skin that supports and separates the epidermis from adipose tissue. Interdigitating papillae secure the epidermis to the dermis and provide nourishment to the epidermal cells. Elastin, collagen, and reticular fibers provide resilience, strength, and stability. Sensory nerve fibers located in the dermis form a complex network that provides sensations of pain, touch, and temperature. The dermis also contains autonomic motor nerves that innervate blood vessels, glands, and the arrector pili muscles.

Hypodermis

The dermis is connected to underlying tissues by the hypodermis, a subcutaneous layer that consists of loose connective tissue filled with adipose. This adipose layer generates heat and provides insulation, shock absorption, and a reserve of calories.

Appendages

Cutaneous appendages are outgrowths of the skin and include eccrine sweat glands, apocrine sweat glands, sebaceous glands, hair, and nails.

The eccrine sweat glands open directly onto the surface of the skin and help regulate body temperature through sweat secretion. These glands are distributed throughout the body except at the lip margins, eardrums, nail beds, inner surface of the prepuce, and glans penis.

The apocrine glands are specialized structures found only in the axillae, nipples, areolae, anogenital area, eyelids, and external ears. Apocrine glands secrete an oily fluid containing protein, carbohydrate, and other substances. Secretions from these glands are odorless. Body odor is produced by bacterial decomposition of apocrine sweat.

The sebaceous glands secrete sebum, a lipid-rich substance that acts as a lubricant and moisturizer for skin and hair. Secretory activity, which is stimulated by sex hormones (primarily testosterone), varies according to hormonal levels throughout the life cycle.

A strand of hair consists of a root and a shaft, which sit in a follicle. At the base of the follicle the papilla contains a loop of capillaries supplying nourishment for growth. Melanocytes in the follicle synthesize pigment, which gives hair its color. Adults have both vellus and terminal hair. Vellus hair is short, fine, soft, and nonpigmented. Terminal hair is coarser, longer, thicker, and usually pigmented. Each hair goes through cyclic changes: anagen (growth), catagen (atrophy), and telogen (rest), after which the hair is shed (exogen). Males and females have about the same number of hair follicles with differential stimulation by hormones. The shape of the hair follicle directly relates to the shape of the hair itself (straight vs. curly). This shape does vary by skin type.

The nails are appendages of the skin, which are composed of epidermal cells converted to hard plates of keratin. They protect the fingertips and are important in dexterity. The nail plate sits on the highly vascular nail bed, which lies on the periosteum. The white crescent-shaped area extending beyond the proximal nail fold marks the end of the nail matrix, the site of nail growth. The layer of skin covering the nail root is the cuticle, or eponychium, which pushes up and over the lower part of the nail body. The paronychium is the soft tissue surrounding the nail border (Fig. 9.2).

Infants and Children

The skin of infants and children is smoother than adults' skin due to the absence of coarse terminal hair and diminished exposure to the elements, particularly ultraviolet (UV) radiation. Desquamation of the stratum corneum may be present at birth or shortly thereafter. It may vary from mild flakiness to coarse shedding of large sheets of skin, but postterm infants often have cracked, peeling skin. Vernix caseosa, a mixture of sebum and cornified epidermis, covers the infant's body at birth. The subcutaneous fat layer is poorly developed in newborns, predisposing them to hypothermia. The newborn's body, particularly the shoulders and back, can be covered with fine, silky hair called *lanugo*. More commonly seen in preterm infants, this hair is shed within 10 to 14 days. Some newborns are bald, whereas others have a large amount of head hair. Most of the hair is shed by about 2 to 3 months of age, to be replaced by more permanent hair with a new texture and often a different color.

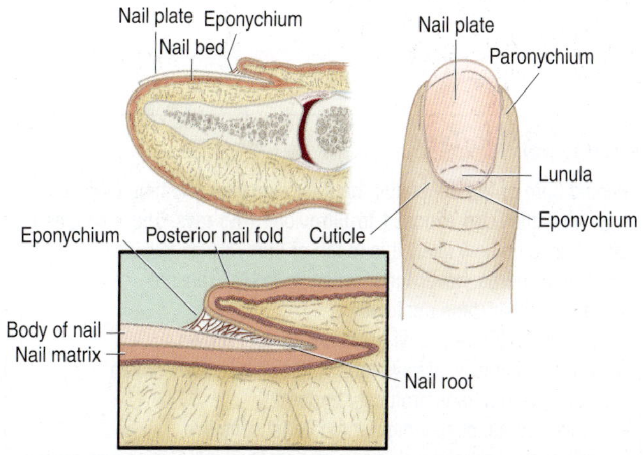

FIG. 9.2 **Anatomic structures of the nail.** (From Swartz, M. H. (2021). *Textbook of physical diagnosis* (8th ed.). Philadelphia: Elsevier.)

The eccrine sweat glands begin to function after the first month of life, whereas apocrine function does not begin until puberty; thus children lack offensive perspiration.

Adolescents

During adolescence, the apocrine glands enlarge and become active, causing increased axillary sweating and sometimes body odor. Sebaceous glands increase sebum production in response to increased hormone levels, primarily androgen, giving the skin an oily appearance and predisposing the individual to acne.

Coarse terminal hair appears in the axillae and pubic areas of all adolescents and on the faces of adolescents assigned male at birth. Hair production is one response to changing androgen levels. (Refer to Chapter 8 for a more thorough discussion of maturational changes during adolescence.)

Pregnant Patients

Increased blood flow to the skin, especially to the hands and feet, results from peripheral vasodilation and increased numbers of capillaries. Acceleration of sweat and sebaceous gland activity occurs as well. Both processes assist in dissipating the excess heat caused by increased metabolism during pregnancy. Spider angiomas and cherry hemangiomas that are present may increase in size.

The skin thickens, and fat is deposited in the subdermal layers. Because of increased fragility of connective tissues, separation may occur with stretching. Most pregnant patients have some degree of increased pigmentation that is seen on the face, nipples, areolae, axillae, vulva, perianal skin, and umbilicus. During pregnancy, nevi may grow and change color, and new nevi may appear.

Older Adults

Sebaceous and sweat gland activity decreases in older adults, and, as a result, the skin becomes drier with less perspiration produced. With aging and increased sun exposure, the epidermis thins and becomes more fragile, with decreased resistance to trauma. Epidermal permeability is increased, reducing the efficiency of the barrier function of the stratum corneum, causing skin to become dry.

Aging and sun exposure also contribute to decreasing elasticity and collagen loss in the dermis. The dermis shrinks, causing the epidermis to fold and become wrinkled. This effect is increased in lighter skin, which has earlier onset and greater skin wrinkling and sagging signs than darker skin.

Subcutaneous tissues also decrease, particularly in the extremities, giving joints and bony prominences a sharp, angular appearance. The hollows in the thoracic, axillary, and supraclavicular regions deepen as well.

Gray hair results from a decrease in the number of functioning melanocytes. Axillary and pubic hair production declines because of a reduction in hormones. The density and rate of scalp hair growth (anagen phase) decline with age. The size of hair follicles also changes, and terminal scalp hair progressively transitions into vellus hair, causing age-associated baldness in both males and females. The opposite transition, from vellus to terminal, occurs in the hair of the nares and on the tragus of male ears. Both sexes experience overall loss of hair from the trunk and extremities. Peripheral extremity hair loss may also occur when peripheral vascular disease is present.

Nail growth slows, and nails become more brittle because of decreased peripheral circulation. The nails, particularly the toenails, become thick, brittle, hard, and yellowish. They develop longitudinal ridges and are prone to splitting into layers.

REVIEW OF RELATED HISTORY

For each of the symptoms or conditions discussed in this section, targeted topics to include in the history of the present illness are listed. Responses to questions about these topics provide clues to focus the physical examination and develop an appropriate diagnostic evaluation. Questions regarding medication use (prescription and over-the-counter preparations) as well as complementary, alternative, and integrative therapies are relevant for each.

History of Present Illness

Skin

- Changes in skin: dryness, pruritus, sores, rashes, growths, color, texture, odor, amount of perspiration; changes in wart or nevus; lesion that does not heal or is chronically irritated (see Risk Factors boxes)
- Temporal sequence: date of initial onset; time sequence of occurrence and development; intermittent; sudden or gradual onset; date of recurrence, if any
- Symptoms: itching, pain, exudate, bleeding, color changes, seasonal or climate variations
- Location: skin folds, extensor or flexor surfaces, localized or generalized, sun exposed or protected, mucosal involvement
- Associated symptoms: recent illness, presence of systemic disease or fever, relationship to stress or leisure activities
- Recent exposure to environmental or occupational toxins or chemicals, new skin or personal care products, new household cleaning products (aerosols)
- Recent exposure to persons with similar skin condition
- Apparent cause of problem, patient's perception of cause
- Travel history: where, when, length of stay, exposure to diseases, contact with travelers
- What the patient has been doing for the problem, response to treatment, what makes the condition worse or better
- How the patient is adjusting to the problem
- Medications: antibiotics, any new medications; either over-the-counter or prescription, topical preparations to treat—supplements, powders, teas, steroids, antifungals

You can use the National Cancer Institute's Melanoma Risk Assessment Tool to estimate a person's absolute risk of developing invasive melanoma at https://mrisktool.cancer.gov.

Risk Factors

Melanoma

- Exposure to sunlight or ultraviolet radiation (UVA and UVB), including:
  - Severe blistering sunburns, even as a child
  - Indoor tanning device usage
  - Geographic exposure (people who live in areas that get large amounts of UV radiation from the sun, e.g., higher altitude)
- Previous personal history of melanoma
- Family history of melanoma (first-degree relative)
- Atypical nevi
- Large congenital nevus (>15 cm)
- Immune suppression
- Skin type, relative inability to tan (Box 9.1)

Risk Factors

Basal and Squamous Cell Cancer

- Age (older than 50 years)
- Exposure to sunlight or ultraviolet radiation (UVA and UVB)
  - Indoor tanning device usage
  - Blistering sunburns
  - Chronic and cumulative exposure—squamous cell carcinoma
  - Intermittent exposure—basal cell carcinoma
  - Geographic location: near equator or at high altitudes
- Skin type, relative inability to tan (see Box 9.1)
- Exposure to arsenic, creosote, coal tar, and/or petroleum products
- Overexposure to radium, radioisotopes, or x-rays
- Repeated trauma or irritation to skin
- Precancerous dermatoses
- Large scars

BOX 9.1 Skin Type

People burn or tan depending on their skin type, the time of year, and how long they are exposed to ultraviolet (UV) rays. The six types of skin, based on how likely it is to tan or burn, are as follows:

I: Always burns, never tans, sensitive to UV exposure
II: Burns easily, tans minimally
III: Burns moderately, tans gradually to light brown
IV: Burns minimally, always tans well to moderately brown
V: Rarely burns, tans profusely to dark
VI: Never burns, deeply pigmented, least sensitive

Although everyone's skin can be damaged by UV exposure, people with skin types I and II are at the highest risk.

Hair

- Changes in hair: loss or growth, distribution, texture, color
- Occurrence: sudden or gradual onset, symmetric or asymmetric pattern, recurrence
- Associated symptoms: pain, itching, lesions, presence of systemic disease or high fever, recent stress, hair-pulling, infection
- Exposure to drugs, environmental or occupational toxins or chemicals, commercial hair care chemicals
- Nutrition: dietary changes, dieting
- What the patient has been doing for the problem, response to treatment, what makes the problem worse or better
- How the patient is adjusting to the problem
- Medications: drugs or preparations for hair loss (minoxidil, finasteride, dihydrotestosterone [DHT] inhibitors)

Nails

- Changes in nails: splitting, breaking, discoloration, ridging, thickening, markings, separation from nail bed
- Recent history: systemic illness, high fever, trauma, stress, biting
- Associated symptoms: pain, swelling, exudate
- Temporal sequence: sudden or gradual onset, relationship to injury of nail or finger
- Recent exposure to drugs, environmental or occupational toxins or chemicals; frequent immersion in water
- What the patient has been doing for the problem, response to treatment, what makes the problem worse or better
- Medications: chemotherapy (taxanes, anthracyclines), psoralens, retinoids, tetracyclines, antimalarials

Past Medical History

Skin

- Previous skin problems: sensitivities, allergic skin reactions, skin disorders (e.g., atopic dermatitis), congenital or acquired lesions, treatment
- Tolerance to sunlight (see Box 9.1)
- Diminished or heightened sensitivity to touch
- Cardiac, respiratory, liver, endocrine, or other systemic diseases

Hair

- Previous hair problems: loss, thinning, unusual growth or distribution, brittleness, breakage, treatment
- Systemic problems: thyroid disorder, rheumatologic disease, any severe illness, malnutrition, associated skin disorder

Nails

- Previous nail problems: injury; bacterial, fungal, or viral infection
- Systemic problems: associated skin disorder; congenital anomalies; respiratory, cardiac, endocrine, hematologic, or other systemic disease

Family History

- Current or past dermatologic diseases or disorders in family members; melanoma and other skin cancers; dermatoses (e.g., psoriasis); infestations; bacterial, fungal, or viral infections
- Allergic hereditary diseases such as asthma or allergic rhinitis
- Autoimmune disorders such as systemic lupus erythematosus
- Familial hair loss or pigmentation patterns

Personal and Social History

- Skin care habits: cleansing routine; soaps, oils, emollients, or local applications used; cosmetics; home remedies or preparations used; sun exposure patterns and history; sunburn history; use of sunscreen agents; recent changes in skin care habits (see Patient Safety, "Sunscreen")
- Skin self-examination (Box 9.2)
- Hair care habits: cleansing routine, shampoos and oils and moisturizers, coloring preparations used, permanents, applied heat, hair straightening, extensions,

BOX 9.2 Patient Instructions for Skin Self-Examination

- Always use a good light positioned to minimize distracting glare. Look for a new growth or any skin change.
- Be aware of the locations and appearance of nevi and birthmarks.
- Examine your back and other hard-to-see areas of the body using full-length and handheld mirrors. Ask a friend or relative to help inspect those areas that are difficult to see, such as the scalp and back.
- Begin with your face and scalp using one or more mirrors. Proceed downward, focusing on the neck, chest, and torso. Check under the breasts. With the back to the mirror, use a hand mirror to inspect the back of the neck, shoulders, upper arms, back, buttocks, and legs. Concentrate especially on areas where atypical nevi (those with unexpected changes) are most common—the shoulders and back—and areas where ordinary nevi are rarely found—the scalp, breast, and buttocks. Check hands, including nails. In a full-length mirror, examine elbows, arms, and underarms. Sitting down, check the legs and feet, including the soles, heels, nails, and between the toes. Use a hand mirror to examine the genitals. See as well as feel any early signs of a nevus change. Use a cell phone to take photos of nevi, and compare the photographs of the same nevi over a period of several months. Monitor change in size by measuring. It can be done simply with a small ruler or even by comparing the nevi to the size of your thumb or fingernail.
- Patients of color should pay particular attention to nail beds for any change of character.
- Consult your primary care provider promptly if any pigmented skin spots look like melanoma, if new nevi have appeared, or if any existing nevi have changed. See also the ABCDE changes in nevi ("Melanoma" in the "Abnormalities" section).

recent changes in hair care habits. Note that hair care practices can often vary by hair type.

- Nail care habits: any difficulty in clipping or trimming nails, instruments used; biting nails; use of artificial nail overlays
- Exposure to environmental or occupational hazards: dyes, chemicals, plants, toxic substances, frequent immersion of hands in water, frequent sun exposure, hand sanitizers
- Recent psychological or physiologic stress
- Use of alcohol, tobacco
- Sexual history: sexually transmitted infections (syphilis, gonorrhea, human immunodeficiency virus [HIV])
- Use of illicit drugs

Patient Safety

Sunscreen

Do you ask if your patients use sunscreen? Keep this in mind when they respond: Skin should be the same color all year long. Those who use sunscreen with a protection factor of 30 or higher are still at risk for significant sunburn. Why? People often don't use enough sunscreen. They think they are protected, but they are in fact getting significant UV exposure. It is necessary to apply sunscreen generously (about 1 to 2 ounces over the entire body) and frequently. Apply minutes before exposure and then reapply after swimming, bathing, or sweating and after every 2 hours of sun exposure.

Other recommendations include:

- Do not sunbathe.
- Avoid unnecessary sun exposure, especially between 10:00 AM and 4:00 PM, the peak hours for harmful UV radiation; seek shade if you must be outdoors during these hours.
- When exposed to sunlight, wear protective clothing such as long pants, long-sleeved shirts, broad-brimmed hats, and UV-protective sunglasses. Look for SPF-containing clothing, which offers the benefit of not needing reapplication.
- Never use tanning booths.
- Teach children good sun protection habits at an early age; the damage that leads to adult skin cancers starts in childhood.

Infants

- Birth history: term or premature
- Feeding history: breast or formula, type of formula, what foods introduced and when (see Clinical Pearl, "Carotenemia")
- Diaper history: type of diapers used, skin cleansing routines, and methods of cleaning
- Types of clothing and washing practices: soaps and detergents used, new blanket or clothing
- Bathing practices: frequency, types of soap, oils, shampoos or emollients used
- Dress habits: amount and type of clothing in relation to environmental temperature
- Temperature and humidity of the home environment: air conditioning, heating system (drying or humidified)

CLINICAL PEARL

Carotenemia

Carotenemia, or xanthoderma, common in infants who have started eating baby foods, is characterized by yellow pigmentation of the skin and increased beta-carotene levels in the blood. Carotenemia does not cause orange discoloration of the sclerae and is thus typically easy to distinguish from jaundice. In most cases, it is a benign condition that follows increased consumption of carotene-rich foods, such as carrots, squash, and sweet potatoes. If parental anxiety is high, provide reassurance and counsel that after discontinuation of carotene-rich foods, the skin color will normalize in weeks or months.

Children and Adolescents

- Eating habits and types of food
- Food allergies. Some children with eczema have worsening with specific foods.
- Exposure to infectious diseases in childcare settings, school: impetigo; viruses that produce skin rashes (Coxsackie); measles, mumps, rubella, varicella in unvaccinated children, sexual activity
- Allergic disorders: eczema, urticaria, pruritus, allergic rhinitis, asthma, other chronic respiratory disorders
- Pets or animal exposure
- Activities: sports, use of musical instruments
- Outdoor exposures such as hiking, camping, picnics, gardening
- Skin injury history: frequency of falls, cuts, abrasions; repeated history of unexplained injuries
- Chronic hair-pulling or manipulation
- Nail-biting

Pregnant Patients

- Weeks of gestation or postpartum
- Prior pregnancies
- Hygiene practices
- Presence of skin problems before pregnancy (e.g., acne may worsen)
- Effects of pregnancy on preexisting conditions (e.g., autoimmune disorders may remit; condylomata acuminata commonly become larger and more numerous)

Older Adults

- Increased or decreased sensation to touch or to the environment
- Generalized chronic itching; exposure to skin irritants, detergents, lotions (any moisturizer that comes in a pump has a high alcohol content), woolen clothing, humidity of environment
- Susceptibility to skin infections

- Healing response: delayed or interrupted
- Frequent falls resulting in multiple cuts or bruises
- Risk for pressure ulcers secondary to immobilization or nonambulatory status
- History of chronic medical conditions (e.g., diabetes mellitus, vascular disease)
- Medications and polypharmacy

EXAMINATION AND FINDINGS

Equipment

- Centimeter ruler (flexible, clear)
- Flashlight or penlight
- Handheld magnifying lens or dermatoscope
- Wood's lamp (to view fluorescing or depigmented lesions)

Skin

Use inspection and palpation to examine the skin, and remember, the most important tools you have are your own eyes and powers of observation. When gross inspection leaves you uncertain, sometimes a handheld magnifying glass or dermatoscope will help.

Inspection

Adequate lighting is essential. Direct, overhead lighting should be used when examining patients. Tangential lighting is helpful in assessing contour. Inadequate lighting can result in inadequate assessment.

Although the skin is commonly observed as each part of the body is examined, it is important to make a brief but careful overall visual sweep of the entire body. This "bird's-eye view" gives a good idea of the distribution, extent, and symmetry of any lesions. It also allows for identification of "ugly duckling" lesions that stand out. The gross view will allow the practitioner to know where to pay particular attention during the remainder of the examination (Box 9.3).

Adequate exposure of the skin is also necessary. It is essential to remove clothing and to fully remove drapes or coverings as each section of the body is examined, while respecting patient privacy and having a chaperone when examining sensitive areas. Make sure that the room temperature is comfortable. Look carefully at all areas, remembering to inspect areas that are usually not exposed, such as the axillae, buttocks, perineum, backs of thighs, and inner upper thighs. Ask patients to remove shoes and socks to look at the feet, and pay careful attention to intertriginous surfaces (areas where two skin surfaces may touch, e.g., axillae and groin), especially in infants and older adults. As you complete the examination for each area, redrape or cover the patient. When inspecting the skin, it is important to have a systematic routine in place to ensure that no areas are forgotten or overlooked. Skin thickness varies over the body, with the thinnest skin being on the eyelids and the thickest present in areas subject to increased pressure or rubbing—most notably the soles, palms, and elbows. Make note of calluses on the hands or feet and look for corns on pressure points. Corns are flat or slightly elevated, circumscribed, painful lesions with a central core and a smooth, hard surface (Fig. 9.3). A superficial area of hyperkeratosis is called a *callus*. Calluses usually occur on the weight-bearing areas of the feet and on the palmar surface of the hands. Calluses are not as well demarcated as corns and are usually not as tender, if at all (Fig. 9.4).

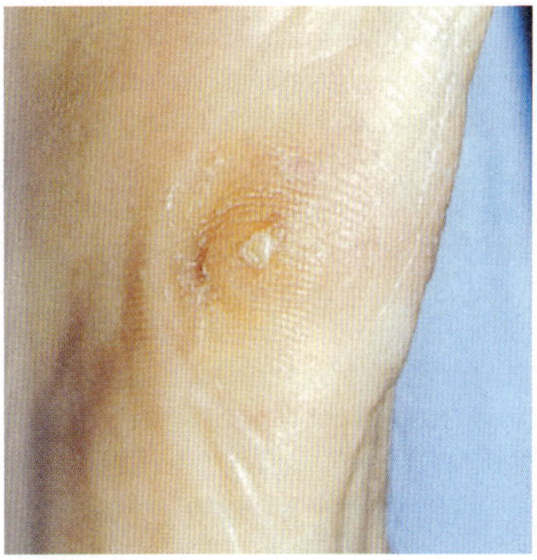

FIG. 9.3 Corn. (From Ferri, F. F. (2021). *Ferri's clinical advisor 2021*. Philadelphia: Elsevier.)

BOX 9.3 Cutaneous Manifestations of Traditional Health Practices

The use of certain traditional health practices by various cultural groups can produce cutaneous manifestations that could be wrongly confused with disease or physical abuse. Two such practices are coining and cupping as used by some Asian subcultures. In coining, a coin dipped in mentholated oil is vigorously rubbed across the skin in a prescribed manner, causing a mild dermabrasion. This practice is believed to release excess force from the body and hence restore balance. In cupping, a series of small heated glasses are placed on the skin, forming a suction that leaves a red or purpuric circular mark, drawing out the bad force. The skin markings may alarm the clinician who is unaware of such practices. The lesson: in the history, ask about home remedies or practices.

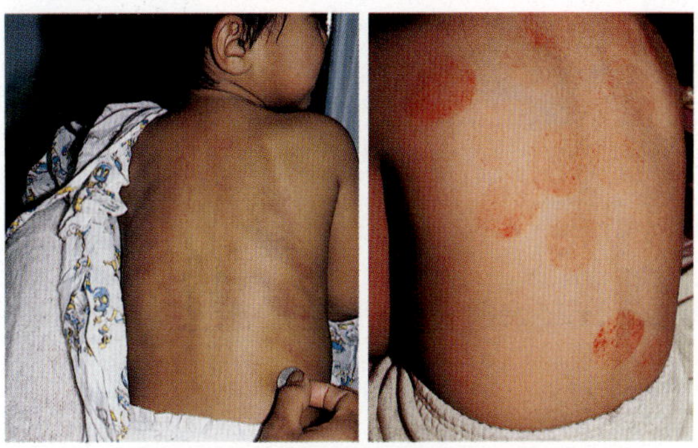

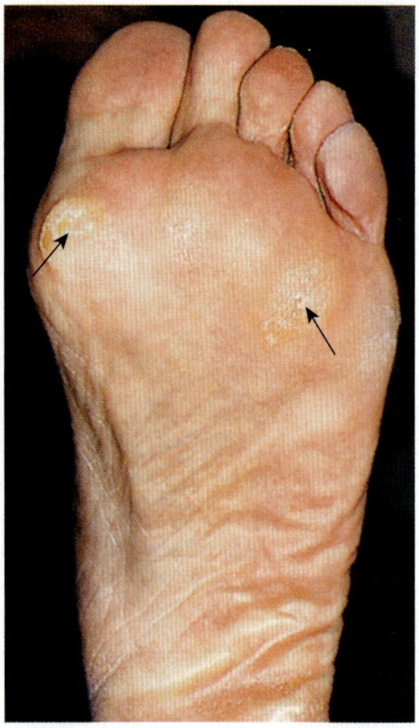

FIG. 9.4 Callus under the metatarsophalangeal joints. (From Lawrence, C. M., & Cox, N. H. (1993). *Physical signs in dermatology: Color atlas and text.* St. Louis: Mosby.)

The range of expected skin color varies from dark brown to white with pink or yellow overtones. Although color should assume an overall uniformity, there is often pigment variation that may be sun related, trauma induced, or simply normal (e.g., knuckles may be darker in dark-skinned patients). Callused areas may appear yellow. Vascular flush areas (e.g., cheeks, neck, upper chest, and genital area) may appear pink or red, especially with anxiety or excitement. Be aware that skin color may be masked by cosmetics and tanning agents. Look for localized areas of discoloration. Notably, erythema may be more difficult to appreciate in darker skin. It is important to ask the patient if their skin is more red than normal, itchy, or otherwise changed.

Individuals with dark skin may show pigmentary demarcation lines. These lines, a normal variation, mark the border between deeply pigmented skin and lighter pigmented skin. They are most commonly seen on the arms, legs, chest, and back and have been reported most often in Black and Japanese populations. Accentuation of preexisting lines or appearance of new lines may occur during pregnancy.

Nevi (moles) occur in forms that vary in size and degree of pigmentation. Nevi are present on most persons regardless of skin color and may occur anywhere on the body. They may be flat, raised, dome shaped, smooth, rough, or hairy. Their color ranges from pink, tan, gray, blue, and shades of brown to black. Table 9.1 describes the features and occurrence of various types of pigmented nevi.

Nevi occur more often in lighter-skinned than in darker-skinned individuals. There is a strong association between sun exposure and the number of nevi. They increase in number throughout infancy and childhood, with peak incidence in the fourth to fifth decades. Nevi frequently involute and diminish in number with advancing age and rarely develop after 40 years of age.

Although most nevi are harmless, some may be atypical or develop into melanoma. Table 9.2 describes differences in the features of normal and atypical nevi. Atypical nevi tend to occur on heavily sun damaged skin, classically the upper back in males and on the legs in females (Box 9.4).

Several variations in skin color occur in almost all healthy adults and children, including nonpigmented striae (i.e., silver or pink "stretch marks" that occur during pregnancy, adolescent growth spurts, or weight gain); freckles in sun-exposed areas; birthmarks; and nevi (Fig. 9.5). Adult females (and sometimes males) will commonly have melasma (Fig. 9.6), areas of hyperpigmentation on the face and neck that are associated with pregnancy or hormonal variation. This condition is more noticeable in darker-skinned patients. The absence

TABLE 9.1 Features and Occurrence of Various Types of Pigmented Nevi

TYPE	FEATURES	OCCURRENCE	COMMENTS
Halo nevus	Sharp, oval, or circular; depigmented halo around nevus; may undergo many morphologic changes; usually disappears and halo repigments (may take years)	Usually on back in young adult	Usually benign; biopsy indicated because same process can occur around melanoma
Intradermal nevus	Dome shaped; raised; flesh to black color; may be pedunculated or hair bearing	Cells limited to dermis	No indication for removal other than cosmetic
Junction nevus	Flat or slightly elevated; dark brown	Nevus cells lining dermoepidermal junction	Should be removed if exposed to repeated trauma
Compound nevus	Slightly elevated, brownish papule; indistinct border	Nevus cells in dermis and lining dermoepidermal junction	Should be removed if exposed to repeated trauma
Congenital nevus	May be present at birth; may cover large area; hair growth may occur after several years		Should be removed if changes occur
Blue nevus	Blue to blue-gray in color	Nevus cells in dermis	Typically benign, but should be removed if changes occur

TABLE 9.2 Features of Normal and Atypical Nevi

FEATURE	NORMAL NEVUS	ATYPICAL NEVUS
Color	Uniformly tan or brown; all nevi on one person tend to look alike	Mixture of tan, brown, black, and red/pink; nevi on one person often do not look alike
Shape	Round or oval with a clearly defined border that separates the nevus from surrounding skin	Irregular borders may include notches; may fade into surrounding skin and include a flat portion level with the skin
Surface	Begins as a flat, smooth spot on the skin; becomes raised; forms a smooth bump	May be smooth, slightly scaly, or have a rough, irregular, "pebbly" appearance
Size	Usually less than 6 mm (size of a pencil eraser)	Often larger than 6 mm and sometimes larger than 10 mm
Number	Typical adult has 10–40 nevi scattered over the body	Many persons do not have increased number; however, persons severely affected may have more than 100 nevi
Location	Usually above the waist on sun-exposed surfaces of the body; scalp, breast, and buttocks rarely have normal nevi	May occur anywhere on the body, but most commonly on the back; may also appear below the waist and on the scalp, breast, and buttocks

BOX 9.4 Atypical Nevus or Melanoma?

Atypical nevi occur predominantly on the trunk. They tend to be large, usually greater than 5 mm, with a flat component. The border is typically ill defined. The shape can be round, oval, or irregular. The color is usually brown but can be mottled with dark brown, pink, and tan. Some individuals have only 1 to 5 nevi; others have more than 100.

In melanoma, the border is more irregular. Lesions tend to be larger, often greater than 6 mm. Color variation within the lesion is characteristic, ranging from tan-brown, dark brown, or black to pink, red, gray, blue, or white. Any lesion suggestive of a melanoma must be biopsied.

of melanin produces patches of unpigmented skin or hair, such as with vitiligo (Fig. 9.7).

Alterations in color in dark-skinned persons are best seen in the sclera, conjunctiva, buccal mucosa, tongue, lips, nail beds, and palms. Particular variations in skin color may be the result of physiologic pigment distribution. The palms and soles are lighter in color than the rest of the body and should be assessed when concerned for diffuse skin changes such as erythroderma, which is an intense, widespread reddening of the skin. Hyperpigmented lentigos on the palms and soles of the feet are common in darker-skinned patients. These are small pigmented spots on the skin with a clearly demarcated edge that is surrounded by normal-appearing skin. It is a harmless (benign) hyperplasia of melanocytes. Freckling of the buccal cavity, gums, and tongue commonly occurs and is benign. The sclera may appear yellowish brown (often described as "muddy") or may contain brownish pigment that resembles nevi. A bluish hue of the lips and gums can be a normal finding in persons with dark skin tone, giving a false impression of cyanosis.

Systemic disorders can produce generalized or localized color changes; these are described in Table 9.3. Localized redness often results from an inflammatory process. Pale, shiny skin of the lower extremities may reflect peripheral changes that occur with systemic diseases such as diabetes mellitus and peripheral vascular disease. Injury, steroids, vasculitis, stasis, and several systemic disorders

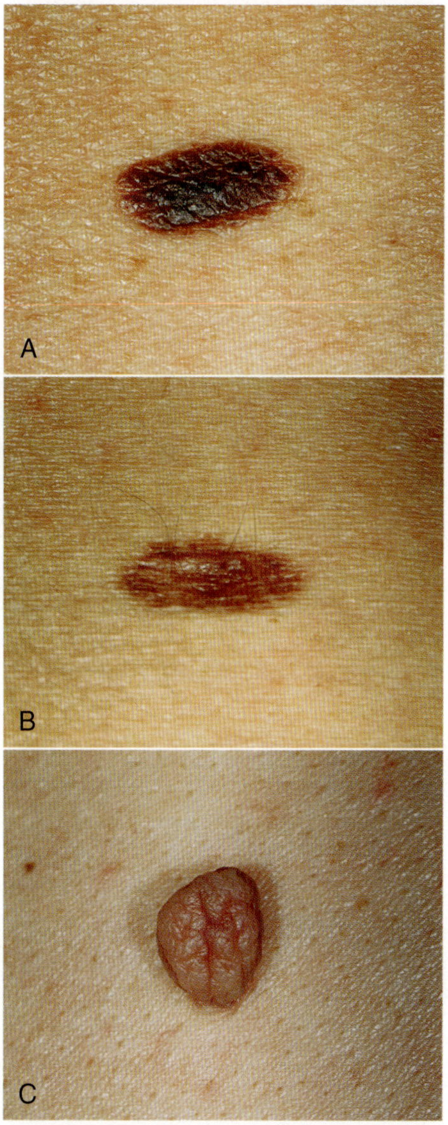

FIG. 9.5 Commonly occurring nevi. (A) Junction nevus. The color and shape of this black lesion are uniform. (B) Compound nevus. The center is elevated and the surrounding area is flat, retaining the features of a junction nevus. (C) Dermal nevus. Papillomatous with soft, wrinkled surface.

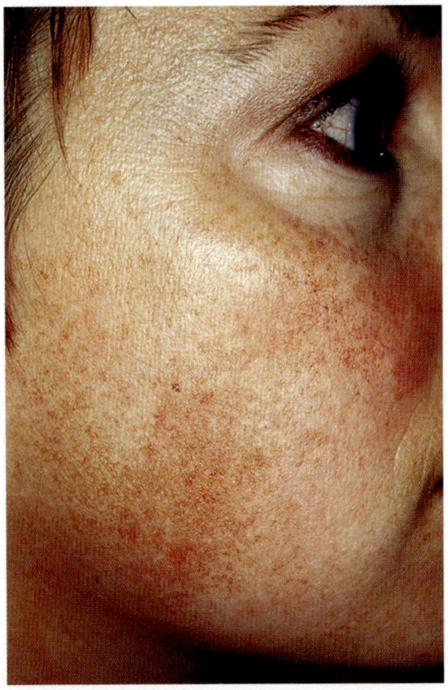

FIG. 9.6 Facial hyperpigmentation: chloasma (melasma). (From Bolognia, J., & Jorizzo, J. (2012). *Dermatology* (3rd ed.). Elsevier.)

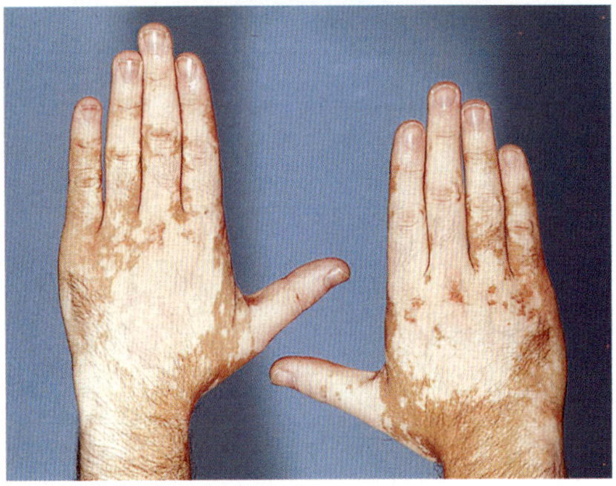

FIG. 9.7 Vitiligo. (From Kumar, P., & Clark, M. L. (2017). *Kumar and Clark's clinical medicine* (9th ed.). Edinburgh: Elsevier.)

can cause localized hemorrhage into the skin, producing red-purple discolorations. Bleeding into the skin results in ecchymoses (i.e., bruising); pinpoint bleeding from capillaries is called *petechiae* (smaller than 0.5 cm in diameter; Fig. 9.8) or purpura (larger than 0.5 cm in diameter; Fig. 9.9). Vascular skin lesions are characterized in Fig. 9.10 (see Clinical Pearl, "Telangiectasias: Spider Angioma"). Box 9.5 describes some characteristic odors that you may note as you examine the skin.

CLINICAL PEARL

Telangiectasias: Spider Angioma

Telangiectasias are small, permanently dilated blood vessels consisting of venules or arterioles. Spider angiomas are arterial. Blanch the center, and they will refill in an organized way from the center out and evenly in all directions (see Fig. 9.10).

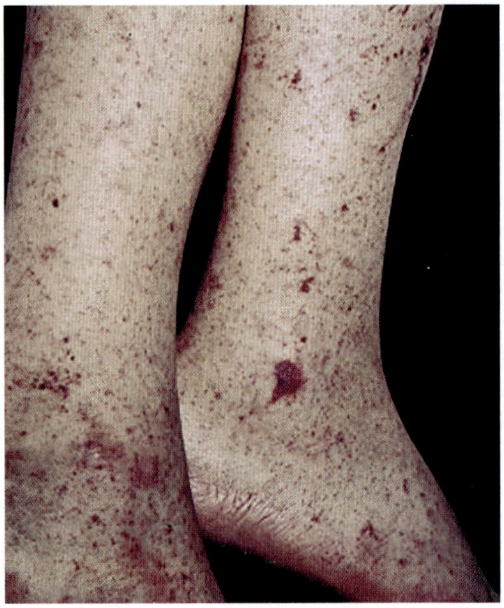

FIG. 9.8 Petechiae. (From Dinulos, J. (2021). *Habif's clinical dermatology* (7th ed.). St. Louis: Elsevier.)

TABLE 9.3 Cutaneous Color Changes

COLOR	CAUSE	DISTRIBUTION	SELECT CONDITIONS
Brown	Darkening of melanin pigment	Generalized	Pituitary, adrenal, liver disease
		Localized	Nevi, neurofibromatosis
White	Absence of melanin	Generalized	Albinism
		Localized	Vitiligo
Red (erythema)	Increased cutaneous blood flow	Localized	Inflammation
		Generalized	Fever, viral exanthem, urticaria
	Increased intravascular red blood cells	Generalized	Polycythemia
Yellow	Increased bile pigmentation (jaundice)	Generalized	Liver disease
	Increased carotene pigmentation	Generalized (except sclera)	Hypothyroidism, increased intake of vegetables containing carotene
Blue	Increased unsaturated hemoglobin secondary to hypoxia	Lips, mouth, nail beds	Cardiovascular and pulmonary diseases
Violaceous	Damage to blood vessels or extravasation of blood into skin	Localized	Vasculitis, vasculopathy, bruising

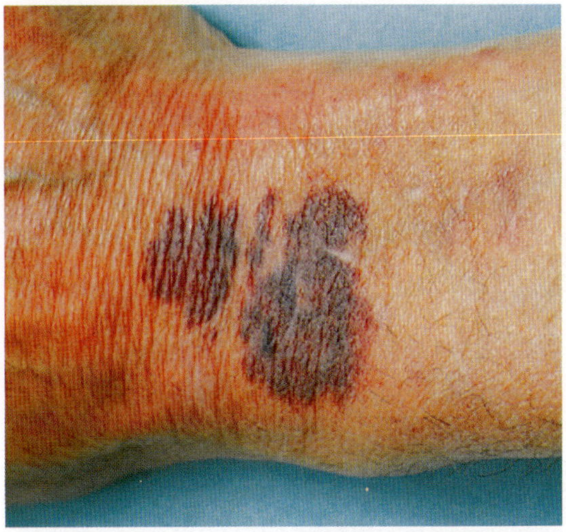

FIG. 9.9 **Senile purpura.** (From Hoffbrand, A. V., Pettit, J. E., & Vyas, P. (2010). *Color atlas of clinical hematology* (4th ed.). Philadelphia: Mosby.)

Palpation

As you inspect, palpate the skin for moisture, temperature, texture, turgor, and elasticity. Palpation may yield additional data for describing lesions, particularly in relation to elevation or depression.

Minimal perspiration or oiliness should be present. Increased perspiration may be associated with activity, a warm environment, obesity, anxiety, or excitement; it may be especially noticeable on the palms, scalp, and forehead, and in the axillae. The intertriginous areas, or skin in body folds, may also be damp, leading to development of intertrigo (Fig. 9.11).

The skin should range in temperature from cool to warm to the touch. Use the dorsal surface of your hands or fingers in this case because these areas are most sensitive to temperature perception. At best, this assessment is a rough estimate of skin temperature; what you are really looking for is bilateral symmetry. Environmental conditions, including the temperature of the examining room, as well as body location may affect surface temperature.

The texture should feel smooth, soft, and even. Roughness on exposed areas or areas of pressure (particularly the elbows, soles, and palms) may be caused by dry skin or irritation. Extensive or widespread roughness may be the result of a keratinization disorder or damaged skin. Hyperkeratosis, especially of the palms and soles, may be a sign of a systemic disorder such as exposure to arsenic, other toxins, or a sign of internal malignancy.

Assessment of skin elasticity can be helpful in detecting certain conditions. Gently pinch a small section of skin on the forearm or sternal area between the thumb and forefinger and then release the skin (Fig. 9.12). The skin should move easily when pinched and return to place immediately when released. Poor skin turgor can indicate severe dehydration. In this case, the skin is very slow to return to normal and "tents" up. This may occur with excessive vomiting, diarrhea, or dehydration from another cause. Skin that is firm or cannot be pinched may suggest an underlying connective tissue disease such as scleroderma.

Skin Lesions

As you assess the skin, pay particular attention to any lesions that may be present. *Skin lesion* is a general term that collectively describes any pathologic skin change or occurrence. Lesions may be primary (i.e., those that occur as initial spontaneous manifestations of a pathologic process) or secondary (i.e., those that result from later evolution of or external trauma to a primary lesion).

Tables 9.4 and 9.5 show the characteristics of primary and secondary lesions. The nomenclature is often used inaccurately; if you are uncertain about a lesion, use the descriptors rather than the name. Be aware that several types of lesions may occur concurrently and that secondary changes may obscure primary characteristics.

Describe lesions according to characteristics (Table 9.6), exudates, configuration, and location and distribution.

Characteristics

- Size (measure all dimensions)
- Shape
- Color
- Texture
- Elevation or depression
- Attachment at base: pedunculated (having a stalk) or sessile (without a stalk)
- Exudates
- Color
- Odor
- Amount
- Consistency
- Configuration
- Annular (rings)
- Grouped
- Linear
- Arciform (bow-shaped)
- Diffuse
- Location and distribution
- Generalized or localized
- Region of the body (Box 9.6)
- Patterns (Figs. 9.13–9.15)
- Discrete or confluent

A small, clear, flexible ruler is necessary for measuring the size of lesions. Examiners often use comparisons to common objects, such as coins, to estimate the size or shape of lesions. Subjective estimates should not be used as measures of size; instead, use the ruler and report sizes in centimeters. Try to measure size in all dimensions (i.e., height, width, and depth) when possible.

Use a light for closer inspection of a particular lesion to detect its nuances of color, elevation, and borders. Transillumination may be used to determine the presence of fluid in cysts or bullae. Darken the room and place the tip of the transilluminator against the side of the cyst or

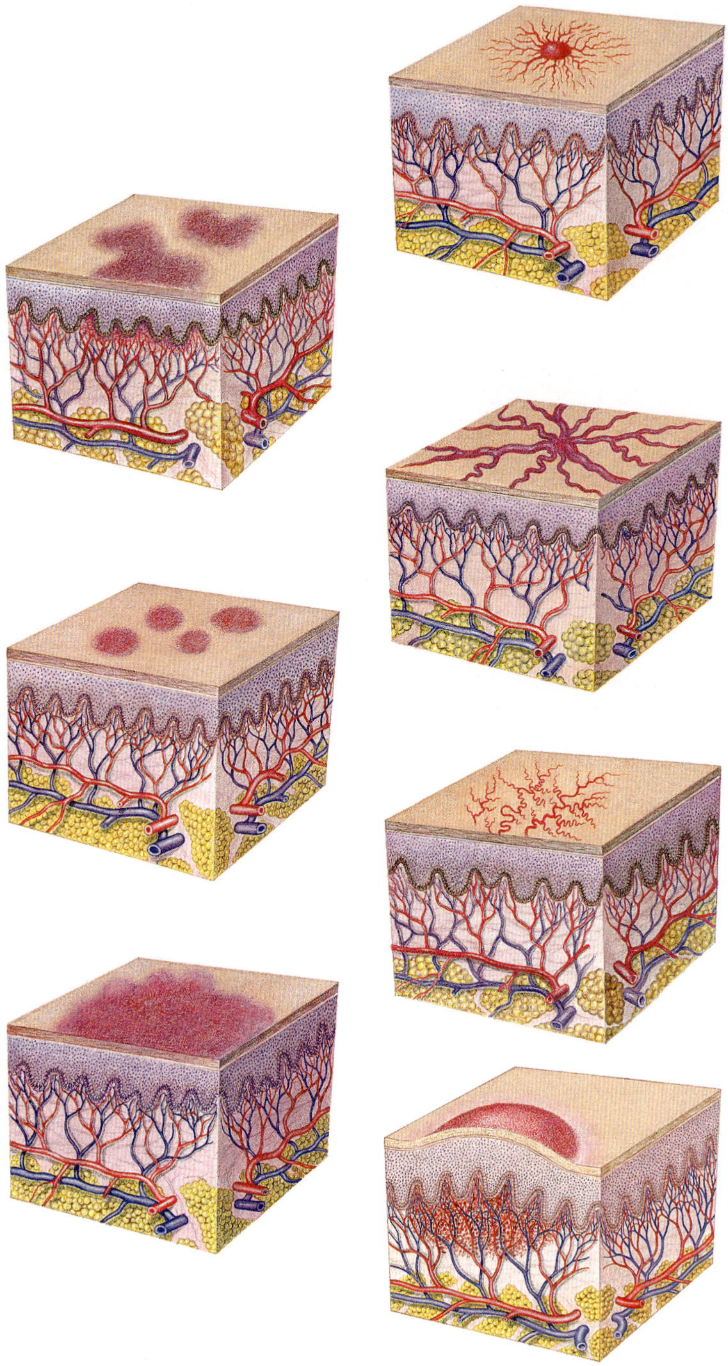

FIG. 9.10 Characteristics and causes of vascular skin lesions.

mass. Fluid-filled lesions will transilluminate with a red glow, whereas solid lesions will not.

A dermatoscope is a handheld magnifying lens that is useful in evaluating the subtle details of a lesion. It provides polarized light to allow for visualization of deeper skin structures and nonpolarized light for the assessment of superficial skin lesions.

The Wood's lamp can be used to evaluate epidermal hypopigmented areas and to distinguish fluorescing lesions. Depigmented lesions will enhance, whereas hypopigmented lesions will not. Darken the room and shine the light on the area to be examined. Look for the enhancement of depigmented lesions like vitiligo, hyperpigmentation of café au lait spots, and the yellow-green fluorescence that indicates the presence of some types of fungal infection.

Hair

Palpate the hair for texture while inspecting it for color, distribution, and quantity. The scalp hair may be coarse or

BOX 9.5 Smell the Skin

Even the skin may have odors suggesting a variety of problems, whether infectious, metabolic, or neurologic. Sweatiness intensifies the odor.

CAUSE OF ODOR	TYPE OF ODOR
Clostridium gas gangrene	Rotten apples
Proteus infection	Mousy
Pseudomonas infection (especially burns)	Grapelike
Tuberculous lymphadenitis (scrofula)	Stale beer
Anaerobic infection; scurvy	Putrid
Intestinal obstruction, peritonitis	Feculent
Phenylketonuria	Mousy, musty

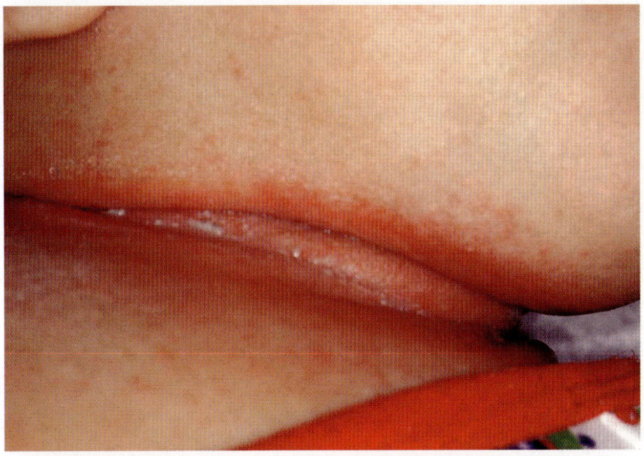

FIG. 9.11 Examining an intertriginous area. (From Kliegman, R. M., & Stanton, B. M. D. (2016). *Nelson textbook of pediatrics* (20th ed.). Philadelphia: Elsevier.)

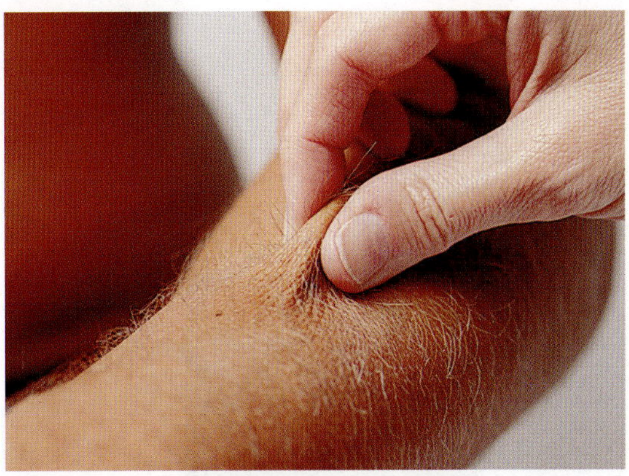

FIG. 9.12 Testing skin turgor.

fine, curly or straight, and should be shiny, smooth, and resilient. Palpate the scalp hair for dryness and brittleness that could indicate a systemic or genetic disorder. Color will vary from very light blonde, to black, to gray and may show alterations with rinses, dyes, or permanents.

The quantity and distribution of hair vary according to individual genetic makeup. Hair is commonly present on the scalp, lower face, neck, nares, ears, chest, axillae, back and shoulders, arms, legs, toes, and pubic area, and around the nipples. Note hair loss, which can be either generalized or localized. Inspect the lower legs and feet for hair loss that may indicate poor circulation or nutritional deficit. Look for any inflammation or scarring that accompanies hair loss, particularly when it is localized. Diffuse hair loss usually occurs without inflammation and scarring. Note whether the hair shafts are completely absent or simply broken off.

Genetically predisposed males often display a gradual symmetric hair loss on the frontal or vertex of the scalp during adulthood. Asymmetric hair loss may indicate a pathologic condition. Females in their 20s and older may also develop adrenal androgenic female-pattern alopecia (hair loss), with a gradual loss of hair from the vertex of the scalp in a Christmas tree distribution.

Fine vellus hair covers the body, whereas coarse terminal hair occurs on the scalp, pubic, and axillary areas; on the arms and legs (to some extent); and in the beard of males. The male pubic hair configuration is an upright triangle with the hair extending midline to the umbilicus (see Chapter 8, Fig. 8.13). The female pubic configuration is an inverted triangle; the hair may extend midline to the umbilicus (see Chapter 8, Fig. 8.11). Look for hirsutism in females—growth of terminal hair in a male distribution pattern on the face, body, and pubic area. Hirsutism, whether by itself or associated with other signs of virilization, may be a sign of an endocrine disorder.

Nails

Inspection

Inspect the nails for color, length, configuration, symmetry, and cleanliness. The condition of the fingernails can provide important insight to the patient's sense of self, as the condition of the hair and nails gives a clue about the patient's level of self-care and some sense of emotional state and social integration. The nails also can demonstrate physical examination signs that may indicate an underlying systemic disease.

Nail edges should be smooth and rounded. Jagged, broken, or bitten edges or cuticles are indicators of poor care habits and may predispose the patient to localized infection. Ragged cuticles are also a classic sign of dermatomyositis. Peeling nails (from the plate splitting into layers) are usually found in individuals whose hands are subject to repeated water immersion or those who have underlying psoriasis.

Examine the proximal and lateral nail folds for redness, swelling, pus, warts, cysts, and tumors. Pain usually accompanies ingrown nails and infections.

Color. The shape and opacity of nails vary considerably among individuals. Nail bed color should consist of variations of pink. Pigment deposits or bands may be present

TABLE 9.4 Primary Skin Lesions

DESCRIPTION	EXAMPLES		
Macule A flat, circumscribed area that is a change in the color of the skin; less than 1 cm in diameter	Freckles, flat nevi, petechiae	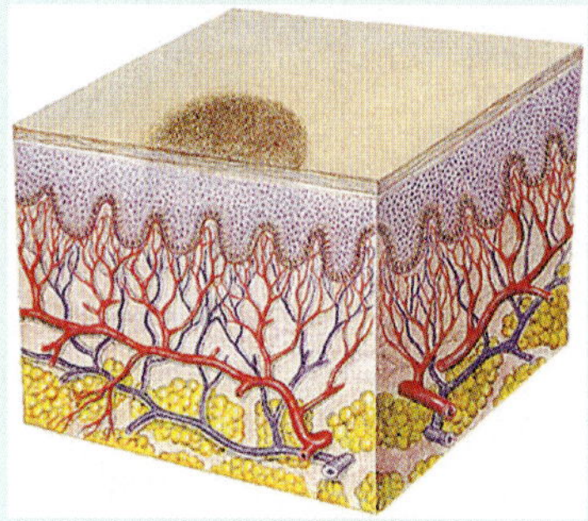	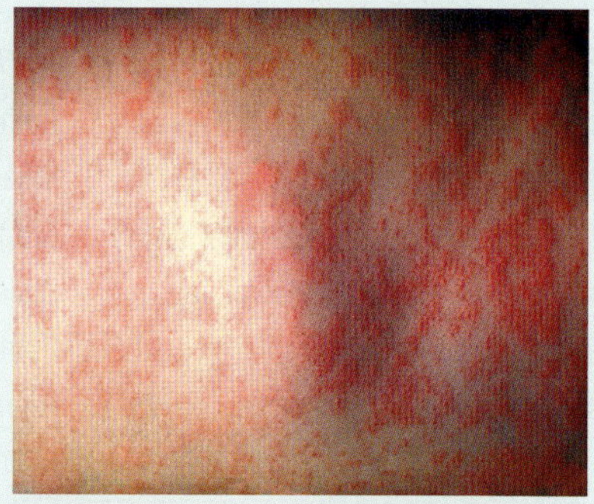 *Measles*
Papule An elevated, firm, circumscribed area; less than 1 cm in diameter	Wart (verruca), lichen planus	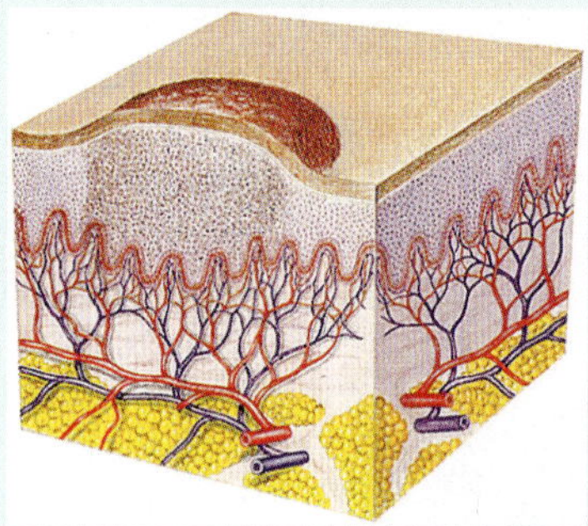	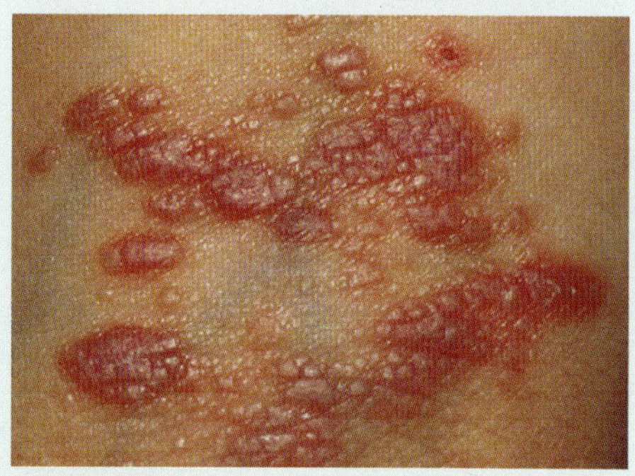 *Lichen planus*
Patch A flat, nonpalpable, irregularly shaped macule greater than 1 cm in diameter	Vitiligo, port-wine stains, café au lait patch	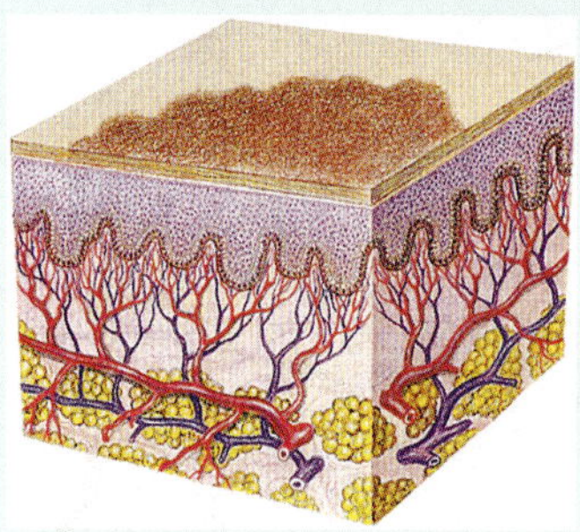	 *Vitiligo*
Plaque Elevated, firm, and rough lesion with flat surface greater than 1 cm in diameter	Psoriasis, atopic dermatitis	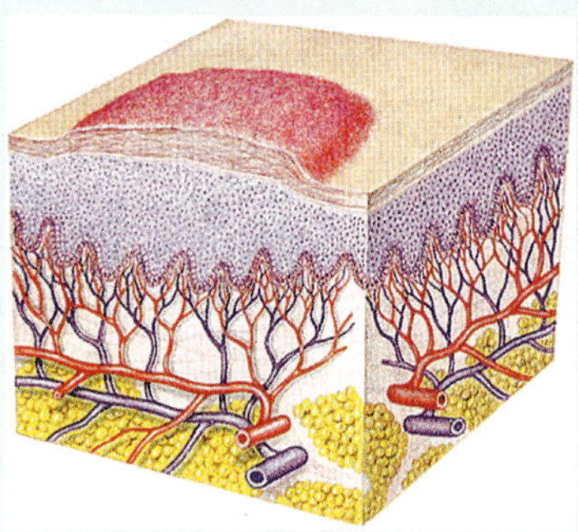	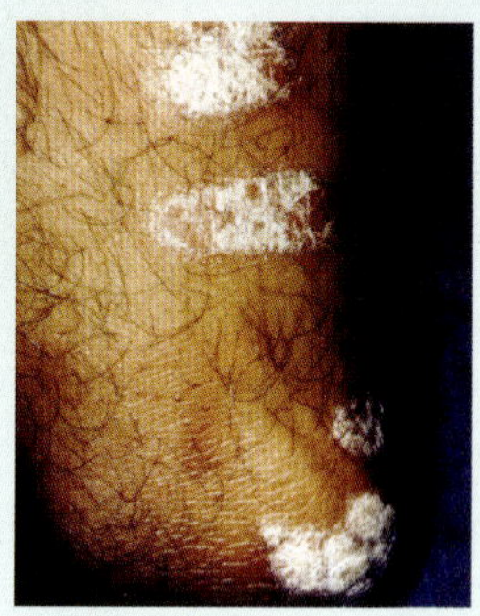 *Psoriasis*

TABLE 9.4 Primary Skin Lesions—cont'd

DESCRIPTION	EXAMPLES	
Wheal Elevated, irregular-shaped area of cutaneous edema; solid, transient, variable diameter	Insect bites, urticaria, allergic reaction	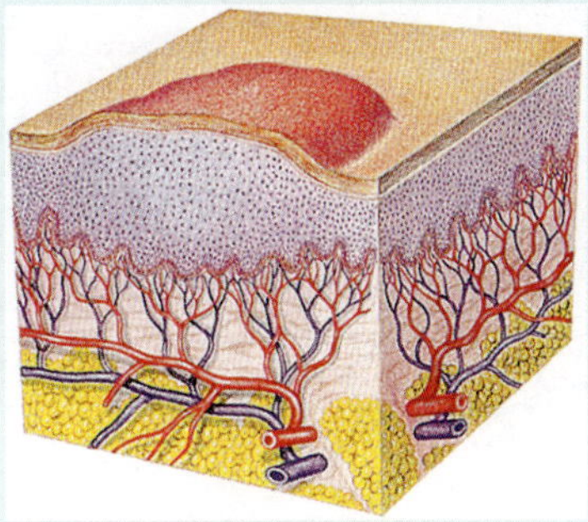 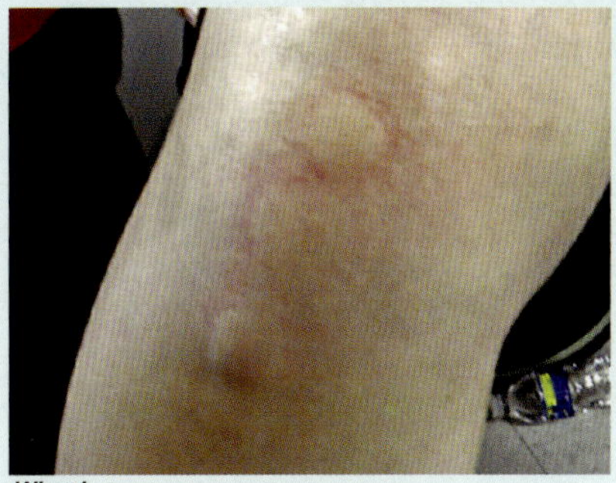 *Wheal*
Nodule Elevated, firm, circumscribed lesion; deeper in dermis than a papule; 1–2 cm in diameter	Erythema nodosum, dermatofibroma	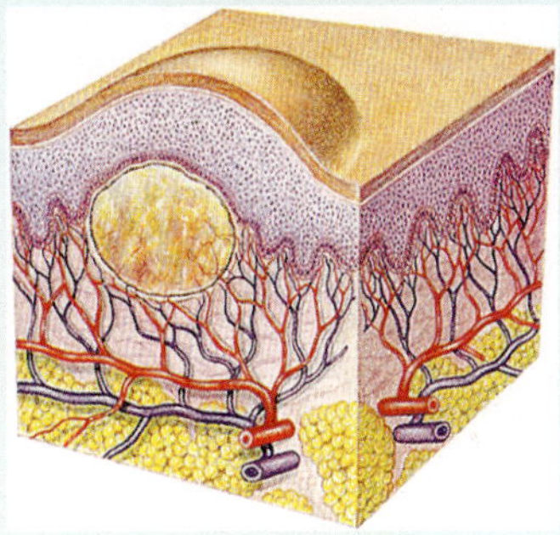 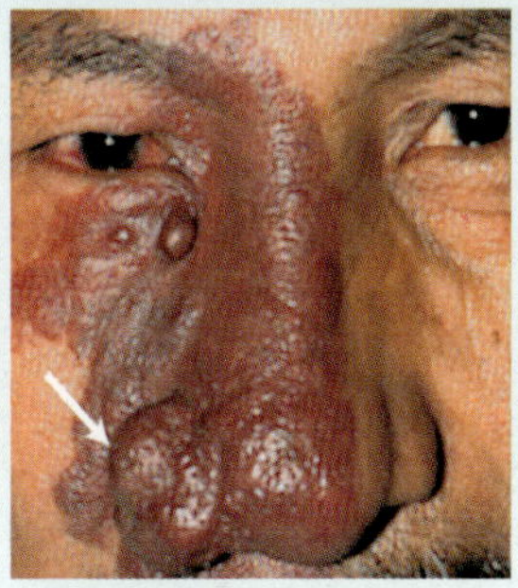 *Dermatofibroma*
Tumor Elevated and solid lesion; may or may not be clearly demarcated; deeper in dermis; greater than 2 cm in diameter	Neoplasms, benign tumor, lipoma	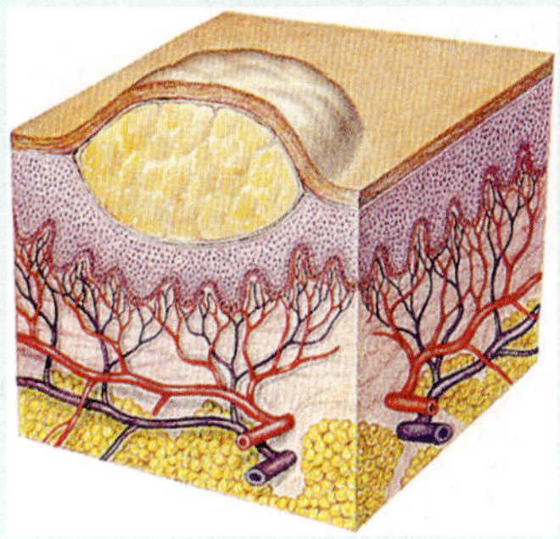 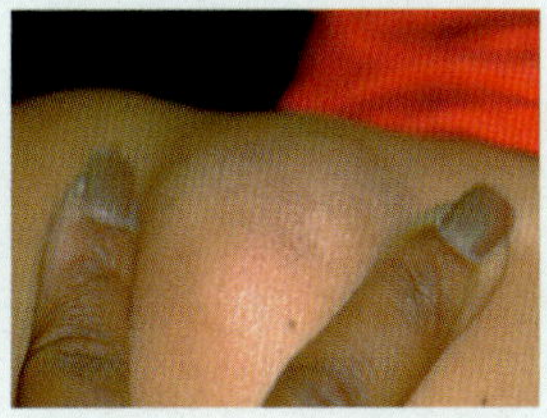 *Lipoma*
Vesicle Elevated, circumscribed, superficial, not into dermis; filled with serous fluid; less than 1 cm in diameter	Varicella (chickenpox), herpes zoster (shingles)	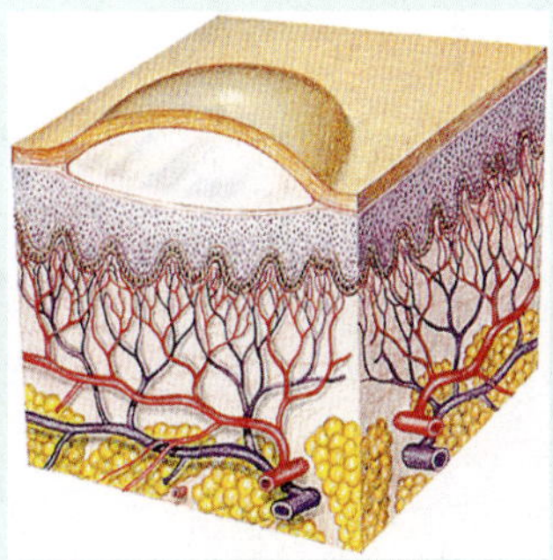 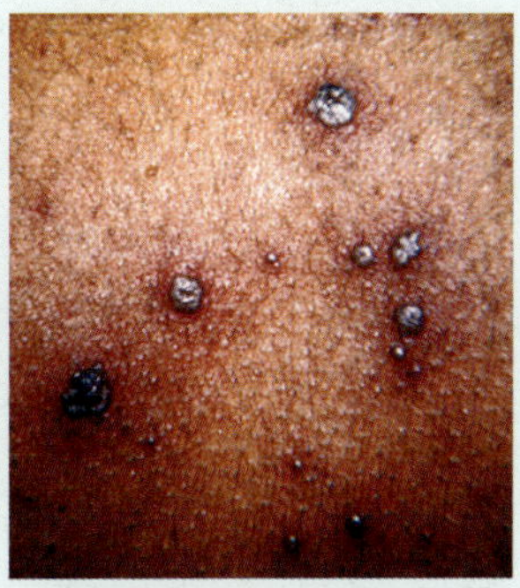 *Vesicles caused by varicella*

Continued

TABLE 9.4 Primary Skin Lesions—cont'd

DESCRIPTION	EXAMPLES		
Bulla Vesicle greater than 1 cm in diameter	Bullous pemphigus, pemphigus vulgaris	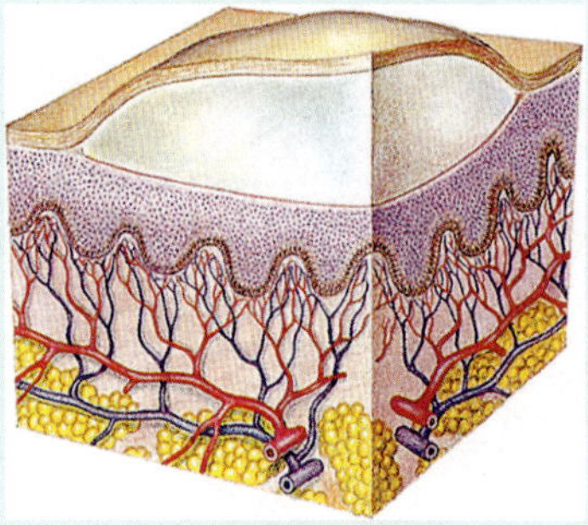	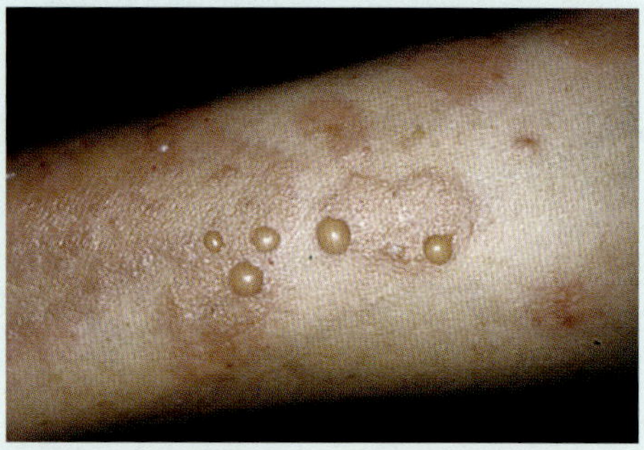 *Bullous pemphigoid*
Pustule Elevated, superficial lesion; similar to a vesicle but filled with purulent fluid	Impetigo, acne	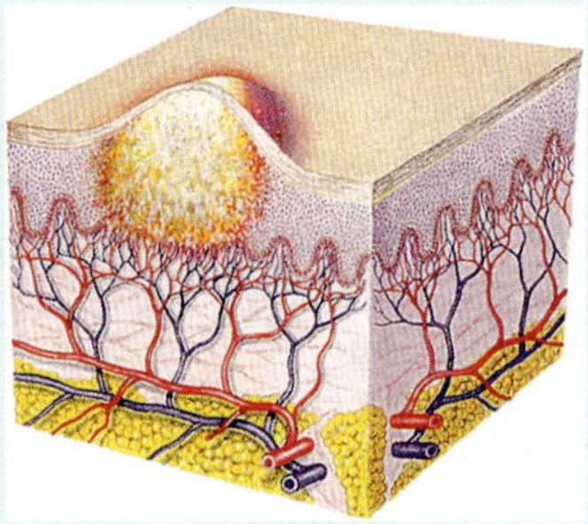	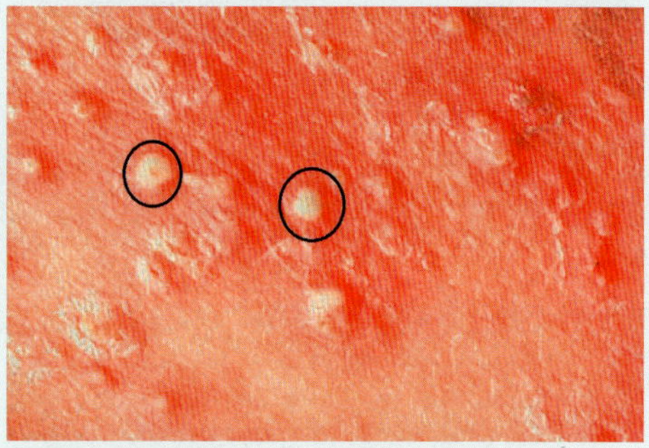 *Acne*
Cyst Elevated, circumscribed, encapsulated lesion; in dermis or subcutaneous layer; filled with liquid or semisolid material	Epidermal inclusion cyst, cystic acne	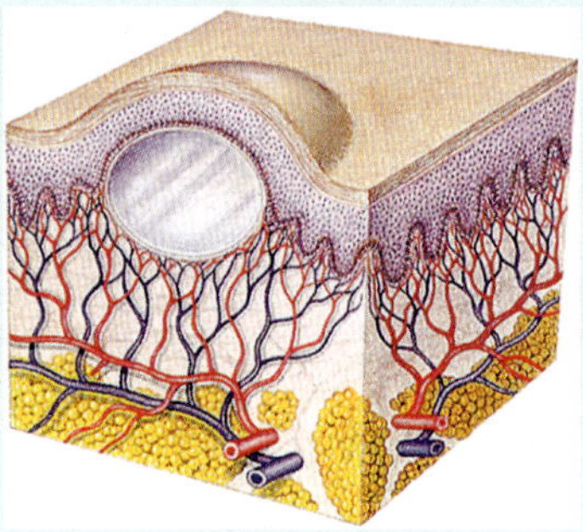	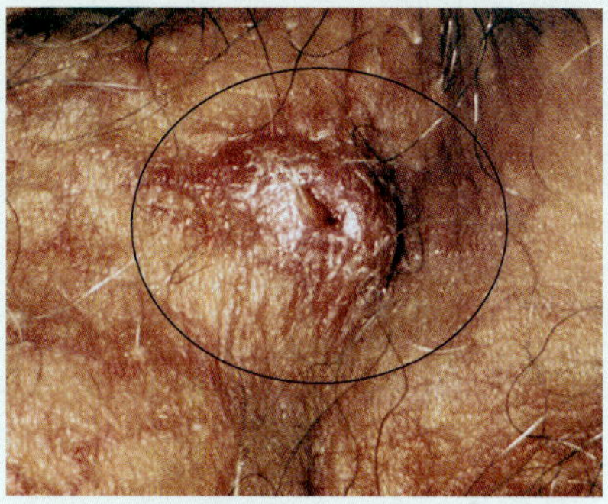 *Epidermal inclusion cyst*
Telangiectasia Fine, irregular, red lines produced by capillary dilation	Telangiectasia in rosacea	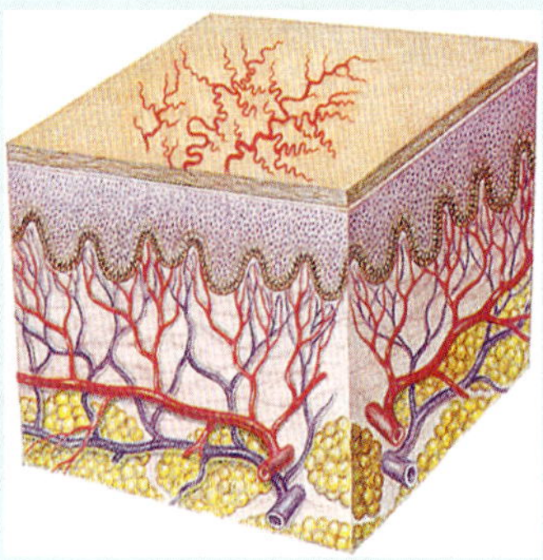	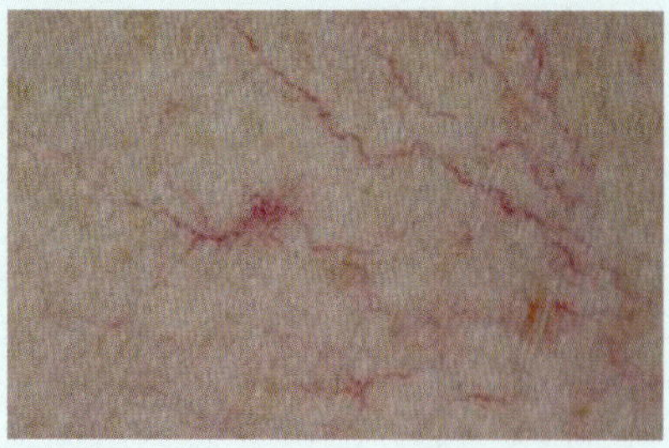 *Telangiectasia*

TABLE 9.5 Secondary Skin Lesions

DESCRIPTION	EXAMPLES
Scale Heaped-up, keratinized cells; flaky skin; irregular; thick or thin; dry or oily; variation in size	Flaking of skin with seborrheic dermatitis or after a drug reaction; dry skin 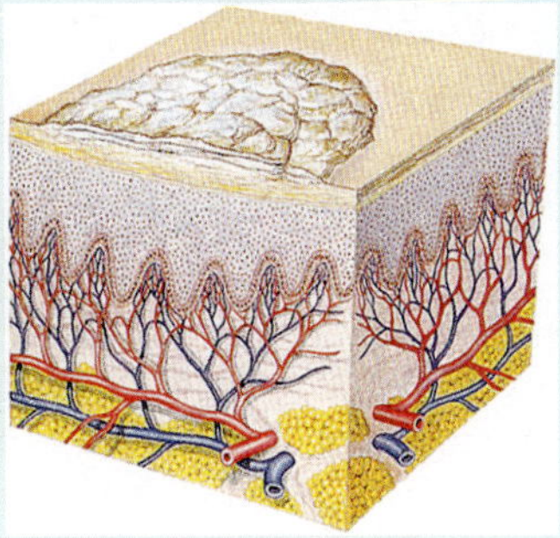 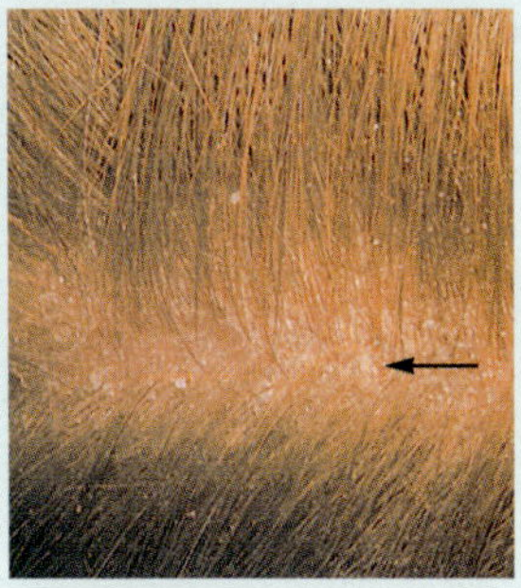 *Fine scaling*
Lichenification Rough, thickened epidermis secondary to persistent rubbing, itching, or skin irritation; often involves flexor surface of extremity	Chronic atopic dermatitis 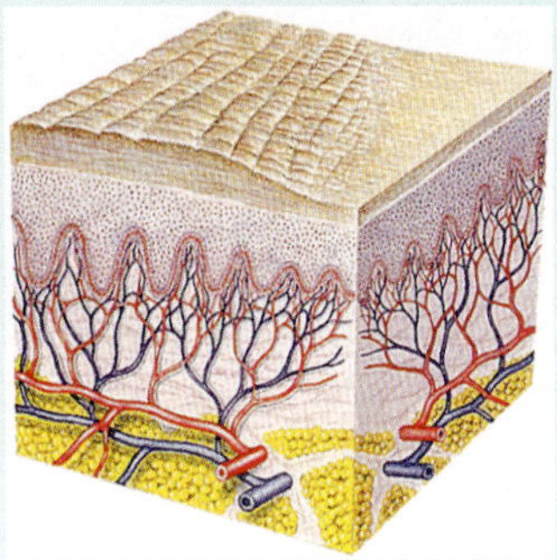 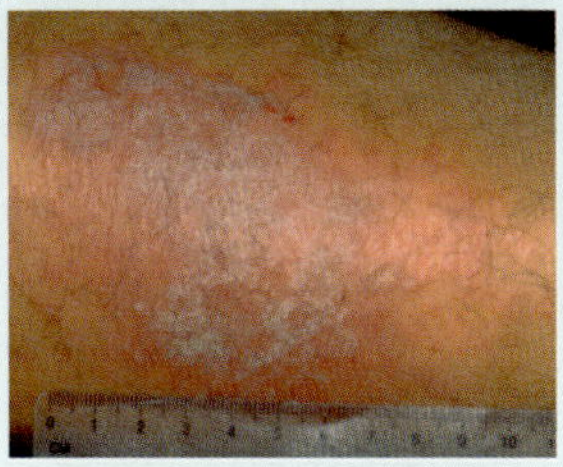 *Lichenification (chronic atopic dermatitis)*
Keloid Irregularly shaped, elevated, progressively enlarging scar; grows beyond the boundaries of the wound; caused by excessive collagen formation during healing	Keloid formation after surgery 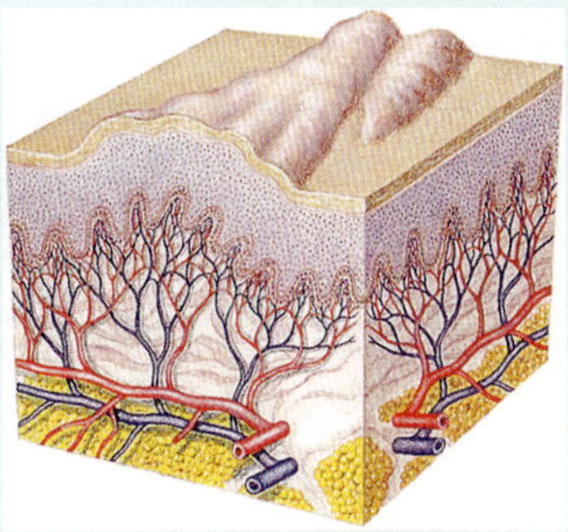 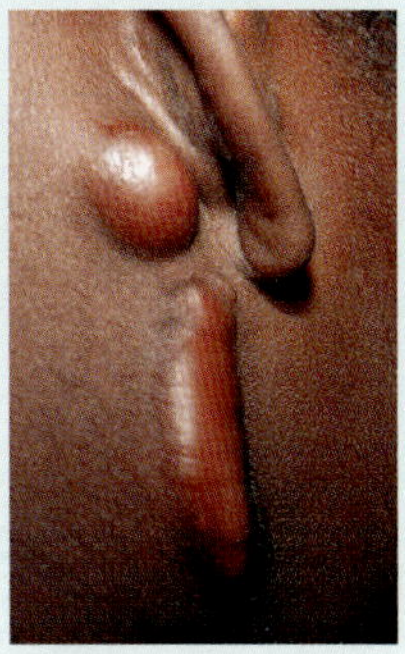 *Keloid*
Scar Thin to thick fibrous tissue that replaces normal skin after injury or laceration to the dermis	Healed wound or surgical incision 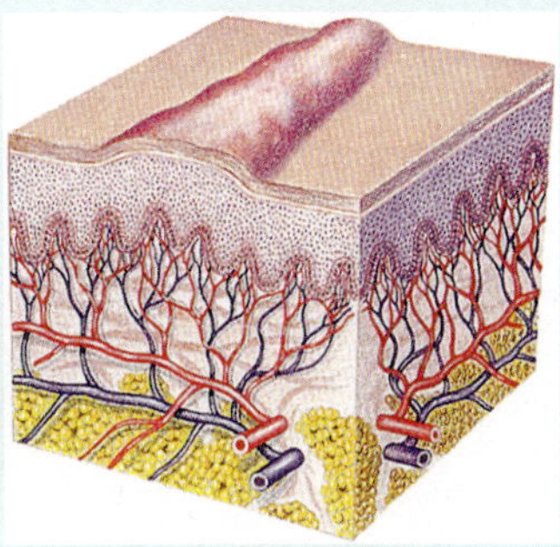 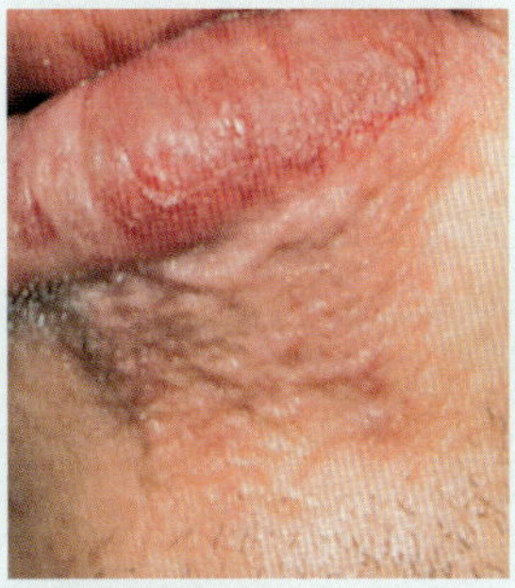 *Hypertrophic scar*

Continued

TABLE 9.5 Secondary Skin Lesions—cont'd

DESCRIPTION	EXAMPLES
Excoriation Loss of the epidermis; linear hollowed-out, crusted area	Abrasion or scratch, scabies 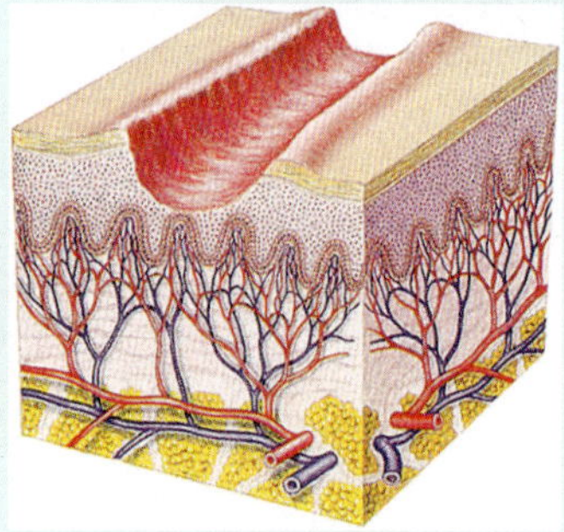 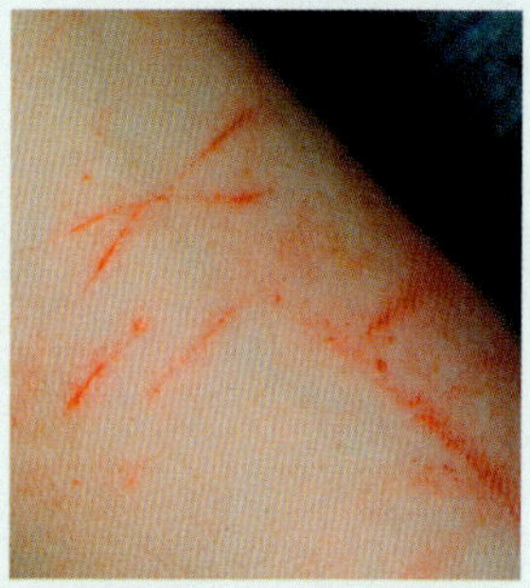 *Excoriation from tree branch*
Fissure Linear crack or break from the epidermis to the dermis; may be moist or dry	Athlete's foot, cracks at the corner of the mouth 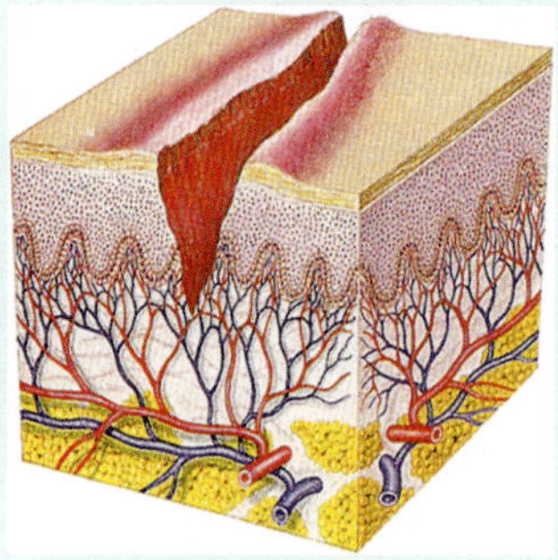 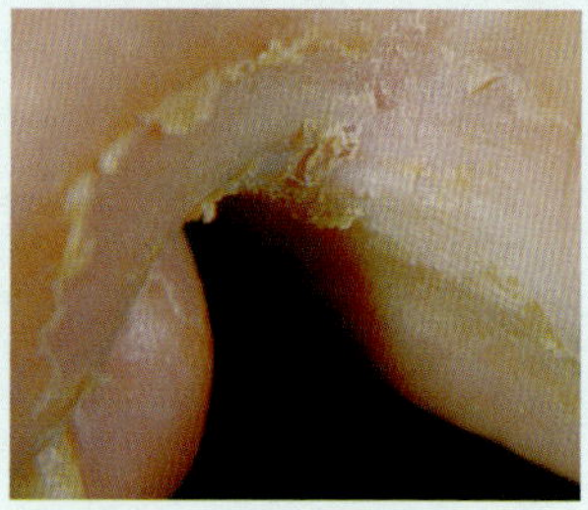 *Scaling and fissures from tinea pedis*
Erosion Loss of part of the epidermis; depressed, moist, glistening; follows rupture of a vesicle or bulla	Varicella, variola after rupture 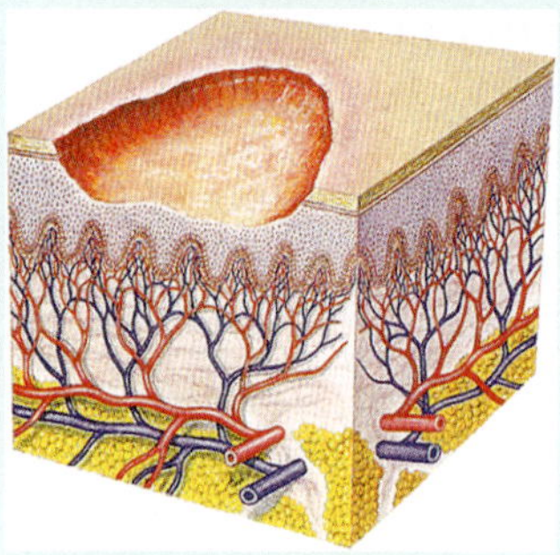 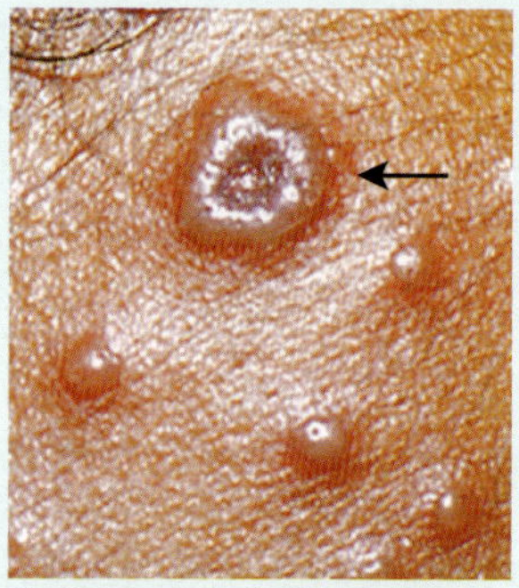 *Erosion in varicella (chickenpox after rupture of a blister)*
Ulcer Loss of epidermis and dermis; concave; varies in size	Decubitus, stasis ulcers 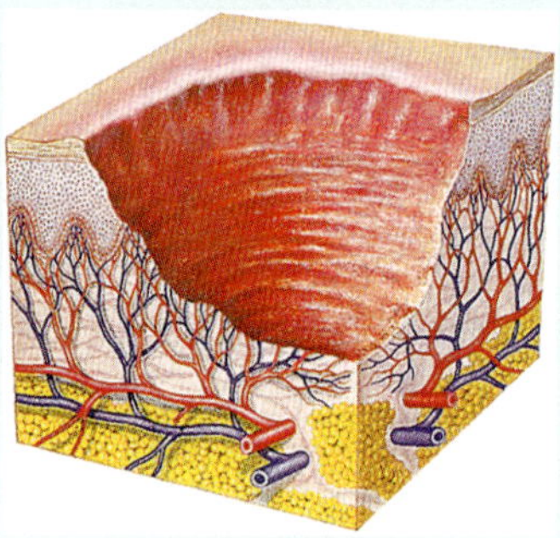 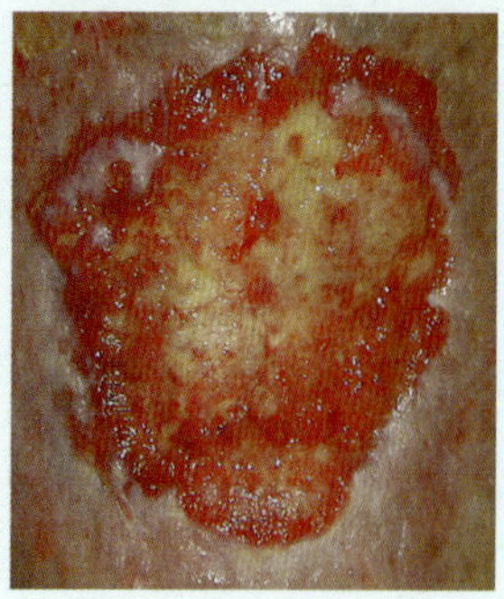 *Stasis ulcer*

TABLE 9.5 Secondary Skin Lesions—cont'd

DESCRIPTION	EXAMPLES
Crust Dried serum, blood, or purulent exudates; slightly elevated; size varies; brown, red, black, tan, or straw-colored	Scab on abrasion, eczema 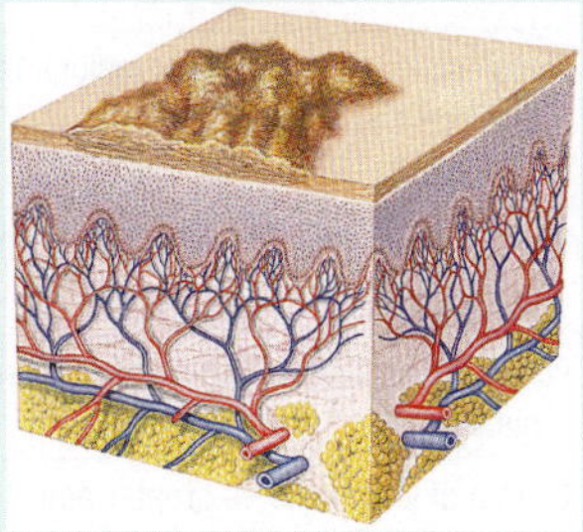 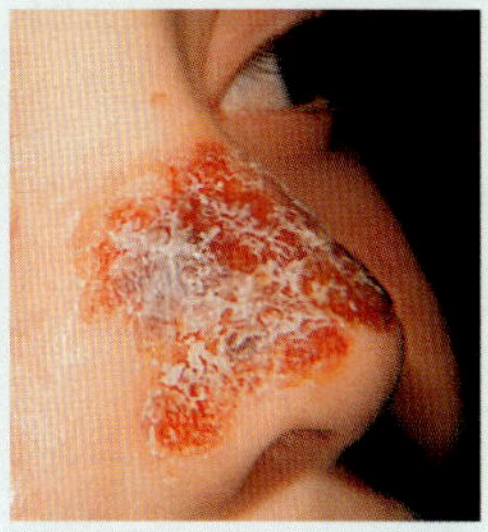 *Scab*
Atrophy Thinning of skin surface and loss of skin markings; skin translucent and paperlike	Striae; aged skin 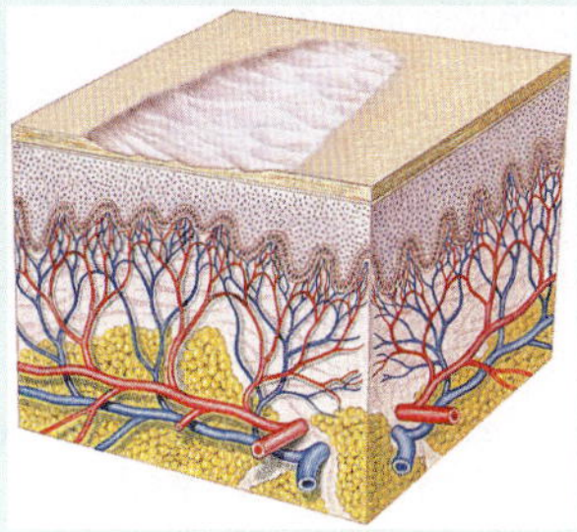 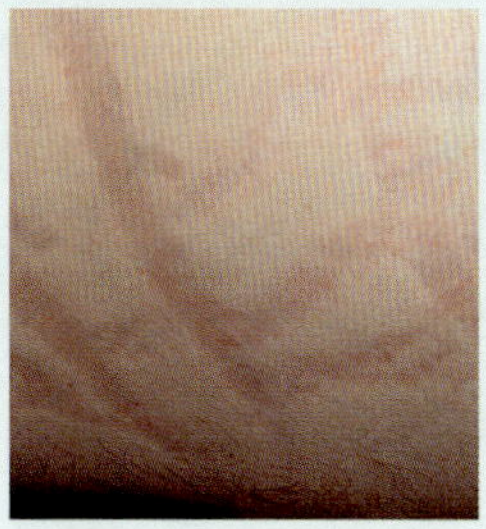 *Striae*

Photos from Public Health Image Library (PHIL), Centers for Disease Control and Prevention: macule/measles, Heinz F. Eichenwald, MD, Bob Craig; Patch/Vitiligo, Brian Hill, New Zealand; Plaque/psoriasis, Richard S. Hibbets; Vesicle/varicella, Dr. John Noble, Jr.; sebaceous cyst, Dr. Gavin Hart; fissure/tinea pedis, Dr. Lucille K. Georg.
Hypertrophic nodule; hypertrophic scar, from Goldman, M. P., & Fitzpatrick, R. E. (1994). *Cutaneous laser surgery: The art and science of selective photothermolysis.* St. Louis: Mosby.
Bulla/blister; papule/lichen planus; keloid, from Weston, W. L., Lane, A. T., & Morelli, J. G. (2007). *Color textbook of pediatric dermatology* (4th ed.). St. Louis: Mosby.
Pustule/acne, from Ferri, F. F. (2009). *Ferri's color atlas and text of clinical medicine.* Philadelphia: Saunders.
Tumor/lipoma; telangiectasia; excoriation; lichenification, from Lemmi, F. O., & Lemmi, C. A. E. (2000). *Physical assessment findings CD-ROM.* Philadelphia: Saunders.
Scaling, from Baran, R., Dawber, R. P. R., & Levene, G. M. (1991). *Color atlas of the hair, scalp, and nails.* St. Louis: Mosby.
Stasis ulcer, from Pozez, A. L., Aboutanos, S. Z., & Lucas, V. S. (2007). Diagnosis and treatment of uncommon wounds. *Clinics in Plastic Surgery*, 34(4), 749–764.
Striae, courtesy Antoinette Hood, MD, Department of Dermatology, Indiana University School of Medicine, Indianapolis.

TABLE 9.6 Morphologic Characteristics of Skin Lesions

CHARACTERISTIC	DESCRIPTION	EXAMPLES
Distribution		
Localized	Lesion appears in one small area	Impetigo, herpes simplex (e.g., labialis), tinea corporis (ringworm)
Regional	Lesions involve a specific region of the body	Acne vulgaris (pilosebaceous gland distribution), herpes zoster (nerve dermatomal distribution), psoriasis (flexural surfaces and skin folds)
Generalized	Lesions appear widely distributed or in numerous areas simultaneously	Urticaria, disseminated drug eruptions
Shape/Arrangement		
Round/discoid/nummular	Coin-shaped (no central clearing)	Nummular eczema
Oval	Ovoid shape	Pityriasis rosea
Annular	Round, active margins with central clearing	Tinea corporis, sarcoidosis
Zosteriform (dermatomal)	Following a nerve or segment of the body	Herpes zoster
Polycyclic	Interlocking or coalesced circles (formed by enlargement of annular lesions)	Psoriasis, urticaria
Linear	In a line	Contact dermatitis, poison ivy
Iris/target lesion	Pink macules with purple central papules	Erythema multiforme
Stellate	Star-shaped	Meningococcal septicemia
Serpiginous	Snakelike or wavy line track	Cutanea larva migrans

Continued

TABLE 9.6 Morphologic Characteristics of Skin Lesions—cont'd

CHARACTERISTIC	DESCRIPTION	EXAMPLES
Reticulate	Netlike or lacy	Polyarteritis nodosa, lichen planus, lesions of erythema infectiosum
Morbilliform	Measleslike: maculopapular lesions that become confluent on the face and body	Measles, roseola, drug eruptions
Border/Margin		
Discrete	Well demarcated or defined, able to draw a line around it with confidence	Psoriasis
Indistinct	Poorly defined, have borders that merge into normal skin or outlying ill-defined papules	Nummular eczema
Active	Margin of lesion shows greater activity than center	Tinea capitis
Irregular	Nonsmooth or notched margin	Malignant melanoma
Border raised above	Center of lesion depressed compared with the edge	Basal cell carcinoma center
Advancing	Expanding at margins	Cellulitis
Associated Changes Within Lesions		
Central clearing	An erythematous border surrounds lighter skin	Tinea eruptions
Desquamation	Peeling or sloughing of skin	Rash of toxic shock syndrome
Keratotic	Hypertrophic stratum corneum	Calluses, warts
Punctation	Central umbilication or dimpling	Basal cell carcinoma, molluscum contagiosum
Telangiectasias	Dilated blood vessels within lesion blanch completely, may be markers of systemic disease	Basal cell carcinoma, actinic keratosis
Pigmentation		
Flesh	Same tone as the surrounding skin	Neurofibroma, some nevi
Pink	Light red undertones	Eczema, pityriasis rosea
Erythematous	Dark pink to red	Tinea eruptions, psoriasis
Salmon	Orange-pink	Psoriasis
Tan-brown	Light to dark brown	Most nevi, pityriasis versicolor
Black	Black or blue-black	Malignant melanoma
Pearly	Shiny white, almost iridescent	Basal cell carcinoma
Purple	Dark red-blue-violet	Purpura, Kaposi sarcoma
Violaceous	Light violet	Erysipelas
Yellow	Waxy	Lipoma
White	Absent of color	Lichen planus

BOX 9.6 Regional Distribution of Skin Lesions

Sun-Exposed Areas
- Sunburn
- Lupus erythematosus
- Pellagra
- Porphyria

Cloth-Covered Areas
- Irritant contact dermatitis
- Miliaria

Flexural Aspects of Extremities
- Atopic dermatitis
- Intertrigo
- Candidiasis
- Tinea cruris

Extensor Aspects of Extremities
- Psoriasis
- Dermatomyositis

Stocking and Glove (Acrodermatitis)
- Parvovirus/atopic dermatitis
- Tinea pedis with "id" reaction[a]
- Poststreptococcal infection
- Child abuse burns

Truncal
- Pityriasis rosea (Christmas tree pattern)
- Atopic dermatitis
- Drug reaction

Face, Shoulder, Back
- Acne vulgaris
- Folliculitis
- Cushing syndrome

[a]An "id" reaction is a generalized acute cutaneous reaction, probably immunologic in origin, to a variety of stimuli, including fungal infection.

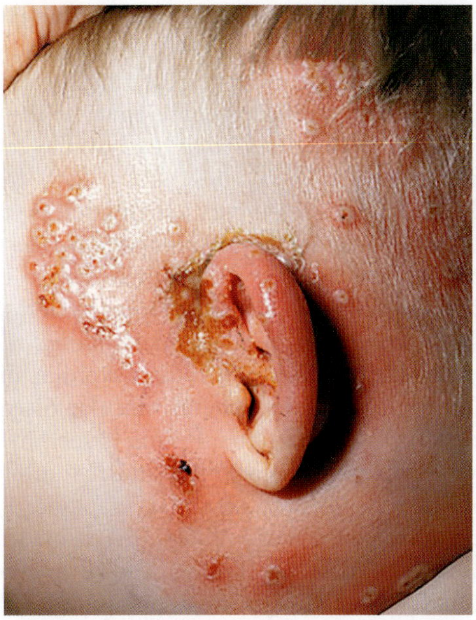

FIG. 9.13 **Clustering of lesions due to varicella.** (From Zitelli, B. J., & Davis, H. W. (2018). *Zitelli and Davis' atlas of pediatric physical diagnosis* (7th ed.). Philadelphia: Elsevier.)

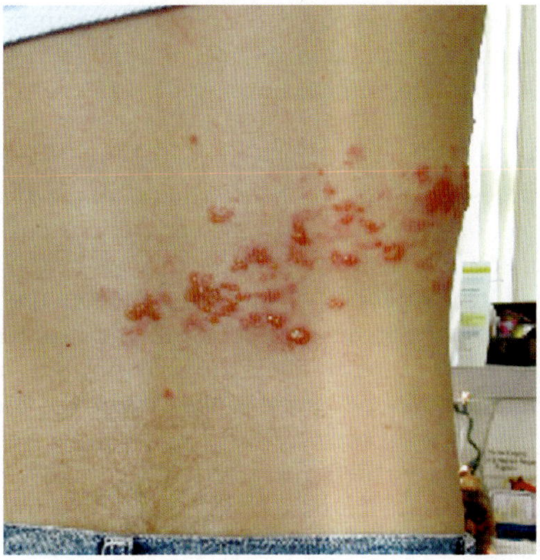

FIG. 9.14 **Linear formation of lesions (herpes zoster).** (From Morse, S., Ballard, R., et al. (2010). *Atlas of sexually transmitted diseases and AIDS* (4th ed.). St. Louis: Elsevier.)

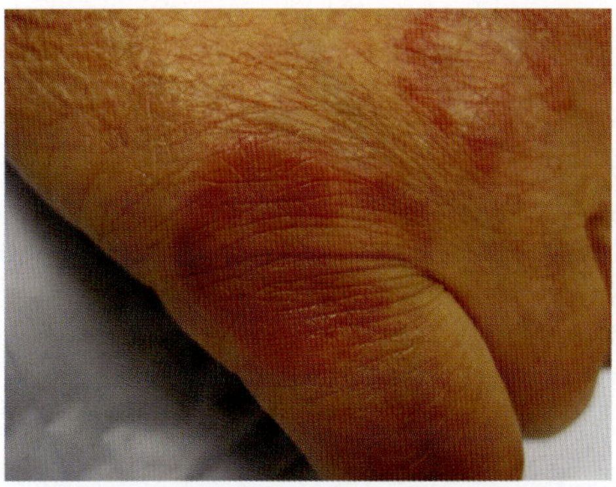

FIG. 9.15 **Annular formation of lesions (granuloma annulare).** An annular plaque or plaques may occur on the dorsa of the feet or hands as a manifestation of granuloma annulare. (From Keimig, E. L. (2015). Granuloma annulare. *Dermatologic Clinics, 33*(3), 315–329.)

in the nail beds of persons with dark skin (Fig. 9.16). Yellow discoloration occurs with several nail diseases, including psoriasis and fungal infections, and may also occur with chronic respiratory disease. Proximal subungual fungal infection is associated with HIV. Diffuse darkening of the nails may arise from antimalarial drug therapy, candidal infection, hyperbilirubinemia, and chronic trauma, such as occurs from tight-fitting shoes. Green-black discoloration, which is associated with *Pseudomonas* infection, may be confused with a similar discoloration caused by injury to the nail bed (subungual hematoma). Pain accompanies a subungual hematoma, whereas *Pseudomonas* infection is painless. Nail beds that are blue may be a transient response to a cold examining room. A single blue or black nail may indicate melanoma or bruising/bleeding from trauma. Generalized blue nails may be caused by conditions that produce cyanosis such as asthma, cardiac disorders, or severe anemia. Other causes of blue nails include silver poisoning, medication side effects, and Wilson disease, an inherited disorder of copper metabolization. Splinter hemorrhages—longitudinal red or brown streaks—may occur in endocarditis or vasculitis, with severe psoriasis of the nail matrix, or as the result of minor injury to the proximal nail fold (habit-tic deformity). White spots in the nail plate (leukonychia punctate), a common finding, result from cuticle manipulation or other forms of mild trauma that injure the nail matrix (Fig. 9.17).

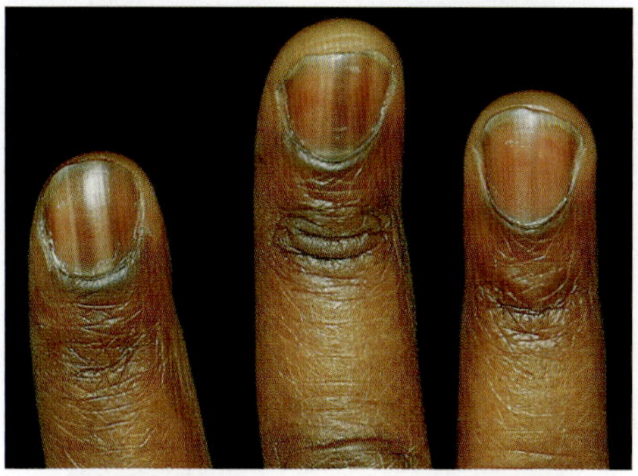

FIG. 9.16 **Pigmented bands in nails are expected in persons with dark skin.**

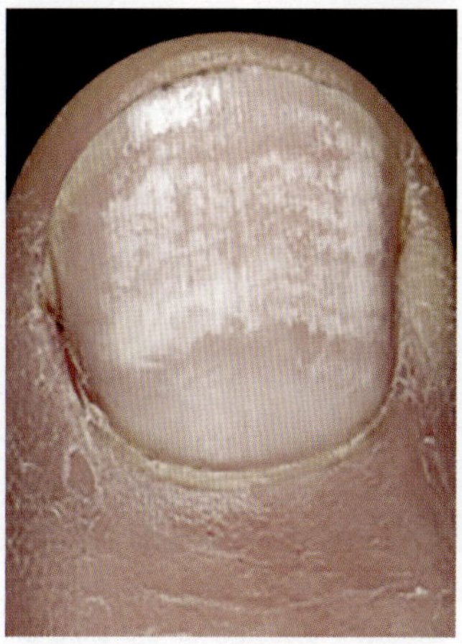

FIG. 9.17 **Leukonychia.** (From Dinulos, J. (2021). *Habif's clinical dermatology* (7th ed.). St. Louis: Elsevier.)

These spots need to be differentiated from longitudinal white streaks or transverse white bands that are indicative of a systemic disorder. Separation of the nail plate from the bed produces a white, yellow, or green tinge on the nonadherent portion of the nail.

Nail Plate. The nail plate should appear smooth and flat or slightly convex. Complete absence of the nail (anonychia) may occur as a congenital condition. Look for nail ridging, grooves, depressions, and pitting. Longitudinal ridging and beading are common expected variants (Fig. 9.18). Longitudinal ridges and grooves may also occur with lichen planus of the nail. Transverse grooves result from repeated injury to the nail, usually the thumb, as with chronic manipulation of the proximal nail fold (Fig. 9.19). The most common cause is picking at the thumb with the index finger (habit-tic deformity). Chronic inflammation, such as occurs with chronic paronychia or chronic eczema, produces transverse rippling of the nail plate. Transverse depressions that appear at the base of the lunula occur after stress that temporarily interrupts nail formation.

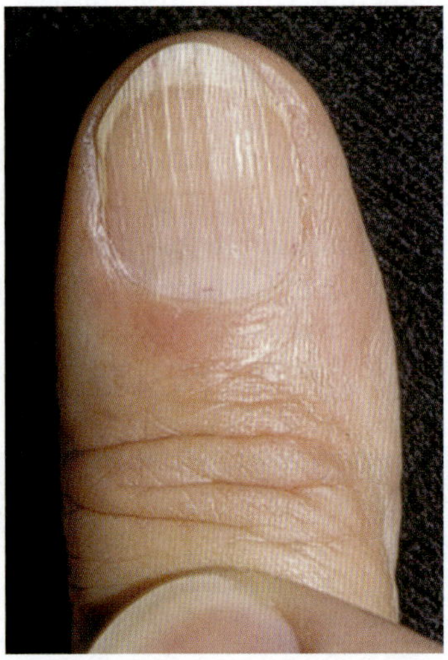

FIG. 9.18 Aging nails. (Longitudinal ridging of the nail is a common expected variation.)

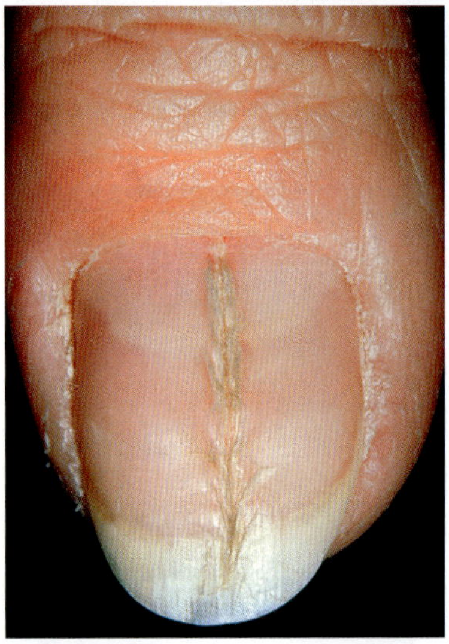

FIG. 9.19 Median nail dystrophy. (From James, W. D., Berger, T., Elston, D., et al. (2016). *Andrews' diseases of the skin: Clinical dermatology* (12th ed.). Philadelphia: Elsevier.)

Involvement of a single nail usually points to an injury to the nail matrix. Assure the patient that the nail will grow out and assume normal appearance in about 6 months for fingernails and 12 months for toenails. Depressions that occur in all the nails are usually a response to systemic disease, including syphilis, disorders producing high fevers, peripheral vascular disease, and uncontrolled diabetes mellitus. Pitting is seen most commonly with psoriasis. Broadening and flattening of the nail plate may be seen in secondary syphilis. Fig. 9.20 illustrates unexpected nail findings. Pigmented deposits or bands may be present in the nail beds of persons with dark skin. The sudden appearance of such a band may indicate melanoma. Extension of the pigment backward onto the proximal nail fold is a worrisome sign of possible melanoma.

Inward folding of the lateral edges of the nail causes the nail bed to draw up; this often becomes painful. Curvature is most common in the toenails and is thought to be caused by shoe compression.

Nail Base Angle. The nail base angle should measure 160 degrees. One way to observe this is to place a ruler or a sheet of paper across the nail and dorsal surface of the finger and examine the angle formed by the proximal nail fold and nail plate. In clubbing, the angle increases and approaches or exceeds 180 degrees. Another method of assessment is the Schamroth technique (Fig. 9.21). Have the patient place together the nail (dorsal) surfaces of the thumbs from both the right and left hands. When the nails are clubbed, the diamond-shaped window at the base of the nails disappears and the angle between the distal tips increases. Clubbing is associated with a variety of respiratory and cardiovascular diseases, cirrhosis, colitis, and thyroid disease (Fig. 9.22).

Palpation

The nail plates should feel hard and smooth with a uniform thickness. Thickening of the nail may occur from tight-fitting shoes, chronic trauma, and some fungal infections. Thinning of the nail plate may also accompany some nail diseases. Pain in the area of a nail groove may be secondary to ischemia.

Gently squeeze the nail between your thumb and the pad of your finger to test for adherence of the nail to the nail bed. Separation of the nail plate from the bed is common with psoriasis, trauma, candidal or *Pseudomonas* infections, and some medications. The nail base should feel firm (Fig. 9.23). A boggy nail base accompanies clubbing.

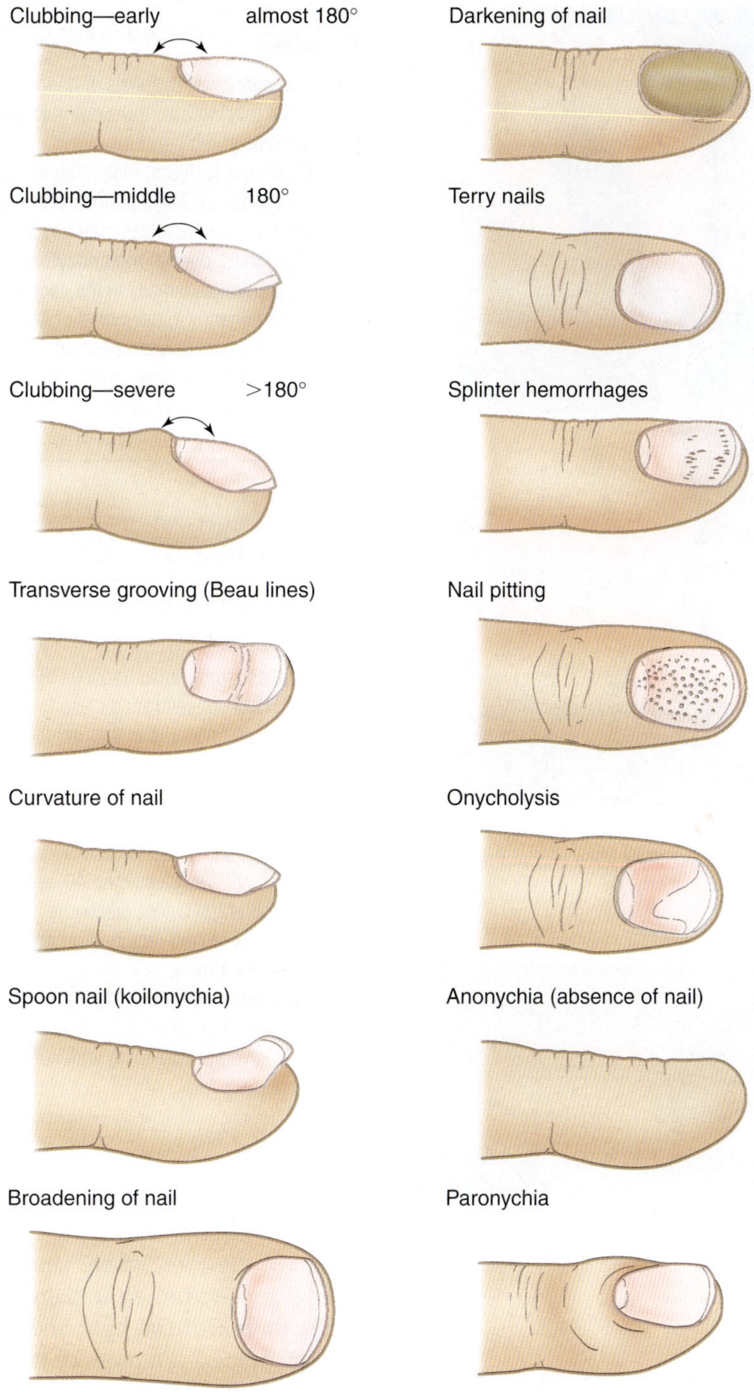

FIG. 9.20 Nails: Unexpected findings and appearance.

Infants and Children

In the first few hours of life, an infant's skin may look very red. The gentle pink coloring that predominates in infancy usually surfaces on the first day after birth. Skin color is partly determined by the amount of subcutaneous fat; the less subcutaneous fat, the redder and more transparent the skin. Dark-skinned newborns do not always manifest the intensity of melanosis that will be readily evident during the first year of life. The exceptions in this regard are the nail beds and skin of the scrotum. The expected color changes in newborns are described in Box 9.7.

Physiologic jaundice may be present to a mild degree in many newborn infants. It usually starts after the first day of life and disappears by the eighth to tenth day but may persist for as long as 3 to 4 weeks. Intense and persistent jaundice suggests liver disease, a hemolytic process, or severe, overwhelming infection. Risk factors for hyperbilirubinemia and causes of jaundice in newborns are listed in the Risk Factors box.

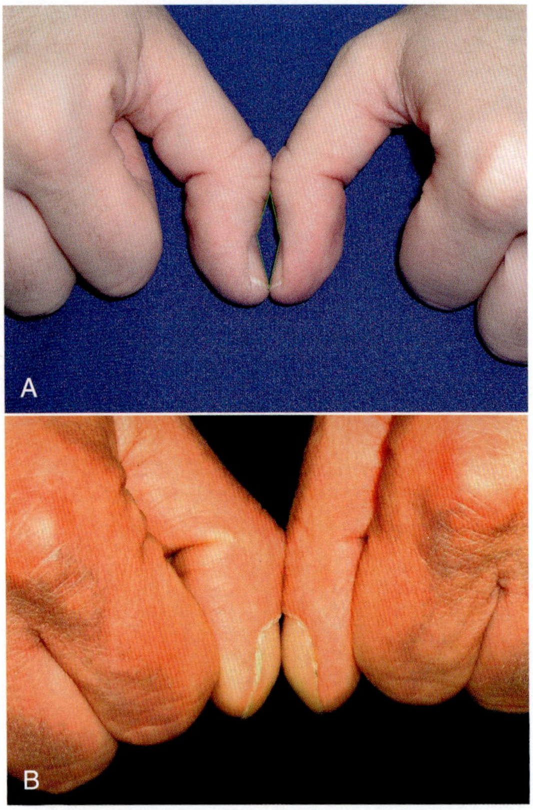

FIG. 9.21 **Schamroth technique.** (A) Patient with healthy nails, illustrating window. (B) Patient with nail clubbing, illustrating loss of the window and prominent distal angle.

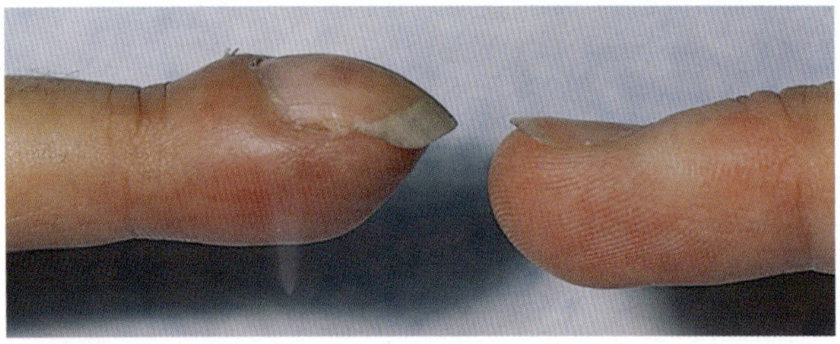

FIG. 9.22 A normal finger *(right)* is compared with a finger with nail clubbing. (From Swartz, M. H. (2021). *Textbook of physical diagnosis* (8th ed.). Philadelphia: Elsevier.)

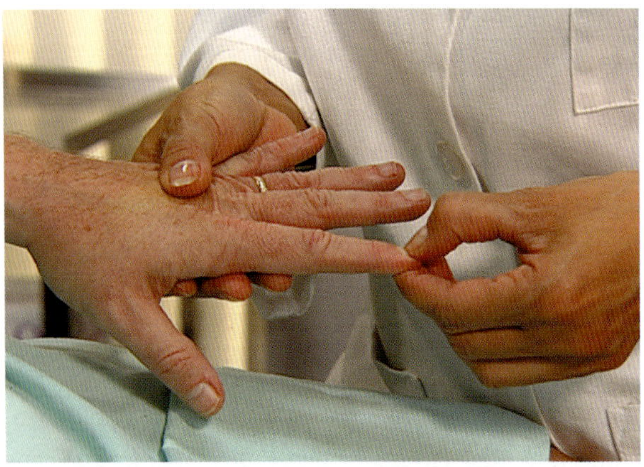

FIG. 9.23 Testing nail bed adherence.

BOX 9.7 Expected Color Changes in the Newborn

- **Acrocyanosis:** Cyanosis of hands and feet
- **Cutis marmorata:** Transient mottling when infant is exposed to decreased temperature
- **Erythema toxicum:** Pink papular rash with vesicles superimposed on the thorax, back, buttocks, and abdomen; may appear in 24 to 48 hours and resolves after several days
- **Congenital dermal melanocytosis:** Irregular areas of deep blue pigmentation, usually in the sacral and gluteal regions; seen predominantly in newborns of African, Native American/American Indian, Asian, or Latin descent
- **Nevus simplex (also called salmon patches, stork bites, or angel kisses):** Flat, deep pink localized areas usually seen on the midforehead, eyelids, upper lip, and back of the neck

Risk Factors

Major Risk Factors for Severe Hyperbilirubinemia in Infants of 35 or More Weeks' Gestation

- Predischarge transcutaneous bilirubin (TcB) or total serum bilirubin (TSB) concentration close to the phototherapy threshold
- Jaundice observed in the first 24 hours
- Family history or genetic ancestry suggestive of inherited red blood cell disorders, including glucose-6-phosphate dehydrogenase (G6PD) deficiency
- Gestational age 35 to 36 weeks (i.e., risk increases with each additional week less than 40 weeks)
- Phototherapy before discharge
- Parent or sibling requiring phototherapy or exchange transfusion
- Down syndrome
- Cephalohematoma or significant bruising (e.g., from vacuum-assisted delivery)
- Exclusive breastfeeding with suboptimal intake and weight loss is excessive

In examining a newborn for hyperbilirubinemia, look at the whole body. Be sure to examine the oral mucosa and sclera of the eyes, where jaundice can be detected more easily, and examine the baby in natural daylight if possible. Both artificial light and environmental colors (e.g., orange drapes) can produce false colors.

Check the skin of the newborn carefully for small defects, especially over the entire length of the spine, the vertex of the scalp, from the nape of the neck to the bridge of the nose, and the neck extending to the ear. This may indicate brachial sinus tracts or brachial cleft cysts. The skin should feel soft and smooth. Also look for skin findings that may signal underlying systemic conditions (Box 9.8).

Inspect the skin for distortions in contour suggestive of congenital vascular malformations, any nodules, congenital birth marks, and/or tumors. Transillumination may help if there is a question about the density of the mass or the amount of fluid contained therein. With more density and less fluid, there is a diminished tendency to glow with transillumination.

BOX 9.8 Skin Lesions: External Clues to Internal Problems

Many systemic conditions or disorders may present congenital external clues that are apparent on physical examination. The following are a few examples of cutaneous markers that may signal underlying disease. A thorough evaluation is necessary, although some clues may be isolated findings and may require no intervention, follow-up, or treatment.

- **Faun tail nevus:** Tuft of hair overlying the spinal column at birth, usually in the lumbosacral area; may be associated with spina bifida occulta.
- **Café au lait macules:** Flat, evenly pigmented spots varying in color from light brown to dark brown or black in darker skin; larger than 5 mm in diameter; present at birth or shortly thereafter; may be associated with neurofibromatosis or miscellaneous other conditions, including pulmonary stenosis, temporal lobe dysrhythmia, and tuberous sclerosis.
- **Freckling in the axillary or inguinal area:** Multiple flat pigmented macules associated with neurofibromatosis; may occur in conjunction with café au lait macules.
- **Facial port-wine stain:** Usually at least one eyelid and/or the forehead of one side of the face are affected. It may be associated with ocular defects, most notably glaucoma, or may be accompanied by angiomatous malformation of the meninges (Sturge-Weber syndrome), resulting in atrophy and calcification of the adjacent cerebral cortex.
- **Port-wine stain of limb and/or trunk:** When accompanied by varicosities and hypertrophy of underlying soft tissues and bones, may be associated with orthopedic problems (Klippel-Trenaunay-Weber syndrome).
- **Supernumerary nipples:** Congenital accessory nipples with or without glandular tissue, located along the mammary ridge (see Chapter 17); may be associated with renal abnormalities, especially in the presence of other minor anomalies.
- **"Hair collar" sign:** A ring of long, dark, coarse hair surrounding a midline scalp nodule in infants is usually an isolated cutaneous anomaly that may indicate neural tube closure defects of the scalp.

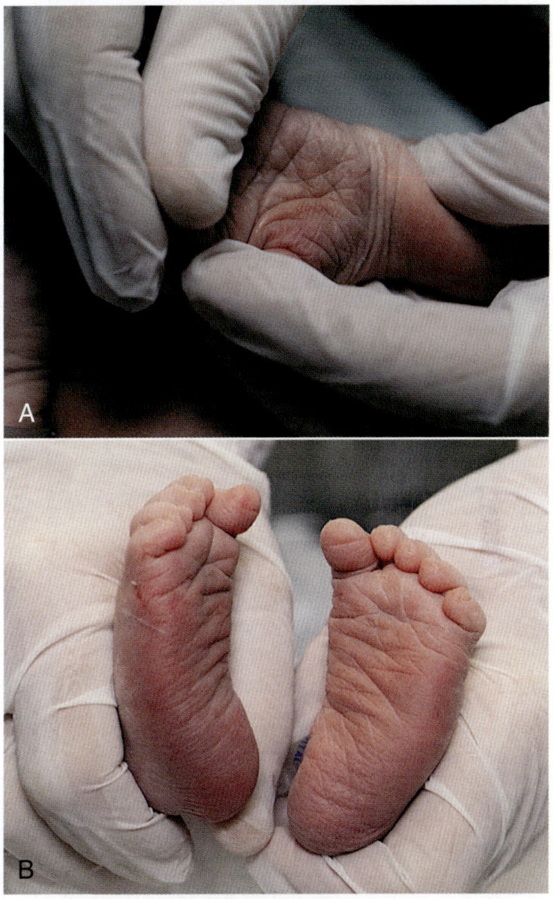

FIG. 9.24 **Expected creases of a newborn's hands (A) and feet (B).**

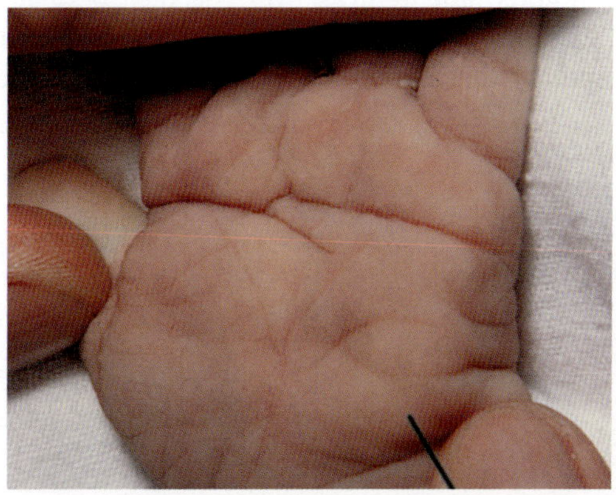

FIG. 9.25 **Unexpected palmar crease.** Single transverse crease in a child with Down syndrome. Compare with Fig. 9.24A. (From Zitelli, B. J., McIntire, S. C., & Nowalk, A. J. (2012). *Zitelli and Davis' atlas of pediatric physical diagnosis* (6th ed.). Philadelphia: Saunders.)

Examine the hands and feet of newborns for skin creases. Flexion causes creases that are readily discernible on the fingers, palms, and soles (Fig. 9.24). One indicator of maturity is the number of creases; the older the baby, the more creases there will be. Examine the crease patterns of the fingers and palms, as abnormalities are associated with specific patterns. The most commonly recognized pattern is a single transverse crease in the palm that is commonly seen in children with Down syndrome (trisomy 21), but this may also be a typical finding (Fig. 9.25).

All newborn infants are covered, to some degree, by vernix caseosa—a whitish, moist, cheeselike substance. Transient puffiness of the hands, feet, eyelids, legs, pubis, or sacrum occurs in some newborns, but it has no discernible cause, and it should not create concern if it disappears within 2 to 3 days.

Newborn infants are particularly susceptible to hypothermia, partly because of their poorly developed subcutaneous fat. In addition, infants have a relatively large body surface area, providing greater area for heat loss. Combined with an inability to shiver, these factors cause term newborns to lose heat. Care should be taken to use a warm surface or heat lamp when uncovering the newborn for examination.

Cutis marmorata, a mottled appearance of the body and extremities, is part of a newborn's response to changes in ambient temperature, whether cooling or heating. It is more common in premature infants and children with Down syndrome or hypothyroidism (Fig. 9.26). Cyanosis of the hands and feet (acrocyanosis) may be present at birth and may persist for several days or longer if the newborn is kept in cool ambient temperatures. It often recurs when the baby is chilled. If cyanosis persists, suspect an underlying cardiac or pulmonary defect (Fig. 9.27).

Bluish-black to slate gray spots (congenital dermal melanocytosis) are sometimes seen on the back, buttocks, shoulders, and legs of healthy babies. These hyperpigmented patches occur most often in babies with dark skin and usually disappear in the preschool years. Hyperpigmented patches may be mistaken for bruises by the inexperienced examiner (Fig. 9.28).

The appearance of several vascular lesions is common in infancy. Infantile hemangiomas are true neoplasms, which develop in the first 1 to 2 months of life, grow for 2 to 6 months, and regress over the next 5 to 10 years (Fig. 9.29). A nevus simplex ("stork bite") represents a common capillary vascular formation, found most frequently on the midforehead, eyelids, upper lip, and back of the neck. A port wine stain is also a capillary malformation that may be associated with underlying arteriovenous malformations in Sturge-Weber syndrome.

Coffee-colored patches (café au lait macules) may be either harmless or indicative of underlying disease. Be suspicious of neurofibromatosis (NF-1) if six or more café au lait macules more than 5 mm in diameter at the greatest are found in prepubertal individuals or if they present more than 15 mm in greatest diameter after puberty (Fig. 9.30).

Milia are small, whitish, discrete papules on the face commonly found during the first 2 to 3 months of life. The sebaceous glands function in an immature fashion at this age and are easily clogged by sebum (Fig. 9.31).

Sebaceous hyperplasia produces numerous tiny, yellow macules and papules in the newborn, probably the result of androgen stimulation from the parent. It commonly occurs on the forehead, cheeks, nose, and chin of a full-term

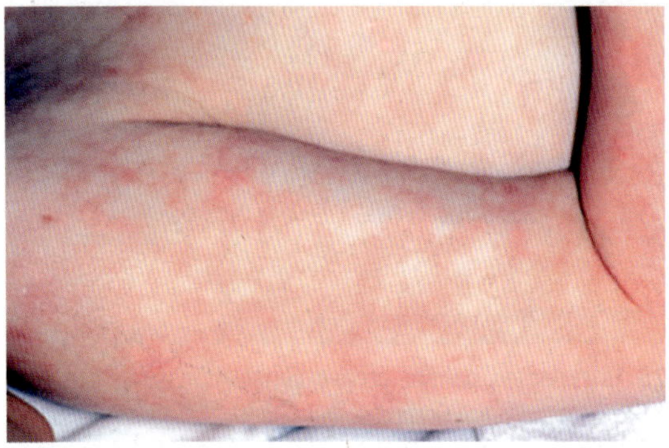

FIG. 9.26 **Mottling (cutis marmorata).** (From O'Connor, N. R., McLaughlin, M. R., & Ham, P. (2008). Newborn skin: Part I: Common rashes. American Family Physician, 77, 47–52.)

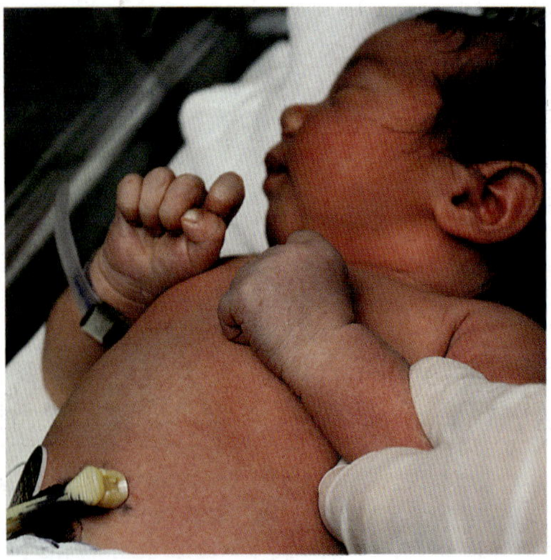

FIG. 9.27 **Acrocyanosis of hands in a newborn.**

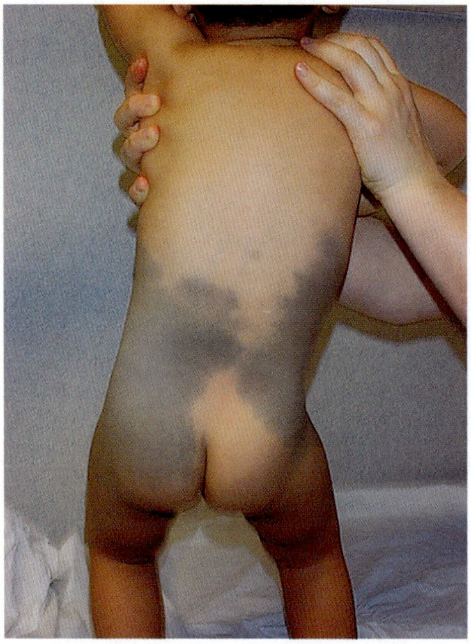

FIG. 9.28 **Hyperpigmented patches are common in babies with dark skin.** (From Taïeb, A., & Boralevi, F. (2007). Hypermelanoses of the newborn and of the infant, *Dermatologic Clinics*, *25*(3), 327–336.)

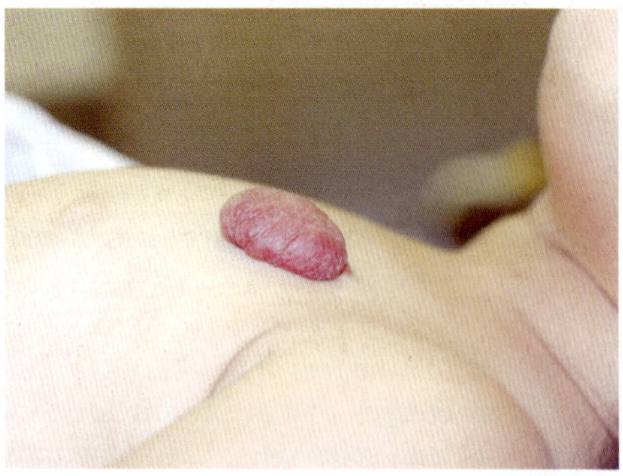

FIG. 9.29 **Hemangioma.** (From Kliegman, R. M., & Stanton, B. M. D. (2016). *Nelson textbook of pediatrics* (20th ed.). Philadelphia: Elsevier.)

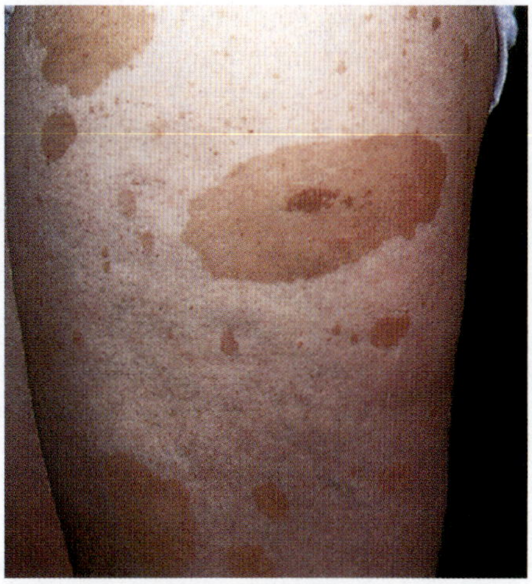

FIG. 9.30 Café au lait patches. (From Epstein, O., Perkin, G. D., & Cookson, J. (2008). *Clinical examination* (4th ed.). Elsevier.)

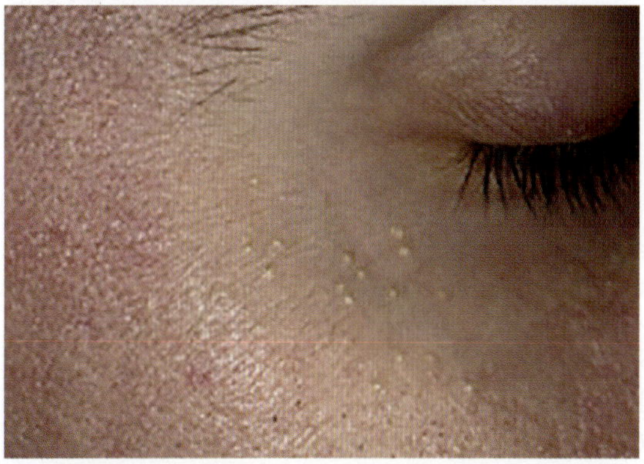

FIG. 9.31 Milia. (From Dinulos, J. (2021). *Habif's clinical dermatology* (7th ed.). St. Louis: Elsevier.)

infant. Sebaceous hyperplasia disappears quickly within 1 to 2 months of life but may recur in later life in patients with rosacea or chronic sun damage.

The skin and subcutaneous tissues of an infant and young child, more readily than in the older child and adolescent, can give an important indication of the state of hydration and nutrition (Table 9.7). The tissue turgor is best evaluated by gently pinching a fold of the abdominal skin between the index finger and thumb. As with the adult, resiliency allows it to return to its undisturbed state when released. A child with severe dehydration (i.e., more than 10% of body weight) or very poorly nourished will have skin that retains "tenting" after it is pinched. How quickly the tent disappears helps to determine the degree of dehydration or malnutrition (Fig. 9.32).

Because the normal range of skin moisture is broad, look at other factors that may suggest a problem. Excessive sweating or dryness alone rarely has pathologic significance in infants or children.

Children with atopic dermatitis or chronic skin changes involving the face will commonly rub their eyes, sufficiently sometimes to cause an extra crease or pleat of skin below the eye. This is known as the *Dennie-Morgan fold* and often referred to as the *allergic salute;* it is secondary to chronic rubbing and inflammation. Also see the Clinical Pearl, "Bald Spots in Infants and Children."

TABLE 9.7 Estimating Dehydration

RETURN TO NORMAL AFTER THE PINCH	DEGREE OF DEHYDRATION
<2 seconds	<5% loss of body weight
2–3 seconds	5%–8% loss of body weight
3–4 seconds	9%–10% loss of body weight
>4 seconds	>10% loss of body weight

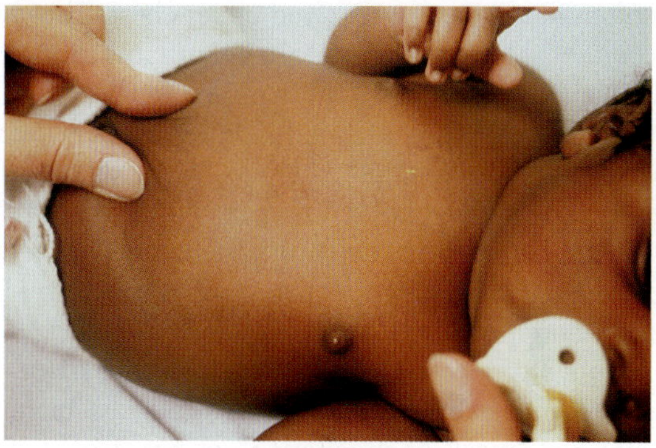

FIG. 9.32 Testing skin turgor in an infant.

CLINICAL PEARL

Bald Spots in Infants and Children

Bald spots in children? History is important. The differential diagnosis includes tinea capitis, alopecia areata, or trichotillomania (compulsive hair-pulling). Infants who sleep on their backs may develop areas of alopecia from pressure on the occiput. Supine sleeping reduces the risk for sudden infant death syndrome (SIDS). Providing tummy time while the infant is awake can promote motor development and decrease the likelihood of developing a bald spot.

Adolescents

The examination of an adolescent's skin is the same as it would be for an adult. The adolescent's skin may have increased oiliness and perspiration, and hair oiliness may also be increased. Increased sebum production predisposes the adolescent to develop acne and seborrheic dermatitis.

As a reflection of maturing apocrine gland function, increased axillary perspiration occurs, and the characteristic adult body odor develops during adolescence. Hair on the extremities darkens and becomes coarser. Over time pubic and axillary hair develops and assumes adult characteristics. Adolescents assigned male at birth develop facial and chest hair that varies in quantity and coarseness. Chapter 8 provides a more thorough discussion of the maturational changes that occur during adolescence.

Pregnant Patients

Striae gravidarum (stretch marks) may appear over the abdomen, thighs, and breasts during the second trimester of pregnancy. They fade after delivery but never fully disappear (Fig. 9.33). There is an increase in telangiectasias, which may be found on the face, neck, chest, and arms; these appear during the second to fifth months of pregnancy and usually resolve after delivery. Hemangiomas that were present before pregnancy may increase in size, or new ones may develop. Cutaneous tags (molluscum fibrosum gravidarum) are either pedunculated or sessile skin tags that are most often found on the neck and upper chest. They result from epithelial hyperplasia and are not inflammatory. Most resolve spontaneously or can be removed easily.

An increase in pigmentation is common and is found to some extent in all pregnant patients. The areas usually affected include the areolae and nipples, vulvar and perianal regions, axillae, and linea alba. Pigmentation of the linea alba is called the *linea nigra*. It extends from the symphysis pubis to the top of the fundus in the midline (Fig. 9.34). Preexisting pigmented nevi and freckles may darken, with some nevi increasing in size. New nevi may form also. Melasma, or "mask of pregnancy," occurs frequently in pregnant patients. The darkened, blotchy skin is usually symmetric and found on the forehead, cheeks, bridge of the nose, and chin (see Fig. 9.6).

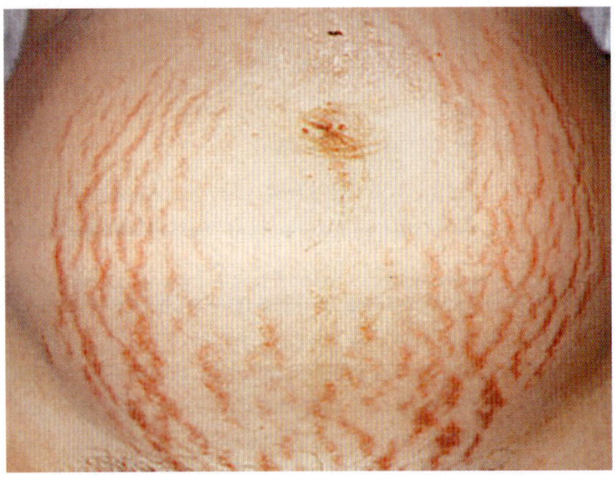

FIG. 9.33 Striae. (From Symonds, I., & Arulkumaran, S. (2013). *Essential obstetrics and gynaecology e-book* (5th ed.). Edinburgh: Churchill Livingstone.)

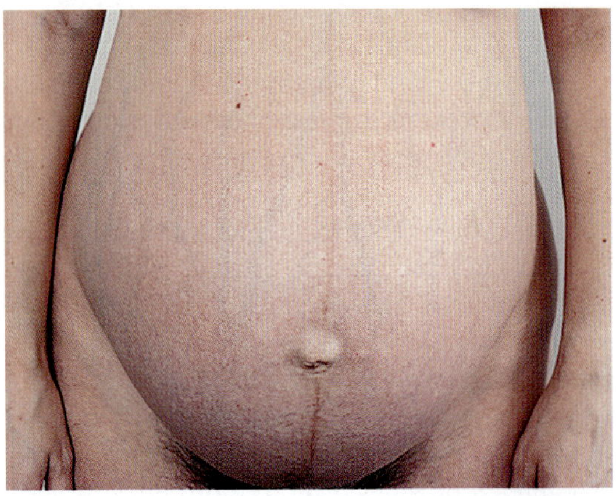

FIG. 9.34 Linea nigra on abdomen during pregnancy.

Palmar erythema is a common finding in pregnancy. A diffuse redness covers the entire palmar surface or the thenar and hypothenar eminences. The cause is unknown but is likely related to estrogens, and it usually disappears after delivery.

Itching over the abdomen and breasts resulting from skin stretching is common and not a cause for concern; however, itching accompanied by a rash may signal a pregnancy-specific dermatosis, which requires further investigation. Itching during pregnancy can also be caused by impaired flow of bile from the liver, which may also produce jaundice. The itching is generalized but may be more severe on the palms and soles. Be alert for these serious manifestations of underlying pathology. Hair growth is altered in pregnancy by the circulating hormones. The growing phase of the hair is lengthened, and hair loss is decreased. Two to six months after delivery, increased hair shedding occurs (telogen effluvium). Regrowth will occur in 6 to 12 months. Acne vulgaris may be aggravated during the first trimester of pregnancy but often improves in the third trimester.

Older Adults

The skin of an older adult may appear more transparent and paler in light-skinned individuals. Pigment deposits, increased freckling, and hypopigmented patches may develop, causing the skin to take on a less uniform appearance.

Flaking or scaling, associated with the drier skin that comes with aging, occurs most commonly over the extremities. The skin also thins (especially over bony prominences, the dorsal surface of hands and feet, forearms, and lower legs) and takes on a parchmentlike appearance and texture (Fig. 9.35).

The skin often appears to hang loosely on the bony frame as a result of a general loss of elasticity, loss of

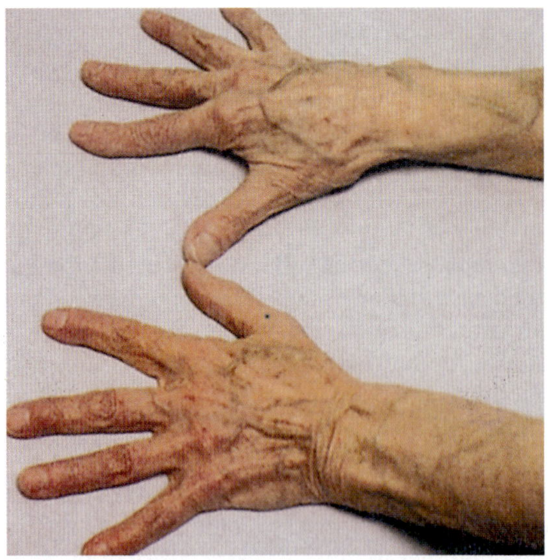

FIG. 9.35 Hands of an older adult. Note prominent veins and thin appearance of the skin.

underlying adipose tissue, and years of gravitational pull (Fig. 9.36). You may observe tenting of the skin when testing for turgor (Fig. 9.37; see Clinical Pearl, "Hydration Status in Older Adults").

CLINICAL PEARL

Hydration Status in Older Adults

Because loss of skin turgor is a common finding in older adults, it is not a good indicator of hydration status. To determine hydration status, use other assessments, such as amount of saliva, urine output, and urine specific gravity.

The immobility of some older adults, especially when combined with decreased peripheral vascular circulation, increases their risk for pressure ulcers (decubitus ulcers). During examination, pay particular attention to bony prominences and areas subject to persistent pressure or shearing forces. Heels and the sacrum are common sites for this occurrence in patients who are confined to bed. Do not neglect to examine less obvious areas such as the elbows, scapulae, and back of the head. Assess the diameter and depth of the ulcer, and stage it accordingly. The staging criteria are described in Table 9.8.

Increased wrinkling is evident, especially in areas exposed to the sun and in expressive areas of the face. Sagging or drooping is most obvious under the chin; beneath the eyes; and in the earlobes, breasts, and scrotum. Senile purpura (bruises), particularly on the dorsal surfaces of the hands and lower arms that get tapped or bumped more frequently, is commonly seen in older adults, especially when on anticoagulant or antiplatelet therapy.

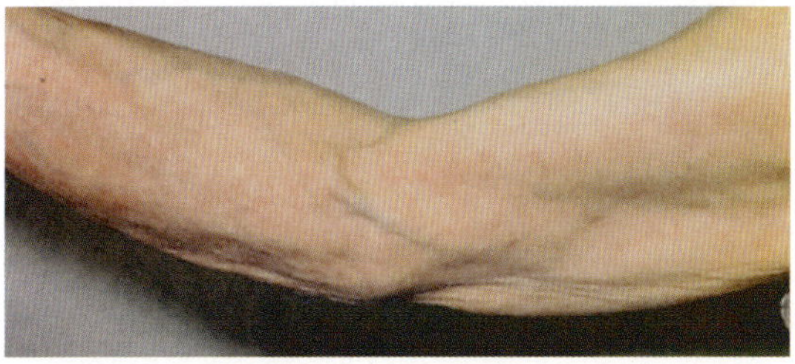

FIG. 9.36 Skin hanging loosely, especially around bony prominences.

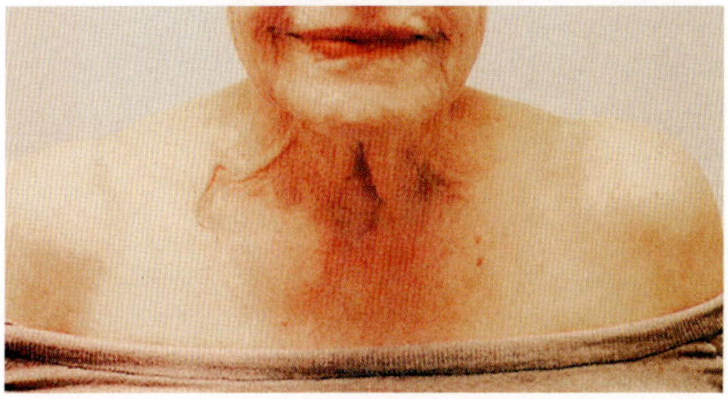

FIG. 9.37 Skin turgor in an older adult. Note tenting.

TABLE 9.8 Staging of Pressure Ulcers (Decubitus Ulcers)

STAGE	CHARACTERISTICS
Suspected deep tissue injury	Localized area of discolored intact skin (purple or maroon) or blood-filled blister due to damage of underlying soft tissue from pressure and/or shear. The area may be preceded by tissue that is painful, firm, mushy, boggy, warmer, or cooler compared with adjacent tissue.
I	Intact skin with nonblanchable redness of a localized area, usually over a bony prominence. Darkly pigmented skin may not have visible blanching; its color may differ from the surrounding area. The area may be painful, firm, soft, warmer, or cooler compared with adjacent tissue. Category/stage I may be difficult to detect in individuals with dark skin tones. May indicate "at-risk" individuals (a heralding sign of risk).
II	Partial-thickness loss of dermis presenting as a shallow open ulcer with a red-pink wound bed, without slough. May also present as an intact or open/ruptured serum-filled blister. Presents as a shiny or dry shallow ulcer without slough or bruising.[a] This category/stage should not be used to describe skin tears, tape burns, perineal dermatitis, maceration, or excoriation.
III	Full-thickness tissue loss. Subcutaneous fat may be visible, but bone, tendon, or muscle is not exposed. Slough may be present but does not obscure the depth of tissue loss. May include undermining and tunneling. The depth of a category/stage III pressure ulcer varies by anatomic location. The bridge of the nose, ear, occiput, and malleolus do not have subcutaneous tissue, and category/stage III ulcers can be shallow. In contrast, areas of significant adiposity can develop extremely deep category/stage III pressure ulcers. Bone/tendon is not visible or directly palpable.
IV	Full-thickness tissue loss with exposed bone, tendon, or muscle. Slough or eschar may be present on some parts of the wound bed. Often includes undermining and tunneling. The depth of a category/stage IV pressure ulcer varies by anatomic location. The bridge of the nose, ear, occiput, and malleolus do not have subcutaneous tissue, and these ulcers can be shallow. Category/stage IV ulcers can extend into muscle and/or supporting structures (e.g., fascia, tendon, or joint capsule), making osteomyelitis possible. Exposed bone/tendon is visible or directly palpable.
Unstageable	Full-thickness tissue loss in which the base of the ulcer is covered by slough (yellow, tan, gray, green, or brown) and/or eschar (tan, brown, or black) in the wound bed. Until enough slough and/or eschar is removed to expose the base of the wound, the true depth, and therefore category/stage, cannot be determined. Stable (dry, adherent, intact without erythema or fluctuance) eschar on the heels serves as "the body's natural (biologic) cover" and should not be removed.

[a] Bruising indicates suspected deep tissue injury.

From *National Pressure Ulcer Advisory Panel*. (2014). http://www.npuap.org/wp-content/uploads/2014/08/Quick-Reference-Guide-DIGITAL-NPUAP-EPUAP-PPPIA-Jan2016.pdf.

SKIN, HAIR, AND NAILS

Several types of lesions may occur on the skin of healthy older adults. The following lesions are considered expected findings:

- Cherry angiomas are tiny, bright ruby-red to dark blue/black, round papules that may become brown with time. They occur in virtually everyone older than 30 years and increase numerically with age (Fig. 9.38).
- Seborrheic keratoses are pigmented, raised, warty lesions, usually appearing on the trunk. These must be distinguished from other growths such as nevi or actinic keratoses, which may have malignant potential. Because the lesions may look similar, seek the assistance of an experienced practitioner for evaluation (Fig. 9.39).
- Sebaceous hyperplasia presents as a yellowish, flattened papule with a central depression that is often difficult to discern from a basal cell carcinoma (Fig. 9.40).
- Cutaneous tags (acrochordons) are small, soft, skin-colored, pedunculated (narrow stalk) papules of skin, usually appearing on the neck and upper chest (Fig. 9.41).
- Cutaneous horns are small, hard projections of the epidermis, usually occurring on the forehead and face, and can be the manifestation of an underlying squamous cell carcinoma or a wart (Fig. 9.42).
- Solar lentigines (singular: lentigo) are irregular, gray-brown macules that occur in sun-exposed areas that can range in size from a few millimeters to over a centimeter. These are often referred to as *age spots* or, incorrectly, as *liver spots* (Fig. 9.43). Note that "liver spots" have no relationship to the liver. They are epidermal proliferations and are signs of photoaging of the skin.

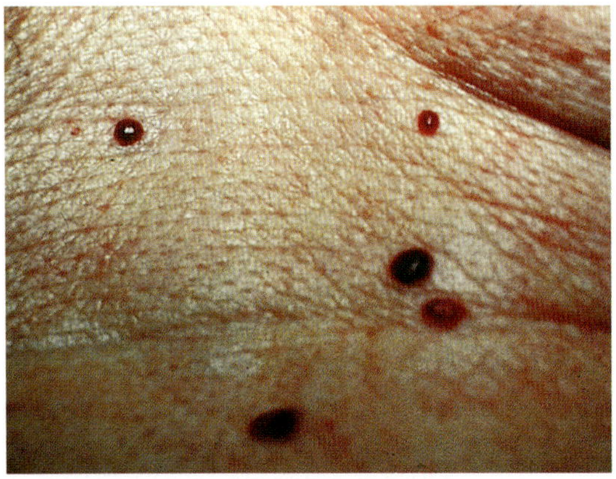

FIG. 9.38 Cherry angioma in an older adult. (From Ignatavicius, D. D., & Workman, M. L. (2016). *Medical-surgical nursing: Patient-centered collaborative care.* St. Louis: Elsevier.)

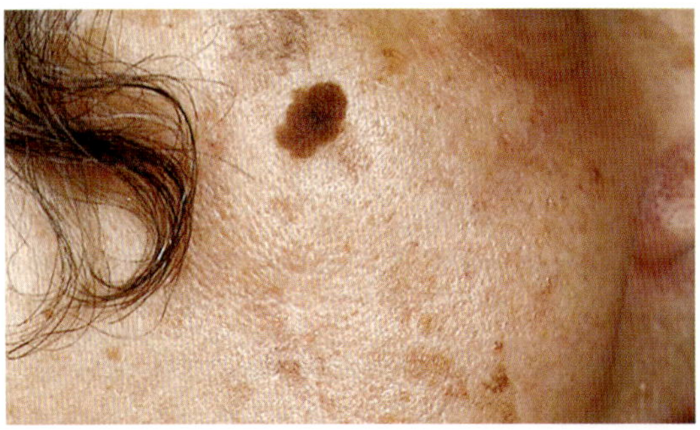

FIG. 9.39 Seborrheic keratoses in an older adult. (From Glynn, M., & Drake, W. M. (2012). *Hutchison's clinical methods: An integrated approach to clinical practice* (23rd ed.). Edinburgh: Saunders.)

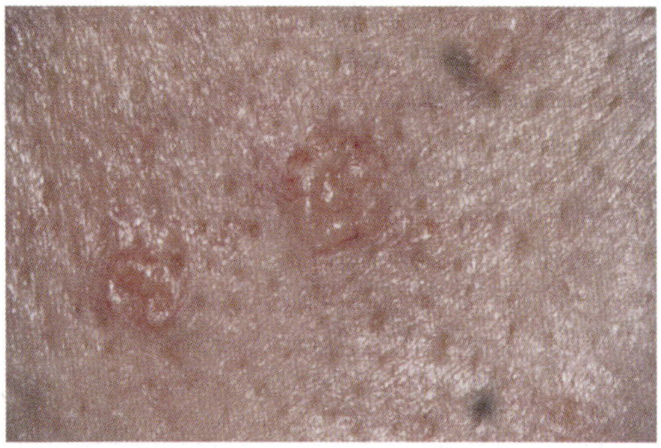

FIG. 9.40 Sebaceous hyperplasia. (From Damm, D. D., Allen, C. M., & Chi, A. C. (2024). *Oral and maxillofacial pathology* (5th ed.). Elsevier Inc)

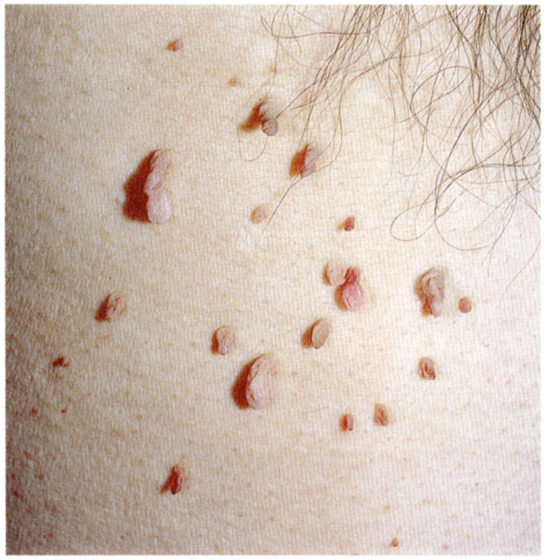

FIG. 9.41 Multiple cutaneous tags in axilla. (From Salvo, S. (2014). *Mosby's pathology for massage therapists* (3rd ed.). St. Louis: Mosby.)

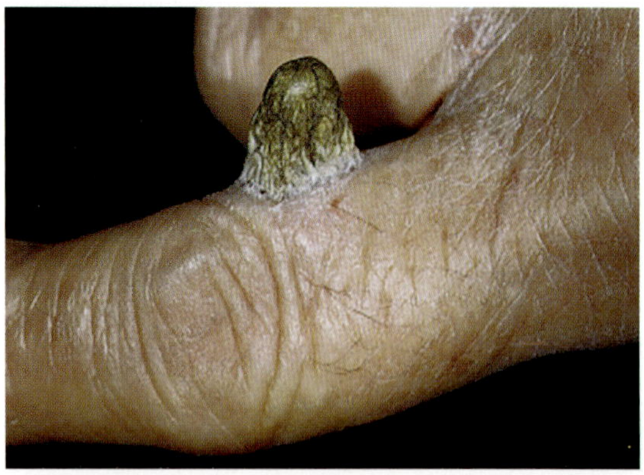

FIG. 9.42 Cutaneous horn. (From Dinulos, J. (2021). *Habif's clinical dermatology* (7th ed.). St. Louis: Elsevier.)

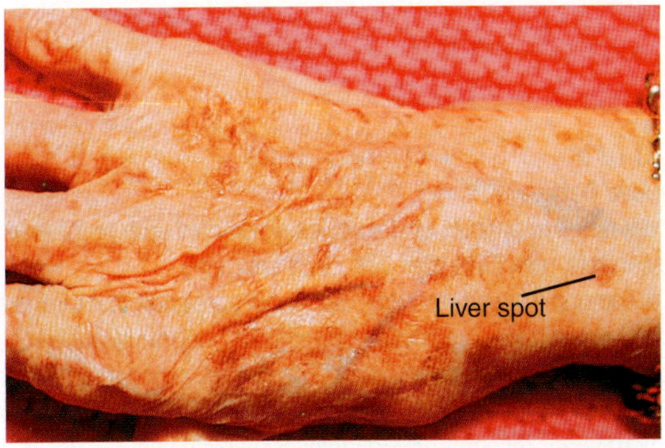

FIG. 9.43 **Lentigo, a brown macule that appears in sun-exposed areas.** (From Ignatavicius, D. D., & Workman, M. L. (2016). *Medical-surgical nursing: Patient-centered collaborative care.* St. Louis: Elsevier.)

The hair turns gray or white as melanocytes cease functioning. Head, body, pubic, and axillary hair thins and becomes sparse and drier. Males may show an increase in coarse aural, nasal, and eyebrow hair; females tend to develop coarse facial hair. Symmetric balding, usually frontal or occipital, often occurs in males.

The nails thicken; become more brittle; and may be deformed, misshapen, striated, distorted, or peeling. They can take on a yellowish color and may lose their transparency. These changes occur most often in the toenails.

ABNORMALITIES

SKIN, HAIR, AND NAILS

Skin: Inflammatory and Infectious Conditions

Eczematous Dermatitis

Most common inflammatory skin disorder; several forms, including irritant contact dermatitis, allergic contact dermatitis, and atopic dermatitis

PATHOPHYSIOLOGY

- Common factor of the various forms are intercellular edema and epidermal breakdown
- Eczematous dermatitis has three stages: acute, subacute, and chronic
- Itch-scratch cycle perpetuates the rash
- Excoriation from scratching predisposes to infection and causes crust formation (Fig. 9.44)

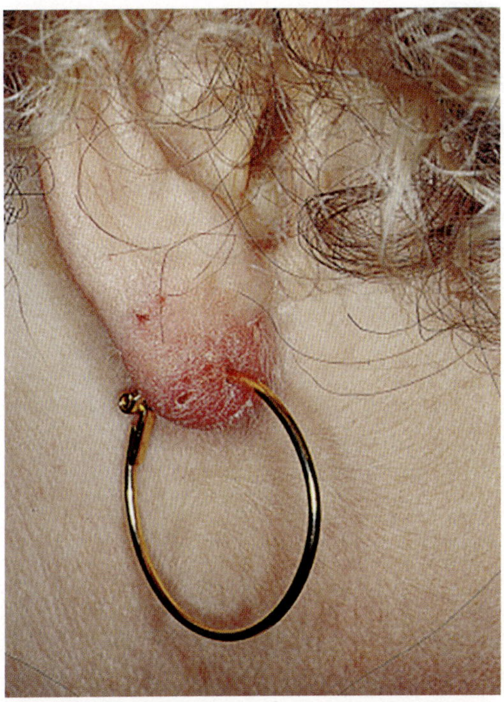

FIG. 9.44 **Contact dermatitis due to nickel allergy.** (From Dinulos, J. (2021). *Habif's clinical dermatology* (7th ed.). St. Louis: Elsevier.)

PATIENT DATA

Subjective Data

- Itching is typically present
- Those with atopic dermatitis often report allergy history (allergic rhinitis, asthma)
- For irritant or allergic contact, exposure history is important

Objective Data

- Acute phase characterized by erythematous, pruritic, weeping vesicles
- Subacute eczema characterized by erythema and scaling
- Chronic stage characterized by thick, lichenified, pruritic plaques
- Atopic dermatitis: during childhood, lesions involve the flexures, nape, and dorsal aspects of the limbs; in adolescence and adulthood, lichenified plaques affect the flexures, head, and neck

Folliculitis

Inflammation and infection of the hair follicle and surrounding dermis

PATHOPHYSIOLOGY

- Presence of inflammatory cells within the wall and ostia of the hair follicle creates a follicular-based pustule
- Inflammation can be either superficial or deep; deep folliculitis can result from chronic lesions of superficial folliculitis or from lesions that are manipulated
- Persistent or recurrent lesions may result in scarring and permanent hair loss
- Sometimes due to a bacterial (e.g., *Staphylococcus*) or yeast infection

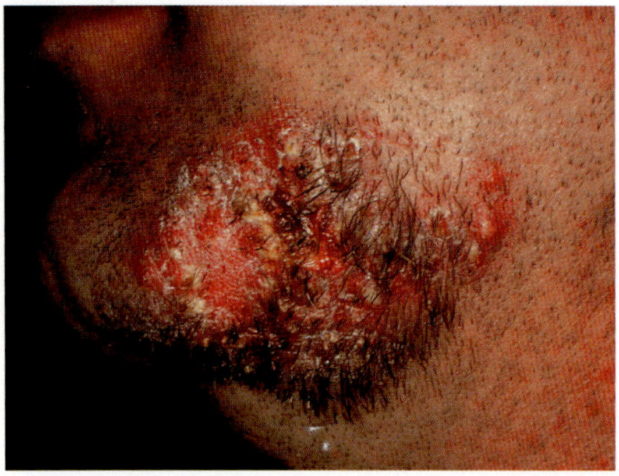

FIG. 9.45 Beard folliculitis. (From Bolognia, J., & Jorizzo, J. (2012). *Dermatology* (3rd ed.). Elsevier.)

PATIENT DATA

Subjective Data

- Acute onset of papules and pustules associated with pruritus or mild discomfort; may have pain with deep folliculitis
- Risk factors: frequent shaving, immunosuppression, hot tubs without adequate chlorine, preexisting dermatoses, long-term antibiotic use, occlusive clothing and/or occlusive dressings, exposure to hot and humid temperatures, diabetes mellitus, obesity, and use of epithelial growth factor receptor (EGFR) inhibitor medications

Objective Data

- Primary lesion is a small pustule 1–2 cm in diameter that is located over a pilosebaceous orifice and may be perforated by a hair
- Pustule may be surrounded by inflammation or nodular lesions; after the pustule ruptures, a crust forms (Fig. 9.45)
- May have suppurative drainage with deep folliculitis
- Any hair-bearing site can be affected; the sites most often involved are the face, scalp, thighs, axilla, and inguinal area

Furuncle (Boil)

A deep-seated infection of the pilosebaceous unit

PATHOPHYSIOLOGY

- *Staphylococcus aureus* is the most common organism
- Initially, a small perifollicular abscess that spreads to the surrounding dermis and subcutaneous tissue
- May occur singly or in multiples; when infection involves several adjacent follicles, a coalescent purulent mass or carbuncle forms

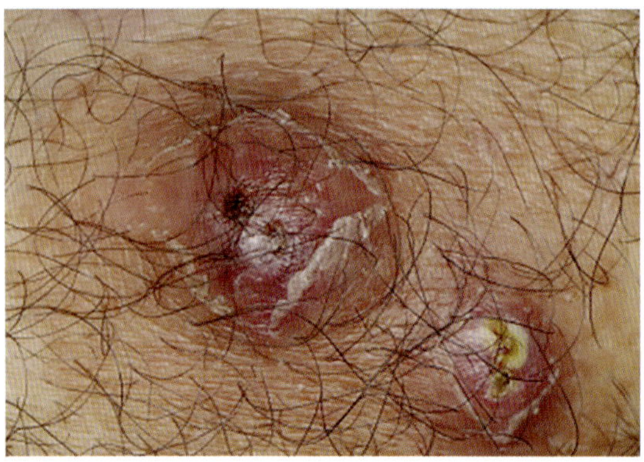

FIG. 9.46 Furuncle. (From Dinulos, J. (2021). *Habif's clinical dermatology* (7th ed.). St. Louis: Elsevier.)

PATIENT DATA

Subjective Data

- Acute onset of tender, red nodule with center filled with pus

Objective Data

- Skin is red, hot, and tender
- Center of the lesion is purulent and forms a core that may rupture spontaneously or require surgical incision (Fig. 9.46)
- Sites commonly involved are the face and neck, arms, axillae, breasts, thighs, and buttocks

Cellulitis

Diffuse, acute infection of the skin and subcutaneous tissue

PATHOPHYSIOLOGY

- Majority of cases caused by *Streptococcus pyogenes* or *Staphylococcus aureus*

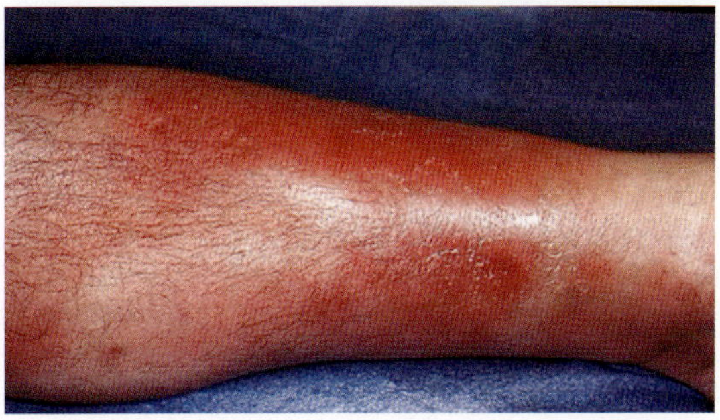

FIG. 9.47 **Cellulitis of the leg.** (From Gawkrodger, D., & Ardern-Jones, M. R. (2017). *Dermatology: An illustrated color text* (6th ed.). Edinburgh: Elsevier.)

PATIENT DATA

Subjective Data

- Break in the skin, such as a fissure, cut, laceration, insect bite, or puncture wound
- Pain and swelling at the site
- May have fever

Objective Data

- Skin is red, hot, tender, and indurated; borders are not well demarcated (Fig. 9.47)
- Lymphangitic streaks and regional lymphadenopathy may be present
- If it appears in a bilateral distribution, then consider stasis dermatitis instead

Tinea (Dermatophytosis)

Group of noncandidal fungal infections that involve the stratum corneum, nails, or hair

PATHOPHYSIOLOGY

- Infection by dermatophytes, typically acquired by direct contact with infected humans or animals; invade the skin and survive on dead keratin
- Lesions are usually classified according to anatomic location and can occur on nonhairy parts of the body (tinea corporis), on the groin and inner thigh (tinea cruris), on the scalp (tinea capitis), on the feet (tinea pedis), and on the nails (tinea unguium)

PATIENT DATA

Subjective Data

- May report pruritus
- May report hair breaking
- Nail changes accompany onychomycosis

Objective Data

- Although often annular, lesions can vary in appearance and may be papular, pustular, vesicular, erythematous, or scaling (Fig. 9.48)
- Secondary bacterial infection may be present
- Microscopic examination of skin scraping with potassium hydroxide (KOH) solution shows presence of hyphae
- Infected nails are yellow and thick and may separate from the nail bed

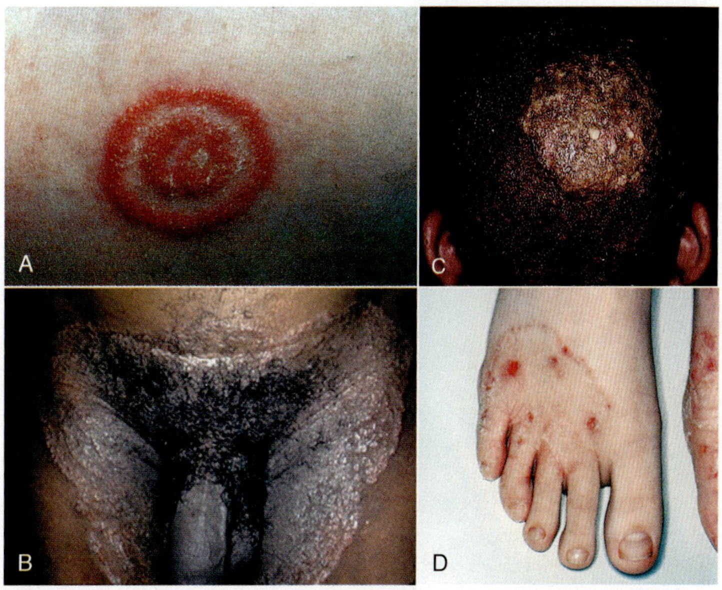

FIG. 9.48 (A) Tinea corporis. (B) Tinea cruris. (C) Tinea capitis. (D) Tinea pedis. (A, C, and D, From Callen, J. P., Greer, K. E., Paller, A. S., et al., (2000). *Color atlas of dermatology* (2nd ed.). Philadelphia: Saunders; B, from Courtesy Kenneth E. Greer. From Marchetti, M. A.,Wilson, B. Dermatologic conditions, In: DeLee & Drez's Orthopaedic Sports Medicine, Pages 285–297, Fig. 26-8. Copyright 2015 by Saunders, an imprint of Elsevier Inc.)

Pityriasis Rosea

Self-limiting inflammation of unknown cause

PATHOPHYSIOLOGY

- Possible infectious etiology, likely human herpesvirus (HHV)-6 or HHV-7
- Not contagious

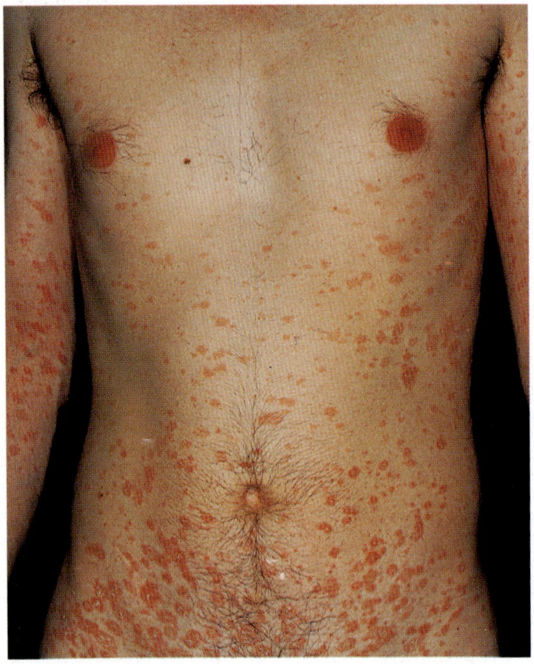

FIG. 9.49 **Pityriasis rosea.** (From Salvo, S. (2014). *Mosby's pathology for massage therapists* (3rd ed.). St. Louis: Mosby.)

PATIENT DATA

Subjective Data

- Sudden onset with occurrence of a primary (herald) oval or round plaque
- Herald lesion is often missed
- Eruption occurs 1–3 weeks later and lasts for several weeks
- Pruritus may be present with the generalized eruption
- Often occurs in young adults during the springtime

Objective Data

- Lesions are usually oval, pale, erythematous, flat-topped papules and plaques with fine scaling (Fig. 9.49)
- Lesions develop on the extremities and trunk; palms and soles are not involved, and facial involvement is rare
- Trunk lesions are characteristically distributed in parallel alignment following the skin tension lines in a Christmas tree–like pattern

Psoriasis

Chronic and recurrent disease of keratinocyte proliferation

PATHOPHYSIOLOGY

- Multifactorial origin with genetic component and immune regulation
- Characterized by increased epidermal cell turnover, increased numbers of epidermal stem cells, and abnormal differentiation of keratin expression leading to thickened skin with copious scale
- Related to tumor necrosis factor (TNF)-alpha

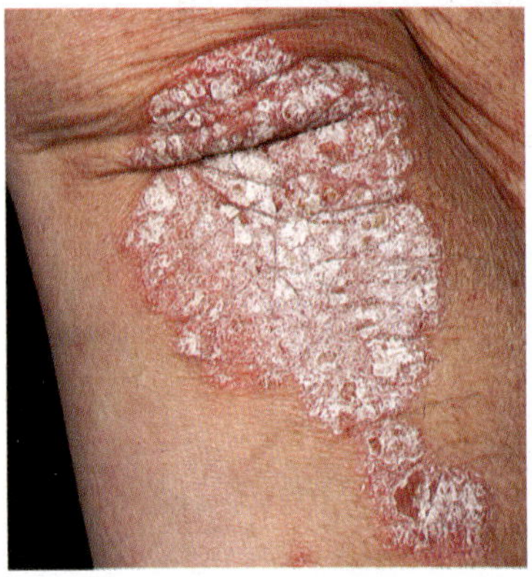

FIG. 9.50 **Psoriasis.** Note characteristic silver scaling. (From Glynn, M., & Drake, W. M. (2012). *Hutchison's clinical methods: An integrated approach to clinical practice* (23rd ed.). Edinburgh: Saunders.)

PATIENT DATA

Subjective Data

- May have pruritus
- Concerns about appearance
- Does not typically get superinfected

Objective Data

- Characterized by well-circumscribed, dry, silvery, scaling papules and plaques (Fig. 9.50)
- Lesions commonly occur on the back, buttocks, extensor surfaces of the extremities, and scalp
- Can be associated with psoriatic arthritis in up to 30% of patients
- May have pitting nail involvement

Rosacea

Chronic inflammatory skin disorder

PATHOPHYSIOLOGY

- Cause unknown; occurs most often in persons with a fair complexion
- Lasts for years, with episodes of activity followed by quiescent periods of variable length

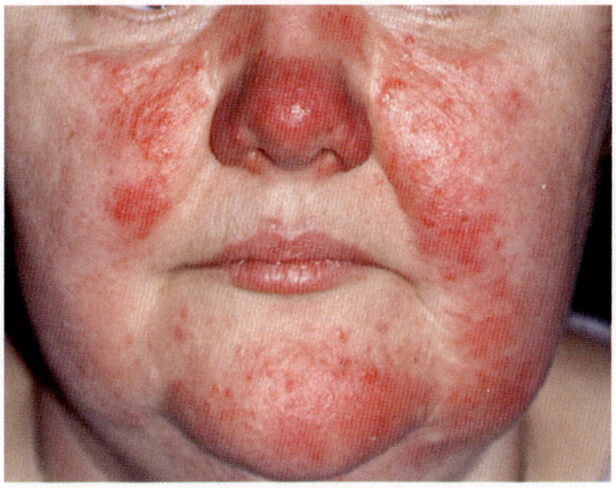

FIG. 9.51 Rosacea. (From Wollina, U. (2011). Rosacea and rhinophyma in the elderly. *Clinics in Dermatology*, 29(1), 61–68.)

PATIENT DATA

Subjective Data

- Itching is absent
- Many patients report a stinging pain associated with flushing episodes
- As erythema may not be as evident in darker skin tones, ask about burning sensation and skin sensitivity
- Common triggers are exposure to the sun, cold weather, sudden emotion (e.g., laughter or embarrassment), hot beverages, spicy foods, and alcohol consumption

Objective Data

- Eruptions appear on the forehead, cheeks, nose, and occasionally around the eyes
- Characterized by telangiectasia, erythema, papules, and pustules that occur particularly in the central area of the face (Fig. 9.51)
- Although rosacea resembles acne, comedones are not present
- Tissue hypertrophy of the nose (rhinophyma) may occur, characterized by sebaceous hyperplasia, redness, prominent vascularity, and swelling of the skin of the nose (Fig. 9.52)

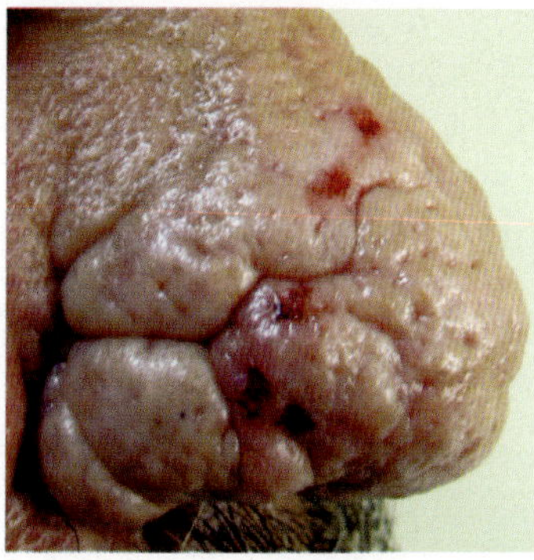

FIG. 9.52 Rhinophyma. (From Tüzün, Y., Wolf, R., Kutlubav, Z., et al. (2014). Rosacea and rhinophyma. *Clinics in Dermatology*, *32*(1), 35–46.)

Herpes Zoster (Shingles)

Varicella-zoster viral (VZV) infection.

PATHOPHYSIOLOGY

- VZV is morphologically and antigenically identical to the virus causing varicella (chickenpox)
- Dormant viral particles (since the original episode of varicella) in the posterior spinal ganglia or cranial sensory ganglia become activated and spread along the nerve

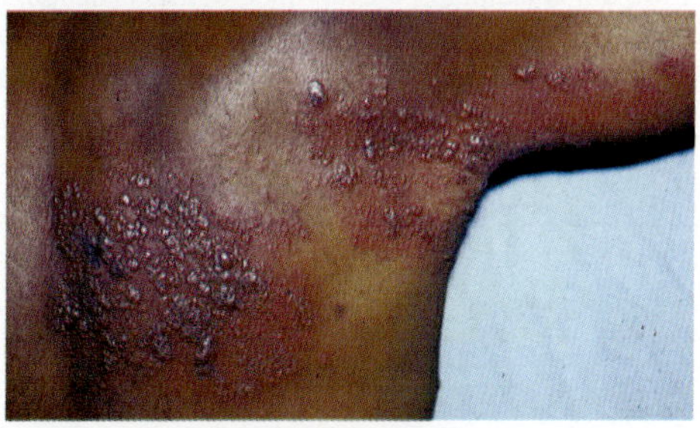

FIG. 9.53 Herpes zoster (shingles) confined to one dermatome. (From Busam, K. J. (2016). *Dermatopathology: A volume in the series: Foundations in diagnostic pathology* (2nd ed.). Philadelphia: Saunders.)

PATIENT DATA

Subjective Data

- Pain, itching, or burning of the dermatome area usually precedes eruption by 4–5 days
- After eruption resolves, there may be persistent pain called *postherpetic neuralgia*

Objective Data

- Single dermatome that consists of red, swollen plaques or vesicles that become filled with purulent fluid (Fig. 9.53)
- Does not cross midline
- Can still occur in immunized patients
- Disseminated lesions in immunosuppressed or older adults

Herpes Simplex

Infection by herpes simplex virus (HSV)

PATHOPHYSIOLOGY

- Two virus types cause the infection: type 1, usually associated with oral infection, and type 2, usually associated with genital infection
- Crossover infections are becoming common

PATIENT DATA

Subjective Data

- Tenderness, pain, paresthesia, or mild burning at the infected site before onset of the lesions

Objective Data

- Grouped vesicles appear on an erythematous base and then erode, forming a crust (Fig. 9.54)
- Lesions last 2–6 weeks
- Can occur anywhere on the body

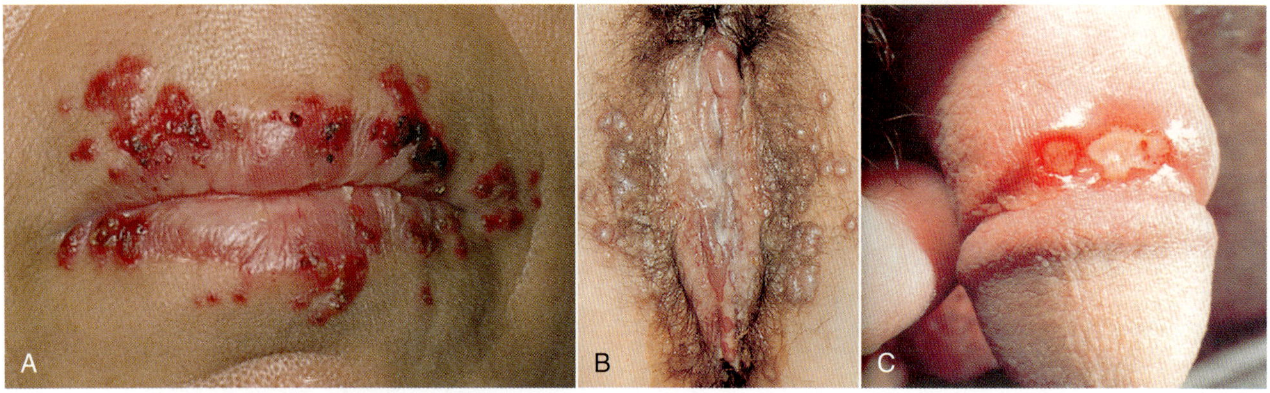

FIG. 9.54 **Herpes simplex.** (A) Oral. (B) Female genital. (C) Male genital. (A, from Salvo, S. (2014). *Mosby's pathology for massage therapists* (3rd ed.). St. Louis: Mosby; B, from Swartz, M. H. (2010). *Textbook of physical diagnosis* (6th ed.). Philadelphia: Saunders; C, from Bennett, J. E., Dolin, R., & Blaser, M. J. (2020). *Mandell, Douglas, and Bennett's principles and practice of infectious diseases* (9th ed.). Elsevier.)

Lyme Disease

A tick-borne disease that can lead to multisystemic infection

PATHOPHYSIOLOGY

- Spirochetal infection caused by *Borrelia burgdorferi*
- Most common tick-borne disease in the United States
- The spirochete is deposited by the tick into the skin rather than directly into the bloodstream
- Three phases of the disease are recognized: early localized, early disseminated, and late disease
- The objective clinical manifestations are thought to be due to an inflammatory response to live spirochetes or to their antigens

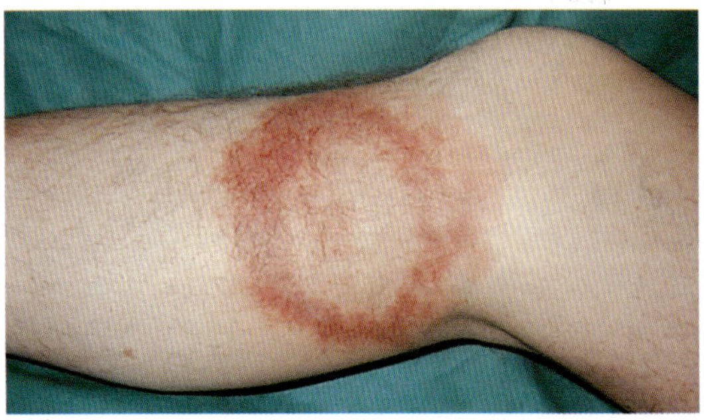

FIG. 9.55 **Erythema migrans (Lyme disease).**

PATIENT DATA

Subjective Data

- Exposure to ticks
- Constitutional symptoms of fatigue, anorexia, and headache may develop
- Expanding rash

Objective Data

- Early localized infection typically manifested by a single erythema migrans skin lesion: a flat to slightly raised, erythematous skin lesion (usually $\geq$5 cm in diameter) that is round or oval in shape, with central clearing (Fig. 9.55; classic target or bull's-eye appearance)
- Early disseminated infection is usually manifested by multiple erythema migrans skin lesions; by neurologic symptoms such as facial palsy, meningitis, or encephalitis; or by symptoms of carditis such as lightheadedness, palpitations, dyspnea, chest pain, or syncope
- Late disease can be manifested by a chronic arthritis or acrodermatitis chronica atrophicans

Skin: Cutaneous Reactions

Drug Eruptions

Cutaneous reactions to medications

PATHOPHYSIOLOGY

- Immunologically mediated cutaneous reactions to medications include immunoglobulin E (IgE)–dependent, cytotoxic, immune complex, and cell-mediated hypersensitivity reactions
- Nonimmunologically mediated reactions include direct release of mast cell mediators and idiosyncratic reactions

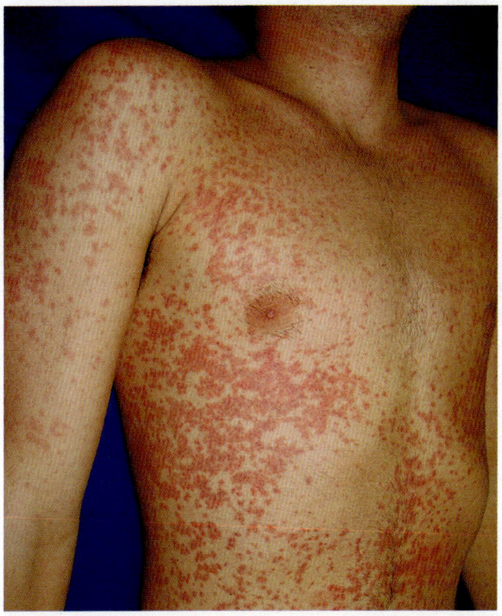

FIG. 9.56 **Drug eruption.** (From Zaoutis, L. B., & Chiang, V. W. (2007). *Comprehensive pediatric hospital medicine.* Philadelphia: Mosby.)

PATIENT DATA

Subjective Data

- Rash appears from one to several weeks after taking a drug
- Pruritus may be present
- Offending drug often difficult to find; do not forget about supplements or over-the-counter treatments

Objective Data

- Most common: discrete to confluent erythematous macules and papules on the trunk, face, extremities, palms, or soles of the feet (Fig. 9.56)
- Rash fades in 1–3 weeks and may desquamate

Acanthosis Nigricans

A nonspecific reaction pattern associated with obesity, certain endocrine syndromes, or malignancies or as an inherited disorder

PATHOPHYSIOLOGY

- Insulin resistance and hyperinsulinism may lead to an activation of insulin-like growth factor receptors, promoting epidermal growth
- Inherited form: rare, autosomal dominant trait with no obesity or associated endocrinopathies
- Malignant form: results from secretion of tumor products with insulin-like activity or transforming growth factor alpha, which stimulates keratinocytes to proliferate

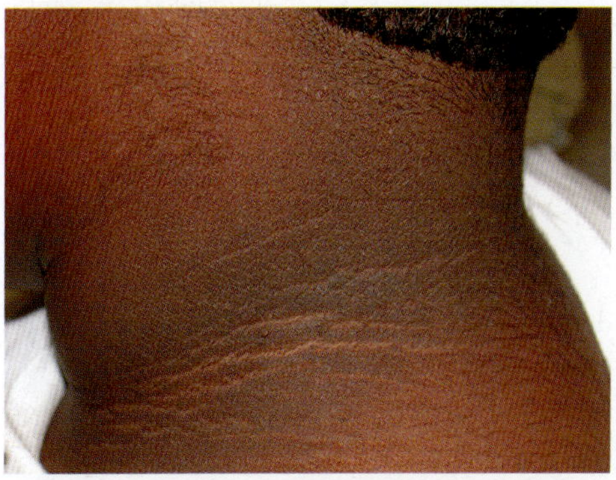

FIG. 9.57 **Acanthosis nigricans.** (From Scheinfeld, N. S. (2004). Obesity and dermatology. *Clinics in Dermatology*, 22(4):303–309.)

PATIENT DATA

Subjective Data

- May have history of obesity, endocrine disorders
- With a rise in childhood obesity, this is seen more often in children and adolescents
- Appearance in older adults associated with malignancy

Objective Data

- Symmetric, brown thickening of the skin with plaques or patches of thickened skin with a velvety or slightly verrucous texture (Fig. 9.57)
- Lesions range in severity from slight discoloration of a small area to extensive involvement of wide areas
- Most common site of involvement is the axillae, but the changes may be observed in other flexural areas of the neck, groin, and arms
- Involvement of the dorsal and palmar hands or mucosal surfaces may indicate malignant association

Skin: Malignant/Neoplastic Abnormalities

Basal Cell Carcinoma

The most common form of skin cancer

PATHOPHYSIOLOGY

- Arises from the basal layer of the epidermis
- Occurs in various clinical forms including nodular, pigmented, cystic, sclerosing, and superficial
- Occurs most frequently on exposed parts of the body—the face, ears, neck, scalp, and shoulders

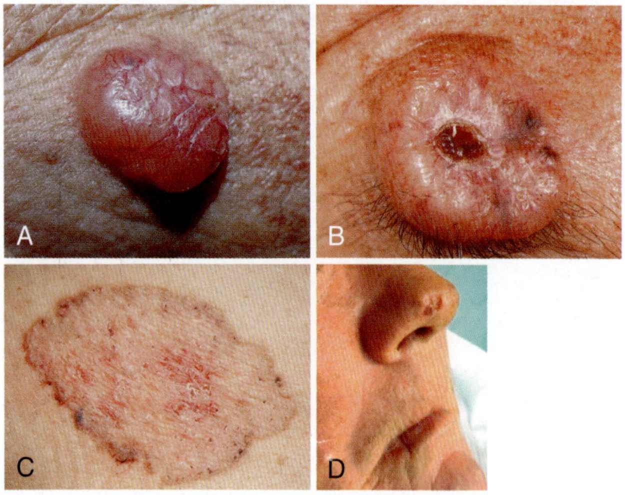

FIG. 9.58 Common presentations of basal cell carcinoma. (From Fitzsimons Army Medical Center, Scholes, M., & Ramakrishnan, V. (2016). *ENT secrets* (4th ed.). Elsevier.)

PATIENT DATA

Subjective Data

- Persistent sore or lesion that has not healed
- May have crusting
- May itch

Objective Data

- Shiny nodule that is pearly or translucent; may be pink, red, or white or tan, black, or brown (Fig. 9.58)
- Open sore; may have crusting; may bleed
- Reddish patch or irritated area, frequently occurring on the face, chest, shoulders, arms, or legs
- Pink growth with a slightly elevated, rolled border and a crusted indentation in the center; as the growth slowly enlarges, tiny blood vessels may develop on the surface
- Scarlike area that is white, yellow, or waxy and often has poorly defined borders; the skin appears shiny and taut

Squamous Cell Carcinoma

Second most common form of skin cancer

PATHOPHYSIOLOGY

- This malignant tumor arises in the epithelium and has squamous differentiation
- Lesions occur most commonly in sun-exposed areas, particularly the scalp, back of hands, lower lip, and ear; the rim of the ear and the lower lip are especially vulnerable

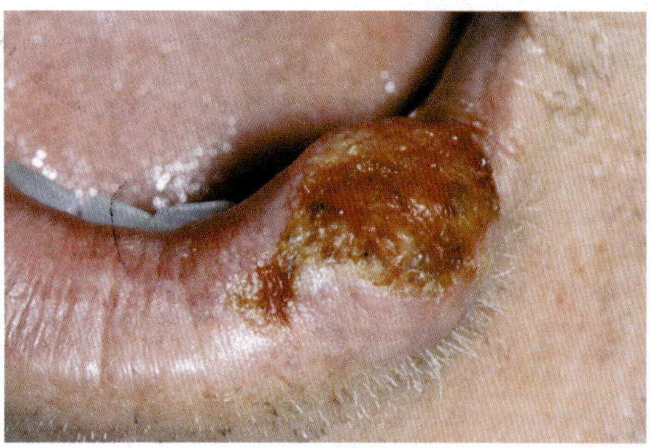

FIG. 9.59 Squamous cell carcinoma. (From Neville, B. W., Damm, D. D., Allen, C. M., et al. (2016). *Oral and maxillofacial pathology* (4th ed.). St. Louis: Elsevier.)

PATIENT DATA

Subjective Data

- Persistent sore or lesion that has not healed or that has grown in size
- May have crusting and/or bleeding

Objective Data

- Elevated growth with volcano-type pattern (Fig. 9.59)
- Wartlike growth; may have crusting, may bleed
- Scaly red patch with irregular borders; may have crusting and may bleed
- Open sore; may have crusting

Malignant Melanoma

Lethal form of skin cancer that develops from melanocytes

PATHOPHYSIOLOGY

- Melanocytes migrate into the skin, eye, central nervous system, and mucous membrane during fetal development
- Less than half of the melanomas develop from nevi; the majority arise de novo from melanocytes
- More likely to involve acral sites (hands, feet, and nail beds) in darker-skinned patients
- The exact cause of malignancy is not known; heredity, hormonal factors, UV light exposure, or an autoimmunologic effect may contribute to causation

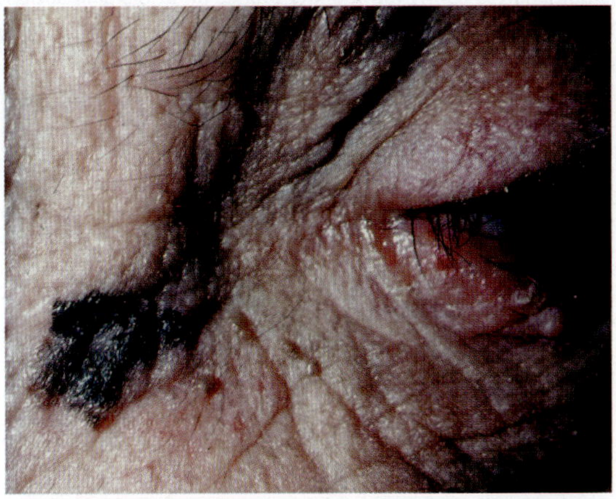

FIG. 9.60 Malignant melanoma. (From Goldman, L. *Golman-Cecil medicine* (26th ed.). Copyright © 2020 by Elsevier, Inc. All rights reserved.)

PATIENT DATA

Subjective Data

- New nevus or preexisting nevus that has changed or is changing
- New pigmented lesion that has irregularities (Fig. 9.60)
- History of melanoma
- History of atypical nevi
- Family history of melanoma (first-degree relative)
- Significant sunlight or tanning bed use

Objective Data

- ABCDE changes in nevi (Fig. 9.61)
- *A* Asymmetry of lesion: one-half of a nevus or birthmark does not match the other
- *B* Borders: edges are irregular, ragged, notched, or blurred; pigment may be streaming from the border
- *C* Color: the color is not the same all over and may have differing shades of brown or black, sometimes with patches of red, white, or blue
- *D* Diameter: the diameter is >6 mm (about the size of a pencil eraser) or is growing larger
- *E* Evolution: changes seen in existing pigmented lesions, particularly in a nonuniform, asymmetric manner

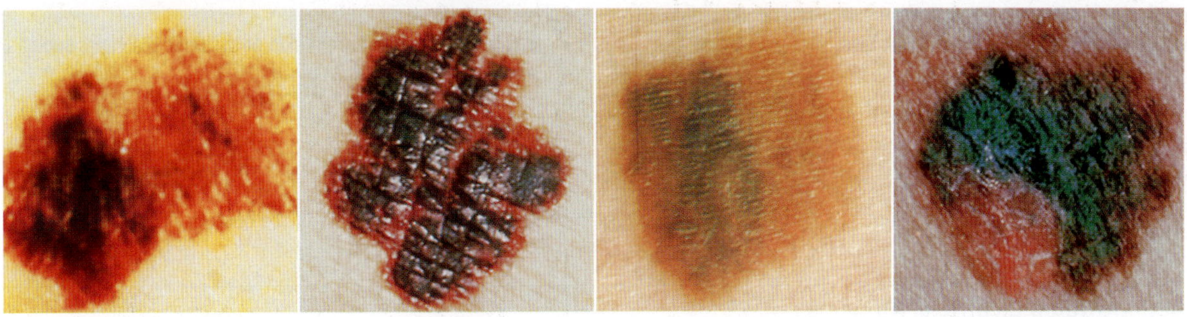

Asymmetry Border Color Diameter

FIG. 9.61 ABCD changes in nevi. (Reproduced with permission from the American Academy of Dermatology, 2010. All rights reserved.)

Hair Disorders

Alopecia Areata

Sudden, rapid, coin-shaped loss of hair, usually from the scalp or face

PATHOPHYSIOLOGY

- Cause unknown; autoimmune phenomenon from a genetic-environmental interaction may trigger the disease
- Any hair-bearing surface may be affected
- Regrowth begins in 1–3 months; the prognosis for total regrowth is excellent in cases with limited involvement

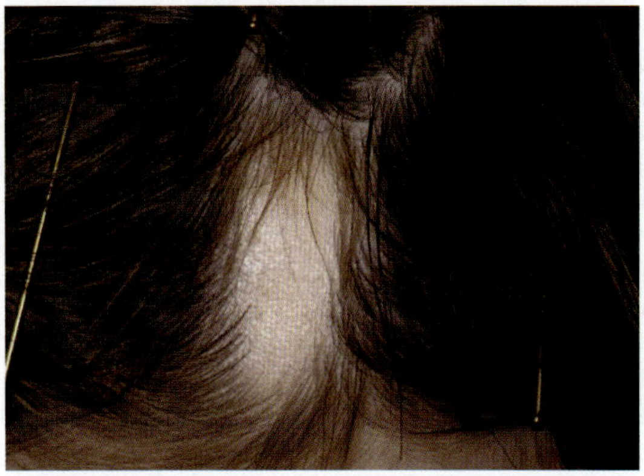

FIG. 9.62 Alopecia areata. (From Champagne, C., & Farrant, P. (2015). Hair loss in infancy and childhood. *Paediatrics and Child Health*, *25*(2):66–71.)

PATIENT DATA

Subjective Data

- Sudden, rapid, round patches of hair loss
- May also report nail pitting
- May have family history

Objective Data

- Hair loss is in sharply defined, round patches (Fig. 9.62)
- Nonscarring
- The hair shaft is poorly formed and breaks off at the skin surface
- Small vellus hair, often white before regaining its pigment, indicates hair regrowth

Scarring Alopecia

Replacement of hair follicles with scar tissue

PATHOPHYSIOLOGY

- Skin disorders of the scalp or follicles result in scarring and destruction of hair follicles and permanent hair loss

PATIENT DATA

Subjective Data

- May have other concurrent skin or systemic disorders such as systemic lupus erythematosus

Objective Data

- Patchy, irregular hair loss
- Scalp may be inflamed
- Hair follicles are lost and may be pustular or plugged

Central Centrifugal Cicatricial Alopecia

The most common cause of alopecia or hair loss in Black females

PATHOPHYSIOLOGY

- Presumed due to mutations in PADI3 gene, leading to defects in the hair shaft
- Scalp biopsy shows premature desquamation of the inner root sheath of the hair follicle with inflammation in the early phases and scarring in the late phase around the hair follicles

PATIENT DATA

Subjective Data

- Itching or tenderness may develop and is largely confined to the zone of hair loss

Objective Data

- Hair loss typically starts in the central crown and/or vertex of the scalp before spreading out centrifugally over time (Fig. 9.63)
- The area of alopecia is typically symmetrical with the most severe hair loss in the center and less peripherally

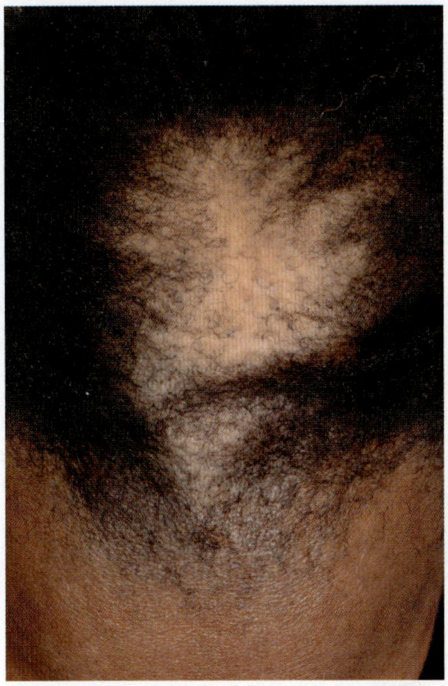

FIG. 9.63 **Permanent hair loss with centrifuge extension from the vertex.** (Gerami, P., & Busam, K. J. (2026). *Dermatopathology: A volume in the series foundations in diagnostic pathology* (3rd ed.). Elsevier Inc.)

Hirsutism

Growth of terminal hair in females in the male distribution pattern on the face, body, and pubic areas

PATHOPHYSIOLOGY

- Caused by high androgen levels (from ovaries or adrenal glands) or by hair follicles that are more sensitive to normal androgen levels; free testosterone is the androgen that causes hair growth
- Many causes, including genetic, physiologic, endocrine, drug related, and systemic disorders

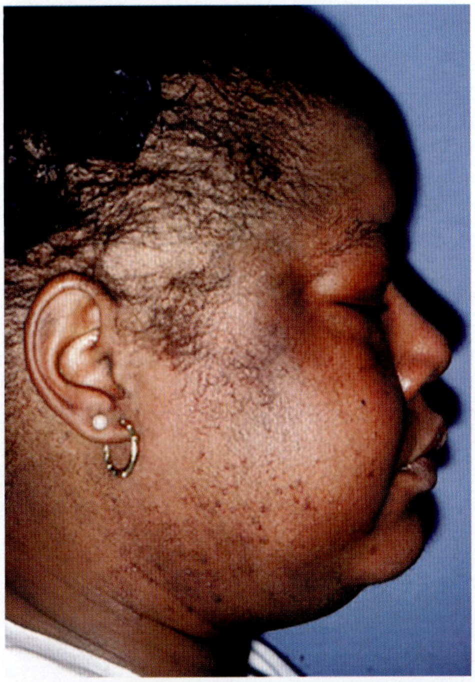

FIG. 9.64 **Facial hirsutism.** Patient with Cushing disease with a round face, thin hair, hirsutism, and acne. (From James, W., Elston, D., & Mcmahon, P. J. (2018). *Andrew's diseases of the skin clinical atlas.* Elsevier.)

PATIENT DATA

Subjective Data

- Excessive hair growth on the face or body
- Onset, severity, and rate depend on underlying cause

Objective Data

- Presence of thick, dark terminal hairs in androgen-sensitive sites: face, chest, areola, external genitalia, upper and lower back, buttocks, inner thigh, and linea alba (Fig. 9.64)
- Hirsutism may or may not be accompanied by other signs of virilization

Nails: Infection

Paronychia

Inflammation of the paronychium

PATHOPHYSIOLOGY

- Invasion of bacteria or yeast between the nail fold and the nail plate
- Can occur as an acute or chronic process

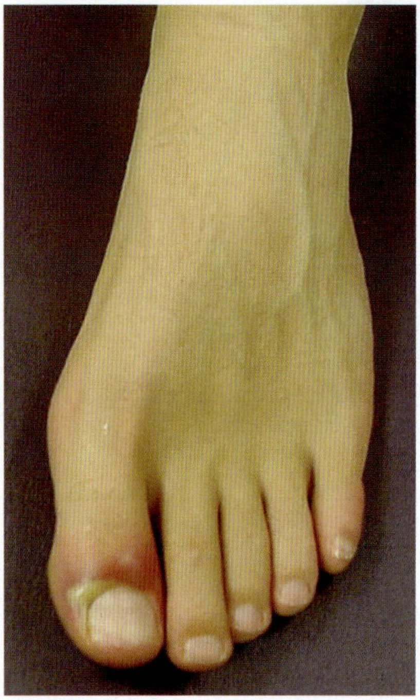

FIG. 9.65 **Paronychia.** (From Cuppett, M., & Walsh, K. (2012). *General medical conditions in the athlete* (2nd ed.). St Louis: Mosby.)

PATIENT DATA

Subjective Data

- Acute: usually bacterial with a history of nail trauma or manipulation
- Chronic: usually fungal with a history of repeated exposure to moisture (e.g., through hand washing); evolves slowly initially, with tenderness

Objective Data

- Redness and swelling at the lateral and proximal nail folds
- Purulent drainage often accumulates under the cuticle (Fig. 9.65)
- Chronic paronychia can produce rippling of the nails

Onychomycosis

Fungal infection of the nail.

PATHOPHYSIOLOGY

- The fungus grows in the nail plate, causing it to crumble

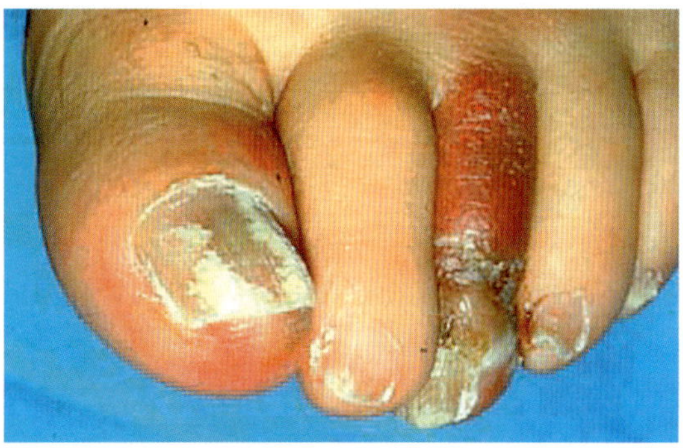

FIG. 9.66 **Onychomycosis.** (From Hay, R. J., & Baran, R. (2011). Onychomycosis: a proposed revision of the clinical classification. *Journal of the American Academy of Dermatology*, 65(6), 1219–1227.)

PATIENT DATA

Subjective Data

- Characteristic nail changes include discoloration, thickening, brittleness, and separation from the nail bed
- May report associated discomfort, paresthesia, loss of manual dexterity; may interfere with ability to exercise or walk

Objective Data

- In the most common form, the distal nail plate turns yellow or white as hyperkeratotic debris accumulates, causing the nail to separate from the nail bed (onycholysis)
- Pitting does not occur, distinguishing it from psoriasis (Fig. 9.66)
- Often associated with tinea pedis

Nails: Injury

Ingrown Nails

Nail pierces the lateral nail fold and grows into the dermis

PATHOPHYSIOLOGY

- Caused by lateral pressure of poorly fitting shoes, improper or excessive trimming of the lateral nail plate, or trauma

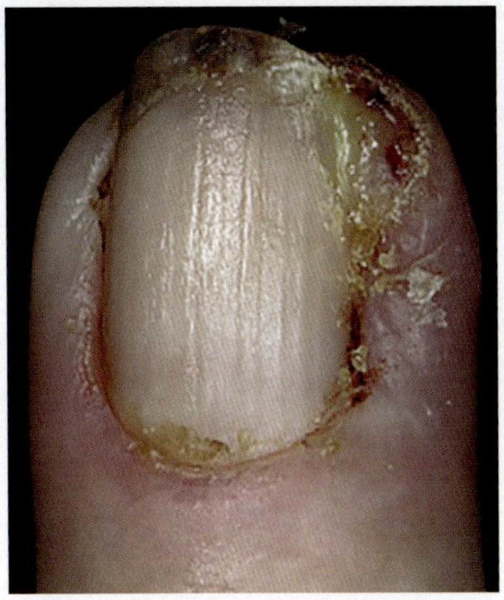

FIG. 9.67 **An ingrown nail has stimulated the formation of granulation tissue.** (From Dinulos, J. (2021). *Habif's clinical dermatology* (7th ed.). St. Louis: Elsevier.)

PATIENT DATA

Subjective Data

- Pain and swelling
- History related to cause: tight shoes, excessive trimming, trauma

Objective Data

- Redness and swelling at the area of nail penetration (Fig. 9.67)
- Commonly involves the large toe

Subungual Hematoma

Trauma to the nail plate severe enough to cause immediate bleeding and pain

PATHOPHYSIOLOGY

- Amount of bleeding may be sufficient to cause separation and loss of the nail plate
- Trauma to the proximal nail fold may also cause bleeding that is not apparent for several days
- Hematoma remains until the nail grows out or is decompressed to release the blood and relieve the pressure

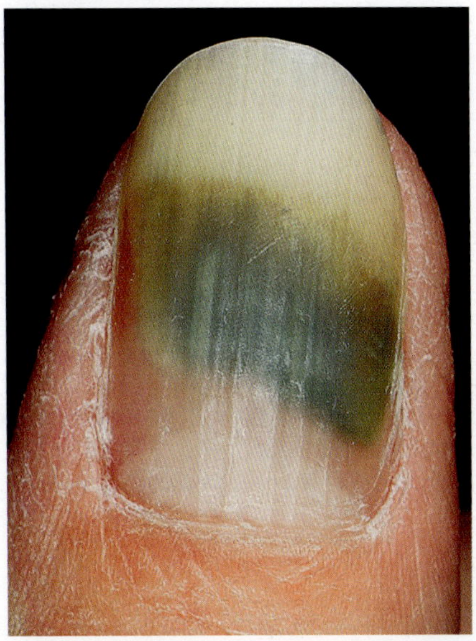

FIG. 9.68 **Subungual hematoma.** (From Baren, J. M., Rothrock, S. G., Brennan, J., et al. (2008). *Pediatric emergency medicine*. Philadelphia: Saunders.)

PATIENT DATA

Subjective Data

- Trauma to the nail
- May be very painful

Objective Data

- Discolored dark nail (Fig. 9.68)
- Color is typically red to purple as opposed to truly brown or black that might indicate a subungual melanoma

Onycholysis

Loosening of the nail plate with separation from the nail bed that begins at the distal groove

PATHOPHYSIOLOGY

- Associated most commonly with minor trauma to long fingernails
- Other causes include psoriasis, *Candida* or *Pseudomonas* infection, medications, allergic contact dermatitis, and hyperthyroidism

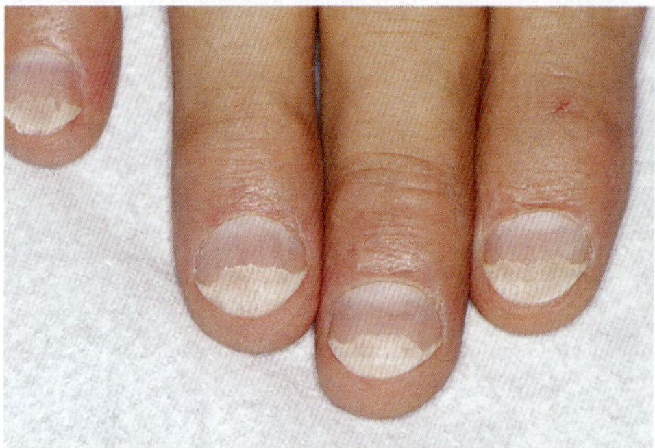

FIG. 9.69 Onycholysis. Separation of nail plate starts at the distal groove. (From Scher, R. K., & Daniel, C. R. (2005). *Nails: Diagnosis, therapy, surgery* (3rd ed.). Philadelphia: Saunders.)

PATIENT DATA

Subjective Data

- Painless separation of the plate from the bed
- May report history of nail trauma

Objective Data

- Nonadherent portion of the nail opaque with a white, yellow, or green tinge (Fig. 9.69)

Nails: Changes Associated With Systemic Disease

Koilonychia (Spoon Nails)

Central depression of the nail with lateral elevation of the nail plate

PATHOPHYSIOLOGY

- Associated with iron deficiency anemia, syphilis, fungal dermatoses, hemochromatosis, and hypothyroidism

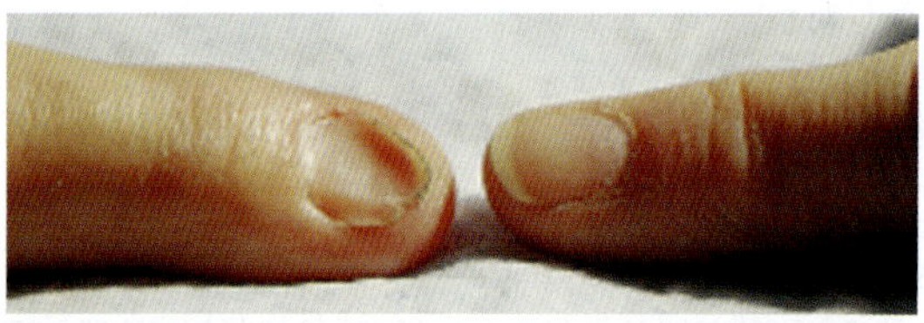

FIG. 9.70 A normal fingernail in comparison with koilonychia secondary to iron deficiency anemia. (From Swartz, M. H. (2021). *Textbook of physical diagnosis* (8th ed.). Philadelphia: Elsevier.)

PATIENT DATA

Subjective Data

- History consistent with associated disorders

Objective Data

- Concave curvature and spoon appearance (Fig. 9.70; see also Fig. 9.19)

Beau Lines

Transverse depression in the nail bed

PATHOPHYSIOLOGY

- Temporary interruption of nail formation due to systemic disorders
- Associated with coronary occlusion, hypercalcemia, and skin disease

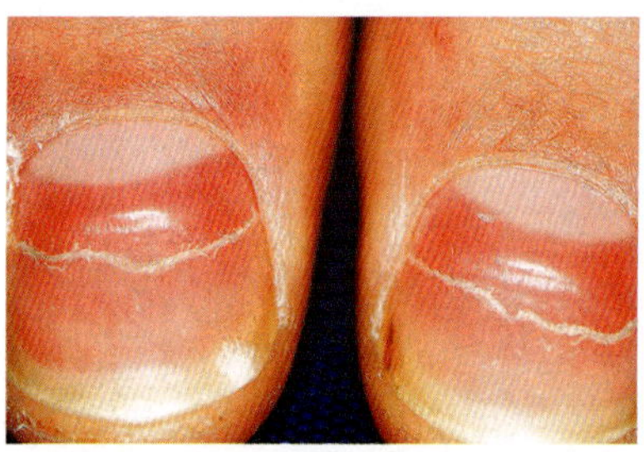

FIG. 9.71 Beau lines following systemic disease. (From Hansen, R. C., & Schachner, L. A. (2011). *Pediatric dermatology* (4th ed.). Elsevier Ltd.)

PATIENT DATA

Subjective Data

- History consistent with associated disorders

Objective Data

- Transverse depressions at the bases of the lunulae (crescent-shaped "moon") in all of the nails
- Grooves disappear when the nails grow out (Fig. 9.71)

Infants and Children

Seborrheic Dermatitis

Chronic, recurrent, erythematous scaling eruption localized in areas where sebaceous glands are concentrated (e.g., scalp, back, and intertriginous and diaper areas)

PATHOPHYSIOLOGY

- Cause is unknown, though it is thought likely related to the development of sebaceous glands; also thought to be due to overgrowth of commensal flora *(Malassezia)*
- Condition most commonly occurs in infants within the first 3 months of life

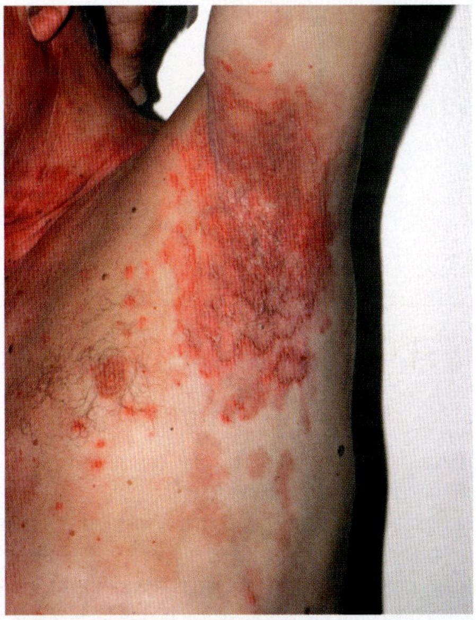

FIG. 9.76 Pustular seborrheic dermatitis. (From James, W., Elston, D., & Mcmahon, P. J. (2018). *Andrew's diseases of the skin clinical atlas.* Elsevier.)

PATIENT DATA

Subjective Data

- Parent reports thick, greasy scalp scales or body rash
- No associated symptoms

Objective Data

- Scalp lesions are scaling, adherent, thick, yellow, and crusted ("cradle cap") and can spread over the ear and down the nape of the neck (Fig. 9.76)
- Lesions elsewhere are erythematous, scaling, and fissured, typically on central body or in diaper area

Miliaria Rubra ("Prickly Heat")

PATHOPHYSIOLOGY

- Caused by sweat retention from occlusion of sweat ducts during periods of heat and high humidity
- Results from immaturity of skin structures
- Overdressed babies are susceptible to this condition in the summer

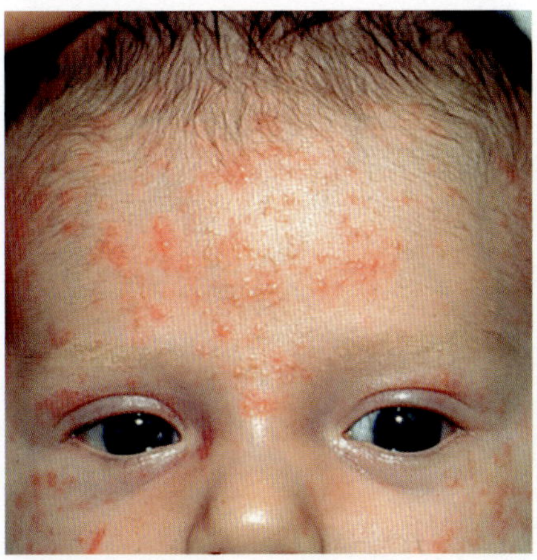

FIG. 9.77 Miliaria in an infant. (From Fitzpatrick, J., & High, W. (2018). *Urgent care dermatology.* Philadelphia: Elsevier.)

PATIENT DATA

Subjective Data

- Parent reports rash noted when undressing the infant

Objective Data

- Irregular, red, macular rash, usually on covered areas of the skin (Fig. 9.77)

Impetigo

Common, contagious superficial skin infection

PATHOPHYSIOLOGY

- Caused mostly by staphylococcal or streptococcal infection of the epidermis

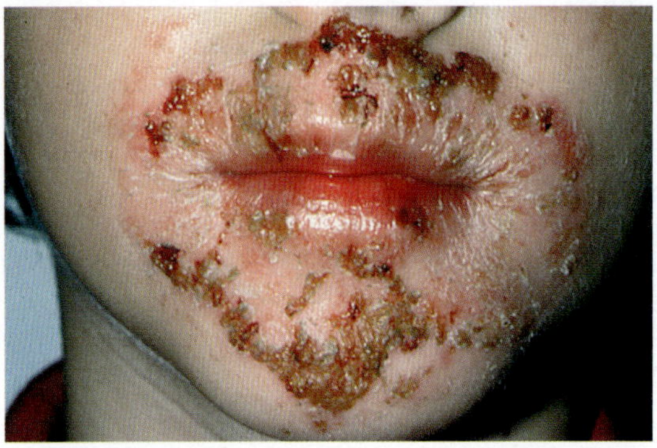

FIG. 9.78 Impetigo. Note characteristic crusting. (From Neville, B. W., Damm, D. D., Allen, C. M., et al. (2016). *Oral and maxillofacial pathology* (4th ed.). St Louis: Elsevier.)

PATIENT DATA

Subjective Data

- Lesion, typically on the face, that itches and burns
- Also on other parts of the body associated with minor injuries or insect bites

Objective Data

- Initial lesion is a small erythematous macule that changes into a vesicle or bulla with a thin roof
- Lesion crusts, with a characteristic honey color from the exudate as the vesicles or bullae rupture (Fig. 9.78)
- May have regional lymphadenopathy

Acne Vulgaris

Common condition due to plugging of hair follicles

PATHOPHYSIOLOGY

- Androgens stimulate the pilosebaceous units at the time of puberty to enlarge and produce large amounts of sebum
- Simultaneously, the keratinization process in the pilosebaceous canal is disrupted, with impaction and obstruction of the outflow of sebum resulting in comedo formation—open blackheads and closed whiteheads
- Wall of the closed comedo may rupture, spilling the follicular contents into the dermis, leading to the development of inflammatory papules
- Presence of *Cutibacterium acnes* brings in neutrophils, which cause the inflammatory response

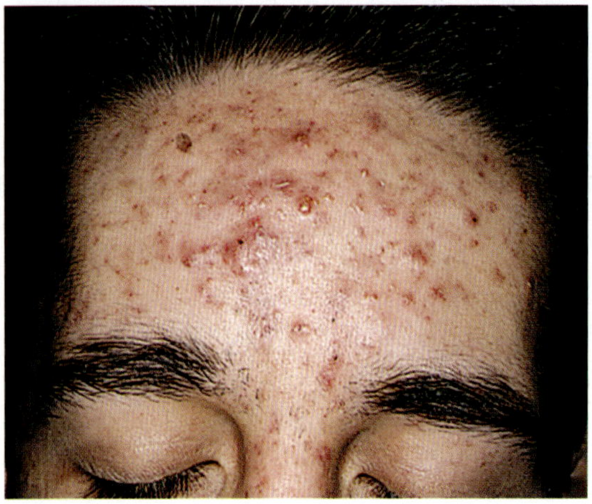

FIG. 9.79 Acne in an adolescent. (From Swartz, M. H. (2014). *Textbook of physical diagnosis* (7th ed.). Philadelphia: Saunders.)

PATIENT DATA

Subjective Data

- Most commonly reported by adolescents
- May occur initially as an adult or continue into the adult years
- Patient reports comedones (plugged follicles—blackheads and whiteheads), papules, and pustules over the forehead, nose, cheeks, lower face, chest, and back that evolve on the face, chest, and back

Objective Data

- Noninflammatory acne: open (whiteheads) and closed (blackheads) comedones
- Inflammatory acne: papules, nodules, or cystic lesions (Fig. 9.79)
- Characteristic "ice pick" scarring may be present from previous lesions

Chickenpox (Varicella)

Acute, highly communicable disease common in children and young adults

PATHOPHYSIOLOGY

- Caused by the varicella-zoster virus (VZV)
- VZV is communicable by direct contact, droplet transmission, and airborne transmission
- Incubation period is 2–3 weeks; the period of communicability lasts from 1 to 2 days before onset of the rash until lesions have crusted over
- Routine childhood immunization has resulted in a significant decline in incidence
- After primary infection, VZV remains dormant in sensory nerve roots for life
- Can reactivate to cause shingles

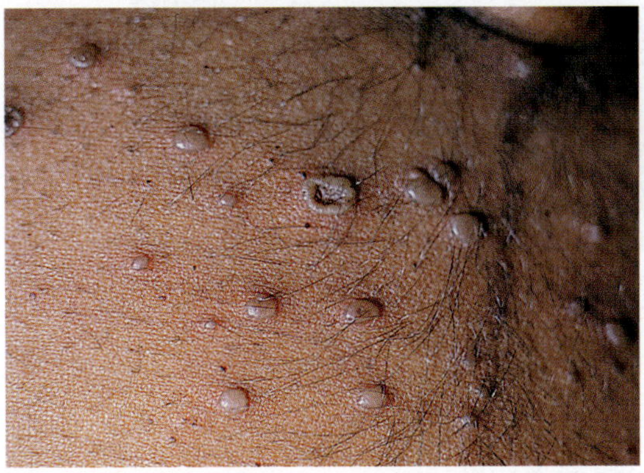

FIG. 9.80 **Varicella (chickenpox).** Note vesicular lesions. (From Swartz, M. H. (2014). *Textbook of physical diagnosis* (7th ed.). Philadelphia: Saunders.)

PATIENT DATA

Subjective Data

- Fever, headache, sore throat, mild malaise
- Pruritic rash that started on scalp and then moved to extremities
- Started as papular and in a few hours became vesicular
- Child has not had varicella vaccine

Objective Data

- Papular and vesicular lesions on trunk, extremities, face, buccal mucosa, palate, or conjunctivae (Fig. 9.80)
- Lesions usually occur in successive clusters, eventually spreading to entire body, with several stages of maturity present at one time
- Complications include conjunctival involvement, secondary bacterial infection, viral pneumonia, encephalitis, aseptic meningitis, myelitis, Guillain-Barré syndrome, and Reye syndrome

Measles (Rubeola)

Also called hard measles or red measles

PATHOPHYSIOLOGY

- Measles virus infects by invasion of the respiratory epithelium
- Local multiplication at the respiratory mucosa leads to a primary viremia, during which the virus spreads in leukocytes to the reticuloendothelial system
- Both endothelial and epithelial cells are infected; infected tissues include thymus, spleen, lymph nodes, liver, skin, conjunctiva, and lung
- Incubation period is commonly 18 days; the period of communicability lasts from a few days before the fever to 4 days after appearance of the rash
- Disease is preventable by immunization

PATIENT DATA

Subjective Data

- Fever, conjunctivitis, stuffy nose, and cough, followed by a red, blotchy rash first on the face and then spreading to trunk and extremities
- Child has not had measles vaccine
- International travel or exposure to individuals from endemic areas

Objective Data

- Koplik spots (discrete white macular lesions) on the buccal mucosa
- Macular rash on the face and neck
- Maculopapular lesions on trunk and extremities in irregular confluent patches
- Rash lasts 4–7 days (Fig. 9.81)
- Symptoms may be mild or severe
- Complications involve infection of the respiratory tract and central nervous system

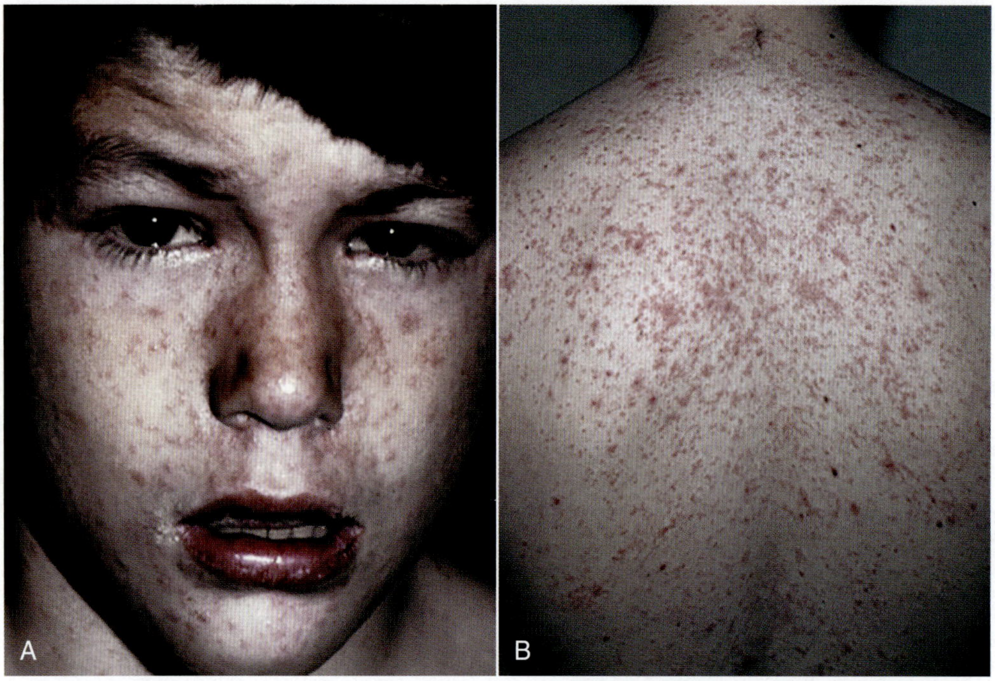

FIG. 9.81 Rubeola. (A) A maculopapular rash appears on the face and becomes confluent. (B) The rash then appears on the trunk. (From Dinulos, J. (2021). *Habif's clinical dermatology* (7th ed.). St. Louis: Elsevier.)

German Measles (Rubella)

Mild, febrile, highly communicable viral disease

PATHOPHYSIOLOGY

- Spread in droplets that are shed from respiratory secretions of infected persons
- Patients are most contagious while the rash is erupting, but they may shed virus from the throat from 10 days before until 15 days after the onset of the rash
- Incubation period is 14–23 days
- Disease is preventable by immunization

PATIENT DATA

Subjective Data

- Low-grade fever, stuffy nose, sore throat, and cough
- This is followed by a macular rash on the face and trunk that rapidly becomes papular

Objective Data

- Generalized light pink to red morbilliform rash
- By the second day, rash spreads to the upper and lower extremities; it fades within 3 days
- Reddish spots occur on the soft palate during the prodrome or on the first day of the rash (Forchheimer spots; Fig. 9.82)
- Infection during the first trimester of pregnancy may lead to infection of the fetus and may produce a variety of congenital anomalies (congenital rubella syndrome)

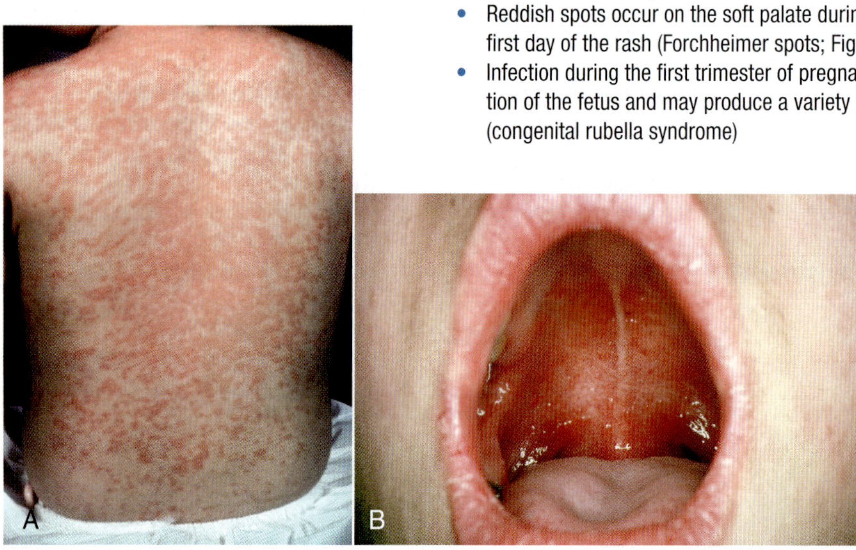

FIG. 9.82 Rubella (German measles). (A) Note the pinkish red, maculopapular eruption. (B) Red palatal lesions (Forchheimer spots) are seen in some patients on day 1 of the rash. (From James, W., Elston, D., & Mcmahon, P. J. (2018). *Andrew's diseases of the skin clinical atlas.* Elsevier.)

Hair-Pulling (Trichotillomania)

Loss of scalp hair can be caused by physical manipulation

PATHOPHYSIOLOGY

- Hair is twisted around the finger and pulled or rubbed until it breaks off; the act of manipulation is usually an unconscious habit

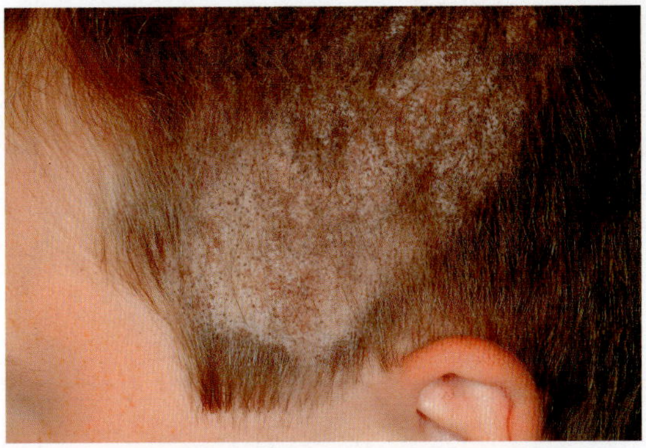

FIG. 9.83 Trichotillomania. (From Paller, A. S., & Mancini, A. J. (2016). *Hurwitz clinical pediatric dermatology: A textbook of skin disorders of childhood and adolescence* (5th ed.). Edinburgh: Elsevier.)

PATIENT DATA

Subjective Data

- May report tension, anxiety, emotional stressors

Objective Data

- The affected area has an irregular border, and hair density is greatly reduced, but the site is not bald (Fig. 9.83)

Patterns of Injury in Physical Abuse

Physical findings in children who have been physically abused include bruises, burns, lacerations, scars, bony deformities, alopecia, retinal hemorrhages, dental trauma, and head and abdominal injuries. Skin and hair abnormalities may be the most visible clues in detecting this problem. It is important to examine the skin that is usually covered by clothing. Some skin and hair findings commonly associated with physical abuse are described in the following paragraphs.

- *Bruises:* These may be patterned consistent with the implement used, such as belt marks (Fig. 9.84), marks from a looped electrical cord, and oval or fingertip grab marks. Bruising associated with abuse occurs over soft tissue; toddlers and older children who bruise themselves accidentally do so over bony prominences. Any bruise in an infant who is not yet developmentally able to be mobile should be cause for concern.
- *Lacerations:* Lacerations of the frenulum and lips are associated with forced feeding. Human bites can cause breaks in the skin and leave a characteristic bite mark.
- *Burns:* Patterns that are common include scald burns in stocking and glove distribution (when hands or feet are placed on a hot surface or immersed); buttock burns consistent with immersion (Fig. 9.85); and cigarette burns (Fig. 9.86), a characteristic small, round burn, often on areas hidden by clothing. The absence of splash marks or a pattern consistent with spills of hot liquids may be helpful in differentiating accidental from deliberate burns.
- *Hair loss:* Patchy hair loss or bald spots, in the absence of a scalp disorder such as ringworm, may indicate repeated hair-pulling.
- Presence of anogenital warts in a child under 2 years should also raise suspicion of physical and/or sexual abuse, although these can be autoinoculated.

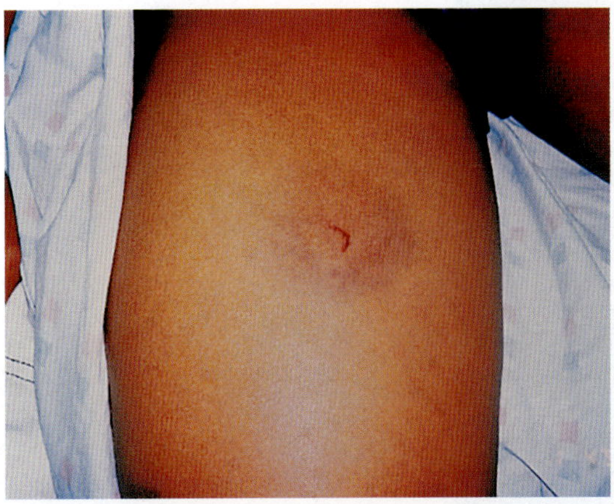

FIG. 9.84 This contusion in the configuration of a closed horseshoe with a central linear abrasion was inflicted with a belt buckle. (From Zitelli, B. J., McIntire, S. C., & Nowalk, A. J. (2012). *Zitelli and Davis' atlas of pediatric physical diagnosis* (6th ed.). Philadelphia: Saunders.)

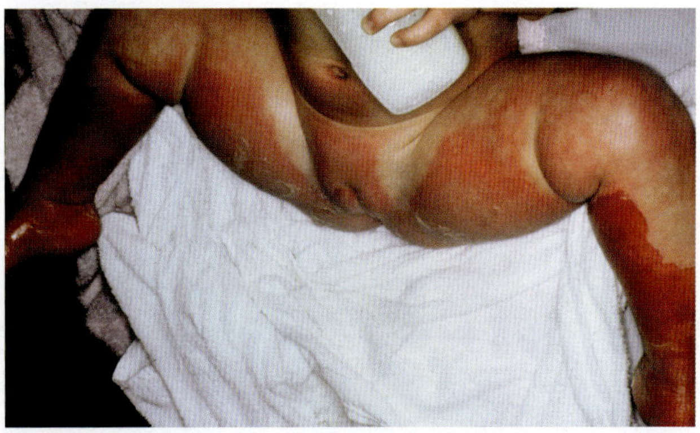

FIG. 9.85 Burns on the perineum, thighs, legs, and feet. (Courtesy Dr. Thomas Layton, Mercy Hospital, Pittsburgh; from Zitelli, B. J., McIntire, S. C., & Nowalk, A. J. (2012). *Zitelli and Davis' atlas of pediatric physical diagnosis* (6th ed.). Philadelphia: Saunders.)

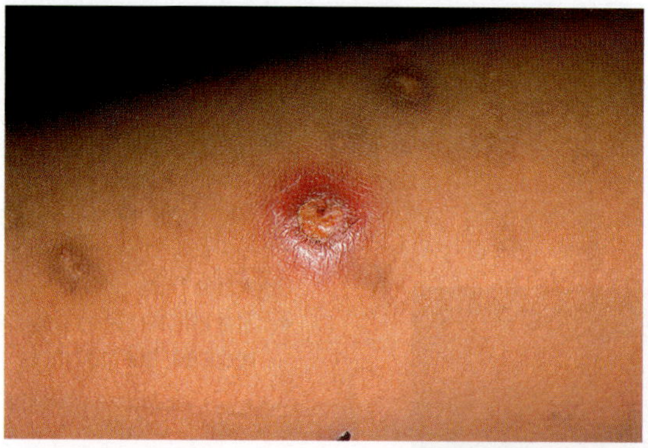

FIG. 9.86 Cigarette burns. These burns demonstrate various stages of healing. (From Paller, A. S., & Mancini, A. J. (2016). *Hurwitz clinical pediatric dermatology: A textbook of skin disorders of childhood and adolescence* (5th ed.). Edinburgh: Elsevier.)

Older Adults

Stasis Dermatitis

Skin inflammation resulting from chronic edema

PATHOPHYSIOLOGY

- Occurs on the lower legs in some patients with venous insufficiency
- Incompetent venous valves, inadequate tissue support, and postural hydrostatic pressure contribute to the development of venous stasis
- Dermatologic changes secondary to the effects of extravasated blood, which induces a mild inflammatory response in the dermis and subcutaneous fat
- May occur as an allergic response to an epidermal protein antigen created through increased hydrostatic pressure or because the skin has been compromised and is more susceptible to irritation and trauma

PATIENT DATA

Subjective Data

- Sense of fullness or dull aching in the lower legs and ankles
- Gradual increase in pigmentation and redness
- Area may be itchy and/or painful

Objective Data

- Erythematous, scaling, weeping patches on lower extremity; ulceration may be present (Fig. 9.87)
- Dermatitis may be acute, subacute, or chronic and recurrent

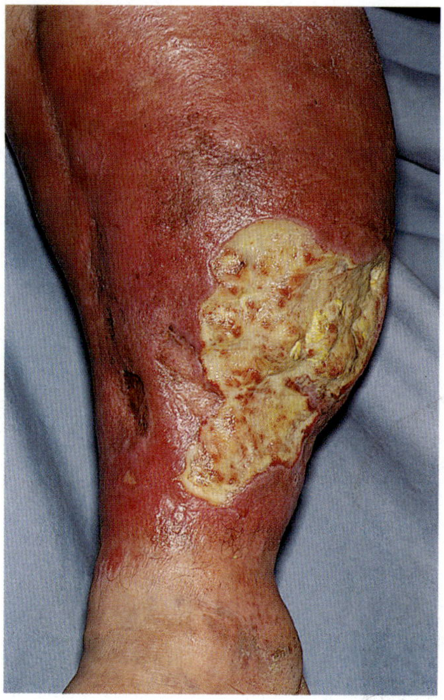

FIG. 9.87 Severe stasis dermatitis in an older adult. (From Swartz, M. H. (2014). *Textbook of physical diagnosis* (7th ed.). Philadelphia: Saunders.)

Actinic Keratosis

Atypical squamous cells confined to the upper layers of epidermis

PATHOPHYSIOLOGY

- Occurs secondary to chronic sun damage
- Most lesions remain superficial; lesions can progress into squamous cell carcinoma over time

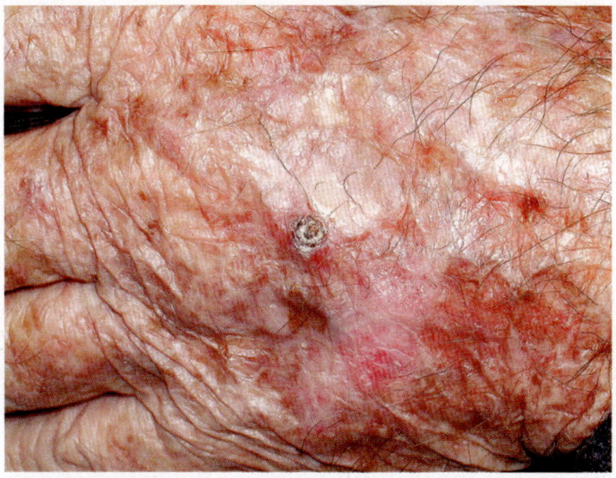

FIG. 9.88 **Actinic keratosis in an older adult in an area of sun exposure.** (From Busam, K. J. (2016). *Dermatopathology: A volume in the series: Foundations in diagnostic pathology* (2nd ed.). Philadelphia: Saunders.)

PATIENT DATA

Subjective Data

- History of chronic sun exposure
- Increasing number of lesions with age

Objective Data

- Raised, gritty, erythematous lesion that usually has an irregular, rough surface
- Lesion is most common on the dorsal surface of the hands, arms, neck, and face (Fig. 9.88)

Physical Abuse in Older Adults

Abuse in older adults can assume the form of physical abuse, neglect, sexual abuse, psychological abuse, financial abuse, or violation of rights. Physical neglect is probably the most common type of abuse encountered by health care professionals. However, be aware that when one form of abuse is present, it is typically accompanied by other forms.

Physical abuse and neglect may present clues that aid in detection. Assessment of general appearance may indicate poor hygiene, emaciation, healed fractures with deformity, and unexplained trauma. Carefully inspect the skin, particularly on hidden areas such as the axillae, inner thighs, soles of the feet, palms, and abdomen; look for bruising, burns, abrasions, or areas of tenderness. Bruising on extensor surfaces is common and usually occurs accidentally; bruising at various stages of resolution located on inner soft surfaces is more likely to indicate abuse.

Careful history taking is essential. When abuse is suspected, it is important to ask direct questions, such as "Is anyone hurting or harming you?" or "Have you been confined against your will?" This questioning should occur in a private setting away from accompanying family members or caregivers. Determination of mental status is also essential (see Chapter 5), because unintended self-neglect or abuse is also possible. If the patient is cognitively impaired, abuse by another may still be present but needs to be corroborated.

CHAPTER

10 Lymphatic System

The lymphatic system is examined region by region during the examination of other body systems (i.e., head and neck, breast and axillary, genitalia, and extremities) and by palpating the spleen. Sometimes you may perform a comprehensive lymphatic examination, exploring all the areas in which the lymph nodes are accessible. Individual chapters in this book discuss the lymphatic system in specific body areas.

Physical Examination Components

1. Inspect the visible nodes and surrounding area for:
   - Edema
   - Erythema
   - Red streaks
2. Palpate the superficial lymph nodes and compare side to side for:
   - Size
   - Consistency
   - Mobility
   - Discrete borders or matting
   - Tenderness
   - Warmth

   If you discover an enlarged node, consider the associated region drained by the node to suggest possible sources for a presenting problem or clinical concern.

ANATOMY AND PHYSIOLOGY

The lymphatic system consists of lymph fluid; the collecting lymphatic ducts; and various tissues, including the lymph nodes, spleen, thymus, tonsils, adenoids, and Peyer patches in the small intestine. Bits of lymph tissue are found in other parts of the body, including the mucosa of the stomach and appendix, bone marrow, and lungs (Fig. 10.1). Functions of the lymphatic system include conserving fluid and plasma that leak from capillaries, defending the body against disease as part of the immune system, and absorbing lipids from the intestinal tract.

The immune system protects the body from the antigenic substances of invading organisms, removes damaged cells from the circulation, and provides a partial barrier to the maturation of malignant cells within the body. When it functions well, the individual has a competent immune system with an intact immune response to antigen exposure. Tissue rejection of transplanted organs is an unwelcome manifestation of immunocompetence. When the immune system fails, the individual may experience a variety of conditions or illnesses, such as an allergic reaction or an immunodeficiency (either congenital or acquired; e.g., infection with human immunodeficiency virus [HIV]), or an autoimmune disease—that is, a pathogenic response to oneself, frequently with the creation of autoantibodies (e.g., systemic lupus erythematosus). An integral part of the immune system, the lymphatic system supports a network of defenses against microorganisms.

Except for the placenta and the brain, every tissue supplied by blood vessels has lymphatic vessels. This wide-ranging presence is essential to the system's role in immunologic and metabolic processes. That role involves the following:

- Movement of lymph fluid within the cardiovascular system, a major factor in the maintenance of fluid balance. Without lymphatic drainage, fluid would build up in interstitial spaces because more fluid leaves capillaries than veins can absorb.
- Filtration of fluid before it is returned to the bloodstream, filtering out substances that could be harmful to the body and filtering microorganisms from the blood.
- Phagocytosis—the ingestion and digestion by cells of solid substances such as other cells, bacteria, and bits of dead tissue or foreign particles—which is a specific function of cells in lymph nodes.
- Production of lymphocytes within the lymph nodes, tonsils, adenoids, spleen, and bone marrow.
- Production of antibodies.
- Absorption of fat and fat-soluble substances from the intestinal tract.

In addition, the lymphatic system plays an undesirable role in providing at least one pathway for the spread of malignancy.

Lymph is a clear, sometimes milky-colored, or yellow-tinged fluid. It contains a variety of white blood cells (mostly lymphocytes) and, occasionally, red blood cells. The lymphatic and cardiovascular systems are intimately related. The fluids and proteins that constitute lymph move from the bloodstream into the interstitial spaces. They are then collected throughout the body by a profusion of microscopic tubules (Fig. 10.2). These tubules

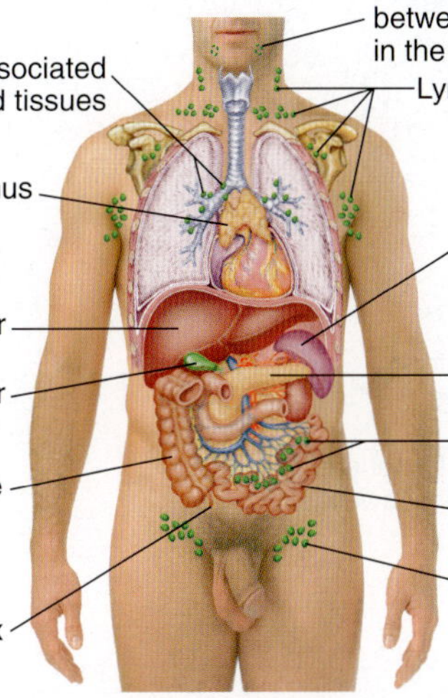

FIG. 10.1 Lymphatic system (lymphoreticular system). Lymphatic system of the human shows labels as follows: tonsils, bilaterally, between palatine arches in the pharynx; lymph nodes; spleen, pancreas, intestinal-associated lymphoid tissues, small intestine, lymph nodes, appendix, large intestine, gallbladder, liver, thymus, and bronchial-associated lymphoid tissues.

unite, forming larger ducts that collect lymph and carry it to the lymph nodes around the body.

The lymph nodes receive lymph from the collecting ducts in the various regions (Figs. 10.3 to 10.11), passing it on through efferent vessels. Ultimately, the large ducts merge into the venous system at the subclavian veins.

The drainage point for the right upper body is a lymphatic trunk that empties into the right subclavian vein. The thoracic duct, the major vessel of the lymphatic system, drains lymph from the rest of the body into the left subclavian vein. It returns the various fluids and proteins to the cardiovascular system, forming a closed but porous circle.

The lymphatic system has no built-in pumping mechanisms of its own. Lymph fluid is propelled by muscle movement and peristaltic contraction of the lymph-collecting vessels. Because of this, the movement of lymph is sluggish compared with that of blood. As lymph fluid volume increases, it flows faster in response to mounting capillary pressure, greater permeability of the capillary walls of the cardiovascular system, increased bodily or metabolic activity, and mechanical compression. Conversely, mechanical

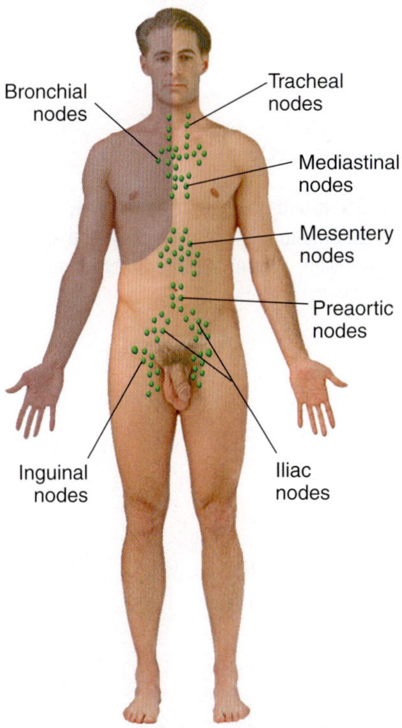

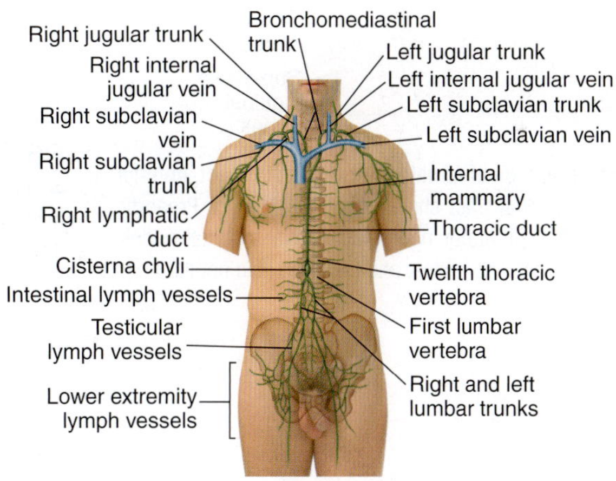

FIG. 10.2 Lymphatic drainage pathways. Shaded area of the body is drained via the right lymphatic duct, which is formed by the union of three vessels: right jugular trunk, right subclavian trunk, and right bronchomediastinal trunk. Lymph from the remainder of the body enters the venous system by way of the thoracic duct.Anterior view of human shows labels as follows: Tracheal nodes, mediastinal nodes, mesentery nodes, preaortic nodes, iliac nodes, inguinal nodes, and bronchial nodes. Right side of chest, shoulder, arm, and right side of face is shaded. Anterior view of human body from neck to pelvic region shows labels as follows: Left jugular trunk, left internal jugular vein, left subclavian trunk, left subclavian vein, internal mammary, thoracic duct, twelfth thoracic vertebra, first lumbar vertebra, right and left lumbar trunks, lower extremity lymph vessels, testicular lymph vessels, intestinal lymph vessels, cisterna chyli, right lymphatic duct, right subclavian trunk, right subclavian vein, right internal jugular vein, and right jugular trunk.

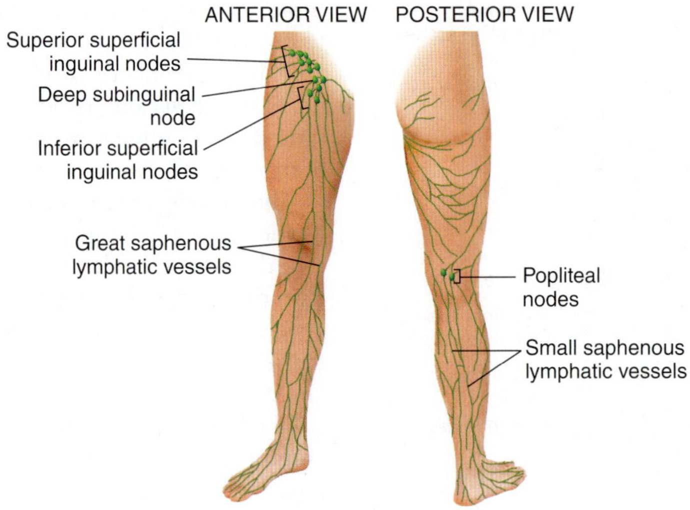

FIG. 10.3 Lymphatic drainage of lower extremity. Anterior view of leg shows labels for superior superficial inguinal nodes, deep subinguinal node, inferior superficial inguinal nodes, and great saphenous lymphatic vessels. Posterior view of leg shows labels for popliteal nodes and small saphenous lymphatic vessels.

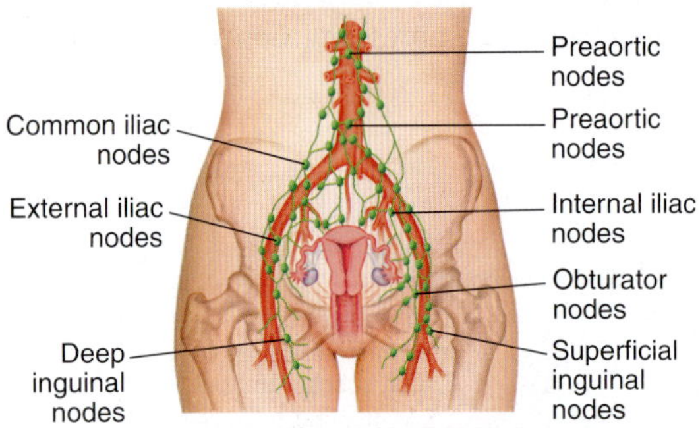

FIG. 10.4 Lymphatic drainage of female internal genital tract. Anterior view of female internal genital tract shows labels as follows: Preaortic nodes, internal iliac nodes, obturator nodes, superficial inguinal nodes, deep inguinal nodes, external iliac nodes, and common iliac nodes.

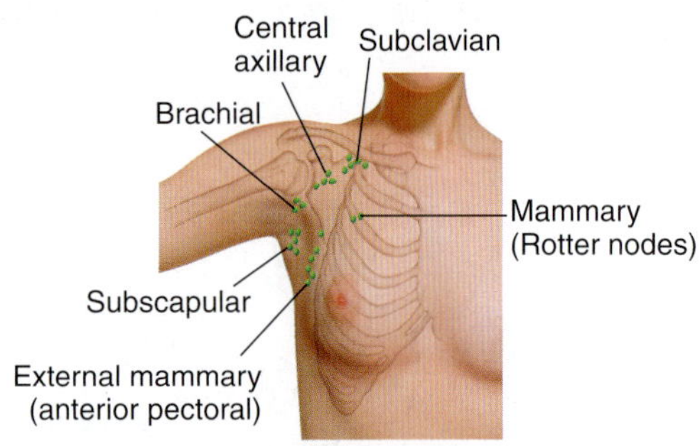

FIG. 10.6 Six groups of lymph nodes may be distinguished in the axillary fossa. Anterior view of right chest and shoulder shows labels as follows: Subclavian, central axillary, brachial, subscapular, and external mammary (anterior pectoral).

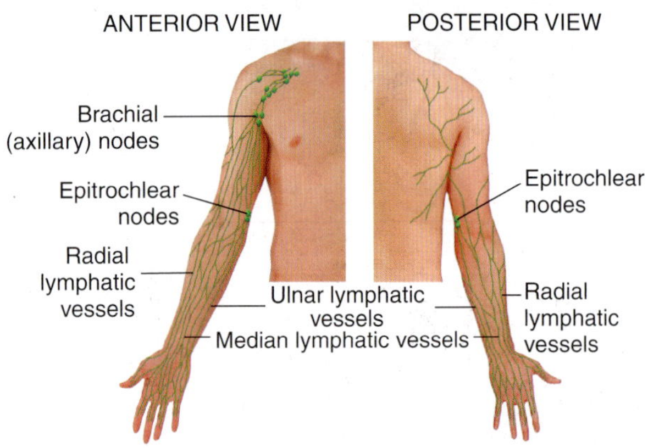

FIG. 10.5 Systems of deep and superficial collecting ducts, carrying lymph from upper extremity to subclavian lymphatic trunk. The only peripheral lymph center is the epitrochlear, which receives some of the collecting ducts from the pathway of the ulnar and radial nerves. Anterior view of arm shows labels for brachial (axillary) nodes, epitrochlear nodes, radial lymphatic vessels, ulnar lymphatic vessels, and median lymphatic vessels. Posterior view of arm shows labels for epitrochlear nodes, radial lymphatic vessels, median lymphatic vessels, and ulnar lymphatic vessels.

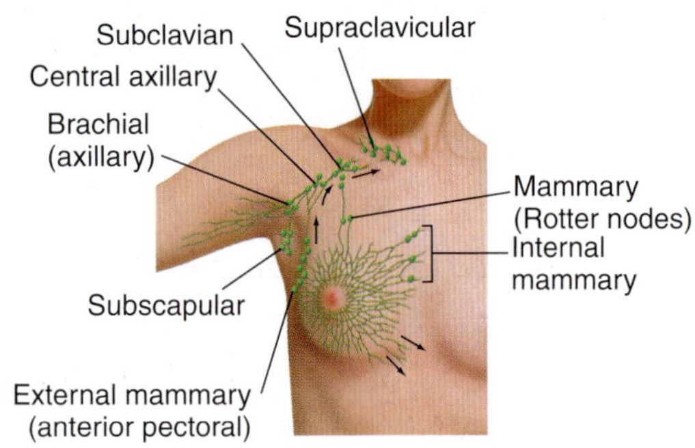

FIG. 10.7 Lymphatic drainage of the breast. Close-up view of the breast shows labels as follows: Mammary (Rotter nodes), internal mammary, external mammary (anterior pectoral), subscapular, brachial (axillary), central axillary, subclavian, and supraclavicular.

obstruction will slow or stop the movement of lymph, dilating the system. The permeability of the lymphatic system is protective; if it is obstructed, lymph may diffuse into the vascular system, or collateral connecting channels may develop.

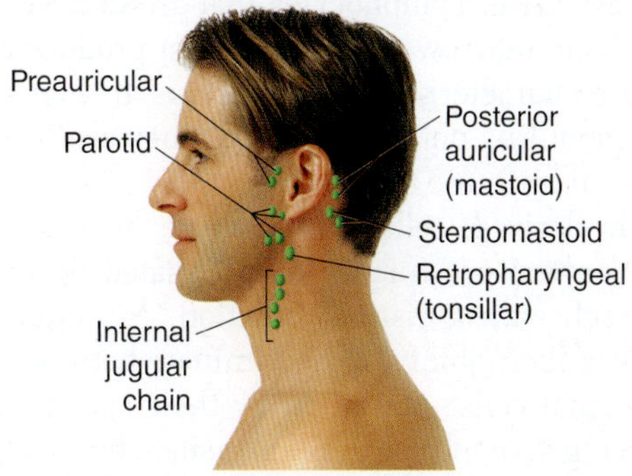

FIG. 10.8 **Lymph nodes involved with the ear.** Side view of head shows labels as follows: Posterior auricular (mastoid), sternomastoid, retropharyngeal (tonsillar), internal jugular chain, parotid, and preauricular.

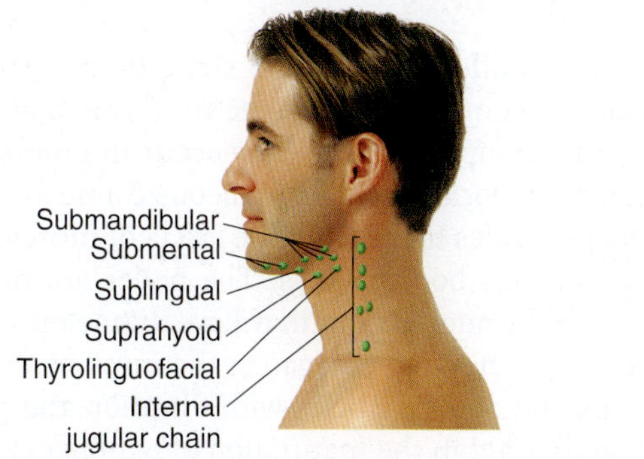

FIG. 10.9 **Lymph nodes involved with the tongue.** Side view of neck shows labels as follows: Submandibular, submental, sublingual, suprahyoid, thyrolinguofacial, and internal jugular chain.

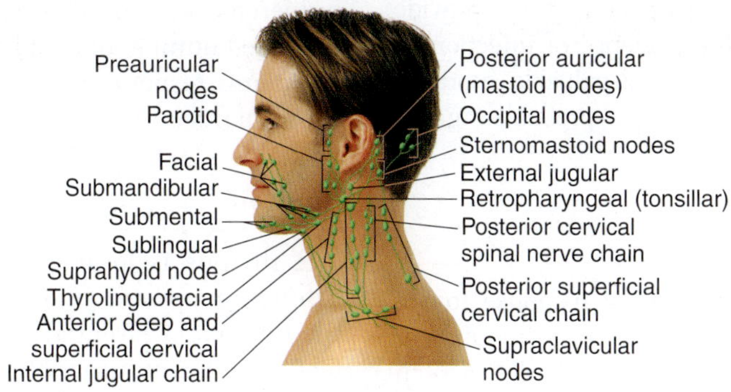

FIG. 10.10 **Lymphatic drainage system of head and neck.** If the group of nodes is commonly referred to by another name, the second name appears in parentheses. Side view of neck and head shows labels as follows: Posterior auricular (mastoid nodes), occipital nodes, sternomastoid nodes, external jugular, retropharyngeal (tonsillar), posterior cervical spinal nerve chain, posterior superficial cervical chain, supraclavicular nodes, internal jugular chain, anterior deep and superficial cervical, thyrolinguofacial, suprahyoid node, sublingual, submental, submandibular, facial, parotid, and preauricular nodes.

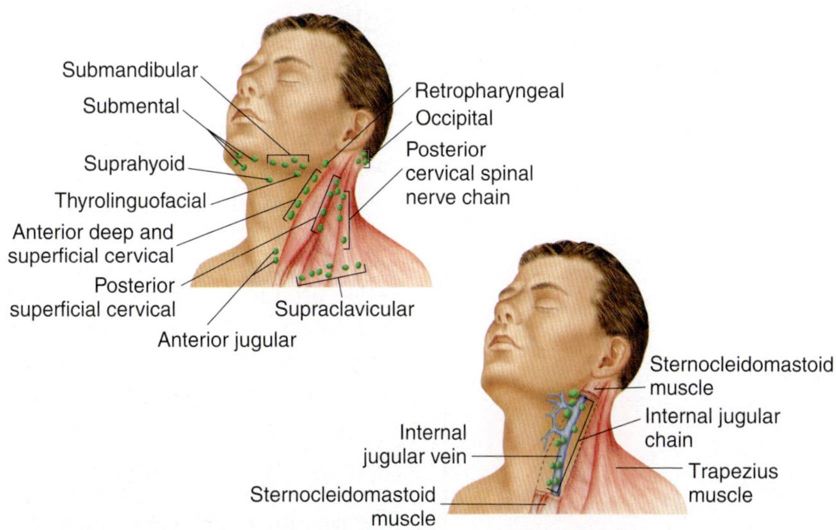

FIG. 10.11 **Lymph nodes of neck.** Note relationship to the sternocleidomastoid muscle. Side view of face and neck at the top shows labels as follows: Retropharyngeal, occipital, posterior cervical spinal nerve chain, supraclavicular, anterior jugular, posterior superficial cervical, anterior deep and superficial cervical, thyrolinguofacial, suprahyoid, submental, and submandibular. Side view of face and neck at the bottom shows labels as follows: Sternocleidomastoid muscle, internal jugular chain, trapezius muscle, sternocleidomastoid muscle, and internal jugular vein.

Lymph Nodes

Lymph nodes are discrete structures surrounded by a capsule composed of connective tissue and a few elastic fibrils. Lymph nodes usually occur in groups. Superficial nodes are located in subcutaneous connective tissues, and deeper nodes lie beneath the fascia of muscles and within the various body cavities. The nodes are numerous and tiny, but some of them may have diameters as large as 0.5 to 1 cm. They defend against the invasion of microorganisms and other particles with filtration and phagocytosis, and they aid in the maturation of lymphocytes and monocytes. Most lymph carried by the lymphatic vessels passes through at least one lymph node before entering the blood circulation.

The superficial lymph nodes are the gateway to assessing the health of the entire lymphatic system. Readily accessible to inspection and palpation, they provide some of the earliest clues to the presence of infection or malignancy (Box 10.1). For example, a palpable supraclavicular node should be suspected as a probable sign of malignancy.

Lymphocytes

Lymphocytes are central to the body's response to antigenic substances. They are not uniform in size or function. Some are small, approximately 7 to 8 μm in diameter; others range in size to as much as five times that. They arise from a number of sites in the body, including the lymph nodes, tonsils, adenoids, and spleen, but are primarily produced in the bone marrow, where early cells (stem cells) capable of developing in a variety of pathways arise. Lymphocytes that are derived primarily from bone marrow (B lymphocytes) produce antibodies and are characterized by the various arrangements of immunoglobulins on their surface. They are involved in the humoral immune response.

Marrow-derived cells that mature in the thymus (T lymphocytes) are further differentiated into types of T cells, each with a distinct function. A unique feature of T cells is their ability to discriminate between healthy and abnormal cells. Activation by their specific antigen (e.g., a living virus, bacterium, parasite, chemical, malignant change) elicits an immune response. T lymphocytes also have an important role in controlling the immune responses brought about by B lymphocytes.

Among lymphocytes, B cells have a relatively short life span of 3 to 4 days. T cells, which are four or five times as numerous as B cells, have a life span of 100 to 200 days. An increased number of lymphocytes in the blood represents a systemic response to most viral infections and to some bacterial infections.

BOX 10.1 Lymph Nodes Most Accessible to Inspection and Palpation

The more superficial the node, the more accessible it is.

The "Necklace" of Nodes

- Parotid and retropharyngeal (tonsillar)
- Submandibular
- Submental
- Sublingual (facial)
- Superficial anterior cervical
- Superficial posterior cervical
- Preauricular and postauricular
- Sternocleidomastoid
- Occipital
- Supraclavicular

The Arms

- Axillary
- Epitrochlear (cubital)

The Legs

- Superficial superior inguinal
- Superficial inferior inguinal
- Occasionally, popliteal

Thymus

The thymus is located in the superior mediastinum, extending upward into the lower neck. In early life, the thymus is essential to the development of the protective immune function (Fig. 10.12). It is the site for production of T lymphocytes, the cells responsible for cell-mediated immunity reactions and the controlling agent for the humoral immune responses generated by B lymphocytes. It is largest and most active during the neonatal and preadolescent periods and atrophies after puberty.

Spleen

The spleen is situated in the left upper quadrant of the abdominal cavity between the stomach and the diaphragm. A highly vascular organ, it is composed of two systems: (1) the white pulp, made up of lymphatic nodules and diffuse lymphatic tissue, and (2) the red pulp, made up of venous sinusoids. The spleen has several functions including destroying old red blood cells, producing antibodies, storing red blood cells, and filtering microorganisms from the blood. Its examination therefore is essential to the evaluation of the immune system (see Chapter 18).

Tonsils and Adenoids

The palatine tonsils are commonly referred to as "the tonsils." Small and diamond-shaped, they are set between the palatine arches on either side of the pharynx just beyond the base of the tongue. Composed principally of lymphoid tissue, the tonsils are organized as follicles and crypts; both are covered by mucous membrane. The pharyngeal tonsils, or adenoids, are located at the nasopharyngeal border; the

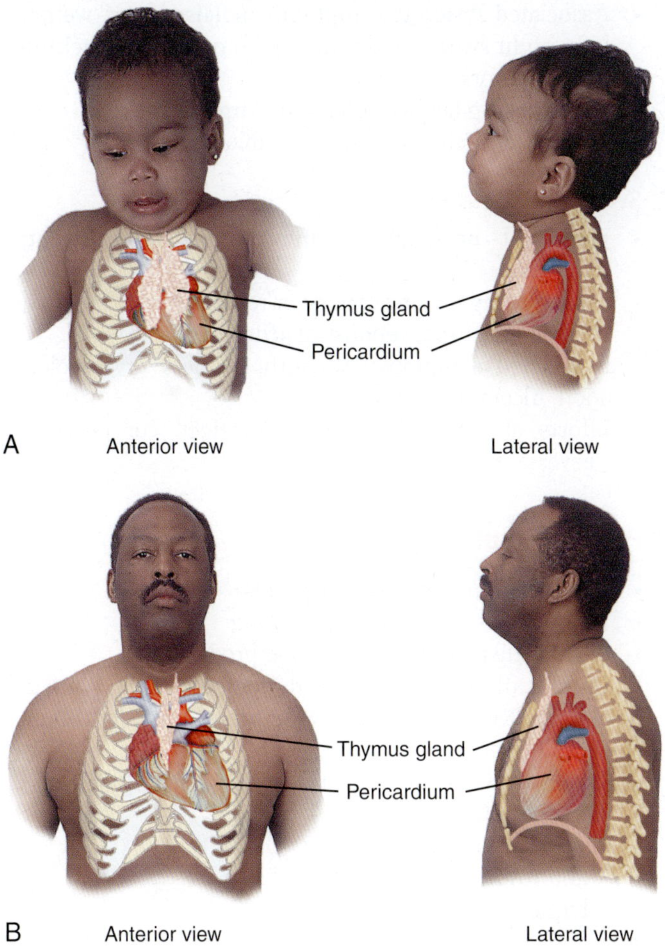

FIG. 10.12 Location of the thymus gland and its size relative to the rest of the body. (A) During infancy. (B) During adult life. (A) Anterior and lateral view of infant shows large thymus gland and small pericardium. (B) Anterior and lateral view of adult shows small thymus gland and large pericardium.

lingual tonsils are located near the base of the tongue. Defensive responses to inhaled and intranasal antigens are activated in these tissues. When enlarged, the adenoids and tonsils can obstruct the nasopharyngeal passageway.

Peyer Patches

Peyer patches are small, raised areas of lymph tissue on the mucosa of the small intestine and consist of many clustered lymphoid nodules. Peyer patches are important in immune surveillance in the intestinal tract. They facilitate an immune response when pathogenic microorganisms are detected.

Infants, Children, Pregnant Patients, and Older Adults

Infants and Children

The immune system and the lymphoid system begin developing at about 20 weeks of gestation. The ability to produce antibodies is still immature at birth, increasing the infant's vulnerability to infection during the first few months of life (see Clinical Pearl, "Umbilical Cord"). The mass of lymphoid tissue is relatively plentiful in infants; increases during childhood, especially between 6 and 9 years of age; and then regresses to adult levels by puberty (see Chapter 8, Fig. 8.2).

> **CLINICAL PEARL**
>
> **Umbilical Cord**
>
> The umbilical cord should drop off by 1 to 2 weeks after birth. Delayed umbilical cord separation is associated with leukocyte adhesion deficiency, an autosomal recessive disorder that causes recurrent infections.

The thymus is at its largest relative to the rest of the body shortly after birth but reaches its greatest absolute weight at puberty. Then it involutes, replacing much of its tissue with fat and becoming a rudimentary organ in the adult.

The palatine tonsils, like much lymphoid tissue, are much larger during early childhood than after puberty. An enlargement of the tonsils in children is not necessarily an indication of problems. They also appear larger relative to the smaller size of the pediatric mouth and throat.

The lymph nodes have the same distribution in children that they do in adults. The finding of small 2- to 3-mm, discrete, palpable, mobile nodes in the neonate is not unusual. Before 2 years of age, inguinal, occipital, and postauricular nodes are common; after 2 years of age, they are more indicative of a problem. On the other hand, cervical and submandibular nodes are uncommon during the first year and much more common in older children. Supraclavicular nodes are not usually palpable; their presence, associated with a high incidence of malignancy, is always a cause for concern. Circumcision does not increase the likelihood of inguinal nodes. It is possible that the infant's relatively large mass of lymphoid tissue is needed to compensate for an immature ability to produce antibodies, thus adding to the demand for filtration and phagocytosis.

The lymphatic system gradually reaches adult competency during childhood (Fig. 10.13).

Pregnant Patients

Pregnancy is a state of altered immune function. The complex changes are not fully understood and reflect multiple mechanisms to achieve and maintain fetal tolerance during pregnancy while still allowing for normal immune defense in the pregnant patient. The immune changes in pregnancy can lead to temporary remission of the pregnant individual's autoimmune/inflammatory diseases (e.g., rheumatoid arthritis).

Older Adults

The number of lymph nodes may diminish and size may decrease with advanced age; some of the lymphoid structures are lost. The nodes of older patients are more likely to be fibrotic and fatty than those of the young, a contributing factor to impaired ability to resist infection.

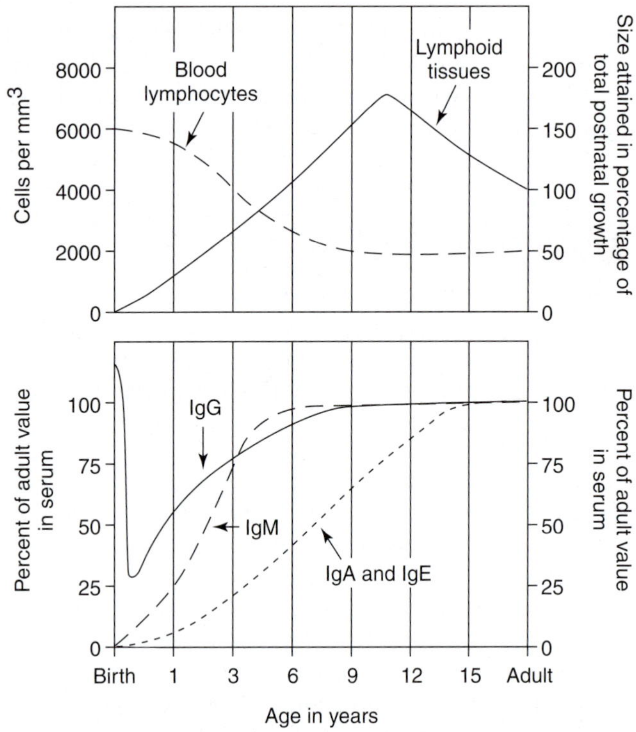

FIG. 10.13 **Relative levels of presence and function of the immune factors.** *Top graph:* The left vertical axis represents cells per millimeter cubed ranging from 0 to 8000, in increments of 2000. The right vertical axis represents size attained in percentage of total postnatal growth ranging from 0 to 200, in increments of 50. The horizontal axis represents age in years. A curve marked "Lymphoid tissues" starts at 0 of the left vertical axis and reaches 7000 on the left and 180 on the right vertical axes in 11 years. A dashed curve marked "Blood lymphocytes" starts at 6000 on the left vertical axis, decreases in a concave-up manner, and ends at 50 on the right vertical axis. *Bottom graph:* The left and right vertical axes represent percentage of adult value in serum ranging from 0 to 100, in increments of 25. The horizontal axis represents age in year ranges as follows: Birth, 1, 3, 6, 9, 12, 15, and adult. A dashed curved arrow marked "IgA" and "IgE" starts at (Birth, 0), increases, reaches (15, 100 of both axes), and ends at (Adult, 0). Another dashed curve marked "IgM" starts at (Birth, 0), increases in a concave-up manner, reaches (6, 100), and ends at (Adult, 100). A curve starts near the top of the vertical axis, reaches 24 on the left vertical axis after birth, reaches (8, 100), and ends at (Adult, 100). All data are approximate.

REVIEW OF RELATED HISTORY

For each of the symptoms or conditions discussed in this section, targeted topics to include in the history of the present illness are listed. Responses to questions about these topics provide clues for focusing the physical examination and the development of an appropriate diagnostic evaluation. Questions regarding medication use (prescriptions and over-the-counter preparations) as well as complementary, alternative, and integrative therapies are relevant for each.

History of Present Illness

Enlarged Node(s) (Lumps, Knots, Bumps, Kernels, Swollen Glands)

- Character: onset, location, duration, number, tenderness
- Associated local symptoms: pain, redness, warmth, red streaks
- Associated systemic symptoms: malaise, fever, weight loss, night sweats, abdominal pain or fullness, itching (some tumors cause pruritus)
- Predisposing factors: infection, surgery, trauma
- Medications: chemotherapy, antibiotics

Swelling of Extremity

- Unilateral or bilateral, intermittent or constant, duration
- Predisposing factors: cardiac or renal disorder, surgery, infection, trauma, venous insufficiency
- Associated symptoms: warmth, redness or discoloration, ulceration
- Efforts at treatment and their effect: compression sleeves or stockings, elevation

Past Medical History

- Chest imaging; reason and results
- Tuberculosis and other skin testing
- Blood transfusions, use of blood products
- Chronic illness: cardiac, renal, malignancy, HIV infection (see Risk Factors box: "Human Immunodeficiency Virus Infection")
- Surgery: trauma to regional lymph nodes, organ transplant, lymph node biopsy
- Recurrent infections
- Autoimmune disorder
- Allergies

Risk Factors

Human Immunodeficiency Virus Infection

Adolescents and Adults

- Sexual activity
  - Professional sex workers
  - Unprotected anal or vaginal sex
  - Sex with persons infected with HIV
- Injection drug use
  - Parenteral exposure to HIV blood–contaminated needles and/or syringes
  - Sex with injection drug users
- Hepatitis, tuberculosis (TB), or sexually transmitted infection (STI)
  - Diagnosis of, or been treated for, hepatitis, TB, or an STI such as syphilis, herpes, chlamydia, gonorrhea, or bacterial vaginosis
- Blood or clotting factor transfusion
  - Transfusion with infected blood or blood concentrates (e.g., factor VIII, factor IX) between 1978 and 1985
- Work related (rare)
  - Puncture of the skin with needles or other sharp objects contaminated with the blood of an HIV-infected patient

Infants and Children

- Mother with HIV infection
  - Antiretroviral treatment during pregnancy
  - During gestation
  - At birth
  - During breastfeeding
- Sexual abuse

Family History

- Malignancy
- Anemia
- Recent infectious diseases
- Tuberculosis
- Immune disorders
- Hemophilia

Personal and Social History

- Travel, especially to areas with insufficient sanitation or insect control
- Use of illicit or recreational drugs, especially injected
- Sexual history (risk factors for HIV exposure)

Infants and Children

- Recurrent infections: pharyngitis; bacterial infections (e.g., acute otitis media, cutaneous abscesses, sinus and pulmonary infections); oral candidiasis; chronic diarrhea; chronic severe eczema
- Present or recent infections, trauma distal to nodes
- Poor growth, failure to thrive
- Loss of interest in playing or eating
- Immunization history
- Maternal HIV infection

Pregnant Patients

- Weeks of gestation
- Exposure to infections
- Presence of pets in household (exposure to cat feces or litter)
- Immunization status: influenza, pneumonia, meningococcal, tetanus/diphtheria/pertussis

Older Adults

- Presence of an autoimmune disease
- Present or recent infection or trauma distal to nodes
- Delayed healing
- Immunization status: influenza, pneumococcal, tetanus/diphtheria/pertussis, shingles (herpes zoster)

BOX 10.2 Terms

Conditions

Lymphadenopathy (adenopathy)—enlarged lymph node(s)
Lymphadenitis—inflamed and enlarged lymph node(s)
Lymphangitis—inflammation of the lymphatics that drain an area of infection; tender erythematous streaks extend proximally from the infected area; regional nodes may also be tender
Lymphedema—edematous swelling due to excess accumulation of lymph fluid in tissues caused by inadequate lymph drainage
Lymphangioma—congenital malformation of dilated lymphatics

Nodes

Shotty—small, nontender nodes that feel like BBs under the skin
Fluctuant—wavelike motion that is felt when the node is palpated
Matted—group of nodes that feel connected and seem to move as a unit

EXAMINATION AND FINDINGS

Equipment

- Centimeter ruler
- Skin-marking pencil

Inspection and Palpation

Disorders of the lymph system present with three possible physical signs: enlarged lymph nodes (lymphadenopathy), red streaks on the overlying skin (lymphangitis), or lymphedema (Box 10.2). Inspect each area of the body for apparent lymph nodes, edema, erythema, red streaks, and skin lesions. Using the pads of the second, third, and fourth fingers, gently palpate for superficial lymph nodes (see Box 10.1 and Fig. 10.14). Try to detect any hidden enlargement, and note the consistency, mobility, tenderness, size, and warmth of the nodes. In areas where the skin is more mobile, move the skin over the area of the nodes. Press lightly at first, then gradually increase pressure. Heavier pressure alone can displace nodes before you have had a chance to recognize their presence. Superficial nodes are accessible to palpation but in healthy adults are not large or firm enough to be felt. You may detect small, movable, discrete, "shotty" nodes (multiple small nodes that feel like BBs under the skin) less than 1 cm in diameter that move under your fingers. Shotty nodes are generally of no clinical consequence and usually represent transient enlargement of the lymph nodes after viral infection. However, even shotty nodes in the epitrochlear or supraclavicular regions require additional evaluation. A node fixed to surrounding tissues is cause for concern.

When enlarged lymph nodes are encountered, explore the accessible adjacent areas and regions drained by those nodes for signs of possible infection or malignancy. Examine other regions for enlargement. Enlarged lymph nodes in any region should be characterized according to location, size, shape, consistency (fluctuant, soft, firm, hard), tenderness, mobility or fixation to surrounding tissues, and discreteness. Lymph nodes that are enlarged and juxtaposed so that they feel like a large mass rather than discrete nodes are described as "matted." Marking with a skin pencil at the periphery of the node at the 12, 3, 6, and 9 o'clock positions defines the extent of the node and helps guide the assessment of change (see Clinical Pearl, "Reminders About Nodes").

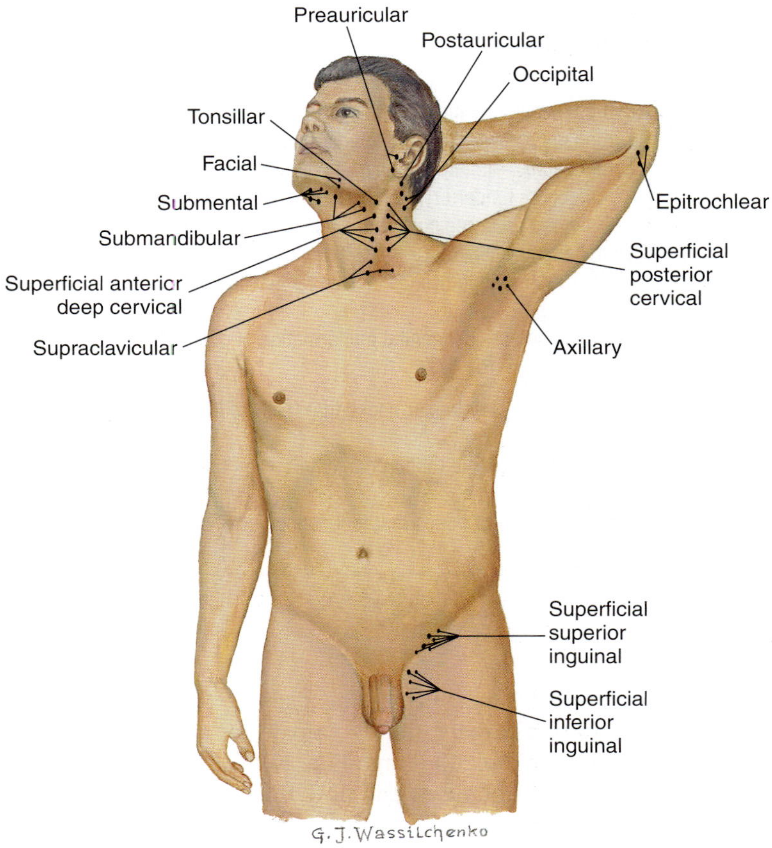

FIG. 10.14 Some of the accessible lymph nodes. Anterior view of human body shows labels as follows: preauricular, postauricular, occipital, epitrochlear, superficial posterior cervical, axillary, superficial superior inguinal, superficial inferior inguinal, supraclavicular, superficial anterior deep cervical, submandibular, submental, facial, and tonsillar.

CLINICAL PEARL

Reminders About Nodes

- A hard, fixed, painless node suggests a malignant process.
- The more tender a node, the more likely it is an inflammatory process.
- Nodes do not pulsate; arteries do.
- A palpable supraclavicular node is highly suggestive of thoracic or abdominal malignancy.
- Slow nodal enlargement over weeks and months suggests a benign process; rapid enlargement without signs of inflammation suggests malignancy.

If there is tenderness on touch, note the degree of discoloration or redness and any unusual increase in vascularity, heat, or pulsations. If bruits are audible with the stethoscope, it is a blood vessel, not a lymph node. When you are uncertain of the nature of the findings, check whether any large mass transilluminates; as a rule, nodes do not and fluid-filled cysts do.

Lymph nodes that are large, fixed or matted, inflamed, or tender indicate a problem. With bacterial infection, nodes may become warm or tender to the touch, matted, and much less discrete, particularly if the infection persists. It is possible to infer the site of an infection from the pattern of lymph node enlargement. For example, infections of the ear usually drain to the preauricular, retropharyngeal, and deep cervical nodes (see Fig. 10.8).

Lymph nodes to which a malignancy has spread vary greatly in size, from tiny to many centimeters in diameter. They are sometimes discrete, sometimes matted and firmly fixed to underlying tissues; they tend to be harder than expected. Involvement is often asymmetric; contralateral nodes in similar locations may not be palpable.

Fluctuant nodes—nodes that feel like they contain fluid—suggest suppuration from infection. Fixation of the nodes to underlying tissue is most common in metastatic cancer but can also occur with chronic inflammation (see Clinical Pearl, "Not Always Pathology").

CLINICAL PEARL

Not Always Pathology

Palpable lymph nodes do not always have a pathologic cause; a submandibular or cervical node less than 1 cm in diameter or an inguinal node less than 2 cm in diameter in an adult may be considered normal. Solitary nodes in other areas are more likely to have a pathologic cause. The supraclavicular node that warns of malignancy lies anterior to the sternocleidomastoid muscle.

In tuberculosis, the lymph nodes, often felt in the cervical chains, are usually body temperature, soft, matted, and not tender or painful.

Lymphadenopathy that is widespread, involving several lymph node regions, indicates systemic disease or disorder. Also see Clinical Pearl, "Drugs and Nodes."

> **CLINICAL PEARL**
>
> **Drugs and Nodes**
>
> Diphenylhydantoin in particular can cause nodal enlargement. So too, on occasion, can aspirin, barbiturates, penicillin, tetracycline, potassium iodide, cephalosporin, sulfonamide, allopurinol, atenolol, captopril, carbamazepine, hydralazine, phenytoin, primidone, pyrimethamine, and quinidine, among others.

The differentiation of an enlarged lymph node from other masses depends on many variables; for example, some sites are incompatible with the distribution of nodes, and some palpable sensations (e.g., thrill, consistency) are not possible with the basic structure of nodes (see the Differential Diagnosis box "Conditions Simulating Lymph Node Enlargement").

> **DIFFERENTIAL DIAGNOSIS**
>
> ***Conditions Simulating Lymph Node Enlargement***
>
> - Lymphangioma (transilluminates; hemangiomas do not)
> - Cystic hygroma (thin-walled, contains clear lymph fluid)
> - Hemangioma (tends to feel spongy; appears reddish blue, with color depending on size and extent of blood vessel involvement; Valsalva maneuver may enlarge the mass)
> - Branchial cleft cyst (sometimes accompanied by a tiny orifice in the neck along the lower third of the anteromedial border of the sternocleidomastoid muscle between the muscle and the overlying skin; may fluctuate in size when inflamed)
> - Thyroglossal duct cyst (midline in the neck; may retract when tongue is protruded)
> - Granular cell tumor
> - Laryngocele
> - Esophageal diverticulum
> - Thyroid goiter
> - Graves disease
> - Hashimoto thyroiditis
> - Parotid swelling (e.g., from parotitis or tumor)
> - Femoral hernia (below inguinal ligament; protrudes with cough; reducible)

Head and Neck

Lightly palpate the entire neck for nodes. The anterior border of the sternocleidomastoid muscle is the dividing line for the anterior and posterior triangles of the neck and is a useful landmark for describing location. The muscles and bones of the neck together create these "triangles" (Fig. 10.15).

Bending the patient's head slightly forward or to the side will ease taut tissues and allow better accessibility to palpation. Feel for nodes on the head in the following six-step sequence (Fig. 10.16):

1. The occipital nodes at the base of the skull
2. The postauricular nodes located superficially over the mastoid process
3. The preauricular nodes just in front of the ear (Fig. 10.17)
4. The parotid and retropharyngeal (tonsillar) nodes at the angle of the mandible
5. The submandibular nodes halfway between the angle and the tip of the mandible
6. The submental nodes in the midline behind the tip of the mandible

Then move down to the neck, palpating in the following four-step sequence:

1. The superficial cervical nodes at the sternocleidomastoid muscle
2. The posterior cervical nodes along the anterior border of the trapezius muscle (Fig. 10.18)
3. The cervical nodes deep to the sternocleidomastoid (the deep cervical nodes may be difficult to feel if you press too vigorously; probe gently with your thumb and fingers around the muscle)
4. The supraclavicular areas, probing deeply in the angle formed by the clavicle and the sternocleidomastoid muscle, the area of Virchow nodes (Fig. 10.19)

On occasion, postauricular nodes associated with ear infection (particularly external otitis) may be surrounded by some cellulitis; this may cause the ears to protrude.

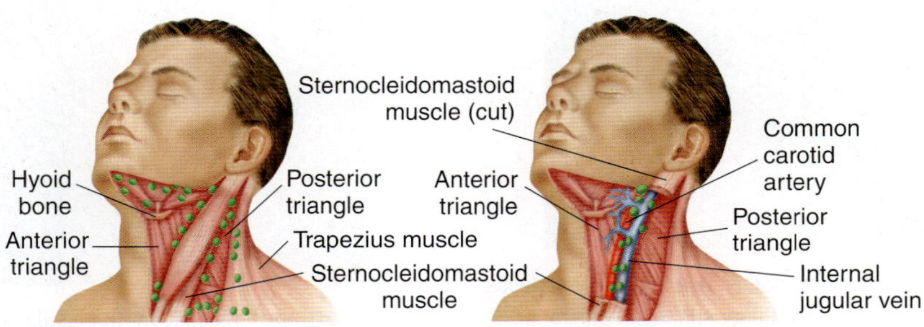

FIG. 10.15 The triangles of the neck. Side view of neck on the left shows labels for posterior triangle, trapezius muscle, sternocleidomastoid muscle, anterior triangle, and hyoid bone. Side view of neck on the right shows labels for common carotid artery, posterior triangle, internal jugular vein, sternocleidomastoid muscle, anterior triangle, and sternocleidomastoid muscle (cut).

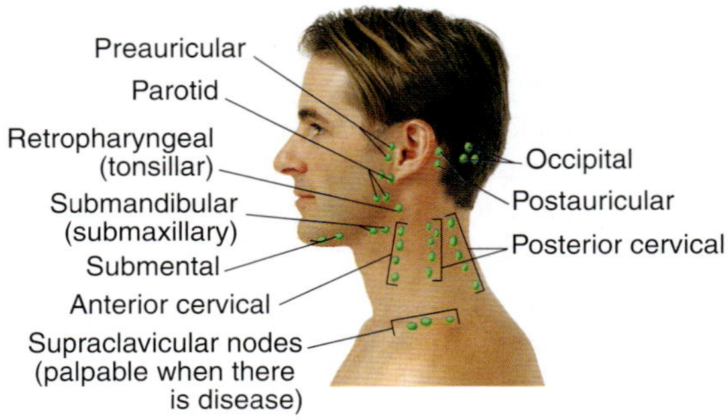

FIG. 10.16 Palpable lymph nodes of the head and neck. Side view of head and neck shows labels as follows: occipital, postauricular, posterior cervical, supraclavicular nodes (palpable when there is disease), anterior cervical, submental, submandibular (submaxillary), retropharyngeal (tonsillar), parotid, and preauricular.

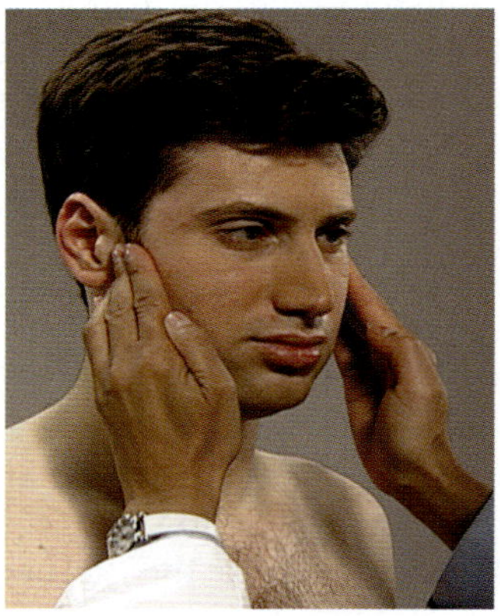

FIG. 10.17 Palpation of preauricular lymph nodes. Compare the nodes bilaterally.Close-up shows health care professional's hands checking palpation close to the ears on the face of a patient using the index and middle fingers.

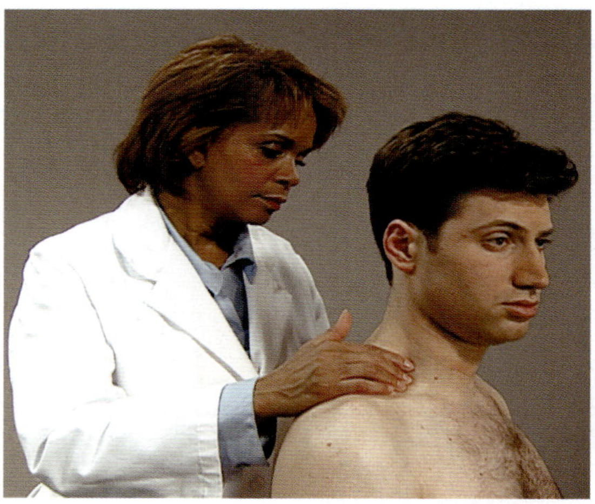

FIG. 10.18 Palpation of posterior cervical nodes. Use the dorsal surfaces (pads) of the fingertips to palpate along the anterior surface of the trapezius muscle and then move slowly in a circular motion toward the posterior surface of the sternocleidomastoid muscle. A health care professional pressing the right trapezius muscle of a patient using the fingertips.

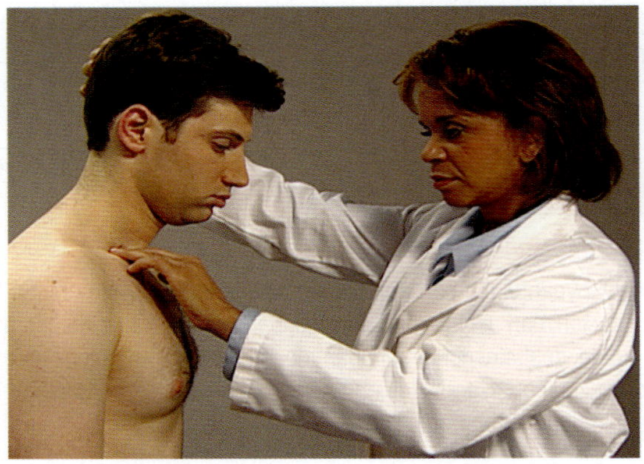

FIG. 10.19 Palpation for supraclavicular lymph nodes. Encourage the patient to relax the musculature of the upper extremities so that the clavicles drop. The examiner's free hand is used to flex the patient's head forward to relax the soft tissues of the anterior neck. The fingers are hooked over the clavicle lateral to the sternocleidomastoid muscle. A health care professional placing her hand on the back of the head while checking the palpation on the anterior side of the neck of a patient.

Axillae

Think of the axillary examination by imagining a pentagonal structure: the pectoral muscles anteriorly, the back muscles (i.e., latissimus dorsi and subscapularis) posteriorly, the rib cage medially, the upper arm laterally, and the axilla at the apex. Let the soft tissues roll between your fingers, the chest wall, and muscles as you palpate. A firm, deliberate, yet gentle touch may feel less ticklish to the patient.

On palpation of the axillary lymph nodes, support the patient's forearm with your contralateral arm and bring the palm of your examining hand flat into the axilla; alternatively, let the patient's forearm rest on that of your examining hand (Fig. 10.20). Rotate your fingertips and palm, feeling the nodes; if they are palpable, attempt to glide your fingers beneath the nodes (see Clinical Pearl,

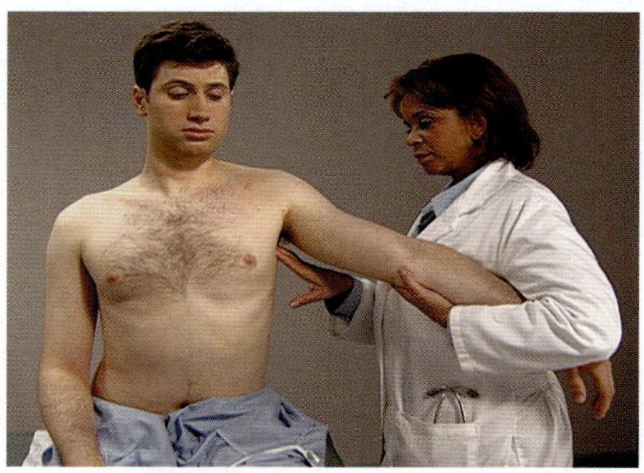

FIG. 10.20 Soft tissues of the axilla are gently rolled against the chest wall and the muscles surrounding the axilla. A health care professional holding the lower arm of a patient against her chest wall while feeling the nodes near the armpit of the patient.

"Vaccinations and Nodes"). A more complete examination of the breast, the axilla, and adjacent areas is described in Chapter 17.

CLINICAL PEARL

Vaccinations and Nodes

Immunizations, particularly BCG (bacillus Calmette-Guérin), MMR (measles/mumps/rubella), smallpox, and COVID-19, administered in the upper arm may cause transient reactive axillary node enlargement. Rarely, human papillomavirus (HPV) vaccination may cause node enlargement in the axilla or head and neck region.

Think About It

If you find a palpable lymph node, consider not only that finding but also the patient's history and other possible findings. For example, if there is an enlarged and tender axillary node, the patient reports having been scratched by a cat, and there is an infected wound on that extremity, then the cause is inflammatory. On the other hand, if there is an enlarged inguinal node in the absence of an obvious wound or infection and the patient also reports night sweats and unintentional weight loss, consider malignancy as a cause.

Epitrochlear Lymph Nodes

To palpate the epitrochlear nodes, support the arm in one hand as you explore the elbow with the other. Grasp the patient's right wrist, palm facing up, with your left hand. The elbow should be in a relaxed position at approximately 90 degrees. Place your right hand under the patient's right elbow, and cup your fingers around the elbow to find the area that is proximal and slightly anterior to the medial epicondyle of the humerus. There is a groove between the triceps and biceps muscles. Palpate that groove with your fingers using a circular motion (Fig. 10.21). Repeat using your left hand for the patient's left elbow. An enlarged node can indicate local infection or systemic illness.

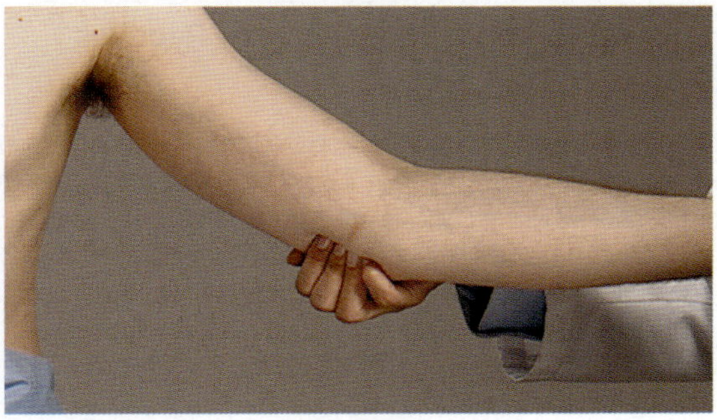

FIG. 10.21 Palpation for epitrochlear lymph nodes is performed in the depression above and posterior to the medial condyle of the humerus. Close-up view of a health care professional's hand under the elbow of a patient.

Inguinal and Popliteal Lymph Nodes

Use a systematic approach when palpating sites of lymph node clusters. Move the hand in a circular fashion, probing gently without pressing hard. Relieve tension by flexing the extremity.

To palpate the inguinal and popliteal area, have the patient lie supine with the knee slightly flexed. The superior superficial inguinal (femoral) nodes are close to the surface over the inguinal canals. The inferior superficial inguinal nodes lie deeper in the groin (Fig. 10.22).

The lymphatic drainage of the testes is into the abdomen. Enlarged nodes there are not accessible to inspection and palpation. Nodes in the inguinal area enlarge if there are lesions of the penile and scrotal surfaces. Similarly, the internal genital organs drain into the iliac and para-aortic nodes and are not accessible to inspection and palpation; however, the vulva and lower third of the vagina drain into the inguinal nodes. Enlargement of the inguinal nodes suggests infection or metastatic carcinoma in the associated anatomic area. To examine the popliteal nodes, relax the posterior popliteal fossa by flexing the knee. Wrap your hand around the knee and palpate the fossa with your fingers.

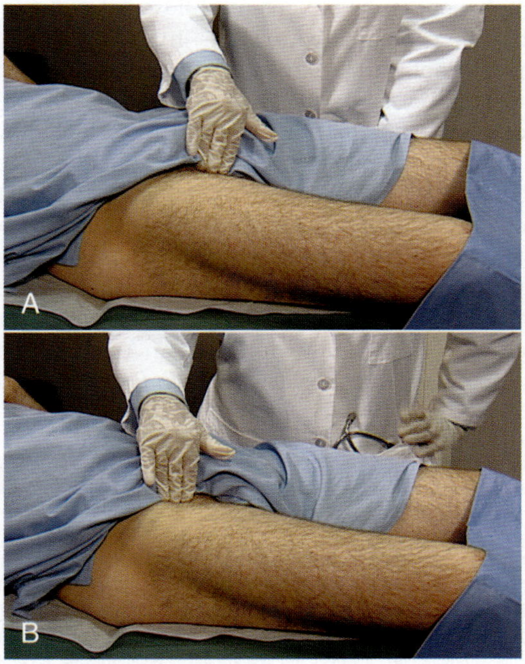

FIG. 10.22 (A) Palpation of inferior superficial inguinal (femoral) lymph nodes. (B) Palpation of superior inguinal lymph nodes.

Patient Safety

Hold Back on Invasive Procedures

One way to promote patient safety is to judiciously limit the number of invasive tests and procedures ordered. Psychological discomfort and physical discomfort are frequent companions to invasive procedures. The best way to avoid the unnecessary discomfort is to perform a knowledgeable and skilled history and physical examination. There are many indications in this chapter for the biopsy of suspicious lymph nodes, but just as important—perhaps more so—there are indications to resist biopsy.

Spleen

Examination of the spleen is detailed in Chapter 18. The spleen is involved in all systemic inflammations, generalized hematopoietic disorders, and many metabolic disturbances. In each of these situations, the spleen enlarges. When sufficiently enlarged, the patient may report pain or a heavy sensation in the left upper quadrant. Massive splenomegaly may cause early satiety or discomfort after eating.

Infants and Children

The technique of examination is similar for all ages. You may find small, firm, discrete, and movable nodes that are neither warm nor tender located in the occipital, postauricular, cervical, and inguinal chains. Inguinal nodes may even be readily visible in a very thin child. In children, such nodes are not as worrisome as in the adult. Their shape is usually globular or ovoid, sometimes flatter or more cylindrical.

Lymph node enlargement in children is a more common finding compared with adults. In the well child, they are typically not warm, tender, or fluctuant; are not matted together; are not associated with erythema; and have not been demonstrated to be associated with serious illness. It is not unusual to find enlarged postauricular and occipital nodes in children younger than 2 years of age. Past that age, such enlargement is relatively uncommon and may be significant (see the Differential Diagnosis boxes for mumps and for immune deficiency disease in a child). Conversely, cervical and submandibular nodal enlargement is relatively less common in children younger than 1 year of age and much more common in older children (see Clinical Pearl, "Cervical Nodes"). These age distributions should be considered in your decision to further evaluate lymph node enlargement. The discovery of small lymph nodes in the inguinal, cervical, or axillary chains of neonates may not in itself require further investigation (Box 10.3). In general, laboratory tests are not indicated in otherwise well children who have cervical lymphadenopathy.

The palatine tonsils may be enlarged in children; this in itself is not a problem. Excessive enlargement may obstruct the nasopharynx, increasing the risk of sleep apnea and, on rare occasions, pulmonary hypertension (see Chapter 13, Fig. 13.37).

DIFFERENTIAL DIAGNOSIS

Mumps Versus Cervical Adenitis

Mumps, or epidemic parotitis, is characterized by a painful swelling of the parotid glands unilaterally or bilaterally and, occasionally, by swelling and tenderness of the other salivary glands along the mandible. The swelling can obscure the angle of the jaw and may appear on inspection as a cervical adenitis. On palpation, however, the two are easily distinguished. A cervical adenitis does not ordinarily obscure the angle of the jaw. Your fingers can separate the node from the angle so that you can feel the hard sharpness of the bone, a finding generally not associated with parotid swelling.

DIFFERENTIAL DIAGNOSIS

How to Discover an Immune Deficiency Disease in a Child

Begin with a thorough history:
- Family history
- Risk factors for HIV infection
- Illness in siblings
- Previous infections, type of infection (e.g., mucosal), and the age of onset of frequent infection
- Previous hospitalizations
- Serious recurring infections and infections that are uncommon (e.g., infection with *Pneumocystis jirovecii;* other infections, particularly fungal, that do not yield to therapy)

Note unusual findings on the physical examination (e.g., generalized lymphadenopathy and enlargement of the liver and/or spleen). The child who is not growing well, who has recurrent infection, and in whom unusual examination findings persist could have an immune deficiency. HIV infection in the young can have a long clinical latency. Suspicion in a child at risk should lead to testing.

CLINICAL PEARL

Cervical Nodes

The childhood diseases of rubella, rubeola, and varicella often present with obvious cervical nodes, usually posterior rather than anterior. Hepatitis A or B and infectious mononucleosis have the same pattern of cervical node involvement.

BOX 10.3 When Lymphadenopathy Requires Further Investigation

Although the detection of lymphadenopathy is common and the number of associated diseases is great, it is not often necessary to perform a biopsy or other laboratory tests. Yet there are situations that indicate a risk for malignancy and require consideration for further investigation:
- Older patients with localized and persistent lymphadenopathy, without evidence of infection or inflammation, might have cancer unless a biopsy proves otherwise
- Young adults and children with localized supraclavicular lymphadenopathy
- Posterior cervical lymphadenopathy adds a risk for malignancy, more than lymphadenopathy that occurs in the anterior cervical chain
- Any lump that grows rapidly at any age

ABNORMALITIES

Lymphatic System

ACUTE LYMPHANGITIS

Inflammation of one or more lymphatic vessels

PATHOPHYSIOLOGY

- Pathogenic organisms enter the lymphatic vessels directly through a wound or as a complication of infection and produce a local inflammatory response
- Inflammation or infection then extends proximally toward regional lymph nodes

PATIENT DATA

Subjective Data

- Enlarged lymph node
- Pain, malaise, possibly fever
- Minor trauma to the skin distal to the area of infection

Objective Data

- Red streaks in the skin after the course of the lymphatic collecting duct
- Appears as a tracing of rather fine lines streaking up the extremity
- Sometimes indurated and palpable to gentle touch
- Look distal to the inflammation for sites of infection, particularly between digits

ACUTE SUPPURATIVE LYMPHADENITIS

Infection and inflammation of a lymph node; may affect a single or localized group of nodes

PATHOPHYSIOLOGY

- Most commonly caused by group A beta-hemolytic streptococci and coagulase-positive staphylococcal infection
- Other pathogens may include actinomycotic adenitis as a result of dental disease, mycobacterial lymphadenitis in the presence of the tuberculosis organism, and *Pasteurella multocida* infection at the site of a scratch or bite from a dog or cat
- Lymph nodes enlarge because of the cellular infiltration and edema.
- Nodes are tender because of distention of the capsule
- Acute lymphadenitis most often seen in the cervical region because of microbial drainage from infections of the teeth or tonsils and in the axillary or inguinal regions secondary to infections in the extremities
- Systemic viral infections (particularly in children) and bacteremia often produce generalized lymphadenopathy

PATIENT DATA

Subjective Data

- Enlarged lymph nodes
- Pain from enlarged lymph nodes

Objective Data

- Involved node usually firm and tender
- Overlying tissue edematous; skin appears erythematous, usually within 72 hours
- When abscess formation is extensive, nodes are fluctuant
- Mycobacterial adenitis characterized by an inflammation without warmth that may or may not be slightly tender

LYMPHEDEMA

Edematous swelling due to excess accumulation of lymph fluid in tissues caused by inadequate lymph drainage

PATHOPHYSIOLOGY

- Result of protein-rich interstitial volume overload secondary to lymph drainage failure
- Four major physiologic mechanisms: increased blood capillary hydrostatic pressure, decreased plasma protein concentration, increased blood permeability, and blockage of lymph return
- Primary lymphedema: hypoplasia and maldevelopment of the lymphatic system; can manifest in infants or later; termed *praecox* in adolescence and *tarda* in patients approaching 40 years of age
- Secondary: acquired damage to regional lymph nodes—pressure from tumors, scar tissue after radiation, or surgical removal of lymph nodes

PATIENT DATA

Subjective Data

- Painless swelling of a limb; unilateral or bilateral
- Onset usually gradual
- History of trauma, surgery, or radiation to a regional area
- Travel to areas where filariasis is common
- Family history of leg swelling

Objective Data

- Swelling and often grotesque distortion of the extremities (Fig. 10.23)
- Lymphedema may or may not pit
- Overlying skin eventually thickens and feels tougher than usual
- Primary lymphedema often apparent at birth and most often involves the legs, particularly the dorsum of the foot; the degree varies with the severity and distribution of the abnormality and may not appear until young adulthood
- See Table 10.1 for grading of lymphedema

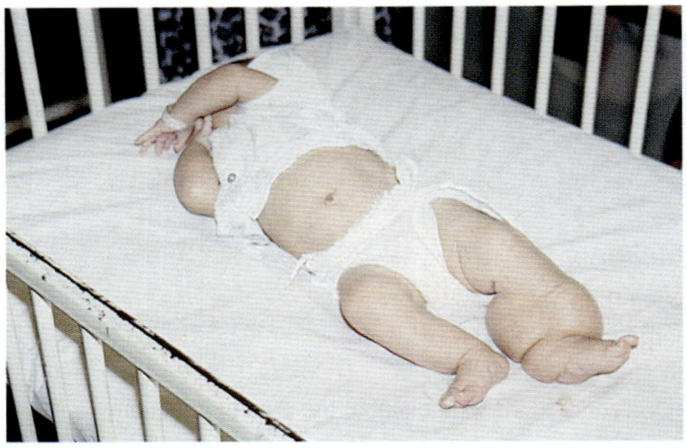

FIG. 10.23 Lymphedema. Close-up view of a baby lying supine on the hospital bed shows excessive swelling on the right lower leg and foot.

DIFFERENTIAL DIAGNOSIS

Lymphedema or Edema?

- Both can be either pitting or nonpitting.
- Except in early stages, lymphedema does not resolve with elevation of the affected area. Edema secondary to increased capillary filtration (e.g., chronic venous insufficiency) usually improves.
- Diuretics do not help lymphedema. They may help edema.
- Be aware that some patients may have both edema and lymphedema.

TABLE 10.1 Grading of Lymphedema by the International Society of Lymphology Criteria

STAGING	DESCRIPTION
Stage 0	Latent or subclinical
	Swelling is not evident despite impaired lymph transport.
Stage I	Pitting may occur.
	There is early accumulation of fluid relatively high in protein content (e.g., in comparison with "venous" edema), and it subsides with limb elevation.
Stage II	Tissue fibrosis is present.
	Limb elevation alone rarely reduces tissue swelling.
	Pitting may be present. Late in stage II, the limb may or may not pit as excess subcutaneous tissue or fibrosis develops.
Stage III	Pitting is absent.
	Trophic skin changes are present (acanthosis nigricans, fat deposits, and warty overgrowths).

Stages refer only to the physical condition of the extremities.
From Executive Committee of the International Society of Lymphology. (2020). The diagnosis and treatment of peripheral lymphedema: 2020 Consensus Document of the International Society of Lymphology. *Lymphology, 53*(1), 3–19.

LYMPHANGIOMA/CYSTIC HYGROMA

Congenital malformation of dilated lymphatics

PATHOPHYSIOLOGY

- Results from a failure of complete development and subsequent obstruction of the lymphatic system; commonly found in the neck

PATIENT DATA

Subjective Data

- Painless cystic masses
- Usually manifest during the first year of life and are often enlarged after an upper respiratory infection
- Asymptomatic when in the posterior triangle of the neck, but if found anteriorly, may cause airway or swallowing problems

Objective Data

- Soft, nontender, and easily compressible spongy fluid-containing mass without discrete margins
- Most present at birth and apparent early in life, usually in the neck or axilla, less commonly in the chest or extremities
- May be large enough to distort face and neck
- Diagnosis through physical examination and imaging studies (ultrasound, computed tomography, or magnetic resonance imaging), which show a thin-walled, multiloculated cystic mass

LYMPHATIC FILARIASIS (ELEPHANTIASIS)

Massive accumulation of lymphedema throughout the body; the most common cause of secondary lymphedema worldwide

PATHOPHYSIOLOGY

- Results from widespread inflammation and obstruction of the lymphatics by the filarial worms *Wuchereria bancrofti* or *Brugia malayi;* transmitted by mosquitoes
- Adequate drainage is prevented, and the patient becomes more susceptible to infection, cellulitis, and fibrosis
- The term *elephantiasis* is often incorrectly used to describe the result of any obstruction, congenital or acquired
- See Differential Diagnosis box

PATIENT DATA

Subjective Data

- Swelling of limb or body area
- Travel to infected areas: Asia, Africa, the Western Pacific, India, Philippines
- Many patients are asymptomatic, but some may develop fever with lymphangitis and lymphadenitis, chronic pulmonary infection, and progressive lymphedema

Objective Data

- Lymphedema of the entire arm or leg; the genital regions (vulva, scrotum, breasts)
- Diagnosis can be made by identification of microfilariae microscopically in blood

DIFFERENTIAL DIAGNOSIS

When the Body Swells

A number of pathologic processes can cause swelling of the extremities and other areas in the body. These can stem from, but are not limited to, the cardiovascular system (e.g., congestive heart failure or constrictive pericarditis); diseases of the liver (e.g., obstruction of the hepatic vein [Chiari syndrome] and portal vein thrombosis); and kidney malfunction. The most common cause, particularly of the feet and the ankles, is stasis. This may occur in otherwise well individuals who must stand or sit for long periods. The failure to move with some regularity increases orthostatic pressure in the legs. Pregnancy is also a common contributor, even in the absence of venous abnormality in the legs. Significant disruption of lymphatic circulation in the arms after breast surgery can occur as a consequence of damage to the lymph system. Myxedema, a finding associated with hypothyroidism, is typified by a dry, waxy swelling (see Chapter 11, Fig. 11.10). The edema in this condition can cause a typical facies, with swollen lips and a thick nose; it also does not pit.

NON-HODGKIN LYMPHOMA

Malignant neoplasm of the lymphatic system and the reticuloendothelial tissues

PATHOPHYSIOLOGY

- Non-Hodgkin lymphomas occur most often in lymph nodes in the chest, neck, abdomen, tonsils, and skin; they may also develop in sites other than lymph nodes such as the digestive tract, central nervous system, and around the tonsils
- Most arise in B cells; the rest occur in T cells
- Histologically, their cells are often undifferentiated but resemble lymphocytes, histiocytes, or plasma cells

PATIENT DATA

Subjective Data

- Painless enlarged lymph node(s)
- Fever, weight loss, night sweats, abdominal pain, or fullness
- Family history of non-Hodgkin lymphomas

Objective Data

- Nodes may be localized in the posterior cervical triangle or may become matted, crossing into the anterior triangle
- Nodes usually well defined and solid
- Cannot distinguish the findings of these conditions from those in Hodgkin lymphoma through physical examination alone

HODGKIN LYMPHOMA

Malignant lymphoma

PATHOPHYSIOLOGY

- Unknown etiology, several subtypes
- Starts in a single node or chain and spreads to contiguous lymph nodes, spleen, liver, and bone marrow
- Neoplastic giant cells release factors that induce the accumulation of reactive lymphocytes, macrophages, and granulocytes.
- Occurs in all races, generally in late adolescence and young adulthood, although it also occurs in people older than 50 years; most often, Hodgkin lymphoma starts in B-cell lymphocytes located in lymph nodes in the neck area, although any lymph node may be the site of initial disease

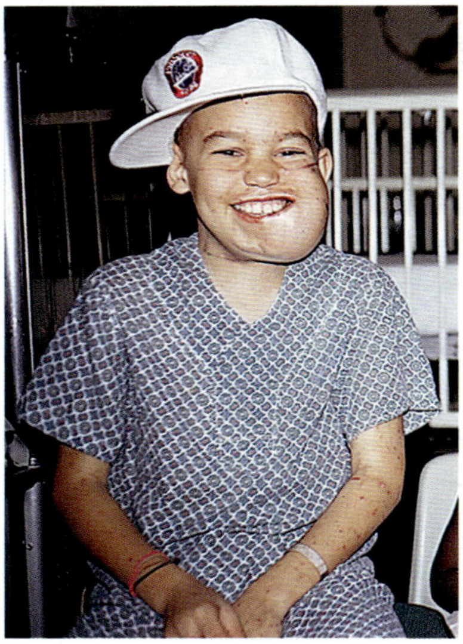

FIG. 10.24 **Hodgkin disease.** Note the impressive extent of the enlargement. Close-up view of a patient with excessive swelling in the left mandible.

PATIENT DATA

Subjective Data
- Painless enlarged lymph nodes
- May have abdominal pain, sometimes fever
- May have history of infectious mononucleosis

Objective Data
- Clinical presentation variable
- Most commonly, painless enlargement of the cervical lymph nodes, often in the posterior triangle, that is generally asymmetric and progressive (Fig. 10.24)
- Nodes sometimes matted and firm, almost rubbery
- Usually asymmetric; may occasionally be enlarged in similar patterns on both sides of the body
- Nodal size may fluctuate

EPSTEIN-BARR VIRUS MONONUCLEOSIS

Infectious mononucleosis

PATHOPHYSIOLOGY

- Initially infects oral epithelial cells; after intracellular viral replication and cell lysis with release of new virions, virus spreads to contiguous structures such as the salivary glands, with eventual viremia and infection of the entire lymphoreticular system, including the liver and spleen
- Incubation period of infectious mononucleosis in adolescents is 30–50 days

PATIENT DATA

Subjective Data
- Malaise, fatigue, acute or prolonged (longer than 1 week) fever, headache, sore throat, nausea, abdominal pain, and myalgia
- Prodromal period may last 1–2 weeks

Objective Data
- Generalized lymphadenopathy most commonly in the anterior and posterior cervical nodes and the submandibular lymph nodes and less commonly in the axillary and inguinal lymph nodes
- Epitrochlear lymphadenopathy is particularly suggestive of infectious mononucleosis
- Hepatomegaly; symptomatic hepatitis or jaundice is uncommon, but elevated liver enzymes are common
- Splenomegaly to 2–3 cm below the costal margin is typical; massive enlargement is uncommon
- Moderate to severe pharyngitis with tonsillar enlargement, occasionally with exudates
- Petechiae at the junction of the hard and soft palate frequently seen
- Diagnosis with mononucleosis spot test

TOXOPLASMOSIS

Zoonosis, caused by the parasite *Toxoplasma gondii*

PATHOPHYSIOLOGY

- Ingestion or inhalation of oocysts in soil/fomites, undercooked meat, or raw eggs; cat feces or litter
- Infection persists for life without signs of disease
- In immunosuppressed persons, quiescent parasites multiply, resulting in neurologic disease or other organ manifestations
- May cause serious congenital infection if exposed during pregnancy, particularly in the first trimester; transmitted directly from pregnant mother to fetus

PATIENT DATA

Subjective Data

- No significant symptoms
- History of eating raw or rare meat or uncooked eggs
- History of direct contact with cat feces, cleaning the litter box, gardening in feces-contaminated soil

Objective Data

- Single node, chronically enlarged and nontender
- Node is usually in the posterior cervical chain

ROSEOLA INFANTUM

Infection by human herpes virus 6 (HHV-6)

PATHOPHYSIOLOGY

- Common in infancy with peak age of acquisition 2 years
- Virus present in the saliva of most adults and is readily transmitted by oral secretions
- Latency permits persistence of the virus in the presence of a fully developed immune response and allows lifelong infection of the host.
- Through periodic reactivation of latent virus and the production of recurrent infection, virus shedding occurs at intervals throughout life, allowing the virus to be spread to new susceptible hosts

PATIENT DATA

Subjective Data

- Fever—usually high grade and persistent over 3–4 days
- Sometimes associated with a mild respiratory illness and lymphadenopathy

Objective Data

- Adenopathy, discrete and not tender, involves the occipital and postauricular chains and may last for some time
- When the fever diminishes, a morbilliform fine maculopapular rash occurs, spreading from the trunk to the extremities; the child begins feeling much better

HERPES SIMPLEX VIRUS

Infection by human herpes simplex virus 1 (HSV-1) or HSV-2

PATHOPHYSIOLOGY

- Transmitted by oral secretions, genital secretions, and close contact
- HSV causes lytic infection of fibroblasts and epithelial cells and establishes latent infection in neurons
- Alternates between being inactive and active
- HSV-1 spread by oral contact; causes both oral and genital infection
- HSV-2 spread by sexual contact; causes genital infection
- Both viruses can infect and produce latent infection at either site; reactivation of each is most common at the preferred site
- Most adults are infected by HSV-1

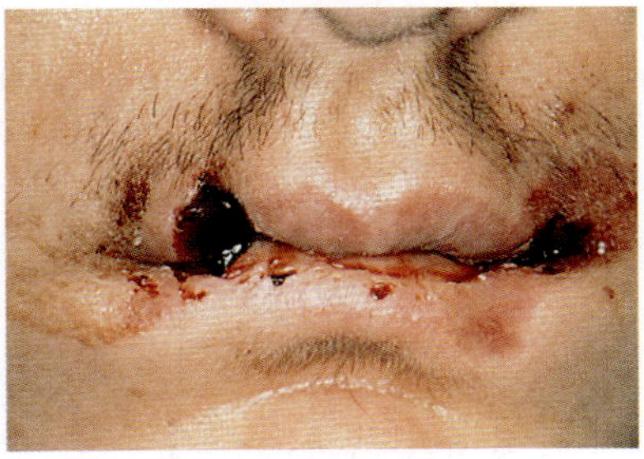

FIG. 10.25 Herpes simplex. Close-up view of a closed mouth shows inflammation and sores of dried dark red blood on the lips.

PATIENT DATA

Subjective Data

- Burning, itching lesions
- May report enlarged lymph nodes
- Periods of time with no symptoms

Objective Data

- Discrete labial and gingival vesicles or ulcers (Fig. 10.25)
- May have enlargement of the anterior cervical and submandibular nodes
- These nodes tend to be somewhat firm, quite discrete, movable, and tender; the frequency of this condition and the symptoms are generally sufficient to establish the diagnosis; a viral culture or molecular testing can be obtained if necessary

CAT SCRATCH DISEASE

A common cause of subacute or chronic lymphadenitis in children

PATHOPHYSIOLOGY

- Caused mainly by *Bartonella henselae* and *Bartonella clarridgeiae;* usually follows a bite, scratch, or other penetrating injury from a kitten or cat; the organisms, however, rarely cause illness in the cat

PATIENT DATA

Subjective Data

- Bite, scratch, or wound from cat or kitten
- Inoculation lesion: a papule or pustule lasts 3–5 days and then becomes vesicular and crusts in 2–3 days
- Painful enlarged lymph nodes

Objective Data

- Inoculation lesion; may be healing
- Lymphadenopathy develops in 1–2 weeks in the region that drains the primary lesion
- Single lymph node most often, but multiple nodes are involved occasionally
- Tender nodes commonly in head, neck, and axillae; the accessible nodal areas in the arms and legs are less often involved
- Nodes can be very large—up to several centimeters; often red and tender and occasionally suppurate
- Diagnosis can be made in the presence of a nodal enlargement lasting longer than 3 weeks, accompanied by an inoculation lesion of the skin and after an interaction with a cat, a cat scratch, or a cat lick on a break in the skin
- Lymphadenopathy can last for 2–4 months or even longer

HUMAN IMMUNODEFICIENCY VIRUS/ACQUIRED IMMUNE DEFICIENCY SYNDROME

Viral infection that attacks the body's immune system

PATHOPHYSIOLOGY

- HIV is a retrovirus of the Retroviridae family in the *Lentivirus* genus.
- The virus targets CD4+ T-lymphocyte helper cells and impairs cell-mediated immunity
- HIV seropositivity (HIV+): antibodies to HIV present, but sequelae of recurrent infections and neoplastic disease have not yet occurred
- AIDS manifested clinically as the development of recurrent, often severe, opportunistic infections
- Common life-threatening diseases associated with full-blown AIDS include Kaposi sarcoma, *Pneumocystis jiroveci* pneumonia, pulmonary tuberculosis, recurrent pneumonia, invasive cervical cancer, a parotid enlargement simulating mumps, anemia and thrombocytopenia, chronic diarrhea, and recurrent infections

PATIENT DATA

Subjective Data

- Enlarged lymph nodes
- Initial symptoms include severe fatigue, malaise, weakness, persistent unexplained weight loss, fevers, arthralgias, and persistent diarrhea

Objective Data

- Generalized lymphadenopathy
- Lymphadenopathy may be absent in patients undergoing antiretroviral therapy
- In children there may be a prolonged clinical latent period, but initial signs may include neurodevelopmental problems with loss of developmental milestones
- Progressive infection characterized by decreasing CD4+ T-lymphocyte count and increasing viral load level
- Progression to AIDS is defined by
  - The number of CD4 cells below 200 cells per cubic millimeter of blood (200 cells/mm^3) OR
  - Development of one or more opportunistic infections regardless of the CD4 count

SERUM SICKNESS (TYPE III HYPERSENSITIVITY REACTION)

An immune complex disease

PATHOPHYSIOLOGY

- Systemic type III hypersensitivity reaction in response to antigens
- Mediated by the tissue deposition of circulating immune complexes, the activation of complement, and the ensuing inflammatory response
- Patient can react similarly to repeated exposure to the stimuli; subsequent reactions may be more severe and even fatal

PATIENT DATA

Subjective Data

- Enlarged lymph nodes
- Pain, pruritus, and erythematous swelling at the injection site
- Urticaria, other rashes, lymphadenopathy, joint pain, fever, and at times facial edema
- Medications: beta-lactam antibiotics (especially cefaclor), sulfonamide antibiotics, minocycline
- Organ transplant

Objective Data

- Findings become apparent about 7–10 days after administration of the provoking substance
- Urticaria, maculopapular or purpuric lesions
- Lymphadenopathy most prominent in the area draining the injection site; can be generalized
- Facial and neck edema
- Symptoms subside slowly, recurring at times over several weeks

LATEX ALLERGY TYPE IV DERMATITIS

Delayed hypersensitivity reaction

PATHOPHYSIOLOGY

- T-cell–mediated, delayed response
- Allergic contact dermatitis that involves the immune system and is caused by the chemicals used in latex products

PATIENT DATA

Subjective Data

- Exposure to latex products
- Rash at area of contact

Objective Data

- Skin reaction usually begins 48–72 hours after contact.
- Vesicular lesions, erythema localized to area of contact
- Reaction may progress to oozing skin blisters

LATEX ALLERGY TYPE I REACTION

True allergic reaction caused by protein antibodies

PATHOPHYSIOLOGY

- Immunoglobulin E antibodies form as a result of interaction between a foreign protein and the body's immune system
- Antigen-antibody reaction causes release of histamine, leukotrienes, prostaglandins, and kinins

PATIENT DATA

Subjective Data

- Exposure to latex
- Allergy to cross-sensitizing foods (e.g., banana, avocado, potato, tomato, kiwi)

Objective Data

- Local: urticaria (skin wheals)
- Systemic: generalized urticaria with angioedema (tissue swelling), asthma, eye/nose itching and gastrointestinal symptoms, anaphylaxis (cardiovascular collapse)

CHAPTER

11

Head and Neck

The head provides the bony housing and protective cover for the brain, including the organs that provide senses of vision, hearing, smell, and taste. The neck provides stability and support for the head and holds vital vessels, the trachea, the esophagus, and the spinal cord. A flexible cervical spine is necessary for head movement, balance adaptation, and increasing extent of vision.

ANATOMY AND PHYSIOLOGY

The skull is composed of seven bones (two frontal, two parietal, two temporal, and one occipital) that are fused together and covered by the scalp. Bones of the skull are helpful when it comes to identifying landmarks on the head (Fig. 11.1). The bony structure of the face is formed from the fused frontal, nasal, zygomatic, ethmoid, lacrimal, sphenoid, and maxillary bones and the movable mandible. The face has cavities for the eyes, nose, and mouth.

Major facial landmarks are the palpebral fissures and the nasolabial folds (Fig. 11.2). Facial muscles are innervated by cranial nerve (CN) V and CN VII. The temporal artery is the major accessible artery of the face, passing just anterior to the ear, over the temporal muscle, and onto the forehead.

The paired parotid, submandibular, and sublingual salivary glands produce saliva, which moistens the mouth, inhibits formation of dental caries, and starts the digestion of carbohydrates. The parotid glands are located anterior to the ear and above the mandible, the submandibular glands are located medial to the mandible at the angle of the jaw, and the sublingual glands are located anteriorly in the floor of the mouth.

Physical Examination Components

Head

1. Observe head position:
   - Tilted
   - Tremor
2. Inspect skull and scalp for:
   - Size
   - Shape (molding)
   - Symmetry
   - Lesions
   - Trauma
3. Inspect facial features, including:
   - Symmetry
   - Shape
   - Unusual features
   - Tics
   - Characteristic facies
   - Pallor or pigmentation variations
4. Palpate head and scalp, noting:
   - Symmetry
   - Tenderness (particularly over areas of frontal and maxillary sinuses)
   - Scalp movement
   - Sutures/fontanels
   - Hair texture, color, and distribution
5. When appropriate, auscultate the temporal arteries and palpate, noting:
   - Thickening
   - Hardness
   - Tenderness
6. Inspect and palpate the salivary glands.
7. Transilluminate the skull of infants with rapidly increasing head circumference.

Neck

1. Inspect the neck for:
   - Symmetry
   - Alignment of trachea
   - Fullness
   - Masses, webbing, and skinfolds
2. Palpate the neck, noting the following:
   - Tracheal position
   - Tracheal tug
   - Movement of hyoid bone and cartilages with swallowing
   - Lymph nodes
   - Paravertebral musculature and spinous processes
3. Palpate the thyroid gland for the following:
   - Size
   - Shape
   - Configuration
   - Consistency
   - Tenderness
   - Nodules
   - If gland is enlarged, auscultate for bruits.
4. Evaluate range of motion of the neck (also see Chapter 22).

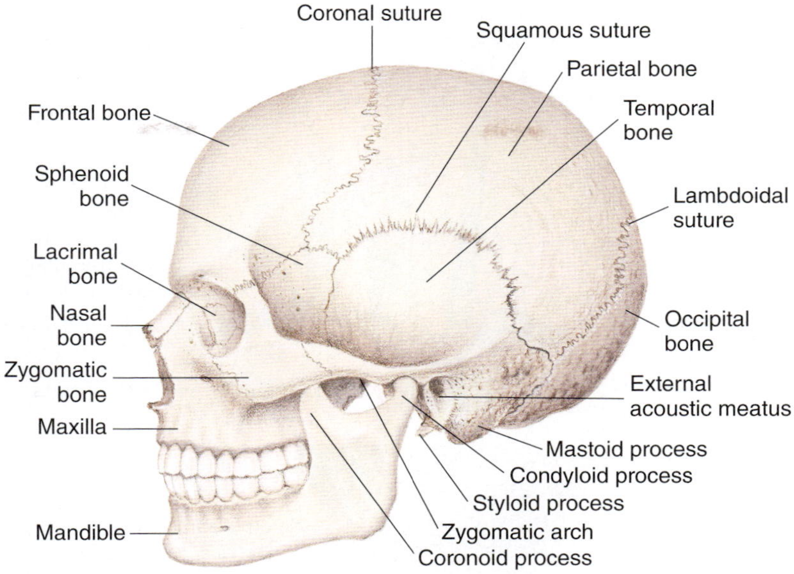

FIG. 11.1 Bones of the skull. Side view of skull shows labels as follows: Coronal suture, squamous suture, parietal bone, temporal bone, lambdoidal suture, occipital bone, external acoustic meatus, mastoid process, condyloid process, styloid process, zygomatic arch, coronoid process, mandible, maxilla, zygomatic bone, nasal bone, lacrimal bone, sphenoid bone, and frontal bone.

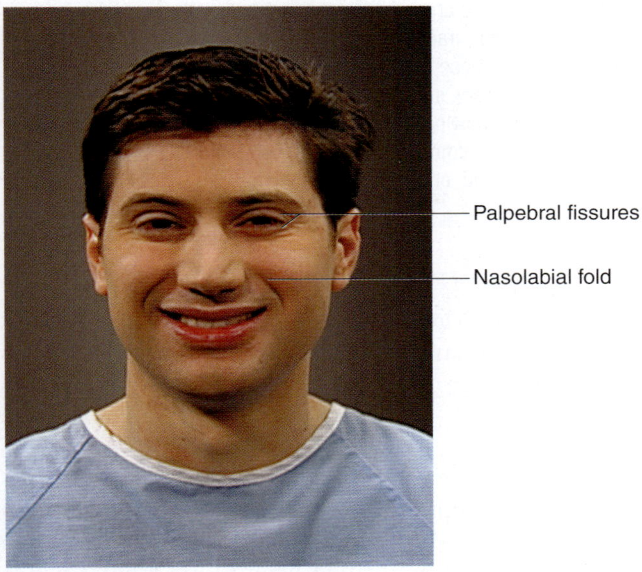

FIG. 11.2 Landmarks of the face. Anterior view of a patient's face shows palpebral fissures and nasolabial fold.

The neck is formed by the cervical vertebrae, ligaments, and sternocleidomastoid and trapezius muscles, which give it support and facilitate movement. The neck begins at the clavicles and sternum inferiorly and at the base of the skull superiorly. It contains the trachea, esophagus, internal and external jugular veins, common carotid, internal and external carotid arteries, and thyroid gland (Fig. 11.3). Horizontal mobility is greatest between cervical vertebrae 4 and 5 or 5 and 6 in adults. The sternocleidomastoid muscle extends from the upper sternum and medial third of the clavicle to the mastoid process (see Fig. 22.2C). The trapezius muscle extends from the scapula, the lateral third of the clavicle, and the vertebrae to the occipital prominence (see Fig. 22.2C and D).

The relationship of these muscles to each other and to adjacent bones creates triangles used as anatomic landmarks. The anterior triangle is formed by the medial border of the sternocleidomastoid muscles, the mandible, and the midline (Fig. 11.4). The posterior triangle is formed by the trapezius and sternocleidomastoid muscles and the clavicle (see Fig. 11.4) and contains the posterior cervical lymph nodes (Fig. 11.5). For a complete description of the lymph nodes of the head and neck, see Chapter 10 and Figs. 10.8 to 10.11, 10.14, and 10.15.

The hyoid bone, cricoid cartilage, trachea, thyroid, and anterior cervical lymph nodes lie inside these triangles (see Fig. 11.3). The common carotid artery and internal jugular vein are deep and run parallel to the sternocleidomastoid muscle along its medial margin. The external jugular vein crosses the surface of the sternocleidomastoid muscle diagonally. The hyoid bone lies just below the mandible. The thyroid cartilage is shaped like a shield; its notch on the upper edge marks the level of bifurcation of the common carotid artery. The cricoid cartilage is the uppermost ring of the tracheal cartilages.

The thyroid is the largest endocrine gland in the body, producing two hormones, thyroxine (T_4) and triiodothyronine (T_3). The two lateral lobes are butterfly

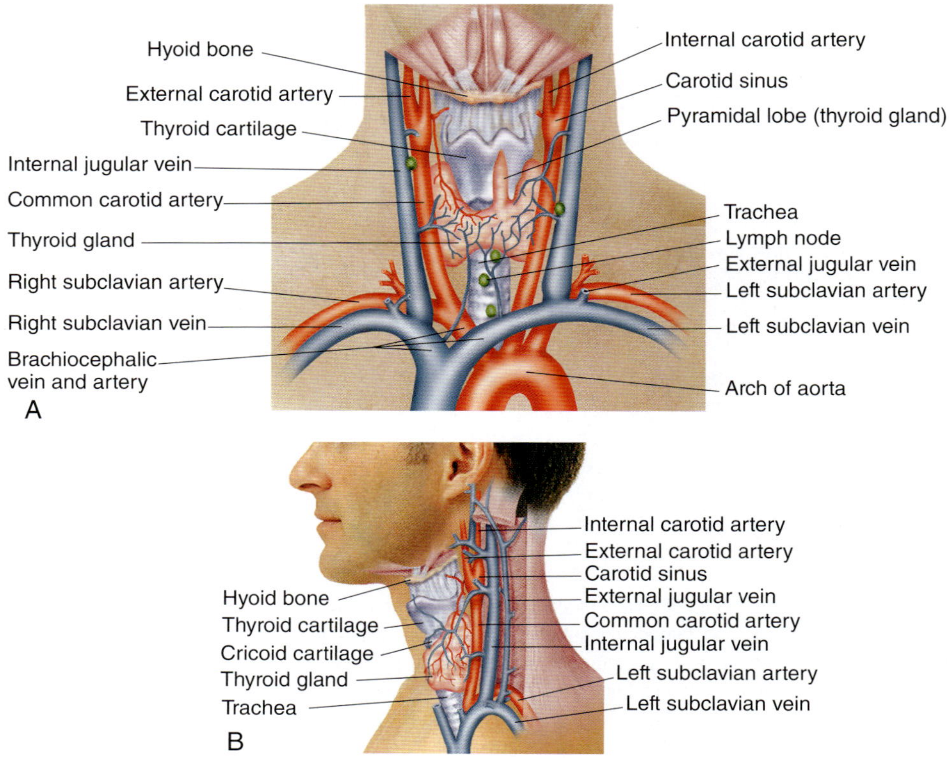

FIG. 11.3 Underlying structures of the neck. (A) Anterior view of underlying area of neck shows labels as follows: internal carotid artery, carotid sinus, pyramidal lobe (thyroid gland), trachea, lymph node, external jugular vein, left subclavian artery, left subclavian vein, arch of aorta, brachiocephalic vein and artery, right subclavian vein, right subclavian artery, thyroid gland, common carotid artery, internal jugular vein, thyroid cartilage, external carotid artery, and hyoid bone. (B) Lateral view of neck showing labels as follows: internal carotid artery, external carotid artery, carotid sinus, external jugular vein, common carotid artery, internal jugular vein, left subclavian artery, left subclavian vein, trachea, thyroid gland, cricoid cartilage, thyroid cartilage, and hyoid bone.

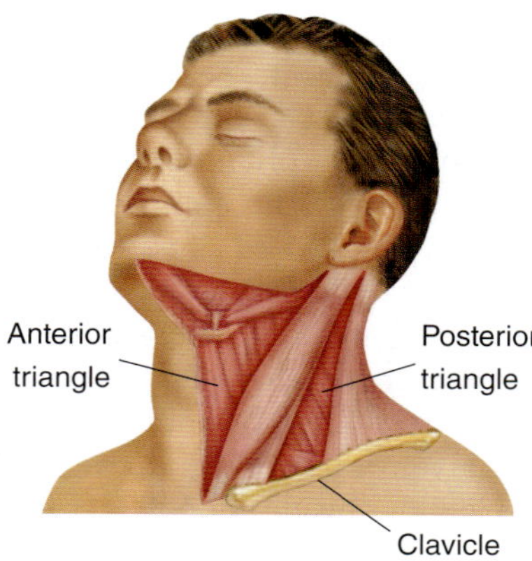

FIG. 11.4 Anterior and posterior triangles of the neck. Side view of neck shows labels for posterior triangle, clavicle, and anterior triangle.

shaped and are joined by an isthmus at their lower aspect (see Fig. 11.3). This isthmus lies across the trachea below the cricoid cartilage. A pyramidal lobe, extending upward from the isthmus and slightly to the left of midline, is present in about one-third of the population. The lobes curve posteriorly around the cartilages and are largely covered by the sternocleidomastoid muscles.

Infants

In infants, the seven cranial bones are soft and separated by the sagittal, coronal, and lambdoid sutures (Fig. 11.6). The anterior and posterior fontanels are the membranous spaces formed where four cranial bones meet and intersect. Spaces between the cranial bones permit the expansion of the skull to accommodate brain growth. Ossification of the sutures begins after completion of brain growth, at about 6 years of age, and is finished by adulthood. The fontanels ossify earlier, with the posterior fontanel usually closing by 2 months of age and the anterior fontanel closing by 12 to 15 months of age.

The process of birth through the vaginal canal often causes molding of the newborn skull, during which the cranial bones may shift and overlap. Within days, the newborn skull usually resumes its appropriate shape and size.

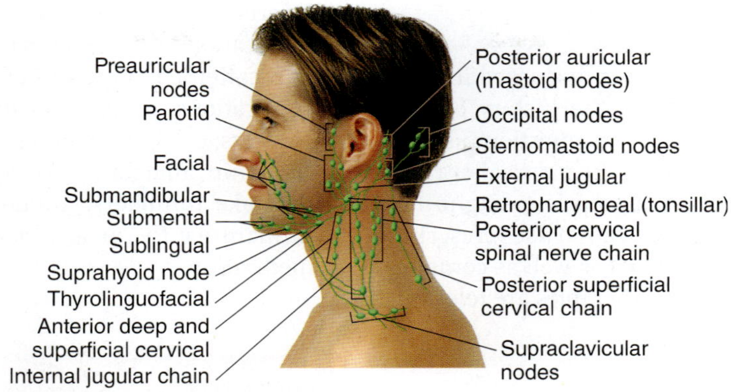

FIG. 11.5 Lymphatic drainage system of head and neck. (If the group of nodes is often referred to by a second name, that name appears in parentheses.) Side view of head and neck shows labels as follows: posterior auricular (mastoid nodes), occipital nodes, sternomastoid nodes, external jugular, retropharyngeal (tonsillar), posterior cervical spinal nerve chain, posterior superficial cervical chain, supraclavicular nodes, internal jugular chain, anterior deep and superficial cervical, thyrolinguofacial, suprahyoid node, sublingual, submental, submandibular, facial, parotid, and preauricular nodes.

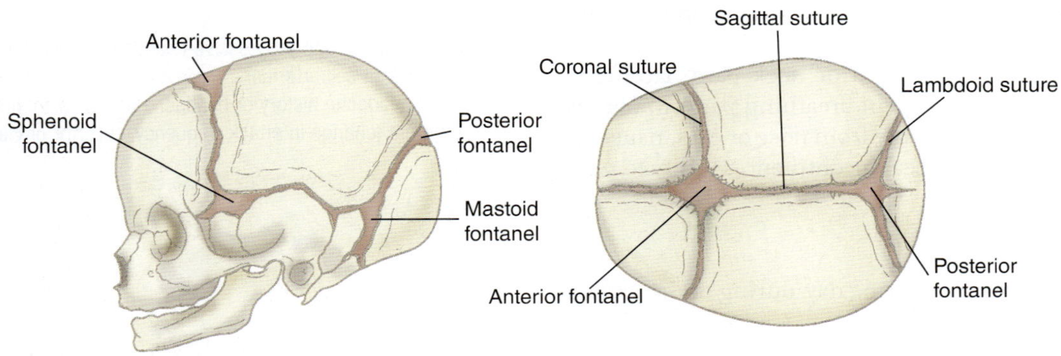

FIG. 11.6 Fontanels and sutures on the infant's skull. Side view of skull shows labels for sphenoid fontanel, anterior fontanel, posterior fontanel, and mastoid fontanel. Top view of skull shows labels for coronal suture, sagittal suture, lambdoid suture, posterior fontanel, and anterior fontanel.

Children and Adolescents

Subtle changes in facial appearance occur throughout childhood. In adolescents assigned male at birth, the nose and thyroid cartilage enlarge and facial hair develops, emerging first on the upper lip, then the cheeks, lower lip, and chin.

Pregnant Patients

The fetal thyroid gland becomes functional in the second trimester. Before this time, the pregnant patient is the source of thyroid hormone for the fetus and thus requires increased iodine intake.

As long as adequate iodine intake is maintained, the size of the thyroid will not detectably change on physical examination; however, a slight enlargement may be detectable on ultrasound (Fig. 11.7).

Older Adults

The rate of T_4 production and degradation gradually decreases with aging, and the thyroid gland becomes more fibrotic.

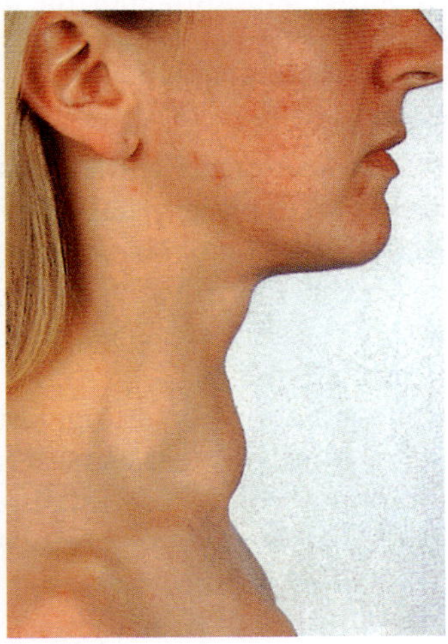

FIG. 11.7 Thyroid enlargement in pregnancy. Note the large nodule in the patient's left lobe. Thyroid size increases in pregnancy in areas of iodine deficiency but not in those with sufficient iodine. Side view of neck of a person shows a large lump. (From Gaw, A., & Murphy, M., et al. (2013). *Clinical biochemistry: an illustrated colour text* (5th ed.). Philadelphia: Elsevier.)

REVIEW OF RELATED HISTORY

For each of the symptoms or conditions discussed in this section, targeted topics to include in the history of the present illness are listed. Responses to questions about these topics provide clues for focusing the physical examination and the development of an appropriate diagnostic evaluation. Questions regarding medication use (prescription and over-the-counter preparations) as well as complementary, alternative, and integrative therapies are relevant for each.

History of Present Illness

Traumatic Brain Injury

- Independent observer's description of event
- State of consciousness after injury: immediately and 5 minutes later; duration of unconsciousness; combative, confused, alert, or dazed (see Chapter 23)
- Predisposing factors: seizure disorder, hypoglycemia, poor vision, lightheadedness, syncope, sports participation
- Associated symptoms: head or neck pain, laceration, local tenderness, change in breathing pattern, blurred or double vision, discharge from nose or ears, nausea or vomiting, urinary or fecal incontinence, ability to move all extremities

Headache

- Onset: early morning, during day, during night; gradual versus abrupt
- Duration: minutes, hours, days, weeks; relieved by medication or sleep; resolves spontaneously; occurs in clusters; headache-free periods
- Location: entire head, unilateral, specific site (neck, sinus region, behind eyes, hatband distribution)
- Character: throbbing, pounding, boring, dull, nagging, constant pressure, aggravated with movement
- Severity: grade each event's severity on a scale from 1 (mild) to 10 (severe)
- Visual prodrome: scotoma; hemianopia (decreased vision or blindness takes place in half the visual field of one or both eyes); distortion of size, shape, or location
- Pattern: worse in the morning or evening, worse or better as day progresses, awakens patient from or occurs only during sleep
- Episodes closer together or worsening, lasting longer
- Change in level of consciousness as pain increases
- Associated symptoms: confusion, impaired alertness, nausea, vomiting, diarrhea, photophobia, visual disturbance, difficulty falling asleep, increased lacrimation, nasal discharge, tinnitus, paresthesia, weight loss, mobility impairment
- Precipitating factors: fever, fatigue, stress, food additives, prolonged fasting, alcohol, seasonal allergies, menstrual cycle, sexual intercourse, oral contraceptives, amount of caffeine intake
- Efforts to treat: sleep, pain medication, need for daily medications, rebound if pain medications are not taken or if caffeine not consumed
- Medications: antiepileptic drugs, antiarrhythmics, beta-blockers, calcium channel blockers, oral contraceptives, serotonin antagonists or agonists, selective serotonin reuptake inhibitors, antidepressants, nonsteroidal antiinflammatory drugs, narcotics, caffeine-containing medication

> **CLINICAL PEARL**
>
> History red flags that can indicate serious pathology causing a headache can be remembered using the "SSNOOP" headache mnemonic:
>
> **S**ystemic symptoms (fever, weight loss)
>
> **S**econdary headache risk factors (HIV, cancer, pregnancy)
>
> **N**eurologic symptoms or abnormal signs (confusion, impaired alertness, or consciousness)
>
> **O**nset: sudden, abrupt, or split-second (subarachnoid hemorrhage, venous sinus thrombosis, arterial dissection, or increased intracranial pressure)
>
> **O**lder: new-onset and progressive headache, especially in middle age >50 (giant cell arteritis)
>
> **P**revious headache history or headache progression: first headache or different (change in attack frequency, severity, or clinical features)

Adapted from Dodick, D. W. (2006). Chronic daily headache. *New England Journal of Medicine, 354*,158–165.

Stiff Neck

- Neck injury or strain, traumatic brain injury, neck swelling
- Fever, associated headache, other symptoms of meningitis (confusion, drowsiness/lethargy, photophobia, cranial nerve deficits, and seizure)
- Character: limitation of movement; pain with movement, pain relieved by movement; continuous or cramping pain; radiation patterns to arms, shoulders, hands, or down the back
- Predisposing factors: unilateral vision or hearing loss, work position (e.g., long hours in front of a computer)
- Efforts to treat: heat, physical therapy, complementary medicine (e.g., chiropractor)
- Medications: analgesics, muscle relaxants
- Symptoms of thyroid disease
- Change in temperature preference: more or less clothing than worn by other members of the household
- Neck swelling; difficulty swallowing; redness; pain with touch, swallowing, or hyperextension of the neck
- Change in texture of hair, skin, or nails; increased pigmentation of skin at pressure points
- Change in mood and energy, irritability, nervousness or lethargy, disinterest
- Increased prominence of eyes (exophthalmos), periorbital swelling, blurred or double vision
- Tachycardia, palpitations

- Change in menses
- Change in bowel habits
- Medications: thyroid preparations

Past Medical History

- Traumatic brain injury
- Subdural hematoma
- Recent lumbar puncture
- Radiation treatment around head and neck
- Headaches (see "Differential Diagnosis")
- Surgery for tumor, goiter
- Seizure disorder
- Thyroid dysfunction
- Neck arthritis

Family History

- Headaches: type, character, similarity to that of the patient
- Thyroid dysfunction
- Hydrocephalus

Personal and Social History

- Employment: job type, risk of traumatic brain injury, use of hard hat or other protective headgear, exposure to toxins or chemicals
- Stress; tension; demands at home, work, or school
- Potential risk of injury: handrails available; use of seat belts, car seats, and booster seats; unsafe environment
- Nutrition: recent weight gain or loss, food intolerances, eating habits (e.g., skipping meals)
- Alcohol or substance use
- Sports participation, weight training, use of protective padding and helmet, if necessary

Infants

- Prenatal history: maternal use of drugs or alcohol, uterine abnormalities, treatment of hyperthyroidism
- Birth history: birth order (firstborn more likely to experience torticollis); vaginal or cesarean section delivery; presentation, difficulty of delivery, use of forceps or other assist device (associated with caput succedaneum, cephalohematoma, facial nerve palsy, molding)
- Unusual head shape: bulging or flattening (congenital anomaly or positioning in utero), preterm infant, head held at angle, preferred position at rest, frequency of supine position (see Patient Safety, "Back to Sleep")
- Strength of head control
- Acute illness: diarrhea, vomiting, fever, limited neck movement, irritability (associated with meningitis)
- Congenital anomalies: craniofacial abnormalities (e.g., Pierre Robin sequence, encephalocele, microcephaly, hydrocephalus)
- Neonatal screening for congenital hypothyroidism

Pregnant Patients

- Weeks of gestation or postpartum
- Presence of preexisting disease (e.g., hypothyroidism, hyperthyroidism), access to iodine-rich foods or use of antithyroid medication
- History of pregnancy-induced hypertension (PIH)
- Alcohol and substance use

Older Adults

- Dizziness or vertigo with head or neck movement
- Weakness or impaired balance (increases risk of falling and head injury)

EXAMINATION AND FINDINGS

Equipment

- Tape measure (primarily for infants)
- Stethoscope
- Cup of water (for evaluation of thyroid gland)
- Transilluminator (or flashlight) for infants

Head and Face

Inspection

Begin examining the head and neck by inspecting the head position and facial features. The patient's head should be upright and still. A horizontal jerking or bobbing motion may be associated with a tremor; a nodding movement may be associated with aortic insufficiency, especially if the nodding is synchronized with the pulse. Holding the head tilted to one side to favor a good eye or ear often occurs with unilateral hearing or vision loss, but it is also associated with torticollis (shortening or excessive contraction of the sternocleidomastoid muscle; see Fig. 11.36).

Inspect facial features (i.e., eyelids, eyebrows, palpebral fissures, nasolabial folds, and mouth) for shape and symmetry with rest (some slight asymmetry is common); movement; and expression. By doing this, the integrity of CN V and VII (trigeminal and facial, respectively) has been partially tested. Complete evaluation of the cranial nerves is detailed in Chapter 23.

Facies is defined as an expression or appearance of the face and features of the head and neck that, when considered together, is characteristic of a clinical condition or syndrome. Once a facies is recognized, the examiner may be able to diagnose the condition or syndrome even before completing the examination. Note any change in the shape of the face or any unusual features, such as edema, bruising, coarsened features, exophthalmos, hirsutism, lack of expression, excessive perspiration, pallor, or pigmentation variations. Facies may develop slowly, and the health care clinician should be alert to early changes suggestive of a developing facies. For example, a patient with early changes of acromegaly is shown in Fig. 11.14. One way to better appreciate these changes is to ask the patient to provide an older photograph of themselves. Figs. 11.8 to 11.22 demonstrate some facies and their associated disorders.

When facial asymmetry is present, note whether all features on one side of the face are affected or only a portion of the face, such as the forehead, lower face, or mouth. Suspect facial nerve damage near or in the brainstem when the entire side of the face is affected, and suspect peripheral facial nerve weakness when the lower face is affected (see Fig. 11.13). If only the mouth

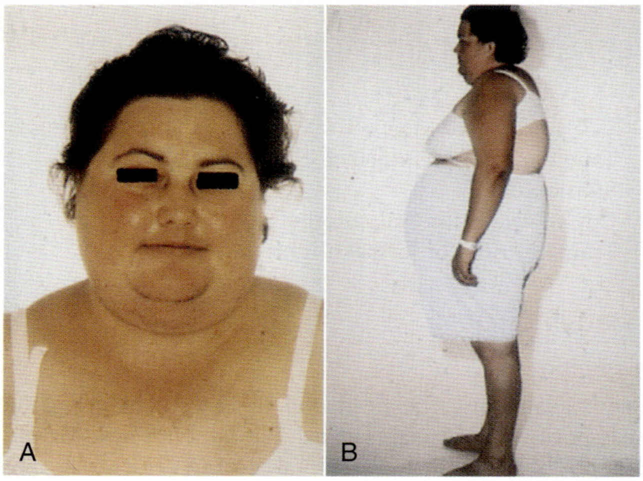

FIG. 11.8 (A) Cushing syndrome facies, a rounded or moon-shaped face with thin erythematous skin. (B) Side view of the same patient with upper thoracic fat pad (buffalo hump). (From Melmed, S., Koenig, R., Rosen, C. J., Auchus, R. J., & Goldfine, A. B. (2019). *Williams textbook of endocrinology* (14th ed.).)

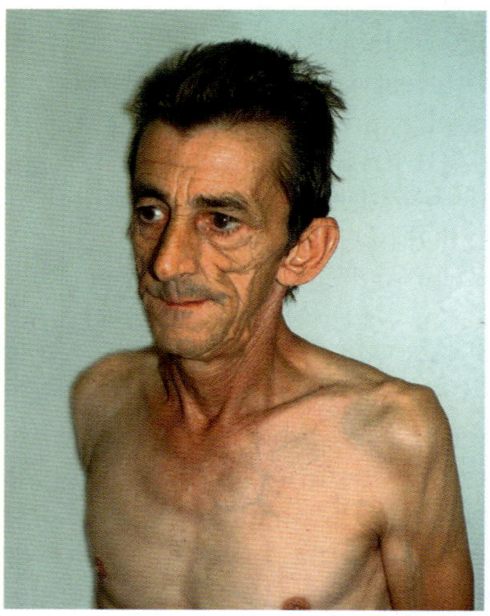

FIG. 11.9 Hippocratic facies. Note sunken appearance of the eyes, cheeks, and temporal areas; sharp nose; and dry, rough skin seen in this patient in the terminal stages of throat cancer. Side view of patient's face and chest area shows prominent bones mainly on the shoulder, neck, and face. (From Lemmi, F. O., & Lemmi, C. A. E. (2001). *Physical assessment findings [CD-ROM].* Philadelphia: Saunders.)

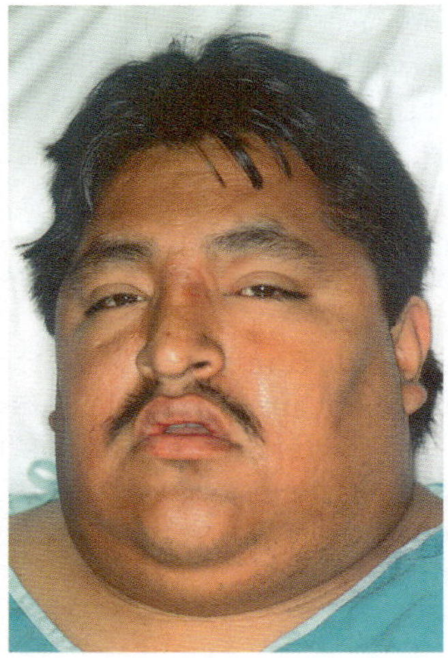

FIG. 11.10 Myxedema facies. Note dull, puffy, yellowed skin; coarse, sparse hair; temporal loss of eyebrows; periorbital edema; and prominent tongue. Close-up view of face of a patient shows excess fat under the chin and neck. (From Lemmi, F. O., & Lemmi, C. A. E. (2001). *Physical assessment findings [CD-ROM].* Philadelphia: Saunders.)

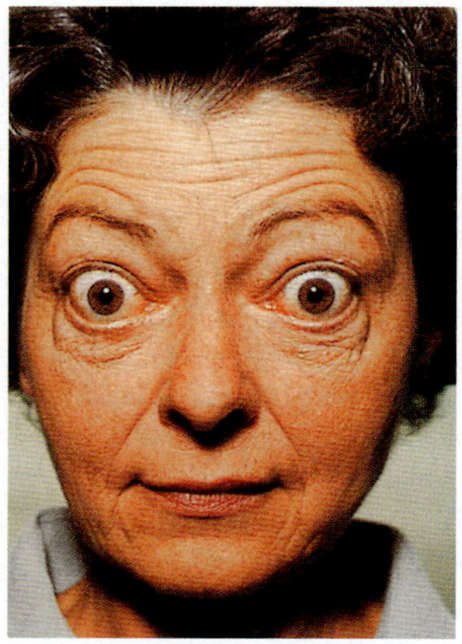

FIG. 11.11 Hyperthyroid facies. Note fine, moist skin with fine hair, prominent eyes and lid retraction, and staring or startled expression. Close-up view of face of a patient shows large protruding eyes and wrinkles on the forehead, under eyes, and at the mouth corners. (From Gaw, A., & Murphy, M., et al. (2013). *Clinical biochemistry: an illustrated colour text* (5th ed.). Philadelphia: Elsevier.)

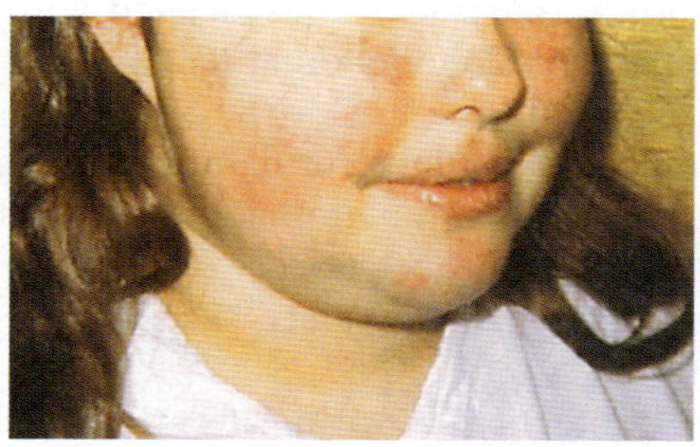

FIG. 11.12 Butterfly rash of systemic lupus erythematosus. Note butterfly-shaped rash over malar surfaces and bridge of nose. Either a blush with swelling or scaly, red, maculopapular lesions may be present. Close-up view of patient's cheek shows red patches. (Courtesy Walter Tunnessen, MD, Chapel Hill, NC.)

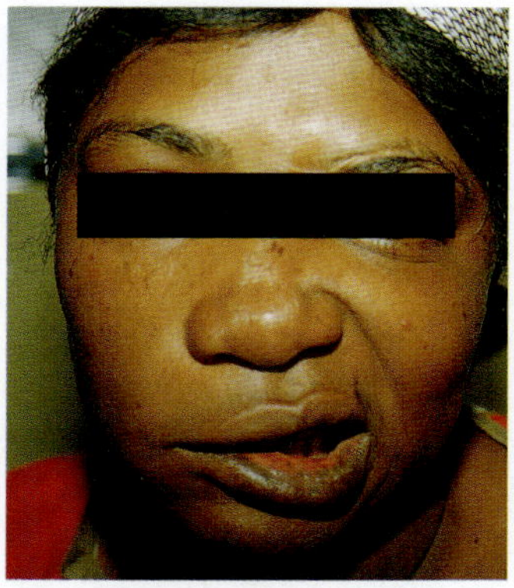

FIG. 11.13 Bell palsy. Left facial palsy (cranial nerve VII). Facies include asymmetry of one side of the face, eyelid not closing completely, drooping lower eyelid and corner of mouth, and loss of nasolabial fold. Close-up of woman's face shows asymmetry and mouth turned to the left side with lower lip slightly hanging. (From Mancall, E. L., & Brock, D. G. (2011). Gray's clinical neuroanatomy: The anatomic basis for clinical neuroscience.)

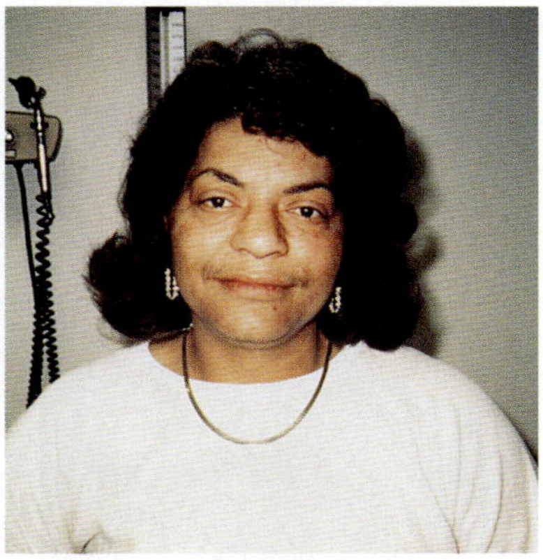

FIG. 11.14 Early acromegaly. Note the coarsening of features with broadening of the nasal alae and prominence of the zygomatic arches. Close-up of a woman's face and region above best shows a broad nose and wrinkles under the eyes. (Courtesy Gary Wand, MD, Johns Hopkins University and Hospital, Baltimore, MD.)

is involved, suspect a problem with the peripheral trigeminal nerve.

Tics—spasmodic muscular contractions of the face, head, or neck—should be noted. They may be associated with pressure on or degenerative changes of the facial nerves, a feature of Tourette syndrome, or possibly psychogenic in origin (functional neurologic disorder).

Inspect the skull for size, shape, and symmetry. Examine the scalp by systematically parting the hair from the frontal to occipital region, noting any lesions, scabs, tenderness, nits, or scaliness (Fig. 11.23). Pay special attention to the areas behind the ears, at the hairline, and at the crown of the head. Note any hair loss (alopecia) pattern, such as bitemporal recession of hair or balding over the crown of the head (more common in males than in females), or hair loss associated with tight braiding. In children, a common cause of hair loss is tinea capitis (fungal infection of the scalp).

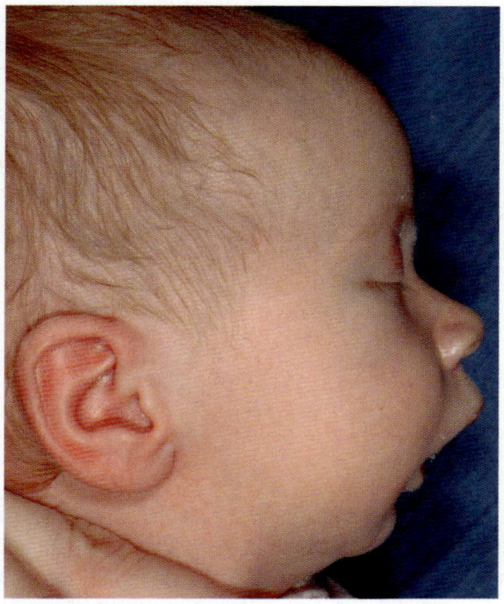

FIG. 11.15 Pierre Robin sequence; a triad of micrognathia, glossoptosis, and palatal clefting. Shows a lateral view with severe micrognathia and cleft palate. Note the small retruded mandible. Side view of infant's face shows underdeveloped lower jaw and chin. (From Neligan, P. C., & Buck, D. W. (Eds.). (2013). Core procedures in plastic surgery.)

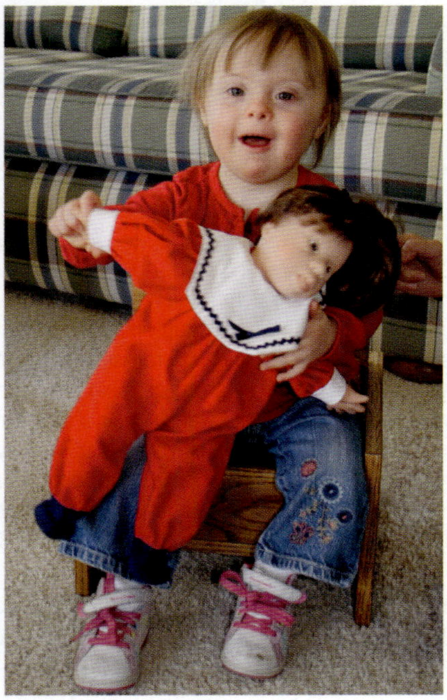

FIG. 11.16 Down syndrome. Note depressed nasal bridge, epicanthal folds, mongoloid slant of eyes, and low-set ears. Close-up view of a child suffering from Down syndrome sitting on a chair with a doll in their hands. (From Hockenberry, M. J., & Wilson, D. (2012). *Wong's essentials of pediatric nursing* (9th ed.).)

Palpation

Palpate the skull in a gentle rotary movement, progressing systematically from front to back. The skull should be symmetric and smooth. The bones should be indistinguishable, as the sites of fusion are not generally palpable after 6 months of age; however, the ridge of the sagittal

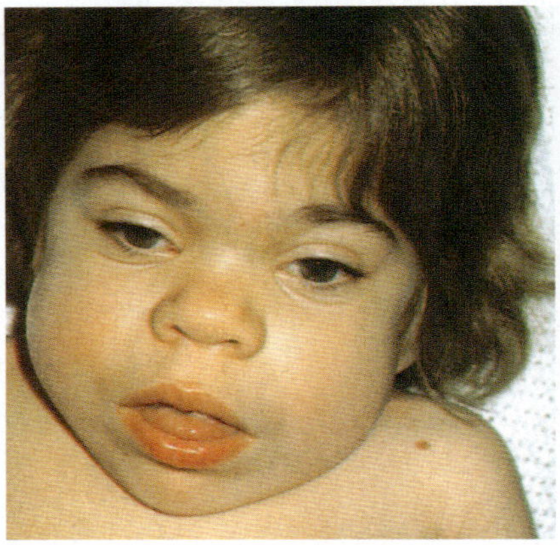

FIG. 11.17 **Hurler syndrome.** Facies includes enlarged skull with low forehead, corneal clouding, and short neck. Close-up view of child's face shows chin touching the region below the neck and the tongue slightly protruding outward. (From Ansell, B. M., et al. (1992). Color atlas of pediatric rheumatology. London: Mosby-Wolfe.)

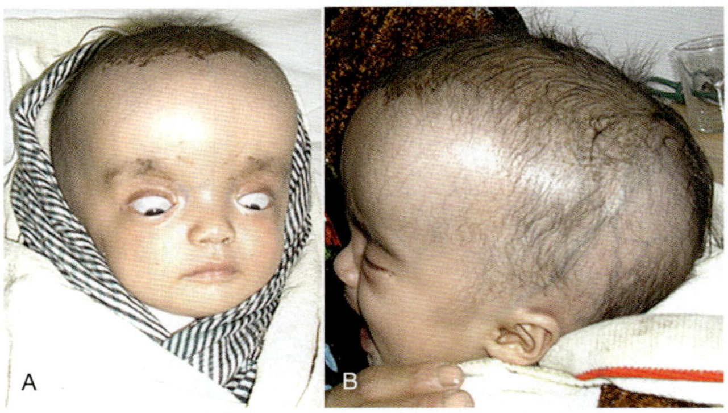

FIG. 11.18 **Hydrocephalus.** (A) Coronal view with characteristic enlarged head, thinning of the scalp with dilated scalp veins, and bossing of the skull. (B) Anteroposterior view demonstrating sclera visible above the iris. In this case the infant has paresis of upward gaze. This phenomenon is often termed the *sunsetting sign.* (A) Front view of child's face shows enlarged forehead, loss of hair on eyebrows, and only small portion of eyeballs visible near the lower eyelid. (B) Side view of child's face shows enlarged head with veins clearly visible and less density of hair. (From Amelot, A., et al. (2013). Resolution of the sunset sign. *Pediatr Neurol, 49*(5):383-384.)

suture may be felt on some individuals. The scalp should move freely over the skull, and no tenderness, swelling, or depressions on palpation are expected. Tenderness with an indentation or a depression of the skull may indicate a skull fracture.

Palpate the patient's hair, noting its texture, color, and distribution. Hair should be smooth and symmetrically distributed with no splitting or cracked ends. Coarse, dry, and brittle hair may be associated with hypothyroidism. Fine, silky hair may be associated with hyperthyroidism or may be inherited.

Palpate the temporomandibular joint space bilaterally, as described in Chapter 22, Figs. 22.26 and 22.27.

Inspect for any asymmetry or growth of the salivary glands. If noted, palpate for possible discrete growth (see Fig. 11.33), noting whether the gland is fixed or movable,

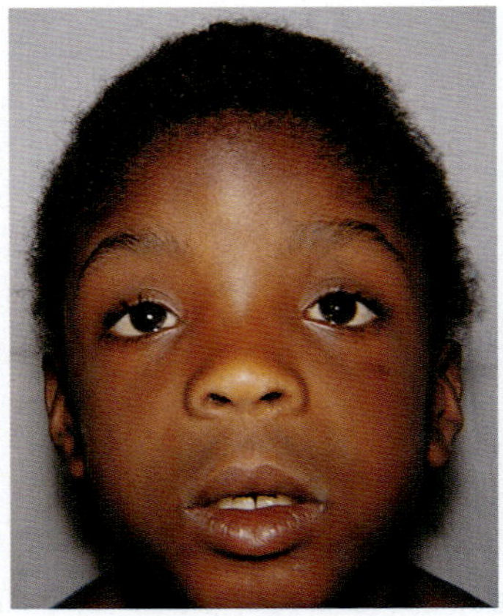

FIG. 11.19 **Fetal alcohol syndrome.** This is one of the most common causes of acquired intellectual disability. Note the poorly formed philtrum; widespread eyes, with inner epicanthal folds and mild ptosis; hirsute forehead; short nose; and relatively thin upper lip. Front view of young boy's face shows small forehead with hair and a large gap between the base of the nose and upper lip. (From Zitelli, B. J., & Davis, H. W. (2002). *Atlas of pediatric physical diagnosis* (4th ed.). St. Louis: Mosby.)

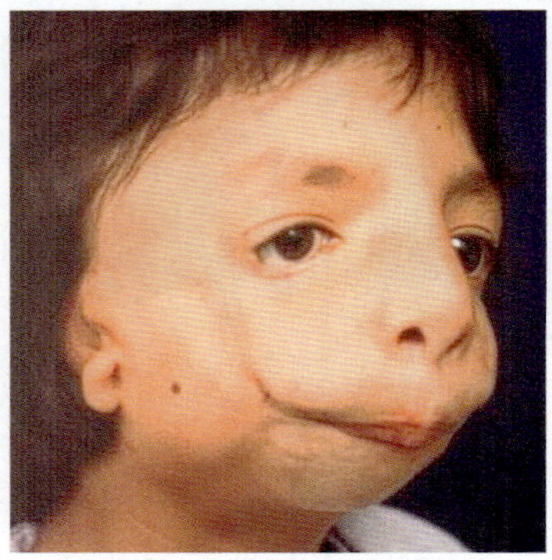

FIG. 11.20 **Treacher Collins syndrome.** Note the maxillary hypoplasia, micrognathia, and auricular deformity. Side view of a child's face shows deformed ear, protruding upper lip, very small lower jaw, and underdeveloped chin. (From Neligan P. C., & Buck D. W., II. (Eds.). (2013). Core procedures in plastic surgery.)

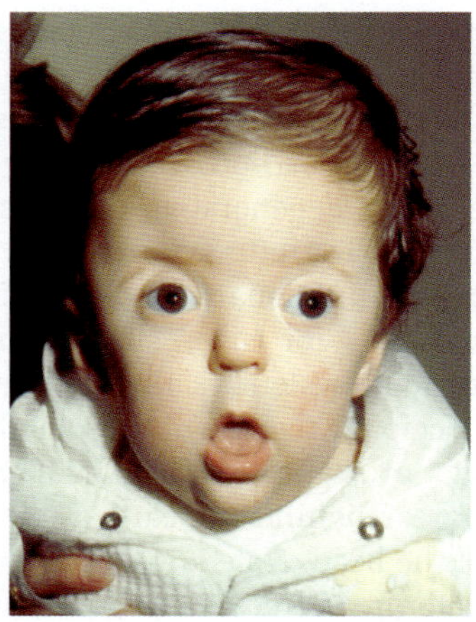

FIG. 11.21 **Apert syndrome.** Note the severe maxillary and midfacial hypoplasia. Front view of a child's face shows sunken appearance on forehead and open mouth with lower lip larger than the upper lip. (From Jones, K. L., & Jones, M. C. (2013). Smith's recognizable patterns of human malformation.)

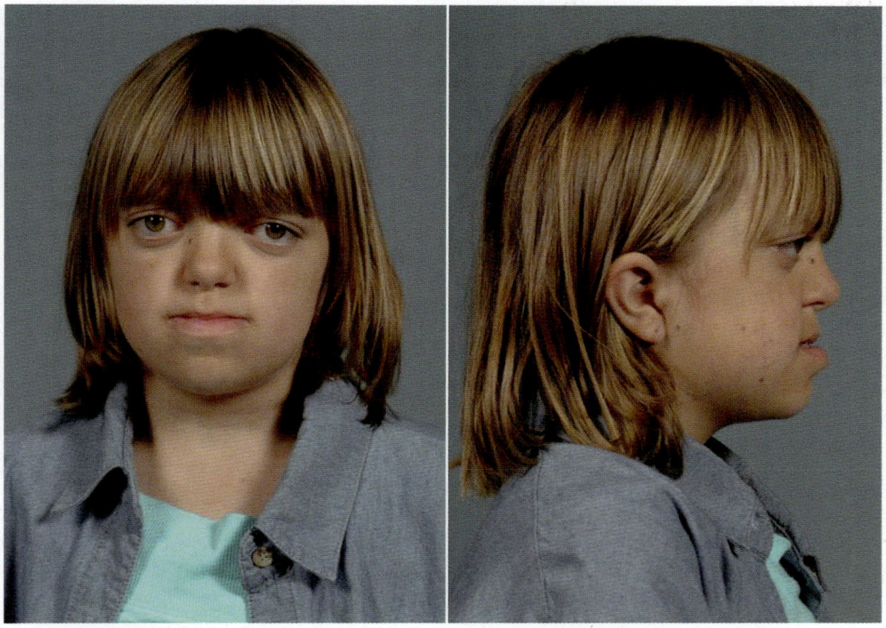

FIG. 11.22 Crouzon syndrome. Observe the severe maxillary and midfacial hypoplasia with low-set ears. Front and side views of a young girl's face show underdeveloped upper lip. (From Dicus Brookes, C., et al. (2014). Craniosynostosis syndromes. *Atlas Oral Maxillofac Surg Clin North Am*, *22*(2):103-110.)

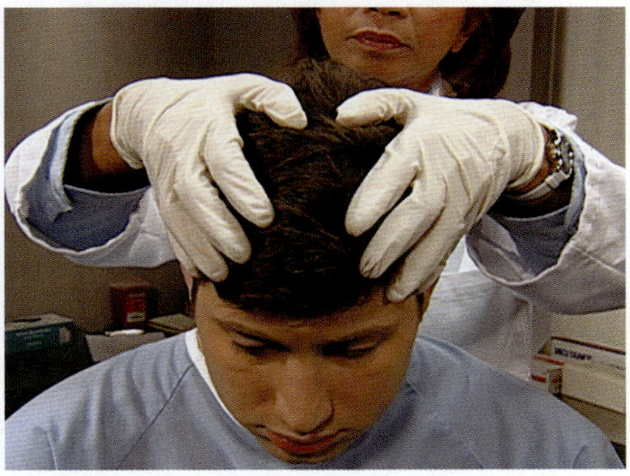

FIG. 11.23 Inspection of the scalp. Close-up view of gloved hands of a health care professional standing behind and examining the scalp of a patient.

soft or hard, tender or nontender. With the patient's mouth open, try to squeeze out substances through the salivary ducts by pressing on the glands. The parotid duct, also known as the *Stensen duct,* opens into the mouth next to the maxillary second molar tooth. The submandibular duct (Wharton duct) opens in a small papilla at the sides of the frenulum. An enlarged, tender gland may suggest either viral or bacterial infection or a ductal stone preventing saliva from exiting the gland. A discrete nodule may represent a cyst or tumor that is either benign or malignant.

Percussion

Percussion of the head and neck is not routinely performed. One exception is when evaluating for hypocalcemia; percussion on the masseter muscle may produce a hyperactive masseteric reflex: the Chvostek sign.

Auscultation

Auscultation of the skull is not routinely performed. However, intracranial bruits are considered uncommon in neonates but common in childhood. For example, in individuals who develop diplopia, a bruit or blowing sound over the orbit may be rarely heard and suggests an expanding cerebral aneurysm. If you suspect a vascular anomaly of the brain, use the bell of the stethoscope and listen over the temporal region, over the eyes, and below the occiput (Fig. 11.24). A bruit is highly suggestive of a vascular anomaly. Ultrasound is also a valuable tool for

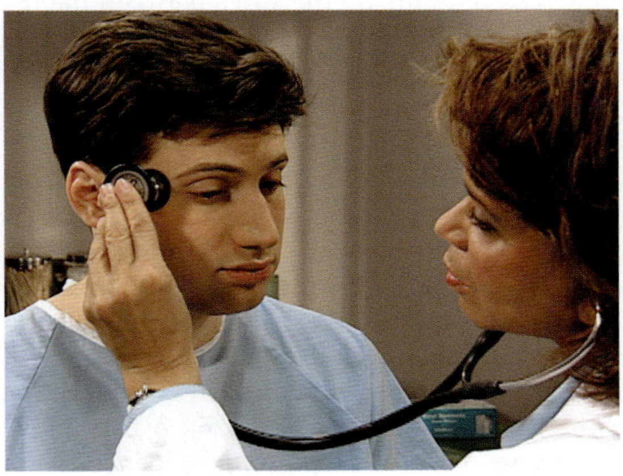

FIG. 11.24 Auscultation for a temporal bruit. A health care professional wearing a stethoscope and placing the diaphragm on one side of the eyebrow close to the right ear of a patient.

evaluating an infant's brain for intracranial vascular abnormalities. A bruit can also be associated with temporal arteritis, along with tenderness along the temporal artery.

Neck

Inspection

Inspect the neck in the usual anatomic position, in slight hyperextension, and as the patient swallows. Look for bilateral symmetry of the sternocleidomastoid and trapezius muscles, alignment of the trachea, landmarks of the anterior and posterior triangles, and any subtle fullness at the base of the neck. Note any apparent masses, webbing, excess skinfolds, unusual shortness, or asymmetry. Observe for any distention of the jugular vein or prominence of the carotid arteries. Carotid artery and jugular vein examinations are described in Chapter 16.

Webbing, excessive posterior cervical skin, or an unusually short neck may be associated with chromosomal abnormalities (e.g., Turner syndrome). The transverse portion of the omohyoid muscle in the posterior triangle can sometimes be mistaken for a mass. Marked edema of the neck may be associated with local infections (e.g., cervical lymphadenitis). A mass filling the base of the neck or visible thyroid tissue that glides upward when the patient swallows may indicate an enlarged thyroid or goiter (see Fig. 11.7).

Evaluate range of motion by asking the patient to flex, extend, rotate, and laterally turn the head and neck (see Chapter 22). Movement should be smooth and painless and should not cause dizziness. Nuchal rigidity—resistance to flexion of the neck—may be associated with meningeal irritation. CN XI (spinal accessory nerve) may also be examined (see Chapter 23, Table 23.3, Figs 23.24A and 23.24B).

Palpation

The ability to palpate and identify structures in the neck varies with the patient's habitus.

Palpate the trachea for midline position. Place a thumb along each side of the trachea in the lower portion of the neck (Fig. 11.25). Compare the space between the trachea and the sternocleidomastoid muscle on each side. An unequal space indicates displacement of the trachea from the midline and may be associated with a mass or pathologic condition in the chest.

Identify the hyoid bone and the thyroid and cricoid cartilages. They should be smooth and nontender and should move under your finger when the patient swallows. On palpation, the cartilaginous rings of the trachea in the lower portion of the neck should be distinct and nontender.

With the patient's neck extended, position the index finger and thumb of one hand on each side of the trachea below the thyroid isthmus (Fig. 11.26). A tugging sensation, synchronous with the pulse, is evidence of the tracheal tug sign (Cardarelli sign or Oliver sign), suggesting the presence of an aortic aneurysm (see Clinical Pearl, "Cardarelli Sign and Oliver Sign").

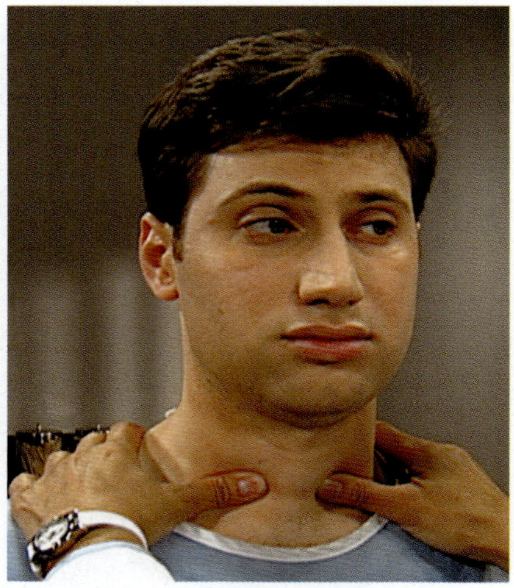

FIG. 11.25 Position of the thumbs to evaluate the midline position of the trachea. Close-up view of health care professional's hands pressing around the trachea of a patient using their thumbs.

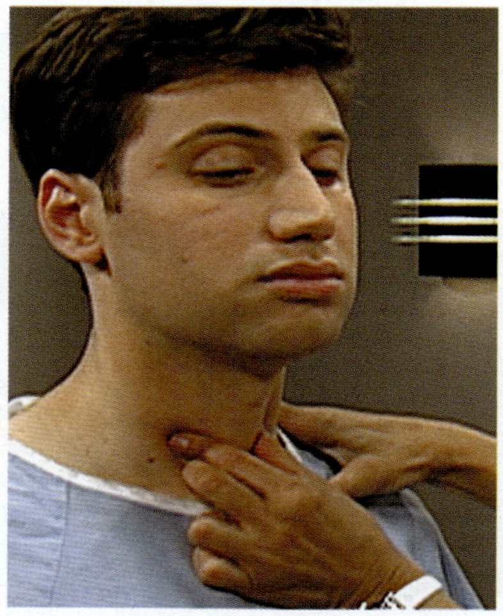

FIG. 11.26 Position of the thumb and finger to detect tracheal tugging. Close-up view of one hand being placed on the shoulder of a patient while gripping the skin around the trachea using the thumb and index finger of the other hand.

The paravertebral muscles and posterior spinous processes should be palpated for tenderness. This examination coupled with neck range of motion is useful in the evaluation of a stiff neck. See Chapter 22.

> **CLINICAL PEARL**
>
> **Cardarelli Sign and Oliver Sign**
>
> The Cardarelli sign can be felt by pressing on the thyroid cartilage and displacing it to the patient's left. This increases contact between the left bronchus and the aorta, allowing systolic pulsations from the aorta to be felt at the surface if an aneurysm is present. The Oliver sign is elicited by gently grasping the cricoid cartilage and applying upward pressure while the patient stands with their chin extended upward. Because of the anatomic position of the aortic arch, which overrides the left main bronchus, a downward tug of the trachea may be felt if an aneurysm is present.

Lymph Nodes

Inspect and palpate the head and neck for lymph nodes. A description of the sequence is given in Chapter 10.

Thyroid Gland

Examination of the thyroid gland involves inspection, palpation, and occasionally auscultation. Begin by asking patients to gently extend their neck. (Hyperextension can actually make the examination more difficult.) Ask them to swallow, which often permits visualization of the gland's size, symmetry, and contour because it moves with swallowing. An enlarged thyroid gland may be visible only when observing from the lateral aspect. A glass of water can be indispensable for examining the thyroid, as it helps the patient swallow multiple times.

Palpation of the thyroid gland requires a gentle touch. Nodules and asymmetry will be more difficult to detect if pressing too hard. Palpate the thyroid for size, shape, configuration, consistency, tenderness, and the presence of any nodules. Although the thyroid gland may be palpated from in front of or behind the patient, facing the patient facilitates the correlation of inspection with palpation findings. It is also more convenient in examining rooms where the table is against a wall. Choose one approach to use consistently.

Evidence-Based Practice in Physical Examination

Thyroid Examination

Estimates of thyroid size tend to be exaggerated when the gland is small and underestimated when the gland is markedly enlarged (more than twice the normal size). Evaluations were made by comparing the estimated size on physical examination with the size measured by ultrasound or after surgical excision. The estimation of thyroid size by lateral inspection is the most sensitive test for determining the presence of a goiter; a thyroid that is not visible on lateral inspection rules out a goiter.

For both approaches, position the patient to relax the sternocleidomastoid, with the neck flexed slightly forward and laterally toward the side being examined. Ask the patient to hold a sip of water in the mouth until you have your hands positioned, and then instruct the patient to swallow.

To palpate the thyroid using the frontal approach, have the patient sit on the examining table. First place your thumb over the trachea approximately 3 cm beneath the prominence of the thyroid cartilage, and during a swallow, attempt to identify the isthmus. To examine the right lobe of the thyroid, use your left thumb to press the trachea toward the patient's right. Such pressure helps move the right lobe out of the tracheoesophageal groove for easier palpation. Then place the first three fingers of your right hand in the right thyroid bed with your fingertips medial to the margin of the sternocleidomastoid muscle. Leave your fingers still while the patient again swallows, thus allowing the gland to move beneath your fingers (Fig. 11.27). To examine the left lobe, move your hands to the reverse corresponding positions. By palpating above the cricoid cartilage, you may be able to feel the pyramidal lobe of the thyroid, if present.

To examine the thyroid from behind, have the patient sit with the neck at a comfortable level. Position two fingers of each hand on the sides of the trachea just beneath the cricoid cartilage. Ask the patient to swallow, feeling for movement of the isthmus. Then displace the trachea to the left (using your fingers of your right hand), and with the first three fingers of your left hand medial to the left sternocleidomastoid, palpate the left lobe as the patient swallows again. To palpate the right lobe, repeat using your hands in the reverse corresponding positions (Fig. 11.28).

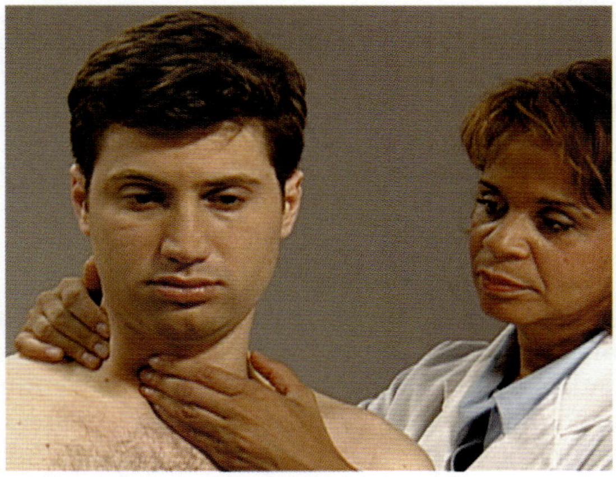

FIG. 11.27 Palpation of the right thyroid lobe and lateral border from in front of the patient. A health care professional feeling the right thyroid lobe of a patient using the fingertips of both hands.

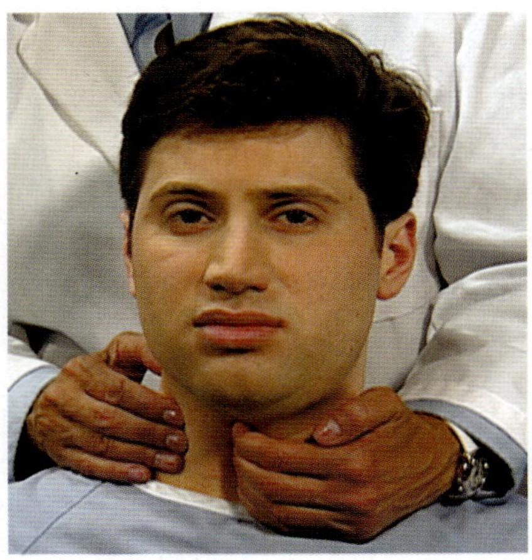

FIG. 11.28 Palpation of the right thyroid lobe from behind the patient. Displace the trachea to the patient's right and palpate the right lobe as the patient again swallows. Close-up view of a health care professional standing behind and checking the right thyroid lobe of a patient using the fingertips of one hand and the nails of the other hand.

CLINICAL PEARL

Is It the Thyroid Gland?

The thyroid gland moves with swallowing; subcutaneous fat that mimics a goiter does not.

The thyroid lobes, if felt, should be small, smooth, and free of nodules. The gland should rise freely with swallowing. The thyroid at its broadest dimension is approximately 4 cm, and the right lobe is often 25% larger than the left. The consistency of the thyroid tissue should be firm yet pliable. Coarse tissue or a gritty sensation suggests an inflammatory process. If nodules are present, they should be characterized by number, whether they are smooth or irregular, and whether they are soft or hard. An enlarged, tender thyroid may indicate thyroiditis (see Clinical Pearl, "Is It the Thyroid Gland?").

If the thyroid gland is enlarged, auscultate for vascular sounds with the bell of the stethoscope. In a hypermetabolic state, the blood supply is dramatically increased, and a vascular bruit may be heard.

Infants

Inspection

Measure the infant's head circumference and compare it with expected size for age and previous points on the growth chart, as detailed in Chapter 8. Inspect the infant's head from all angles for symmetry of shape, noting any prominent bulges or depressions (see Clinical Pearl, "Examining the Head"). Inspect the scalp for scaling and crusting, birthmarks or skin lesions, dilated scalp veins, the presence of excessive hair, or unusual hairline. Dilated scalp veins and a head circumference increasing faster than expected may indicate increased intracranial pressure (hydrocephalus; see Fig. 11.18).

CLINICAL PEARL

Examining the Head

Examining the head from above is helpful for evaluating head shape.

Birth trauma may cause swelling of the scalp. Caput succedaneum is subcutaneous edema over the presenting part of the head at delivery (Fig. 11.29). It is the most common form of birth trauma of the scalp and usually occurs over the occiput, and the edema crosses suture lines. The affected part of the scalp feels soft, and the margins are poorly defined. Generally, the edema resolves in a few days.

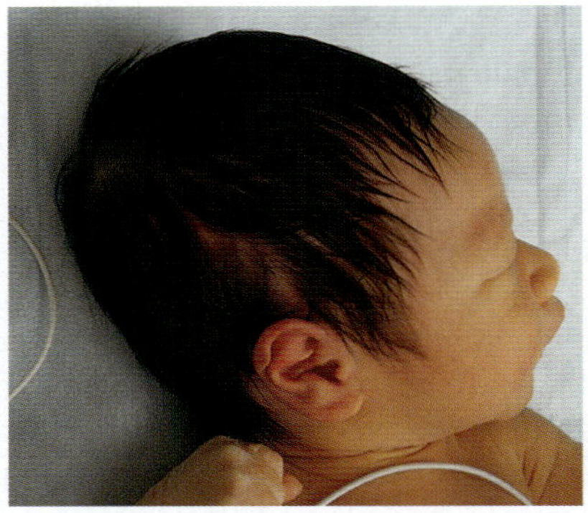

FIG. 11.29 Caput succedaneum. Significant scalp edema as a result of compression during transit through the birth canal. Edema does cross suture lines. Side view of the large head and face of an infant, lying in supine position, shows protruded upper lip. (From Price, D. L. (2012). *Pediatric nursing: an introductory text* (11th ed.). Elsevier.)

Cephalohematoma is a subperiosteal collection of blood and is therefore bound by the suture lines. It is commonly found in the parietal region and, unlike caput, may not be immediately obvious at birth. A cephalohematoma is firm, and its edges are well defined; it does not cross suture lines. As it ages, the cephalohematoma may liquefy and become fluctuant on palpation (Fig. 11.30).

Inspect the face for spacing of the features, symmetry, paralysis, skin color, and texture. Uterine positioning can cause some facial asymmetry in the newborn.

Head shape with an unusual contour may be related to premature or irregular closing of suture lines. Preterm infants often have long, narrow heads (brachycephaly) because their soft cranial bones become flattened with positioning and the weight of the head. Note any skull asymmetry or a particularly flattened spot on the back or one side of the head (plagiocephaly).

Think About It

On examination, when skull deformation, or asymmetrical distortion, reveals a flat spot on one side of the head or the whole back of the head (plagiocephaly), think about what could cause the infant to lie in the same position most of the time; these include the following: torticollis (see Fig 11.36), prematurity, and back sleeping.

Plagiocephaly can result from premature fusion of one of the sutures (craniosynostosis; see Fig. 11.39) or from external deformation (positional plagiocephaly). Positional plagiocephaly is common among infants with torticollis or those who prefer one head position for sleep. Bossing (bulging of the skull) of the frontal areas is associated with prematurity, thalassemia, Paget disease, and rickets. Bulging in other areas of the skull may indicate cranial defects or intracranial masses.

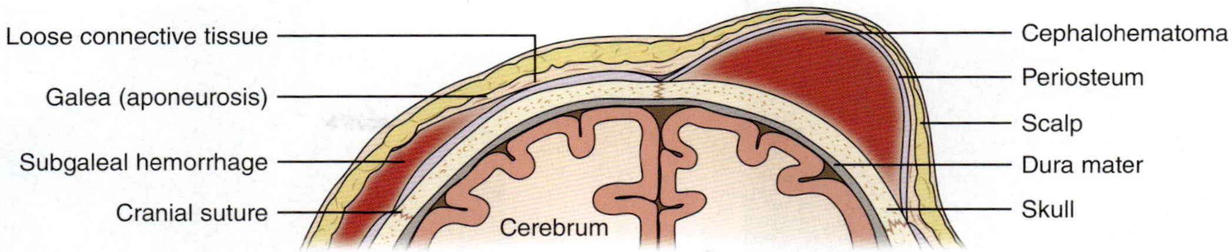

FIG. 11.30 **Cephalohematoma.** Swelling does not cross suture lines. Upper part of skull with inflammation shows labels as follows: cephalohematoma, periosteum, scalp, dura mater, skull, cerebrum, cranial suture, subgaleal hemorrhage, galea (aponeurosis), and loose connective tissue. (From Martin et al. (2015). Fanaroff and Martin's neonatal-perinatal medicine e-book: Diseases of the fetus and infant.)

Patient Safety

Back to Sleep

The American Academy of Pediatrics recommendations focus on a safe sleep environment to reduce the risk of all sleep-related infant deaths, including sudden infant death syndrome (SIDS). The recommendations include supine positioning ("Back to Sleep"); use of a firm, noninclined sleep surface; breastfeeding (unless contraindicated); room sharing without bed sharing; routine immunizations; consideration of pacifier use; and avoidance of soft bedding (a wearable blanket is preferable to blankets to reduce the risk of head covering or entrapment), overheating (to decrease risk of overheating, it is advised not to place hats on infants when indoors), and exposure to tobacco smoke, nicotine, alcohol, marijuana, opioids, and illicit drug use. In addition, there are no data that other commercial devices that are designed to monitor infant vital signs reduce the risk of SIDS, and there is concern that use of these monitors will lead to parent complacency and decreased adherence to safe sleep guidelines. Although "Back to Sleep" greatly reduced the incidence of SIDS, there has been a dramatic increase in positional plagiocephaly. The risk of positional plagiocephaly can be reduced by supervised, awake tummy time to facilitate development and to minimize the formation of positional plagiocephaly. In addition, beginning at birth, alternate the supine head position (i.e., left or right occiput) during sleep nightly. For infants who prefer to face an open door, alternate the infant's position between the head and foot of the crib. Additionally, periodically changing the orientation of the infant to outside activity can also be beneficial for prevention (From Moon, R. Y., Carlin, R. F., Hand, I.; The Task Force on Sudden Infant Death Syndrome and the Committee on Fetus and Newborn. [2022]. Sleep-related infant deaths: Updated 2022 recommendations for reducing infant deaths in the sleep environment. *Pediatrics, 150*[1], e2022057991.)

Observe the infant's head control, position, and movement. Note any jerking, tremors, or inability to move the head in one direction. Chapters 22 and 23 provide further details.

Inspect the infant's neck for symmetry, size, and shape. Note the presence of edema, distended neck veins, pulsations, masses, webbing, or excessive nuchal skin. To observe the newborn's neck, which is usually not easily visible in the supine position, elevate the upper back of the infant and permit the head to fall back into extension. The neck appears short during infancy and lengthens by 3 to 4 years of age. Marked edema may indicate a localized infection. A cystic mass high in the neck may be a thyroglossal duct cyst or a branchial cleft cyst. A mass over the clavicle, changing size with crying or respiration, suggests a cystic hygroma.

Palpation

Palpate the infant's head, identifying suture lines and fontanels. Note any tenderness over the scalp. Suture lines feel ridgelike until about 6 months of age, after which they are usually no longer palpable. Vaginally delivered newborns may have molding with prominent ridges from overriding sutures. Fontanels may be small or not palpable at birth. A third fontanel (the mastoid fontanel), located between the anterior and posterior fontanels, may be an expected variant and is common in infants with Down syndrome. Any palpable ridges in addition to the expected suture lines may indicate skull fractures.

Measure the size of the anterior and posterior fontanels using two dimensions (anteroposterior and lateral). In infants younger than 6 months, the anterior fontanel diameter should not exceed 4 to 5 cm. It should get progressively smaller beyond that age, closing completely by 12 to 15 months of age.

CLINICAL PEARL

Resolution of Molding

Molding of the head at delivery can be highly distressing for parents. Reassure the parents that the abnormal shape generally resolves relatively quickly (Fig. 11.31). Drawings can help you explain that the infant's cranial bones overlap and that their relative lack of development is a protective device for the brain. Symmetry of the head is usually regained within 1 week of birth, with fontanels and suture lines resuming their appropriate shape and size.

With the infant in a supported sitting position, palpate the anterior fontanel for bulging or depression. It should feel slightly depressed, and some pulsation is expected. A bulging fontanel protrudes above the level of the bones of the skull when the infant is sitting and feels tense, similar to the fontanel of an infant during the expiratory phase of crying. A bulging fontanel with marked pulsations may

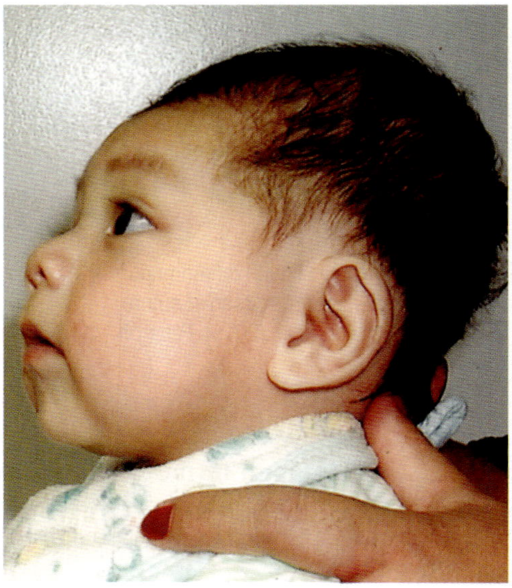

FIG. 11.31 Molding of the newborn head. Side view of the oblong head of an infant. (From Graham, J. M., & Sanchez-Lara, P. A. (2016). *Smith's recognizable patterns of human deformation* (4th ed.). Elsevier.)

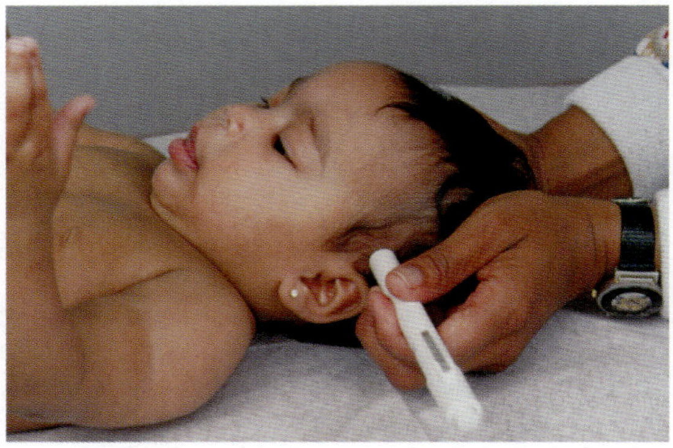

FIG. 11.32 Transillumination of the infant's scalp. Close-up view of a health care professional's hand placing the tip of the transilluminator on one side of the infant's head above the left ear.

indicate increased intracranial pressure from a space-occupying mass or meningitis.

> **CLINICAL PEARL**
>
> **Craniotabes**
>
> Palpate the scalp firmly above and behind the ears to detect craniotabes (German word *crani* for "skull" and the Latin word *tabes* for "wasting"), a softening of the outer table of the skull. A snapping sensation, similar to the feeling of pressing on a ping-pong ball, indicates craniotabes that may be associated with prematurity, rickets, hydrocephalus, marasmus, syphilis, or thalassemia.

Palpate the sternocleidomastoid muscle, noting its tone and the presence of any masses. A mass in the lower third of the muscle may indicate a hematoma. Palpate the trachea. The thyroid is difficult to palpate in an infant unless it is enlarged. The presence of a goiter, which may cause respiratory distress, results from intrauterine deprivation of thyroid hormone. Palpate the clavicles; a crunch is indicative of fracture that occurred at the time of birth in newborns.

Transillumination

You can transilluminate the skull of infants who have suspected intracranial lesions or a rapidly increasing head circumference. Although transillumination is rarely performed because of the availability of radiologic imaging, it is less expensive and can be helpful. Perform the procedure in a completely darkened room, allowing a few minutes to elapse for your eyes to adjust. The transilluminator is placed firmly against the infant's scalp so that no light escapes (Fig. 11.32). Begin at the midline frontal region and inch the transilluminator over the entire head. Observe the ring of illumination through the scalp and skull around the light, noting any asymmetry. A ring of 2 cm or less beyond the rim of the transilluminator is expected with all regions of the head except the occiput, where the ring should be 1 cm or less. Illumination beyond these parameters suggests excess fluid or decreased brain tissue in the skull.

Children

Cranial bruits are common in children up to 5 years of age or in children with anemia. After age 5 years, their presence may suggest vascular anomalies or increased intracranial pressure.

The thyroid of the young child may be palpable. Using techniques described for adults, note the size, shape, position, mobility, and any tenderness. No tenderness should be present. An enlarged, tender thyroid may indicate thyroiditis.

Pregnant Patients

Beginning after 16 weeks of gestation, many pregnant patients develop blotchy, brownish hyperpigmentation of the face, particularly over the malar prominences and the forehead (see Chapter 9, Fig. 9.34). This chloasma, also called *mask of pregnancy*, may further darken with sun exposure, but generally it fades after delivery.

The thyroid gland may hypertrophy and become palpable (see Fig. 11.7). The hypertrophy is caused by hyperplasia of the glandular tissue and increased vascularity. Because of increased vascularity, a thyroid bruit may be heard. The presence of a goiter is not an expected finding. Pregnancy can make the diagnosis of hyperthyroidism difficult. The presence of weight loss, tachycardia, and bruit over the thyroid is highly suggestive. Confirmation of the diagnosis is made by measuring blood levels of thyroid-stimulating hormone (TSH) and free T_4.

Older Adults

The facies of older adults vary with their nutritional status. The eyes may appear sunken with soft bulges underneath, and the eyelids may appear wrinkled and hang loose.

Use caution when evaluating range of motion in an older adult's neck. Rather than have the patient perform an entire rotational maneuver, go slowly and evaluate each movement separately. Note any pain, crepitus, dizziness, jerkiness, or limitation of movement.

With aging, the thyroid becomes more fibrotic, feeling more nodular or irregular on palpation.

DIFFERENTIAL DIAGNOSIS

Comparison of Various Types of Headaches

CHARACTERISTIC	MIGRAINE	MEDICATION REBOUND	CLUSTER	HYPERTENSIVE	MUSCULAR TENSION	TEMPORAL ARTERITIS	SPACE-OCCUPYING LESION
Age at onset	Childhood	Any	Adulthood	Adulthood	Adulthood	Older adulthood	Any
Location	Unilateral or generalized	Generalized or diffuse	Unilateral	Bilateral or occipital	Unilateral or bilateral	Unilateral or bilateral	Localized
Duration	Hours to days	Hours to days	0.5–2 hours	Hours	Hours to days	Hours to days	Rapidly increasing duration
Time of onset	Morning or night	Predictably begins within hours to days of the last dose of the medication or caffeine	Night	Morning	Anytime, commonly in afternoon or evening	Anytime	Steady pain worse upon waking and better within a few hours
Quality of pain	Pulsating or throbbing	Dull or throbbing	Intense burning, boring, searing, knifelike	Throbbing	Bandlike, constricting	Throbbing	Aching
Prodromal event	Vague neurologic changes, personality changes, fluid retention, appetite loss to well-defined neurologic event, scotoma, aphasia, hemianopsia, aura	Daily analgesic use and/or daily caffeine use	Personality changes, sleep disturbances	None	None	None	Aggravated by coughing or bending forward
Precipitating event	Menstrual period, missing meals, birth control pills, letdown after stress	Abrupt discontinuation of analgesics or caffeine	Alcohol consumption	None	Stress, anger, bruxism	None	Develops in temporal relation to the neoplasm

Continued

DIFFERENTIAL DIAGNOSIS—cont'd

Comparison of Various Types of Headaches

CHARACTERISTIC	MIGRAINE	MEDICATION REBOUND	CLUSTER	HYPERTENSIVE	MUSCULAR TENSION	TEMPORAL ARTERITIS	SPACE-OCCUPYING LESION
Frequency	Twice a week	Gradual increase in headache frequency to daily	Several times nightly for several nights, then none	Daily	Daily	Daily	Progressive
Gender predilection	Females	Females	Males	Equal	Equal	Equal	Equal
Other symptoms	Nausea, vomiting	Alternate or preventive medications fail to control the headache	Increased lacrimation and nasal discharge	Generally remits as day progresses	None	None	Vomiting, confusion, abnormal neurologic findings, gait abnormality, papilledema and nystagmus

ABNORMALITIES

Head

Salivary Gland Tumor

Tumor in any of the salivary glands, but most commonly in the parotid (Fig. 11.33)

PATHOPHYSIOLOGY

- Exact mechanism by which tumor growth occurs is incompletely understood

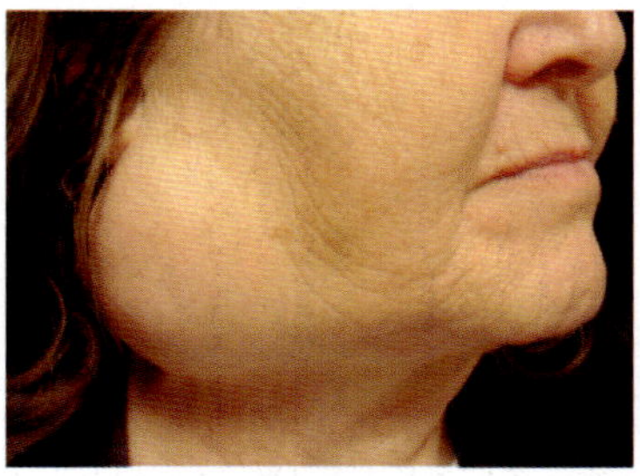

FIG. 11.33 Malignant right parotid gland tumor. Side view of swollen parotid gland below the ear of a female patient. (From Shah, J. P., Patel, S. G., & Singh, B. (2012). Head and neck surgery and oncology.)

PATIENT DATA

Subjective Data

- Slow-growing painless lumps, either in front of ear or under jaw
- Difficulty opening the mouth
- Tongue numbness or weakness

Objective Data

- Benign tumors usually smooth, malignant often irregular
- Facial weakness, fixation of the lump, sensory loss, and ulceration

Thyroid

ADULTS

Hypothyroidism

Underactive thyroid

PATHOPHYSIOLOGY

- Primary: thyroid gland produces insufficient amounts of thyroid hormone
- Secondary: insufficient secretion of thyroid hormone because of inadequate secretion of either thyroid-stimulating hormone (TSH) from the pituitary gland or thyrotropin-releasing hormone (TRH) from the hypothalamus
- More common than hyperthyroidism

PATIENT DATA

Subjective Data

- Weight gain, constipation, fatigue, and cold intolerance (Table 11.1)

Objective Data

- Normal-size thyroid, goiter, or nodule(s)

TABLE 11.1 Hyperthyroidism Versus Hypothyroidism

SYSTEM OR STRUCTURE AFFECTED	HYPERTHYROIDISM	HYPOTHYROIDISM
Constitutional		
Temperature preference	Cool climate	Warm climate
Weight	Loss	Gain
Emotional state	Nervous, easily irritated, highly energetic	Lethargic, complacent, disinterested
Hair	Fine, with hair loss; failure to hold a permanent wave	Coarse, with tendency to break
Skin	Warm, fine, hyperpigmentation at pressure points	Coarse, scaling, dry
Fingernails	Thin, with tendency to break; may show onycholysis	Thick
Eyes	Bilateral or unilateral exophthalmos, lid retraction, double vision	Puffiness in periorbital region
Neck	Goiter, change in shirt neck size, pain over the thyroid	No goiter
Cardiac	Tachycardia, dysrhythmia, palpitations	No change noted
Gastrointestinal	Increased frequency of bowel movements; diarrhea rare	Constipation
Menstrual	Scant flow, amenorrhea	Menorrhagia
Neuromuscular	Increasing weakness, especially of proximal muscles	Lethargic, but good muscular strength

Hyperthyroidism

Overactive thyroid

PATHOPHYSIOLOGY

- Excess thyroid hormone causes an increase in metabolic rate
- Associated with increased total body heat production and increased heart contractility, heart rate, and vasodilation
- Multinodular goiter (Plummer disease)

PATIENT DATA

Subjective Data

- Weight loss
- Tachycardia
- Diarrhea
- Heat intolerance
- See Table 11.1

Objective Data

- Normal-size thyroid, goiter, or nodule(s)
- Fine hair
- Brittle nails
- Exophthalmos
- Tachycardia

Myxedema

Skin and tissue disorder usually caused by severe prolonged hypothyroidism (see Fig. 11.10)

PATHOPHYSIOLOGY

- Decrease in metabolic rate, resulting in accumulation of hyaluronic acid and chondroitin sulfate in the dermis
- Deposition of glycosaminoglycan in all organ systems leading to mucinous edema of facial features

PATIENT DATA

Subjective Data

- Cognitive impairment, slowed mentation, poor concentration, decreased short-term memory, social withdrawal, psychomotor retardation, depressed mood, and apathy
- Constipation
- Muscle pains
- Hearing problems, deafness

Objective Data

- Coarse thick skin, thickening nose, swollen lips, puffiness around eyes
- Slow speech
- Mental dullness, lethargy, mental problems
- Weight gain
- Thin brittle hair, with bald patches

Graves Disease

Overactive thyroid caused by autoimmune antibodies to TSH receptor

PATHOPHYSIOLOGY

- More common in females during third and fourth decades

PATIENT DATA

Subjective Data

- Palpitations
- Heat intolerance
- Weight loss
- Fatigue
- Increased appetite
- Tachycardia
- See Table 11.1

Objective Data

- Diffuse thyroid enlargement; most commonly with prominent eyes (exophthalmos; see Fig. 11.11)
- Dermatologic, constitutional, menstrual, and musculoskeletal abnormalities; nonpitting edema (pretibial myxedema)

Hashimoto Disease

Underactive thyroid caused by autoimmune antibodies against thyroid gland

PATHOPHYSIOLOGY

- Often causes hypothyroidism
- More common in children and females between 30 and 50 years
- Progresses slowly over a number of years

PATIENT DATA

Subjective Data

- Weight gain
- Nausea
- Fatigue
- See Table 11.1

Objective Data

- Enlarged, nontender, smooth thyroid

INFANTS

Thyroglossal Duct Cyst

Palpable cystic mass in the neck

PATHOPHYSIOLOGY

- Remnant of fetal development
- Rises from the foramen cecum at junction of anterior two-thirds and posterior third of tongue (Fig. 11.34)
- Any part can persist, causing a sinus, fistula, or cyst

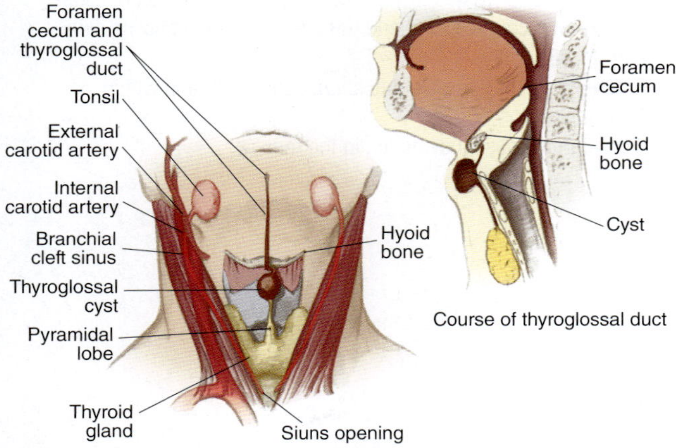

FIG. 11.34 Thyroglossal duct cyst location. Front view of neck shows labels as follows: hyoid bone, sinus opening, thyroid gland, pyramidal lobe, thyroglossal cyst, branchial cleft sinus, internal carotid artery, external carotid artery, tonsil, and foramen cecum and thyroglossal duct. Side view of neck marking the course of a thyroglossal duct shows labels as follows: foramen cecum, hyoid bone, and cyst. (From Rothrock, J. C., & Alexander, S. (2011). Alexander's surgical procedures. Elsevier.)

PATIENT DATA

Subjective Data

- Tenderness, redness, swelling in midline of neck
- Difficulty swallowing or breathing

Objective Data

- Freely movable cystic mass in neck midline
- Moves upward with tongue protrusion and swallowing
- May have small opening in skin, with drainage of mucus

Branchial Cleft Cyst

Congenital lesion formed by incomplete involution of branchial cleft

PATHOPHYSIOLOGY

- Epithelium-lined cyst with or without a sinus tract to overlying skin (Fig. 11.35)

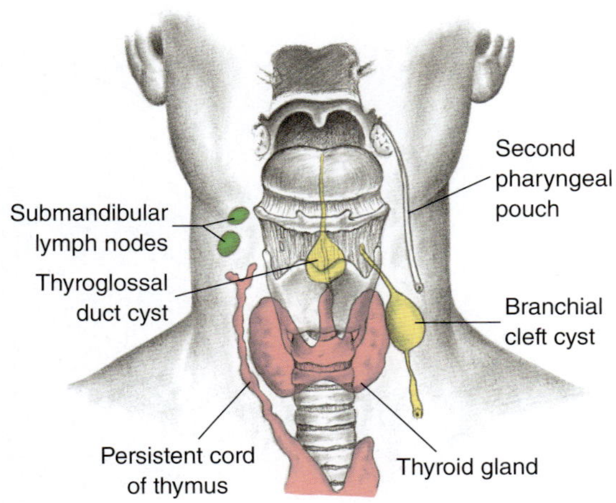

FIG. 11.35 Branchial cleft cyst location in relation to other neck masses. Internal structure of neck shows associated labels as follows: second pharyngeal pouch, branchial cleft cyst, thyroid gland, persistent cord of thymus, thyroglossal duct cyst, and submandibular lymph nodes.

PATIENT DATA

Subjective Data

- Painless mass in lateral neck
- May have intermittent swelling and tenderness
- Discharge if associated with a sinus tract

Objective Data

- Oval, moderately movable, smooth, nontender, fluctuant mass along anteromedial border of sternocleidomastoid muscle
- Usually asymptomatic
- If infected, tenderness and erythema

Torticollis (Wry Neck)

Excessive contraction of the sternocleidomastoid muscle

PATHOPHYSIOLOGY

- Often result of birth trauma or intrauterine malposition
- Acquired torticollis is result of tumors, trauma, cranial nerve IV palsy, muscle spasms, infection, or drug ingestion

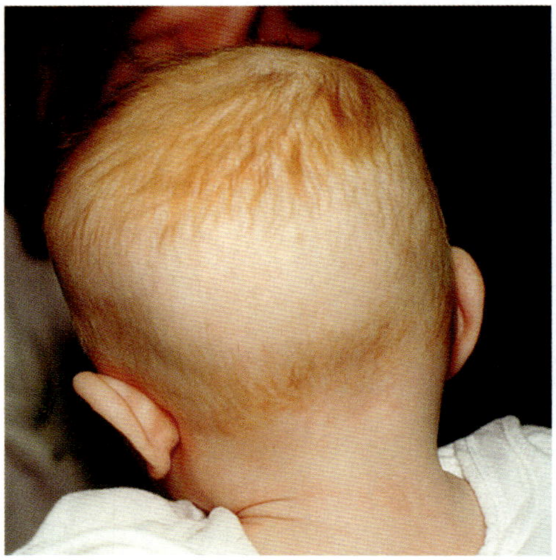

FIG. 11.36 Torticollis, or wry neck. Posterior view of an infant's head slightly tilted to the left. (From Graham, J. M., & Sanchez-Lara, P. A. (2023). *Smith's recognizable patterns of human deformation* (5th ed.).)

PATIENT DATA

Subjective Data

- Circumstances surrounding birth, trauma, medications
- Stiff neck, decreased range of motion of neck
- Possible vision problem

Objective Data

- Head tilted and twisted toward the affected sternocleidomastoid muscle with chin elevated and turned toward the opposite side (Fig. 11.36)
- A hematoma may be palpated shortly after birth and within 2–3 weeks
- Firm, fibrous mass may be felt in the muscle

Encephalocele

Neural tube defect with protrusions of brain and membranes that cover it through openings in the skull

PATHOPHYSIOLOGY

- Failure of the neural tube to close completely during fetal development, can occur any place on the scalp (Fig. 11.37)
- Genetic component; often occurs in families with a history of spina bifida or anencephaly

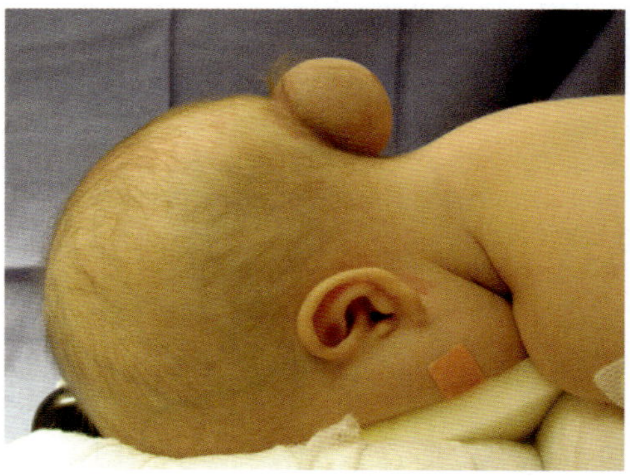

FIG. 11.37 Encephalocele. Close-up view of infant lying prone shows a large lump behind the head. (From Winn, H. R. (Ed.). (2012). Youmans and Winn neurological surgery. Elsevier.)

PATIENT DATA

Subjective Data

- Before birth are visible only by intrauterine ultrasound or seen immediately after birth

Objective Data

- Visible sac of tissue protruding through skull
- Craniofacial abnormalities or other brain malformations, hydrocephalus

Hydrocephalus

A problem in the formation, flow, or absorption of cerebrospinal fluid (CSF), which leads to an increase in the volume of the CSF. See Risk Factors box, "Hydrocephalus in Infants."

PATHOPHYSIOLOGY

- Abnormalities in the CSF circulation can arise from:
    - Congenital malformations, congenital infections (e.g., toxoplasmosis)
    - Acquired abnormalities (e.g., intracranial mass, intracranial hemorrhage, meningitis, and trauma)

Risk Factors

Hydrocephalus in Infants

- Genetic abnormalities: X-linked hydrocephalus is caused by an X chromosome mutation.
- Developmental disorders: Spina bifida and other neural tube defects
- Premature birth: Complications from premature birth, such as intraventricular hemorrhage (bleeding within the brain's ventricles)
- Infections during pregnancy: Infections like cytomegalovirus, toxoplasmosis, mumps, rubella, or syphilis can cause inflammation in fetal brain tissue, increasing the risk.
- Injuries: Trauma to the head during birth or shortly after can result in hydrocephalus.

PATIENT DATA

Subjective Data

- Poor feeding
- Irritability
- Decreased activity
- Vomiting

Objective Data

- Head enlargement (see Fig. 11.18)
- Separation of cranial sutures
- Dilated scalp veins
- Tense anterior fontanelle
- Sunsetting sign (see Fig. 11.18)
- Increased muscle tone (spasticity)
- Macewen sign

Microcephaly

Head circumference is smaller than normal because the brain has not developed properly or has stopped growing (Fig. 11.38)

PATHOPHYSIOLOGY

- Present at birth or may develop in first few years of life
- Multiple causes including congenital infections (e.g., Zika virus) and neuroanatomic abnormalities (e.g., cerebral dysgenesis or craniostenosis)
- Failure of brain to develop normally

PATIENT DATA

Subjective Data

- Associated with intellectual disability

Objective Data

- Head circumference is 2–3 standard deviations below mean for age

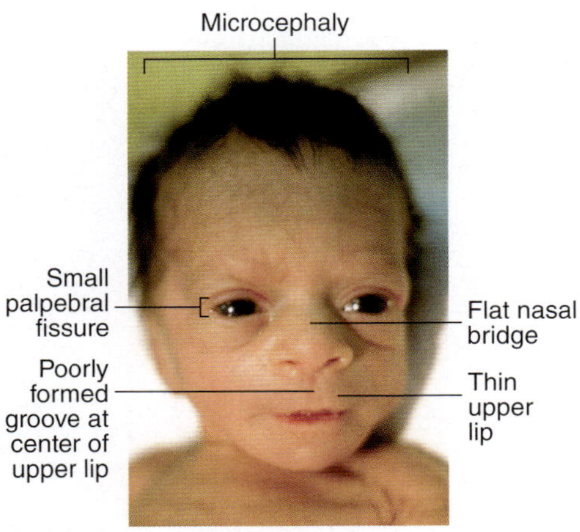

FIG. 11.38 Microcephaly. The facial features of an infant with fetal alcohol syndrome (FAS) include short palpebral (eye) fissures; a flat nasal bridge; a thin, flat upper lip; a poorly formed groove at the center of the upper lip; and a small head (microcephaly). Close-up view of infant's head and face with labels as follows: microcephaly, flat nasal bridge, thin upper lip, poorly formed groove at center of upper lip, and small palpebral fissure. (From Leifer, G. (2011). *Maternity nursing: An introductory text* (11th ed.). Saunders.)

Craniosynostosis

Premature closure of one or more cranial sutures before brain growth is complete

PATHOPHYSIOLOGY

- Leads to misshapen skull (Fig. 11.39)
- Involved sutures determine shape of the head

PATIENT DATA

Subjective Data

- Abnormally shaped skull, usually not accompanied by intellectual disability

Objective Data

- Skull growth restricted perpendicular to fused suture
- If multiple sutures fuse while brain is still growing, intracranial pressure can increase (see signs of increased cranial pressure in Chapter 26)

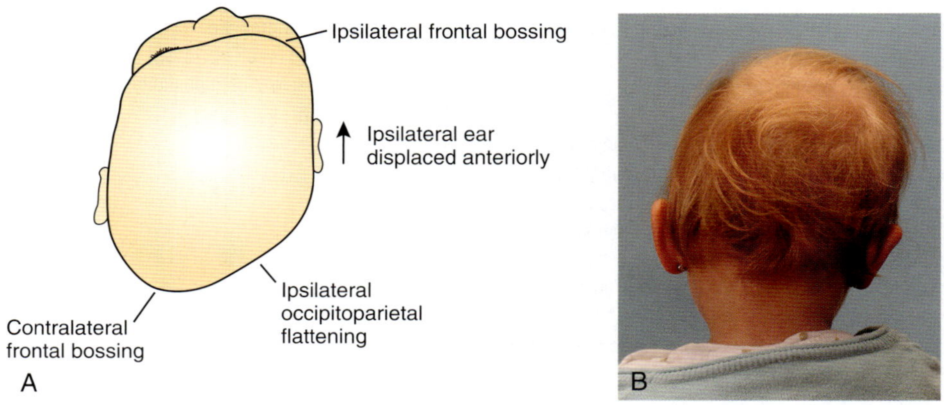

FIG. 11.39 (A) Vertex view of right sided lambdoid craniosynostosis exhibiting a trapezoid-like head shape showing: ipsilateral frontal bossing, ipsilateral ear displaced anteriorly, ipsilateral occipitoparietal flattening, and contralateral frontal bossing. (B) Posterior view of a child's head which is slightly tilted to once side. (A, From Flint P. W., Haughey, B. H., Lund, V. J., Robbins, K. T., Thomas, J. R., Lesperance, M. M., & Francis, H. W. (2020). *Cummings otolaryngology: Head and neck surgery* (7th ed.).; B, from Wilbrand, et al. (2016). Flint, P. W., & Haughey, B. H., et al. (2015). *Cummings otolaryngology—head & neck surgery* (6th ed.). Elsevier.)

CHAPTER

12

Eyes

The comprehensive eye examination involves a series of tests evaluating vision as well as the general health of the eyes and includes screening for ophthalmologic diseases or ocular manifestation of systemic diseases.

ANATOMY AND PHYSIOLOGY

The eye is the sensory organ that transmits visual stimuli to the brain for interpretation (Fig. 12.1). It occupies the orbital cavity; only its anterior aspect is exposed. The eye itself is a direct embryologic extension of the brain.

Four rectus and two oblique muscles are attached to the eye (Fig. 12.2). Cranial nerve (CN) II, the optic nerve, connects the eye to the brain.

External Eye

The external eye is composed of the eyelid, conjunctiva, lacrimal gland, eye muscles, and bony orbit. The orbit also contains fat, blood vessels, nerves, and supporting connective tissue (see Fig. 12.1).

Eyelid

The eyelid is composed of skin, striated muscle, the tarsal plate, and conjunctivae. Meibomian glands in the eyelid provide oils to the tear film. The tarsus provides a skeleton for the eyelid. The eyelid distributes tears over the surface of the eye, limits the amount of light entering it, and protects the eye from foreign bodies. Eyelashes extend from the anterior border of each lid.

Physical Examination Components

1. Measure visual acuity, noting:
    - Near vision
    - Distant vision
    - Peripheral vision
2. Inspect the eyebrows for:
    - Hair texture
    - Size
    - Extension to temporal canthus
3. Inspect the orbital area for:
    - Edema
    - Redundant tissues or edema
    - Lesions
4. Inspect the eyelids for:
    - Ability to open wide and close completely
    - Eyelash position
    - Ptosis
    - Fasciculations or tremors
    - Flakiness
    - Redness
    - Swelling
5. Palpate the eyelids for nodules.
6. Inspect the orbits.
7. Pull down the lower lids and inspect palpebral conjunctivae, bulbar conjunctivae, and sclerae for:
    - Color
    - Discharge
    - Lacrimal gland punctum
    - Pterygium
8. Inspect the external eyes for:
    - Corneal clarity
    - Corneal sensitivity
    - Corneal arcus
    - Color of irides
    - Pupillary size and shape
    - Pupillary response to light and accommodation, afferent pupillary defect
    - Nystagmus
9. Palpate the lacrimal gland in the superior temporal orbital rim.
10. Evaluate muscle balance and movement of eyes:
    - Corneal light reflex
    - Cover-uncover test
    - Six cardinal fields of gaze
11. Ophthalmoscopic examination:
    - Lens clarity
    - Retinal color and lesions
    - Characteristics of blood vessels
    - Disc characteristics
    - Macula characteristics
    - Depth of anterior chamber

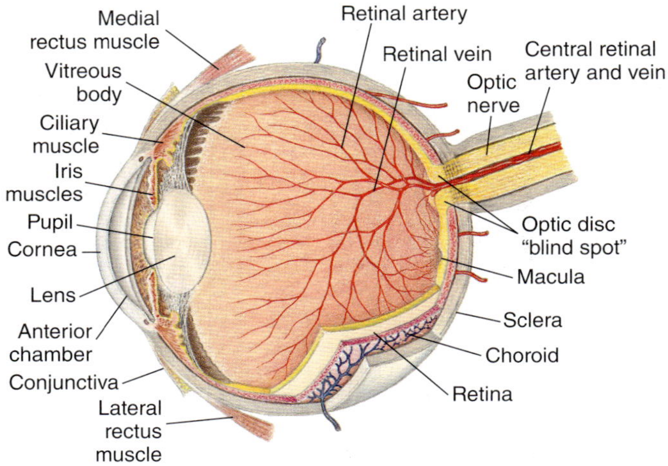

FIG. 12.1 **Anatomy of the human eye.**

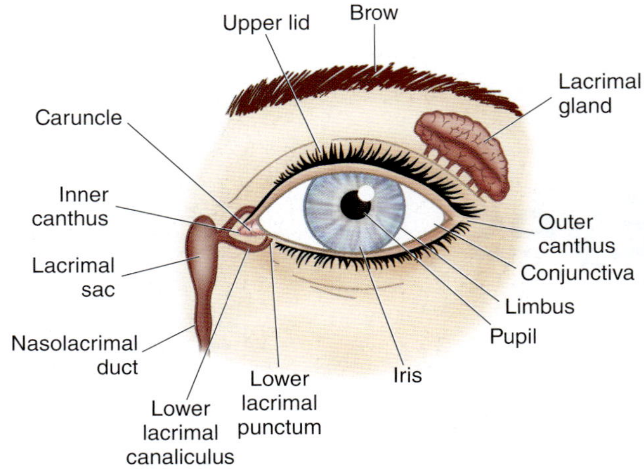

FIG. 12.3 **Important landmarks of the left external eye.** (From Thompson, J. M. (1997). *Mosby's clinical nursing* (4th ed.). St. Louis: Mosby.)

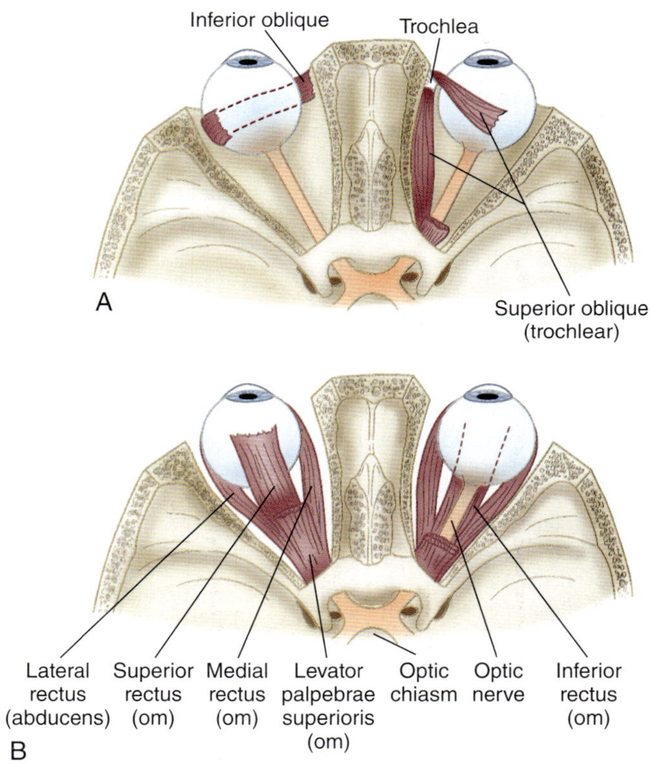

FIG. 12.2 **Extraocular muscles of the eye as viewed from above.** (A) The oblique muscles. (B) The recti muscles (*om,* oculomotor). The cranial nerves, which innervate the muscles, are listed in Fig. 12.22.

Conjunctiva

The conjunctiva is a clear, thin mucous membrane. The palpebral conjunctiva coats the inside of the eyelids. The bulbar (or ocular) conjunctiva covers the outer surface of the eye. The bulbar conjunctiva protects the anterior surface of the eye with the exception of the cornea and the surface of the eyelid in contact with the globe.

Lacrimal Gland

The lacrimal gland is located in the temporal region of the superior eyelid and produces tears that moisten the eye (Fig. 12.3). Tears flow over the cornea and drain via the canaliculi to the lacrimal sac and duct and then into the nasal meatus.

Eye Muscles

Each eye is moved by six muscles—the superior, inferior, medial, and lateral rectus muscles and the superior and inferior oblique muscles (see Figs. 12.2 and 12.22). They are innervated by CNs III (oculomotor), IV (trochlear), and VI (abducens). The oculomotor nerve controls the levator palpebrae superioris (which elevates and retracts the upper eyelid) and all extraocular muscles, except for the superior oblique muscle and the lateral rectus muscle. The superior oblique is the only muscle innervated by the trochlear nerve, and the lateral rectus muscle is the only muscle innervated by the abducens nerve.

Internal Eye

The internal structures of the eye are composed of three separate layers. The outer wall of the eye is composed of the sclera posteriorly and the cornea anteriorly. The middle layer, or uvea, consists of the choroid posteriorly and the ciliary body and iris anteriorly. The inner layer of nerve fibers is the retina (see Fig. 12.1).

Sclera

The sclera is the dense, avascular structure that appears anteriorly as the white of the eye. It physically supports the internal structure of the eye.

Cornea

The cornea constitutes the anterior sixth of the globe and is continuous with the sclera. It is optically clear, has rich sensory innervation, and is avascular. It is a major part of the refractive power of the eye.

Uvea

The iris, ciliary body, and choroids comprise the uveal tract (see Fig. 12.1). The iris is a circular, contractile muscular disc containing pigment cells that produce the color of the eye. The central aperture of the iris is the pupil, through which light travels to the retina. By dilating and contracting, the iris controls the amount of light reaching the retina. The ciliary body produces the aqueous humor (fluid that circulates between the lens and cornea) and contains the muscles controlling accommodation. The choroid is a pigmented, richly vascular layer that supplies oxygen to the outer layer of the retina.

Lens

The lens is a biconvex, transparent structure located immediately behind the iris (see Fig. 12.1). It is supported circumferentially by fibers arising from the ciliary body. The lens is highly elastic, and contraction or relaxation of the ciliary body changes its thickness, thereby permitting images from varied distances to be focused on the retina.

Retina

The retina is the sensory network of the eye. Photoreceptors and neurons transform light impulses into electrical impulses, which are transmitted through the optic nerve, optic tract, and optic radiation to the visual cortex in the brain and then to interpretation in the cerebral cortex. The optic nerve passes through the optic foramen along with the ophthalmic artery and vein. The optic nerve communicates with the brain and the autonomic nervous system of the eye. Accurate binocular vision is achieved when an image is fused on the retina by the cornea and the lens. An object may be perceived in each visual cortex, even when one eye is covered, if the light impulse is cast on both the temporal and nasal retinas. Fibers located on the nasal retina decussate in the optic chiasm (Fig. 12.4).

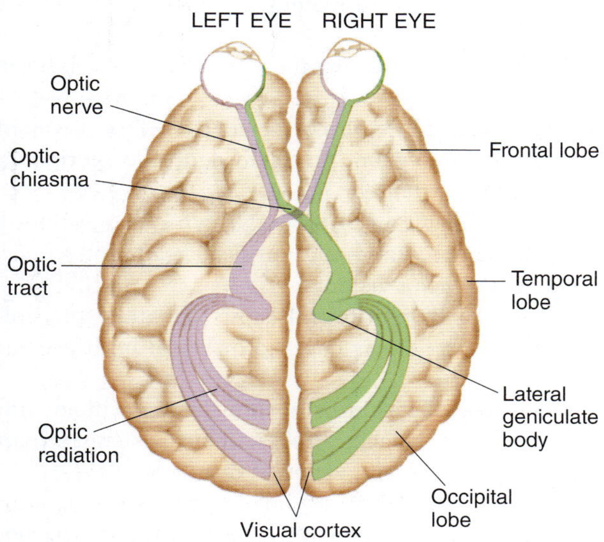

FIG. 12.4 **The optic chiasm.** (Modified from Thompson, J. M. (1997). *Mosby's clinical nursing* (4th ed.). St. Louis: Mosby.)

Accurate binocular vision also requires the synchronous functioning of the extraocular muscles.

Major landmarks of the retina include the optic disc, from which the optic nerve originates, together with the central retinal artery and vein. The macula, or fovea, is the site of central vision (see Fig. 12.1).

Infants and Children

The eyes develop during the first 8 weeks of gestation and may become malformed as a result of prenatal drug and alcohol exposure or infection. The development of vision, which is dependent on maturation of the nervous system, occurs over a longer period (Table 12.1). Term infants are

TABLE 12.1 Chronology of Visual Development

AGE	LEVELS OF DEVELOPMENT
Birth	Awareness of light and dark; infant closes eyelids in bright light Visual acuity 20/670 (6/200)
Neonatal	Rudimentary fixation on near objects; able to regard mother's face
2 weeks	Transitory fixation, usually monocular at a distance of roughly 3 feet Follows large, conspicuously moving objects
4 weeks	Visual acuity 20/550 (6/160) Moving objects evoke binocular fixation briefly
6 weeks	Follows moving objects with jerky eye movements
8 weeks	Visual following now achieved by a combination of head and eye movements Visual acuity 20/150 (6/45)
12 weeks	Visual acuity 20/230 (6/70) Enjoys light objects and bright colors Beginning of depth perception Fusion of images begins to appear
16 weeks	Visual acuity 20/60 (6/18) Fixates immediately on moving target; visually pursues dropped toy
20 weeks	Shows interest in stimuli more than 3 feet away Retrieves a dropped 1-inch cube Can maintain voluntary fixation of stationary object even in the presence of competing moving stimulus
24 weeks	Visual acuity reaches healthy adult level of 20/100 (6/30) Can maintain voluntary fixation of stationary object even in the presence of competing moving stimulus Hand-eye coordination appearing Will fixate on a string Binocular fixation clearly established
26 weeks	Marked interest in tiny objects
28 weeks	Tilts head backward to gaze up
40 weeks	Discriminates simple geometric forms (squares and circles) Looks at pictures with interest
1 year	Visual acuity 20/60 (6/20) Convergence well established Localization in distance crude—runs into large objects
3 years	Visual acuity 20/50 (6/15)

From Courage, M. L., & Adams, R. J. (1990). Visual acuity assessment from birth to three years using the acuity card procedure: Cross-sectional and longitudinal samples. *Optometry and Vision Science, 67*(9), 713–718; and Sokol, S. (1978). Measurement of infant visual acuity from pattern reversal evoked potentials. *Vision Research, 18*(1), 33–39.

hyperopic, with a visual acuity of less than 20/400 (see "Visual Acuity Testing"). Although peripheral vision is fully developed at birth, central vision matures later. One of the earliest visual responses is the infant's regard for the mother's face. By 2 to 3 weeks of age, many infants will show an interest in large objects. Lacrimal drainage is complete at the time of term birth, and by 2 to 3 weeks of age, the lacrimal gland begins producing a full volume of tears. By 3 to 4 months of age, binocular vision development is complete. By 6 months, vision has developed sufficiently so that the infant can differentiate colors.

Young children become less hyperopic with growth. The globe of the eye grows as the child's head and brain grow, and adult visual acuity is achieved at about 4 years of age.

Pregnant Patients

The eyes undergo several changes during pregnancy because of physiologic and hormonal adaptations. These changes can result in hypersensitivity and can change the refractive power of the eye. Tears contain an increased level of lysozyme, resulting in a greasy sensation and perhaps blurred vision for contact lens wearers. Diabetic retinopathy may worsen significantly. Mild corneal edema and thickening associated with blurred vision may occur, especially in the third trimester. Intraocular pressure falls most notably during the latter half of pregnancy.

Older Adults

The major physiologic eye change that occurs with aging is a progressive weakening of accommodation (focusing power) known as *presbyopia*. In general, by 45 years of age, the lens becomes more rigid and the ciliary muscle becomes weaker. The lens also continues to form fibers throughout life. Old fibers are compressed centrally, forming a denser central region that may cause loss of clarity of the lens and contribute to cataract formation (clouding of the lens that can become partially or totally opaque; see Fig. 12.41). See Risk Factors, "Cataract Formation."

Risk Factors

Cataract Formation

- Family history of cataracts
- Steroid medication use
- Exposure to ultraviolet light
- Cigarette smoking
- Diabetes mellitus
- Aging

REVIEW OF RELATED HISTORY

For each of the symptoms or conditions discussed in this section, targeted topics to include in the history of the present illness are listed. Responses to questions about these topics provide clues for focusing the physical examination and the development of an appropriate diagnostic evaluation. Questions regarding medication use (prescription and over-the-counter preparations) in addition to complementary, alternative, and integrative therapies are relevant for each.

History of Present Illness

Red Eye (Presence of Conjunctival Injection or Redness)

- Difficulty with vision: one or both eyes, corrected by lenses
- Recent injury or foreign bodies; sleeping in contact lenses
- Pain: with or without loss of vision, in or around the eye, superficial or deep, insidious or abrupt in onset; burning, itching, or nonspecific uncomfortable or gritty sensation
- History of swelling, infections, or eye surgery
- History of recent illness or similar symptoms in the household
- Allergies: type, seasonal, associated symptoms
- Eye secretions: color (clear or yellow), consistency (watery or purulent), duration, tears that run down the face, decreased tear formation (with sensation of gritty eyes)
- Medications: eye drops or ointments, antibiotics, artificial tears, mydriatics; glaucoma medications, antioxidant vitamins (to prevent macular degeneration), steroids (which promote cataract formation), inhaled anticholinergics (which can worsen glaucoma)

Vision Problem(s)

- Eyelids: recurrent hordeola (stye; acute infection of sebaceous glands of Zeis), chalazion (chronic blockage of meibomian gland), ptosis of the lids so that they interfere with vision (unilateral or bilateral), growths or masses, itching
- Double vision: oculomotor, trochlear, or abducens nerve deficit
- Unilateral or bilateral, corrected by lenses, involving near or distant vision, primarily central or peripheral, transient or sustained
- Cataracts (bilateral or unilateral), types (e.g., infantile, senile, diabetic, traumatic, surgical treatment)
- Adequacy of color vision
- Presence of halos around lights, floaters, or diplopia (when one eye is covered or when both eyes are open)
- Sudden loss of vision or portion of visual field: transient ischemic attack, stroke, amaurosis fugax (painless temporary loss of vision in one or both eyes)
- Trauma: to the eye as a whole or a specific structure (e.g., cornea) or supporting structures (e.g., the floor of the orbit); events surrounding the trauma; efforts at correction and degree of success

Think About It

A person presents with an isolated unilateral sixth nerve (abducens nerve) palsy. The inability to adduct the affected eye causes horizontal binocular diplopia that resolves on closing the affected eye. Consider microvascular disease, the most common cause. Contributing factors include diabetes, hypertension, hypercholesterolemia, and anemia. Typically, in these cases, the palsy resolves within 3 months. Further workup may be pursued if symptoms do not resolve or worsen in 3 months.

From Erdal Y, Gunes T, Emre U. Isolated abducens nerve palsy: Comparison of microvascular and other causes. North Clin Istanb. 2022;9(4):353-357. doi:10.14744/nci.2021.15483.

Past Medical History

- Eye surgery: condition requiring surgery, cataract removal, laser vision correction, date of surgery, outcome
- Chronic illness that may affect eyes or vision: glaucoma, diabetes, atherosclerotic cardiovascular disease (ASCVD), hypertension, thyroid dysfunction, autoimmune diseases, human immunodeficiency virus (HIV), inflammatory bowel diseases
- Medications: steroids, hydroxychloroquine, antihistamines, antidepressants, antipsychotics, antiarrhythmics, immunosuppressants, glaucoma eye drops, beta-blockers, anticholinergics

Family History

- Retinoblastoma (often an autosomal dominant disorder)
- Glaucoma, macular degeneration, diabetes, hypertension, or other diseases that may affect vision or eye health
- Cataracts
- Color blindness, retinal detachment, retinitis pigmentosa, or allergies affecting the eye
- Nearsightedness, farsightedness, strabismus, or amblyopia

Personal and Social History

- Employment: exposure to irritating gases, chemicals, foreign bodies, or high-speed machinery
- Activities: participation in sporting activities that might endanger the eye (e.g., boxing, lacrosse, hockey, basketball, football, paintball, martial arts, rifle shooting, racquetball, fencing, motorcycle riding)
- Use of protective equipment during work or activities that might endanger the eye
- Corrective lenses: type (glasses or contact lenses), when last changed, how long worn, adequacy of corrected vision; methods of cleaning and storage or frequency of disposal, insertion and removal procedures of contact lenses; sleeping with contact lenses in
- Date of last eye examination, history of corrective surgery (e.g., laser-assisted in situ keratomileusis [LASIK])
- History of cigarette smoking (a risk factor for vascular disease, cataract formation, glaucoma, macular degeneration, thyroid eye disease)

Infants and Children

- Preterm: resuscitative efforts, mechanical ventilation or oxygen use, retinopathy of prematurity (ROP), birth weight, gestational age, sepsis, intracranial hemorrhage
- Maternal history of sexually transmitted infections, Zika virus, TORCH (toxoplasmosis, other [syphilis, varicella-zoster, parvovirus B-19], rubella, cytomegalovirus, and herpes) infections
- Congenital abnormalities of the eye or surrounding structures (e.g., hemangioma)
- Symptoms of congenital abnormalities including failure of infant to gaze at mother's face or other objects; failure of infant to blink when bright lights or threatening movements are directed at the face
- White area in the pupil on examination or on a photograph (leukocoria); inability of one eye to reflect light properly (may indicate retinoblastoma or other serious intraocular problem)
- Excessive tearing or discharge, erythema
- Strabismus some or all of the time; frequency; when first noted; occurring when fatigued, sick, or otherwise stressed; head tilt or turn when focusing on objects; associated with frequent blinking or squinting, nystagmus
- Young children: excessive rubbing of the eyes, frequent hordeola, inability to reach for and pick up small objects, night vision difficulties
- School-age children: necessity of sitting near the front of the classroom; poor school performance not explained by intellectual ability; headaches

Pregnant Patients

- Presence of disorders that can cause ocular complications such as pregnancy-induced hypertension (PIH) or gestational diabetes; symptoms indicative of PIH: diplopia, scotomata, blurred vision, or amaurosis fugax
- Use of topical eye medications (may cross the placental barrier)

Older Adults

- Visual acuity: decrease in central vision, distortion of central vision, use of dim or bright light to increase visual acuity, difficulty with glare; difficulty in performing near work without lenses
- Excess tearing
- Dry eyes
- Nocturnal eye pain (sign of subacute angle closure and a symptom of glaucoma)
- Difficulty with depth perception

EXAMINATION AND FINDINGS

Equipment

- Snellen or Sloan chart (adults and children age 6 or more years of age); LEA Cards, or HOTV chart (children ages 3 to 5 years) (see Chapter 3, Fig. 3.17A and B)
- Rosenbaum or Jaeger near vision card (see Chapter 3)
- Penlight
- Cotton wisp
- Ophthalmoscope (see Chapter 3, Figs. 3.13 and 3.15)
- Eye cover, gauze, or opaque card

Visual Acuity Testing

Measurement of visual acuity—the discrimination of small visual details—tests CN II (optic nerve) and is essentially a measurement of central vision. This important assessment is often inappropriately neglected by examiners who are not ophthalmologists. Position the patient 20 feet (6 m) away from the Snellen or Sloan chart (see Fig. 3.17). Make sure the chart is well lighted. Alternatively, special charts for use 10 feet (3 m) away from the patient are available. Test each eye individually by covering one eye with an opaque card or gauze, being careful to avoid applying pressure to the eye. If you test the patient with and without corrective lenses, record the readings separately. Always test vision without glasses first.

Ask the patient to identify all of the letters, beginning at any line. Determine the smallest line in which the patient can identify all of the letters and record the visual acuity designated by that line. (For more information, see Chapter 3.) When testing the second eye, you may want to ask the patient to read the line from right to left to reduce the chance of recall influencing the response. Conduct the test rapidly enough to prevent the patient from memorizing the chart. However, avoid going too quickly when asking that the lines on the chart be read. It is wise to pace the assessment slowly for patient comfort and to allow time for the patient to reason out a response. Visual acuity is recorded as a fraction in which the numerator indicates the distance of the patient from the chart (e.g., 20 feet or 6 m), and the denominator indicates the distance at which the average eye can read the line. Thus 20/200 (6/60) means that the patient can read at 20 feet (6 m) what the average person can read at 200 feet (60 m). The smaller the fraction, the worse the vision. Vision not correctable to better than 20/200 is considered legal blindness (see Clinical Pearl, "Is It Blurry or Is It Double?").

Perform a pinhole test if the visual acuity is recorded at a fraction less than 20/20 (or 6/6) to see if the observed decrease in acuity was caused by a refractive error. Ask the patient to hold a pinhole occluder (or a piece of paper with a small hole in it) over the uncovered eye. This maneuver permits light to enter only the central portion of the lens. Expect an improvement in visual acuity by at least one line on the chart if refractive error is responsible for the diminished acuity (see Clinical Pearl, "Factors That Affect Visual Acuity Testing").

> **CLINICAL PEARL**
>
> **Is It Blurry or Is It Double?**
>
> Blurred vision and diplopia are sometimes confused by the patient. Blurred vision represents a problem with visual acuity, and there are many causes. Diplopia is the perception of two images and may be monocular or binocular. Monocular diplopia is an optical problem; binocular diplopia is an alignment problem.

> **CLINICAL PEARL**
>
> **Factors That Affect Visual Acuity Testing**
>
> Testing of visual acuity involves many complex factors not necessarily related to the ability to see the test object. Motivation and interest, as well as literacy, language, intelligence, and attention span, can modify the results of sensory testing.

Measurement of near vision should be tested in each eye separately with a handheld card such as the Rosenbaum Pocket Vision Screener. Have the patient hold the card at a comfortable distance (about 35 cm, or 14 inches) from the eyes and read the smallest line possible.

Peripheral vision can be accurately measured with sophisticated instruments but is generally estimated by the confrontation test. Sit or stand opposite the patient at eye level at a distance of about 1 m (3 feet). Ask the patient to cover the right eye while you cover your left eye, so the open eyes are directly opposite each other (Fig. 12.5). Both you and the patient should be looking at each other's eye. Fully extend your arm midway between the patient and yourself and then wiggle your fingers as you move your arm slowly centrally. Have the patient tell you when the fingers are first seen. Compare the patient's response to

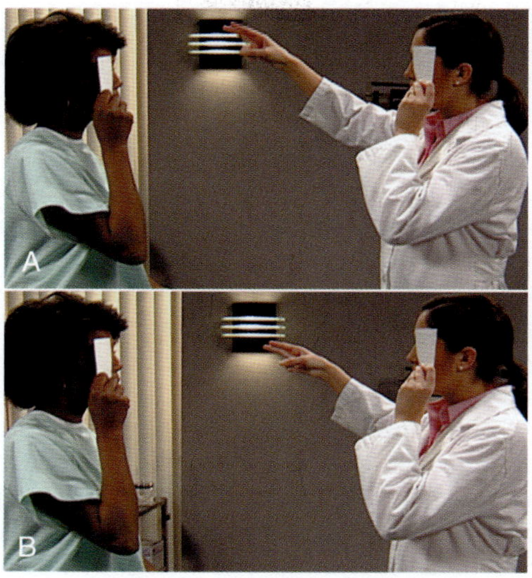

FIG. 12.5 Evaluation of peripheral fields of vision. (A) Temporal field. (B) Nasal field.

the time you first note the fingers. Test the nasal, temporal, superior, and inferior fields. Remember that the nose itself interferes with the nasal portion of the visual field. Unless you are aware of a problem with your vision, you can feel comfortable that the fields are full if they correspond with yours. The confrontation test is imprecise and can be considered significant only when it is abnormal. Lesions most likely to produce confrontation abnormalities include stroke, retinal detachment, optic neuropathy, pituitary tumor compression at the optic chiasm, and central retinal vascular occlusion.

Color vision is rarely tested in the routine physical examination. Color plates are available in which numerals are produced in primary colors and surrounded by confusing colors. The patient is asked to read the numbers. The tests vary in degree of difficulty. For routine testing, check the patient's ability to appreciate primary colors. Red testing may be particularly helpful in determining subtle optic nerve disease, even when visual acuity remains nearly normal. An afferent pupillary defect (discussed later in the chapter) often coexists with a red defect.

External Examination

Carry out examination of the eyes in a systematic manner, beginning with the appendages (i.e., the eyebrows and surrounding tissues) and moving inward.

Surrounding Structures

Inspect the eyebrows for size, extension, and texture of the hair. Note whether the eyebrows extend beyond the eye itself or end short of it. If the patient's eyebrows are coarse or do not extend beyond the temporal canthus, the patient may have hypothyroidism. If the brows appear unusually thin, ask if the patient waxes or plucks them.

Inspect the orbital and periorbital area for edema, puffiness, or redundant tissue below the orbit. Although puffiness may represent the loss of elastic tissue that occurs with aging, periorbital edema is always abnormal; the significance varies directly with the amount. It may represent the presence of thyroid eye disease, allergies, or the presence of renal disease (nephrotic syndrome) or heart disease (congestive heart failure). You may see flat to slightly raised, oval, irregularly shaped, yellow-tinted lesions on the periorbital tissues that represent depositions of lipids and may suggest that the patient has abnormal lipid metabolism. These lesions, called *xanthelasma* (Fig. 12.6), are an elevated plaque of cholesterol deposited in macrophages, most commonly in the nasal portion of the upper or lower lid.

Eyelids

Examine the patient's lightly closed eyes for fasciculations or tremors of the lids, a sign of hyperthyroidism. Inspect the eyelids for their ability to close completely and open widely. Observe for flakiness, redness, or swelling on the eyelid margin. Eyelashes should be present on both lids and should curve away from the globe.

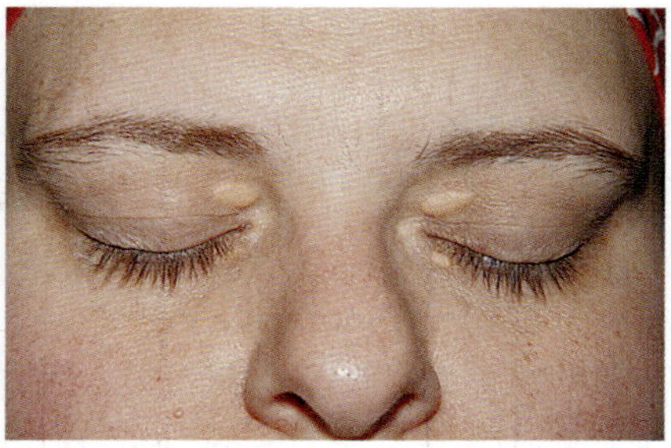

FIG. 12.6 Xanthelasma. (Courtesy John W. Payne, MD, The Wilmer Ophthalmological Institute, The Johns Hopkins University and Hospital, Baltimore, MD.)

When the eye is open, the superior eyelid should cover a portion of the iris but not the pupil itself. If one superior eyelid covers more of the iris than the other or extends over the pupil, then ptosis of that lid is present. Ptosis indicates a congenital or acquired weakness of the levator muscle or a paresis of a branch of the third cranial nerve (Fig. 12.7). Record the difference between the two lids in millimeters. The average upper lid position is 2 mm below the limbus (the border of the cornea and the sclera), and the average lower lid position is at the lower limbus.

You should also note whether the lids evert or invert. When the lower lid is turned away from the eye, it is called *ectropion* and may result in excessive tearing (Fig. 12.8). The inferior punctum, which serves as the tear-collecting system, is pulled outward, and the lower lid cannot collect the secretions of the lacrimal gland.

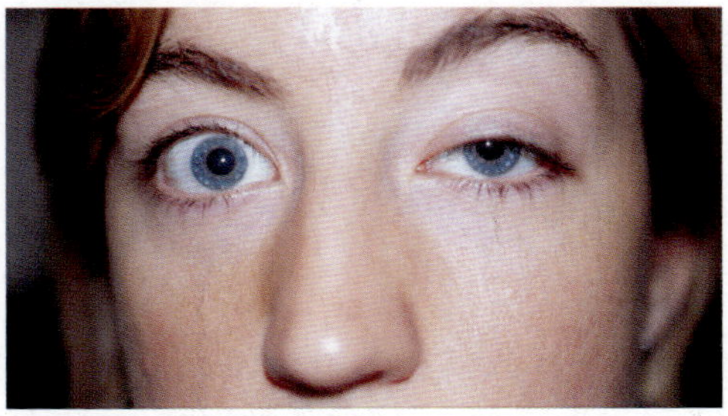

FIG. 12.7 Ptosis, a drooping of the upper eyelid. (From Patzelt, J. (2009). *Basics augenheilkunde* (2nd ed.). Germany: Urban & Fischer.)

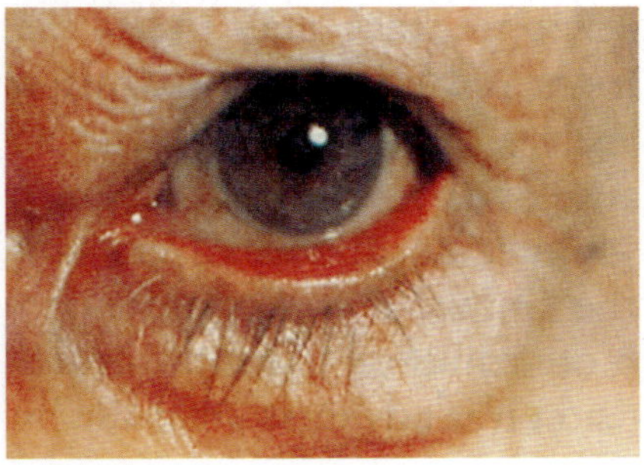

FIG. 12.8 Ectropion. (From Stein, H. A. (1988). *The ophthalmic assistant: Fundamentals and clinical practice* (5th ed.). St. Louis: Mosby.)

When the lid is turned inward toward the globe, a condition known as *entropion* (Fig. 12.9), the lid's eyelashes may cause corneal and conjunctival irritation, increasing the risk of a secondary infection. The patient often reports a foreign body sensation.

An acute suppurative inflammation of the follicle of an eyelash can cause an erythematous or yellow lump. This hordeolum, or stye, is generally caused by a staphylococcal infection (Fig. 12.10).

Crusting along the eyelashes may represent blepharitis caused by bacterial infection, seborrhea, psoriasis, a manifestation of rosacea, or an allergic response (Fig. 12.11).

Ask the patient to close their eyes, and note whether the eyelids meet completely. If the closed lids do not completely cover the globe (a condition called *lagophthalmos*), the cornea may become dried and be at increased risk of infection. Thyroid eye disease, seventh nerve palsy (Bell palsy), and overaggressive ptosis or blepharoplasty surgical repair are common causes.

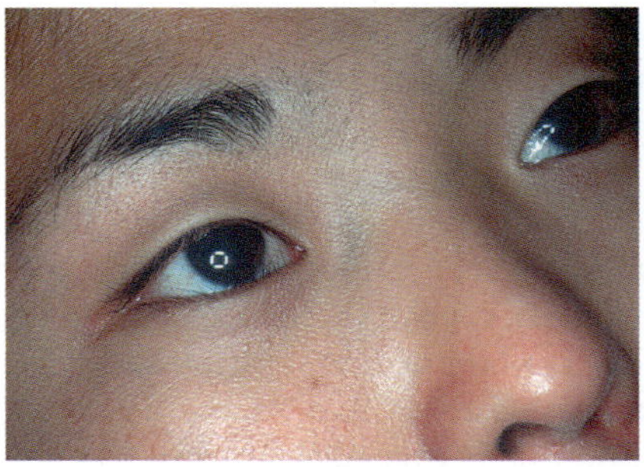

FIG. 12.9 Entropion. Note that this patient has undergone corneal transplantation. (From Palay, D. A., & Krachmer, J. H. (1997). *Ophthalmology for the primary care physician.* St. Louis: Mosby.)

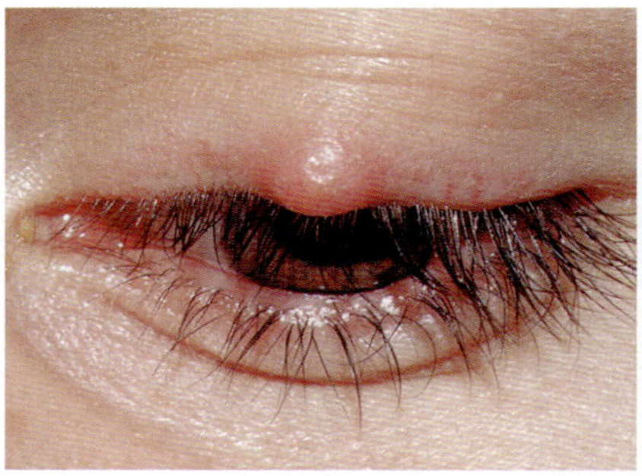

FIG. 12.10 Acute hordeolum of upper eyelid. (From Palay, D. A., & Krachmer, J. H. (1997). *Ophthalmology for the primary care physician.* St. Louis: Mosby.)

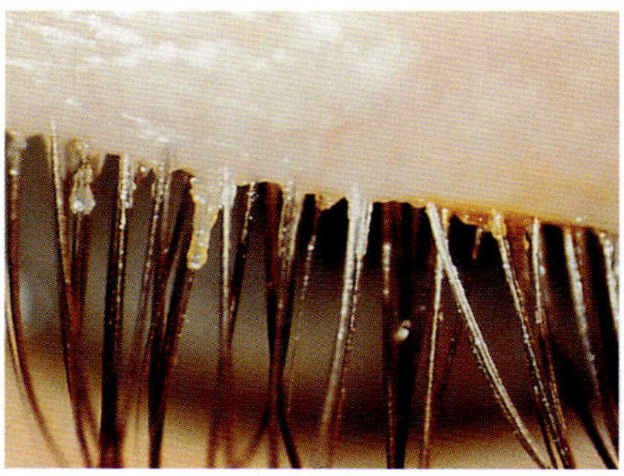

FIG. 12.11 Blepharitis. (From Zitelli, B. J., Davis, H. W. (2017). Zitelli and Davis' atlas of pediatric physical diagnosis, (7th ed.). Philadelphia, Elsevier.)

Palpation

Palpate the eyelids for nodules. Palpation of the eye is one of the simplest methods for intraocular pressure assessment. Gentle palpation through closed lids (digital palpation tonometry) can confirm that the involved eye is much harder than the uninvolved eye. Determine whether the eye can be gently pushed into the orbit without discomfort. Pain on palpation is consistent with scleritis, orbital cellulitis, and cavernous sinus thrombosis. An eye that feels very firm and resists palpation may indicate severe glaucoma or a retrobulbar tumor.

Conjunctiva

The conjunctivae are usually translucent and free of erythema. Inspect the palpebral conjunctiva by having the patient look upward while you draw the lower lid downward, noting translucency and vascular pattern (Fig. 12.12).

Inspect the upper tarsal conjunctiva only when there is a suggestion that a foreign body may be present. Ask the patient to look down while you pull the eyelashes gently downward and forward to break the suction between the lid and globe. Next, evert the lid on a small cotton-covered applicator (Fig. 12.13). After you inspect and remove any foreign body that may be present, return the eyelid to its regular position by asking the patient to look up while you apply downward pressure against the eyelid.

Observe the conjunctiva for erythema or exudate. An erythematous or cobblestone appearance, especially on the tarsal conjunctiva, may indicate an allergic (Fig. 12.14) or infectious conjunctivitis (Fig. 12.15). Bright red blood in a sharply defined area surrounded by healthy-appearing conjunctiva indicates subconjunctival hemorrhage (Fig. 12.16). The blood stays red because of direct diffusion of oxygen through the conjunctiva. Subconjunctival hemorrhages may occur with violent coughing, powerful sneezing, straining as during a constipated bowel movement, intractable vomiting, and spontaneously in

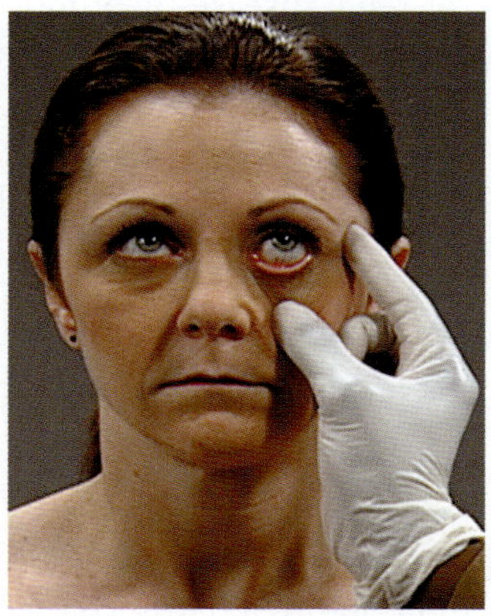

FIG. 12.12 Pulling lower eyelid down to inspect the conjunctiva.

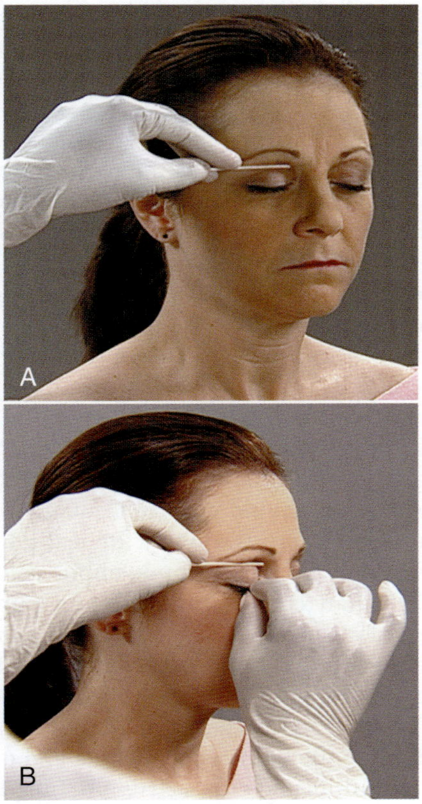

FIG. 12.13 Everting the upper eyelid. (A) Placing applicator above the globe. (B) Withdrawing the lid from the globe.

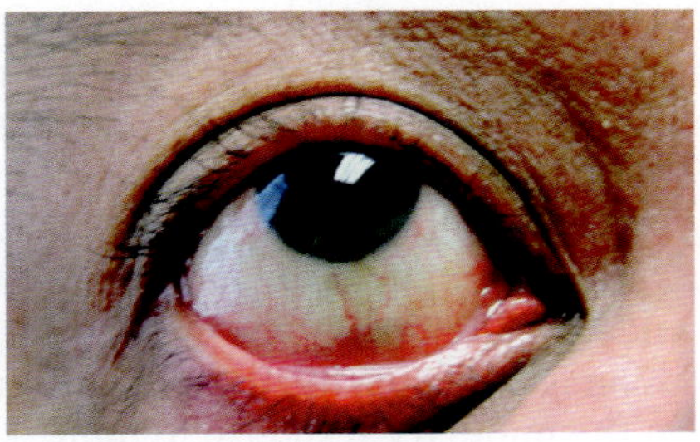

FIG. 12.14 Erythematous eye from a chemical allergy. (From Bielory, L. (2007). Differential diagnoses of conjunctivitis for clinical allergist-immunologists. *Annals of Allergy, Asthma & Immunology*, *98*(2), 105–115.)

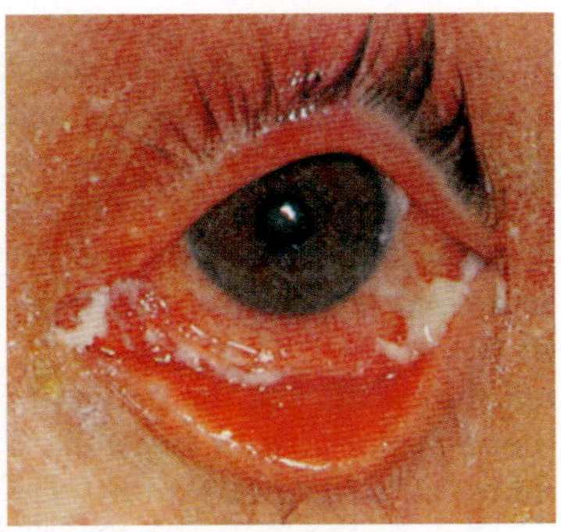

FIG. 12.15 Acute purulent conjunctivitis. (From Newell, F. W. (1996). *Ophthalmology: Principles and concepts* (8th ed.). St. Louis: Mosby.)

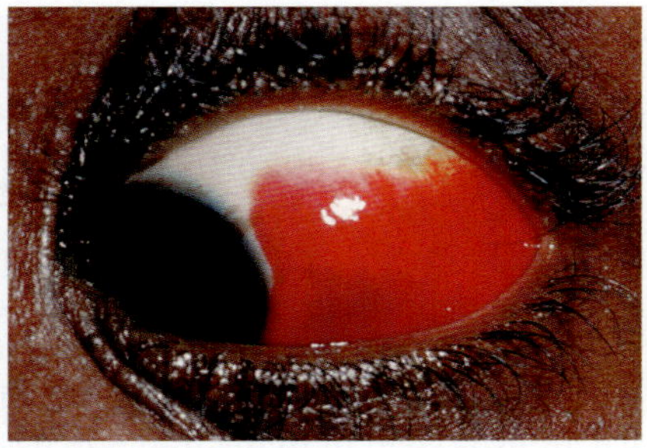

FIG. 12.16 Subconjunctival hemorrhage. (From Krachmer, J. H., & Palay, D. A. (2014). *Cornea atlas* (3rd ed.). Elsevier.)

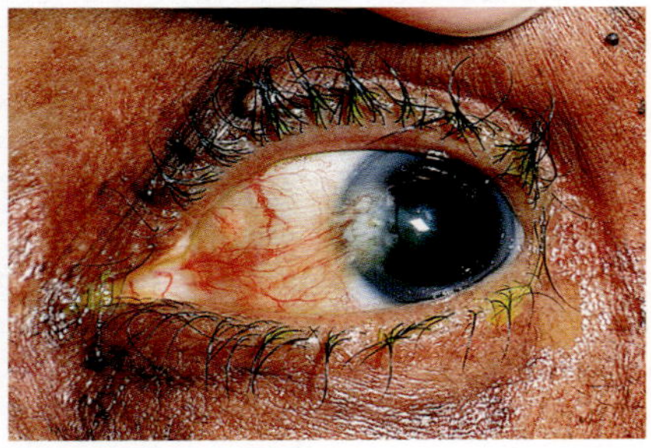

FIG. 12.17 Pterygium. (Courtesy John W. Payne, MD, The Wilmer Ophthalmological Institute, The Johns Hopkins University and Hospital, Baltimore, MD.)

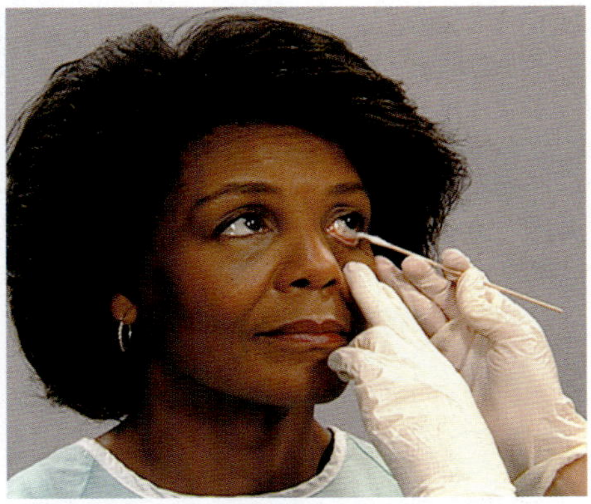

FIG. 12.18 Testing corneal sensitivity.

pregnancy or during labor. Other causes include trauma, foreign objects, and aggressive rubbing of the eye. The hemorrhages resolve spontaneously.

A pterygium is an abnormal growth of conjunctiva that extends over the cornea from the limbus. It occurs more commonly on the nasal side (Fig. 12.17) but may arise temporally as well. A pterygium is more common in people heavily exposed to ultraviolet light. It can interfere with vision if it advances over the pupil.

Cornea

Examine the cornea for clarity by shining a light tangentially on it. Because the cornea is normally avascular, blood vessels should not be present. Corneal sensitivity, controlled by CN V (trigeminal nerve), is tested by touching a wisp of cotton to the cornea (Fig. 12.18). The expected response is a blink, which indicates intact sensory fibers of CN V and motor fibers of CN VII (facial nerve). Decreased corneal sensation is often associated with diabetes, herpes simplex, and herpes zoster viral infections or is a sequela of trigeminal neuralgia or ocular surgery.

You may note a corneal arcus (arcus senilis), which is composed of lipids deposited in the periphery of the cornea. It may in time form a complete circle (circus senilis; Fig. 12.19). Note the subtle clear area between the limbus and the arcus. An arcus is seen in many individuals older than 60 years. If present before age 40, arcus senilis may indicate a lipid disorder. It is possible to have more than one process; Fig. 12.20 demonstrates both corneal circus senilis and a pterygium.

Iris and Pupil

The iris pattern should be clearly visible. In general, the irides are the same color. Note any irregularity in the shape of the pupils. Expect them to be round, regular, and equal in size. Bilateral and unilateral pupil abnormalities are listed in Table 12.2.

Estimate the pupillary sizes and compare them for equality. Pupils may show size variation in a number of ways. Miosis is pupillary constriction to less than 2 mm. The miotic pupil fails to dilate in the dark. It is commonly caused by opioids such as morphine, but drugs to treat glaucoma may also cause miosis. Pupillary dilation of more than 6 mm and failure of the pupils to constrict with light characterize mydriasis. Mydriasis is an accompaniment of coma (e.g., because of diabetes, alcohol, uremia, epilepsy, or brain trauma) or may be caused by some eye drops (e.g., some glaucoma medications,

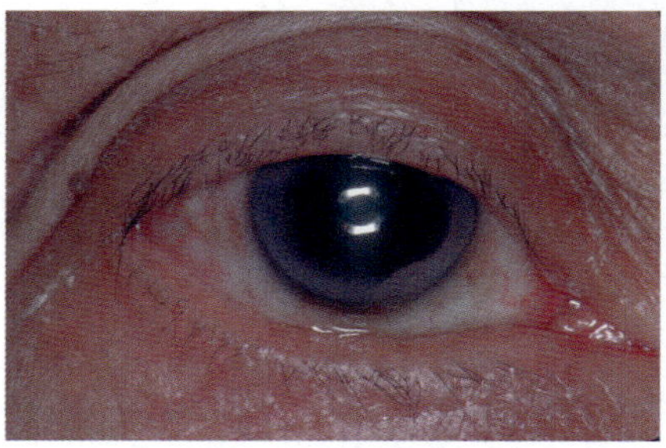

FIG. 12.19 **Corneal arcus senilis.** (From Palay, D. A., & Krachmer, J. H. (1997). *Ophthalmology for the primary care physician.* St. Louis: Mosby.)

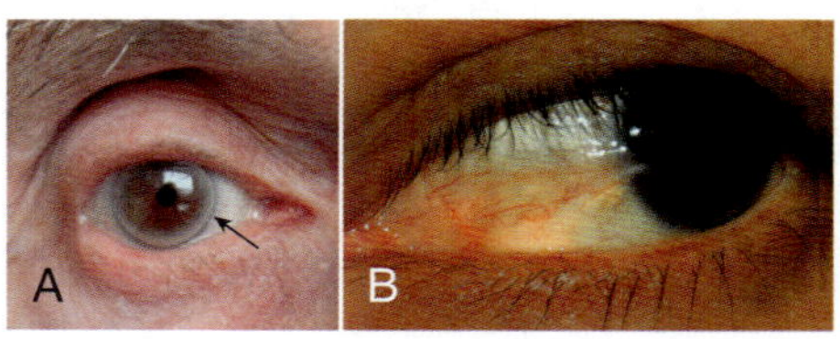

FIG. 12.20 (A) Arcus senilis. (B) Pterygium. (A, From Christoffersen, M., & Tybjærg-Hansen, A. (2016). Visible aging signs as risk markers for ischemic heart disease: Epidemiology, pathogenesis and clinical implications. *Ageing Research Reviews,* 25, 24–41; B, from Holland, E. J., Mannis, M. J., & Lee, W. B. (2013). *Ocular surface disease: Cornea, conjunctiva and tear film.* Elsevier.)

atropine, or strabismus management in children) or opioid withdrawal. Anisocoria, inequality of pupillary size, is a common variation but may also occur in a large range of disease states.

Test the pupils for response to light both directly and consensually. Dim the lights in the room so that the pupils dilate. Shine a penlight directly into one eye and note whether the pupil constricts. Note also the consensual response of the opposite pupil constricting simultaneously with the tested pupil. Repeat the test by shining the light in the other eye.

To evaluate the health of the optic nerve, look for an afferent pupillary defect by performing the swinging flashlight test. Shine the light in one eye and then rapidly swing to the other. There should be a slight dilation in the second eye while the light is crossing the bridge of the nose, but it should constrict equally to the first eye as the light enters the pupil. Repeat going in the other direction. If the second pupil continues to dilate rather than constrict, an afferent pupillary defect is present, also called a *Marcus-Gunn pupil.* This is an important sign of optic nerve disease and can be present in any eye with poor vision from severe retinal disease. There are many causes of afferent pupillary defect, including optic neuritis, glaucoma and optic nerve tumor, and multiple sclerosis. It is possible for an eye to have good visual acuity and an afferent defect. The eye, however, is not normal and the cause must be investigated.

Test the pupils for constriction to accommodation as well. Ask the patient to look at a distant object and then at a test object (either a pencil or your finger) held 10 cm from the bridge of the nose. Expect the pupils to constrict when the eyes focus on the near object. With some patients, especially those with dark irides, it may be easier to observe pupillary dilation when the patient looks from near to far. Testing for pupillary response to accommodation is of diagnostic importance only if there is a defect in the pupillary response to light. A failure to respond to direct light but retaining constriction during accommodation is sometimes seen in patients with diabetes or syphilis.

Lens

Inspect the lens, which should be transparent. Shining a light on the lens may cause it to appear gray or yellow, but light should still pass through. Later examination of the lens with the ophthalmoscope will help judge the clarity.

Sclera

The sclera should be examined primarily to ensure that it is white. The sclera should be visible above the iris only when the eyelids are wide open. If liver disease or a hemolytic disease is present, the sclera may become pigmented and appear either yellow or green. Senile hyaline plaque appears as a dark, slate gray pigment

TABLE 12.2 Descriptions of Various Pupil Abnormalities

ABNORMALITY	CONTRIBUTING FACTORS	APPEARANCE
Bilateral		
Miosis (pupillary constriction; usually less than 2 mm in diameter)	Iridocyclitis; miotic eye drops (e.g., pilocarpine given for glaucoma); opioid abuse	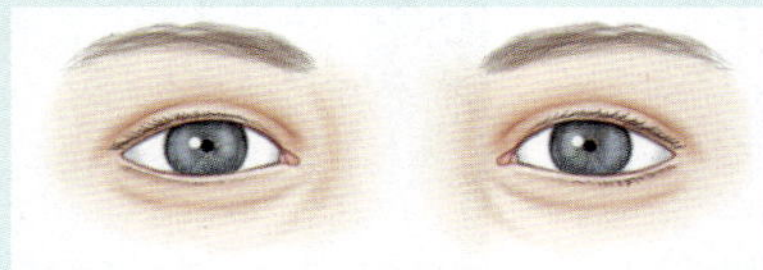
Mydriasis (pupillary dilation; usually more than 6 mm in diameter)	Iridocyclitis; mydriatic or cycloplegic drops (e.g., atropine); midbrain (reflex arc) lesions or hypoxia; oculomotor (cranial nerve [CN] III) damage; acute-angle glaucoma (slight dilation); stimulant (cocaine, amphetamines) abuse	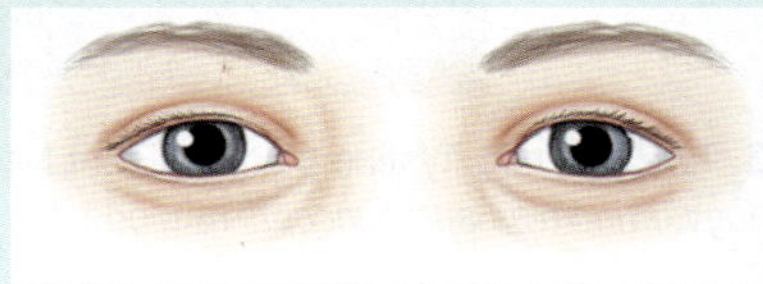
Failure to respond (constrict) with increased light stimulus	Iridocyclitis; retinal degeneration; optic nerve (CN II) destruction; midbrain synapses involving afferent papillae fibers or oculomotor nerve (CN III) (consensual response is also lost); impairment of efferent fibers (parasympathetic) that innervate sphincter pupillae muscle; mydriatics; brain herniation (fixed dilated pupils)	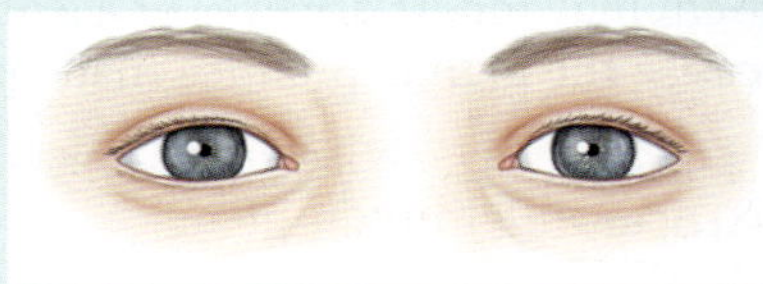
Argyll Robertson pupil	Bilateral, miotic, irregularly shaped pupils that fail to constrict with light but retain constriction with convergence; pupils may or may not be equal in size; commonly caused by neurosyphilis or lesions in midbrain where afferent pupillary fibers synapse	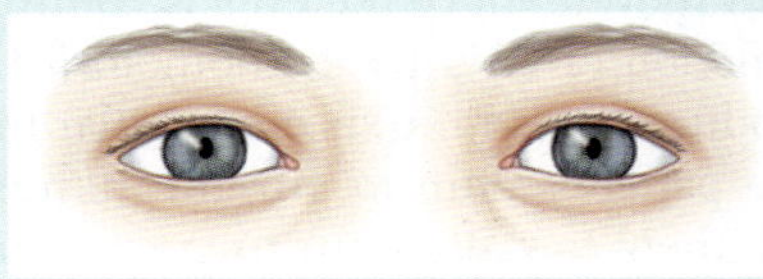
Unilateral		
Anisocoria (unequal size of pupils)	Congenital (approximately 20% of healthy people have minor or noticeable differences in pupil size, but reflexes are normal) or caused by local eye medications (constrictors or dilators) or unilateral sympathetic or parasympathetic pupillary pathway destruction (Note: Examiner should test whether pupils react equally to light; if response is unequal, examiner should note whether larger or smaller eye reacts more slowly [or not at all], because either pupil could represent the abnormal size.)	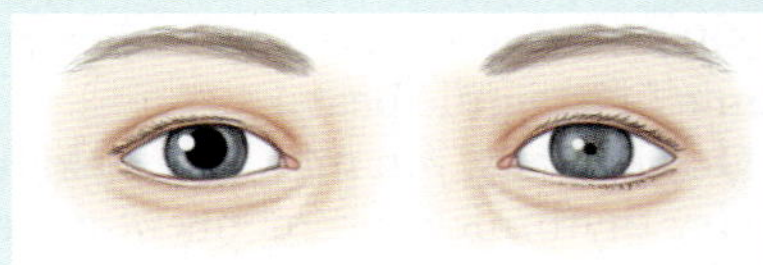
Iritis (anterior uveitis) constrictive response	Acute uveitis is commonly unilateral; constriction of pupil accompanied by pain and reddened eye, especially adjacent to the iris	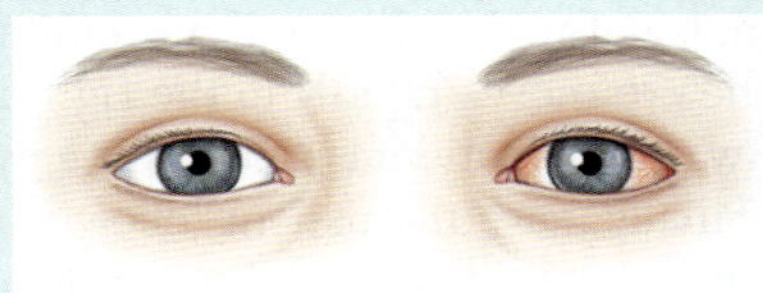
Oculomotor nerve (CN III) damage	Pupil dilated and fixed; eye deviated laterally and downward; ptosis	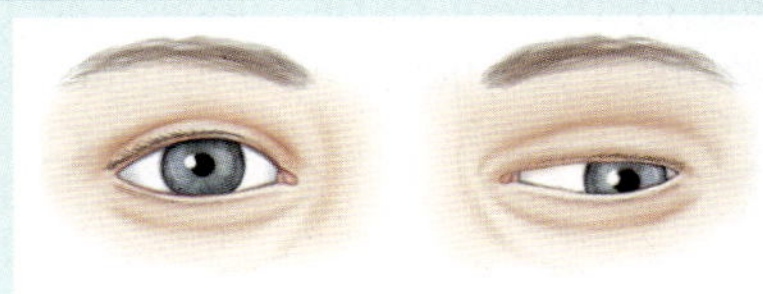
Adie pupil (tonic pupil)	Affected pupil dilated and reacts slowly or fails to react to light; responds to convergence; caused by impairment of postganglionic parasympathetic innervation to sphincter pupillae muscle or ciliary malfunction; often accompanied by diminished tendon reflexes (as with diabetic neuropathy or alcoholism)	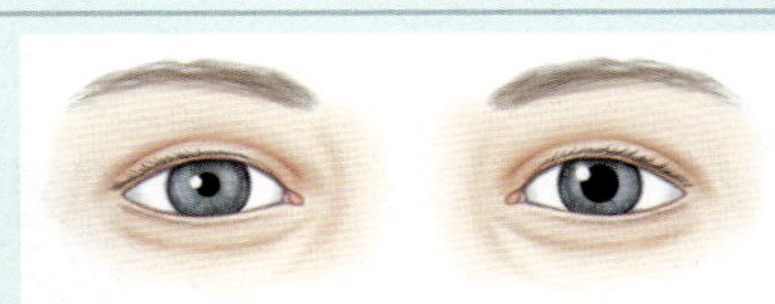

just anterior to the insertion of the medial rectus muscle (Fig. 12.21). Its presence does not imply disease but should be noted.

Lacrimal Apparatus

Inspect the region of the lacrimal gland and palpate the lower orbital rim near the inner canthus. The puncta should be seen as slight elevations with a central depression on both the upper and lower lid margins nasally. If the temporal aspect of the upper lid feels full, evert the lid and inspect the gland. The lacrimal glands are rarely enlarged but may become enlarged in some conditions such as tumors, lymphoid infiltration, sarcoid disease, and Sjögren syndrome. Despite the enlargement, the

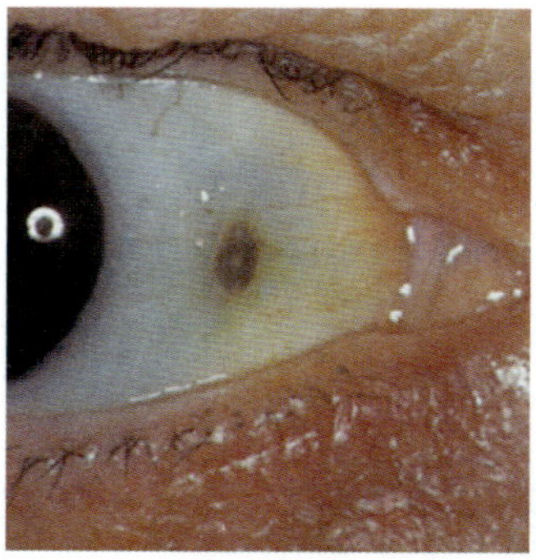

FIG. 12.21 **Senile hyaline plaque.** (From Newell, F. W. (1996). *Ophthalmology: Principles and concepts* (8th ed.). St. Louis: Mosby.)

patient may report dry eyes or a gritty feeling in the eyes because the glands produce inadequate tears.

Extraocular Muscles

Full movement of the eyes is controlled by the integrated function of CNs III (oculomotor), IV (trochlear), and VI (abducens) and the six extraocular muscles. You may hold the patient's chin to prevent movement of the head and ask them to watch your finger as it moves through the six cardinal fields of gaze (Fig. 12.22). Then ask the patient to look to the extreme lateral (temporal) positions. Do not be surprised to observe a few horizontal rhythmic movements (nystagmic beats).

Occasionally, you may note sustained nystagmus, involuntary rhythmic movements of the eyes that can occur in a horizontal, vertical, rotary, or mixed pattern. Jerking nystagmus, characterized by faster movements in one direction, is defined by its rapid movement phase. For example, if the eye moves rapidly to the right and then slowly drifts leftward, the patient is said to have nystagmus to the right.

Finally, have the patient follow your finger in the vertical plane, going from ceiling to floor. Observe the coordinated movement of the globes and the superior lids. The movement should be accomplished smoothly and without exposure of the sclera. Full movements indicate integrity of muscle strength and CNs. Lid lag, the exposure of the sclera above the iris when the patient is asked to follow your finger as you direct the eye in a smooth movement from ceiling to floor, may indicate thyroid eye disease.

Use the corneal light reflex to test the balance of the extraocular muscles. Direct a light source at the nasal bridge from a distance of about 30 cm. Ask the patient to look at a nearby object (but not the light source). This will encourage both eyes to converge. The light should be reflected symmetrically from both eyes. If you find an imbalance with the corneal light reflex test, perform the cover-uncover test (Fig. 12.23) or use a StrabismoScope or photo screening (see Chapter 3, Fig. 3.16) to evaluate. To perform the cover-uncover test, ask the patient to stare straight ahead at a near fixed point. Cover one eye and observe the uncovered eye for movement as it focuses on the designated point. Remove the cover and watch for movement of the newly uncovered eye as it fixes on the object. Repeat the process, covering the other eye. If the eye being tested is the strabismic eye (crossed eye; both eyes not looking at the same place at the same time), then it will fixate on the object by moving after the "straight" eye is covered as long as the vision in this eye is good enough (Fig. 12.24). If the "straight" eye is being tested, there will be no movement because it is already fixated. Depending on the direction that the strabismic eye deviates, the direction of deviation may be assessed. *Exotropic* is outward (away from the midline), and *esotropic* is inward (toward the nose). Movement of the covered or uncovered eye mandates referral to an ophthalmologist.

Ophthalmoscopic Examination

Ophthalmoscopic (funduscopic) examination of the eyes can be a tiring process for the patient. Give the patient brief intervals of rest from the bright light to reduce fatigue and improve comfort.

Inspection of the interior of the eye permits visualization of the optic disc, arteries, veins, and retina. Adequate

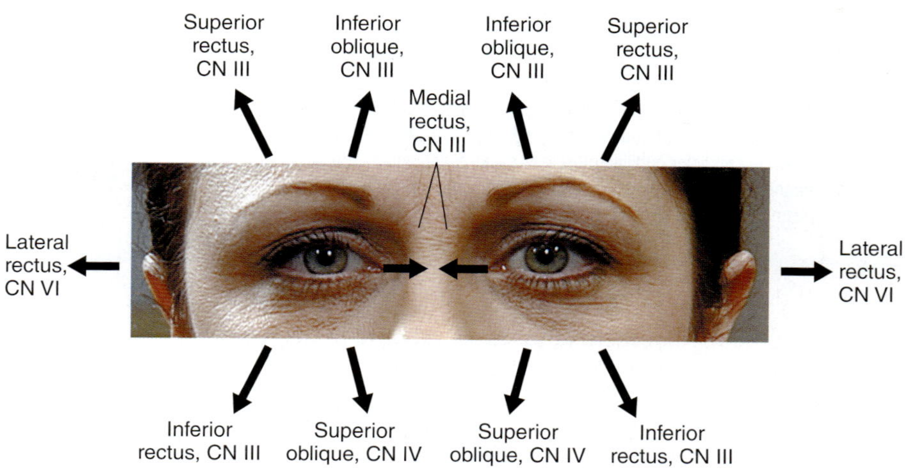

FIG. 12.22 **Cranial nerves and extraocular muscles associated with the six cardinal fields of gaze.**

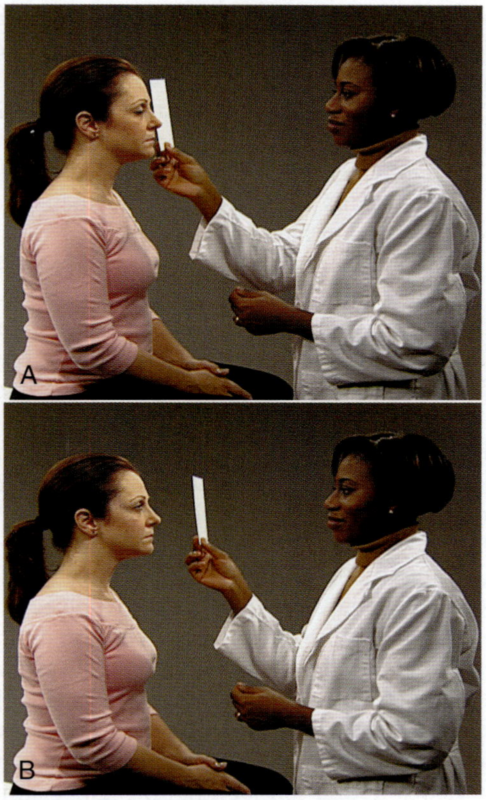

FIG. 12.23 **Evaluating eye fixation by the cover-uncover test.** (A) Patient focuses on near object. (B) Examiner evaluates movement of covered eye as cover is removed.

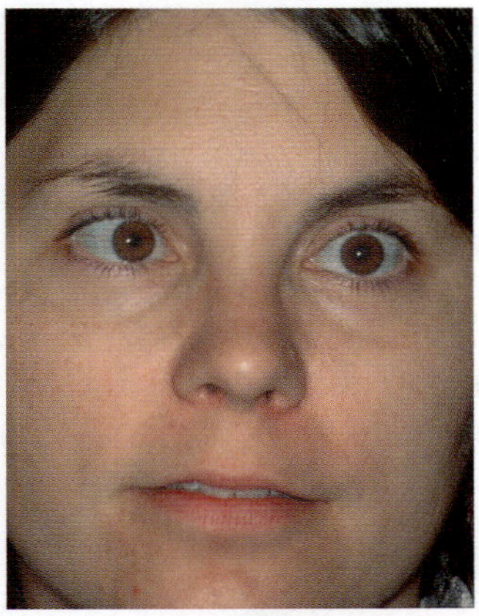

FIG. 12.24 **Strabismus.** (Courtesy Lemmi, F. O., & Lemmi, C. A. E. (2009). *Physical assessment findings CD-ROM.* Philadelphia: Saunders.)

pupillary dilation is necessary and can often be achieved by dimming the lights in the examining room. Instillation of medications that cause mydriasis is used in some cases (Box 12.1).

Examine the patient's right eye with your right eye and the patient's left eye with your left to prevent unintentional nose-to-nose contact. Hold the ophthalmoscope in the hand that corresponds to the examining eye. (The structure of the ophthalmoscope is detailed in Chapter 3.) Change the lens of the ophthalmoscope with your index finger. Start with the lens on the 0 setting, and stabilize yourself and the patient by placing your free hand on the patient's shoulder or head (Fig. 12.25). If using an indirect ophthalmoscope (see Chapter 3, Fig. 3.15), you can use your dominant eye to examine both of the patient's eyes

BOX 12.1 Test for Applying Mydriatics

Before instillation of a mydriatic, inspect the patient's anterior chamber by shining a focused light tangentially at the limbus (the union of the conjunctiva and the sclera). Note the illumination of the iris nasally. This portion of the iris is not lighted when the patient has a shallow anterior chamber, indicating a risk of acute-angle glaucoma. Mydriatics should be avoided in these patients.

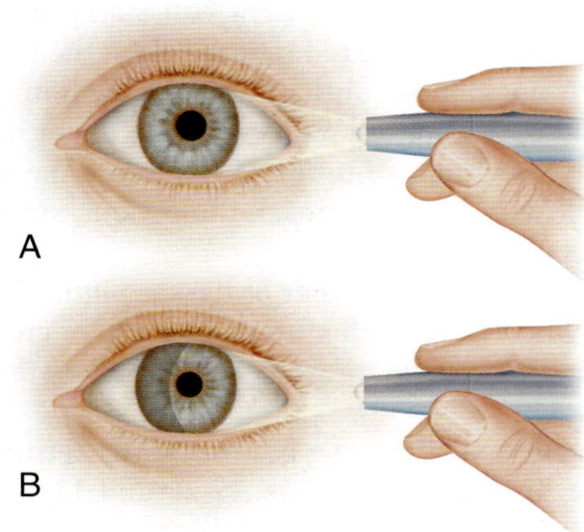

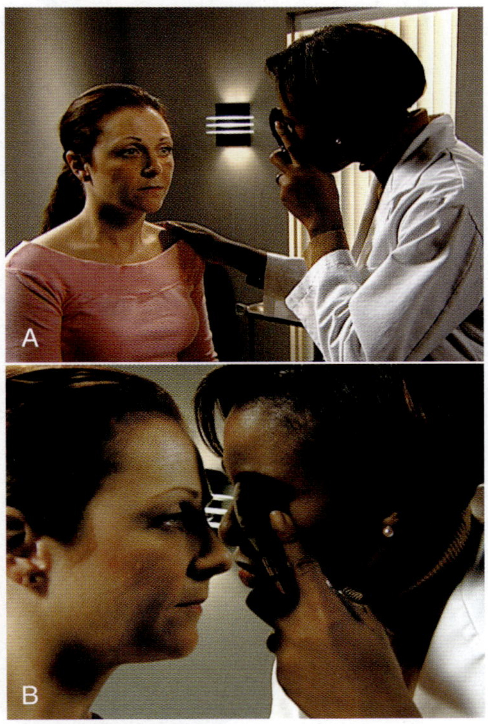

FIG. 12.25 (A) Visualization of the red reflex. (B) Examination of the optic fundus.

because of the increased distance between the patient and examiner. The focus wheel is adjusted with your thumb.

With the patient looking at a distant fixation point, direct the light of the ophthalmoscope at the pupil from about 30 cm (12 inches) away. If using an indirect ophthalmoscope, have the patient focus on an object 15 to 20 feet away, then slowly position the eye cup over the patient's eye. With either scope, visualize a red reflex first. The red reflex is caused by the light illuminating the retina. Any opacities in the path of the light will stand out as black densities. Absence of the red reflex is often the result of an improperly positioned ophthalmoscope, but it may also indicate total opacity of the pupil by a cataract or by hemorrhage into the vitreous humor. If you locate the red reflex and then lose it as you approach the patient, simply move back and start again.

No discrete areas of lighter or darker pigmentation are expected when viewing the fundus, except for crescents or dots at the disc margin, most commonly along the temporal edge.

As you approach the eye gradually, the retinal details should become apparent (Figs. 12.26 and 12.27). At any one time, you will see only a small portion of the retina.

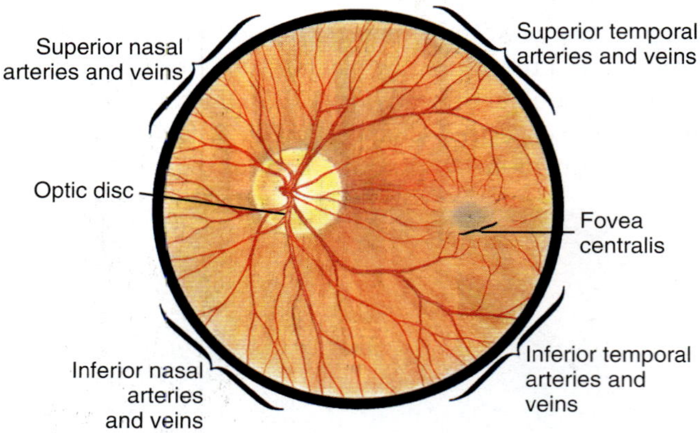

FIG. 12.26 Retinal structures of the left eye.

A blood vessel will probably be the first structure seen when you are about 3 to 5 cm from the patient. You may have to adjust the ophthalmoscope lens to be able to see the retinal details. If your patient is myopic, you will need to use a minus (red) lens; if the patient is hyperopic or lacks a lens (aphakic), you will need a plus lens (see Chapter 3). When fundus details come into focus, you will note the branching of blood vessels. Because they always branch away from the optic disc, you can use these landmarks to find the optic disc. The optic disc is where the retina converges to the optic nerve, and because there are no photoreceptors (rods and cones) in this part of the retina and it cannot respond to light stimulation, it is called a *blind spot*.

Next, look at the vascular supply of the retina. The blood vessels on the disc divide into superior and inferior branches and then into nasal and temporal ones. Venous pulsation may be seen on the disc and should be noted. Arterioles are smaller than venules, generally by a ratio of 3:5 to 2:3. The light reflected from arterioles is brighter than that from venules, and the oxygenated blood is a brighter red. Follow the blood vessels distally as far as you can in each of the four quadrants. Note especially the sites of crossing of the arterioles and venules, because their characteristics may change when hypertension is present. Characteristics found on ophthalmologic examination in a patient with hypertension include narrowing of vessels, increased vascular tortuosity, copper wiring (diffuse red-brown reflex), arteriovenous nicking, and retinal hemorrhages (see Fig. 12.34).

Finally, examine the optic disc itself. The disc margin should be sharp and well defined, especially in the temporal region. The disc is generally yellow to creamy pink, but the color varies with race, being darker in individuals whose skin is dark (Fig. 12.28; see Clinical Pearl, "Fundus Pigmentation"). It is about 1.5 mm in diameter and is the unit of measurement in describing lesion size and location on the fundus. For example, an abnormality of a blood vessel may occur two disc diameters from the optic nerve at the two o'clock position (Fig. 12.29).

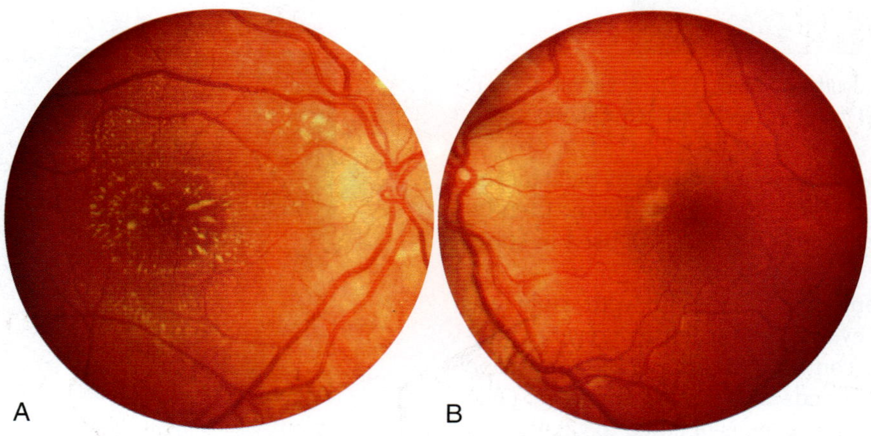

FIG. 12.27 (A) Normal right fundus in a White patient. (B) Normal left fundus. (From Agarwal, A. (2012). *Gass' atlas of macular diseases* (5th ed.). Elsevier.)

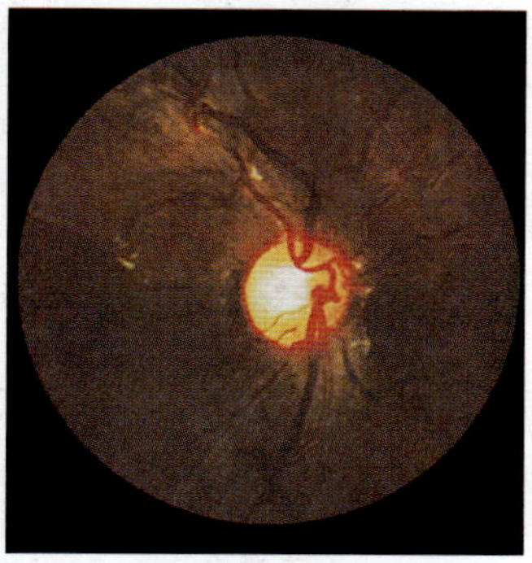

FIG. 12.28 **Fundus of a Black patient.** (From Medcom. (1983). *Selected topics in ophthalmology: Medcom clinical lecture guides.* Garden Grove, CA: Medcom.)

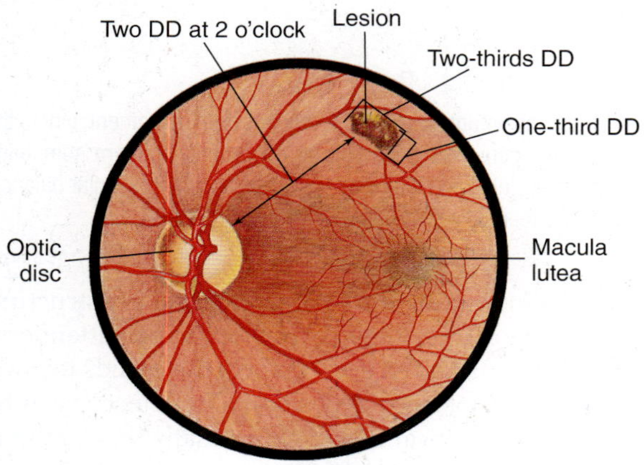

FIG. 12.29 **Method of describing the position and dimension of a lesion in terms of disc diameter.** The lesion in this illustration is described as being two disc diameters (*DD*) from the optic disc at the two o'clock position. The lesion is two-thirds DD long and one-third DD wide.

CLINICAL PEARL

Fundus Pigmentation

The fundus, or retina, appears as a yellow or reddish pink background, depending on the amount of melanin in the pigment epithelium. The pigment generally varies with the skin color of the patient (see Fig. 12.28).

Next examine the macula, also called the *fovea centralis* or *macula lutea*. The site of central vision, it is located approximately two disc diameters temporal to the optic disc. It may be impossible to examine when the pupil is not dilated, because shining light on it induces strong pupillary constriction. To bring it into your field of vision, ask the patient to look directly at the light of the ophthalmoscope. No blood vessels enter the fovea, and it appears as a lighter dot surrounded by an avascular area.

Unexpected Findings

Occasionally, you may see unexpected findings such as myelinated nerve fibers, papilledema (Fig. 12.30), glaucomatous cupping, drusen bodies, cotton-wool bodies, or hemorrhages (Table 12.3).

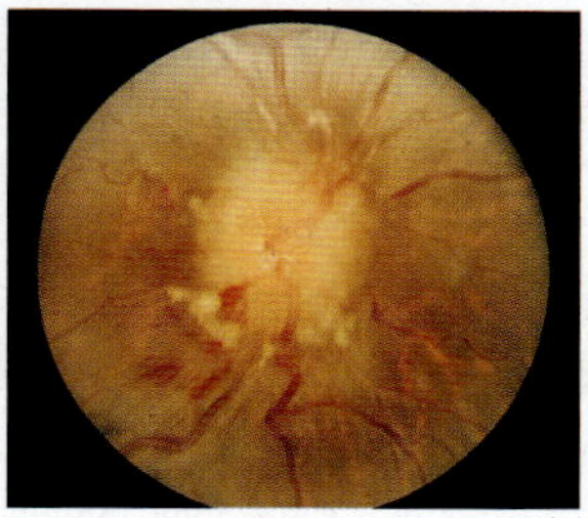

FIG. 12.30 **Severe papilledema.** (Courtesy John W. Payne, MD, The Wilmer Ophthalmological Institute, The Johns Hopkins University and Hospital, Baltimore, MD.)

TABLE 12.3 Unexpected Retinal Findings

UNEXPECTED FINDING	DESCRIPTION	SIGNIFICANCE
Myelinated retinal nerve fibers (see Fig. 12.30)	White area with soft, ill-defined peripheral margins usually continuous with the optic disc Absence of pigment, feathery margins, and full visual fields help distinguish this benign condition from chorioretinitis. Contrast with Fig. 12.47. Nerve fiber layer is the innermost retinal surface; the vessels lie deeper in the retina. Note how the myelinated nerve fibers obscure areas of the retinal blood vessels, particularly inferiorly.	No physiologic significance
Papilledema (see Fig. 12.30)	Loss of definition of optic disc margin initially occurs superiorly and inferiorly, then nasally and temporally central vessels are pushed forward, and veins are markedly dilated. Venous pulsations are not visible and cannot be induced by pressure applied to the globe. Venous hemorrhages may occur.	Caused by increased intracranial pressure transmitted along the optic nerve. Initially, vision is not altered.
Glaucomatous optic nerve head cupping (see Fig. 12.46)	Physiologic disc margins are raised with a lowered central area. Blood vessels may disappear over the edge of the physiologic disc and may be seen again deep within the disc. Occasionally atrophy occurs unilaterally; always compare cupping on the two retinas. Compare with healthy vessels as seen in Figs. 12.26 and 12.27. Impairment of blood supply may lead to optic atrophy, causing the disc to appear much whiter than usual. The cup is usually not particularly enlarged in contrast to glaucomatous atrophy.	Result of increased intraocular pressure with loss of nerve fibers and death of ganglion cells. Peripheral visual fields are constricted.
Cotton-wool spot (see Fig. 12.42)	Ill-defined yellow areas caused by infarction of nerve layer of the retina.	Vascular disease secondary to hypertension or diabetes mellitus is a common cause.

Hemorrhages in the retina vary in color and shape, depending on the cause and location. A hemorrhage at the disc margin often indicates poorly controlled or undiagnosed glaucoma (Fig. 12.31A). Also note the loss of the vessels at the inferior margin of the disc. Flame-shaped hemorrhages occur in the nerve fiber layers, and the blood spreads parallel to the nerve fibers (see Fig. 12.31B). Round hemorrhages tend to occur in the deeper layers and may appear as a dark color instead of the bright red that is characteristic of flame hemorrhages. Dot hemorrhages may actually represent microaneurysms, which are common in diabetic retinopathy. The direct ophthalmoscope does not permit the distinction between dot hemorrhages and microaneurysms. Vascular changes that suggest systemic hypertension may be observed in the retina and are described in Box 12.2.

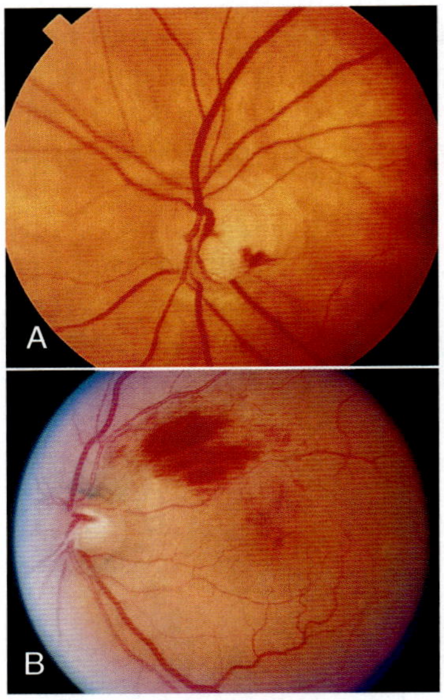

FIG. 12.31 (A) Hemorrhage at the disc margin. (B) Flame hemorrhages. (A, Courtesy John W. Payne, MD, The Wilmer Ophthalmological Institute, The Johns Hopkins University and Hospital, Baltimore, MD. B, Courtesy Robert P. Murphy, MD, Glaser Murphy Retina Treatment Center, Baltimore, MD.)

Infants

Infants often shut their eyes tightly when an eye examination is attempted. It is difficult to separate the eyelids, and often the lids evert when too much effort is exerted. If a parent is present, have the parent hold the infant over a shoulder, and position yourself behind the parent. Turning off the overhead lights can also be helpful (see Clinical Pearl, "Examining an Infant's Eyes").

CLINICAL PEARL

Examining an Infant's Eyes

Even when the infant is crying, there is often a moment when the infant's eyes open. This gives you an opportunity to learn something about the eyes, including their symmetry, extraocular muscular balance, and whether there is a symmetric red reflex.

Begin by inspecting the infant's external eye structures. Note the size of the eyes, paying particular attention to small or differently sized eyes. Inspect the eyelids for swelling, epicanthal folds, and position. To detect epicanthal folds, look for a vertical fold of skin nasally that covers the lacrimal caruncle (Fig. 12.32). Prominent epicanthal folds are an expected variant in Asian infants and may be seen in infants of other racial and ethnic backgrounds, but they may also be suggestive of Down syndrome or other congenital anomalies. Observe the alignment and slant of the palpebral fissures of the infant's eyes. Draw an imaginary

BOX 12.2 Hypertensive Retinopathy

- Retinal changes associated with hypertension have historically been classified according to the Keith-Wagener-Barker (KWB) system of four groups of increasing severity. They described changes in the vascular supply, the retina itself, and the optic disc. Criticism of this system argues that the retinopathy grades are not closely correlated with severity of hypertension, and early stages of hypertensive retinopathy were not well delineated. A simplified prognosis-based classification was subsequently developed (Harjasouliha et al., 2016).
- The arteriole-venule size ratio is usually 3:5. That ratio decreases as arterioles become smaller because of smooth muscle contraction, hyperplasia, or fibrosis. Venules do not have a smooth muscle coat, but share the adventitia of the arteriole where the arteriole and venule cross. Thickening of the arteriolar coat results in apparent nicking of the venule where the venule passes beneath the arteriole, or the venule may appear elevated when it passes over the arteriole.

GRADE OF RETINOPATHY	RETINAL SIGNS	SYSTEMIC ASSOCIATIONS
None	No detectable changes	None
Mild	Retinal arteriolar narrowing, arteriovenous nicking, opacity (copper wiring) of arteriolar wall	Modest association with risk of clinically significant stroke, subclinical stroke, coronary heart disease, and death
Moderate	Hemorrhage (blot, dot, or flame-shaped); cotton-wool spots, hard exudates; and microaneurysms	Strong association with clinically significant stroke, cognitive decline, and death from cardiovascular causes
Malignant or Severe	Some or all of the preceding signs, plus optic disc edema (papilledema)	Strong association with death; presence of papilledema mandates rapid lowering of blood pressure

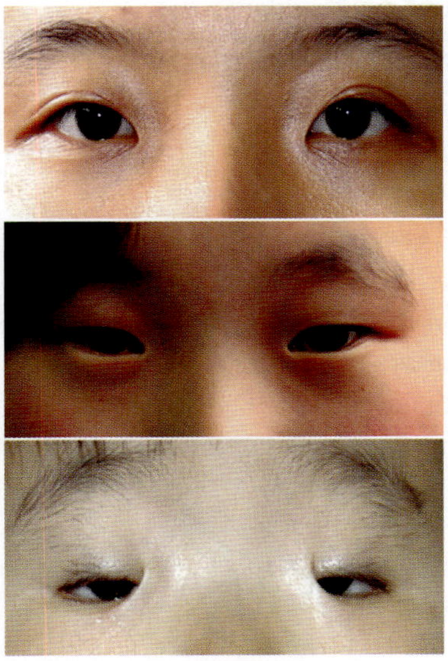

FIG. 12.32 Epicanthal folds. (From Wang, S., Shi, F., Luo, X., Liu, F., Zhou, X., Yang, J., Yang, Q., & Wang, X. (2013). Epicanthal fold correction: Our experience and comparison among three kinds of epicanthoplasties. *Journal of Plastic, Reconstructive & Aesthetic Surgery*, *66*(5), 682–687. https://doi.org/10.1016/j.bjps.2013.01.028.)

line through the medial canthi, and extend the line past the outer canthi of the eyes. The medial and lateral canthi are usually horizontal. When the outer canthi are above the line, an upward slant is present. When the outer canthi are below the line, a downward slant is present (Fig. 12.33).

Inspect the level of the eyelid covering the eye. If hydrocephalus is suspected, evaluate for the sunsetting sign, rapidly lowering the infant from upright to supine position. Look for sclera above the iris (see Fig. 9.18). This sign may be an expected variant in newborns; however, it also may be observed in infants with hydrocephalus and brainstem lesions.

Observe the distance between the eyes, looking for a wide spacing, or hypertelorism, which may be associated with craniofacial defects, including some with intellectual disability. Pseudostrabismus is the false appearance of strabismus caused by a flattened nasal bridge or epicanthal folds. Pseudostrabismus generally disappears by about 1 year of age. Use the corneal light reflex to distinguish pseudostrabismus from strabismus. An asymmetric light reflex may indicate a true strabismus.

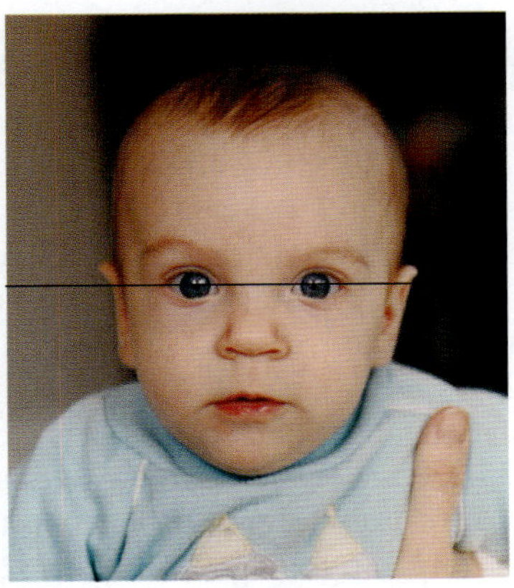

FIG. 12.33 Drawing a line between the two medial canthi and extending it temporally to determine whether a upward (outercorner higher than the inner corner) or downward plapebral slant (outer corner is lower than the inner corner). (Courtesy Matthew Watson.)

Inspect the sclera, conjunctiva, pupil, and iris of each eye. Inspect and compare corneal sizes. Enlarged corneas may be a sign of congenital glaucoma. The newborn's eyelids may be swollen or edematous from birth trauma (Fig. 12.34) but, if accompanied by conjunctival inflammation and drainage, may represent ophthalmia neonatorum (neonatal bacterial conjunctivitis). Any redness, hemorrhages, discharge, or granular appearance beyond the newborn period may indicate infection, allergy, or trauma. Inspect each iris and pupil for any irregularity in shape. A coloboma, or keyhole pupil, is often associated with other congenital anomalies. White specks scattered in a linear pattern around the entire circumference of the iris, called *Brushfield spots,* strongly suggest Down syndrome (trisomy 21).

Test CNs II, III, IV, and VI in the following manner:

- Examine vision grossly by observing the infant's preference for looking at certain objects. Expect the infant to focus on and track a light or face through 60 degrees.
- Elicit the optical blink reflex by shining a bright light at the infant's eyes, noting the quick closure of the eyes and dorsiflexion of the head.
- Perform the corneal reflex as in adults.

Assess for a symmetric red reflex in every newborn. Observe for any opacities, dark spots, or white spots. Opacities or interruption of the red reflex may indicate congenital cataracts, retinoblastoma, or other serious intraocular pathology (Table 12.4).

A funduscopic examination is difficult to conduct on a newborn or young infant and is generally deferred until the child is 3 years old, unless there is concern about a congenital eye abnormality, suspicion of physical abuse (shaken baby syndrome), trauma, or need for an assessment for ROP.

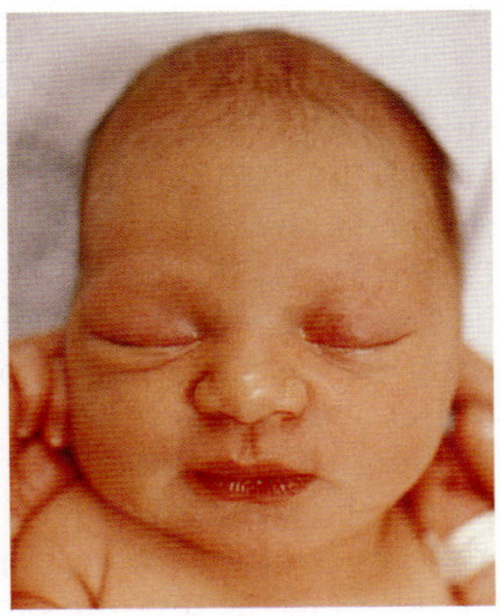

FIG. 12.34 Swollen eyelids in a newborn.

TABLE 12.4 Pediatric Eye Evaluation Screening Recommendations for Health Care Providers

RECOMMENDED AGE FOR SCREENING	SCREENING METHOD	CRITERIA FOR REFERRAL TO AN OPHTHALMOLOGIST
Newborn to 3 months	Red reflex	Abnormal or asymmetric
	Inspection for constant strabismus	Structural abnormality
6 months to 1 year	Fix and follow with each eye	Failure to fix and follow in cooperative infant
	Alternate occlusion	Failure to object equally to the covering of each eye
	Corneal light reflex	Asymmetric
	Red reflex	Abnormal or asymmetric
	Inspection for strabismus	Structural abnormality
	Photo screening*	Failure to meet screening criteria
3–5 years	Visual acuity	20/50 (age 3), 20/40 (age 4), 20/30 (age 5) or worse or two lines of difference between the eyes
	Corneal light reflex/cover-uncover	Asymmetric/ocular fixation movements
	Stereoacuity	Failure to appreciate asymmetric random dot or Titmus stereogram
	Red reflex	Abnormal or asymmetric
	Inspection	Structural abnormality
6 years and older	Visual acuity	20/30 or worse or two lines of difference between the eyes
	Corneal light reflex/cover-uncover	Asymmetric/ocular fixation movements
	Stereoacuity	Failure to appreciate stereopsis
	Red reflex	Abnormal or asymmetric
	Inspection	Structural abnormality

*Photoscreening offers an alternative to traditional visual acuity screening and is useful with preverbal children (under age 3 years), young children (ages 3 to 5 years), and older, noncooperative or nonverbal children. Visual acuity screening should be done when a child is sufficiently mature to respond to this testing (usually ages 4 to 6 years).

From American Academy of Ophthalmology Pediatric Ophthalmology/Strabismus Panel. (2007). *Preferred practice pattern guidelines: Pediatric eye evaluations.* San Francisco, CA; and American Academy of Pediatrics Section on Ophthalmology. (2012). Committee on Practice and Ambulatory Medicine, American Academy of Ophthalmology, American Association for Pediatric Ophthalmology and Strabismus, American Association of Certified Orthoptists: Instrument-based pediatric vision screening policy statement. *Pediatrics, 130*(5), 983–986. http://dx.doi.org/10.1542/peds.2012-2548

Children

Perform the inspection of the young child's external eye structures as described for the infant.

Assessment of visual function of infants is best done evaluating the ability of the child to fixate on and follow an object. This evaluation should be done first binocularly and then with each eye alternately covered. If poor binocular fixation and following are noted after 3 months of age or eye movement is asymmetric (dysconjugate gaze) in children of any age, further evaluation is needed.

Test visual acuity (when the child is awake and cooperative) with the LEA or HOTV for children ages 3 to 5 years. Use the Snellen or Sloan chart for verbal and English-speaking children ages 6 years and older (Loh & Chiang, 2018; see Fig 3.17A and B). Have one examiner point to the line on the chart and another assist the child with covering one eye. Children up to 5 years of age should stand 10 feet away with eye charts calibrated for use at 10 feet. Children 6 years and older may be tested at either 10 feet or at the standard 20 feet, as long as the chart is properly calibrated for the testing distance. To help the child understand the test, the eye chart should be first reviewed with both eyes open. After testing with both eyes, one eye is occluded (preferably with a patch or tape to prevent peeking), and the test is presented to each eye independently. If the child wears glasses, vision should be tested both with and without corrective lenses and recorded separately.

The anticipated visual acuity for children aged 36 to 47 months should be 20/50 or better, 20/40 for children aged 48 to 59 months, and 20/30 or better for children 60 months (5 years) of age or older. A child with vision that falls outside this range should be referred to a specialist for evaluation. Photoscreening is recommended as an alternative to visual acuity screening with vision charts from 3 to 6 years of age; after age 6, visual acuity screening with vision charts becomes more efficient and less costly (American Academy of Pediatrics, 2012; Donahue & Baker, 2015; U.S. Preventive Services Task Force, 2017).

When you are testing visual acuity in the child, any difference in the scores between the eyes should be noted. A child with a two-line difference between the eyes even within the passing range (e.g., 20/25 and 20/40) should also be referred to a specialist.

Examine extraocular movements and CNs III, IV, and VI as performed with adults. You may need to hold the child's head still and use an appealing toy or object for

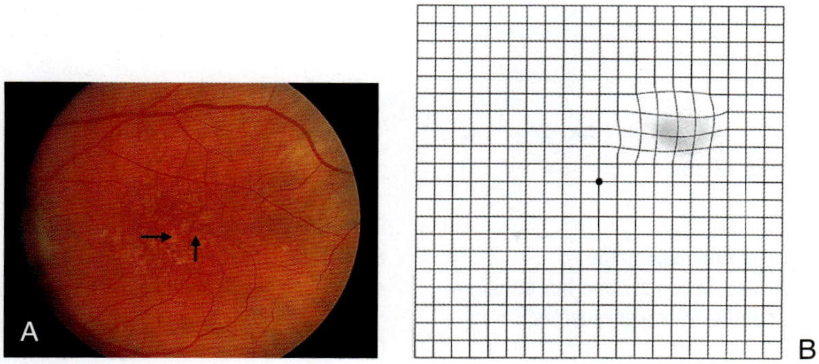

FIG. 12.35 (A) Drusen bodies. (B) Amsler grid showing visual changes caused by fluid leakage under the retina. (A, Courtesy Robert P. Murphy, MD, Glaser Murphy Retina Treatment Center, Baltimore, MD; B, Courtesy Brent A. Bauer, MFA, The Wilmer Ophthalmological Institute, The Johns Hopkins University and Hospital, Baltimore, MD.)

the child to follow through the six cardinal fields of gaze. Peripheral vision can be tested in cooperative children; the young child may prefer to sit on the parent's lap while these tests are performed.

Patience is often needed to gain the child's cooperation for the funduscopic examination. The young child is often unable to keep the eyes still and focused on a distant object. Do not hold the child's eyelids open forcibly because this may lead to some resistance. Rather than move the ophthalmoscope to visualize all retinal fields, inspect the optic disc, the fovea, and the vessels as they pass by. Often the results are better when the child sits on the parent's lap. If this position is used, examine the child as you would an adult.

Pregnant Patients

Retinal examination in pregnant patients can help differentiate between chronic hypertension and PIH. Vascular tortuosity, angiosclerosis, hemorrhage, and exudates may be seen in patients with a long-standing history of hypertension. In a patient with PIH, however, there is segmental arteriolar narrowing with a wet, glistening appearance indicative of edema. This finding is not exclusive to pregnant patients and may be seen with other causes of retinal edema. Hemorrhages and exudates are rare. Detachment of the retina may occur with spontaneous reattachment after hypertension is successfully controlled.

Because of systemic absorption, cycloplegic and mydriatic agents should be avoided unless there is a need to evaluate for retinal disease. Use of nasolacrimal duct occlusion after instillation of topical eye medications may reduce systemic absorption.

Older Adults

Lacrimal glands begin to involute and tear production decreases. The most common causes of decreased visual function include glaucoma, cataracts, and macular degeneration.

Drusen bodies can appear as small, discrete spots that are slightly more yellow than the retina. With time, the spots enlarge. Similar-appearing lesions may occur in many conditions that affect the pigment layers of the retina, but most commonly they are a consequence of the aging process and, depending on size and number, are a precursor of senile macular degeneration (Fig. 12.35A).

When drusen bodies are noted to be increasing in number or in intensity of color, use an Amsler grid to evaluate the patient's central vision. Instruct the patient to observe the grid with each eye, using reading glasses if needed, and to note any distortion of the grid pattern. Distortion could represent macular degeneration (see "Abnormalities"). Fig. 12.35B shows the grid of an individual with drusen bodies who has developed fluid leakage in the area of the macula.

ABNORMALITIES

External Eye

EXOPHTHALMOS

Bulging of eye anteriorly out of orbit (Fig. 12.36).

PATHOPHYSIOLOGY

- Can be from an increase in volume of orbital contents
- Most common cause is Graves disease, in which abnormal connective tissue is deposited in the orbit and extraocular muscles
- Bilateral or unilateral
- When unilateral, a retro-orbital tumor must be considered

PATIENT DATA

Subjective Data

- Change in eye position or Valsalva maneuver

Objective Data

- Apparent eye protrusion; lids do not reach the pupil
- Measurement of degree of exophthalmos is performed using an exophthalmometer, usually by an ophthalmologist

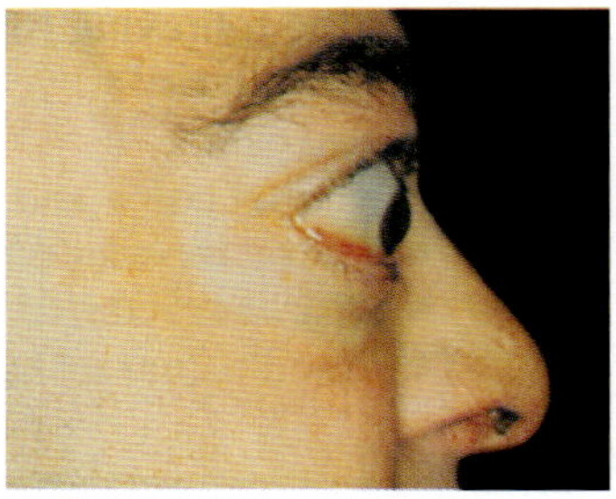

FIG. 12.36 Thyroid exophthalmos. See also Fig. 11.11. (From Stein, H. A., Stein, R. M., & Slatt, B. J. (1994). *Ophthalmic assistant: Fundamentals and clinical practice* (6th ed.). St. Louis: Mosby.)

EPISCLERITIS

Inflammation of the superficial layers of the sclera anterior to the insertion of the rectus muscles (Fig. 12.37).

PATHOPHYSIOLOGY

Pathophysiology is poorly understood. There are two kinds:

- Simple—intermittent episodes of moderate-to-severe inflammation, often recurring at 1- to 3-month intervals, lasting 7–10 days, and resolving after 2–3 weeks
- Nodular—prolonged attacks of inflammation, typically more painful than simple episcleritis

Most cases are idiopathic; may have an underlying systemic condition such as autoimmune disorders, including Crohn disease, rheumatoid arthritis, systemic lupus erythematosus, polyarteritis nodosa, psoriatic arthritis, gout, atopy, foreign bodies, chemical exposure, or infection

PATIENT DATA

Subjective Data

- Acute onset of mild-to-moderate discomfort or photophobia
- Painless injection (redness) and/or watery discharge without crusting

Objective Data

- Diffuse or localized injection of the bulbar conjunctiva
- Purplish elevation of a few millimeters
- Watery discharge

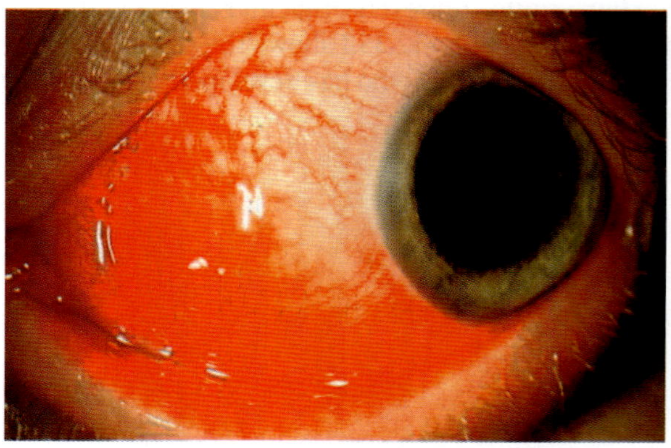

FIG. 12.37 Episcleritis. (From Hegde, V., Mitrut, I., Bennett, H., & Singh, J. (2009). *Episcleritis: An association with IgA nephropathy. Contact Lens & Anterior Eye, 32*(3), 141–142.)

BAND KERATOPATHY

Deposition of calcium in the superficial cornea (Fig. 12.38).

PATHOPHYSIOLOGY

- Most commonly in patients with chronic corneal disease
- May occur in patients with hypercalcemia, hyperparathyroidism, and occasionally in individuals with trauma, renal failure sarcoidosis, or syphilis

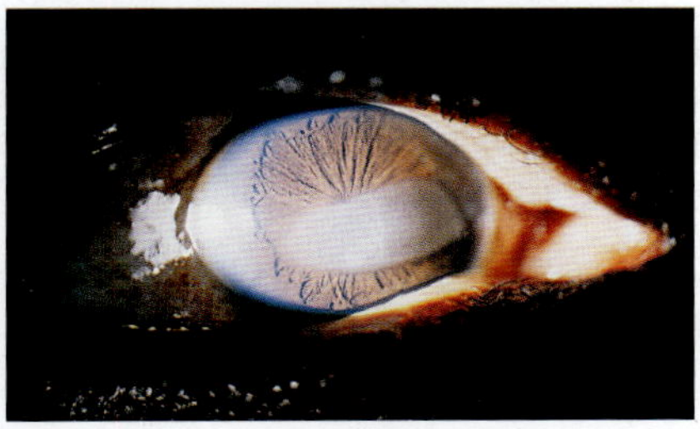

FIG. 12.38 Band keratopathy. (Courtesy John W. Payne, MD, The Wilmer Ophthalmological Institute, The Johns Hopkins University and Hospital, Baltimore, MD.)

PATIENT DATA

Subjective Data

- Decrease in vision as deposition progresses
- Foreign body sensation and irritation

Objective Data

- Line just below the pupil; passes over the cornea rather than around the iris as with arcus senilis
- Horizontal grayish bands interspersed with dark areas that look like holes

CORNEAL ULCER

Disruption of the corneal epithelium and stroma (Fig. 12.39).

PATHOPHYSIOLOGY

Causes:

- Connective tissue disease, such as rheumatoid arthritis, Sjögren syndrome, or a systemic vasculitic disorder (e.g., systemic lupus erythematosus, Wegener granulomatosis, polyarteritis nodosa)
- Infection: viral infection (e.g., herpes simplex virus), bacterial infection
- Extreme dryness: incomplete lid closure or poor lacrimal gland function
- Prolonged use of contact lens

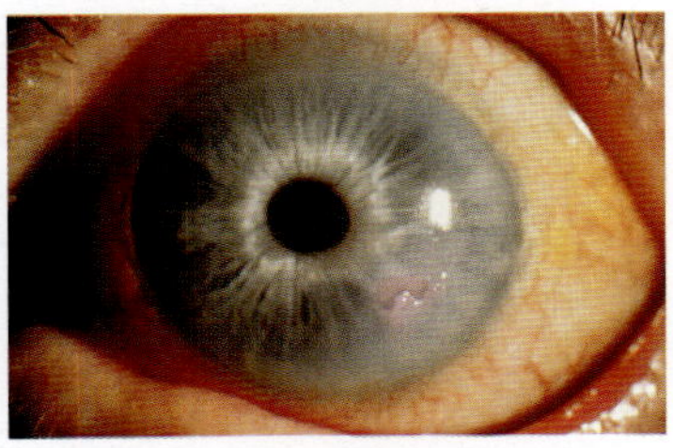

FIG. 12.39 Corneal ulcer in the lower temporal quadrant of the left cornea stained with rose bengal. (Courtesy John W. Payne, MD, The Wilmer Ophthalmological Institute, The Johns Hopkins University and Hospital, Baltimore.)

PATIENT DATA

Subjective Data

- Pain
- Photophobia
- History of wearing contact lenses
- Blurry vision
- Feeling that something is in the eye

Objective Data

- Visual acuity affected variably, depending on ulcer location
- Inflammation and erythema of the lids and conjunctiva
- Purulent exudates
- Ulcer often round or oval and the border sharply demarcated, with the base appearing ragged and gray

Extraocular Muscles

STRABISMUS

Both eyes do not focus on an object simultaneously but can focus with either eye (see Fig. 12.24).

PATHOPHYSIOLOGY

- Paralytic, caused by impairment of one or more extraocular muscles
- Nonparalytic with no primary muscle weakness
- May be a sign of increased intracranial pressure
- Cranial nerve III is particularly vulnerable to damage from brain swelling

PATIENT DATA

Subjective Data

- Poor vision
- May have sudden onset of double vision
- Report of eye deviation

Objective Data

- If an extraocular muscle has become impaired, the eye will not move in the direction controlled by that muscle; for example, if the right sixth nerve is damaged, the right eye does not move temporally
- Detected by the cover-uncover test (see Fig. 12.24) or in children with use of StrabismoScope or photoscreening

Internal Eye

HORNER SYNDROME

Interruption of sympathetic nerve innervation to the eye.

PATHOPHYSIOLOGY

- Can be congenital, acquired, or hereditary (autosomal dominant)
- May result from lesion of the primary neuron, stroke, trauma to the brachial plexus, tumors, dissecting carotid aneurysm, or operative trauma
- Results in triad of ipsilateral miosis, mild ptosis, and loss of hemifacial sweating (Fig. 12.40)

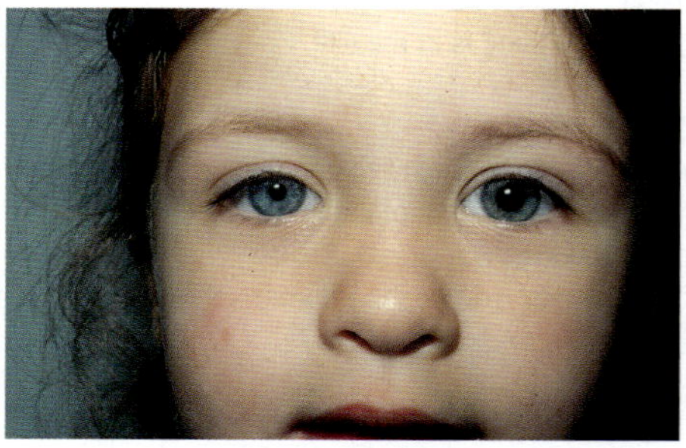

FIG. 12.40 Horner syndrome (right eye). (From Patzelt, J. (2009). *Basics augenheilkunde* (2nd ed.). Germany: Urban & Fischer.)

PATIENT DATA

Subjective Data

- Symptoms depend on the underlying cause

Objective Data

- The ptosis is subtle and appreciated by noting the amount of iris seen superiorly in opposite eye is greater
- Pupil on affected side may be round and constricted
- Anisocoria (difference in pupil size) is greater in darkness
- Affected pupil dilates more slowly than the normal pupil (dilation lag)
- Dry skin is on the same side of their face as the affected pupil

CATARACTS

Opacity in lens (Fig. 12.41).

PATHOPHYSIOLOGY

- Most commonly from denaturation of lens protein caused by aging
- With aging, cataracts are generally central
- Peripheral cataracts may occur in hypoparathyroidism
- Medications such as steroids can cause cataracts
- Congenital cataracts can result from a number of genetic defects, maternal infections such as rubella, or other fetal insults during the first trimester of pregnancy

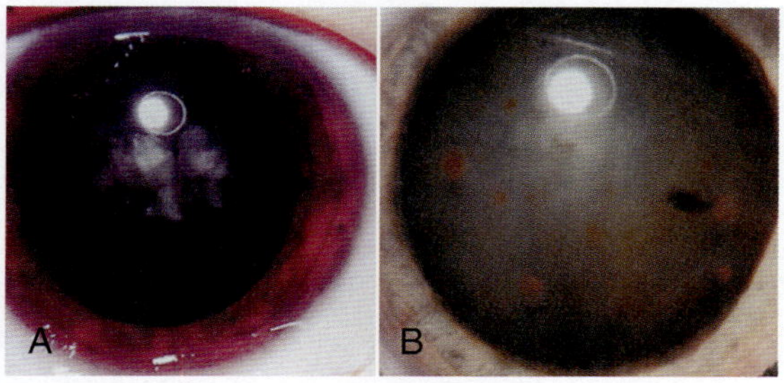

FIG. 12.41 (A) Snowflake cataract of diabetes. (B) Senile cataract. (From Donaldson, D. D. (1976). *Atlas of the eye: The crystalline lens* (Vol. 5). St. Louis: Mosby.)

PATIENT DATA

Subjective Data

- Cloudy or blurry vision
- Faded colors
- Headlights, lamps, or sunlight may appear too bright
- Halo may appear around lights
- Poor night vision or double vision
- Frequent prescription changes

Objective Data

- Cloudiness of the lens, often obvious without special viewing equipment

DIABETIC RETINOPATHY (BACKGROUND OR NONPROLIFERATIVE)

Dot hemorrhages or microaneurysms and the presence of hard and soft exudates

PATHOPHYSIOLOGY

- Hard exudates are the result of lipid transudation through incompetent capillaries
- Soft exudates (also called *cotton-wool spots*) are caused by infarction of the nerve layer (Fig. 12.42)

PATIENT DATA

Subjective Data

- In the initial stages, patient is asymptomatic
- Blurred vision, distortion, or visual acuity loss in more advanced stages

Objective Data

- On ophthalmoscopic examination, blood vessels with balloon-like sacs (microaneurysms)
- Blots of hemorrhages on the retina itself
- Tiny yellow patches of hard exudates

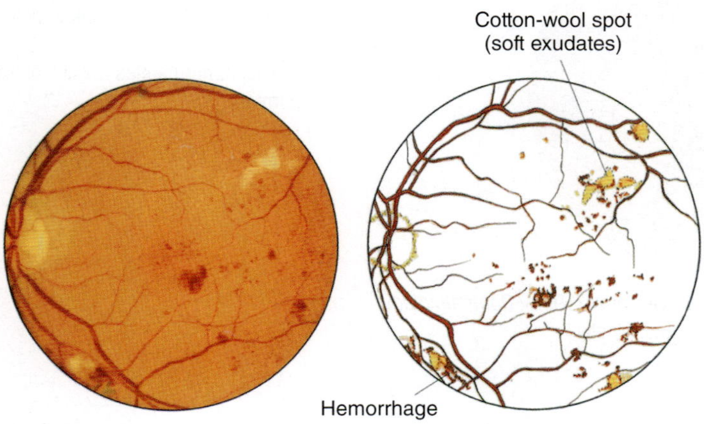

FIG. 12.42 Background diabetic retinopathy. Note flame-shaped and dot-blot hemorrhages, cotton-wool spots, and microaneurysms. (From Yannuzzi et al., 1995; courtesy Drs. George Blankenship and Everett Ai and the Diabetes 2000 Program, St. Louis, MO.)

DIABETIC RETINOPATHY (PROLIFERATIVE)

Development of new vessels as a result of anoxic stimulation (Fig. 12.43).

PATHOPHYSIOLOGY

- Vessels grow out of the retina toward the vitreous humor
- May occur in peripheral retina or on optic nerve itself
- New vessels lack supporting structure of healthy vessels and are likely to hemorrhage
- Bleeding from these vessels is a major cause of blindness in patients with diabetes
- Laser therapy can often control this neovascularization and prevent blindness

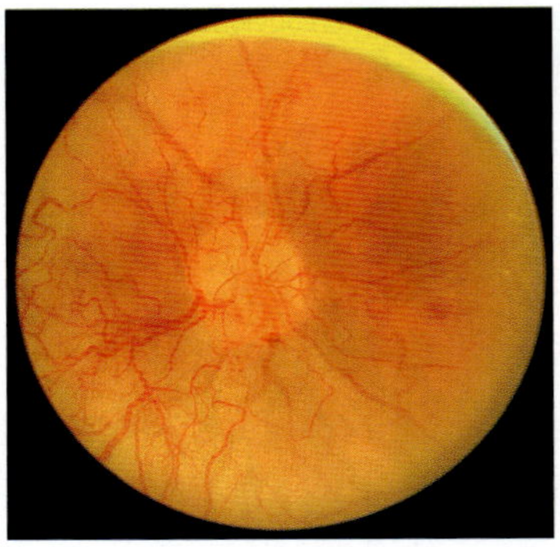

FIG. 12.43 Proliferative diabetic retinopathy. (Courtesy John W. Payne, MD, The Wilmer Ophthalmological Institute, The Johns Hopkins University and Hospital, Baltimore, MD.)

PATIENT DATA

Subjective Data

- Generally asymptomatic
- Floaters, blurred vision, or progressive visual acuity loss in advanced stages

Objective Data

- Visualization of these vessels may require change in the lens setting of the ophthalmoscope
- Vitreous hemorrhage may also be seen, which can obstruct the view of the retina

LIPEMIA RETINALIS

Creamy white appearance of retinal vessels that occurs with excessively high serum triglyceride levels.

PATHOPHYSIOLOGY

- Occurs when the serum triglyceride level exceeds 2000 mg/dL (Fig. 12.44)
- Seen in some of the hyperlipidemic states

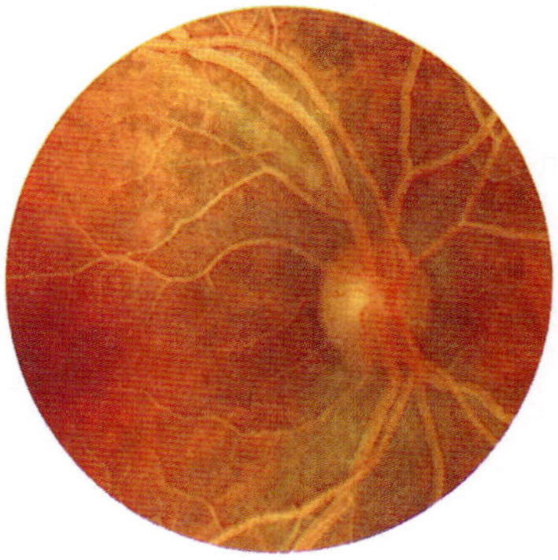

FIG. 12.44 Lipemia retinalis. (From Newell, F. W. (1996). *Ophthalmology: Principles and concepts* (8th ed.). St. Louis: Mosby.)

PATIENT DATA

Subjective Data

- Elevated serum triglyceride levels
- No vision symptoms

Objective Data

- Grade I (early)—white and creamy aspect of peripheral retina vessels
- Grade II (moderate)—the creamy color of the vessels extends toward the optic disc
- Grade III (marked)—retina appears salmon color and all vessels have a milky appearance
- Retinal abnormalities resolve as the triglyceride levels return to normal

RETINITIS PIGMENTOSA

Autosomal recessive disorder in which the genetic defects cause cell death, predominantly in the rod photoreceptors.

PATHOPHYSIOLOGY

- Genetic defect causes cell death (apoptosis) in the photoreceptors. The associated conditions are:
  - Deafness (Usher syndrome)
  - Paralysis of one or more extraocular muscles (ophthalmoplegia), dysphasia, ataxia, and cardiac conduction defects are seen in the mitochondrial DNA disorder (Kearns-Sayre syndrome)
  - Intellectual delay, peripheral neuropathy, acanthotic (spiked) red blood cells, ataxia, steatorrhea, absence of very low-density lipoprotein (VLDL; abetalipoproteinemia is absence of VLDL)

PATIENT DATA

Subjective Data

- Earliest symptom is night blindness
- Tunnel vision or reports of bumping into furniture
- Loss of vision is painless and progresses over years to decades

Objective Data

- Normal examination in the early stages
- Optic atrophy with a waxy pallor, narrowing of the arterioles, and peripheral "bone spicule" pigmentation are hallmarks of advanced disease (Fig. 12.45)

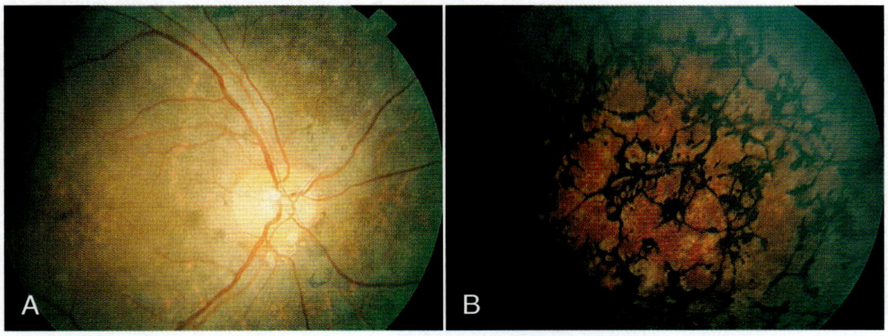

FIG. 12.45 Retinitis pigmentosa. (A) Optic atrophy and narrowing of the arterioles. (B) Classic "bone spicule" pigmentation in the retinal periphery. (Courtesy John W. Payne, MD, The Wilmer Ophthalmological Institute, The Johns Hopkins University and Hospital, Baltimore, MD.)

GLAUCOMA

Disease of the optic nerve wherein the nerve cells die, usually because of excessively high intraocular pressure.

PATHOPHYSIOLOGY

- Acute angle may occur suddenly with dramatically elevated intraocular pressure if the iris blocks the exit of aqueous humor from the anterior chamber
- Open angle caused by decreasing aqueous humor absorption leads to increased resistance and painless buildup of pressure in the eye
- May also be congenital as a result of improper development of the eye's aqueous outflow system

Risk Factors

Glaucoma

- Age: people over 60 years
- Race: increased risk in people of African, Asian, or Hispanic descent
- Family history
- Corneal thickness: people with a thinner cornea
- Medical conditions: diabetes, migraine, hypertension, sickle cell anemia
- Eye injuries: previous eye injury or surgery
- Corticosteroids: especially eye drops

Adapted from https://www.nei.nih.gov/learn-about-eye-health/eye-conditions-and-diseases/glaucoma#:~:text=Am%20I%20at%20risk%20for,a%20family%20history%20of%20glaucoma

PATIENT DATA

Subjective Data

- In open-angle glaucoma, which is more common, symptoms are absent except for gradual loss of peripheral vision over a period of years
- Acute glaucoma is accompanied by intense ocular pain, blurred vision, halos around lights, a red eye, and a dilated pupil
- Occasionally, patients report stomach pain, nausea, and vomiting

Objective Data

- Optic nerve damage can clearly be seen during a dilated eye examination and produces a characteristic appearance of the optic nerve (increased cupping) (Fig. 12.46)
- Visual field tests may show loss of peripheral vision

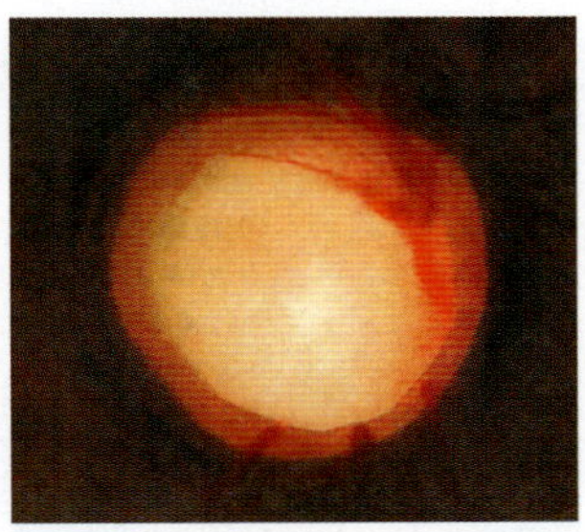

FIG. 12.46 Marked glaucomatous optic nerve head cupping. Compare the disappearance of blood vessels here with the blood vessels of the optic disc in Figs. 12.26 and 12.27. (Courtesy Andrew P. Schachat, MD, The Wilmer Ophthalmological Institute, The Johns Hopkins University and Hospital, Baltimore, MD.)

INTERMEDIATE UVEITIS

Inflammation in the anterior vitreous, ciliary body, and peripheral retina.

PATHOPHYSIOLOGY

- The Standardization of Uveitis Nomenclature's consensus is *intermediate uveitis* should be used for uveitis where the vitreous is the major site of the inflammation and there is an associated infection or systemic disease (e.g., Lyme disease, syphilis, sarcoidosis, or multiple sclerosis)
- Intermediate uveitis may be the presenting feature of an autoimmune disease

PATIENT DATA

Subjective Data

- Blurry vision
- Floaters
- Pain (rare)
- Photophobia (rare)
- Red eye (rare)
- Visual loss due to aggregation of floaters in the vitreous or due to macular edema

Objective Data

- Generally affects patients aged 15–40 years
- Visual acuity is variably affected
- Vitreous snowballs—yellow-white inflammatory aggregates found in the midvitreous and inferior periphery
- Snowbanks—gray-white fibrovascular and/or exudative plaque on the pars plana, usually inferiorly, but may extend around the entire retinal periphery

CHORIORETINITIS (CHORIORETINAL INFLAMMATION, ALSO CALLED POSTERIOR UVEITIS)

Inflammatory process involving both the choroid and the retina.

PATHOPHYSIOLOGY

- Most common cause is laser therapy for diabetic retinopathy but may also be seen in histoplasmosis, cytomegalovirus, toxoplasmosis, or congenital rubella infections

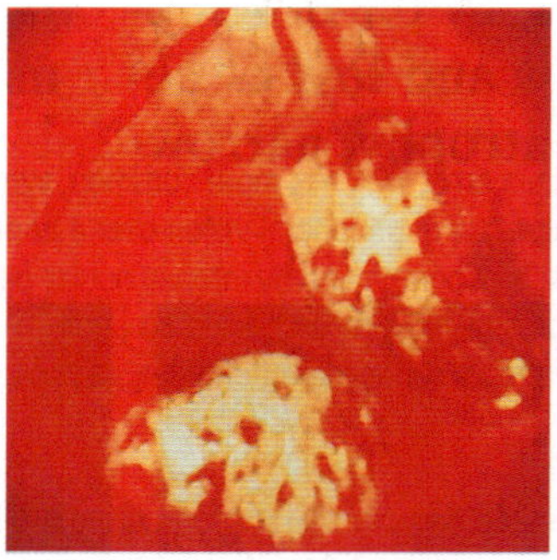

FIG. 12.47 **Patches of chorioretinitis adjacent to the optic disc.** (From Stein, H. A., Stein, R. M., & Slatt, B. J. (1994). *Ophthalmic assistant: Fundamentals and clinical practice* (6th ed.). St. Louis: Mosby.)

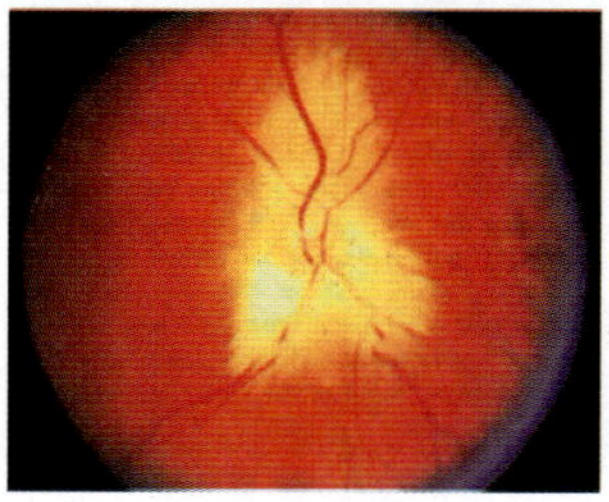

FIG. 12.48 **Myelinated retinal nerve fibers.** (Courtesy Andrew P. Schachat, MD, The Wilmer Ophthalmological Institute, The Johns Hopkins University and Hospital, Baltimore, MD.)

PATIENT DATA

Subjective Data

- History of cleaning cat litter box, laser surgery, or other causal agents
- Pain
- Reduced visual acuity
- Floaters
- Photophobia

Objective Data

- Sharply defined lesion; generally whitish yellow and becomes stippled with dark pigment in later stages ending with a chorioretinal scar (Fig. 12.47)
- Visual field defect can be detected in individuals with a large lesion
- Chorioretinal scar appears; whitish lesions with well-demarcated borders
- May be single or multiple
- Feathery margins contrast with myelinated retinal nerve fibers (Fig. 12.48)

Visual Fields

VISUAL FIELD DEFECTS

Defective vision or blindness.

PATHOPHYSIOLOGY

- May be consequence of degenerative changes within the eye (e.g., cataract) or from a lesion of the optic nerve anterior to its decussation (Figs. 12.49, *1* and 12.50A)
- Most common cause is interruption of the vascular supply to the optic nerve (see Figs. 12.49, *1* and 12.50A)
- Bitemporal hemianopia (see Figs. 12.49, *2* and 12.50B) is caused by a lesion—most commonly a pituitary tumor—interrupting the optic chiasm
- Homonymous hemianopia can be caused by lesions of the optic nerve radiation on either side of the brain occurring after the optic chiasm (see Figs. 12.49, *3* and 12.50C)

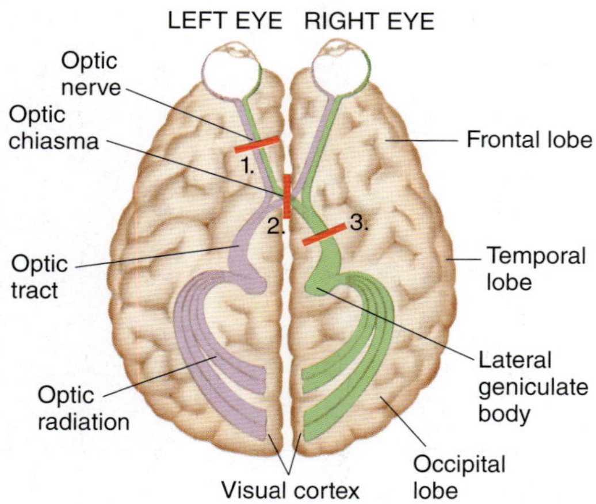

FIG. 12.49 Sites of lesions causing visual loss. (1) Total blindness left eye. (2) Bitemporal hemianopia. (3) Left homonymous hemianopia.

PATIENT DATA

Subjective Data

- Defective vision or blindness

Objective Data

- Visual field defects (see Fig. 12.50)

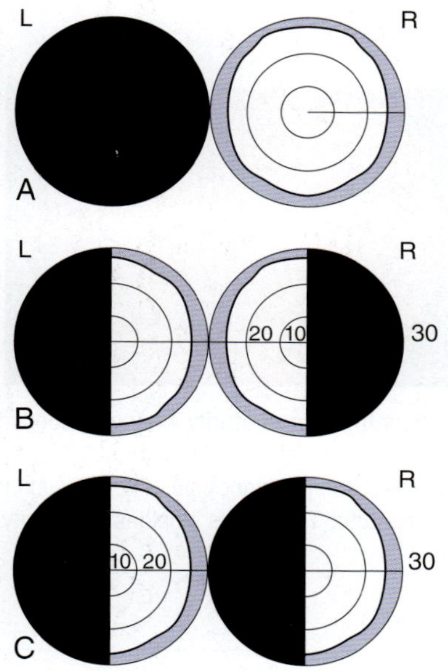

FIG. 12.50 Visual fields corresponding to lesions shown in Fig. 12.49. (A) Total blindness left eye. (B) Bitemporal hemianopia. (C) Left homonymous hemianopia. (Modified from Stein, H. A., Stein, R. M., & Slatt, B. J. (1994). *Ophthalmic assistant: Fundamentals and clinical practice* (6th ed.). St. Louis: Mosby.)

Infants and Children

Retinoblastoma

Embryonic malignant tumor arising from the retina.

PATHOPHYSIOLOGY

- Usually develops during the first 2 years of life
- Transmitted either by autosomal dominant trait or by chromosomal mutation (*RB1* gene on chromosome 13)
- Most common retinal tumor in children

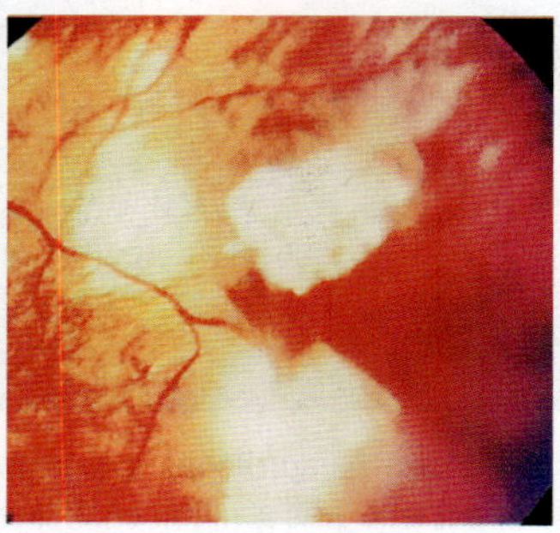

FIG. 12.51 Retinoblastoma. (From Stein, H. A., Stein, R. M., & Slatt, B. J. (1994). *Ophthalmic assistant: Fundamentals and clinical practice* (6th ed.). St. Louis: Mosby.)

PATIENT DATA

Subjective Data

- Family history of retinoblastoma
- White pupil on photographs

Objective Data

- Initial sign is leukocoria, a white reflex (also called a *cat's eye reflex*) rather than the usual red reflex
- Ill-defined mass arising from retina on funduscopic examination; chalky white areas of calcification can be seen (Fig. 12.51)

Retinopathy of Prematurity

Disruption of normal progression of retinal vascular development in preterm infant.

PATHOPHYSIOLOGY

- Results in abnormal proliferation of blood vessels (neovascularization)
- More common in infants with a birth weight of ≤1500 g or gestational age of ≤30 weeks or less
- Some infants with a birth weight 1500–2000 g or a gestational age of >30 weeks who are thought to be at risk for ROP (e.g., infants with hypotension requiring inotropic support, infants with oxygen requirement for several days, or infants who received oxygen without oxygen saturation monitoring; Fierson et al., 2018)

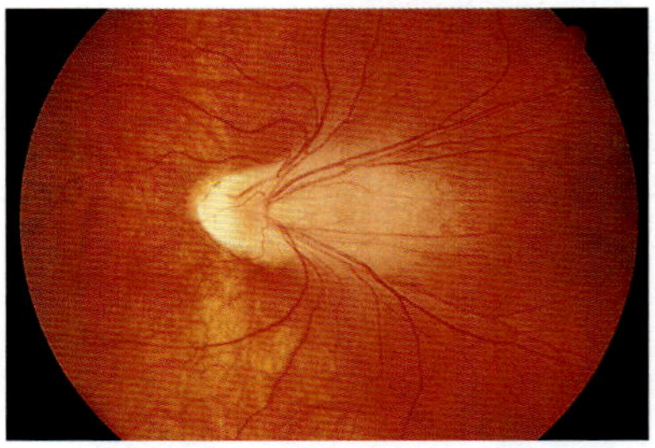

FIG. 12.52 Retinopathy of prematurity. Changes found in posterior pole of the left eye in the cicatricial (scar forming) stage of the disease with traction on the retina in the posterior pole. (Courtesy John W. Payne, MD, The Wilmer Eye Institute, The Johns Hopkins University and Hospital, Baltimore, MD.)

PATIENT DATA

Subjective Data

- Low-birth-weight preterm infants have highest risk for ROP
- Other factors associated with the ROP: anemia, poor weight gain, blood transfusion, respiratory distress, breathing difficulties, and overall health of the infant

Objective Data

- Straight, temporally diverted blood vessels on funduscopic examination (Fig. 12.52)
- Can be mild with no visual defects, or refractive error, amblyopia, or progress to retinal detachment and blindness

Retinal Hemorrhages in Infancy

Abnormal bleeding of the blood vessels in the retina

PATHOPHYSIOLOGY

- Results from acceleration-deceleration impact head injury in abusive head trauma (shaken baby syndrome)
- Usually bilaterally
- Other causes:
  - Vaginal birth
  - Hypertension
  - Bleeding problems/leukemia
  - Meningitis/sepsis/endocarditis
  - Vasculitis
  - Retinal diseases (e.g., infection, hemangioma)
  - Anemia
  - Hypoxia/hypotension

PATIENT DATA

Subjective Data

- Altered responsiveness without good explanation (suspicion of physical abuse)

Objective Data

- Dilated funduscopic examination shows retinal hemorrhages (Fig. 12.53)

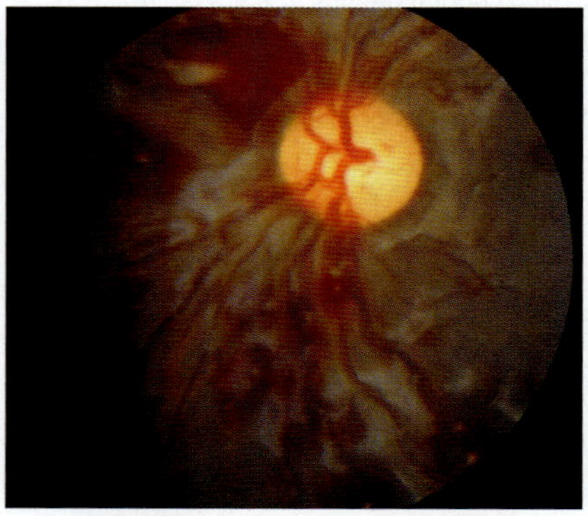

FIG. 12.53 Multiple retinal hemorrhages are seen on funduscopic examination of this infant who was a victim of shaken baby syndrome. (Courtesy Daniel Garibaldi, MD, The Wilmer Ophthalmological Institute, The Johns Hopkins University and Hospital, Baltimore, MD.)

Older Adults

Macular Degeneration

Macular degeneration, also called *age-related macular degeneration* (AMD or ARMD), is caused when part of the retina deteriorates.

PATHOPHYSIOLOGY

Two types:

- Dry (atrophic)—from the gradual breakdown of cells in the macula that results in a gradual blurring of central vision
- Wet (exudative or neovascular)—new abnormal blood vessels grow under the center of the retina. The blood vessels leak, bleed, and scar the retina, distorting or destroying central vision. Vision loss may be rapid
- Leading cause of legal blindness in people older than 55 years in the United States

PATIENT DATA

Subjective Data

- Blurred or decreased central vision
- Blind spots, or scotomas
- Straight lines looking irregular or bent (metamorphopsia)
- Objects appearing a different color or shape in each eye
- Objects appearing smaller in one eye (micropsia)

Objective Data

- Dry form
- Drusen (multiple spots in the macular region); see Fig. 12.35
- Thinning and loss of the retina and the choroid
- Wet form
- Exudates, blood, scarring, and new blood vessel membranes below the retina (see Fig. 12.35B)

CHAPTER

13 Ears, Nose, and Throat

Examination of the ears, nose, and throat provides information about their integrity and function as well as the associated respiratory and digestive tracts. The special senses of smell, hearing, equilibrium, and taste are also associated with the ears, nose, and mouth.

ANATOMY AND PHYSIOLOGY

Ears and Hearing

The ear is a sensory organ that identifies, localizes, and interprets sound and helps to maintain balance. It is divided into the external, middle, and inner ear (Figs. 13.1 and 13.2).

The external ear, including the auricle (or pinna) and external auditory canal, is cartilage covered by skin. The auricle, extending slightly outward from the skull, is positioned on a nearly vertical plane. Note its structural landmarks in Fig. 13.3.

The external auditory canal, an S-shaped pathway leading to the middle ear, is approximately 2.5 cm (1 inch) long in adults. Its skeleton of bone and cartilage is covered with thin, sensitive skin. This canal lining is protected and lubricated with cerumen, a waxy substance secreted by the apocrine glands in the distal third of the canal. Cerumen provides an acidic environment that inhibits the growth of bacteria and fungi.

Physical Examination Components

Ears

1. Inspect the auricles and surrounding areas for:
    - Size, shape, and symmetry
    - Landmarks
    - Color
    - Position
    - Deformities or lesions
2. Palpate the auricles and mastoid areas for tenderness, swelling, and nodules.
3. Inspect the auditory canals with an otoscope, noting:
    - Cerumen
    - Color
    - Lesions
    - Discharge
    - Foreign bodies
4. Inspect the tympanic membranes for:
    - Landmarks
    - Color
    - Contour
    - Perforations
    - Mobility
5. Assess hearing through responses to:
    - Questions
    - Whispered voice
    - Tuning fork for air and bone conduction

Nose and Sinuses

1. Inspect the external nose, noting the shape, size, color, and nares.
2. Palpate the bridge and soft tissues of the nose, noting:
    - Tenderness
    - Displacement of cartilage and bone
    - Masses
3. Evaluate the patency of the nares.
4. Inspect the nasal mucosa and nasal septum for:
    - Color
    - Alignment
    - Discharge
    - Swelling of turbinates
    - Perforation
5. Inspect the frontal and maxillary sinus areas for swelling.
6. Palpate the frontal and maxillary sinuses for tenderness and swelling.

Mouth

1. Inspect and palpate the lips for symmetry, color, and swelling.
2. Inspect the teeth for:
    - Occlusion
    - Caries
    - Loose or missing teeth
    - Surface abnormalities
3. Inspect and palpate the gingiva and buccal mucosa for color, lesions, and tenderness.
4. Inspect the tongue for color, symmetry, swelling, and ulcerations.
5. Assess position and movement of the tongue (cranial nerve XII).
6. Palpate the tongue.
7. Inspect the palate and uvula.
8. Elicit the gag reflex (cranial nerves IX and X).
9. Inspect the oropharyngeal characteristics of the tonsils and posterior wall of the pharynx.

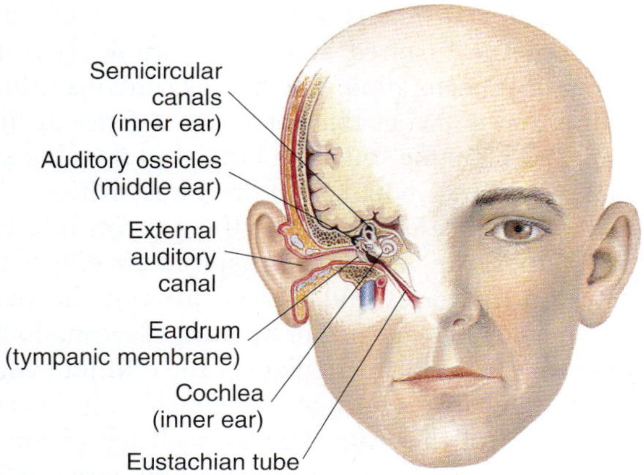

FIG. 13.1 Cross section of the external, middle, and inner ear in relation to other structures of the head and face. Front view of face shows labels for ear and associated regions as follows: semicircular canals (inner ear), auditory ossicles (middle ear), external auditory canal, eardrum (tympanic membrane), cochlea (inner ear), and eustachian tube.

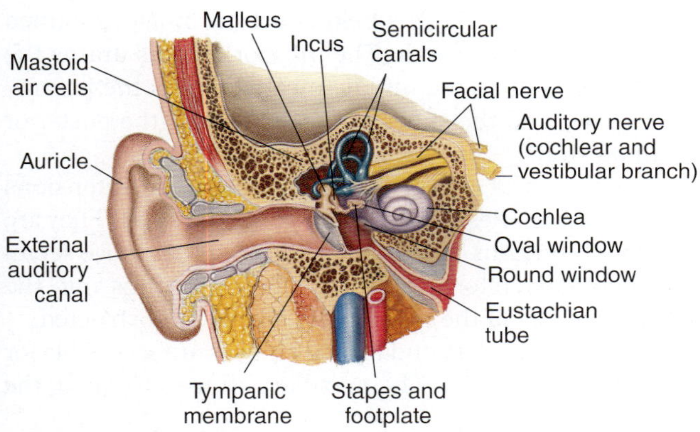

FIG. 13.2 Anatomy of the external, middle, and inner ear. The structure of ear shows labels as follows: malleus, incus, semicircular canals, facial nerve, auditory nerve (cochlear and vestibular branch), cochlea, oval window, round window, eustachian tube, stapes and footplate, tympanic membrane, external auditory canal, auricle, and mastoid air cells.

The middle ear is an air-filled cavity in the temporal bone. It contains the ossicles—three small, connected bones (malleus, incus, and stapes) that transmit sound from the tympanic membrane to the oval window of the inner ear. The air-filled cells of the mastoid area of the temporal bone are continuous with the middle ear. The tympanic membrane, surrounded by a dense fibrous ring (annulus), separates the external ear from the middle ear. It is concave, being pulled in at the center (umbo) by the malleus. The tympanic membrane is translucent, permitting the middle ear cavity and malleus to be visualized. Its conical shape and oblique position to the auditory canal account for the triangular light reflex seen in an otoscopic examination. Most of the tympanic membrane is tense (the pars tensa), but the superior portion (pars flaccida) is more flaccid (Fig. 13.4).

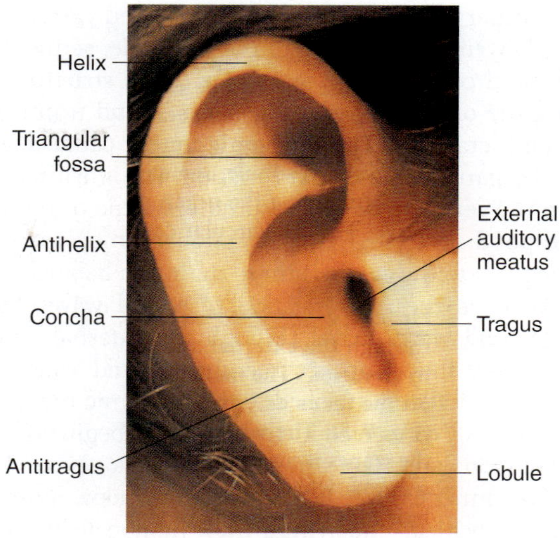

FIG. 13.3 Anatomic structures of the auricle. The helix is the prominent outer rim, whereas the antihelix is the area parallel and anterior to the helix. The concha is the deep cavity containing the auditory canal meatus. The tragus is the protuberance lying anterior to the auditory canal meatus, and the antitragus is the protuberance on the antihelix opposite the tragus. The lobule is the soft lobe on the bottom of the auricle. Close-up view of the ear shows labels as follows: external auditory meatus, tragus, lobule, antitragus, concha, antihelix, triangular fossa, and helix.

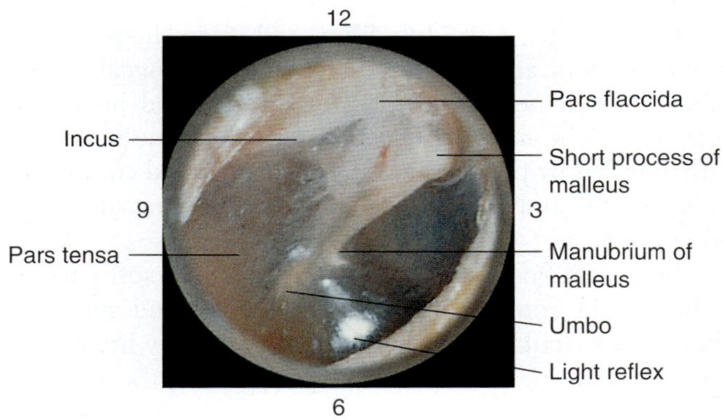

FIG. 13.4 Structural landmarks of the right tympanic membrane in relation to a clock face. Tympanic membrane shows labels as follows: pars flaccida, short process of malleus (between 12 and 3 o'clock position), manubrium of malleus, umbo, light reflex (post 3 o'clock position), pars tensa (at 8 o'clock position), and incus (at 10 o'clock position).

The middle ear mucosa produces a small amount of mucus that is rapidly cleared by the ciliary action of the eustachian tube, a cartilaginous, fibrous, and bony passageway between the nasopharynx and the middle ear. The eustachian tube drains into the posterior aspect of the inferior turbinate of the nose. Muscles briefly open this passage during swallowing, yawning, or sneezing to clear middle ear secretions and equalize the middle ear pressure with atmospheric pressure. The equalized pressure in the middle ear permits the tympanic membrane to vibrate freely with sound waves.

The inner ear is a membranous, curved cavity inside a bony labyrinth consisting of the vestibule, semicircular canals, and cochlea. The cochlea, a coiled structure containing the organ of Corti, transmits sound impulses to the eighth cranial nerve. The semicircular canals contain the end organs for vestibular function. Equilibrium receptors in the semicircular canals and vestibule of the inner ear respond to changes in direction of movement and send signals to the cerebellum to maintain balance.

Hearing is the interpretation of sound waves by the brain. Sound waves travel through the external auditory canal, strike the tympanic membrane, and cause it to vibrate. The malleus, attached to the tympanic membrane, and the serially connected incus and stapes begin vibrating. The vibrations are passed from the stapes to the oval window of the inner ear (see Fig. 13.2). Oval window movement transmits cochlear endolymph fluid motion to the round window, where it dissipates. Hair cells in the organ of Corti detect sound vibrations and send the information to the auditory division of the eighth cranial nerve. These impulses are transmitted to the temporal lobe of the brain for interpretation. Sound may also be transmitted by bone vibrations of the skull that pass to the inner ear.

Nose, Nasopharynx, and Sinuses

The nose and nasopharynx provide a passage for inspired and expired air; humidify, filter, and warm inspired air; identify odors; and provide resonance for laryngeal sound. The external nose is formed by skin-covered bone and cartilage. The nares (anterior openings of the nose) are surrounded by the cartilaginous alae nasi and columella. The frontal and maxillary bones form the nasal bridge (Fig. 13.5).

The nasal floor is formed by the hard and soft palates, whereas the roof is formed by the frontal and sphenoid bones. A vascular mucous membrane, thickly lined with small hairs and mucous secretions, covers the internal nose. The hairs and mucus collect and carry debris and bacteria from the inspired air to the nasopharynx for swallowing or expectoration. The mucus contains immunoglobulins and enzymes that serve as a defense against infection. Receptors for smell are located in the olfactory epithelium that lines about half of the nasal cavities.

The internal nose is divided by the septum into two anterior cavities: the vestibules. Inspired air enters the nose through the nares and passes through the vestibules to the choanae—posterior openings leading to the nasopharynx. The cribriform plate of the ethmoid bone, housing the sensory endings of the olfactory nerve, lies on the roof of the nose. The Kiesselbach plexus, a convergence of small, fragile arteries and veins, is located on the anterior-inferior portion of the septum. The adenoids lie on the posterior wall of the nasopharynx (Fig. 13.6).

Turbinates—parallel, curved bony structures covered by vascular mucous membrane—form the lateral walls of the nose and protrude into the nasal cavity. They increase the nasal surface area to warm, humidify, and filter inspired air. A meatus below each turbinate is named for the turbinate above it. The inferior meatus drains the nasolacrimal duct, the middle meatus drains the paranasal sinuses, and the superior meatus drains the posterior ethmoid sinus.

The paranasal sinuses are air-filled, paired extensions of the nasal cavities within the bones of the skull. They are lined with mucous membranes and cilia that move secretions along excretory pathways. Their openings into the middle meatus of the nasal cavity are easily obstructed.

Only the maxillary and frontal sinuses are accessible for physical examination. The maxillary sinuses lie along the

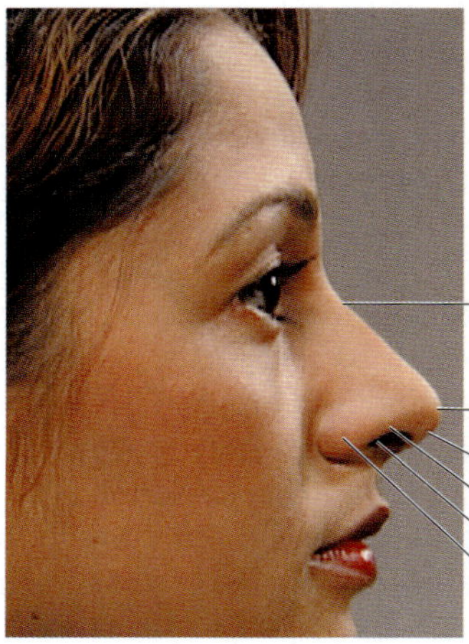

FIG. 13.5 Anatomic structures of the external nose. Side view of the face shows labels for bridge, tip, columella, anterior naris (nostril), vestibule, and ala nasi.

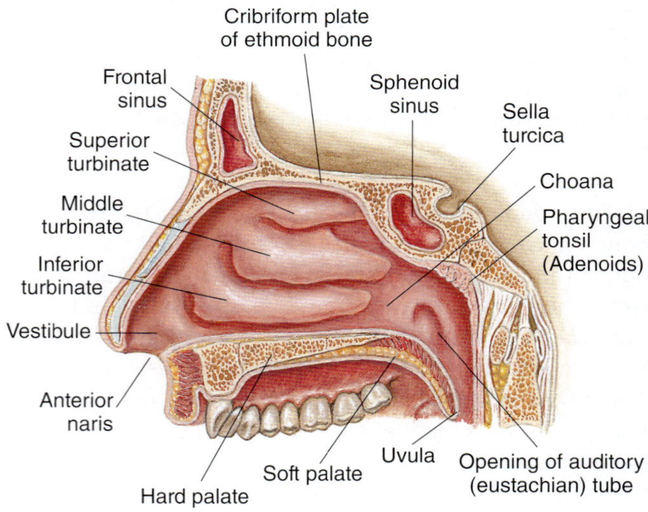

FIG. 13.6 Cross-sectional view of the anatomic structures of the nose and nasopharynx. Cross-sectional view of nose and nasopharynx shows labels as follows: cribriform plate of ethmoid bone, sphenoid sinus, sella turcica, choana, pharyngeal tonsil (adenoids), opening of auditory (eustachian) tube, uvula, soft palate, hard palate, anterior naris, vestibule, inferior turbinate, middle turbinate, superior turbinate, and frontal sinus.

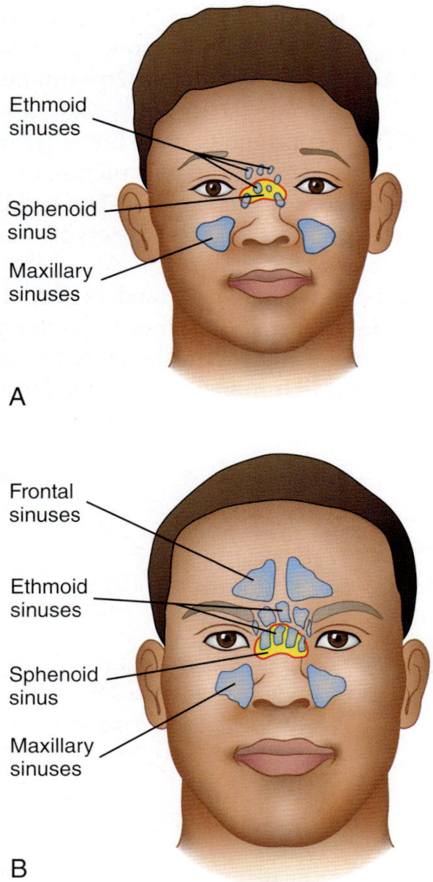

FIG. 13.7 Anterior view of the cranial sinuses. (A) Six-year-old child. (B) Adult. (A) Front view of child's face shows labels for ethmoid sinuses, sphenoid sinus, and maxillary sinuses. (B) Front view of a person's face shows labels for frontal sinuses, ethmoid sinuses, sphenoid sinus, and maxillary sinuses.

lateral wall of the nasal cavity in the maxillary bone. The frontal sinuses that develop during childhood are in the frontal bone superior to the nasal cavities. The ethmoid sinuses lie behind the frontal sinuses and near the superior portion of the nasal cavity. The sphenoid sinuses are deep in the skull behind the ethmoid sinuses (Fig. 13.7).

Mouth and Oropharynx

The mouth and oropharynx release air for vocalization and expiration. They also provide passage for food, liquid, and saliva (either swallowed or vomited); initiate digestion through solid food mastication and salivary gland secretion; and identify taste. The oral cavity is divided into the mouth and the vestibule, the space between the buccal mucosa and the outer surface of the teeth and gums. The mouth, housing the tongue, teeth, and gums, is the anterior opening of the oropharynx. The bony arch of the hard palate and the fibrous soft palate form the roof of the mouth. The uvula hangs from the posterior margin of the soft palate (Fig. 13.8).

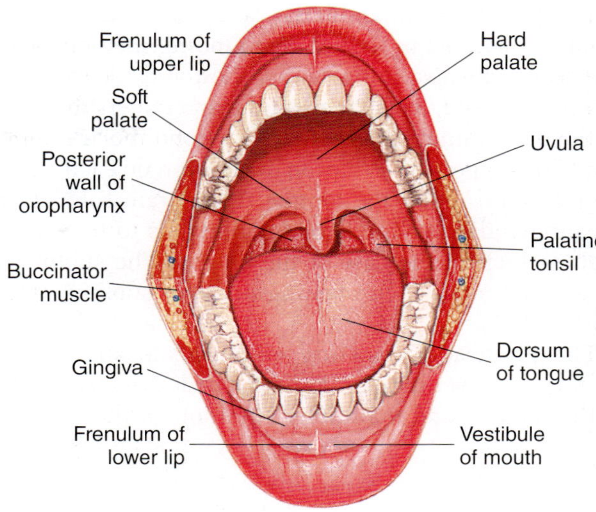

FIG. 13.8 Anatomic structures of the oral cavity. Oral cavity shows labels as follows: hard palate, uvula, palatine tonsil, dorsum of tongue, vestibule of mouth, frenulum of lower lip, gingiva, buccinator muscle, posterior wall of oropharynx, soft palate, and frenulum of upper lip.

Loose, mobile tissue covering the mandibular bone forms the floor of the mouth. The tongue is anchored to the back of the oral cavity by its base and to the floor of the mouth by the frenulum. The dorsal surface of the tongue is covered with thick mucous membrane supporting the filiform papillae. Fungiform papillae (taste receptors) are scattered throughout the filiform papillae of the tongue, and specific areas are sensitive to the five basic taste sensations of sour, sweet, salty, bitter, and umami (savory). The ventral surface of the tongue has visible veins and fimbriated folds (fringelike projections of thin mucous membrane; Fig. 13.9).

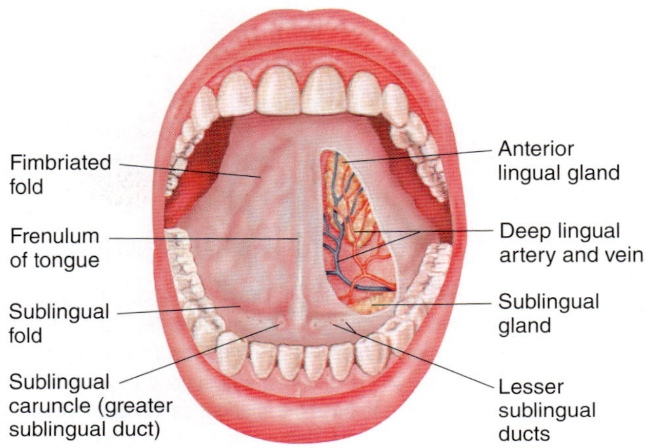

FIG. 13.9 Landmarks of the ventral surface of the tongue. Open mouth shows labels associated with ventral surface of tongue as follows: anterior lingual gland, deep lingual artery and vein, sublingual gland, lesser sublingual ducts, sublingual caruncle (greater sublingual duct), sublingual fold, frenulum of tongue, and fimbriated fold.

The parotid, submandibular, and sublingual salivary glands are located in tissues surrounding the oral cavity. The secreted saliva initiates digestion and moistens the mucosa. Stensen ducts are parotid gland outlets that open on the buccal mucosa opposite the second molar on each side of the upper jaw. Wharton ducts open on each side of the frenulum under the tongue. They drain saliva from the submandibular and sublingual glands to the sublingual caruncle at the base of the tongue. The sublingual glands have many ducts opening along the sublingual fold (see Fig. 13.9).

The gingivae, consisting of fibrous tissue covered by mucous membrane, are attached directly to the teeth, maxilla, and mandible. The roots of the teeth are anchored to the alveolar ridges of the maxilla and mandible. The enamel-covered crown is visible for examination. Adults generally have 32 permanent teeth (Fig. 13.10).

The oropharynx, continuous with but inferior to the nasopharynx, is separated from the mouth by bilateral anterior and posterior tonsillar pillars. The tonsils, lying in the cavity between these pillars, have crypts that collect cell debris and food particles.

Swallowing is initiated when food is forced by the tongue toward the pharynx. Muscles in the pharynx contract and prevent movement of the food into the nasopharynx, and respiration is inhibited as the epiglottis closes. Food is then propelled into the esophagus.

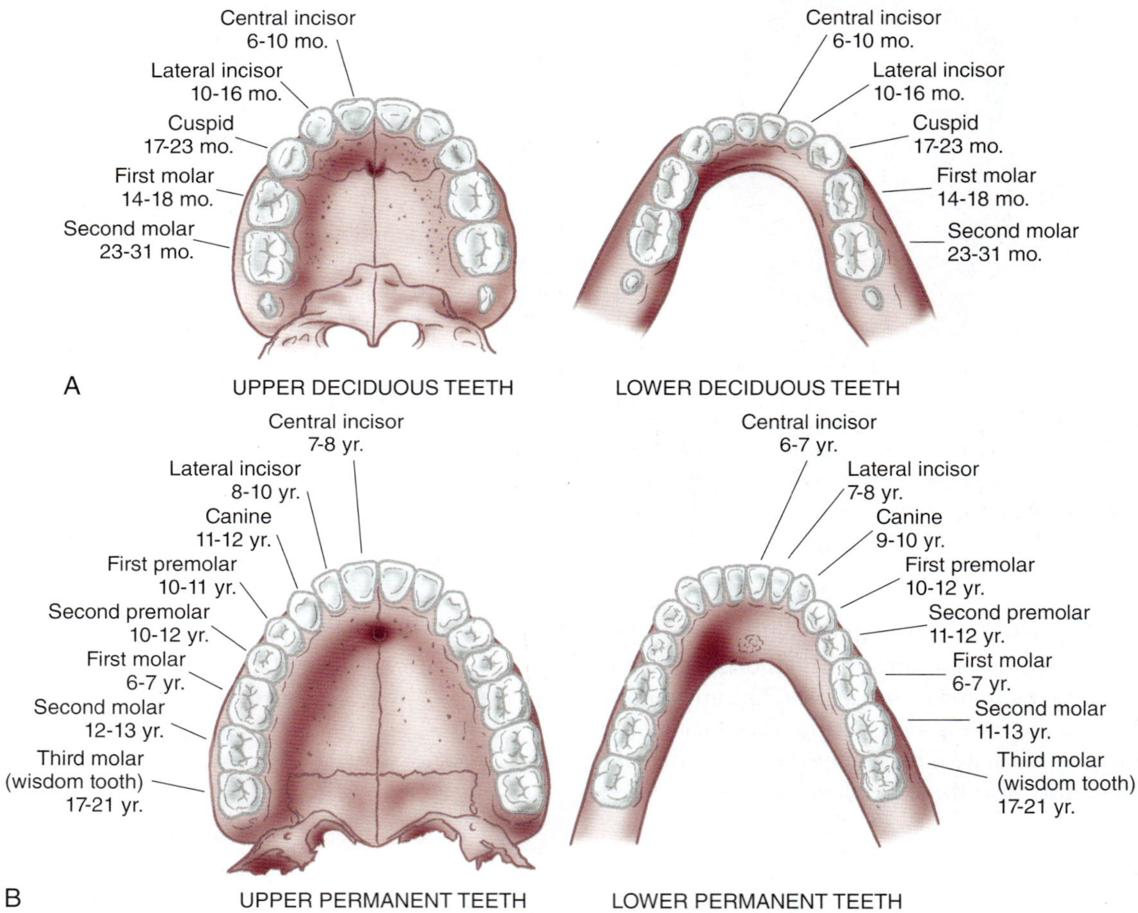

FIG. 13.10 (A) Dentition of deciduous teeth and their sequence of eruption. (B) Dentition of permanent teeth and their sequence of eruption. (A) The upper deciduous teeth in the left quadrant from top to base are marked as follows: central incisor 6–10 months, lateral incisor 10–16 months, cuspid 17–23 months, first molar 14–18 months, and second molar 23–31 months. The lower deciduous teeth in the right quadrant from top to base are marked as follows: central incisor 6–10 months, lateral incisor 10–16 months, cuspid 17–23 months, first molar 14–18 months, and second molar 23–31 months. (B) The upper permanent teeth in left quadrant from top to base are marked as follows: central incisor 7–8 years, lateral incisor 8–10 years, canine 11–12 years, first premolar 10–11 years, second premolar 10–12 years, first molar 6–7 years, second molar 12–13 years, and third molar (wisdom tooth) 17–21 years. The lower permanent teeth in right quadrant from top to base are marked as follows: central incisor 6–7 years, lateral incisor 7–8 years, canine 9–10 years, first premolar 10–12 years, second premolar 11–12 years, first molar 6–7 years, second molar 11–13 years, and third molar (wisdom tooth) 17–21 years.

Fetal Development, Infancy, and Children

Because development of the inner ear occurs during the first trimester of pregnancy, trauma experienced by the fetus during that time may impair hearing. The infant's external auditory canal is shorter than an adult's and has an upward curve. The infant's eustachian tube is wider, shorter, more horizontal, and less stiff than the adult's, which allows easier reflux of nasopharyngeal secretions. As the child grows, the eustachian tube lengthens and its pharyngeal orifice moves inferiorly. Growth of lymphatic tissue, specifically the adenoids, may occlude the eustachian tube and interfere with aeration of the middle ear, predisposing young children to developing middle ear effusions.

Although the maxillary and ethmoid sinuses are present at birth, they are very small. The sphenoid sinuses are present by 5 years of age (see Fig. 13.7). The frontal sinuses begin to develop around 7 to 8 years of age and complete development during adolescence. Infections of the paranasal sinuses can occur during childhood.

Salivation increases by 3 months. Drooling becomes most prominent between 3 and 6 months and slows down by 24 months of age. The 20 deciduous teeth usually erupt between 6 and 24 months of age (see Fig. 13.10). Permanent teeth begin forming in the jaw by 6 months of age. Pressure from these teeth causes resorption of the deciduous teeth roots until the crown is shed. Eruption of the permanent teeth begins at about 6 years of age and is completed around 14 or 15 years of age. Wisdom teeth or third molars are the last and most posteriorly placed permanent teeth to erupt. They usually erupt between 17 and 25 years of age, but this may also occur many years later. Tooth eruption timing may be delayed in cases of poor nutritional status and chronic health conditions.

Pregnant Patients

Elevated levels of estrogen cause increased vascularity of the upper respiratory tract. The capillaries of the nose, pharynx, and eustachian tubes become engorged, leading to symptoms of nasal stuffiness, decreased sense of smell, epistaxis, a sense of fullness in the ears, and impaired hearing. Increased vascularity and proliferation of connective tissue of the gums also may occur. Hormone-induced laryngeal changes may lead to hoarseness, deepening or cracking of the voice, or a persistent cough.

Older Adults

About one-third of people in the United States aged 65 to 74 years report some trouble hearing, and about half of individuals older than 75 years have hearing difficulty (National Institute of Deafness and Other Communication Disorders, 2023). Age-related hearing loss, also called *presbycusis,* is associated with degeneration of hair cells in the organ of Corti, loss of the organ of Corti and cortical auditory neurons, degeneration of the cochlear conductive membrane, and decreased vascularity in the cochlea. Sensorineural hearing loss first occurs with high-frequency sounds and then progresses to tones of lower frequency. Loss of high-frequency sounds usually interferes with the understanding of speech and localization of sound. Conductive hearing loss may result from cerumen impaction and tympanosclerosis or otosclerosis caused by calcification of tissues in the middle ear.

Deterioration of the sense of smell results from the loss of olfactory sensory neurons beginning at about 60 years of age. The sense of taste begins deteriorating at about 50 years of age as salivary gland secretion and the number of papillae on the tongue decrease, reducing the perception of sweet sensations. However, a wide variation in the rate of smell and taste deterioration occurs.

Cartilage formation continues in the ears and nose, making the auricle and nose larger and more prominent. The soft tissues of the mouth change as the granular lining on the lips and cheeks becomes more prominent. The gingival tissue may recede and become more vulnerable to trauma, allowing teeth to erode more easily at the gum line. The tongue becomes more fissured. The older adult may have altered motor function of the tongue, leading to problems with swallowing. Saliva quality and flow may decrease as a result of health conditions or medications (e.g., anticholinergics and diuretics). Lost teeth may contribute to dietary changes or malocclusion and difficulty chewing. Sensitivity to odors and tastes declines. These changes may lead to poor nutrient intake and lower quality of life.

REVIEW OF RELATED HISTORY

For each of the conditions discussed in this section, selected topics to include in the history of the present illness are listed. Responses to questions about these topics help one fully assess the patient's condition and provide clues for focusing the physical examination. Questions regarding medication use (prescription and over-the-counter) as well as complementary, alternative, and integrative therapies are relevant for each area.

History of Present Illness

Ear Pain

- Onset, duration, and course
- Concurrent upper respiratory infection, frequent swimming, head trauma; related complaints in the mouth, teeth, sinuses, throat, or temporomandibular joint
- Associated symptoms: pain, fever, discharge (e.g., waxy, serous, mucoid, purulent, sanguineous); itchiness; reduced hearing, ringing in ear, vertigo; association with diving or flying
- Ear canal cleaning practices; prior cerumen impactions
- Medications: antibiotics, ear drops (e.g., acetic acid, anesthetic, topical steroids, cerumen softeners)

Hearing Loss: One or Both Ears

- Onset: sudden (may indicate vascular or autoimmune process), over a few hours or days (may indicate viral infection), slow or gradual
- Hears best: on telephone, in quiet or noisy environment
- All sounds reduced or some sounds garbled
- Inability to discriminate words
- Reports of people mumbling
- Speech: soft or loud, articulation of speech sounds
- Associated symptoms: tinnitus, ear pain, foreign body, prior cerumen impactions
- Management: hearing aid, when worn, battery change frequency; lipreading, sign language used
- Ototoxic medications: aminoglycosides (gentamicin), chemotherapy (cisplatin), antimalarial (quinine), salicylates, and furosemide

Risk Factors

Hearing Loss

Adults

- Exposure to industrial or recreational noise
- Neurodegenerative and autoimmune disorders
- Otosclerosis
- Syphilis
- Ototoxic medication use
- Radiation therapy for head and neck cancer

Fetuses, Infants, and Children

- Infection, maternal substance use, hypoxia, prematurity
- Assisted ventilation for more than 14 days, hyperbilirubinemia requiring exchange transfusion, or extracorporeal membranous oxygenation (Kraft et al., 2014)
- Infection: bacterial meningitis, recurrent episodes of acute otitis media or otitis media with effusion
- Cleft palate, craniofacial abnormalities, syndromic conditions associated with hearing loss (e.g., Alport, Down, Treacher Collins)
- Ototoxic medications
- Cerumen impaction
- Head trauma
- Family history of child with hearing loss

Vertigo

- Time of onset, duration, circumstances, past episodes
- Description of sensation (to-and-fro movement or rotary motion—room moving around patient or patient spinning); change of sensation with lying down, turning over in bed, or turning head; positions that reduce or exacerbate feeling
- Associated symptoms: nausea, vomiting, tinnitus, hearing loss or change, headache, double vision, ear fullness
- Unsteadiness, loss of balance, falling
- Medications: ototoxic medications such as aminoglycosides (gentamicin), chemotherapy (cisplatin), antimalarial (quinine), salicylates (aspirin), and furosemide; salt-retaining medications such as corticosteroids

Nasal Discharge

- Character (e.g., watery, mucoid, purulent, crusty, bloody); odor, amount, duration, unilateral or bilateral
- Associated symptoms: sneezing, nasal congestion or stuffiness, itching, habitual sniffling, nasal obstruction, mouth breathing, malodorous breath, sore throat, eye burning or itching, cough
- Seasonality of symptoms; allergies or concurrent upper respiratory infection; frequency of occurrence
- Tenderness over face and sinuses, postnasal drip, daytime cough, face pain, headache, recent injury

Snoring

- Change in snoring pattern, reports of snoring loudness by partner or others in household, episodes of apnea (pauses in breathing)
- Daytime sleepiness, behavior challenges, poor academic performance, nocturnal enuresis (associated with obstructive sleep apnea)
- Nosebleed: frequency, duration, amount of bleeding, nasal obstruction, treatment, difficulty stopping the bleeding, site of bleeding, unilateral or bilateral
- Predisposing factors: concurrent upper respiratory infection, dry heat, nose picking, forceful nose blowing, trauma, use of anticoagulants, allergies, dry air or climate

Sinus Pain

- Fever, malaise, cough, headache, maxillary toothache, eye pain
- Nasal congestion, colored nasal discharge
- Pain: tenderness or pressure over sinuses, pain increases when bending forward
- Medications: change in symptoms with decongestants

Dental Problems

- Pain: with chewing, localized to tooth or entire jaw, associated with temporomandibular joint pain, severity, interference with eating, foods no longer eaten, tooth grinding
- Swollen or bleeding gums, mouth ulcers or masses, tooth loss
- Dentures or dental appliances (e.g., braces, retainers): snugness of fit, areas of irritation, length of time dentures or appliances worn daily
- Malocclusion: difficulty chewing, tooth extractions, previous orthodontic work
- Medications: phenytoin, cyclosporine, calcium channel blockers, mouth rinses

Mouth Lesions

- Intermittently or constantly present, duration, painful or painless; excessive dryness of mouth; halitosis
- Associated with stress, foods, seasons, fatigue, tobacco use, alcohol use, dentures
- Variations in tongue character: swelling, size, color, coating, ulceration, difficulty moving
- Mucosal lesions elsewhere (e.g., vagina, urethra, anus)
- Medications: mouth rinses

Risk Factors

Oral Cavity and Oropharyngeal Cancer

- Tobacco use: smoking (cigarettes, cigars, pipes), oral products (chewing tobacco or snuff); risk increases with frequency and duration of use
- Alcohol use disorder: heavy consumption has higher risk, especially when combined with smoking (risk is 30 times higher compared with individuals who do not drink or smoke)
- Chewing betel quid (areca nut and other ingredients) or gutka (combination of betel quid and tobacco); more common in Southeast Asia
- Oral infection with human papillomavirus (HPV type 16 most common)
- Older than 55 years
- Gender: higher rate in males than in females (possibly because of higher alcohol and tobacco use)
- Excess body weight
- Ultraviolet (UV) light exposure associated with cancer of the lip
- Poor nutrition (diet low in fruits and vegetables)
- Inherited genetic syndromes: Fanconi anemia, dyskeratosis congenita

From American Cancer Society. (2021). *Risk factors for oral cavity and oropharyngeal cancers.* https://www.cancer.org/cancer/types/oral-cavity-and-oropharyngeal-cancer/causes-risks-prevention/risk-factors.html

Sore Throat

- Pain with swallowing, associated with upper respiratory infection; exposure to group A streptococcus, gonorrhea, Epstein-Barr virus, or SARS-CoV-2; postnasal drip, mouth breathing, fever
- Exposure to dry heat, smoke, or fumes
- Medications: antibiotics, nonprescription lozenges or sprays

Hoarseness

- Onset: acute, chronic
- Change in voice quality (e.g., breathy, pitch alteration); need to clear throat frequently
- Associated problems: overuse of voice, allergies, inhalation of smoke or other irritants, vaping, gastroesophageal reflux, recent surgery requiring intubation or intensive care treatment

Difficulty Swallowing

- Solids, liquids, or both; progressive difficulty
- Feeling of food in throat, tightness, or substernal fullness
- Drooling, swallowed liquids coming out of nose, coughing or choking when swallowing

Past Medical History

- Systemic disease: hypertension, cardiovascular disease, diabetes mellitus, nephritis, bleeding disorder, gastrointestinal disease, gastroesophageal reflux, asthma
- Ear: frequent ear infections during childhood; trauma, surgery, labyrinthitis; antibiotic use, dosage, and duration
- Nose: trauma, surgery, chronic nosebleeds
- Sinuses: chronic postnasal drip, recurrent or chronic sinusitis, allergies
- Throat: frequent streptococcal throat infections, tonsillectomy, adenoidectomy

Family History

- Hearing problems or hearing loss, Ménière disease, otosclerosis
- Allergies
- Hereditary renal disease

Personal and Social History

- Environmental hazards: exposure to loud, continuous noises (factory, airport, music through headphones—associated with hearing loss); use of protective hearing devices
- Nutrition: excessive sugar intake, foods eaten (associated with caries)
- Oral care patterns: tooth brushing and flossing, last visit to and frequency of dental care, current condition of teeth; braces, dentures, bridges, crowns, mouth guard use
- Tobacco use: pipe, cigarettes, cigars, smokeless; amount, number of pack-years (associated with oral cancer)
- Vaping (use of electronic cigarettes or another vaping device)
- Alcohol use
- Intranasal cocaine use

Fetuses, Infants, and Children

- Prenatal: perinatal infection (e.g., toxoplasmosis, cytomegalovirus, syphilis); irradiation; alcohol and substance use disorders; hypertension; Rh incompatibility; diabetes
- Prematurity: birth weight less than 1500 g, assisted mechanical ventilation for more than 14 days, anoxia, ototoxic medication use
- Hyperbilirubinemia requiring exchange transfusion
- Infection: meningitis, encephalitis, recurrent episodes of acute otitis media with or without tympanostomy tube placement, prolonged episodes of otitis media with effusion, unilateral mumps, persistent nasal discharge or cough for 10 days or more
- Secondary tobacco smoke exposure, out-of-home childcare (associated with occurrence of acute otitis media), siblings in the home
- Congenital abnormalities and syndromes: cleft palate, choanal atresia or stenosis, other craniofacial abnormalities; syndromic condition associated with hearing loss (Waardenburg, Treacher Collins); renal anomalies (branchio-oto-renal syndrome)

- Snoring and daytime somnolence (associated with obstructive sleep apnea)
- Playing with small objects (foreign body in nose or ears)
- Behaviors indicating hearing loss: no reaction to calling name or caregiver's voice, language delay such as no babbling after 6 months of age, no communicative speech and reliance on gestures after 15 months of age, inattention compared with children of the same age
- Failure in language domain on developmental screening tool; failure in newborn hearing screening or screening in childhood
- Dental care: fluoride supplementation or fluoridated water, sleeping with bottle or prolonged bottle use (past 12 months of age), age when first tooth erupted, number of teeth present, thumb sucking, pacifier use

Pregnant Patients

- Weeks of gestation or postpartum
- Presence of symptoms before pregnancy
- Pattern of dental care
- Exposure to infection

Older Adults

- Hearing loss causing any interference with daily life
- Any physical disability: interference with oral care or denture care, problems using hearing aid
- Deterioration of teeth, extractions, difficulty chewing, malnutrition
- Dry mouth (xerostomia)
- Medications decreasing salivation: anticholinergics, diuretics, antihypertensives, antihistamines, antispasmodics, antidepressants, antiemetics; ototoxic drugs

EXAMINATION AND FINDINGS

Equipment

- Otoscope with pneumatic attachment
- Nasal speculum
- Tongue blades
- Tuning forks (512 and 1024 Hz approximate vocal frequencies)
- Gauze
- Gloves
- Penlight or light from otoscope

Ears and Hearing

External Ear

Inspect the auricles for size, shape, symmetry, landmarks, color, and position on the head. Examine the lateral and medial surfaces and surrounding tissue, noting color, presence of deformities, lesions, and nodules. The auricle should have the same color as the facial skin, without moles, cysts or other lesions, deformities, or nodules. No skin tags, openings, or discharge should be present in the preauricular area. A Darwin tubercle, thickening along the upper ridge of the helix, is an expected variation. Preauricular skin tags and preauricular pits, found in front of the ear where the upper auricle originates, are other common variations (Fig. 13.11, A to C).

The auricle color may vary with certain conditions. Blueness may indicate some degree of cyanosis. Pallor or excessive redness may result from vasomotor instability. Frostbite can cause extreme pallor.

An unusual size or shape of the auricle may be a familial trait or indicate abnormality. A cauliflower ear results from blunt trauma and necrosis of the underlying cartilage. Tophi—small, whitish uric acid crystals along the peripheral margins of the auricles—may indicate gout. Sebaceous cysts, elevations in the skin with a punctum indicating a blocked sebaceous gland, are common (see Fig. 13.11, D to F).

To check the auricle's position, draw an imaginary line between the inner canthus of the eye and the most prominent protuberance of the occiput (Fig. 13.12). The top of the auricle should be at or above this line. Draw an imaginary vertical line perpendicular to the previous line, just anterior to the auricle. The auricle's position should be almost vertical, with no more than a 10-degree lateral posterior angle. A low-set position or unusual angle may indicate a genetic syndrome.

Inspect the external auditory canal for discharge and note any odor. A purulent, foul-smelling discharge is associated with otitis externa, perforated acute otitis media, or a foreign body. In cases of head trauma, a bloody or serous discharge is suggestive of a skull fracture.

Palpate the auricles and mastoid area for tenderness, swelling, or nodules. The consistency of the auricle should be firm, mobile, and without nodules. If folded forward, it should readily recoil to its usual position. Pull gently on the lobule; if pain is present, the external auditory canal may be inflamed. Tenderness or swelling in the mastoid area may indicate mastoiditis (Fig. 13.13).

Otoscopic Examination

Otoscopy is the procedure used to inspect the external auditory canal, tympanic membrane, and middle ear (see Fig. 3.18). A handheld otoscope remains the most frequently used tool to perform an ear examination, but new technology using a cell phone attachment has been gaining popularity. When using a traditional otoscope, select the largest speculum that will fit comfortably in the patient's ear. Hold the handle of the otoscope between your thumb and index finger, supported on the middle finger (many examiners use the right hand for the right ear and the left hand for the left ear). Depending on your preference, the bottom of the handle may rest against the palm of the hand or the space between the thumb and index finger. Use the ulnar side of your hand to rest against the

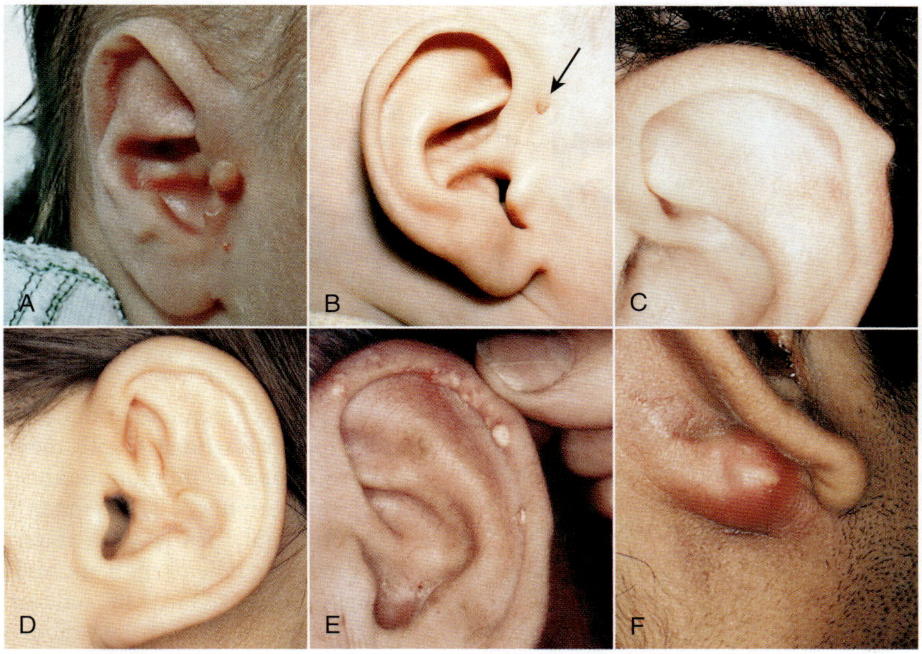

FIG. 13.11 (A) Preauricular skin tag. (B) Auricular sinus. (C) Darwin tubercle. (D) Cauliflower ear. (E) Tophi. (F) Sebaceous cysts. Six close-up views of ears, marked A through F, shows the following: (A) a round lump on tragus. (B) A round lump, indicated by an arrow, in front of the upper part of the ear. (C) A round lump on the helix. (D) Deformed outer ear. (E) Firm deposits on the inner side of the helix. (F) A bump behind the lobule of the ear. (A and B, From Zitelli, B. J., & Davis, H. W. (1997). *Atlas of pediatric physical diagnosis* (3rd ed.). St. Louis: Mosby; C, D, and F, from Bingham, B. J. G., Hawke, M., & Kwok, P. (1992). *Atlas of clinical otolaryngology*. St. Louis: Mosby; E, from American College of Rheumatology. (2009). *Clinical slide collection on the rheumatic diseases*. Atlanta: American College of Rheumatology.)

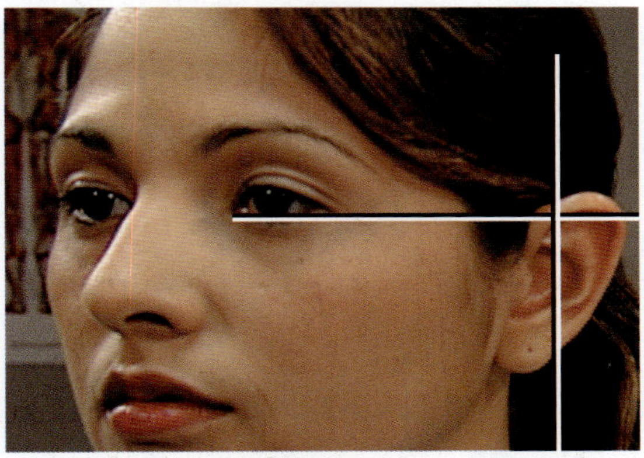

FIG. 13.12 Assessment of auricle alignment showing expected position. Imaginary line extends from inner eye canthus to occiput. Vertical imaginary line just anterior to the auricle. Side view of a face shows a horizontal line across the upper ear and left eye along with a vertical line across the center of the ear intersecting the horizontal line.

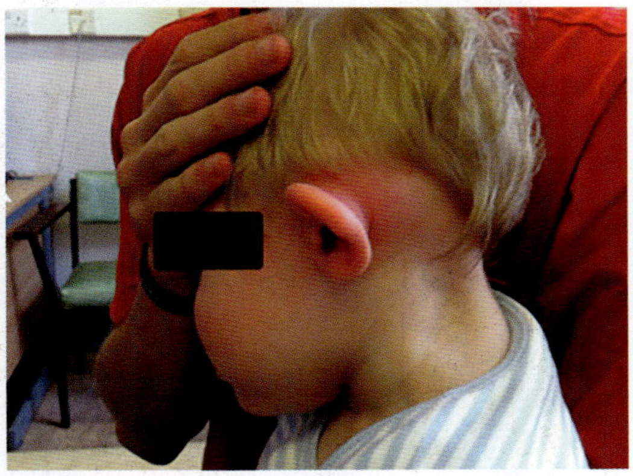

FIG 13.13 Acute mastoiditis in a child. The pinna has been pushed forward because of postauricular swelling over the mastoid bone. Close-up view of a hand holding the head of a child. The child shows inflammation and redness. (From De, M., & Anari, S. (2018). Infections and foreign bodies in ENT. Surgery (Oxford, Oxfordshire), 36(10), 553–559.)

patient's head, stabilizing the otoscope as it is inserted into the canal. Examination of the tympanic membrane with the otoscope requires manipulation of the auricle. Use a firm but gentle grasp to avoid causing discomfort. Tilt the patient's head toward the opposite shoulder, and as the speculum is inserted, pull the patient's auricle upward and back to straighten the auditory canal for the best view (Fig. 13.14).

Slowly insert the speculum to a depth of 1 to 1.5 cm (0.5 inch) and inspect the auditory canal from the meatus to the tympanic membrane, noting discharge, scaling, excessive redness, lesions, foreign bodies, and cerumen. Avoid the speculum tip touching the bony walls of the auditory canal (the inner two-thirds) with the speculum, which will cause pain. Expect to see minimal cerumen and hairs in the outer third of the canal. Cerumen may

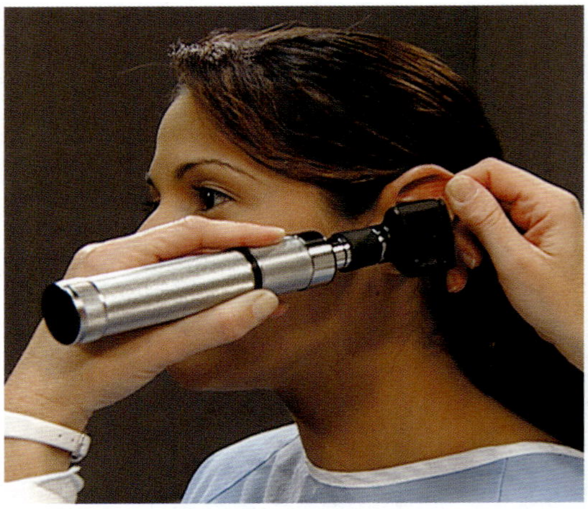

FIG. 13.14 **To examine the adult's ear with the otoscope, straighten the external auditory canal by pulling the auricle up and back.** Close-up view of left hand of an examiner holding an otoscope next to the ear of a patient while pulling the ear from the helix with right hand.

vary in color and texture but should not have an odor. Variation of a single gene determines cerumen consistency (wet, sticky, and brown vs. dry, gray, and flaky). No lesions, discharge, or foreign body should be present (see Clinical Pearl, "Cleaning an Obstructed Auditory Canal").

CLINICAL PEARL

Cleaning an Obstructed Auditory Canal

If a patient with an ear or hearing concern has a tympanic membrane obscured by cerumen, the canal can be cleaned by warm water irrigation or a cerumen spoon. Take care when using a cerumen spoon because the auditory canal is easily abraded, causing pain and bleeding. Irrigation with water at body temperature is preferable for young patients. Do not perform water irrigation in the presence of otitis externa, suspicion of a perforated tympanic membrane, pressure-equalizing tubes, or an opening into the mastoid bone.

Inspect the tympanic membrane for landmarks, color, contour, and perforations. Gently move the otoscope to see the entire tympanic membrane and the annulus (thickening at the periphery). The tympanic membrane should be a translucent, pearly gray color, with visible landmarks (umbo, handle of malleus, and light reflex) and no perforations (Fig. 13.15A). Its contour should be slightly conical with a concavity at the umbo. A bulging tympanic membrane is more conical, usually with a loss of bony landmarks and a distorted light reflex (see Fig. 13.15B). A retracted tympanic membrane is more concave, usually with accentuated bony landmarks and a distorted light

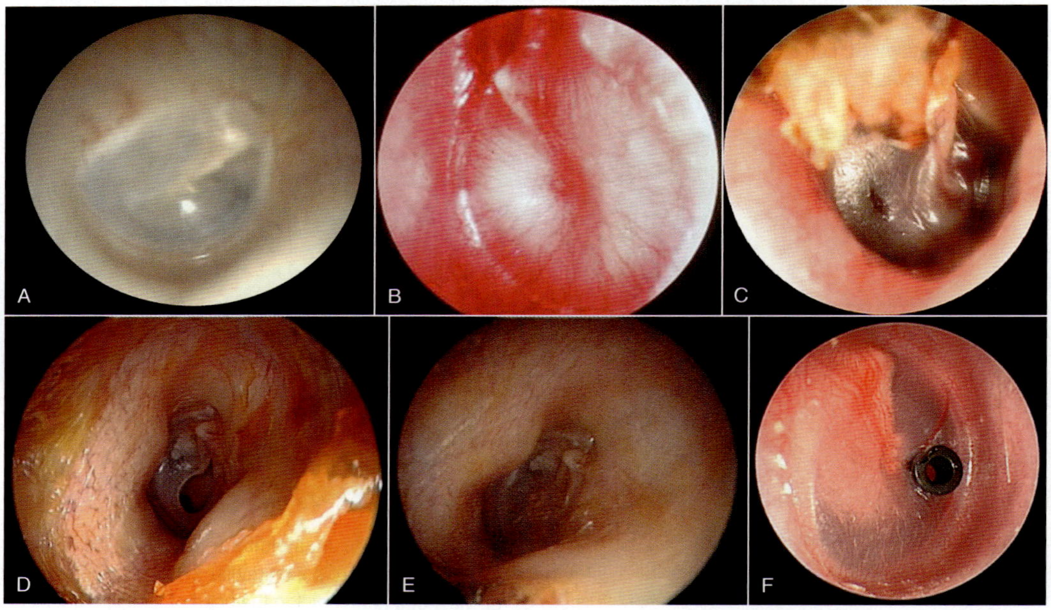

FIG. 13.15 (A) Healthy tympanic membrane. (B) Bulging tympanic membrane with loss of bony landmarks. (C) Tympanic membrane partially obscured by cerumen. (D) Perforated tympanic membrane. (E) Perforated tympanic membrane that has healed. (F) Tympanostomy tube protruding from the right tympanic membrane. Six inside views of ears marked A through F show changes in the appearance of tympanic membrane. (A, From Comunello, E., Wangenheim, A.v, Junior, V. H., Dornelles, C., & Costa, S. S. (2009). A computational method for the semi-automated quantitative analysis of tympanic membrane perforations and tympanosclerosis. *Comput Biol Med*, *39*(10), 889–895; B, from Hammami, B., Chakroun, A., Achour, I., Abid, H., Chakroun, A., Charfeddine, I., & Ghorbel, A. (2010). Transmission deafness and tinnitus: What diagnosis? *Eur Ann Otorhinolaryngol Head Neck Dis*, 127(5), 193–196; C, from Fireman, P. (2006). *Atlas of allergies and immunology* (3rd ed.). St. Louis: Mosby; D and E, from Nassif, N. (2016). Response to the letter to the editor regarding "Tympanic membrane perforation in children: endoscopic type I tympanoplasty, a newly technique, is it worthwhile?" *Int J Pediatr Otorhinolaryngol*, *80*, 110–111; F, from Lambert, E., & Roy, S. (2013). Otitis media and ear tubes. *Pediatr Clin North Am*, *60*(4), 809–826.)

reflex. Fig. 13.15C to F show other variations in appearance of the tympanic membrane, and Table 13.1 shows tympanic membrane characteristics associated with middle ear disorders.

The pneumatic attachment of the otoscope is used to provide information about tympanic membrane mobility and the middle ear space, such as the presence of middle ear effusion. The otoscope should have no air leaks. Make sure the speculum inserted into the canal creates a tight seal with the external auditory canal. Specula that come with the otoscope are sized better for sealing, and they can be cleaned with alcohol swabs between patients. Disposable specula may not be large enough for a tight fit. Gently apply positive pressure (gentle bulb compression) to make the membrane move toward the middle ear. Keep the bulb compressed, unseal and then reseal the speculum, and then apply negative pressure (release compressed bulb) to make the membrane move toward your eye. Movement from positive and negative pressure is expected and is indicated by a change in the cone of light appearance. No movement is expected when the tympanic membrane is perforated or a pressure-equalizing tube is in place. No movement with positive and negative pressure may be a sign of otitis media with effusion (OME) or acute otitis media (AOM). OME results from eustachian tube dysfunction, leading to the development of a transudate in the middle ear. It typically occurs in the setting of an upper respiratory tract infection and is self-limited (4 to 6 weeks).

TABLE 13.1 Tympanic Membrane Signs and Associated Conditions

SIGNS	ASSOCIATED CONDITIONS/CAUSES
Mobility	
Bulging with no mobility	Middle ear effusion caused by acute otitis media
Retracted with no mobility	Obstruction of eustachian tube with or without middle ear effusion
Mobility with negative pressure only	Obstruction of eustachian tube with or without middle ear effusion
Excess mobility in small areas	Healed perforation, atrophic tympanic membrane
Color	
Amber or yellow	Serous fluid in middle ear (otitis media with effusion)
Blue or deep red	Blood in middle ear (hemotympanum)
Chalky white	Infection in middle ear (acute otitis media)
Redness	Infection in middle ear (acute otitis media), prolonged crying
Dullness	Fibrosis, otitis media with effusion
White flecks, dense white plaques	Healed inflammation
Air bubbles	Serous fluid in middle ear
Bullae or vesicles	Bullous myringitis (form of acute otitis media)

In AOM, the effusion typically becomes infected with bacterial pathogens, and the child usually shows symptoms and signs of inflammation (e.g., pain, fever, redness, and bulging of the tympanic membrane; Fig. 13.16). In contrast, otitis externa, often referred to as *swimmer's ear,* is an inflammation of the auditory canal. Water retained in the canal causes tissue maceration, desquamation, and microfissures that favor bacterial or fungal growth (Fig. 13.17). See the Differential Diagnosis table.

Hearing Evaluation

Cranial nerve VIII is tested by evaluating hearing when the patient responds to your questions and directions. Note any behaviors such as cupping a hand behind the ear or tilting an ear toward you when listening. The patient should respond without excessive requests for repetition. Speech with a monotonous tone and erratic volume may indicate hearing loss.

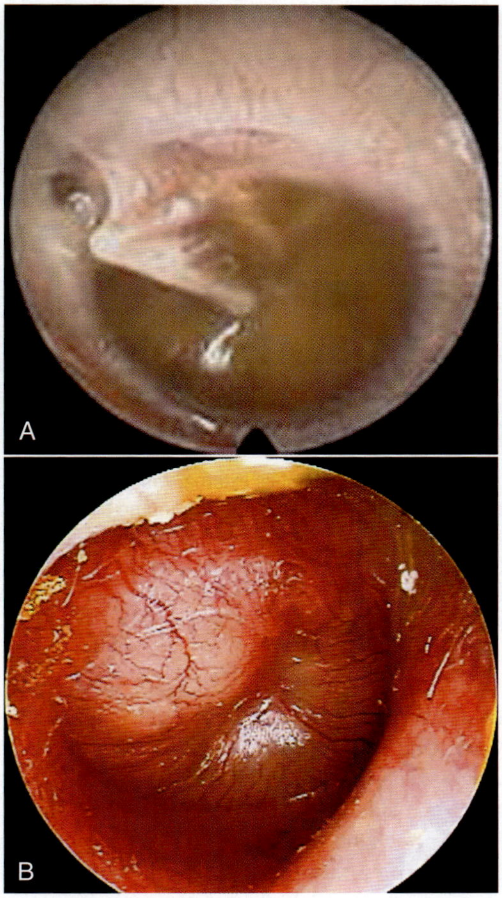

FIG. 13.16 Otitis media with effusion and acute otitis media. (A) The middle ear filled with serous fluid; note the bulging appearance and distorted light reflex. (B) Acute otitis media. Note the red bulging tympanic membrane with obscured bony landmarks and distorted light reflex. (A) Close-up of tympanic membrane shows pale-yellow, watery fluid. (B) Close-up of the tympanic membrane shows inflammation and red lines. (A, From Kliegman, R. M, St Geme III, J. W., Blum, N. J., Tasker, R. C., Wilson, K. M., Schuh, A. M., Mack, C. L. (2025). *Nelston textbook of pediatrics* (22nd ed.). Elsevier.)

DIFFERENTIAL DIAGNOSIS

Otitis Externa, Otitis Media With Effusion, and Acute Otitis Media

SIGNS AND SYMPTOMS	OTITIS EXTERNA	OTITIS MEDIA WITH EFFUSION	ACUTE OTITIS MEDIA
Initial symptoms	Itching in ear canal; typically occurs after swimming	Sticking or cracking sound on yawning or swallowing; no signs of dizziness	Abrupt onset, fever, feeling of blockage, irritability, preceding or concurrent upper respiratory symptoms
Pain	Intense with movement of pinna, chewing	Discomfort, feeling of fullness	Deep-seated earache that interferes with activity or sleep, pulling at ear
Discharge	Watery, then purulent and thick, musty, foul-smelling	None	Only if tympanic membrane ruptures or through tympanostomy tubes; foul-smelling
Hearing	Conductive loss caused by exudate and swelling of ear canal	Conductive loss as middle ear fills with fluid	Conductive loss as middle ear fills with purulent material
Inspection	Canal is red, edematous; tympanic membrane obscured	Tympanic membrane retracted or full, yellowish, mobility impaired; air-fluid level and/or bubbles present	Tympanic membrane with distinct erythema, thickened or clouding; bulging; limited or absent movement from positive or negative pressure, air-fluid level and/or bubbles present; vesicles or bullae may be seen

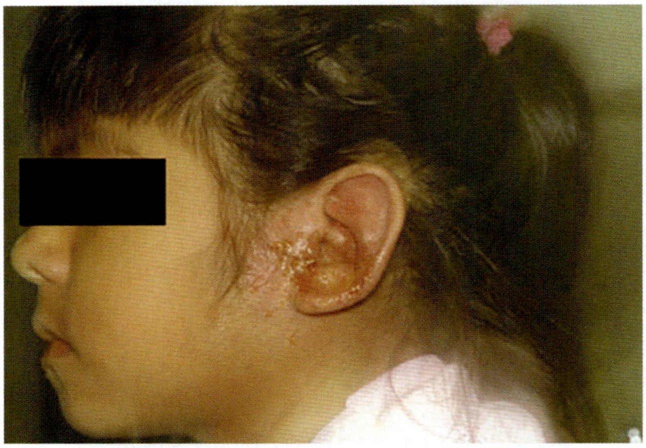

FIG. 13.17 Patient with acute otitis externa, with purulent drainage from the ear canal and mild edema and erythema of the pinna. Side view of a young girl's face shows inflammation and rashes on the pinna, ear canal, and in front of ear. (From Cherry, J., Demmler-Harrison, G. J., Kaplan, S. L., Steinbach, W., & Hotez, P. J. (2019). *Feigin and Cherry's textbook of pediatric infectious diseases* (8th ed.). Philadelphia: Elsevier.)

Whispered Voice Check the patient's response to your whispered voice, one ear at a time. Mask the hearing in the nontested ear by having the patient gently occlude it. Stand behind and to the side of a seated patient at arm's length from the patient's nontested ear. To soften the whisper, exhale fully before whispering a random combination of three to six letters and numbers (e.g., 3, T, 9). Ask the patient to repeat what was heard. Repeat the process with different numbers and letters with the other ear. If the patient is unable to correctly repeat more than 50% of the sounds, they are likely to have hearing impairment and should be referred for formal auditory evaluation. The whispered voice test has been found to have good specificity and sensitivity for detecting hearing loss in adults 50 to 70 years of age (McShefferty et al., 2013).

Weber and Rinne Tests. The tuning fork is used to compare hearing by bone conduction versus that by air conduction. Hold the stem of the tuning fork without touching the tines, and stroke or tap the tines gently to make them vibrate.

The Weber test helps assess unilateral hearing loss. Place the base of the vibrating tuning fork on the midline of the patient's head (Fig. 13.18). Ask the patient whether the sound is heard equally in both ears or is better in one ear (lateralization of sound). Avoid giving the patient a cue

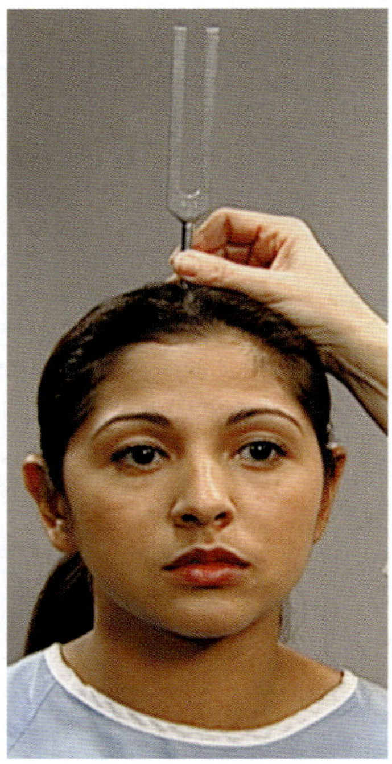

FIG. 13.18 **Weber test.** Touching only the handle, place the base of the tuning fork on the midline of the skull. Avoid touching the vibrating tines. Close-up view of a hand holding a tuning fork and placing it at the center of the skull of a patient.

as to the best response. The patient should hear the sound equally in both ears. If the sound is lateralized, have the patient identify which ear hears the sound better. To test the reliability of the patient's response, repeat the procedure while occluding one ear, and ask which ear hears the sound better. It should be heard best in the occluded ear.

The Rinne test helps distinguish whether the patient hears better by air or bone conduction. Place the base of the vibrating tuning fork against the patient's mastoid bone and ask the patient to tell you when the sound is no longer heard. Time this interval of bone conduction, noting the number of seconds. Quickly position the still-vibrating tines 1 to 2 cm (0.5 to 1 inch) from the auditory canal, and again ask the patient to tell you when the sound is no longer heard. Continue timing the interval of sound caused by air conduction heard by the patient (Fig. 13.19). Compare the number of seconds sound is heard through bone conduction versus air conduction. Air-conducted sound should be heard twice as long as bone-conducted sound (e.g., if bone-conducted sound is heard for 15 seconds, air-conducted sound should be heard for an additional 15 seconds).

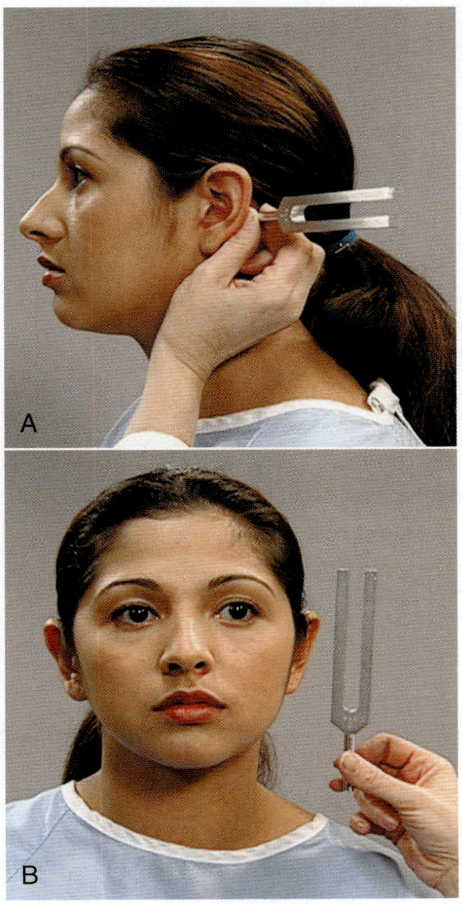

FIG. 13.19 Rinne test. (A) Place the tuning fork on the mastoid bone for bone conduction. (B) To test for air conduction, hold the tuning fork 1 to 2 cm (0.5 to 1 inch) from the ear with the tines facing forward. (A) Close-up view of a hand placing a tuning fork behind the ear of a patient. (B) Close-up view of the same hand holding the tuning fork to one side of the ear.

TABLE 13.2 Interpretation of Tuning Fork Tests

TEST	EXPECTED FINDINGS	CONDUCTIVE HEARING LOSS	SENSORINEURAL HEARING LOSS
Weber	No lateralization, but will lateralize to ear occluded by patient	Sound heard better in affected ear unless sensorineural loss	Sound lateralizes to better ear unless conductive loss
Rinne	Air conduction heard longer than bone conduction by 2:1 ratio (Rinne positive)	Bone conduction heard longer than air conduction in affected ear (Rinne negative)	Air conduction heard longer than bone conduction in affected ear but less than 2:1 ratio

Table 13.2 provides guidelines to help distinguish between conductive and sensorineural hearing loss using the Weber and Rinne tests. Refer all patients with unexpected findings during the hearing screening for a thorough auditory evaluation.

Evidence-Based Practice in Physical Examination

Detection and Treatment of Hearing Loss

In a qualitative synthesis of randomized trials—observational and diagnostic accuracy studies assessing the evidence for benefits and harms of hearing screening in adults 50 years and older—only one large, randomized trial showed benefits of formal hearing screening. In this trial, compared with a control group, a greater proportion of participants screened with a combination of a hearing screening inventory and handheld audiometer reported hearing aid use 1 year later. However, there were no differences in hearing-related function. In another study, quality of life was better for participants using a hearing aid compared with controls. There are currently no clear harms to screening or using hearing aids to treat hearing loss.

From US Preventive Services Task Force, Krist, A. H., Davidson, K. W., Mangione, C. M., Cabana, M., Caughey, A. B., Davis, E. M., Donahue, K. E., Doubeni, C. A., Epling, J. W., Jr, Kubik, M., Li, L., Ogedegbe, G., Pbert, L., Silverstein, M., Stevermer, J., Tseng, C. W., & Wong, J. B. (2021). Screening for Hearing Loss in Older Adults: US Preventive Services Task Force Recommendation Statement. *JAMA*, 325(12), 1196–1201. https://doi.org/10.1001/jama.2021.2566.

Nose, Nasopharynx, and Sinuses

External Nose

Inspect the nose for deviations in shape, size, and color. Observe the nares for discharge and for flaring or narrowing. The skin should be smooth without swelling and conform to the color of the face. The columella, the bridge of tissue separating the nares, should be directly midline, and its width should not exceed the diameter of a naris. The nares are usually oval in shape and symmetrically positioned. A depression of the nasal bridge or saddle nose deformity can result from a fractured nasal bone or previous nasal cartilage inflammation (Fig. 13.20). Nasal flaring is associated with respiratory distress, whereas narrowing of the nares on inspiration may be indicative of chronic nasal obstruction and mouth breathing. A transverse crease at the

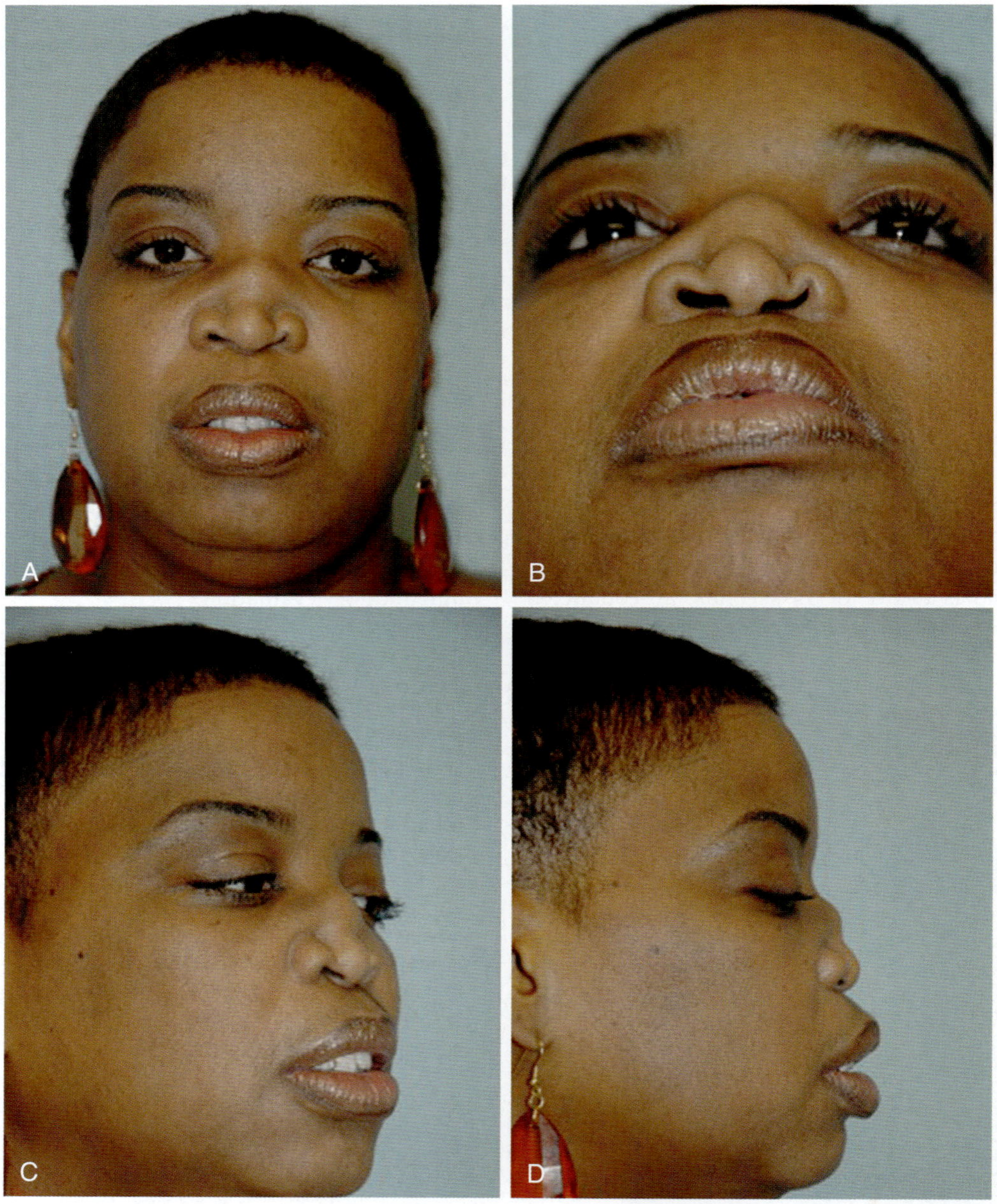

FIG. 13.20 Saddle nose deformity. (A) Progressive loss of septal integrity results in a characteristic saddle nose deformity. (B) Depression and splaying of the middle vault. (C) Collapse of the internal and external valves with widening of the nasal base. (D) Decreased vertical projection, over-rotation of the tip, and retraction of the columella. Four close-up views of the patient's face, marked A through D, from different sides show collapsing of nose bridge.

junction between the cartilage and bone of the nose may indicate frequent upward rubbing of the nose because of chronic nasal itching and allergies (known as the *allergic salute*).

If nasal discharge is present, describe its character (e.g., watery, mucoid, purulent, crusty, or bloody); amount and color; and whether unilateral or bilateral. Potential conditions associated with nasal discharge include the following:

- Allergy—bilateral watery discharge and associated sneezing and nasal congestion
- Epistaxis or trauma—bloody discharge
- Rhinitis or upper respiratory infection—bilateral mucoid or purulent discharge
- Foreign body—unilateral, purulent, thick, greenish, malodorous discharge
- Cerebrospinal fluid leakage—unilateral watery discharge occurring after head trauma

Palpate the bridge and soft tissues of the nose. Note any displacement of bone and cartilage, tenderness, or masses. Place one finger on each side of the nasal arch and gently palpate, moving the fingers from the nasal bridge to the tip. The nasal structures should feel firm and stable to palpation without crepitus (crackling sensation). No tenderness or masses should be present.

Evaluate the patency of the nares. Occlude one naris by placing a finger on the side of the nose, and ask the patient to breathe in and out with the mouth closed. Repeat the procedure with the other naris. Nasal breathing should be noiseless and easy through the open naris.

Nasal Cavity

With the thumb of your nondominant hand, tip the nose upward. Using an otoscope with a large speculum tip in your dominant hand, inspect the nasal cavity. Insert the speculum tip slowly and cautiously. Do not touch the nasal septum to avoid causing pain (Fig. 13.21). Inspect the nasal mucosa for color, discharge, masses, lesions, and turbinate swelling (see Clinical Pearl, "Cocaine Use"). Inspect the nasal septum for alignment, perforation, bleeding, and crusting. Keep the patient's head erect to examine the vestibule and inferior nasal turbinate. Tilt the patient's head back to visualize the middle meatus and middle turbinate, then cautiously move the speculum toward the midline to examine the septum. Only the inferior and middle turbinates will be visible. Repeat in the other naris.

> **CLINICAL PEARL**
>
> **Cocaine Use**
>
> When individuals nasally insufflate ("snort," "sniff") cocaine, signs of recent use include rhinorrhea, hyperemia, and edema of the nasal mucosa. White powder may still be present on the nasal hairs. Signs of chronic use include scabs on the nasal mucosa, decreased perception of taste and smell, and perforation of the nasal septum.

Expect the nasal mucosa to glisten and appear deep pink (pinker than the buccal mucosa). A film of clear discharge is often apparent on the nasal septum. Purulent discharge may be associated with an upper respiratory infection, sinusitis, or a foreign body. Hairs may be present in the vestibule. Increased redness of the mucosa may occur with an infection, whereas localized redness and swelling in the vestibule may indicate a furuncle. Expect the turbinates to be firm and the same color as the surrounding area. Turbinates that appear bluish gray or pale pink with a swollen, boggy consistency may indicate allergies. A rounded, elongated mass projecting into the nasal cavity from boggy mucosa may be a polyp (Fig. 13.22A).

Expect the nasal septum to be close to midline and fairly straight, with the anterior septum thicker than the posterior septum. A nasal septum deviation may be indicated by asymmetric size of the posterior nasal cavities (see Fig. 13.22B). No perforations, bleeding, or crusting should be apparent. Crusting over the anterior portion of the nasal septum (Kiesselbach plexus) may occur at the site of epistaxis.

The sense of smell (cranial nerve I) is often tested with recognition of different odors. This procedure is described in Chapter 23.

Sinuses

Inspect the frontal and maxillary sinus areas for swelling. To palpate the frontal sinuses, use your thumbs to press up under the bony brow on each side of the nose. Then press up under the zygomatic processes, using either your thumbs or index and middle fingers to palpate the maxillary sinuses. Expect no tenderness or swelling over the soft tissue. Swelling, tenderness, and pain over the sinuses may indicate infection.

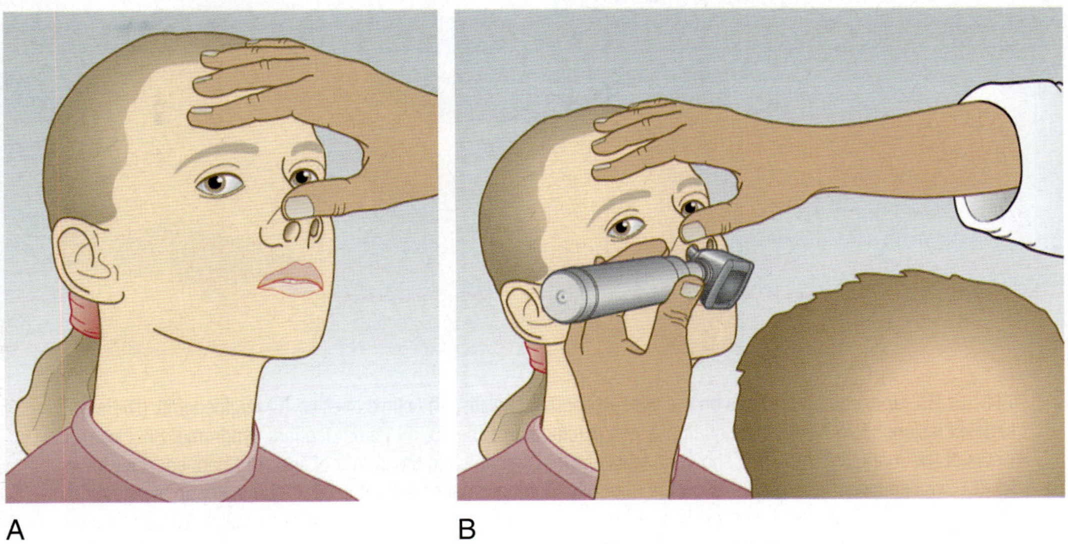

FIG. 13.21 Nasal examination. (A) Elevation of the tip of the nose to give a clear view of the anterior nares. (B) Anterior rhinoscopy using an otoscope with a large speculum. (A) Close-up view of a hand pulling the nose tip up of a patient using thumb while resting the fingers on the forehead. (B) Close-up view of an examiner's hand holding an otoscope and inserting it in one nostril of a patient.

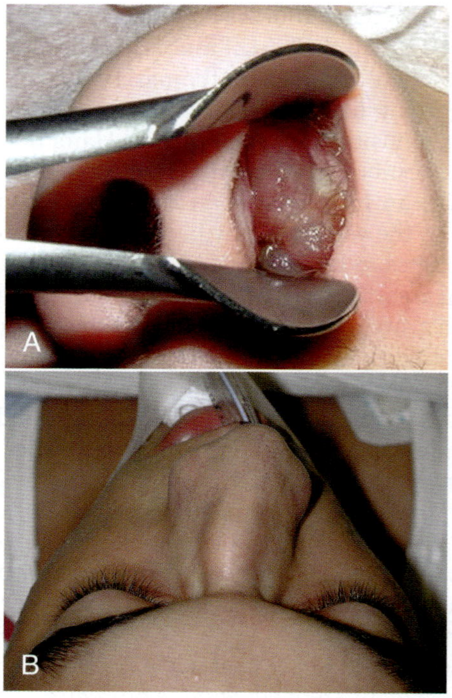

FIG. 13.22 Unexpected findings on nasal examination. (A) Nasal polyps. (B) Deviation of the nasal septum. (A) Close-up view of a nose, held by rhinoscope, shows soft growth along the inner lining. (B) Close-up view of the nose shows slant nasal septum. (A, From Swartz, M. H. (2020). The ear and nose. In M. H. Swartz (Ed.). *Textbook of physical diagnosis: History and examination* (8th ed., pp. 228–248). Elsevier; B, from Cummings et al., 2010.)

Mouth and Oropharynx

Lips

With the patient's mouth closed, inspect and palpate the lips for symmetry, color, swelling, and surface abnormalities. The lip color should be pink on patients with lighter skin and more bluish on individuals with darker skin. Lip symmetry is expected, both at rest and with movement. No lesions should interrupt the distinct vermilion border between the lips and the facial skin. The lip surfaces should be smooth and free of lesions.

Dry, cracked lips (cheilitis) may be caused by dehydration from wind chapping, dentures, braces, or excessive lip licking. Deep fissures at the corners of the mouth (angular cheilitis) may indicate infection, irritation, nutritional deficiencies (iron and B vitamins), or overclosure of the mouth, allowing saliva to macerate the tissue. Swelling of the lips may be caused by infection, trauma, or allergy (angioedema). Lip pallor is associated with anemia, whereas circumoral pallor is associated with scarlet fever caused by group A streptococcus infection. Cyanosis (bluish-purple lips) results from hypoxia associated with a respiratory or cardiovascular condition. Round, oval, or irregular bluish-gray macules on the lips and buccal mucosa are associated with Peutz-Jeghers syndrome. Lesions, plaques, vesicles, nodules, and ulcerations may be signs of infection, irritation, or skin cancer (Fig. 13.23).

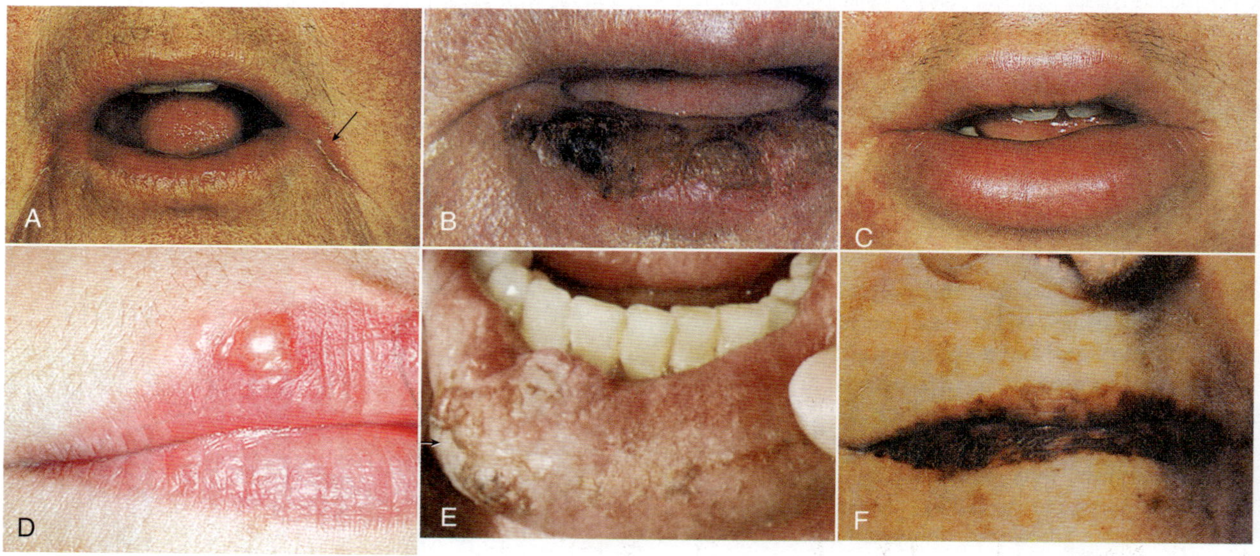

FIG. 13.23 Unexpected findings on the lips. (A) Angular cheilitis. (B) Actinic cheilitis. (C) Angioedema. (D) Herpes simplex lesions (cold sores). (E) Squamous cell carcinoma of the lip. (F) Peutz-Jeghers syndrome. Six close-up views of lips marked A through F show the following: (A) Red patch in the corner of lips. (B) Chapped, scaly lower lip. (C) Swollen lower lip. (D) A lump on the upper lip. (E) Abnormal growth of cells on the lower lip, indicated by an arrow. (F) Black pigmentation on lips. (A, B, and C from Habif, T. P. (2004). *Clinical dermatology* (4th ed.). St. Louis: Mosby; D, from Goldman, L., & Ausiello, D. A. (2008). *Cecil medicine* (23rd ed.). Philadelphia: Saunders; E, from Stewart, J. F., Tattersall, M. H., Woods, R. L., & Fox, R. M. (1978). Unknown primary adenocarcinoma: Incidence of overinvestigation and natural history. *Br Med J, 1*(6177), 1530–1533; F, from Chessell, G. S. J., Jamieson, M. J., Morton, R. A., Petrie, J. C., Towler, H. M. A. (1984). *Diagnostic picture tests in clinical medicine.* London: Wolfe Medical Publications.)

Buccal Mucosa, Teeth, and Gums

Ask the patient to clench their teeth and smile to observe the occlusion of the teeth. The facial nerve (cranial nerve VII) is also tested with this maneuver. Proper tooth occlusion is apparent when the upper molars fit into the grooves on the lower molars and the premolars and canines interlock fully. Indications of malocclusion and problems with the bite include protrusion of the upper incisors (overbite), protrusion of the lower incisors or failure of the upper incisors to overlap with the lower incisors (crossbite), and failure of the back teeth to meet (open bite; Fig. 13.24). Three classes of malocclusion are listed in Table 13.3.

Have the patient remove any dental appliances and open the mouth partially. Using a tongue blade and bright light, inspect the buccal mucosa, gums, and teeth. Expect the mucous membranes to be pinkish red, smooth, and moist. The Stensen duct is a whitish-yellow or whitish-pink protrusion in approximate alignment with the second upper molar. When swelling is noted around the Stensen duct, use gloved hands to milk the tissue toward the Stensen duct. A small amount of clear saliva is expected. Small stones or exudates coming from the Stensen duct are unexpected.

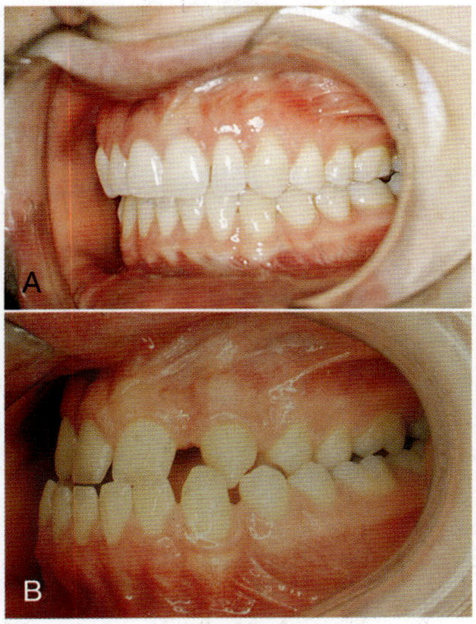

FIG. 13.24 (A) Class I malocclusion. (B) Class III malocclusion. (A) Close-up view of mouth, held by mouth retractor, shows edges of lower incisor teeth behind the upper teeth. (B) Close-up view of mouth, held by mouth retractor, shows one upper tooth missing and lower teeth displaced in forward direction. (Courtesy Drs. Abelson and Cameron, Lutherville, MD.)

TABLE 13.3 Classification of Malocclusion

CLASSIFICATION	CHARACTERISTICS
Class I	Molars have customary relationship, but the line of occlusion is incorrect because of rotated or malpositioned teeth
Class II	Lower molars are distally positioned in relation to the upper molars; the line of occlusion may or may not be correct
Class III	Lower molars are medially positioned in relation to the upper molars; the line of occlusion may or may not be correct

Fordyce spots, an expected variant, are ectopic sebaceous glands that appear on the buccal mucosa and lips as numerous small, yellow-white, raised lesions (Fig. 13.25A). Patchy pigmented mucosa is often found in individuals with dark skin (see Fig. 13.25B). Whitish or pinkish scars are a common result of trauma from poor tooth alignment. A red spot on the buccal mucosa at the opening of the Stensen duct is associated with parotitis (mumps). Aphthous ulcers on the buccal mucosa appear as white, round, or oval ulcerative lesions with a red halo (see Fig. 13.25C). A thickened white patch lesion that cannot be wiped away may be leukoplakia, a premalignant oral lesion most commonly seen in individuals who smoke or use oral tobacco products (see Fig. 13.25D). Leukoedema is a diffuse, filmy, grayish surface with white streaks, wrinkles, or milky alteration (Fig. 13.26). This asymptomatic finding of the buccal mucosa is considered a normal variant. It is found in 90% of Black adults and nearly 50% of Black adolescents. This finding may be seen in White adults, but with much lower frequency than in Black adults (Bhattacharyya & Chehal, 2011).

The gingivae are expected to be coral pink in lighter-skinned patients and may be more hyperpigmented in individuals with darker skin tones. The gingiva usually has a slightly stippled or dotted pink appearance with a clearly defined, tight margin at each tooth. The gum surface beneath dentures should have no inflammation, swelling, or bleeding.

Using gloves, palpate the gums for any lesions, induration, thickening, or masses. Expect the gingiva to feel firm and tightly bound to the underlying bone. No tenderness should be elicited. Epulis, a localized gingival enlargement or granuloma, is usually an inflammatory rather than a neoplastic change (Fig. 13.27). Gingival enlargement occurs with pregnancy, puberty, vitamin C deficiency, certain medications (e.g., phenytoin, cyclosporine, and calcium channel blockers), and leukemia. Easily bleeding, swollen gums with enlarged crevices between the teeth and gum margins or pockets containing debris at tooth margins are associated with gingivitis or periodontal disease (Fig. 13.28).

Inspect and count the teeth, noting wear, notches, caries, and missing teeth. If you are concerned about loose teeth, probe each with a tongue blade to identify those that are not firmly anchored. Loose teeth can be the result of periodontal disease or trauma. The teeth generally have an ivory color, but may be stained yellow from tobacco or brown from coffee or tea. Suspect caries when discolorations are seen on the crown of a tooth.

Oral Cavity

Inspect the dorsum of the tongue, noting any swelling, variation in size or color, coating, or ulcerations. Ask the patient to extend the tongue while you inspect for

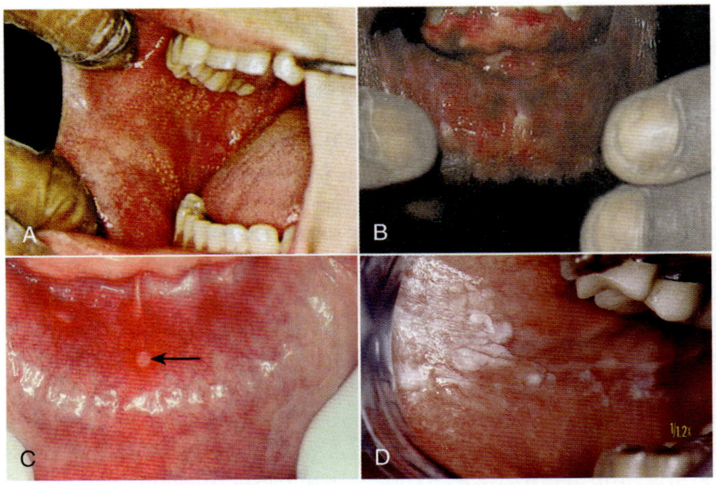

FIG. 13.25 Findings on the buccal mucosa. (A) Fordyce spots. (B) Patchy coloration of mucous membranes in individual of dark skin color. (C) Aphthous ulcer. (D) Leukoplakia. (A) Close-up view of lining of cheek shows tiny pimples. (B) Close-up view of lower lip held by fingers shows gray patches. (C) Inner side of lower lip shows a white lesion, indicated by an arrow. (D) Inside view of mouth shows thick, white growths. (A, From Wood, N. K., & Goaz, P. W. *Differential diagnosis of oral lesions* (4th ed.). St. Louis: Mosby; 1991; B, Hood, A., Dr. Department of dermatology. Indianapolis: Indiana University School of Medicine; C, from Kumar V., Fausto, N., Abbas A. (2006). *Robbins and Cotran pathologic basis of disease* (7th ed.). Philadelphia: Saunders; D, from Richardson, M. R., Flint, P. W., Haughey, B. H., Lund, V. J., Niparko, J. K., Robbins, K. T., Thomas, J. R., Lesperance, M.M. (2013). *Cummings otolaryngology: Head and neck surgery* (5th ed.). St Louis: Mosby.)

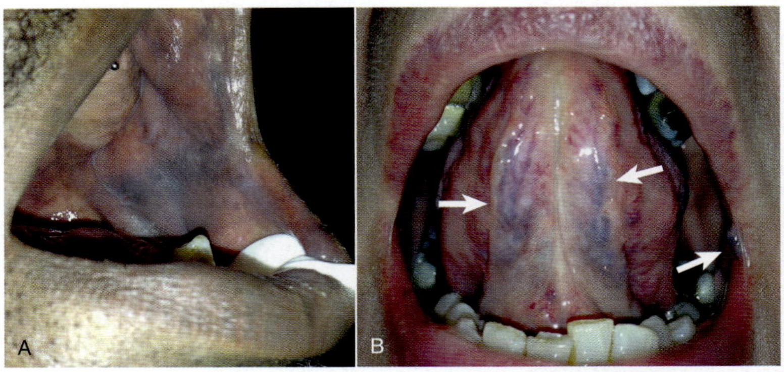

FIG. 13.26 Leukoedema. (A) Inner lining of cheek shows inflammation and whitish-gray patches. (B) Ventral surface of tongue shows whitish-gray patches, indicated by arrows. One arrow points toward a lesion in the cheek area. (From Madani, F. M., & Kuperstein, A. S. (2014). Normal variations of oral anatomy and common oral soft tissue lesions: Evaluation and management. *Med Clin North Am*, *98*(6), 1281–1298.)

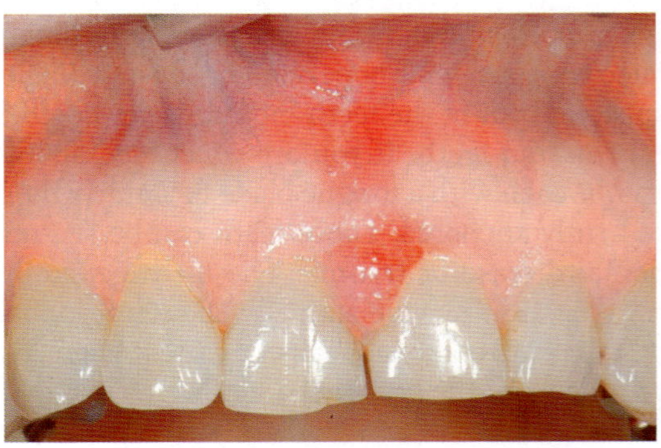

FIG. 13.27 Epulis. Close-up view of upper teeth shows a lump on the gum between two incisors. (From Truschnegg, A., Pichelmayer, M., Acham, S., & Jakse, N. (2016). Nonsurgical treatment of an epulis by photodynamic therapy. *Photodiagnosis Photodyn Ther*, *14*, 1–3.)

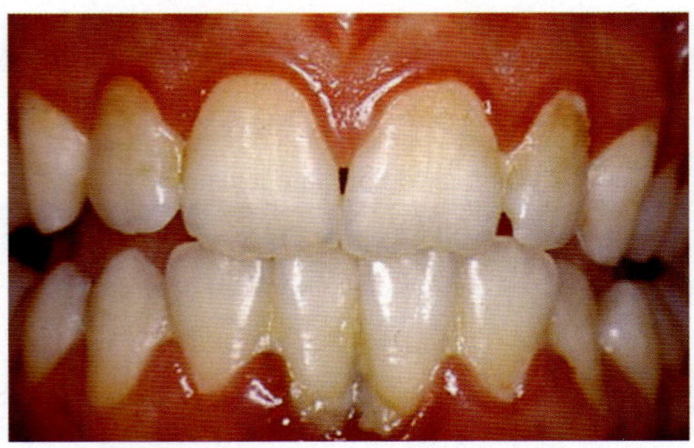

FIG. 13.28 Gingivitis. In the lower incisor teeth, gingivitis progressed to periodontitis characterized by gingival recessions. (From Pizzo, G., Guiglia, R., Lo Russo, L., & Campisi, G. (2010). Dentistry and internal medicine: From the focal infection theory to the periodontal medicine concept. *Eur J Intern Med*, *21*(6), 496–502. doi:10.1016/j.ejim.2010.07.011.)

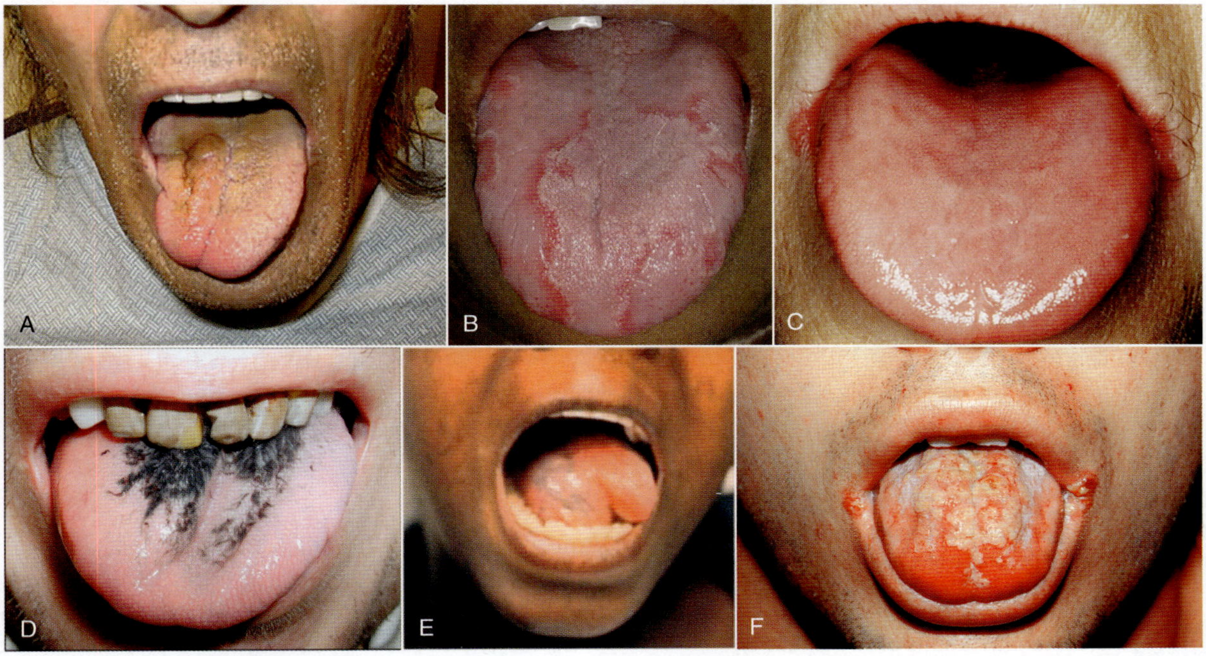

FIG. 13.29 **Findings on the tongue and mouth floor.** (A) Left hypoglossal paralysis. The tongue deviates to the weak side. Note atrophy on the tongue's right side. (B) Geographic tongue. (C) Glossitis, smooth tongue resulting from vitamin deficiency. (D) Black hairy tongue. (E) Ranula (obstructed sublingual salivary gland). (F) Primary gingivostomatitis showing lesions on the tongue. Six close-up views of a tongue, marked A through F, show the following: (A) Yellowish deposits and lumps on the top. (B) White patch with red boundary on the top. (C) Plain tongue with loss of tiny hairlike projections. (D) Black papillae. (E) Large lump under the tongue. (F) White and yellow deposits on the top of the tongue along with inflammation and redness at the corners of the lips. (A, From Yelken, K., Guven, M., Kablan, Y., & Sarikaya, B. (2007). Isolated unilateral hypoglossal nerve paralysis following open septoplasty. *Br J Oral Maxillofac Surg, 46*(4), 308–309; B, from Bakshi, S. S., & Bhattacharjee, S. (2017). Geographic tongue. *J Allergy Clin Immunol Pract, 5*(1), 176; C, from Little, J. W., Falace, D. A., Miller, C. S., Rhodus, N. L. (2013). *Little and Falace's dental management of the medically compromised patient* (8th ed.). St. Louis: Elsevier; D, from Nisa, L., & Giger, R. (2011). Black hairy tongue. *Am J Med, 124*(9), 816–817; E, from Chidzonga MM, et al: Ranula: experience with 83 cases in Zimbabwe, *J Oral Maxillofac Surg, 65*(1):79–82, 2007; F, from White, G. A., & Cox, N. H. (2006). *Diseases of the skin: A color atlas and text* (2nd ed.). St. Louis: Mosby.)

deviation, tremor, and limitation of movement. The procedure also tests the hypoglossal nerve (cranial nerve XII). Expect the protruded tongue to be maintained at the midline. No atrophy or fasciculations should be present. Deviation to one side indicates tongue atrophy and hypoglossal nerve impairment (Fig. 13.29A).

The tongue appears dull red, moist, and glistening. An overall smooth, yet roughened, surface with papillae and small fissures is seen on its anterior portion. The posterior portion should have rugae or a smooth, slightly uneven surface with a thinner mucosa than the anterior portion. The geographic tongue, an expected variant, has superficial denuded circles or irregular areas exposing the tips of papillae. A smooth red tongue with a slick appearance (glossitis) may indicate a vitamin B_{12} deficiency. The hairy tongue with yellow-brown to black elongated papillae on the dorsum sometimes follows antibiotic therapy (see Fig. 13.29B to D).

Ask the patient to touch the tongue tip to the palate area directly behind the upper incisors. Inspect the floor of the mouth and the ventral surface of the tongue for swelling and varicosities, also observing the frenulum, sublingual ridge, and Wharton ducts. Expect the ventral surface of the tongue to be pink and smooth with large veins between the frenulum and fimbriated folds. Wharton ducts are apparent on each side of the frenulum. A ranula (mucocele) may be seen on the floor of the mouth when the duct of a sublingual salivary gland is obstructed (see Fig. 13.29E). Lesions on the tongue may be caused by an infectious process (see Fig. 13.29F).

Wrap the tongue with a piece of gauze and gently pull it to each side while inspecting the lateral borders (Fig. 13.30). Scrape any white or red margins to distinguish between food particles and leukoplakia or another fixed abnormality.

Palpate the tongue and the floor of the mouth for lumps, nodules, or ulceration. Expect the tongue to have a smooth, even texture. Any ulcer, nodule, or thickened white patch on the lateral or ventral surface of the tongue may be suggestive of malignancy (see Clinical Pearl, "Oral Cancer Assessment"). Table 13.4 presents the oral manifestations of human immunodeficiency virus (HIV) infection, and Fig. 13.31 shows oral Kaposi sarcoma.

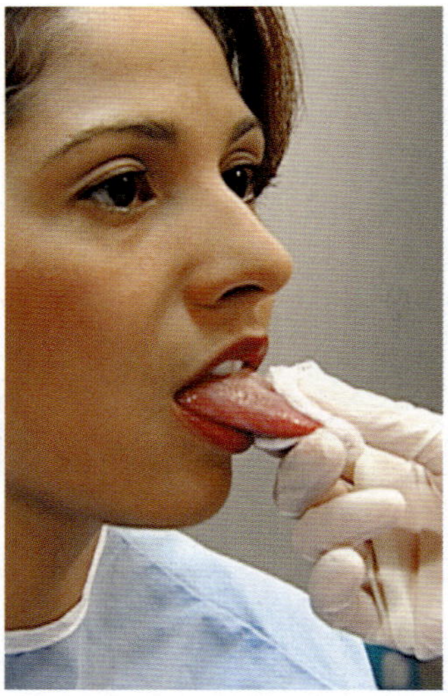

FIG. 13.30 **Inspection of lateral borders of the tongue.** Close-up view of a gloved hand holding the tongue of a patient from the tip.

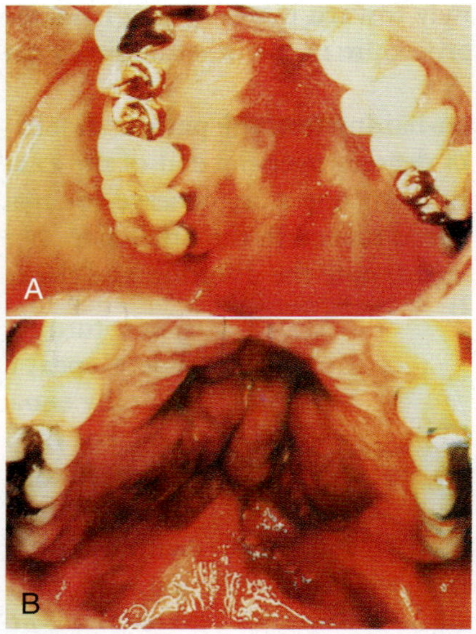

FIG. 13.31 **Oral Kaposi sarcoma.** (Moderately advanced lesion. (B) Advanced lesion. (A) Close-up view of upper jaw shows silver fillings and red, swollen palate. (B) Close-up view of upper jaw shows decayed teeth and large lumps and redness on palate. (From Grimes D: *Infectious diseases*, St Louis, 1991, Mosby; courtesy Silverman, Dr. Sol Jr. University of California, San Francisco.)

TABLE 13.4 **Oral Manifestations of HIV Infection**

LESION	CHARACTERISTICS
Oral hairy leukoplakia	White, irregular lesions on lateral side of tongue or buccal mucosa; may have prominent folds or "hairy" projections
Angular cheilitis	Red, unilateral or bilateral fissures at corners of mouth
Candidiasis	Creamy white plaques on oral mucosa that bleed when scraped
Herpes simplex	Recurrent vesicular, crusting lesions on the vermilion border of the lip
Herpes zoster	Vesicular and ulcerative oral lesions in the distribution of the trigeminal nerve; may also be on gingiva
Human papillomavirus	Single or multiple sessile or pedunculated nodules in the oral cavity
Aphthous ulcers	Recurrent circumscribed ulcers with an erythematous margin
Periodontal disease	In a mouth with little plaque or calculus, gingivitis with bone and soft tissue degeneration accompanied by severe pain
Kaposi sarcoma	In the mouth, incompletely formed blood vessels proliferate, forming lesions of various shades and size as blood extravasates in response to the malignant tumor of the epithelium

CLINICAL PEARL

Oral Cancer Assessment

To screen for signs of oral cancer, carefully examine each of the following areas of the oral cavity, face, and neck. Inspect the vermilion border of the lips (a high-risk site), the labial mucosa, the attached gingival tissues, the alveolar gingival mucosa, and the vestibule by raising and lowering the lips.

Inspect the buccal mucosa and hard palate. Inspect the dorsal surface of the tongue. With the tongue extended right, inspect the left lateral and ventral surfaces of the tongue and lateral floor of the mouth. Extend the tongue to the left to inspect the right tongue surfaces. Inspect the anterior floor of the mouth. Place a gloved finger on the floor of the mouth and a finger of the other hand on the tissue behind the mandible. Compress the tissue between the fingers to palpate the floor of the mouth. Inspect and palpate the throat, neck, and temporomandibular areas.

Ask the patient to tilt the head back for inspection of the palate and uvula. The whitish hard palate should be dome-shaped with transverse rugae. The pinker soft palate is contiguous with the hard palate. The uvula, a midline continuation of the soft palate, varies in length and thickness. The hard palate may have a bony protuberance at the midline, called *torus palatinus,* an expected variant present in 25% to 35% of the population, more commonly seen in females than in males (Silk, 2014; Fig. 13.32A). A nodule on the palate that is not at the midline may indicate a tumor. A bony protuberance, the mandibular torus, occurs bilaterally on the lingual surface of the mandible, near the canine and premolar teeth, and is an expected variant. It occurs in 7% to 10% of the population.

Movement of the soft palate is evaluated by asking the patient to say "ah." Depressing the tongue may be necessary for this maneuver. As the patient vocalizes, observe the soft palate rising symmetrically with the uvula remaining in the midline. This maneuver also tests the glossopharyngeal and vagus nerves (cranial nerves IX and X, respectively). Deviation of the uvula to one side may indicate vagus nerve paralysis or peritonsillar abscess. The uvula deviates toward the unaffected side in both instances. A bifid uvula is often a benign condition and may be a normal variant in some Native Americans; however, it

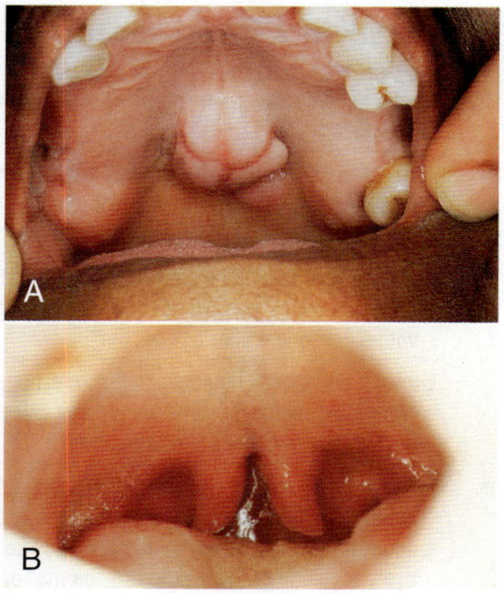

FIG. 13.32 (A) Torus palatinus. (B) Bifid uvula. (A) Inside view of mouth shows bony growth on the hard palate. (B) Inside of the mouth shows uvula split into two. (A, Courtesy Abelson, Dr. Lutherville, MD; B, from Hawke, M., & McCombe, A. W. (1997). *Diseases of the ear: A pocket atlas.* Manticore.)

may indicate a submucous cleft palate (see Fig. 13.32B). A bifid uvula is also associated with Loeys-Dietz syndrome, a disorder in which aortic root dilation and aortic dissection may occur (Van Laer et al., 2014).

Oropharynx

Inspect the oropharynx using a tongue blade to depress the tongue (see Clinical Pearl, "Use of a Tongue Blade"). Observe the tonsillar pillars, noting the size of tonsils, if present, and the integrity of the retropharyngeal wall. The tonsils, usually the same pink color as the pharynx, are expected to fit within the tonsillar pillars. Tonsils may have crypts where cellular debris and food particles collect. If the tonsils are reddened, hypertrophied, and covered with exudate, an infection may be present (Fig. 13.33).

> **CLINICAL PEARL**
>
> **Use of a Tongue Blade**
>
> Most patients dislike the gag reflex associated with use of a tongue blade. Moisten the tongue blade with warm water to help reduce triggering of the gag reflex.

> **Think About It**
>
> If your patient presents with sore throat and has tonsillar enlargement and exudate, before performing a throat swab to rule out streptococcal pharyngitis, review their history and conduct a thorough examination. Fatigue and axillary and inguinal lymphadenopathy should raise your suspicion of infectious mononucleosis from Epstein-Barr virus (EBV). If you find splenomegaly or hepatomegaly on abdominal examination, the likelihood of EBV infection is quite high.

> **Evidence-Based Practice in Physical Examination**
>
> ***Predictors of Streptococcal Pharyngitis***
>
> The Centor clinical prediction rule can help identify streptococcal pharyngitis in pediatric and adult patients. Four clinical signs assessed include tonsil enlargement, tonsillar exudates, tender and enlarged anterior cervical nodes, and absence of cough. The presence of three to four clinical signs increases the probability of streptococcal pharyngitis, which can be confirmed by a rapid strep screen or throat culture. The presence of a measured temperature greater than 38.0°C is another important finding.

From Fine, A. M., Nizet, V., & Mandl, K. D. (2012). Large-scale validation of the Centor and McIsaac scores to predict group A streptococcal pharyngitis. *Archives of Internal Medicine, 172*(11), 847–852.

The posterior wall of the pharynx should be smooth, glistening, pink mucosa with some small, irregular spots of lymphatic tissue and small blood vessels. A red bulge adjacent to the tonsil and extending beyond the midline

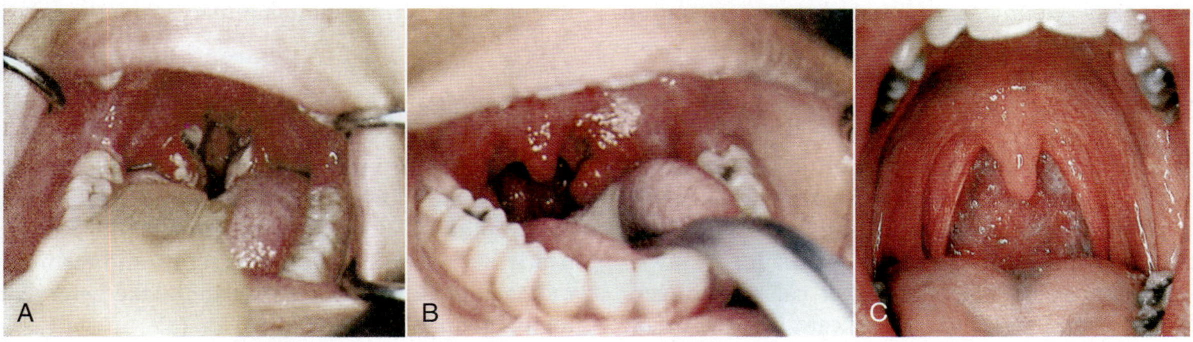

FIG. 13.33 **Findings of the oropharynx.** (A) Tonsillitis and pharyngitis. (B) Acute viral pharyngitis. (C) Postnasal drip. (A) Close-up view of a mouth, held by mouth retractor, and a hand depressing the tongue using a tongue blade. The inside view of the mouth shows inflammation and white growth in the throat. (B) Inside view of the mouth shows inflammation and a red lump in the throat. (C) Inside view of the mouth shows white deposits behind the uvula. (A and B, Courtesy Edward L. Applebaum, MD, Head, Department of Otolaryngology, University of Illinois Medical Center, Chicago.)

may indicate a peritonsillar abscess. A yellowish mucoid film in the pharynx is typical of postnasal drip (see Fig. 13.33C).

After preparing the patient for a gag response, touch the posterior wall of the pharynx. Elicitation of the gag reflex tests the glossopharyngeal and vagus nerves (cranial nerves IX and X, respectively). Expect a bilateral response.

Infants

Ears. The ears, nose, mouth, and throat are common sites of congenital malformations in the newborn and require a thorough examination.

The auricle should be well formed with all landmarks present on inspection (see Fig. 13.3). The newborn's auricle is quite flexible and instantly recoils after bending. The premature infant's auricles may appear flattened with limited incurving of the upper auricle, and ear recoil is slower.

The tip of the auricle should cross the imaginary line between the inner canthus of the eye and the prominent portion of the occiput, varying no more than 10 degrees from vertical (see Fig. 13.12). Auricles that are either poorly shaped or positioned low may be associated with renal disorders and congenital anomalies.

To perform the otoscopic examination, place the infant in a supine or prone position so the head can be turned side to side. Many examiners prefer to hold the otoscope in the right hand for the right ear and left hand for the left ear. Hold the otoscope so that the ulnar surface of your hand rests against the infant's head. The otoscope will move as the infant's head moves, reducing the risk of trauma to the auditory canal. Use your other hand to stabilize the infant's head as the thumb and index finger pull the auricle down to straighten the upward curvature of the canal. The tympanic membrane is usually in an extremely oblique position in the newborn. Because the tympanic membrane does not become conical for several months, the light reflex may appear diffuse. As the middle ear matures during early infancy, the tympanic membrane takes on the expected appearance.

Because the first 3 years of life are critical for speech and language development, universal hearing screening is recommended for all newborns in the United States and around the world. Hearing screening and audiometry should also be performed for infants and children at higher risk of hearing impairment and at regular intervals during health maintenance visits for all infants and children. Knowledge of the sequence of hearing development is necessary to evaluate the infant's hearing (Table 13.5). To conduct an informal hearing assessment during the physical examination, use a bell, whisper, or rub your fingers together as a sound stimulus, taking care that the infant responds to sound rather than to the air movement generated. Remember that responses to repeated sound stimuli will decrease as the infant tunes out the stimulus.

TABLE 13.5 The Sequence of Expected Hearing and Speech Response

AGE	RESPONSE
0–3 months	Turns or looks toward voices; quiets or smiles when hearing caregiver voice; makes different sounds if happy or upset; coos, makes sounds "oh," "ah," or "mm"
4–6 months	Reacts to toys that make sounds; giggles and laughs; vocalizes during play using vowel sounds sometimes with a consonant like "da" or "um"
7–9 months	Looks at person calling name; stops in response to "no"; recognizes names of some people and objects; babbles long strings of sounds like "mamama"
10–12 months	Points, waves, and shows or gives objects; imitates or initiates gestures in play like peek-a-boo; tries to copy sounds; responds to words and phrases like "go bye-bye"; says one or two words like "mama" or "dada"

Modified from American Speech-Language-Hearing Association. (2024). Communication milestones: Birth to 1 year (asha.org). https://www.asha.org/public/developmental-milestones/communication-milestones-birth-to-1-year/

Nose and Sinuses. Expect the external nose to have a symmetric appearance and be positioned midline on the face. Minimal movement of the nares with breathing should be apparent. Deviation of the nose from midline may be related to fetal position. A saddle-shaped nose with a low bridge and broad base; a short, small nose; or a large nose may suggest a chromosomal disorder or congenital anomaly.

Inspect the internal nose by gently tilting the nose tip upward with your thumb and shining a light inside. Small amounts of clear fluid discharge may be seen in crying infants.

Newborns are obligatory nose breathers, so assess nasal patency at birth. With the infant's mouth closed, occlude one naris and then the other, observing the breathing pattern. When obstructed, the infant will be unable to breathe through the open naris. With any breathing difficulty, a small catheter is passed through each naris to the choana, the posterior nasal opening, to assess patency. An obstruction may indicate choanal atresia or stenosis or septal deviation resulting from delivery trauma.

The paranasal sinuses are poorly developed during infancy, and examination is unnecessary.

Mouth. The lips should be well formed with no cleft. The newborn may have sucking calluses on the upper lips, appearing as plaques or crusts, for the first few weeks of life. A smooth philtrum is characteristic of fetal alcohol syndrome. Cleft lip with or without cleft palate is the second most common congenital birth defect, associated with nearly 200 identified gene mutations and environmental risk factors like insufficient folate intake before and during pregnancy (Iwata, 2021).

The crying infant provides an opportunity to examine the mouth. Avoid depressing the tongue because this stimulates a strong reflex protrusion of the tongue, making visualization of the mouth difficult.

The buccal mucosa should be pink and moist. Scrape any white patches on the tongue or buccal mucosa with a tongue blade. Nonadherent patches are usually milk deposits, but adherent patches may indicate candidiasis infection (thrush) (Fig. 13.34A). Copious secretions that accumulate in the newborn's mouth that return after frequent suctioning may indicate esophageal atresia.

Drooling is common between 2 and 6 months of age until infants learn to swallow saliva. Drooling after that age is often attributed to teething and usually disappears by 2 years of age. If drooling persists, be concerned about a potential neurologic or oral motor disorder or an anomaly of the teeth or upper gastrointestinal tract.

The newborn's gums should have no teeth and be smooth with a serrated edge of tissue along the buccal margins. Pearl-like retention cysts along the buccal margin are an expected variant and disappear in 1 to 2 months. If natal teeth are found in a newborn, determine whether they are loose and could be aspirated (see Fig. 13.34B). Such teeth are not usually firmly fixed and may need to be removed. In older infants, count the deciduous teeth, noting any unusual sequence of eruption (see Fig. 13.10A).

Expect the tongue to fit well in the floor of the mouth. The frenulum of the tongue usually attaches at a point midway between the ventral surface of the tongue and its tip. If the tongue does not protrude beyond the alveolar ridge (tongue tie), feeding difficulties may occur (see Fig. 13.34C). Macroglossia is associated with congenital anomalies such as congenital hypothyroidism (see Fig. 13.34D).

The palatal arch should be dome-shaped with no clefts in either the hard or soft palate. A narrow, flat palate or a high, arched palate (associated with congenital anomalies) will affect the tongue's placement and lead to feeding and speech problems. Petechiae are often seen on the newborn's soft palate. Epstein pearls—small, whitish-yellow masses at the juncture between the hard and soft palates—are common and disappear within a few weeks after birth (see Fig. 13.34E). The soft palate is expected to rise symmetrically when the infant cries.

Insert your gloved index finger into the infant's mouth, with the finger pad to the roof of the mouth. Simultaneously evaluate the infant's suck and palpate the hard and soft palates. This maneuver may be performed when quieting the infant to auscultate the heart and lungs. The infant, unless recently fed, is expected to have a strong suck, with the tongue pushing vigorously upward against the finger. Further investigate the absence of a strong suck reflex or disinterest in sucking. Neither the hard nor soft palate should have palpable clefts.

Children

Because the young child often resists otoscopic and oral examinations, most clinicians perform these maneuvers at the end of a visit. Positioning the child on a parent's lap rather than prone or supine on the examining table makes the child feel more secure. One option is to seat the infant

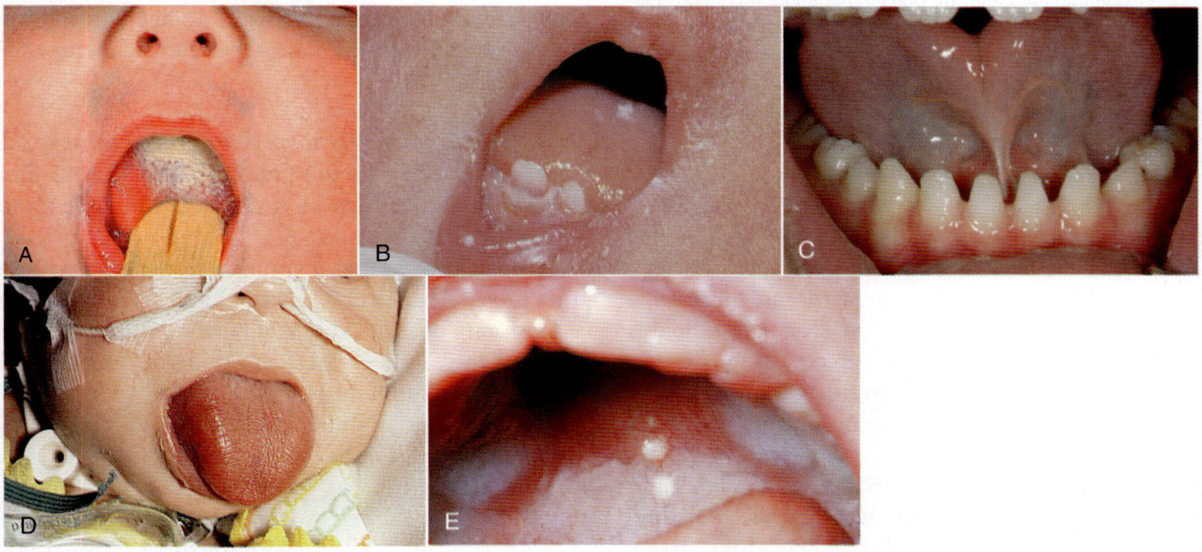

FIG. 13.34 Findings in the infant's mouth. (A) Candidiasis infection (thrush). (B) Natal teeth. (C) Short frenulum. (D) Macroglossia. (E) Epstein pearls. (A) Close-up view of open mouth shows a tongue blade depressing the tongue, which shows white and yellow deposits. (B) Close-up view of infant's mouth shows two teeth in the lower jaw. (C) Close-up view of open mouth shows a small fold of mucous membrane under the tongue. (D) Close-up view of infant's face shows enlarged tongue. (E) Inside view of mouth shows small, white nodules. (A, From Paller, A. S., & Mancini, A. J. (2016). *Hurwitz clinical pediatric dermatology: A textbook of skin disorders of childhood and adolescence* (5th ed.). Edinburgh: Elsevier; B, from Neville, B. W., Damm, D. D., Allen, C. M., & Chi, A. C. (2016). *Oral and maxillofacial pathology* (4th ed.). St. Louis: Elsevier; C, from Guven, Y., Rosti, R. O., Tuna, E. B., Kayserili, H., & Aktoren, O. (2008). Orodental findings of a family with lacrimo-auriculo-dento digital (LADD) syndrome. *Oral Surg Oral Med Oral Pathol Oral Radiol Endod, 106*(6), e33–e44; D, from Eichenfield, L. F., Frieden, I. J., & Zaenglein, A. (2015). *Neonatal and infant dermatology* (3rd ed.). Elsevier; E, from Zitelli, B. J., & Davis, H. W. (2018). *Zitelli and Davis' atlas of pediatric physical diagnosis* (7th ed.). Philadelphia: Elsevier.)

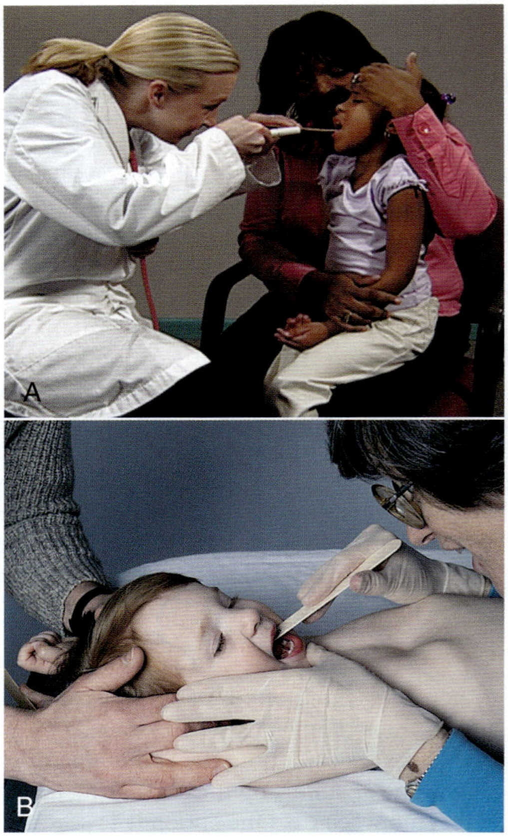

FIG. 13.35 Positioning of toddler for oral examination. (A) Sitting position. (B) Supine position. (A) Close-up view of a child sitting in the lap of her mother. The mother holds her child from the arms and head while the examiner inserts an otoscope in the mouth of the child. (B) Close-up view of an examiner inserting the tongue blade in the child's mouth. Her mother holds him from his head.

or toddler in the parent's lap, with the back to the parent's chest and legs between the adult's legs. The parent can then hold the child's arms with one arm and control the child's head with the other (Fig. 13.35A). If a parent hold is not effective and the child is unable to cooperate, be prepared to move the child to the examining table. Another person, usually the parent, may be needed to effectively hold the child.

To perform the otoscopic examination on an older toddler, face the child sideways with one arm placed around the parent's waist. The parent holds the child firmly against their trunk, using one arm to hold the child's head and the other arm to hold the child's arm and body. Further stabilize the child's head as you insert the otoscope. For the oral examination, face the child forward.

When the child actively resists the examination in other positions, place them in supine position on the examining table. The parent can hold the child's arms extended above the head and assist in immobilizing the head. Lie across the child's trunk and stabilize the child's head with your hands as you insert the tongue blade (Fig. 13.35B).

Ears. When performing the otoscopic examination, pull the auricle either downward and back or upward and back to gain the best view of the tympanic membrane. As the child grows, the shape of the auditory canal changes to the S-shaped curve of the adult. If the child is or has been crying, dilation of blood vessels in the tympanic membrane can cause a pinkish-red appearance. The pneumatic otoscope is especially important for distinguishing a red tympanic membrane caused by crying (the membrane is mobile) from AOM (no mobility). See Differential Diagnosis box.

Assess the toddler's hearing by observing the response to a whispered voice and various noisemakers (e.g., rattle, bell, or tissue paper). Position yourself behind the child while the parent distracts the child. Whisper or use a noisemaker. Expect the child to turn toward the sound consistently. Development of speech provides another indication of hearing acuity.

When testing the hearing of a young child, whisper words that will have more meaning for them (e.g., "Big Bird," "Mickey Mouse," "SpongeBob," "Spider-Man"). Another way to evaluate the young child's hearing is by asking the child to perform tasks using a soft voice. Avoid giving visual cues. The Weber and Rinne tests can be used when the child understands directions and can cooperate with the examiner, usually between 3 and 4 years of age. Audiometry should be performed in all young children at regular intervals and more frequently in those at risk of hearing loss. Regardless of examination findings, any parental concern about a child's hearing warrants further audiologic evaluation (American Academy of Pediatrics, 2023).

Nose and Sinuses. To inspect the internal nose, shine a light while tilting the nose tip upward with your thumb. If a larger area needs to be visualized, the largest otoscope speculum may be used.

Palpate the paranasal sinuses after they have developed (maxillary sinuses at 4 years of age and frontal sinuses at 7 to 8 years of age). Note any periorbital edema or tenderness in the sinus areas. The child with nasal discharge, nasal congestion, and/or cough that has not improved after 10 days after an upper respiratory infection may have a sinus infection if either of these signs is present (DeMuri & Wald, 2010).

Mouth. Engage the child with the oral examination by letting the child hold and manipulate the tongue blade and light. Doing so may reduce the fear of the procedure. Begin with a nonthreatening request, such as "Let me see a big smile," then, "Now open wide so I can see all of your teeth." Flattened edges on the teeth may indicate bruxism (compulsive, unconscious grinding of the teeth). Multiple brown areas or caries on the upper and lower incisors may be the result of a bedtime bottle of juice or formula, commonly called *early childhood caries* (Fig. 13.36). Teeth with a black or gray color may indicate pulp decay or oral iron therapy. Mottled or pitted teeth are often the result of

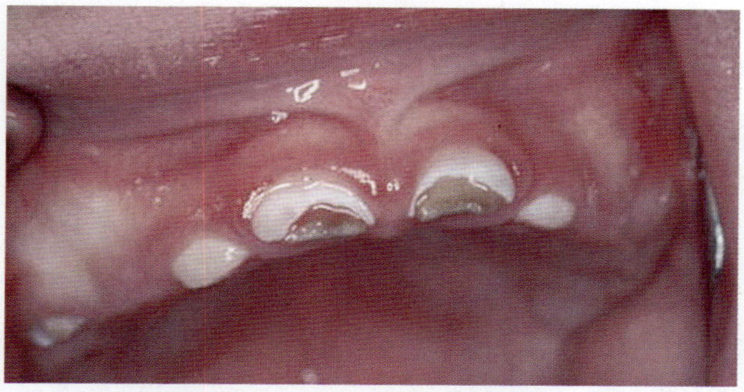

FIG. 13.36 Early childhood caries. Close-up view of upper jaw shows some of the teeth missing and two partially broken teeth. (From Tinanoff, N., & Reisine, S. (2009). Update on early childhood caries since the surgeon general's report. *Academic Pediatrics*, *9*(6), 396–403.)

tetracycline treatment during tooth development or enamel dysplasia. Chalky white lines or speckles on the cutting edges of permanent incisors may result from excessive fluoride intake.

If the child will protrude the tongue and say "ah," the tongue blade is often unnecessary for the oral examination. You could ask the child to "pant like a puppy" to raise the palate. If the child refuses to open the mouth, insert a moistened tongue blade through the lips to the back molars. Gently but firmly insert the tongue blade between the back molars and press the tongue blade to the tongue. This maneuver will stimulate the gag reflex and provide a brief view of the mouth and oropharynx.

Koplik spots, white specks with a red base on the buccal mucosa opposite the first and second molars, occur in the prodromal phase of rubeola (measles).

The tonsils, lying deep in the oral cavity, should match the color of the pharynx. They gradually enlarge to their peak size by about 6 years of age, but the oropharynx should retain an unobstructed passage. Enlarged tonsils are graded to describe their size and potential for airway obstruction (Fig. 13.37). A tonsil pushed backward or forward, possibly displacing the uvula, suggests a peritonsillar abscess or other mass (see "Abnormalities").

When the tongue is depressed, the epiglottis may be visible as a glistening pink structure behind the base of the tongue.

Pregnant Patients

Pregnant patients have increased vascularity of the respiratory tract, resulting in edema and erythema of the nose and pharynx and nasal congestion. Higher estrogen production leads to increased nasal mucous secretions, and often symptoms of a cold occur throughout pregnancy. Nosebleeds may occur. Tympanic membranes may have increased vascularity and be retracted or bulging with serous fluid. The gums may appear reddened, swollen, and spongy, with the hypertrophy resolving within 2 months of delivery.

Older Adults

Ears and Hearing. Inspect the auditory canal of the patient who wears a hearing aid for areas of irritation from the ear mold. Coarse, wirelike hairs are often present along the periphery of the auricle. On otoscopic examination, the tympanic membrane landmarks may appear slightly more pronounced from sclerotic changes.

Some degree of sensorineural hearing loss with advancing age (presbycusis) may be noted (see "Abnormalities"). Conductive hearing loss from otosclerosis and cerumen impaction may also occur.

FUNCTIONAL ASSESSMENT

Ears, Nose, and Throat

The ability to perform activities of daily living (ADLs) is often dependent on the ability to hear, speak, chew food, and swallow. Hearing is important for the personal and social components of the functional assessment. The ability to chew and swallow food is important for adequate nutrition. When the patient has dentures, a hearing aid, or other assistive device, evaluate how effectively the patient uses these devices and is able to care for them, and if they are being checked routinely by health care professionals.

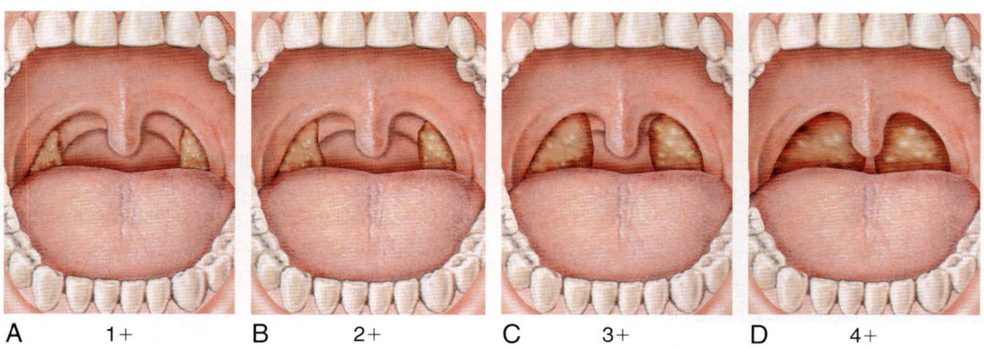

FIG. 13.37 Enlarged tonsils are graded to describe their size. (A) 1+, visible. (B) 2+, halfway between tonsillar pillars and the uvula. (C) 3+, nearly touching the uvula. (D) 4+, touching each other. Four inside views of the mouth, marked A and 1 plus through D and 4 plus show increase in the size of tonsils.

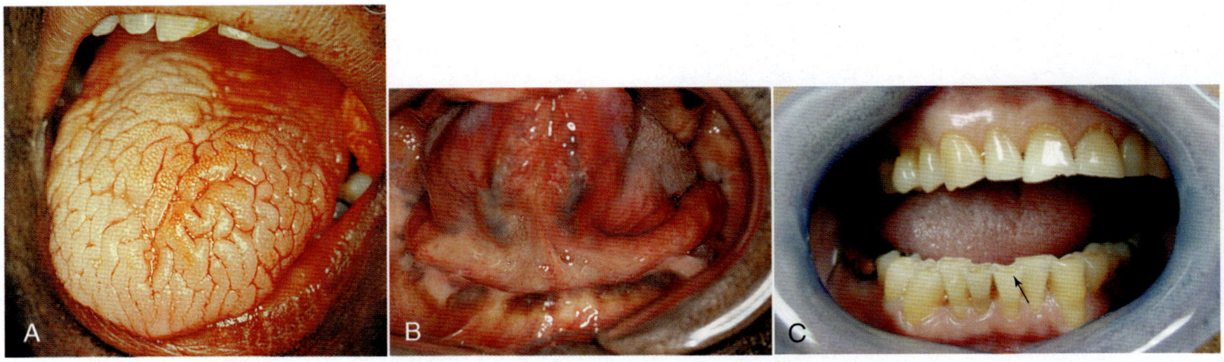

FIG. 13.38 Common findings in the older adult's mouth. (A) Fissured tongue. (B) Varicose veins on tongue. (C) Attrition of teeth and resorption of gums. (A) Close-up view of tongue shows multiple small furrows and clusters of pale yellow deposits. (B) Close-up view of ventral surface shows prominent veins. (C) Close-up view of mouth, held by mouth retractor, shows cutting edges of teeth, indicated by an arrow, in the lower jaw. (A and B, Courtesy Drs. Abelson and Cameron, Lutherville, MD; C, courtesy Daniel M. Laskin, DDS, MS, Medical College of Virginia, Virginia Commonwealth University, Richmond, VA.)

Nose. The nasal mucosa may appear dryer or less glistening. An increased number of bristly hairs in the vestibule is common, especially in males.

Mouth. The lips have increased vertical markings and appear dryer when salivary flow is reduced. The buccal mucosa is thinner, less vascular, and less shiny than that of the younger adult. The tongue may appear more fissured, and veins on its ventral surface may be seen (Fig. 13.38A and B).

The oral tissues may be dryer (xerostomia) when prescribed medications (e.g., anticholinergics or antidepressants) diminish salivary gland secretions or when Sjögren syndrome, a chronic inflammatory condition of the exocrine glands, is present. Decreased saliva may cause an increase in dental caries and oral discomfort.

Natural teeth may be worn down, shortening the crown and altering enamel thickness. Dental caries may be present, and dental restorations may have deteriorated. The teeth may appear longer as resorption of the gum and bone progresses, revealing the teeth roots (see Fig. 13.38C). Many adults older than 65 years have missing teeth. Dental malocclusion may be caused by the migration of remaining teeth after extractions.

ABNORMALITIES

Ear

CHOLESTEATOMA

Abnormal squamous epithelial tissue behind the tympanic membrane.

PATHOPHYSIOLOGY

- As the epithelial tissue enlarges, it can perforate the tympanic membrane, erode the ossicles and temporal bone, and invade the inner ear structures

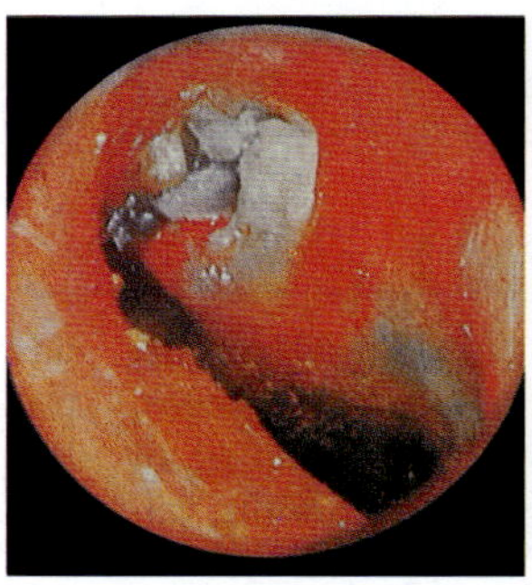

FIG. 13.39 Cholesteatoma. Close-up view of white bony growths trapped behind the tympanic membrane. (Courtesy Richard A. Buckingham, MD, Clinical Professor, Otolaryngology, Abraham Lincoln School of Medicine, University of Illinois, Chicago.)

PATIENT DATA

Subjective Data

- History of recurrent acute otitis media
- Unilateral hearing loss
- Ear fullness or pain
- Tinnitus, mild vertigo
- Discharge from the ear canal (Fig. 13.39)

Objective Data

- Spherical white cyst or pouch behind intact tympanic membrane
- Tympanic membrane may bulge
- Foul-smelling discharge if the tympanic membrane is perforated
- Conductive hearing loss
- Facial nerve paralysis (rare)

HEARING LOSS

Conductive Hearing Loss

Reduced transmission of sound to the middle ear.

PATHOPHYSIOLOGY

- Problem can be in auditory canal, tympanic membrane, or middle ear
- Causes include cerumen impaction, otitis media with effusion, acute otitis media, otitis externa, foreign body, cholesteatoma, stiffening of the ossicles, and otosclerosis (bone deposition immobilizing the stapes)

PATIENT DATA

Subjective Data

- Turns volume louder on television
- Hears better in noisy environment
- Asks to have information repeated
- Speaks softly (hears own voice by bone conduction)

Objective Data

- Bone conduction heard longer than air conduction with Rinne test
- Lateralization to affected ear with Weber test
- Loss of low-frequency sounds

Sensorineural Hearing Loss

Reduced transmission of sound in the inner ear.

PATHOPHYSIOLOGY

- A disorder of the inner ear (cochlea, associated structures, or cranial nerve VIII)
- Causes include damage to cranial nerve VIII, in utero infection (e.g., cytomegalovirus, toxoplasmosis), genetic hearing impairment, genetic syndromes, systemic disease, ototoxic medications, trauma, tumors, or prolonged exposure to loud occupational and recreational noise
- Presbycusis in older adults results from degenerative changes in the inner ear or vestibular nerve

PATIENT DATA

Subjective Data

- Reports that people mumble
- Has difficulty understanding speech
- Speaks more loudly
- Unable to hear in a crowded room

Objective Data

- Air conduction heard longer than bone conduction with Rinne test
- Weber test results—lateralizes to unaffected ear
- Loss of high-frequency sounds (consonants, e.g., *t, p, s*)

Ménière Disease

Inner ear disorder characterized by episodes of hearing loss, vertigo, tinnitus, and ear fullness.

PATHOPHYSIOLOGY

- Likely caused by genetic and environmental factors
- May be caused by excess secretion of endolymph or failure of resorption in the subarachnoid space

PATIENT DATA

Subjective Data

- Sudden onset of severe vertigo (related to moving the head) typically lasting 20 minutes to several hours
- Hearing loss
- Whistling or roaring sounds in affected ear (tinnitus); may be continuous or intermittent
- Sensitivity to sound
- Ear fullness or pressure
- Episodes in clusters with periods of remission

Objective Data

- Hearing loss to low tones initially with fluctuating progression to profound sensorineural hearing loss
- Imbalance
- Nystagmus

Vertigo

Illusion of rotational movement by a patient, most often because of a disorder of the inner ear (see also Ménière disease).

PATHOPHYSIOLOGY

- Acute vestibular neuronitis—inflammation of the vestibular nerve after an acute viral upper respiratory infection
- Benign paroxysmal positional vertigo—otolith fragments gravitate into the semicircular canal, and nerve sensors in the canal cause vertigo with head movements

PATIENT DATA

Subjective Data

- Acute vestibular neuronitis:
  - Spontaneous episode of vertigo that is severe initially and lessens over a few days
  - Difficulty walking
  - Nausea and vomiting
- Benign paroxysmal positional vertigo:
  - Episode of vertigo with head or body movements
  - Lasts less than a minute

Objective Data

- Acute vestibular neuronitis:
  - Spontaneous horizontal nystagmus with or without rotary nystagmus
  - Staggering gait
- Benign paroxysmal positional vertigo:
  - May have no physical findings
  - Rotary nystagmus with Dix-Hallpike maneuver

Sinuses

SINUSITIS

Bacterial infection of one or more of the paranasal sinuses.

PATHOPHYSIOLOGY

- Inflammation, allergies, or structural defect of the nose may block the sinus meatus and prevent the sinus cavity from draining, creating an environment for infection; overproduction of mucus may result from inflammation and increase susceptibility to infection

PATIENT DATA

Subjective Data

- Upper respiratory infection that worsens or persists after 7–10 days
- Frontal headache, facial pain or pressure, or pain in a maxillary tooth
- Purulent nasal discharge or nasal congestion
- Persistent cough, may be worse at night

Objective Data

- May have no physical findings
- Purulent nasal discharge from middle meatus, may be unilateral
- Tenderness over frontal or maxillary sinuses
- Swelling over orbital or involved sinus
- Preadolescent children may have daytime and nighttime cough, halitosis, and fever (DeMuri & Wald, 2010)

Mouth and Oropharynx

ACUTE BACTERIAL PHARYNGITIS

Infection of tonsils or posterior pharynx by microorganisms.

PATHOPHYSIOLOGY

- Microorganisms causing infection often include group A beta-hemolytic streptococci, other streptococcal species, *Neisseria gonorrhoeae, Mycoplasma pneumoniae*

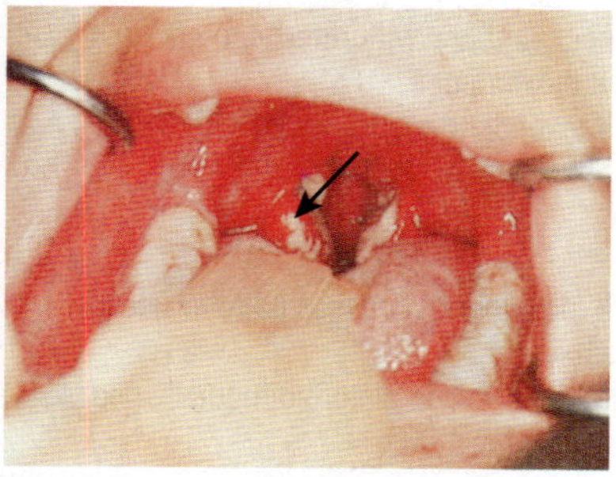

FIG. 13.40 **Tonsillitis and pharyngitis.** Notice the erythema and exudate in crypts of the tonsils. Close-up view of mouth, held by mouth retractor, shows hard, white growths, indicated by an arrow, in the deep oral cavity. (Courtesy Edward L. Applebaum, MD, Head, Department of Otolaryngology, University of Illinois Medical Center, Chicago.)

PATIENT DATA

Subjective Data

- Sore throat, may be referred to pain in ears, dysphagia
- Fever and malaise
- Fetid breath
- May have associated abdominal pain, scarlatiniform rash, and headache

Objective Data

- Red and swollen tonsils
- Crypts filled with purulent exudate (Fig. 13.40)
- Enlarged anterior cervical lymph nodes
- Palatal petechiae

PERITONSILLAR ABSCESS

Deep infection in the space between the palatine tonsil capsule and pharyngeal muscles.

PATHOPHYSIOLOGY

- Thought to develop as a complication of adenotonsillitis or from blockage of the Weber glands, the salivary glands in the space superior to the tonsil in the soft palate
- Peak incidence is in adolescence, with an average age of 13.6 years (Bochner et al., 2017)
- Contributing factors include age (teens to age 40), smoking, periodontal disease, and immunocompromised status (Powell et al., 2013)
- Typically polymicrobial, most commonly including group A beta-hemolytic streptococci and fusobacterium species

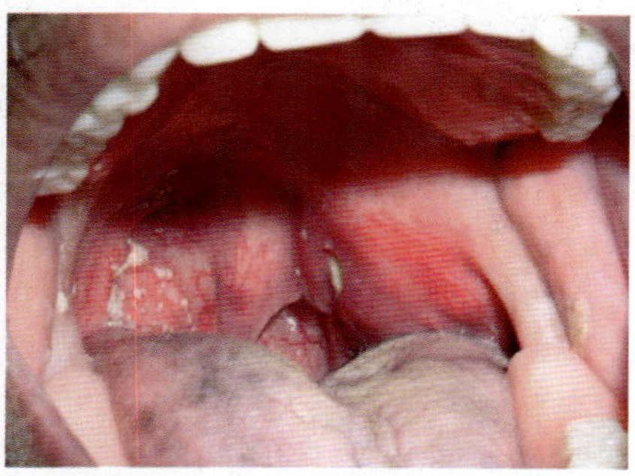

FIG. 13.41 **Swelling of peritonsillar abscess.** Inside view of mouth shows swollen tissue displacing the uvula. The dorsal surface of the tongue has grayish, yellow patches. (From Linkov, G., & Soliman, A. M. (2015). Infections and edema. *Anesthes Clin*, *33*(2), 329–346.)

PATIENT DATA

Subjective Data

- Dysphagia, odynophagia, and drooling
- Severe sore throat with pain radiating to the ear; pain is worse on one side
- Malaise and fever

Objective Data

- Unilateral red and swollen tonsil and adjacent soft palate
- Tonsil may be pushed forward or backward; may displace the uvula to the contralateral side (Fig. 13.41)
- Trismus (spasm of masticator muscles)
- Muffled voice
- Fetid breath
- Cervical and/or submandibular lymphadenopathy

RETROPHARYNGEAL ABSCESS

Life-threatening deep neck space infection that may occlude the airway; occurs in the potential space extending from the base of the skull to the posterior mediastinum between the posterior pharyngeal wall and prevertebral fascia.

PATHOPHYSIOLOGY

- Infection of retropharyngeal space occurs through spread of nasopharyngeal infection or direct inoculation from penetrating trauma
- Most often occurs in pediatric patient after an upper respiratory tract infection with spread to lymph nodes in retropharyngeal space
- Highest incidence is among children under 5 years of age; occurs more frequently in young males (Bochner et al., 2017)
- Predisposing infections include pharyngitis, tonsillitis, sinusitis, and dental infection
- Typically polymicrobial with group A streptococci, *Staphylococcus aureus,* and respiratory anaerobes as common causative organisms

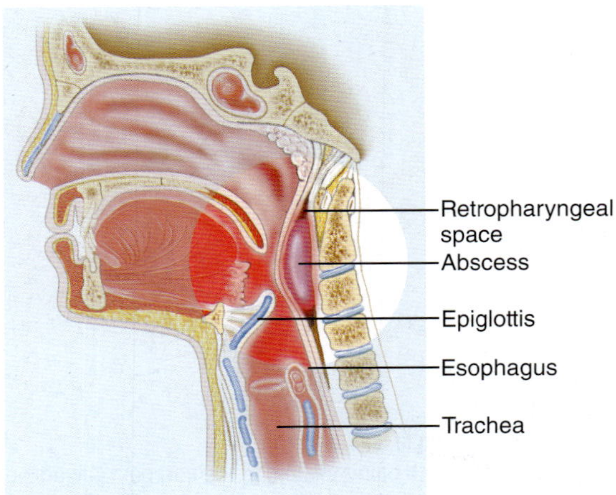

FIG. 13.42 Retropharyngeal abscess. Note the reduced airway size next to the epiglottis. Side view of the face and neck shows labels for retropharyngeal space, abscess, epiglottis, esophagus, and trachea.

PATIENT DATA

Subjective Data

- Recent upper respiratory infection
- Acutely ill, fever
- Drooling
- Anorexia
- Irritable and anxious
- Pain in the neck and jaw with referral to ear
- Limited neck movement
- Chest pain if extends to mediastinum

Objective Data

- Fever
- Lateral neck movement increases pain; torticollis
- Restlessness
- Lateral pharyngeal wall is distorted medially (Fig. 13.42)
- Trismus
- Respiratory distress
- Muffled voice

ORAL CANCER

Cancer involving the oral cavity or related structures.

PATHOPHYSIOLOGY

- Most often, squamous cell carcinoma that originates in the basal cell layer of the oral mucosa
- May occur as a primary lesion, metastasis from a distant site to the jaw or related structure, or extension from a nearby structure (nasal cavity)
- High association with human papillomavirus (HPV): 56% of oropharyngeal squamous cell carcinomas in North America are HPV positive (Marur & Forastiere, 2016)
- Other major risk factors include tobacco use and excessive alcohol use

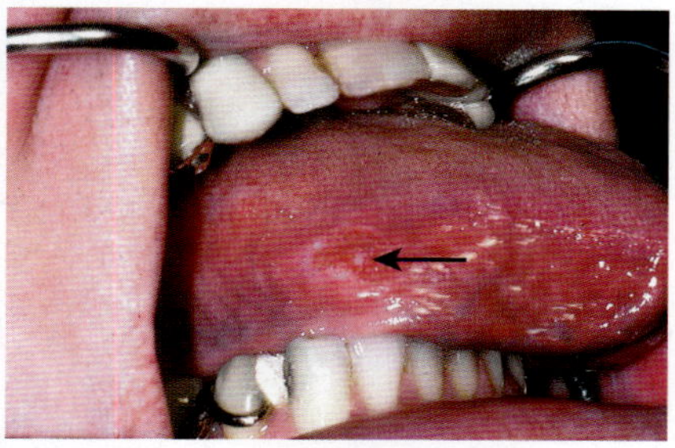

FIG. 13.43 **Squamous cell cancer on the tongue.** Close-up view of mouth, held by mouth retractor, shows protruding tongue and redness along with abnormal growth of cells on the side of tongue, indicated by an arrow. (Courtesy Daniel M. Laskin, DDS, MS, Medical College of Virginia, Virginia Commonwealth University, Richmond, VA.)

PATIENT DATA

Subjective Data

- Painless sore in mouth that does not heal
- Pain with later-stage lesions
- Identified by visit to health care clinician or dentist

Objective Data

- Ulcerative lesion (red or white) appearing as piled-up edges around a core on the lateral border or floor of the mouth (Fig. 13.43)
- Red or white patch on the gums, tongue, tonsil, hard or soft palate, or buccal mucosa
- Firm, nonmobile mass
- Tooth mobility when no periodontal disease is present
- Cervical lymphadenopathy

PERIODONTAL DISEASE (PERIODONTITIS)

Chronic infection of the gums, bones, and other tissues that surround and support the teeth.

PATHOPHYSIOLOGY

- Often results from poor dental hygiene (calculus and hard plaque not removed below the gum line) leading to chronic inflammation and infection of the gingiva and periodontal tissue; underlying bone is reabsorbed and teeth loosen

PATIENT DATA

Subjective Data

- Red and swollen gums that bleed easily with brushing (see Fig. 13.28)
- Tender gums and loose teeth
- Teeth sensitive to temperature or hurt when eating

Objective Data

- Plaque and tartar buildup on teeth; teeth appear long
- Deep pockets between the teeth and gingiva
- Loose or missing teeth
- Halitosis

OROPHARYNGEAL CLEFTS (CLEFT LIP, CLEFT PALATE, CLEFT LIP AND PALATE)

Most common craniofacial congenital malformation.

PATHOPHYSIOLOGY

- Result of the lip or palate failing to fuse during embryonic development before the 12th week of gestation
- Incidence of cleft lip and palate about 1 per 1000 live births; 70% are isolated anomalies (Tan et al., 2016)
- Thought to be caused by interactions between genetic and environmental factors; also occurs in genetic syndromes, fetal exposure to teratogens (e.g., anticonvulsants, alcohol) and conditions present in the mother (e.g., diabetes, folate deficiency, and maternal smoking)

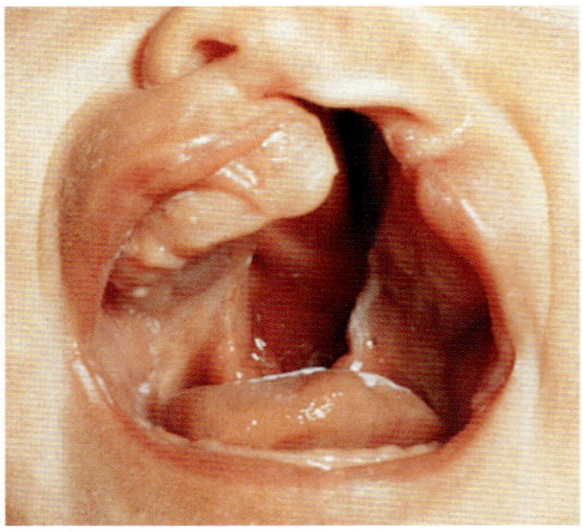

FIG. 13.44 Unilateral cleft lip and palate. Close-up view of mouth shows slit in the palate extending to upper lip and nose. (From Zitelli, B. J., & Davis, H. W. (1997). *Atlas of pediatric physical diagnosis* (3rd ed.). St. Louis: Mosby.)

PATIENT DATA

Subjective Data

- Often diagnosed on prenatal ultrasound
- Difficulty sucking
- Failure to gain weight

Objective Data

- Apparent at birth
- Cleft may be unilateral or bilateral; may involve the lip, hard palate, or soft palate or all three; a partial cleft in any of these tissues may be seen (Fig. 13.44)

CHAPTER

14

Chest and Lungs

The chest and lungs allow for respiration. The purpose of respiration is to keep the body adequately supplied with oxygen and protected from excess accumulation of carbon dioxide. Respiration involves the movement of air back and forth from the alveoli to the outside environment, gas exchange across the alveolar-pulmonary capillary membranes, and circulatory system transport of oxygen to, and carbon dioxide from, the peripheral tissues. This chapter focuses on the examination of the chest and lungs.

Physical Examination Components

1. Inspect the chest—front and back and sides—noting thoracic landmarks for:
   - Size and shape (anteroposterior diameter compared with the lateral diameter)
   - Symmetry
   - Color
   - Superficial venous patterns
   - Prominence of ribs
2. Evaluate respirations for:
   - Rate
   - Rhythm or pattern
3. Inspect chest movement with breathing for symmetry and use of accessory muscles.
4. Note any audible sounds with respiration (e.g., stridor or wheezes).
5. Palpate the chest for:
   - Thoracic expansion
   - Sensations such as crepitus, grating vibrations
   - Tactile fremitus
6. Perform direct or indirect percussion on the chest, comparing sides for:
   - Diaphragmatic excursion
   - Percussion tone intensity, pitch, duration, and quality
7. Auscultate the chest with the stethoscope diaphragm, from apex to base, comparing sides for:
   - Intensity, pitch, duration, and quality of breath sounds
   - Unexpected breath sounds (crackles, rhonchi, wheezes, friction rubs)
   - Vocal resonance

ANATOMY AND PHYSIOLOGY

The chest, or thorax, is a cavitary structure of bone, cartilage, and muscle capable of movement as the lungs expand. It consists anteriorly of the sternum, manubrium, xiphoid process, and costal cartilages; laterally, of the 12 pairs of ribs; and posteriorly, of the 12 thoracic vertebrae (Figs. 14.1 and 14.2). All the ribs are connected to the thoracic vertebrae; the upper 7 are attached anteriorly to the sternum by the costal cartilages, and ribs 8, 9, and 10 join with the costal cartilages just above them. Ribs 11 and 12, sometimes referred to as *floating ribs*, attach posteriorly but not anteriorly. The lateral diameter of the chest generally exceeds the anteroposterior (AP) diameter in adults.

The primary muscles of respiration are the diaphragm and the intercostal muscles. The diaphragm is the dominant muscle. It contracts and moves downward during inspiration, lowering the abdominal contents to increase the intrathoracic space. The external intercostal muscles increase the AP chest diameter during inspiration, and the internal intercostal muscles decrease the lateral diameter during forceful expiration. The sternocleidomastoid, scalene, and trapezius muscles may also contribute to respiratory movements. These "accessory" muscles are used during exercise or when there is pulmonary compromise (Fig. 14.3).

The interior of the chest is divided into three major spaces: the right and left pleural cavities and the mediastinum. The mediastinum, situated between the lungs, contains the heart and major blood vessels. The pleural cavities are lined with serous membranes (parietal and visceral pleurae) that surround the lungs. A tiny space between the parietal and visceral pleura is lined by a small amount of fluid to allow easy lung sliding. The spongy and highly elastic lungs are paired, but not symmetric, with the right having three lobes and the left having two (Fig. 14.4). The left upper lobe has an inferior tonguelike projection, the lingula, which is a counterpart of the right middle lobe. Each lung has a major fissure, known as the *oblique fissure*, that divides the upper and lower portions. In addition, a lesser horizontal fissure divides the upper portion of the right lung into the upper and middle lobes at the level of the fifth rib in the axilla and the fourth rib anteriorly. Each lobe consists of blood vessels, lymphatics, nerves, and an alveolar duct connecting with the alveoli; there can be as many as 300 million in an adult. The entire lung is shaped by an elastic subpleural tissue that limits its expansion. Each lung apex is rounded and extends anteriorly about 4 cm above the first rib into the base of the neck in adults. Posteriorly, the apices of the lungs

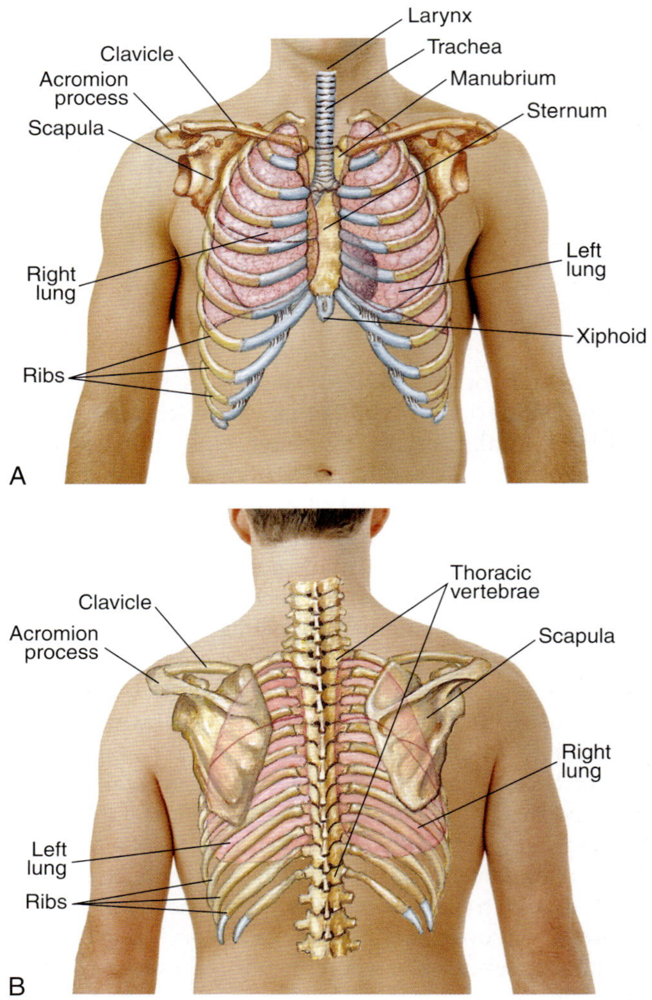

FIG. 14.1 **The bony structures of the chest form a protective expandable cage around the lungs and heart.** (A) Anterior view. (B) Posterior view. (From Thompson, J. M., & Wilson, S. F. (1996). *Health assessment for nursing practice*. St. Louis. Mosby.)

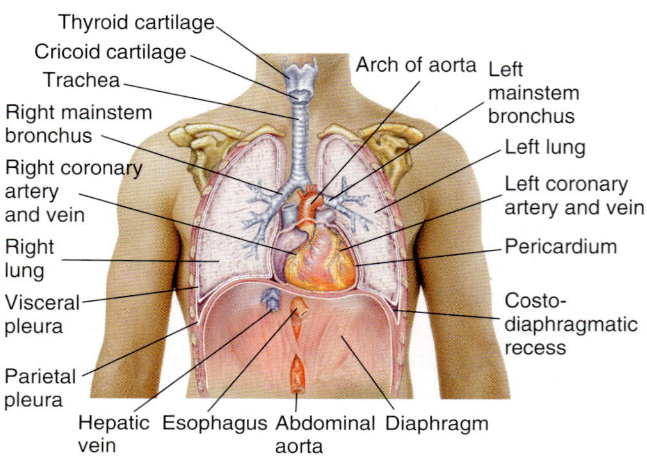

FIG. 14.2 **Chest cavity and related anatomic structures.**

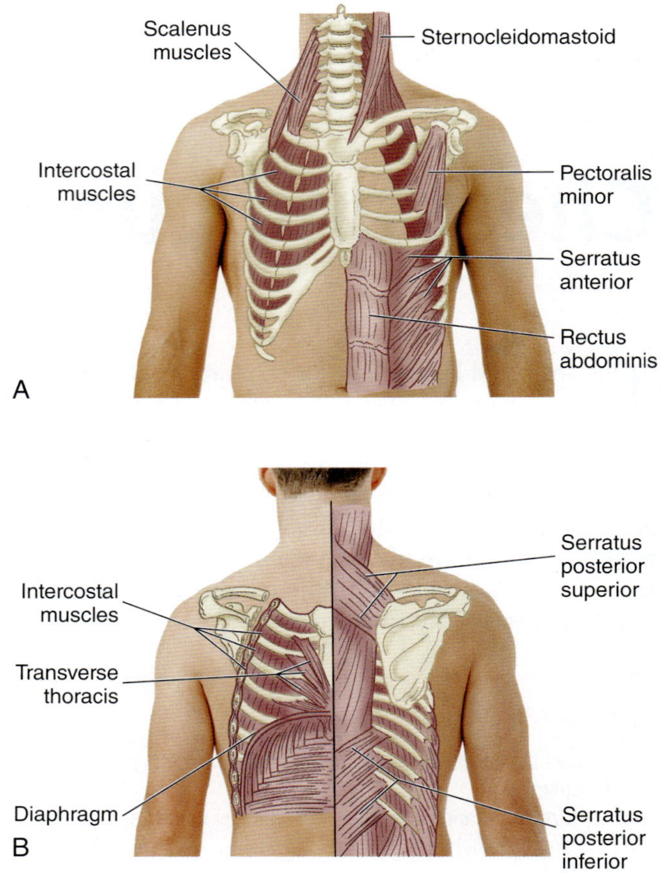

FIG. 14.3 **Muscles of ventilation.** (A) Anterior view. (B) Posterior view.

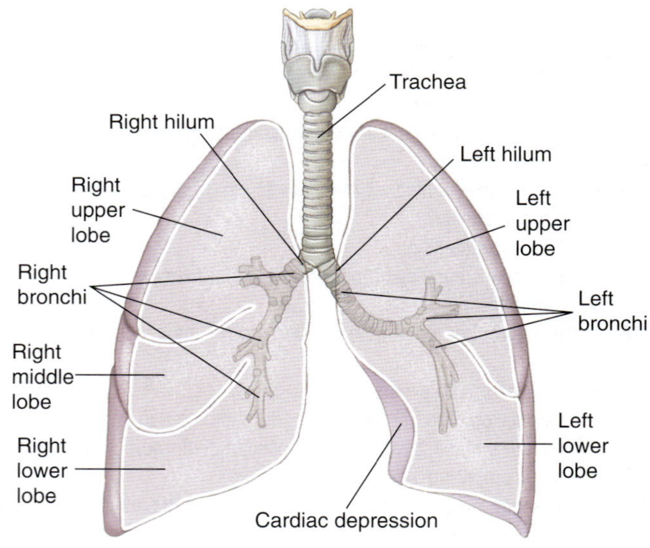

FIG. 14.4 **The lobes of the lungs.**

rise to about the level of T1. The lower borders descend on deep inspiration to about T12 and rise on forced expiration to about T9. The base of each lung is broad and concave, resting on the convex surface of the diaphragm. The medial surfaces of the lung are to some extent concave, providing a cradle for the heart.

The tracheobronchial tree is a tubular system that provides a pathway along which air is filtered, humidified, and warmed as it moves from the upper airway to the alveoli. The trachea is 10 to 11 cm long and about 2 cm in diameter. It lies anterior to the esophagus and posterior to the isthmus of the thyroid. The trachea divides into the right and left main bronchi at about the level of T4 or T5 and just below the manubriosternal joint (Box 14.1), which is called the *sternal angle* or *angle of Louis*.

The right bronchus is wider, shorter, and more vertically placed than the left bronchus (and therefore more susceptible to aspiration of foreign bodies). The main bronchi are divided into three branches on the right and two on the left, each branch supplying one lobe of the lungs. The branches then begin to subdivide into terminal bronchioles and ultimately into respiratory bronchioles.

The bronchial arteries branch from the anterior thoracic aorta and the intercostal arteries, supplying blood to the lung tissue. The bronchial vein is formed at the hilum of the lung, but most of the blood supplied by the bronchial arteries is returned by the pulmonary veins (Fig. 14.5).

BOX 14.1 Visualizing the Lungs From the Surface

Anteriorly

The right lung may ride higher because of the fullness of the dome of the liver. Except for an inferior lateral triangle, the anterior view on the right is primarily the upper and middle lobes, separated by the horizontal fissure at about the fifth rib in the midaxilla to about the fourth at the sternum; on the left as on the right, the lower lobe is set off by a diagonal fissure stretching from the fifth rib at the axilla to the sixth at the midclavicular line.

Posteriorly

Except for the apices, the posterior view is primarily the lower lobe, which extends from about T3 to T10 or T12 during the respiratory cycle.

Right Lateral

The lung underlies the area extending from the peak of the axilla to the seventh or eighth rib. The upper lobe is demarcated at about the level of the fifth rib in the midaxillary line and the sixth rib more anteriorly.

Left Lateral

The lung underlies the area extending from the peak of the axilla to the seventh or eighth rib. The entire expanse is virtually bisected by the oblique fissure from about the level of the third rib medially to the sixth rib anteriorly.

Anatomic Landmarks

The following topographic markers on the chest are used to describe findings (Fig. 14.6):

1. The nipples.
2. The manubriosternal junction (angle of Louis). A visible and palpable angulation of the sternum and the point at which the second rib articulates with the sternum. One can count the ribs and intercostal spaces from this point. The number of each intercostal space corresponds to that of the rib immediately above it.
3. The suprasternal notch. A depression, easily palpable and most often visible at the base of the ventral aspect of the neck, just superior to the manubriosternal junction.
4. Costal angle. The angle formed by the costal margins at the sternum. It is usually no more than 90 degrees, with the ribs inserted at approximately 45-degree angles.
5. Vertebra prominens. The spinous process of C7. It can be more readily seen and felt with the patient's head bent forward. If two prominences are felt, the upper is that of the spinous process of C7 and the lower is that of T1. It is difficult to use this as a guide to counting ribs posteriorly because the spinous processes from T4 down project obliquely, thus overlying the rib below the number of its vertebra.
6. The clavicles.

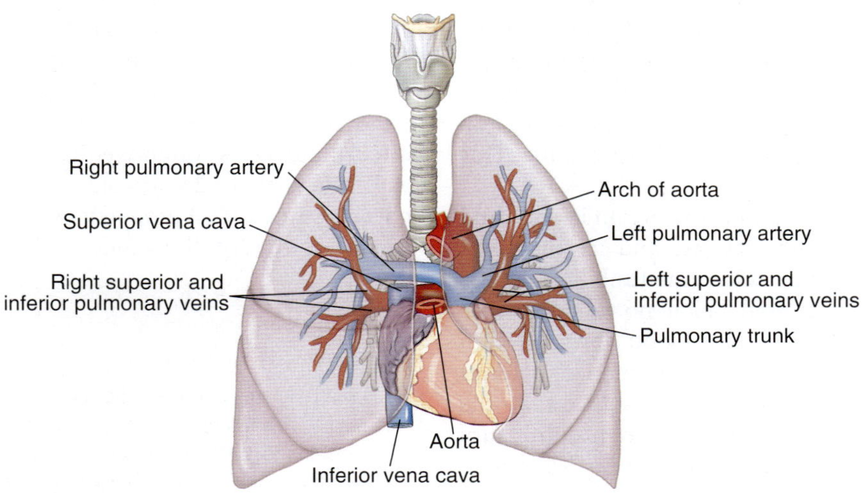

FIG. 14.5 Pulmonary circulation (with ascending aorta removed).

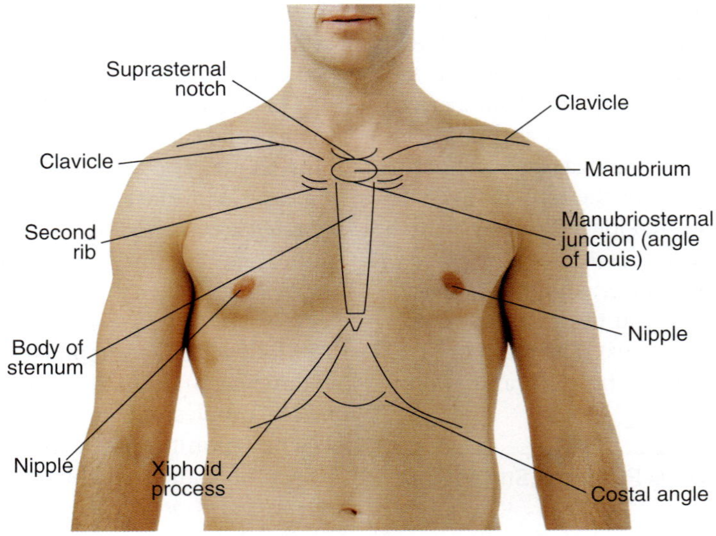

FIG. 14.6 **Topographic landmarks of the chest.**

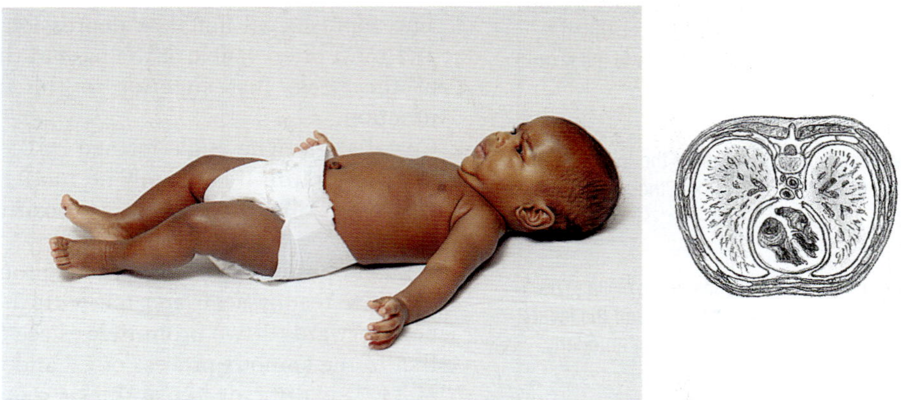

FIG. 14.7 **Chest of healthy infant.** Note that the anteroposterior diameter is approximately the same as the lateral diameter.

Infants and Children

Before birth the lungs contain no air, and the alveoli are collapsed. Fetal gas exchange is mediated by the placenta. Relatively passive respiratory movements occur throughout gestation; they do not open the alveoli or expand the lungs. The lungs are not fully grown at birth. The number of alveoli increases at a rapid rate in the first 2 years of life. This slows down by age 8 years.

At birth, the change in respiratory function is rapid and dramatic. After the infant's initial gasp and cry, the lungs fill with air for the first time. When the umbilical cord is cut shortly thereafter, maternal blood no longer comes through the placenta. At this point blood flows through the infant lungs more vigorously. The pulmonary arteries expand and relax, offering much less resistance than the systemic circulation. This relative decrease in pulmonary pressure most often leads to closure of the heart's foramen ovale within minutes after birth, and the increased oxygen tension in the arterial blood usually stimulates contraction and closure of the ductus arteriosus (see Clinical Pearl, "Patent Ductus Arteriosus"). The pulmonary and systemic circulations adopt their mature configurations, and the lungs are fully integrated for postnatal function.

The chest of the newborn is generally round, with the AP diameter approximating the lateral diameter, and the circumference is roughly equal to that of the head until the child is about 2 years old (Fig. 14.7). With growth, the chest assumes adult proportions, with the lateral diameter exceeding the AP diameter.

CLINICAL PEARL

Patent Ductus Arteriosus

The heart's foramen ovale and the ductus arteriosus do not always close so readily. This failure to close is more common in premature infants born before 30 weeks of gestation. A large patent ductus arteriosus, sometimes appreciated as a "machinelike" continuous murmur on auscultation, can lead to left ventricular overload and heart failure.

The relatively thin chest wall of the infant and young child makes the bony structure more prominent than in the adult. It is more cartilaginous and yielding, and the xiphoid process is often more prominent and more movable.

Pregnant Patients

Mechanical and biochemical factors, including the enlarged uterus and an increased level of circulating progesterone, interact to create changes in the respiratory function of the pregnant patient. Anatomic changes that occur in the chest as the lower ribs flare include an increase in the lateral diameter of about 2 cm and an increase in the circumference of 5 to 7 cm. The costal angle progressively increases from about 68.5 degrees to approximately 103.5 degrees in later months of pregnancy. The diaphragm at rest rises as much as 4 cm above its usual resting position, yet diaphragmatic movement increases so that the major work of breathing is done by the diaphragm. Minute ventilation increases because of increased tidal volume, although the respiratory rate remains relatively unchanged.

Older Adults

The barrel chest that is seen in many older adults results from loss of muscle strength in the thorax and diaphragm (see Fig. 14.9), coupled with the loss of lung elasticity. In addition, skeletal changes of aging tend to emphasize the dorsal curve of the thoracic spine, resulting in an increased AP chest wall diameter, leading to a restrictive pattern of lung function. There may also be stiffening and decreased expansion of the chest wall.

With aging, the alveoli become less elastic and relatively more fibrous. The associated loss of some of the interalveolar folds decreases the alveolar surface available for gas exchange. This and the loss of strength in the muscles of respiration result in underventilation of the alveoli in the lower lung fields and a decreased tolerance for exertion. The net result of these changes is a decrease in vital capacity and an increase in residual volume.

Aging mucous membranes tend to become drier, and older adults are less able to clear mucus. Retained mucus encourages bacterial growth and predisposes the older adult to respiratory infection.

REVIEW OF RELATED HISTORY

For each of the symptoms or conditions discussed in this section, targeted topics to include in the history of the present illness are listed. Responses to questions about these topics provide clues for focusing the physical examination and the development of an appropriate diagnostic evaluation. Questions regarding medication use, prescription and over-the-counter preparations, and complementary, alternative, and integrative therapies are relevant for each.

History of Present Illness

Cough

- Onset: sudden, gradual
- Duration
- Nature of cough: dry, moist, wet, hacking, hoarse, barking, whooping, bubbling, productive, nonproductive
- Sputum production: duration, frequency, with activity, at certain times of day
- Sputum characteristics: amount, color (clear, purulent, blood tinged, mostly blood), foul odor
- Pattern: occasional, regular, paroxysmal; related to time of day, weather, activities (e.g., exercise), talking, deep breaths; change over time
- Severity: tires patient, disrupts sleep or conversation, causes chest pain
- Associated symptoms: shortness of breath, chest pain or tightness with breathing, fever, nasal congestion, noisy respirations, hoarseness, gagging
- Efforts to treat: prescription or nonprescription drugs, vaporizers, lozenges, dry candy, frequent sips of water

Mechanism of Cough

Coughs are a common symptom of a respiratory problem. They are usually preceded by a deep inspiration. This is followed by closure of the glottis and contraction of the chest, abdominal, and even the pelvic muscles, and then a sudden, spasmodic expiration, forcing a sudden opening of the glottis. Air and secretions are exhaled. The causes may be related to localized or more general insults at any point in the respiratory tract. Coughs may be voluntary, but they are usually reflexive responses to an irritant such as a foreign body (microscopic or larger), an inflammatory process like asthma, an infectious agent, an underlying problem in the lung parenchyma such as pulmonary fibrosis, or a mass of any sort compressing the respiratory tree. A habit cough can develop after an upper respiratory infection in children and adolescents. They may also be a clue to an anxiety state.

Describe a cough according to its moisture, frequency, regularity, pitch and loudness, quality, and circumstances. The type of cough may offer some clue to the cause. Although a cough may not have a serious cause, do not ignore it.

Dry or Moist. A moist or productive cough may be caused by viral or bacterial infection and can be accompanied by sputum production. A dry or nonproductive cough can have a variety of causes (e.g., cardiac problems, allergies, gastroesophageal reflux with pharyngeal irritation).

Onset. An acute onset, particularly with fever, suggests infection; in the absence of fever, a foreign body or inhaled irritants can be additional possible causes.

Frequency of Occurrence. Note whether the cough is seldom or often present. An infrequent cough may result from allergens or environmental insults.

Regularity. A regular, paroxysmal cough is heard in pertussis. An irregularly occurring cough may have a variety of causes such as smoking, early congestive heart failure, an inspired foreign body or irritant, or a tumor within or compressing the bronchial tree.

Pitch and Loudness. A cough may be loud and high pitched or quiet and relatively low pitched.

Postural Influences. A cough may occur soon after a person has reclined or assumed an erect position (e.g., with a nasal drip or pooling of secretions in the upper airway).

Quality. A dry cough may sound loud and harsh if it is caused by compression of the respiratory tree (as by a tumor) or hoarse if it is caused by croup. Pertussis produces an inspiratory whoop at the end of a paroxysm of coughing in older children and adults.

Sputum

The production of sputum is generally associated with cough. Sputum in more than small amounts and with any degree of consistency always suggests the presence of disease. When the onset is acute, infection is the most probable cause. A chronic cough can indicate a significant anatomic change (e.g., tumor, cavitation, or bronchiectasis). The Differential Diagnosis table delineates possible pathologic conditions and their accompanying sputum findings.

DIFFERENTIAL DIAGNOSIS

Some Causes of Sputum

CAUSE	POSSIBLE SPUTUM CHARACTERISTICS
Bacterial infection	Yellow, green, rust (blood mixed with yellow sputum), clear, or transparent; purulent; blood streaked; sticky
Viral infection	Blood-streaked (not common)
Chronic infectious disease	All of the above; particularly abundant in the early morning; slight, intermittent blood streaking; occasionally, large amounts of blood[a]
Cancer	Slight, persistent, intermittent blood streaking
Infarction	Blood clotted; large amounts of blood
Tuberculous cavity	Occasional large amounts of blood[a]

[a]Ascertain that the blood is not swallowed from a nosebleed or caused by gastric bleeding.

Shortness of Breath (Box 14.2)

- Onset: sudden or gradual; duration; gagging or choking event before onset
- Pattern
- Position most comfortable, number of pillows used to sleep comfortably

BOX 14.2 Descriptors of Respiration

Dyspnea, or difficult and labored breathing with shortness of breath, is commonly observed with pulmonary or cardiac compromise. A sedentary lifestyle and obesity can cause it in an otherwise well person. In general, dyspnea increases with the severity of the underlying condition. It is important to establish the amount and kind of effort that produces dyspnea:

- Is it present even when the patient is resting?
- How much walking? On a level surface? Upstairs?
- Is it necessary to stop and rest when climbing stairs?
- With what other activities of daily life does dyspnea begin? With what level of physical demand?

Other manifestations of respiratory difficulty include the following:

Orthopnea—shortness of breath that begins or increases when the patient lies down; ask whether the patient needs to sleep on more than one pillow and whether that helps.

Paroxysmal nocturnal dyspnea—a sudden onset of shortness of breath after a period of sleep; sitting upright is helpful.

Platypnea—dyspnea increases in the upright posture.

- Related to extent of exercise, certain activities, time of day, eating, environmental exposure
- Harder to inhale or exhale
- Severity: extent of activity limitation, fatigue with breathing, anxiety about getting air
- Associated symptoms: pain or discomfort (relationship to specific point in respiratory exertion, location), cough, diaphoresis, ankle edema
- Efforts to treat: oxygen use

Chest Pain (see Clinical Pearl, "Chest Pain")

- Onset and duration; associated with trauma, coughing, lower respiratory infection, recent anesthesia or surgery, history of thrombosis, prolonged immobilization increasing risk for pulmonary embolism
- Associated symptoms: shallow breathing, fever, coughing, anxiety about getting air, radiation of pain to neck or arms
- Efforts to treat: heat, splinting, pain medication
- Other medications: illicit drug use (e.g., cocaine)

CLINICAL PEARL

Chest Pain

Chest pain does not generally originate in the heart when:

- There is a constant achiness that lasts all day.
- It does not radiate.
- It is made worse by pressing on the chest wall.
- It is a fleeting, needlelike jab that lasts only a few seconds.
- It is situated in the shoulders or between the shoulder blades in the back.

Think of the heart but, importantly in such circumstances, also think of other possibilities in the chest (e.g., pulmonary embolism, pleurisy, aortic dissection, tumor).

Past Medical History

- Thoracic, nasal, and/or pharyngotracheal trauma or surgery, hospitalizations for pulmonary disorders, dates
- Use of oxygen or ventilation-assisting devices including continuous or bilevel positive airway pressure machines (CPAP or BiPAP, respectively)
- Chronic pulmonary diseases: tuberculosis (date, treatment, compliance), bronchitis, emphysema, bronchiectasis, asthma, cystic fibrosis
- Other chronic disorders: cardiac, cancer, blood clotting disorders
- Testing: allergy, pulmonary function tests, interferon gamma release assay (IGRA), tuberculin skin tests, chest imaging
- Immunization against *Streptococcus pneumoniae,* Tdap, influenza, SARS-CoV-2, respiratory syncytial virus (RSV)

Family History

- Tuberculosis
- Cystic fibrosis
- Emphysema
- Allergy, asthma, atopic dermatitis
- Malignancy
- Bronchiectasis
- Bronchitis
- Clotting disorders (risk of pulmonary embolism)
- Pneumothorax

Personal and Social History

- Employment: nature of work, extent of physical and emotional effort and stress, crowded work conditions, environmental hazards, exposure to chemicals, animals, vapors, dust, pulmonary irritants (e.g., asbestos), allergens, use of protective masks
- Home environment: location, possible allergens, type of heating, use of air conditioning, humidifier, ventilation, exposure to secondhand tobacco smoke, use of smoke and carbon monoxide detectors in the home
- Tobacco use: type of tobacco (cigarettes, e-cigarettes, cigars, pipe, smokeless), duration and amount (Pack-years = Number of years of smoking × Number of packs smoked per day), age started, efforts to quit smoking with factors influencing success or failure, the extent of smoking by others at home or at work (secondhand smoking)
- Exposure to respiratory infections, influenza, tuberculosis, pertussis, SARS-CoV-2, RSV
- Nutritional status: weight loss or obesity
- Use of complementary and alternative therapies
- Exercise tolerance: amount of exercise, diminished ability to perform up to expectations
- Regional or travel exposures (e.g., tuberculosis infection in India, China, Indonesia, South Africa, and Nigeria; histoplasmosis in southeastern and midwestern United States; coccidioidomycosis [valley fever] in southwestern United States, Mexico, Central and South America; schistosomiasis in east and southwest Asia, Africa, and the Caribbean)
- Hobbies: owning birds or other animals, woodworking or welding
- Alcohol or substance use (e.g., cocaine, inhaled methamphetamine); see Clinical Pearl, "Pain From Cocaine"

CLINICAL PEARL

Pain From Cocaine

If an adolescent or adult describes severe, acute chest pain, ask about substance use, particularly cocaine. Cocaine can cause tachycardia, hypertension, coronary arterial spasm (with infarction), and pneumothorax (lung collapse), with severe acute chest pain being the common result.

Infants and Children

- Low birth weight, prematurity and gestational age at birth, use of antenatal steroids for lung maturation, history of intubation, duration of ventilation assistance, respiratory distress syndrome, bronchopulmonary dysplasia (chronic lung disease), transient tachypnea of the newborn
- Coughing or sudden onset of difficulty breathing, possible aspiration of small object, toy, or food
- Possible ingestion of kerosene, antifreeze, or hydrocarbons in household cleaners
- Apneic episodes: associated perioral cyanosis, breath holding, posttussive emesis, history of sudden infant death in sibling
- Swallowing dysfunction or other neuromuscular disorders, recurrent spitting up and gagging, recurrent pneumonia (possible gastroesophageal reflux)
- Immunization status—especially pneumococcal and influenza vaccines

Pregnant Patients

- Weeks of gestation or estimated date of delivery
- Presence of multiple fetuses, polyhydramnios, or other conditions in which a larger uterus displaces the diaphragm farther upward
- Exercise type and energy expenditure
- Exposure to and frequency of respiratory infections, status of influenza immunization

Older Adults

- Exposure to and frequency of respiratory infections, status of pneumococcal, influenza, and pertussis vaccines
- Need for supplemental oxygen
- Effects of weather on respiratory efforts and occurrence of infections

- Immobilization or marked sedentary habits
- Difficulty swallowing or choking/coughing episodes when eating
- Alteration in daily living habits or activities as a result of respiratory symptoms
- Because older adults are at risk for chronic respiratory diseases (lung cancer, chronic bronchitis, emphysema, and tuberculosis), reemphasize the following:
    - Smoking history
    - Cough, dyspnea on exertion, or breathlessness
    - Blood-tinged or yellowish/greenish sputum
    - Fatigue
    - Significant weight changes
    - Fever, night sweats

EXAMINATION AND FINDINGS

Equipment

- Marking pen
- Centimeter ruler and tape measure
- Stethoscope with bell and diaphragm (for infants, you need a smaller stethoscope)
- Drapes

Inspection

Have the patient sit upright, if possible without support, unclothed to the waist. Clothing of any kind is a barrier for inspection, palpation, percussion, and auscultation. A drape should cover the patient when full exposure is not necessary. The room and stethoscope should be comfortably warm, and a bright tangential light is needed to highlight chest movement. Position the patient so that the light source comes at different angles to accentuate findings that are more subtle and otherwise difficult to detect, such as retractions, or the presence of deformity (e.g., pectus excavatum). If the patient is in bed and mobility is limited, you should have access to both sides of the bed. After informing the patient, do not hesitate to raise and lower the bed as needed.

Note the shape and symmetry of the chest from both the back and the front, the costal angle, the angle of the ribs, and the intercostal spaces. The bony framework is obvious, the clavicles are prominent superiorly, and the sternum is usually rather flat and free of an abundance of overlying tissue. Box 14.3 lists thoracic landmarks to use as you record findings. The chest will not be absolutely symmetric, but one side can be used as a comparison for the other. The AP diameter of the chest is ordinarily less than the lateral diameter (Fig. 14.8). The relationship is expressed as the thoracic ratio and is expected to be about 0.70 to 0.75. It does increase with age; however, when the AP diameter approaches or equals the lateral diameter (a ratio of 1.0 or even greater), most often, a chronic condition is present. Barrel chest (Fig. 14.9) results from compromised respiration as in, for example, chronic asthma, emphysema, or

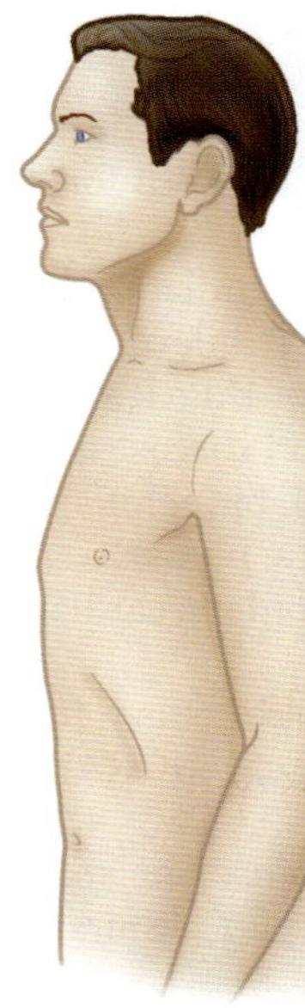

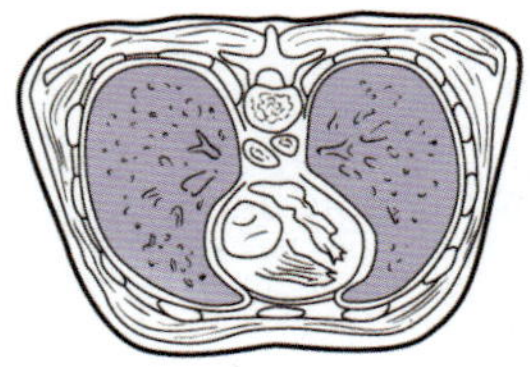

FIG. 14.8 Thorax of healthy adult male with anteroposterior diameter less than lateral diameter.

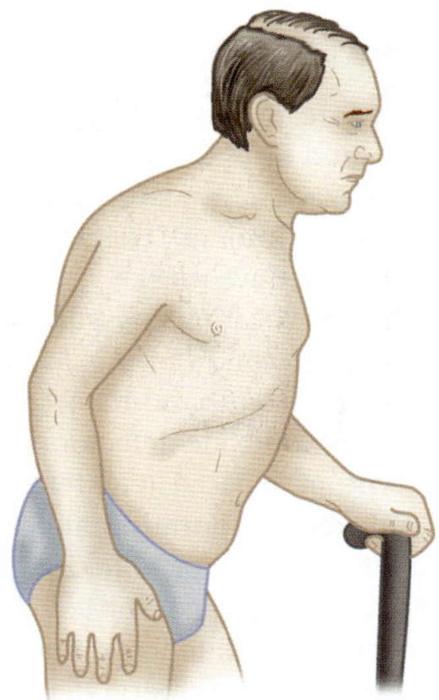

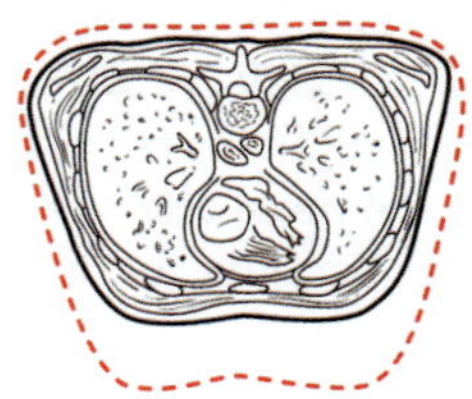

FIG. 14.9 Barrel chest with increased anteroposterior diameter.

BOX 14.3 Thoracic Landmarks

In conjunction with the anatomic landmarks of the chest, the following imaginary lines on the surface will help localize the findings on physical examination (Fig. 14.10):

Midsternal line: vertically down the midline of the sternum

Right and left midclavicular lines: parallel to the midsternal line, beginning at midclavicle; the inferior borders of the lungs generally cross the sixth rib at the midclavicular line

Right and left anterior axillary lines: parallel to the midsternal line, beginning at the anterior axillary folds

Right and left midaxillary lines: parallel to the midsternal line, beginning at the midaxilla

Right and left posterior axillary lines: parallel to the midsternal line, beginning at the posterior axillary folds

Vertebral line: vertically down the spinal processes

Right and left scapular lines: parallel to the vertebral line, through the inferior angle of the scapula when the patient is erect

The spinous process of the seventh cervical vertebra is readily palpated. The thoracic vertebrae can then be counted down from that point (Fig. 14.11).

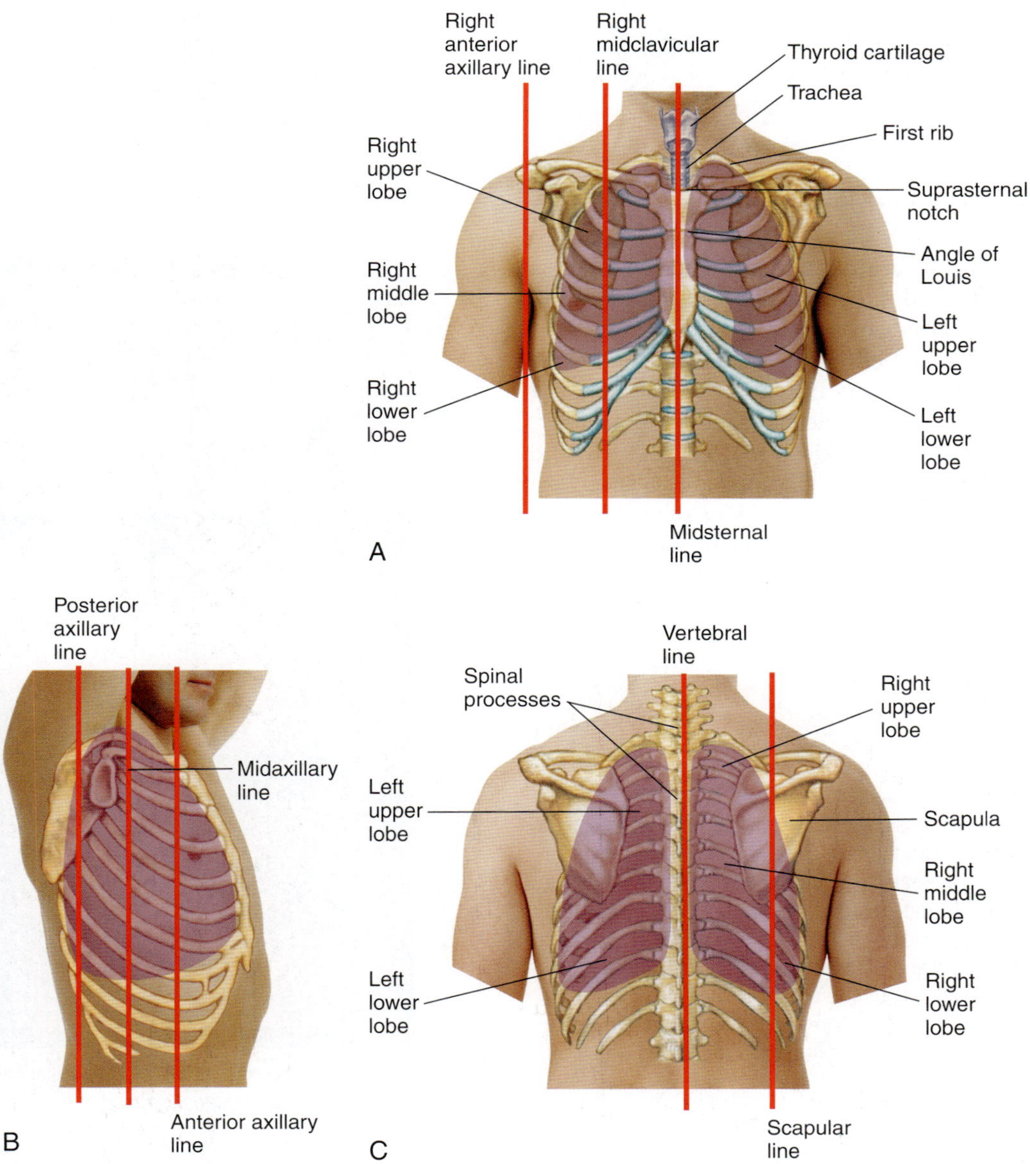

FIG. 14.10 Thoracic landmarks. (A) Anterior thorax. (B) Right lateral thorax. (C) Posterior thorax.

Continued

BOX 14.3 Thoracic Landmarks—cont'd

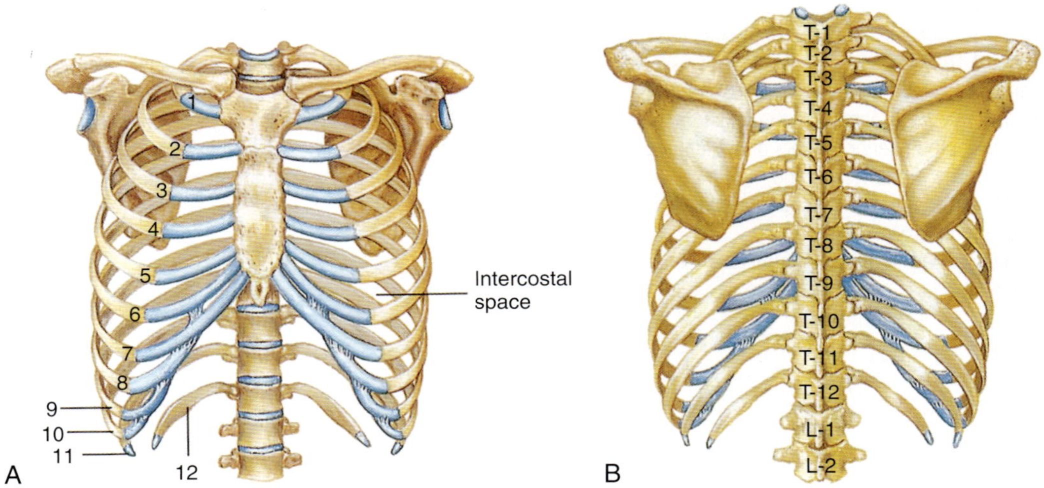

FIG. 14.11 Rib cage. (A) Anterior view. (B) Posterior view.

cystic fibrosis. The ribs are more horizontal, the spine is somewhat kyphotic, and the sternal angle is more prominent. The trachea may be posteriorly displaced.

Other changes in the chest wall contour may be the result of structural problems in the spine, rib cage, or sternum. The spine may be deviated either posteriorly (kyphosis) or laterally (scoliosis; see Figs. 22.31B and 22.72). Two common structural findings are pigeon chest (pectus carinatum), which is a prominent sternal protrusion, and funnel chest (pectus excavatum), which is an indentation of the lower sternum above the xiphoid process (Fig. 14.12). See Clinical Pearl, "The Sequence of Steps."

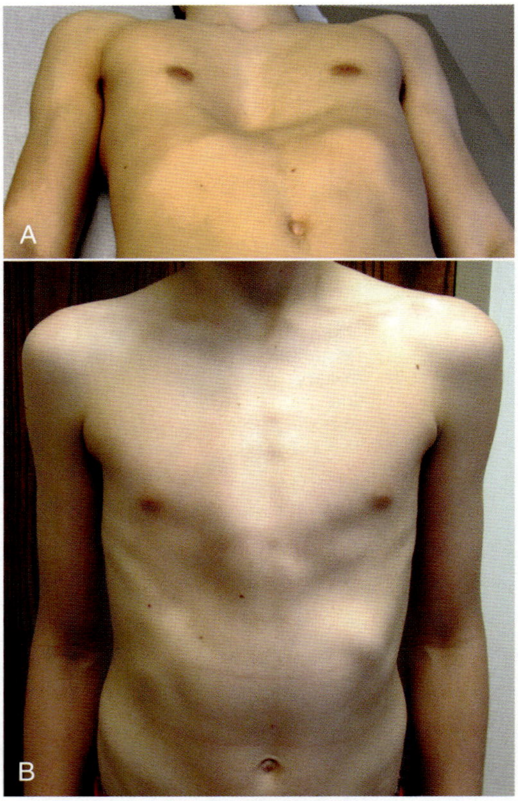

FIG. 14.12 (A) Pectus excavatum. (B) Pectus carinatum. (From Tasker, R. C., et al. (2025). *Nelson textbook of paediatrics* (22nd ed.). Elsevier Inc.)

CLINICAL PEARL

The Sequence of Steps

The sequence of steps in examination of the chest and lungs is inspection, palpation, percussion, and auscultation. The integration of all four steps, together with the history, will often provide adequate information regarding the pathologic process. Listening to the lungs without also inspecting and palpating the chest will deny you the chance to interpret your findings in the most accurate way. Dullness on percussion, for example, is present in both pleural effusion and lobar pneumonia. Breath sounds are absent in the former and may be bronchial in the latter. On palpation you will often find that tactile fremitus is absent when an effusion exists and is increased with lobar pneumonia.

Observing Respiration

Determine the respiratory rate. The adult rate at rest should be 12 to 16 respirations per minute; the ratio of respirations to heartbeats is approximately 1:4. It is best to not tell the patient that you are going to count the respirations to prevent the patient from varying the rate. Count the respiratory rate after palpating the pulse, just as if you were counting the pulse rate for a longer time. Respiratory rates can vary in the different waking and sleep states. The expected rate of respirations (breaths per minute) depends on a number of factors, including the age of the individual and the degree of exertion. Noting the behavior of the

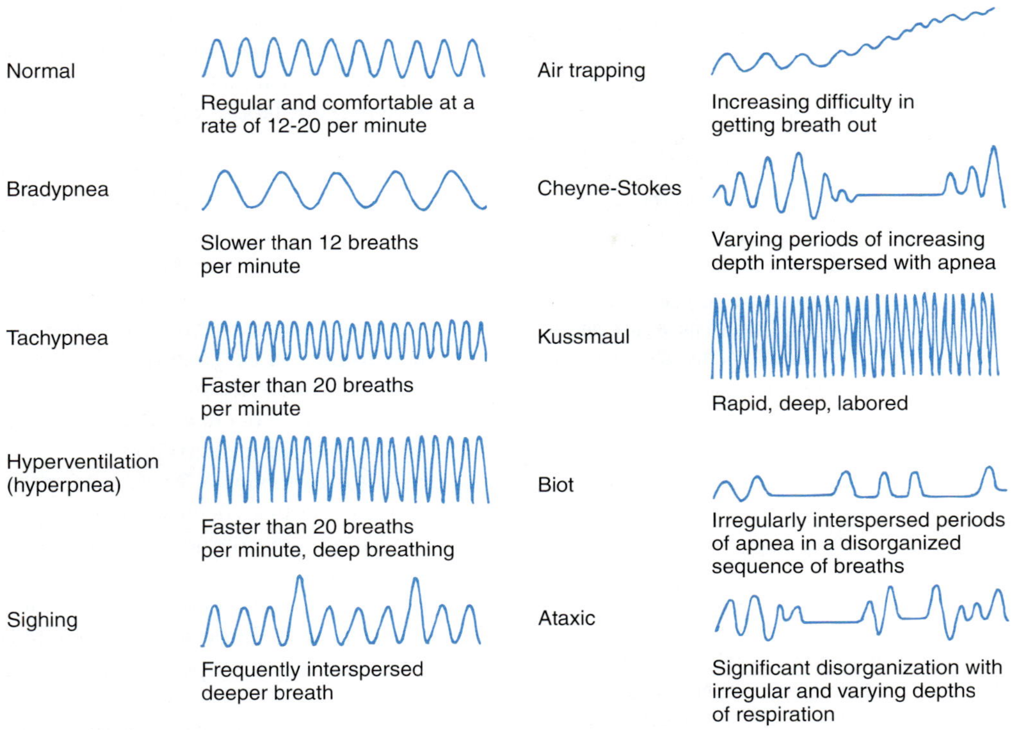

FIG. 14.13 Patterns of respiration. The horizontal axis indicates the relative rates of these patterns. The vertical swings of the lines indicate the relative depth of respiration.

patient relative to the rate is often helpful. Matching your respiratory rate to that of the patient can give you a sense of whether or not the patient is tachypneic or hypopneic.

Note the pattern (or rhythm) of respiration and the way in which the chest moves (Fig. 14.13). Expect the patient to breathe easily, regularly, and without apparent distress. The pattern of breathing should be even, neither too shallow nor too deep. Note the length of the inspiratory and expiratory phases. The inspiratory to expiratory (I:E) ratio is the ratio of the duration of inspiratory and expiratory phases. A normal I:E ratio in a healthy individual is typically 1:2 with exhalation lasting twice as long as inhalation. Note any variations in respiratory rate.

Risk Factors

Respiratory Disability: Barriers to Normal Function

- Age: increases with advancing age
- Family history of asthma, cystic fibrosis, tuberculosis, and other contagious disease; neurofibromatosis
- Smoking
- Sedentary lifestyle or forced immobilization
- Occupational exposure to asbestos, dust, or other pulmonary irritants and toxic inhalants
- Extreme obesity
- Difficulty swallowing for any reason
- Weakened diaphragm and chest muscles (e.g., amyotrophic lateral sclerosis, polymyositis)
- History of frequent respiratory infections

Tachypnea is a persistent respiratory rate above 16 respirations per minute in an adult. Confirm that the respiratory rate is persistent. Rapid breathing may occur during hyperventilation or simply as a self-conscious response to your observation. It is often a symptom of protective splinting from the pain of a broken rib or pleurisy. Massive liver enlargement or abdominal ascites may prevent descent of the diaphragm and produce a similar pattern. Hypopnea, a rate slower than 12 respirations per minute, may indicate neurologic or electrolyte disturbance, infection, or a conscious response to protect against the pain of pleurisy or other irritative phenomena. It may also indicate an excellent level of cardiorespiratory fitness.

Note any variations in respiratory rhythm. It may be difficult to discern abnormalities unless they are quite obvious (Box 14.4). Hyperventilation can be caused by breathing rapidly (tachypnea), breathing deeply (hyperpnea), or both. Exercise and anxiety can cause hyperpnea, but so can central nervous system and metabolic disease. Kussmaul breathing, always deep and most often rapid, is the eponym applied to the respiratory effort associated with metabolic acidosis. Hypopnea, on the other hand, refers to abnormally shallow respirations (e.g., when pleuritic pain limits excursion).

A regular periodic pattern of breathing with intervals of apnea followed by a crescendo/decrescendo sequence of respiration is called *periodic breathing* or *Cheyne-Stokes respiration* (see Fig. 14.13). Children and older adults may exhibit this pattern during sleep, but otherwise it occurs in patients who are seriously ill, particularly those with brain damage at the cerebral level, with drug-associated respiratory compromise, or with severe congestive heart failure (Box 14.5).

BOX 14.4 Influences on the Rate and Depth of Breathing

The rate and depth of breathing will:

INCREASE WITH	DECREASE WITH
Acidosis (metabolic)	Alkalosis (metabolic)
Central nervous system lesions (pons and medulla)	Central nervous system lesions (cerebrum)
Anxiety	Neurologic disorders (e.g., myasthenia gravis and amyotrophic lateral sclerosis)
Aspirin poisoning	Narcotic overdoses
Oxygen need (hypoxemia)	Obesity (extreme)
Pain	

BOX 14.5 Apnea

Apnea, which is the absence of spontaneous respiration, may have its origin in the respiratory system and in a variety of central nervous system and cardiac abnormalities. Common contributors include seizures, central nervous system trauma or hypoperfusion, a variety of infections of the respiratory passageway, drug ingestions, and obstructive sleep disorders.

Primary apnea	A self-limited condition, and not uncommon after a blow to the head. It is especially noted immediately after the birth of a newborn, who will breathe spontaneously when sufficient carbon dioxide accumulates in the circulation.
Secondary apnea	Breathing stops and will not begin spontaneously unless resuscitative measures are immediately instituted. Any event that severely limits the absorption of oxygen into the bloodstream will lead to secondary apnea.
Reflex apnea	When irritating and nausea-provoking vapors or gases are inhaled, there can be an involuntary, temporary halt to respiration.
Sleep apnea	Characterized by periods of an absence of breathing and oxygenation during sleep. Caused by blockage of the airway when the soft tissue in the back of the throat collapses during sleep, and airflow is not maintained through the nose and mouth.
Apneustic breathing	Characterized by a long inspiration and what amounts to expiration apnea. The neural center for control is in the pons and medulla. When it is affected, breathing can become gasping because inspirations are prolonged and expiration constrained.
Periodic apnea of the newborn	A normal condition characterized by an irregular pattern of rapid breathing interspersed with brief periods of apnea that one usually associates with rapid eye movement sleep.

An occasional deep, audible sigh that punctuates an otherwise regular respiratory pattern is associated with emotional distress or an incipient episode of more severe hyperventilation. Sighs may also occur in normal respiration.

If the pulmonary tree is seriously obstructed for any reason, inspired air has difficulty overcoming the resistance and getting out. Air trapping is the result of a prolonged but inefficient expiratory effort. Air trapping can also result from increased resistance (i.e., chronic bronchitis); decreased elastic recoil of the lung (i.e., emphysema); or a drop in the critical closing pressure of the airway (i.e., asthma). Any one of these, or a combination of these conditions, will lead to decreased expiratory flow rates, which ultimately can lead to air trapping. The rate of respiration increases to compensate; as this happens, the effort becomes more shallow, the amount of trapped air increases, and the lungs hyperinflate. On a chronic basis, this can lead to a barrel chest.

Biot or ataxic respiration consists of irregular respirations varying in depth and interrupted by intervals of apnea but lacking the repetitive pattern of periodic respiration. On occasion, the respirations may be regular, but the apneic periods may occur in an irregular pattern. Biot respiration usually is associated with severe and persistent increased intracranial pressure, respiratory compromise resulting from drug poisoning, or brain damage at the level of the medulla and generally indicates a poor prognosis.

Inspect the chest wall movement during respiration. Again, different angles of illumination will aid inspection and help delineate chest wall movement and possible deformities. Expansion should be symmetric, without apparent use of accessory muscles. Chest asymmetry can be associated with unequal expansion and respiratory compromise caused by pneumonia, a collapsed lung, or limited lung expansion from extrapleural air, fluid, or a mass. Unilateral or bilateral bulging can be a reaction of the ribs and interspaces to respiratory obstruction. A prolonged expiration and bulging on expiration are probably caused by airway outflow obstruction or the valvelike action of compression by a tumor, an aneurysm, or an enlarged heart. When this happens, the costal angle widens beyond 90 degrees.

Retractions are seen when the chest wall seems to cave in at the sternum, between the ribs, at the suprasternal notch, above the clavicles, and at the lowest costal margins. This suggests an obstruction to inspiration at any point in the respiratory tract. As intrapleural pressure becomes increasingly negative, the musculature "pulls back" in an effort to overcome blockage. Any significant obstruction makes the retraction observable with each inspiratory effort. The degree and level of retraction depend on the extent and level of obstruction (Box 14.6). When the obstruction is high in the respiratory tree (e.g., with tracheal or laryngeal involvement), breathing is characterized by stridor. With paradoxical breathing, on inspiration the lower thorax is drawn in, and on expiration, the

BOX 14.6 Is the Airway Patent or Obstructed?

Determining the patency of the upper airway is essential to a complete evaluation of pulmonary status. The upper airway is obstructed when there is:

- Inspiratory stridor (with an I/E ratio of more than 2:1)
- A hoarse cough or cry
- Flaring of the alae nasi
- Retraction at the suprasternal notch

The upper airway is severely obstructed when:

- Stridor is inspiratory and expiratory
- Cough has a barking character
- Retractions also involve the subcostal and intercostal spaces
- Cyanosis is obvious even with supplemental oxygen

When the obstruction is above the glottis:

- Stridor tends to be quieter
- The voice is muffled
- Swallowing is more difficult
- Cough is not a factor
- The head and neck may be awkwardly positioned to preserve the airway (e.g., extended with retropharyngeal abscess; head to the affected side with peritonsillar abscess)

When the obstruction is below the glottis:

- Stridor tends to be louder, more rasping
- The voice is hoarse
- Swallowing is not affected
- Cough is harsh, barking
- Positioning of the head is not a factor

opposite occurs. This develops when negative intrathoracic pressure is transmitted to the abdomen by a weakened, poorly functioning diaphragm; obstructive airway disease; or during sleep, in the event of upper airway obstruction.

A foreign body in a bronchus (usually the right because of its larger diameter and more vertical placement) causes unilateral retractions, but they are not seen in the suprasternal notch. Retraction of the lower chest occurs with asthma and bronchiolitis.

Looking for Clues at the Periphery

Observe the lips and nails for cyanosis, the lips for pursing, the fingers for clubbing, and the alae nasi for flaring. Any of these peripheral clues suggests pulmonary or cardiac difficulty. Pursing of the lips can occur with an increased expiratory effort. Patients learn without being taught that it reduces the sensation of dyspnea. Clubbing—enlargement of the terminal phalanges of the fingers and/or toes—is associated with emphysema, lung cancer, the cyanosis of congenital heart disease, cirrhosis, or cystic fibrosis (see Figs. 9.20, 9.21, and 9.22). Flaring of the alae nasi during inspiration is a sign of air hunger. Smell the breath; pulmonary infection may make it malodorous, or the sweet pungent smell of diabetic ketoacidosis may explain tachypnea or Kussmaul respirations. Note whether there are supernumerary nipples; these may be a clue to other congenital abnormalities. Look for any superficial venous patterns over the chest, which may be a sign of heart disorders or vascular obstruction. The underlying fat and relative prominence of the ribs may give some clue to general nutrition.

Palpation

Palpate the thoracic muscles and skeleton, feeling for pulsations, areas of tenderness, bulges, depressions, masses, and unusual movement. Expect bilateral symmetry and some elasticity of the rib cage, but the sternum and xiphoid should be relatively inflexible and the thoracic spine rigid.

Crepitus, a crackly or crinkly sensation, can be both palpated and heard—a gentle, bubbly feeling. It indicates air in the subcutaneous tissue from a rupture somewhere in the respiratory system or by infection with a gas-producing organism. It may be localized (e.g., over the suprasternal notch and base of the neck) or cover a wider area, potentially involving the arms and face, with the associated swelling mimicking an allergic reaction. Crepitus always results from an underlying pathologic process.

A palpable, coarse, grating vibration, usually on inspiration, suggests a pleural friction rub caused by inflammation of the pleural surfaces. Think of it as the feel of leather rubbing on leather.

To evaluate thoracic expansion during respiration, stand behind the patient and place your thumbs along the spinal processes at the level of the 10th rib, with your palms lightly in contact with the posterolateral surfaces (Fig. 14.14). Watch your thumbs diverge during quiet and deep breathing. A loss of symmetry in the movement of the thumbs suggests a problem on one or both sides. A patient who is barrel chested with chronic obstructive pulmonary disease (COPD) may not demonstrate this. The chest is so inflated that it cannot expand farther, and your hands may even come together a bit.

Tactile Fremitus

Note the quality of the tactile fremitus, the palpable vibration of the chest wall that results from speech or other

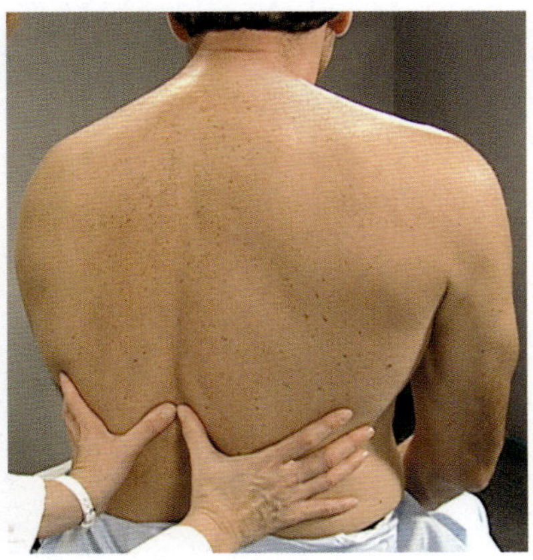

FIG. 14.14 **Palpating thoracic expansion.** The thumbs are at the level of the 10th rib.

verbalizations. Fremitus is best felt posteriorly and laterally at the level of the bifurcation of the bronchi. There is great variability depending on the intensity and pitch of the voice and the structure and thickness of the chest wall. In addition, the scapulae may obscure fremitus.

Evidence-Based Practice in Physical Examination

Is There a Pleural Effusion?

A review of a number of studies indicates that dullness to percussion and decreased tactile fremitus are the most useful findings for pleural effusion. Dullness to chest percussion makes the probability of a pleural effusion more likely. The absence of reduced tactile vocal fremitus makes pleural effusion less likely.

From Hockenberry, M. J. (2009). *Wong's essentials of pediatric nursing* (8th ed.). St. Louis: Mosby/Elsevier.

Ask the patient to recite a few numbers or say a few words ("99" is a favorite, as is "Mickey Mouse," depending perhaps on the age) while you systematically palpate the chest with the palmar surfaces of the fingers or with the ulnar aspects of the hand. Use a firm, light touch, establishing even contact. For comparison, palpate both sides simultaneously and symmetrically; or use one hand, alternating between the two sides. Move about the patient, palpating each area carefully, right side to left side (Fig. 14.15). Some examiners prefer to use their dominant hand, moving it back and forth to make comparisons.

Decreased or absent fremitus may be caused by excess air in the lungs or may indicate emphysema, pleural thickening or effusion, or bronchial obstruction. Increased fremitus, often coarser or rougher in feel, occurs in the presence of fluids or a solid mass within the lungs and may be caused by lung consolidation, heavy but nonobstructive bronchial secretions, or a compressed lung. Gentle, more tremulous fremitus than expected occurs with some lung consolidations and some inflammatory and infectious processes.

Examining the Trachea

Note the position of the trachea. Place an index finger in the suprasternal notch and move it gently, side to side, along the upper edges of each clavicle and in the spaces above to the inner borders of the sternocleidomastoid muscles. These spaces should be equal on both sides, and the trachea should be in the midline directly above the suprasternal notch. This can also be determined by palpating with both thumbs simultaneously (Fig. 14.16). A slight, barely noticeable deviation to the right is not unusual.

The trachea may be deviated because of problems within the chest and may, on occasion, seem to pulsate. Volume loss (from fibrosis or atelectasis) pulls the trachea toward the affected lung. Thyroid enlargement or pleural effusion may cause the trachea to deviate away from the affected side. Pneumothorax can make the trachea go either way, depending on whether there is a tension pneumothorax. In this case pressure builds up on the side of the collapsed lung, and the deviation is away from the affected side. In response to a simple collapsed lung, the trachea deviates to the affected side. Anterior mediastinal tumors may push it posteriorly; with inflammation of the mediastinum (mediastinitis), the trachea may be pushed forward (see Clinical Pearl, "Clue to a Mediastinal Mass").

CLINICAL PEARL

Clue to a Mediastinal Mass

An anterior mediastinal mass may compress the trachea and compromise respiration. Patients may develop the harsh sound of stridor with more difficulty breathing. Instinctively, the patient may sit up and lean forward in an attempt to relieve the compression; this action may serve as a clue to the possibility of such a mass.

Percussion

Percussion tones heard over the chest, as elsewhere, are described in Chapter 3 and summarized in Fig. 14.17

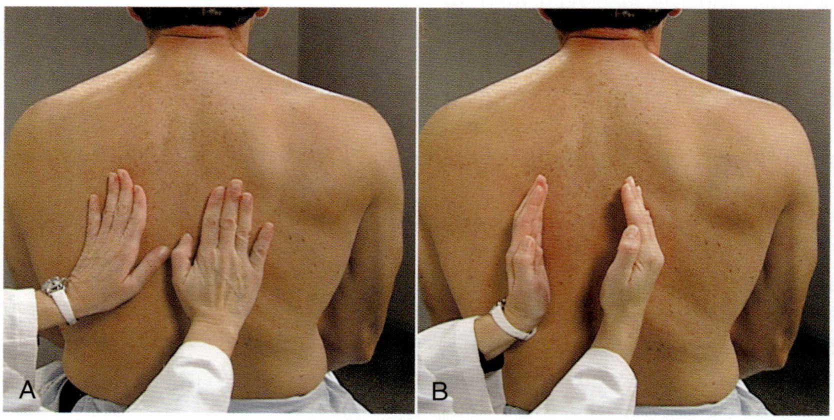

FIG. 14.15 Two methods for evaluating tactile fremitus. (A) With palmar surface of both hands. (B) With ulnar aspect.

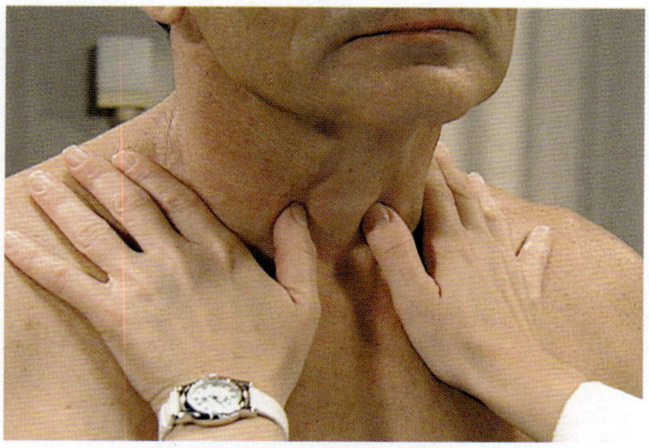

FIG. 14.16 **Palpating to evaluate midline position of the trachea.**

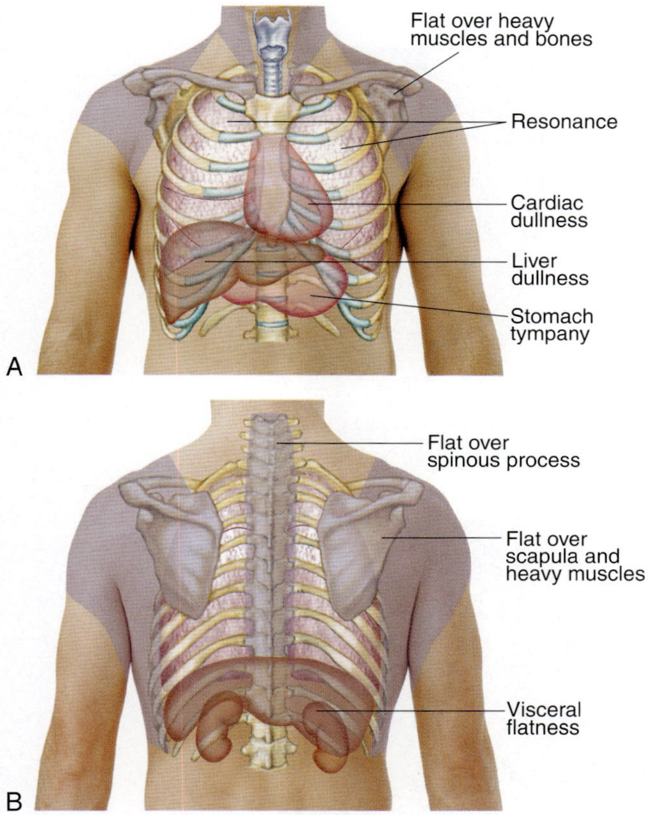

FIG. 14.17 **Percussion tones throughout the chest.** (A) Anterior view. (B) Posterior view.

and Table 14.1. You can percuss directly or indirectly, as described in Chapter 3. Remember that the heavier the stroke you use, the more likely you are to miss a transitional area from resonance to dullness. Tap sharply and consistently from the wrist without excessive force.

Compare all areas bilaterally, using one side as a control for the other. The following sequence serves as one model. First, examine the back with the patient sitting with the head bent forward and arms folded in front. This moves the scapulae laterally, exposing more of the lung. Then ask the patient to raise the arms overhead while you percuss the lateral and anterior chest. For all positions, percuss at 4- to 5-cm intervals over the intercostal spaces, moving systematically from superior to inferior and medial to lateral (Figs. 14.18 and 14.19). This sequence is one of many that you may follow. Adopt the one most comfortable for you and use it consistently. Resonance, the expected sound, can usually be heard over all areas of the lungs. Hyperresonance associated with hyperinflation may indicate emphysema, pneumothorax, or asthma. Dullness or flatness suggests pneumonia, atelectasis, pleural effusion, or asthma.

TABLE 14.1 Percussion Tones Heard Over the Chest

TYPE OF TONE	INTENSITY	PITCH	DURATION	QUALITY
Resonant	Loud	Low	Long	Hollow
Flat	Soft	High	Short	Very dull
Dull	Medium	Medium to high	Medium	Dull thud
Tympanic	Loud	High	Medium	Drumlike
Hyperresonant[a]	Very loud	Very low	Longer	Booming

[a]Hyperresonance is an abnormal sound, the result of air trapping (e.g., in obstructive lung disease). See Chapter 3, Table 3.3, for definitions and a more complete discussion of these tones.

Diaphragmatic Excursion

Measure the diaphragmatic excursion, the movement of the thoracic diaphragm that occurs with inhalation and exhalation.

The following steps suggest one approach to measuring the diaphragmatic excursion:

- Ask the patient to take a deep breath and hold it.
- Percuss along the scapular line until you locate the lower border, the point marked by a change in note from resonance to dullness.
- Mark the point with a marking pen at the scapular line. Allow the patient to breathe, and then repeat the procedure on the other side.
- Ask the patient to take several breaths, to exhale as much as possible, and then to hold (Box 14.7).
- Percuss up from the marked point and make a mark at the change from dullness to resonance.
- Remind the patient to start breathing. Repeat on the other side.
- Measure and record the distance in centimeters between the marks on each side. The excursion distance is usually 3 to 5 cm (Fig. 14.20).

Alternatively, you might use strips of tape, or use one hand as a stationary landmark, percussing directly with the other and estimating the distance. The diaphragm is usually higher on the right than on the left because it sits over the bulk of the liver. Its descent may be limited by several types of pathologic processes: pulmonary (e.g., as a result of emphysema); abdominal (e.g., massive ascites, tumor); or superficial pain (e.g., fractured rib).

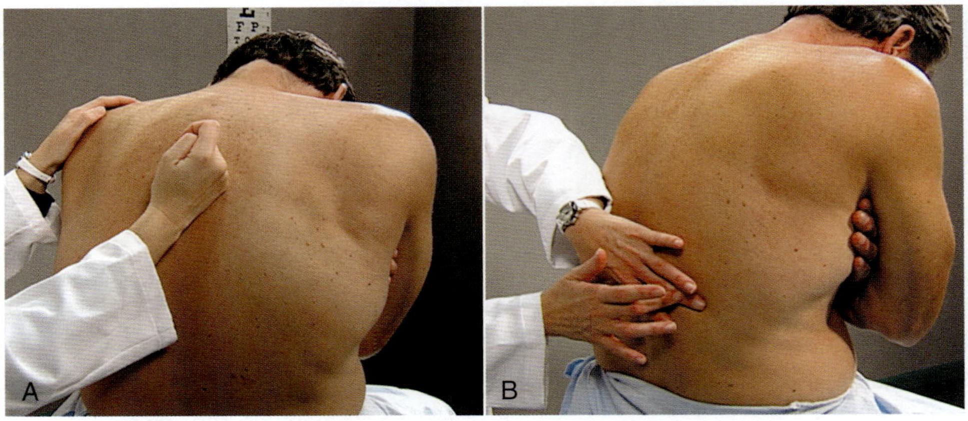

FIG. 14.18 (A) Direct percussion using ulnar aspect of fist. (B) Indirect percussion.

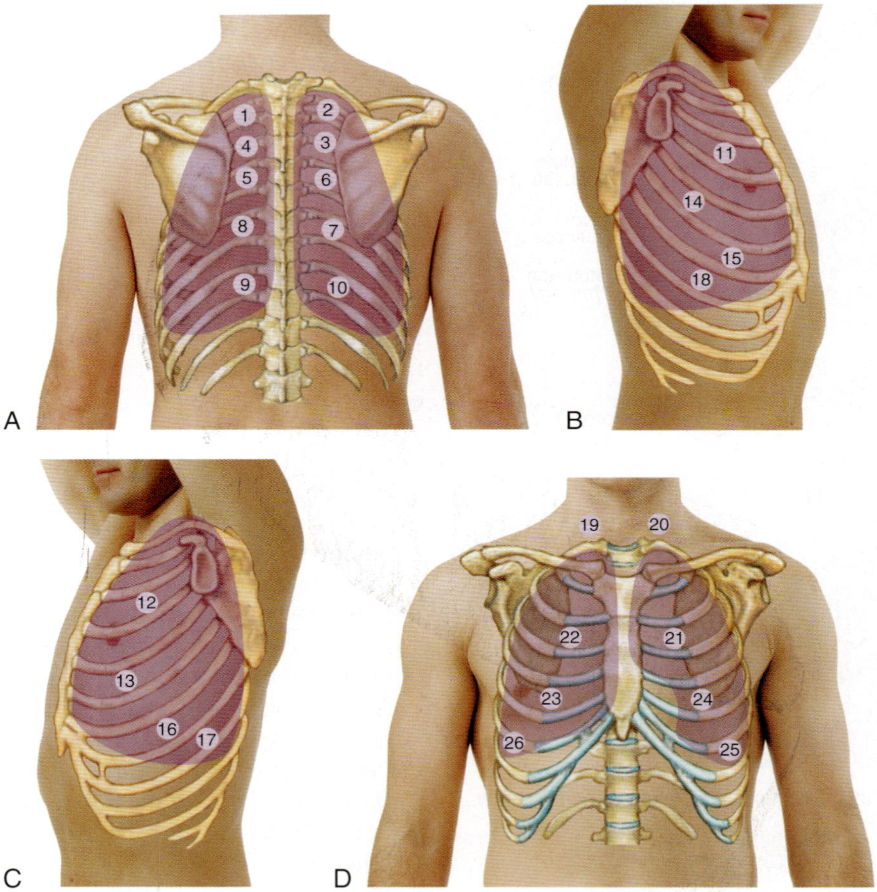

FIG. 14.19 Suggested sequence for systematic percussion and auscultation of the thorax. (A) Posterior thorax. (B) Right lateral thorax. (C) Left lateral thorax. (D) Anterior thorax. The pleximeter finger or the stethoscope is moved in the numeric sequence suggested; however, other sequences are possible. It is beneficial to be systematic.

Auscultation

Auscultation with a stethoscope provides important clues to the condition of the lungs and pleura. All sounds can be characterized in the same manner as the percussion notes: intensity, pitch, quality, and duration.

Have the patient sit upright, if possible, and breathe slowly and deeply through the open mouth, exaggerating normal respiration. Demonstrate this yourself. Caution the patient to keep a pace consistent with comfort; hyperventilation, which occurs more easily than one might think, may cause faintness, and exaggerated breathing

BOX 14.7 Bad Breath: A Possible Sign of Pathology

Smell the Breath

Auscultation of the lungs makes it possible (occasionally, even uncomfortably so) to become aware of a patient's breath odor. Bad breath, even when it is not too distinct, is easily noticed. Infection, either acute or chronic, somewhere in the nasal or oral cavity or deep in the lung, can be the source. An especially foul or putrid odor of breath and/or sputum suggests anaerobic respiratory infections, empyema, bronchiectasis, lung abscess, or a particularly insistent bronchitis. Your nose may provide a significant clue:

Sweet, fruity	Diabetic ketoacidosis; starvation ketosis
Fishy, stale	Uremia (trimethylamines)
Ammonia-like	Uremia (ammonia)
Musty fish, clover	Fetor hepaticus: hepatic failure, portal vein thrombosis, portacaval shunts
Foul, feculent	Intestinal obstruction
Foul, putrid	Nasal/sinus pathology: infection, foreign body, cancer; respiratory infections: empyema, lung abscess, bronchiectasis
Halitosis	Tonsillitis, gingivitis, respiratory infections, Vincent angina, gastroesophageal reflux
Cinnamon	Pulmonary tuberculosis

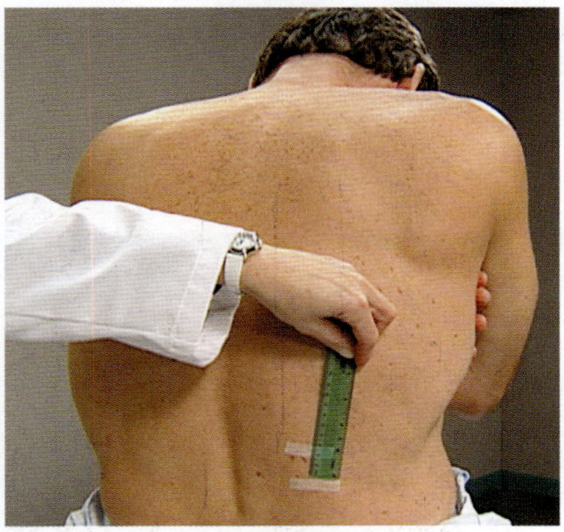

FIG. 14.20 Measuring diaphragmatic excursion. Excursion distance is usually 3 to 5 cm.

can be tiring, especially for frail patients. Because most pulmonary pathologic conditions occur at the lung bases, it is a good idea to examine these first, before the patient becomes too tired.

The diaphragm of the stethoscope is usually preferable to the bell for listening to the lungs because it transmits the ordinarily high-pitched sounds better and because it provides a broader area of sound. Place the stethoscope firmly on the skin, over an intercostal space. When the individual breath sound is being evaluated, there should be no movement of the patient or stethoscope except for the respiratory excursion.

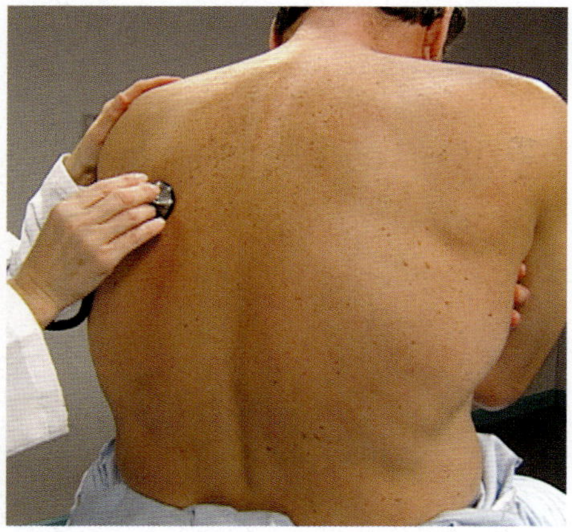

FIG. 14.21 Auscultation with a stethoscope.

To auscultate the back, ask the patient to sit as for percussion, with the head bent forward and arms folded in front to enlarge the listening area (Fig. 14.21). Then have the patient sit more erect with the arms overhead for auscultating the lateral chest. Finally, ask the patient to sit erect with the shoulders back for auscultation of the anterior chest. As with so much else, the exact sequence you adopt is not as important as using the same sequence each time to ensure that the examination is thorough.

Listen systematically at each position throughout inspiration and expiration, taking advantage of a side-to-side comparison as you move downward from apex to base at intervals of several centimeters. Make sure to listen for the presence of crackles at the lung bases in the midaxillary line on the bilateral aspect of the chest. The sounds of the middle lobe of the right lung and the lingula on the left are best heard in the respective axillae.

Breath Sounds

Breath sounds are made by the flow of air through the respiratory tree. They are characterized by pitch, intensity, quality, and relative duration of their inspiratory and expiratory phases and are classified as vesicular, bronchovesicular, and bronchial (tubular) (Fig. 14.22 and Table 14.2).

Vesicular breath sounds are low-pitched, low-intensity sounds heard over healthy lung tissue. Bronchovesicular sounds are heard over the major bronchi and are typically moderate in pitch and intensity. The sounds highest in pitch and intensity are the bronchial breath sounds, which are ordinarily heard only over the trachea. Both bronchovesicular and bronchial breath sounds are abnormal if they are heard over the peripheral lung tissue.

Breathing that resembles the noise made by blowing across the mouth of a bottle is defined as amphoric and

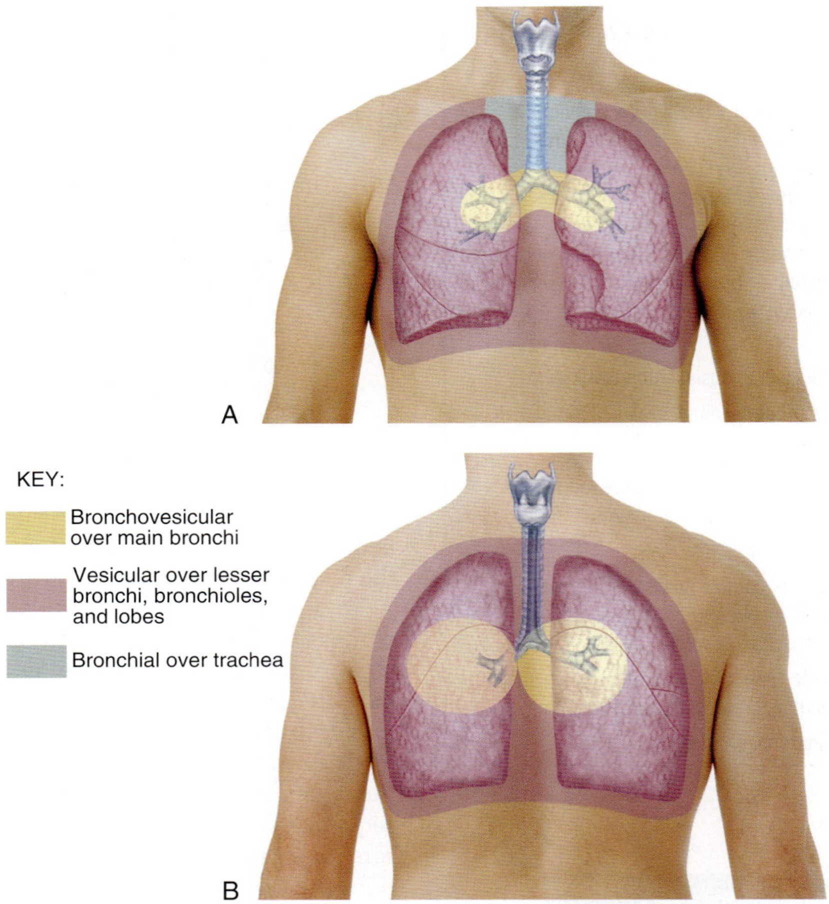

FIG. 14.22 **Expected auscultatory sounds.** (A) Anterior view. (B) Posterior view.

TABLE 14.2 Characteristics of Normal Breath Sounds

SOUND	CHARACTERISTICS	FINDINGS
Vesicular	Heard over most of the lung fields; low pitch; soft and short expirations (see Figs. 14.22 and 14.23); more prominent in a thin person or a child, diminished in the overweight or very muscular patient	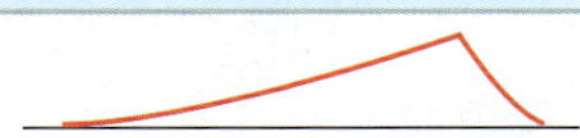
Bronchovesicular	Heard over main bronchus area and over upper right posterior lung field; medium pitch; expiration equals inspiration	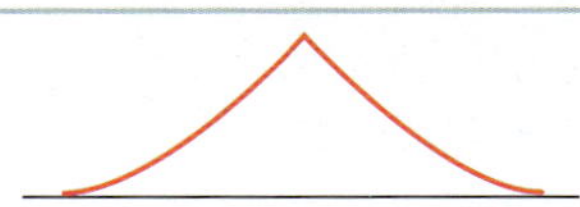
Bronchial/tracheal (tubular)	Heard only over trachea; high pitch; loud and long expirations, sometimes a bit longer than inspiration	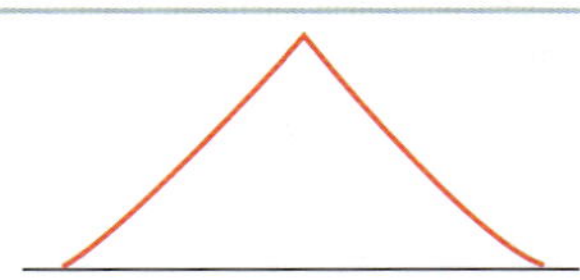

is most often heard with a large, relatively stiff-walled pulmonary cavity or a tension pneumothorax with bronchopleural fistula. Cavernous breathing, sounding as if coming from a cavern, is commonly heard over a pulmonary cavity in which the wall is rigid.

The volume of breath sounds is largely dependent on the speed with which air enters and leaves the mouth. These sounds are relatively more difficult to hear or can be absent in the following situations: fluid or pus has accumulated in the pleural space, secretions or a foreign

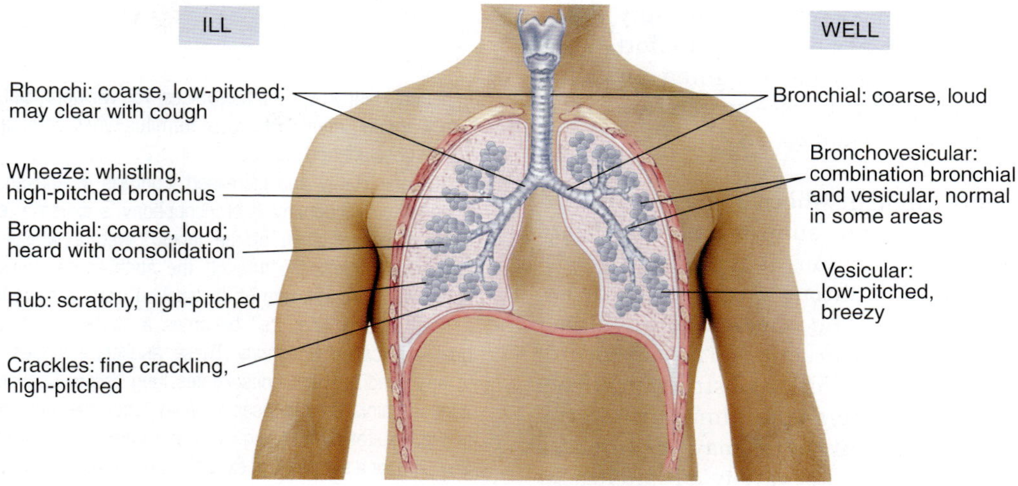

FIG. 14.23 Schema of breath sounds in the ill and well patient.

body obstructs the bronchi, breathing is shallow from splinting caused by pain, or the lungs are hyperinflated such as occurs in severe obstruction from asthma or COPD. Breath sounds are easier to hear when the lungs are consolidated; the fluid-filled alveoli surrounding the tube of the respiratory tree promotes sound transmission better than air-filled alveoli.

Most of the abnormal sounds heard during lung auscultation are superimposed on the breath sounds. Avoid listening through clothing or patient gowns, as this can produce extraneous sounds. Listen directly to the skin overlying the lungs. Extraneous sounds such as the crinkling of chest or back hair must be carefully distinguished from far more significant adventitious sounds. Sometimes it helps to moisten chest hair to minimize this problem. The common terms used to describe adventitious sounds are crackles or rales, rhonchi, wheezes, and friction rub (Fig. 14.23). Crackles are discontinuous; rhonchi and wheezes are continuous. Box 14.8 gives a detailed description of adventitious breath sounds.

BOX 14.8 Adventitious Breath Sounds

Fine crackles: high-pitched, discrete, discontinuous crackling sounds heard during the end of inspiration; not cleared by a cough
Medium crackles: lower, more moist sound heard during the midstage of inspiration; not cleared by a cough
Coarse crackles: loud, bubbly noise heard during inspiration; not cleared by a cough
Rhonchi (sonorous wheeze): loud, low, coarse sounds like a snore most often heard continuously during inspiration or expiration; coughing may clear sound (usually means mucus accumulation in trachea or large bronchi)
Wheeze (sibilant wheeze): musical noise most often heard continuously during inspiration or expiration; usually louder during expiration
Pleural friction rub: dry, rubbing, or grating sound, usually caused by inflammation of pleural surfaces; heard during inspiration or expiration; loudest over lower lateral anterior surface

Crackles. A crackle is an abnormal respiratory sound heard more often during inspiration and characterized by discrete discontinuous sounds, each lasting just a few milliseconds. The individual noise tends to be brief and the interval to the next one similarly brief.

Crackles may be fine, high pitched, and relatively short in duration or coarse, low pitched, and relatively longer in duration. They are caused by the disruptive passage of air through the small airways in the respiratory tree. High-pitched crackles are described as *sibilant;* the more low-pitched crackles are termed *sonorous.* Crackles with a dry quality, more crisp than gurgling, are apt to occur higher in the respiratory tree. These may sound like Velcro being torn open. You might listen for crackles at the open mouth. If their origin is in the upper airways, they will be easily heard; if in the lower, not so easily.

Rhonchi. Rhonchi (sonorous wheezes) are deeper, more rumbling, more pronounced during expiration, more likely to be prolonged and continuous, and less discrete than crackles. They are caused by the passage of air through an airway obstructed by thick secretions, muscular spasm, tumor, or external pressure. The more sibilant, higher-pitched rhonchi arise from the smaller bronchi, as in asthma; the more sonorous, lower-pitched rhonchi arise from larger bronchi, as in tracheobronchitis. Rhonchi may at times be palpable.

At times, it may be difficult to distinguish between crackles and rhonchi. In general, rhonchi tend to disappear after coughing, whereas crackles do not. If such sounds are present, listen to several respiratory excursions: a few with the patient's accustomed effort, a few with deeper breathing, a few before coughing, and a few after. Rhonchi are more likely to have an expiratory component and are usually polyphonic.

Wheezes. A wheeze (sibilant wheeze) is a continuous, high-pitched, musical sound (almost a whistle) heard during inspiration or expiration. It is caused by relatively high-velocity airflow through a narrowed or obstructed airway. The longer the wheeze and the higher the pitch, the worse the obstruction. The absence of wheeze does not mean there is no obstruction. If obstruction is so severe that there is minimal airflow, you may not hear any wheezing. Wheezes may be composed of complex combinations of a variety of pitches or of a single pitch, and they may vary from area to area and minute to minute. If a wheeze is heard bilaterally, it may be caused by the bronchospasm of asthma (reactive airway disease) or acute or chronic bronchitis. Unilateral or more sharply localized wheezing or stridor may occur with a foreign body. A tumor compressing a part of the bronchial tree can create a consistent wheeze or whistle of a single pitch at the site of compression.

Other Sounds. A friction rub occurs outside the respiratory tree. It has a dry, crackly, grating, low-pitched sound and is heard in both expiration and inspiration. It may have a machinelike quality. It may have no significance if heard over the liver or spleen; however, a friction rub heard over the heart or lungs is caused by inflamed, roughened surfaces rubbing together. Over the pericardium, this sound suggests pericarditis; over the lungs, pleurisy. The respiratory rub disappears when the breath is held; the cardiac rub does not.

Mediastinal crunch (Hamman sign) is found with mediastinal emphysema. A great variety of sounds (loud crackles, clicking, and gurgling sounds) are heard over the precordium. They are synchronous with the heartbeat and not particularly so with respiration. These sounds can be more pronounced toward the end of expiration and are easiest to hear when the patient leans to the left or lies down on the left side.

Vocal Resonance

The spoken voice transmits sounds through the lung fields that may be heard with the stethoscope. Ask the patient to recite numbers, names, or other words. These transmitted sounds are usually muffled and indistinct and are best heard medially. Pay particular attention to vocal resonance if there are other unexpected findings during any part of the examination of the lungs, such as dullness on percussion or changes in tactile fremitus. The factors that influence tactile fremitus similarly influence vocal resonance (see Clinical Pearl, "Vocal Resonance").

CLINICAL PEARL

Vocal Resonance

In patients with lower-pitched voices, you will appreciate upon auscultation a greater intensity to vocal fremitus when compared with patients with higher-pitched voices.

Greater clarity and increased loudness of spoken sounds are defined as bronchophony. If bronchophony is extreme (e.g., in the presence of consolidation of the lungs), even a whisper can be heard clearly and intelligibly through the stethoscope (whispered pectoriloquy). When the intensity of the spoken voice is increased and there is a nasal quality (e.g., "e" becomes a stuffy, broad "a"), the auditory quality is called *egophony.* These auditory changes may be present in any condition that consolidates lung tissue. Conversely, vocal resonance diminishes and loses intensity when there is loss of tissue within the respiratory tree (e.g., with the barrel chest of emphysema). See Box 14.9 for a summary of expected findings of a healthy chest and lungs.

Infants

The examination of the chest and lungs of the newborn follows a sequence similar to that for adults. Inspecting without disturbing the baby is important, and for this reason auscultation often occurs at the same time as inspection. Percussion may be unreliable and is typically not performed on infants. The examiner's fingers may be too large for a baby's chest and particularly so for the premature infant.

A newborn's Apgar scores at 1 and 5 minutes after birth tell you a great deal about the infant's condition. Depressed respiration often has its origins in the maternal environment during labor, such as sedatives or compromised blood supply to the newborn or from aspiration of meconium, or it may result from mechanical obstruction by mucus. Table 14.3 explains the Apgar scoring system. This score requires some subjective judgment and cannot be considered absolute.

BOX 14.9 Summary of Expected Findings of the Chest and Lungs

When the lungs are healthy, the respiratory tree clear, the pleurae unaffected by disease, and the chest wall symmetrically and appropriately structured and mobile, the following characteristics will be found:

On inspection:
- Symmetry of movement on expansion
- Absence of retractions

On palpation:
- Midline trachea without a tug
- Symmetric, unaccentuated tactile fremitus

On percussion:
- Range of 3 to 5 cm in the descent of diaphragm
- Resonant and symmetric percussion notes

On auscultation:
- Absence of adventitious sounds
- Vesicular breath sounds, except for bronchovesicular sounds beside the sternum and the more prominent bronchial components in the area of the larger bronchi

TABLE 14.3 Infant Evaluation at Birth: Apgar Scoring System

	0	1	2
Heart rate	Absent	Slow (<100 beats/min)	>100 beats/min
Respiratory effort	Absent	Slow or irregular	Good, crying
Muscle tone	Limp	Some flexion of extremities	Active motion
Response to catheter in nostril (tested after oropharynx is clear)	No response	Grimace	Cough or sneeze
Color	Blue or pale	Body pink, extremities blue	Completely pink

Add the scores of the five individual observations to get the full Apgar score. The lower the total, the more likely it is that there is a problem.

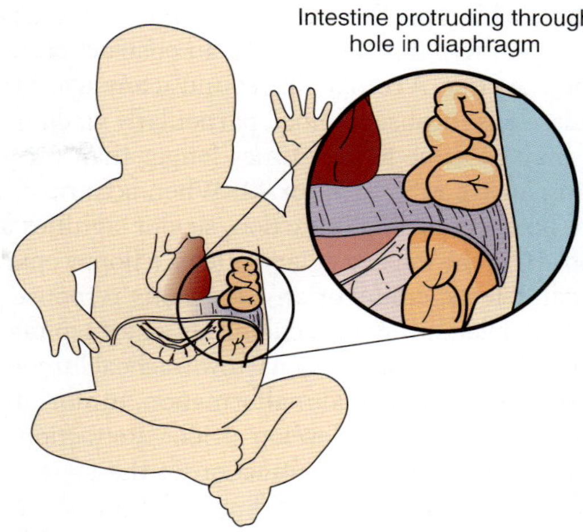

FIG. 14.24 **Diaphragmatic hernia.** (From Phillips, N. (2007). *Berry & Kohn's operating room technique* (11th ed.). St. Louis: Elsevier.)

The newborn's lung function is particularly susceptible to a number of environmental factors. The pattern of respirations will vary with feeding and sleep. In the first few hours after birth, the respiratory effort can be depressed by the passive transfer of medications given to the patient before delivery. Count the respiratory rate for 1 minute. The expected rate varies from 40 to 60 respirations per minute, although a rate of 80 is not uncommon. Babies delivered by cesarean section generally have a more rapid rate than babies delivered vaginally. Note the regularity of respiration. Babies are obligate nose breathers, and at this age, nasal breathing is common. The more premature an infant at birth, the more likely some irregularity in the respiratory pattern will be present. Periodic breathing—a sequence of relatively vigorous respiratory efforts followed by a pause of as long as 10 to 15 seconds—is common. It is cause for concern if the pauses tend to be prolonged and the baby becomes centrally cyanotic (i.e., cyanotic about the mouth, face, and torso). The persistence of periodic breathing episodes in preterm infants is relative to the gestational age of the baby, with the period of breathing cessation diminishing in frequency as the baby approaches term status. In the term infant, periodic breathing should wane in the first days to weeks after birth.

Coughing is rare in the newborn and should be considered a problem. Sneezing, on the other hand, is frequent and expected—it clears the nose. Hiccups are also frequent, although usually silent, particularly after meals. Frequent hiccupping, however, may suggest seizures, drug withdrawal, or encephalopathy, among other possibilities.

Newborns rely primarily on the diaphragm for their respiratory effort, only gradually adding the intercostal muscles. Infants quite commonly also use the abdominal muscles. Paradoxical breathing (the chest wall collapses as the abdomen distends on inspiration) is common, particularly during sleep.

If the chest expansion is asymmetric, suspect some compromise of the baby's ability to fill one of the lungs (e.g., pneumothorax, atelectasis, or diaphragmatic hernia; Fig. 14.24).

Palpate the clavicle, rib cage, and sternum, noting loss of symmetry, unusual masses, or crepitus. Crepitus around a fractured clavicle (with no evidence of pain) is common after a difficult forceps delivery. The newborn's xiphoid process is more mobile and prominent than that of the older child or adult. It has a sharp inferior tip that moves slightly back and forth under your finger.

Auscultate the chest. If the baby is crying and restless, it pays to wait for a quieter moment (see Clinical Pearl, "The Crying Baby"). Localization of breath sounds is difficult, particularly in the very small chest of the preterm infant. Breath sounds are easily transmitted from one segment of the auscultatory area to another; therefore the absence of sounds in any given area may be difficult to detect. Crackles and rhonchi are commonly heard immediately after birth because fetal fluid has not been completely cleared. Whenever auscultatory findings are asymmetric, suspect a problem—for example, with meconium aspiration. Gurgling from the intestinal tract, slight movement, and mucus in the upper airway may all contribute to adventitious sounds, making evaluation difficult. You should suspect a diaphragmatic hernia if a gastrointestinal gurgling sound is persistently heard in the chest of a newborn in respiratory distress.

CLINICAL PEARL

The Crying Baby

Seize the opportunity that a crying child presents. A sob is often followed by a deep breath. The sob itself allows the evaluation of vocal resonance. The crying child may pause occasionally, and the heart sounds may be heard. These pauses may be a bit prolonged as the breath is held, giving the chance to distinguish a murmur from a breath sound.

Stridor is a high-pitched, piercing sound most often heard during inspiration. It is the result of an obstruction high in the respiratory tree. A compelling sound at any age, it cannot be dismissed as inconsequential, particularly when inspiration (I) may be three to four times longer than expiration (E), giving an I/E ratio of 3:1 or 4:1. When accompanied by a cough, hoarseness, and retraction, stridor signifies a serious problem in the trachea or larynx (e.g., a floppy epiglottis; congenital defects; croup; or an edematous response to an infection, an allergen, smoke, chemicals, or an aspirated foreign body). Infants who have a narrow tracheal lumen from compression by a congenital malformation, tumor, abscess, or double aortic arch can develop stridor. Retraction at the supraclavicular notch and contraction of the sternocleidomastoid muscles indicate significant respiratory distress.

Respiratory grunting is a mechanism by which the infant tries to expel trapped air or fetal lung fluid while trying to retain air and increase oxygen levels. When persistent, it is cause for concern. Flaring of the alae nasi is another indicator of respiratory distress at this, or any, age.

Children

Children use the thoracic (intercostal) musculature for respiration by the age of 6 or 7 years. In young children, obvious intercostal exertion (retractions) on breathing suggests an airway problem (e.g., asthma). Usual respiratory rates for children are listed in the following chart. Rates decrease with age, with a greater variation in the first 2 years of life. Sustained rates that exceed the indicated limits should be investigated (Box 14.10).

AGE	RESPIRATIONS PER MINUTE
Newborn	30–80
1 year	20–40
3 years	20–30
6 years	16–22
10 years	16–20
17 years	12–16

BOX 14.10 Assessment of Respiratory Distress in Children

Important observations to be made of the respiratory effort include the following:

Does a loss of synchrony between left and right occur during the respiratory effort? Is there a lag in movement of the chest on one side? If so, consider atelectasis or diaphragmatic hernia.

Is there stridor? If so, consider croup or epiglottitis.

Is there retraction at the suprasternal notch intercostally or at the xiphoid process? Do the nares dilate and flare with respiratory effort? If so, consider respiratory distress.

Is there an audible expiratory grunt? Is it audible with the stethoscope only or without the stethoscope? If so, consider lower airway obstruction or focal atelectasis.

If the roundness of the young child's chest persists past the second year of life, be concerned about the possibility of a chronic obstructive pulmonary problem such as cystic fibrosis.

CLINICAL PEARL

Foreign Body

Think about the possibility of a foreign body when a patient, particularly a child, presents with wheezing for the first time, especially if lung findings are asymmetric. The history may not at first offer a clue.

Children younger than 5 or 6 years may not be able to give enough of an expiration to satisfy you, particularly when you suspect subtle wheezing. Asking them to "blow out" your flashlight or pretend birthday candles or to blow away a bit of tissue in your hand may help bring out otherwise difficult-to-hear end expiratory sounds. It is also easier to hear the breath sounds when the child breathes more deeply after running up and down the hallway (see Clinical Pearl, "Foreign Body").

The child's chest is thinner and ordinarily more resonant than the adult's chest; the intrathoracic sounds are easier to hear, and hyperresonance is common in the young child. With either direct or indirect percussion, it is easy to miss the dullness of an underlying consolidation. If you sense some loss of resonance, give it as much importance as you would give frank dullness in the adolescent or adult. Also, with percussion, your finger can learn to feel the dull areas, a tactile sense that comes in handy at times with a crying child. The dull areas are sensed as having more resistance than resonant areas because they move less.

Because of the thin chest wall, the breath sounds of the young child may sound louder, harsher, and more bronchial than those of the adult. Bronchovesicular breath sounds may be heard throughout the chest.

Pregnant Patients

Pregnant patients experience both structural and ventilatory changes. Dyspnea (shortness of breath) is common in pregnancy and is usually a result of normal physiologic changes. Overall, the pregnant patient increases her ventilation by breathing more deeply, not more frequently. Asthma can have a varied course, getting worse, getting better, or being unaffected by the pregnancy with about equal frequency.

Older Adults

The examination procedure for older adults is the same as that for younger adults, although there may be variations in some expected findings. Chest expansion is often decreased. The older patient may be less able to use the respiratory muscles because of muscle weakness, general physical disability, or a sedentary lifestyle. Calcification of rib articulations may also interfere with chest expansion, requiring the use of accessory muscles. Bony prominences are marked, and there is loss of subcutaneous tissue. The dorsal curve of the thoracic spine is prominent (kyphosis) with flattening of the lumbar curve (Fig. 14.25). The AP diameter of the chest is increased in relation to the lateral diameter.

Older patients may have more difficulty breathing deeply and holding their breath than younger patients, and they may tire more quickly, even when not sick. Adapt the pace and demands of the examination to individual needs.

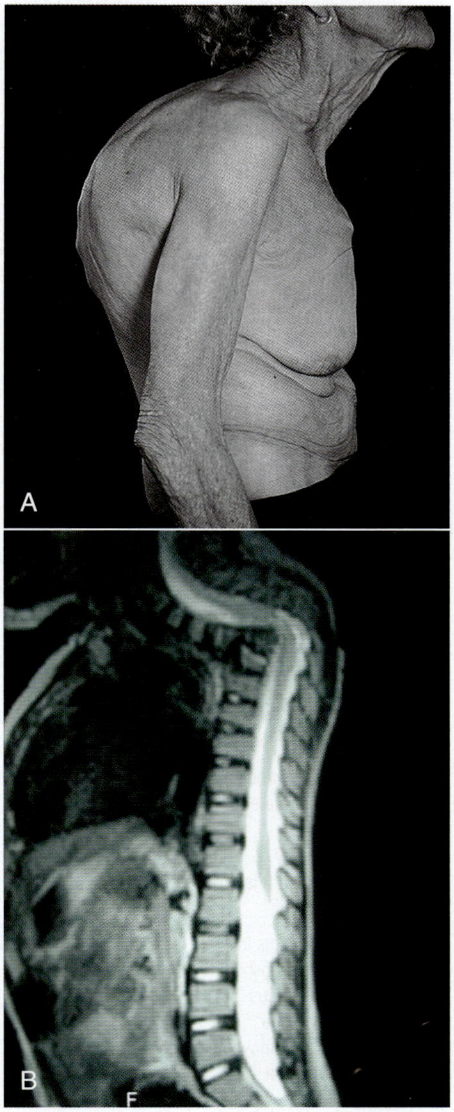

FIG. 14.25 Pronounced dorsal curvature in older adult. (A, From Hochberg, M. C., et al. (2015). *Rheumatology* (6th ed.). Philadelphia: Elsevier; B, from Errico, 2009.)

ABNORMALITIES

Physical findings associated with many common conditions are listed in Table 14.4.

TABLE 14.4 Physical Findings Associated With Common Respiratory Conditions

CONDITION	INSPECTION	PALPATION	PERCUSSION	AUSCULTATION
Asthma	Tachypnea Nasal flaring Intercostal retractions	Tachycardia Diminished fremitus	Occasional hyperresonance Occasional limited diaphragmatic descent; diaphragmatic level lower	Prolonged expiration Wheezes Diminished lung sounds
Atelectasis	Delayed and/or diminished chest wall movement (respiratory lag), narrowed intercostal spaces on affected side Tachypnea	Diminished fremitus Apical cardiac impulse deviated ipsilaterally Trachea deviated ipsilaterally	Dullness over affected lung	Wheezes, rhonchi, and crackles in varying amounts depending on extent of collapse
Bronchiectasis	Tachypnea Respiratory distress Hyperinflation Clubbing (especially cystic fibrosis)	Few, if any, consistent findings	No unusual findings if there are no accompanying pulmonary disorders	A variety of crackles, usually coarse, and rhonchi, sometimes disappearing after cough
Bronchitis	Occasional tachypnea Occasional shallow breathing Often no deviation from expected findings	Tactile fremitus undiminished	Resonance	Breath sounds may be prolonged Occasional crackles, expiratory wheezes and rhonchi
Chronic obstructive pulmonary disease	Respiratory distress Audible wheezing Cyanosis Distention of neck veins, peripheral edema (in presence of right-sided heart failure) Clubbing, rarely	Somewhat limited mobility of diaphragm Somewhat diminished vocal fremitus	Occasional hyperresonance	Postpertussive rhonchi (sonorous wheezes) and sibilant wheezing Inspirational crackles (best heard with stethoscope held over open mouth) Breath sounds somewhat diminished
Emphysema	Tachypnea Deep breathing Pursed lips Barrel chest Thin, underweight	Apical impulse may not be felt Liver edge displaced downward Diminished fremitus	Hyperresonance Limited descent of diaphragm on inspiration Upper border of liver dullness pushed downward	Diminished breath and voice sounds with occasional prolonged expiration Diminished audibility of heart sounds Only occasional adventitious sounds
Pleural effusion and/or thickening	Diminished and delayed respiratory movement (lag) on affected side	Cardiac apical impulse shifted contralaterally Trachea shifted contralaterally Diminished fremitus Tachycardia	Dullness to flatness	Diminished to absent breath sounds Bronchophony, whispered pectoriloquy Egophony and/or crackles in area superior to effusion Occasional friction rub
Pneumonia consolidation	Tachypnea Shallow breathing Flaring of alae nasi Occasional cyanosis Limited movement at times on involved side; splinting	Increased fremitus in presence of consolidation Decreased fremitus in presence of a concomitant empyema or pleural effusion Tachypnea	Dullness if consolidation is large	A variety of crackles with lobar and occasional rhonchi Bronchial breath sounds Egophony, bronchophony, whispered pectoriloquy
Pneumothorax	Tachycardia Cyanosis Respiratory distress Bulging intercostal spaces Respiratory lag on affected side Contralateral tracheal deviation with tension pneumothorax	Diminished to absent fremitus Cardiac apical impulse, trachea, and mediastinum shifted contralaterally Diminished to absent tactile fremitus Tachycardia	Hyperresonance	Diminished to absent breath sounds Succussion splash audible if air and fluid mix Sternal and precordial clicks and crackling (Hamman sign) from pneumomediastinum Diminished to absent whispered voice sounds

Physical findings will vary in intensity depending on the severity of the underlying problem and on occasion may not be present in the early stages.

Adults

Asthma

Small airway obstruction caused by inflammation within the airways

PATHOPHYSIOLOGY

- Acute episodes triggered by allergens, anxiety, cold air, exercise, upper respiratory infections, cigarette smoke, or other environmental agents
- Results in mucosal edema, increased secretions, and bronchoconstriction with increased airway resistance and impeded respiratory flow

PATIENT DATA

Subjective Data

- Episodes of paroxysmal dyspnea
- Chest pain is common and, with it, a feeling of tightness
- Episodes may last for minutes, hours, or days
- May be asymptomatic between episodes
- May only exhibit a chronic cough or coughing only with physical activity

Objective Data

- Tachypnea and paroxysmal coughing with wheezing on expiration and inspiration
- Expiration becomes more prolonged with labored breathing, fatigue, and anxious expression as airway resistance increases
- Hypoxemia by pulse oximetry may develop
- Decreased peak expiratory flow rate

Atelectasis

Incomplete expansion of the lung at birth or the collapse of the lung at any age (Fig. 14.26)

PATHOPHYSIOLOGY

- Collapse caused by compression from outside (e.g., pleural effusion, tumors) or resorption of gas from the alveoli in the presence of airway obstruction
- Loss of elastic recoil of the lung may be caused by thoracic or abdominal surgery, plugging, or foreign body

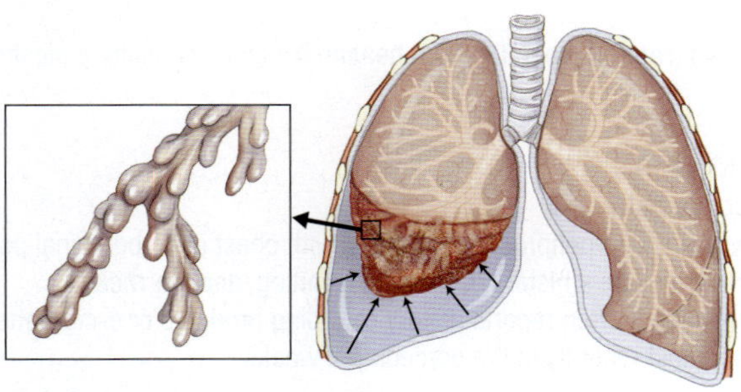

FIG. 14.26 Atelectasis. (From LaFleur Brooks, M. (2009). *Exploring medical language* (7th ed.). St. Louis: Mosby.)

PATIENT DATA

Subjective Data

- Frequently seen in the postoperative setting
- Symptoms of postobstructive pneumonia may develop in the setting of airway obstruction from a foreign body or tumor

Objective Data

- Auscultation dampened or muted in the involved area because the affected area of the lung is airless
- Radiograph may show consolidation associated with a postobstructive pneumonia

Bronchitis

Inflammation of the large airways

PATHOPHYSIOLOGY

- Inflammation of the bronchial tubes leads to increased mucus secretions (Fig. 14.27)
- Acute bronchitis is usually caused by a viral infection, whereas chronic bronchitis is usually caused by irritant exposure, most commonly smoking

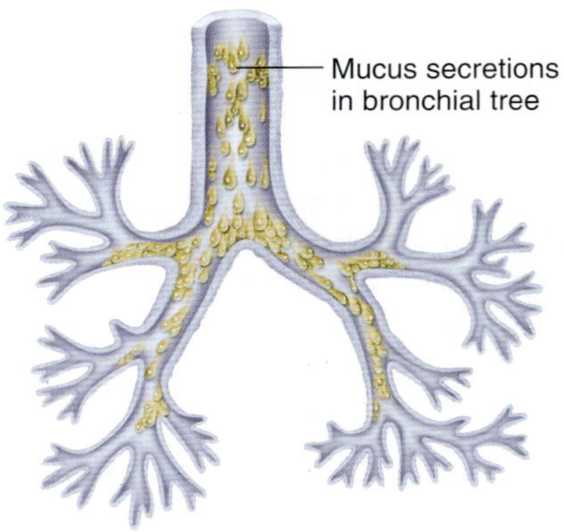

FIG. 14.27 **Acute bronchitis.** (From Wilson, S. F., & Giddens, J. (2013). *Health assessment for nursing practice* (5th ed.). St. Louis: Mosby.)

PATIENT DATA

Subjective Data

- Acute bronchitis may be accompanied by fever and chest pain
- In chronic bronchitis, the cough may be productive

Objective Data

- May have hacking, nonproductive cough with minimal auscultation findings with no respiratory distress
- Greater involvement may lead to wheezing or dampened auscultation in the involved areas

E-Cigarette or Vaping Use–Associated Lung Injury

Respiratory failure with low blood oxygen levels resulting from the inhalation of aerosols (vapors) produced from heating solutions containing nicotine or other substances

PATHOPHYSIOLOGY

- Acute inflammation of the lung tissues involving activation of alveolar macrophages by free radicals
- Vitamin E acetate in vaping products and e-cigarettes containing tetrahydrocannabinol (THC) associated with life-threatening pulmonary inflammation and may cause death

PATIENT DATA

Subjective Data

- Dyspnea with nonproductive cough, with chest and abdominal pain
- There may be a history of nausea, vomiting, and diarrhea
- The patient often reports history of vaping products or e-cigarette use, most recently in the preceding 2 weeks

Objective Data

- Tachypnea, tachycardia, fever at presentation
- Hypoxemia requiring supplemental oxygen or mechanical ventilation is common

Pleurisy

Inflammatory process involving the visceral and parietal pleura (Fig. 14.28)

PATHOPHYSIOLOGY

- Often the result of pulmonary embolism, or infection (bacterial or viral), or connective tissue disease (e.g., lupus)
- Sometimes associated with neoplasm or asbestosis

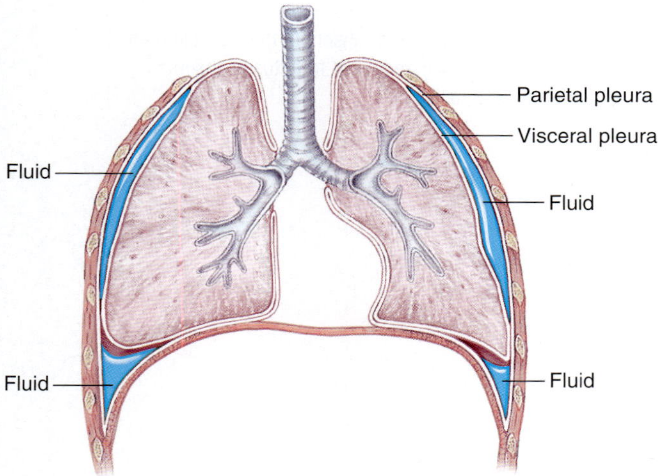

FIG. 14.28 Pleurisy. (From Wilson, S. F., & Giddens, J. (2013). *Health assessment for nursing practice* (5th ed.). St. Louis: Mosby.)

PATIENT DATA

Subjective Data

- Usually sudden onset with chest pain when taking a breath (pleuritic)
- Rubbing of the pleural surfaces can be felt by the patient
- Pain can be referred to the ipsilateral shoulder if the pleural inflammation is close to the diaphragm

Objective Data

- Respirations are rapid and shallow with diminished breath sounds
- A pleural friction rub can be auscultated
- Fever may be present

Pleural Effusion

Excessive nonpurulent fluid in the pleural space (Fig. 14.29)

PATHOPHYSIOLOGY

- Sources of fluid vary and include infection, heart failure, renal insufficiency, connective tissue disease, neoplasm, and trauma

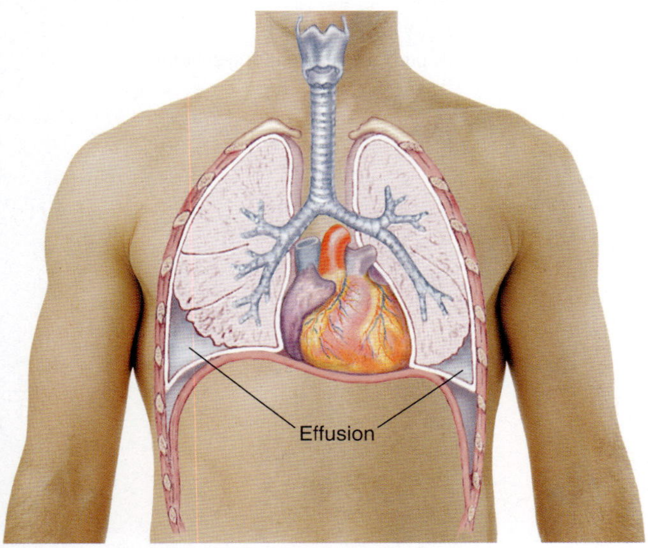

FIG. 14.29 Pleural effusion. (From Wilson, S. F., & Giddens, J. (2013). *Health assessment for nursing practice* (5th ed.). St. Louis: Mosby.)

PATIENT DATA

Subjective Data

- Cough with progressive dyspnea is the typical presenting concern
- Pleuritic chest pain will occur with an inflammatory effusion

Objective Data

- The findings on auscultation and percussion vary with the amount of fluid present and also with the position of the patient
- Dullness to percussion and decreased tactile fremitus are the most useful findings for pleural effusion
- When the fluid is mobile, it will gravitate to the most dependent position
- In the affected areas, the breath sounds are muted and the percussion note is often hyperresonant in the area above the perfusion

Empyema

Purulent exudative fluid collected in the pleural space (Fig. 14.30)

PATHOPHYSIOLOGY

- Non–free-flowing purulent fluid collection develops most commonly from adjacent infected tissues
- May be complicated by pneumonia, simultaneous pneumothorax, or a bronchopleural fistula

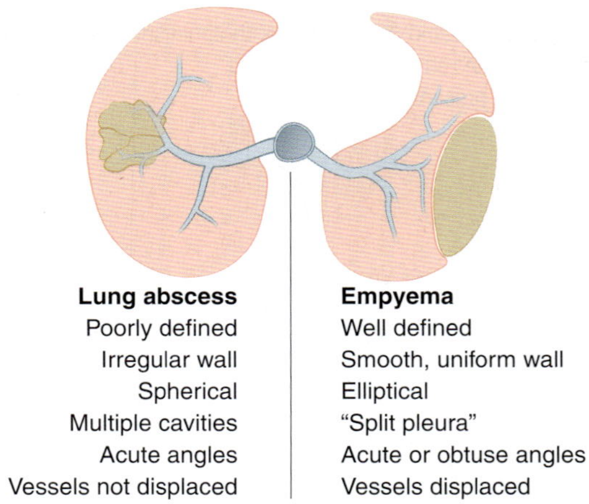

FIG. 14.30 **Empyema and lung abscess.** (From Webb, W. R., Brant, W. E., & Major, N. M. (2015). *Fundamentals of body CT* (4th ed.). Philadelphia: Saunders.)

PATIENT DATA

Subjective Data

- With cough, chest pain, and patient appearing ill
- Progressive dyspnea develops
- Cough may produce blood or sputum

Objective Data

- Breath sounds are distant or absent in the affected area
- Percussion note is dull and vocal fremitus is absent
- Often febrile and tachypneic

Lung Abscess

Usually a well-circumscribed, fluid-containing cavity with an air-fluid interface. Typically unilateral when caused by aspiration (see Fig. 14.30).

PATHOPHYSIOLOGY

- Aspiration of food or infected material from upper respiratory or dental sources of infection are the most common causes
- It may elude diagnosis for some time

PATIENT DATA

Subjective Data

- Malaise, fever, and shortness of breath

Objective Data

- Percussion note is dull, and the breath sounds are distant or absent over the affected area
- Pleural friction rub may be auscultated
- Cough may produce purulent, foul-smelling sputum

Pneumonia

Inflammatory response of the bronchioles and alveoli to an infective agent (bacterial, fungal, or viral; Fig. 14.31)

PATHOPHYSIOLOGY

- Acute infection of the pulmonary parenchyma may be caused by different organisms that are acquired in the community or hospital setting
- Concomitant inflammatory exudates lead to lung consolidation

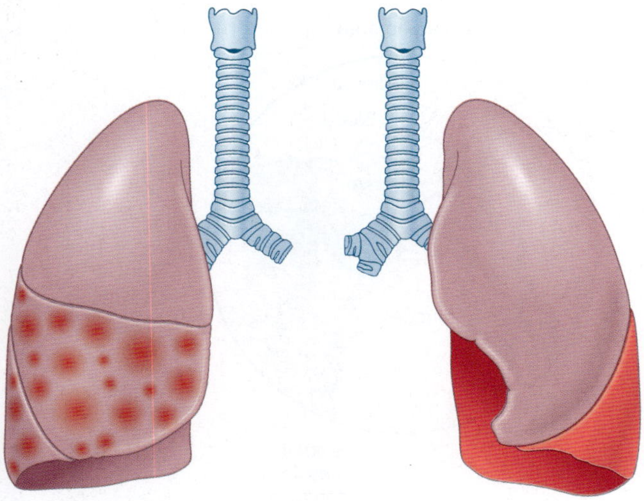

FIG. 14.31 **Lobar pneumonia and lobular or bronchopneumonia.** (From Kumar, V., Abbas, A. K., & Aster, J. C. (2018). *Robbins basic pathology* (10th ed.). Elsevier.)

PATIENT DATA

Subjective Data

- In cases of bacterial infections, can be rapid onset (hours to days) of cough, pleuritic chest pain, and dyspnea
- In the case of mycobacterial, fungal, or atypical infections, onset of symptoms is more insidious
- Sputum production is common with bacterial infection
- Chills, fever, rigors, and nonspecific abdominal symptoms of nausea and vomiting may be present
- Involvement of the right lower lobe can stimulate the 10th and 11th thoracic nerves to cause right lower quadrant pain and simulate an abdominal process

Objective Data

- Febrile, tachypneic, and tachycardic
- Crackles and rhonchi are common with diminished breath sounds
- Egophony, bronchophony, and whispered pectoriloquy in affected areas
- Dullness to percussion and increased fremitus occur over the area of consolidation
- In children particularly, but also in adults, audible crackles are not always heard

Influenza

Viral infection of the lung. Although this originates as a viral respiratory infection, because of alterations in the epithelial barrier, the infected host is more susceptible to secondary bacterial infection (Fig. 14.32).

PATHOPHYSIOLOGY

- Entire respiratory tract may be overwhelmed by interstitial inflammation and necrosis extending throughout the bronchiolar and alveolar tissue
- When mild, it may seem to be just a cold; however, older adults, the very young, and the chronically ill are particularly susceptible to developing more severe symptoms

PATIENT DATA

Subjective Data

- Characterized by cough, fever, malaise, headache, coryza, and mild sore throat, typical of the common cold
- Significant respiratory distress can develop, leading to high morbidity and mortality, especially in the very young, very old, and immunocompromised patients

Objective Data

- Crackles, wheezes, rhonchi, and tachypnea are common

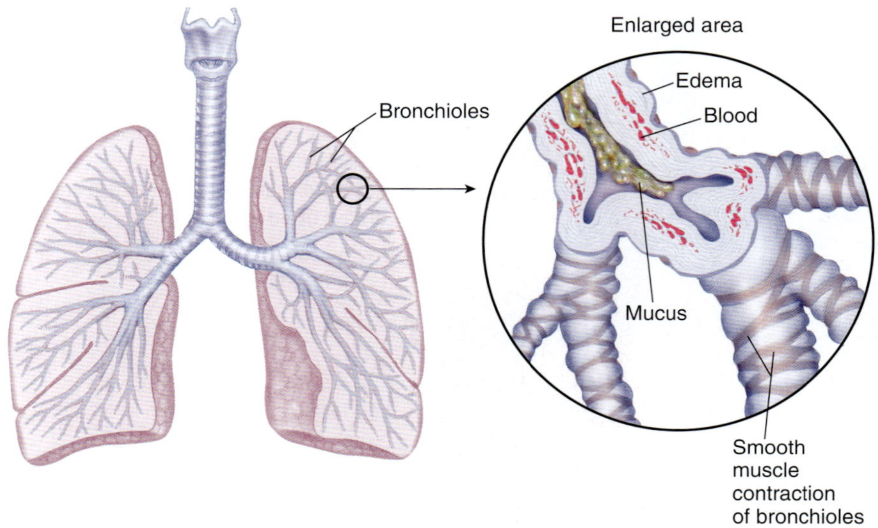

FIG. 14.32 Influenza.

Covid-19

Covid-19 is a viral infection caused by severe acute respiratory syndrome coronavirus 2 (SARS-CoV-2)

PATHOPHYSIOLOGY

- The predominant means of transmission is through person-to-person infection via aerosolized respiratory secretions
- Transmission of SARS-CoV-2 can begin prior to the development of symptoms and peak within several days into the onset of symptoms
- Older adults and the chronically ill are particularly susceptible to developing more severe symptoms

PATIENT DATA

Subjective Data

- Characterized by fever, cough, malaise, headache, dyspnea, smell and taste disorders
- Significant respiratory distress can develop, leading to high morbidity and mortality, especially in the elderly and immunocompromised patients

Objective Data

- Crackles, wheezes, rhonchi, and tachypnea with bilateral pneumonia may occur

Tuberculosis

Chronic infectious disease that most often begins in the lung but may then have widespread manifestations (Fig. 14.33).

PATHOPHYSIOLOGY

- The tubercle bacillus is inhaled from the airborne moisture of the coughs and sneezes of infected persons, infecting the recipient's lung
- Potential for a postprimary spread locally or throughout the body

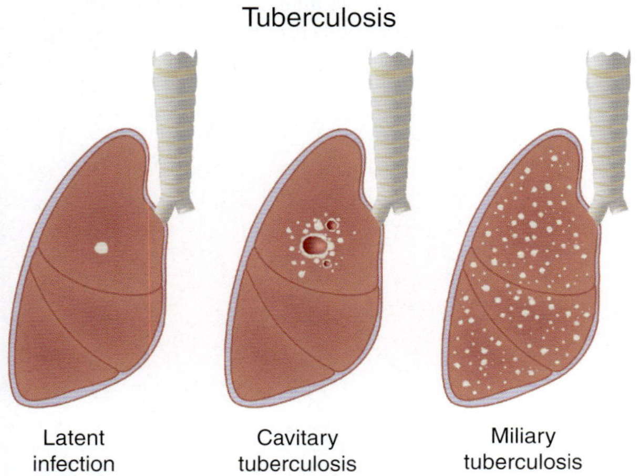

FIG. 14.33 **Tuberculosis.** (From *Tuberculosis*, January 14, 2017. http://www.dovemed.com/diseases-conditions/tuberculosis-tb/.)

PATIENT DATA

Subjective Data

- Latent period: asymptomatic, some regional lymph nodes may be involved
- Active infection: fever, cough, weight loss, night sweats
- History of travel to region with endemic tuberculosis or close contact with infected person

Objective Data

- Latent disease: no pulmonary findings
- Active disease: consolidation and/or pleural effusion may develop with corresponding findings and cough with blood-streaked sputum
- Positive tuberculin skin test, sputum testing for acid-fast bacilli, and IGRA

Pneumothorax

Presence of air or gas in the pleural cavity (Fig. 14.34)

PATHOPHYSIOLOGY

- May result from trauma or may occur spontaneously, perhaps because of rupture of a congenital or acquired bleb
- In *tension pneumothorax,* air leaks continually into the pleural space, resulting in a potentially life-threatening emergency from increasing pressure in the pleural space

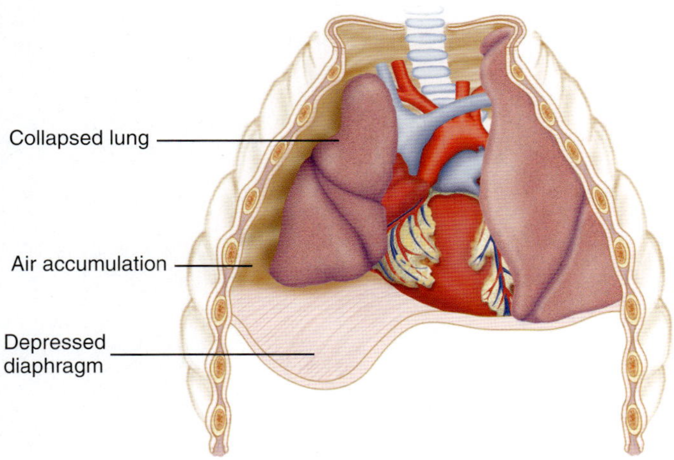

FIG. 14.34 **Pneumothorax.**

PATIENT DATA

Subjective Data

- Minimal collections of air may easily be without symptoms at first, particularly because spontaneous pneumothorax paradoxically has its onset most often when the patient is at rest
- Larger collections provoke dyspnea and chest pain

Objective Data

- The breath sounds over the pneumothorax are distant
- A mediastinal shift with tracheal deviation away from the involved side can be seen with a tension pneumothorax
- An unexplained but persistent tachycardia may be a clue to a minimal pneumothorax

Hemothorax

Presence of blood in the pleural cavity (Fig. 14.35)

PATHOPHYSIOLOGY

- May be the result of trauma or invasive medical procedures (e.g., thoracentesis, central line placement or attempt, pleural biopsy)
- When air is present with the blood, this is called a *hemopneumothorax*

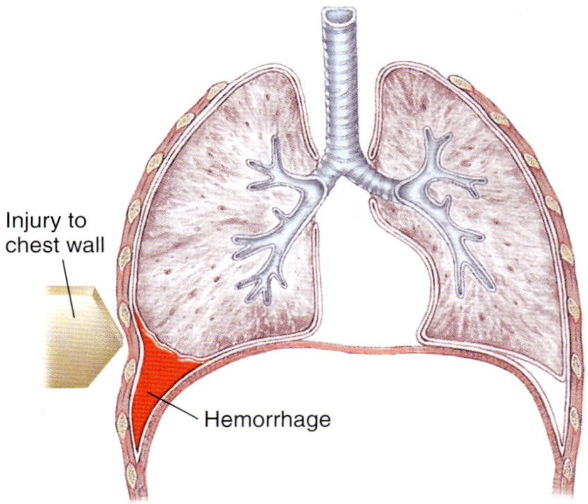

FIG. 14.35 **Hemothorax.** (From Wilson, S. F., & Giddens, J. (2013). *Health assessment for nursing practice* (5th ed.). St. Louis: Mosby.)

PATIENT DATA

Subjective Data

- Dyspnea and lightheadedness may develop depending on the degree and acuity of blood loss and decreased pulmonary function

Objective Data

- Breath sounds will be distant or absent if blood predominates
- Percussion note will be dull, and fremitus will be decreased
- Tachycardia and hypotension with excessive blood loss leading to hemorrhagic shock

Lung Cancer

Generally refers to lung adenocarcinoma, a malignant tumor that evolves from bronchial epithelial structures (Fig. 14.36)

PATHOPHYSIOLOGY

- Etiologic agents include tobacco smoke, asbestos, ionizing radiation, and other inhaled carcinogenic agents

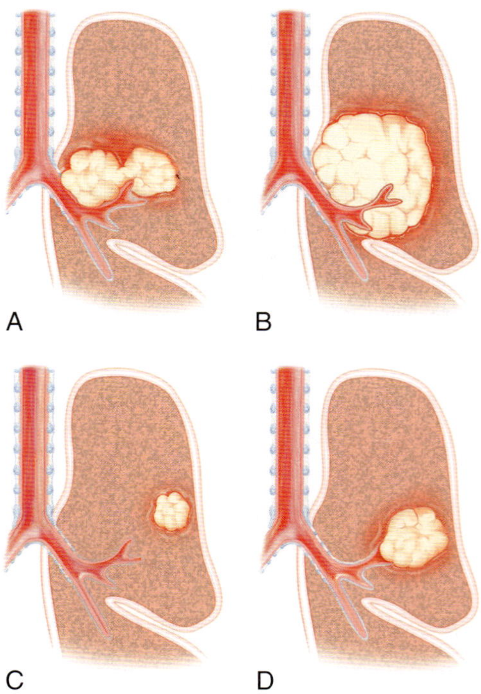

FIG. 14.36 **Cancer of the lung.** (A) Squamous (epidermoid) cell carcinoma. (B) Small cell (oat cell) carcinoma. (C) Adenocarcinoma. (D) Large cell carcinoma.

PATIENT DATA

Subjective Data

- May cause cough, wheezing, and hemoptysis
- Peripheral tumors without airway obstruction may be asymptomatic
- Unintentional weight loss may occur

Objective Data

- Findings are based on the extent of the tumor and the patterns of its invasion and metastasis
- With airway obstruction, a postobstructive pneumonia can develop with consolidation
- A malignant pleural effusion may develop

Pulmonary Embolism

The embolic occlusion of pulmonary arteries typically resulting from dislodged thrombosis within the deep veins of the legs

PATHOPHYSIOLOGY

- Risk factors include, among others, age older than 40 years, a history of venous thromboembolism, surgery with anesthesia longer than 30 min, heart disease, cancer, fracture of the pelvis and leg bones, obesity, and acquired or genetic thrombophilia

PATIENT DATA

Subjective Data

- Pleuritic chest pain with or without dyspnea is a major clue to embolism

Objective Data

- There may be a low-grade fever or an isolated tachycardia
- Hypoxia by pulse oximetry may be evident
- Dullness to percussion and decreased fremitus if there is an effusion
- Pleural friction rub as a possible finding

Epiglottitis

Acute, life-threatening infection involving the epiglottis and surrounding tissues (Fig. 14.37A)

PATHOPHYSIOLOGY

- Acute inflammation of the epiglottis caused by bacterial invasion (*Haemophilus influenzae* type B, group A beta hemolytic *Streptococcus, Staphylococcus*), leading to life-threatening airway obstruction, may cause death
- Immunization against *H. influenzae* type B has greatly reduced the incidence in the United States

PATIENT DATA

Subjective Data

- Begins suddenly and progresses rapidly without cough
- Painful sore throat with difficulty swallowing
- Muffled voice

Objective Data

- Patient sits straight up with neck extended and head held forward, appearing very anxious and ill, unable to swallow and drools from an open mouth; cough is absent
- High fever
- Beefy red epiglottis

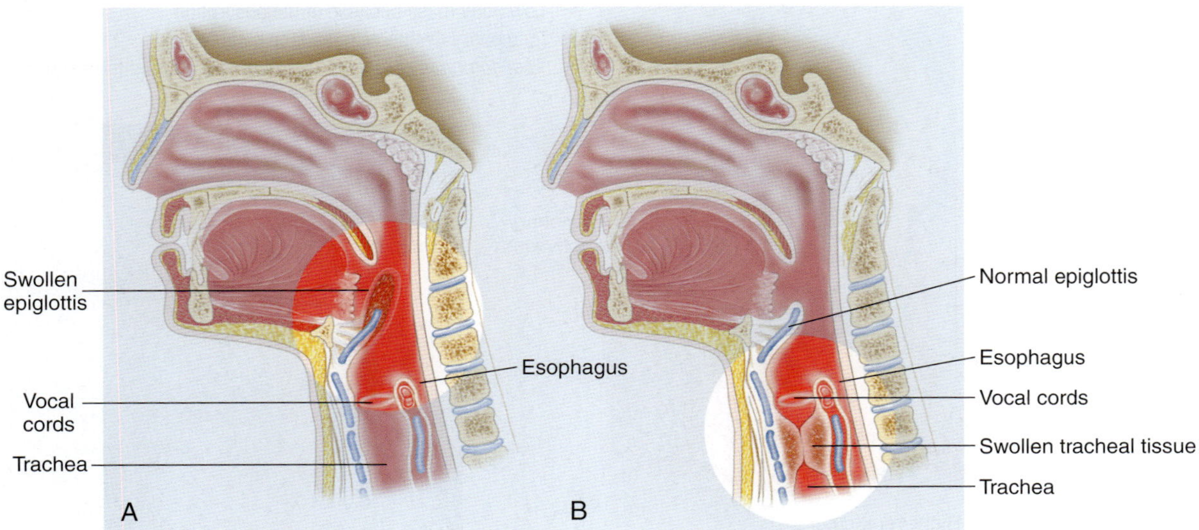

FIG. 14.37 Croup syndrome. (A) Acute epiglottitis. (B) Laryngotracheobronchitis.

Infants, Children, and Adolescents

Diaphragmatic Hernia

Result of an imperfectly structured diaphragm, occurs once in slightly more than 2000 live births (see Fig. 14.24)

PATHOPHYSIOLOGY

- On the left side, at least 90% of the time; the liver is not there to get in the way
- In a Bochdalek hernia, the diaphragm may not develop properly, and the intestine may become trapped in the chest cavity as a result
- In a Morgagni hernia, the tendon that should develop in the middle of the diaphragm does not develop properly

PATIENT DATA

Subjective Data

- The degree of respiratory distress can be slight or very severe depending on the extent to which the bowel has invaded the chest through the defect

Objective Data

- Bowel sounds are heard in the chest with a flat or scaphoid abdomen
- The heart is usually displaced to the right
- Tachypnea, retraction, and grunting

Cystic Fibrosis

Autosomal recessive disorder of exocrine glands involving the lungs, pancreas, and sweat glands (Fig. 14.38)

PATHOPHYSIOLOGY

- Thick mucus causes progressive clogging of the bronchi and bronchioles
- Bronchiectasis results with cyst formation and subsequent pulmonary infection
- Autosomal recessive caused by mutations of *CFTR* (cystic fibrosis transmembrane conductance regulator) gene
- Every U.S. state screens for cystic fibrosis in newborns with an assay for immunoreactive trypsinogen (IRT), a pancreatic enzyme

PATIENT DATA

Subjective Data

- Cough with sputum is a hallmark in children younger than 5 years
- Salt loss in sweat is distinctive such that a parent may notice that the child's skin tastes unusually salty
- There may be a history of malabsorption; large, bulky stools; constipation; poor weight gain; frequent infection requiring antibiotics; meconium ileus; or intestinal obstruction

Objective Data

- Bronchiectasis with the associated findings
- Barrel chest
- Nasal polyps
- Low body mass because of malabsorption
- Pulmonary dysfunction leads to clubbing
- *Pseudomonas aeruginosa* is frequently isolated from sputum cultures

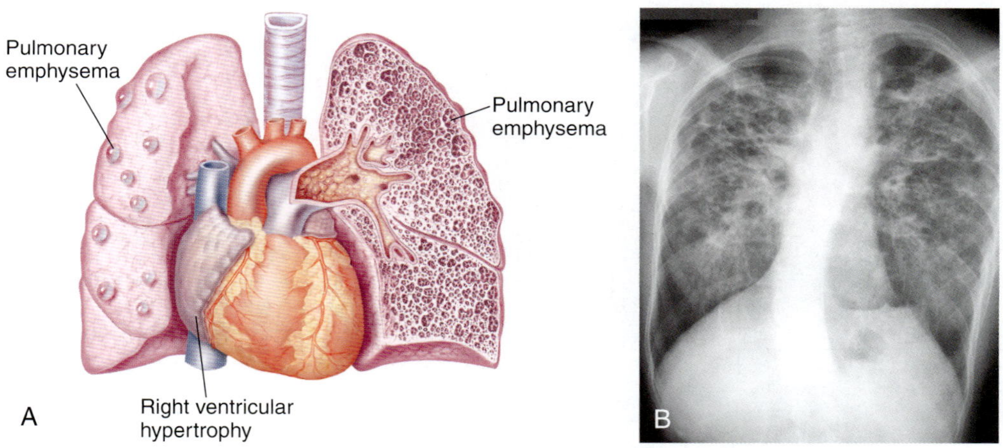

FIG. 14.38 Cystic fibrosis.

Croup (Laryngotracheal Bronchitis)

Syndrome that generally results from infection with a variety of viral agents, particularly the parainfluenza viruses, occurring most often in children from about 1.5 to 3 years of age

PATHOPHYSIOLOGY

- The inflammation is subglottic and may involve areas beyond the larynx (laryngotracheobronchitis; see Fig. 14.37B)
- An aspirated foreign body may mimic croup on occasion

PATIENT DATA

Subjective Data

- An episode begins with upper respiratory symptoms, mild fever
- The child often awakens suddenly after going to bed, often very frightened, with a harsh, barking cough

Objective Data

- Labored breathing, retraction, hoarseness, barking cough, and inspiratory stridor are characteristic
- Restless, irritable
- Fever does not always accompany croup; the child does not have the toxic, drooling facies of persons with epiglottitis

Tracheomalacia

Lack of rigidity or a floppiness of the trachea or airway

PATHOPHYSIOLOGY

- Trachea narrows in response to the varying pressures of inspiration and expiration
- Tends to be benign and self-limited with increasing age
- Need to eliminate the possibilities of fixed lesions (e.g., a vascular lesion), tracheal stenosis, or even a foreign body

PATIENT DATA

Subjective Data

- "Noisy breathing" or wheezing in infancy is often inspiratory stridor

Objective Data

- Stridor, wheezing, and findings of respiratory distress develop with airway collapse or severe compromise

Bronchiolitis

Bronchiolar (small airway) inflammation leading to hyperinflation of the lungs, occurring most often in infants younger than 6 months

PATHOPHYSIOLOGY

- Usual cause is RSV; other viral organisms include adenovirus, parainfluenza virus, and human metapneumovirus
- The virus acts as a parasite, invading small bronchioles
- The virus bursts and invades other cells that die and obstruct and irritate the airway

PATIENT DATA

Subjective Data

- Begins with upper respiratory symptoms
- Poor feeding, vomiting, and diarrhea
- Lethargy
- Expiration becomes difficult, and the infant appears anxious

Objective Data

- Breaths are rapid and short with generalized retractions and perioral cyanosis developing
- Wheezing, grunting, diminished breath sounds
- Lung hyperinflation leads to an increased AP diameter of the thoracic cage and abdomen
- Hyperresonant percussion

Older Adults

Chronic Obstructive Pulmonary Disease

COPD is a nonspecific designation that includes a group of respiratory problems in which coughs, chronic and often excessive sputum production, and dyspnea are prominent features. Ultimately, an irreversible expiratory airflow obstruction occurs. Chronic bronchitis, bronchiectasis, and emphysema are the main conditions that are included in this group.

Emphysema

Condition in which the lungs lose elasticity and alveoli enlarge in a way that disrupts function (Fig. 14.39)

PATHOPHYSIOLOGY

- Most patients have an extensive smoking history
- Alveolar gas is trapped in expiration, and gas exchange is seriously compromised

PATIENT DATA

Subjective Data

- Dyspnea is common even at rest, requiring supplemental oxygen when severe
- Cough is infrequent without much production of sputum

Objective Data

- Chest may be barrel shaped
- Breath sounds are diminished with scattered crackles or wheezes
- Overinflated lungs are hyperresonant on percussion
- Inspiration is limited with a prolonged expiratory effort (i.e., longer than 4 or 5 seconds) to expel air
- When severe, may lead to pulmonary hypertension and cor pulmonale

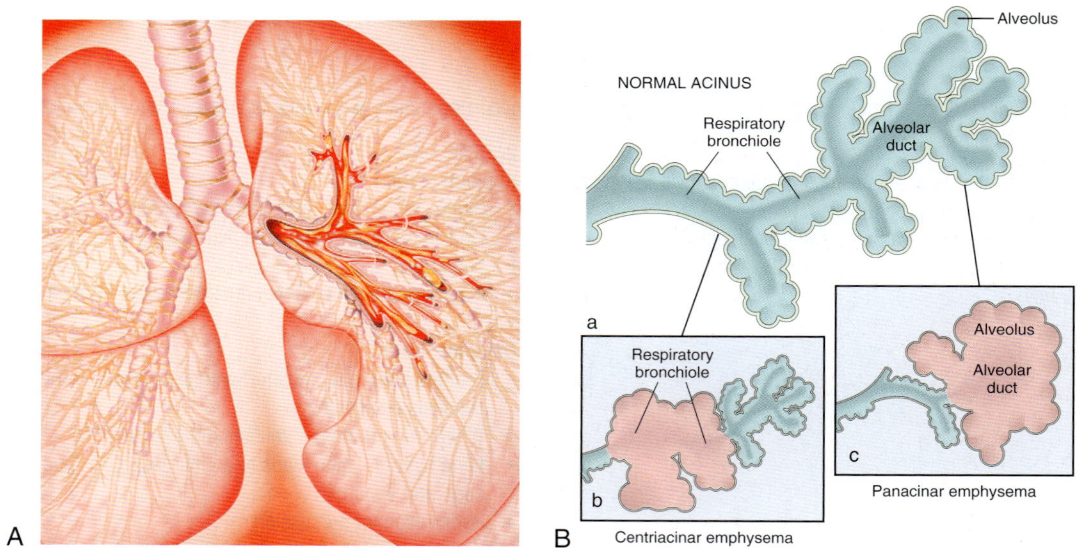

FIG. 14.39 Chronic obstructive pulmonary disease with lobar emphysema. (A, From Barnes, P. J. (2013). Chronic obstructive pulmonary disease: Important advances. *The Lancet. Respiratory Medicine*, *1*(1), e7–e8; B, from Kumar, V., Abbas, A. K., & Aster, J. C. (2018). *Robbins basic pathology* (10th ed.). Elsevier.)

Bronchiectasis

Chronic dilation of the bronchi or bronchioles caused by repeated pulmonary infections and bronchial obstruction (Fig. 14.40)

PATHOPHYSIOLOGY

- Frequently seen in cystic fibrosis
- Malfunction of bronchial muscle tone and loss of elasticity

PATIENT DATA

Subjective Data

- Chronic cough with expectoration of large amounts of sputum is most often the major clue
- Severe hemoptysis may occur

Objective Data

- Tachypnea and clubbing
- Crackles and rhonchi, sometimes disappearing after cough

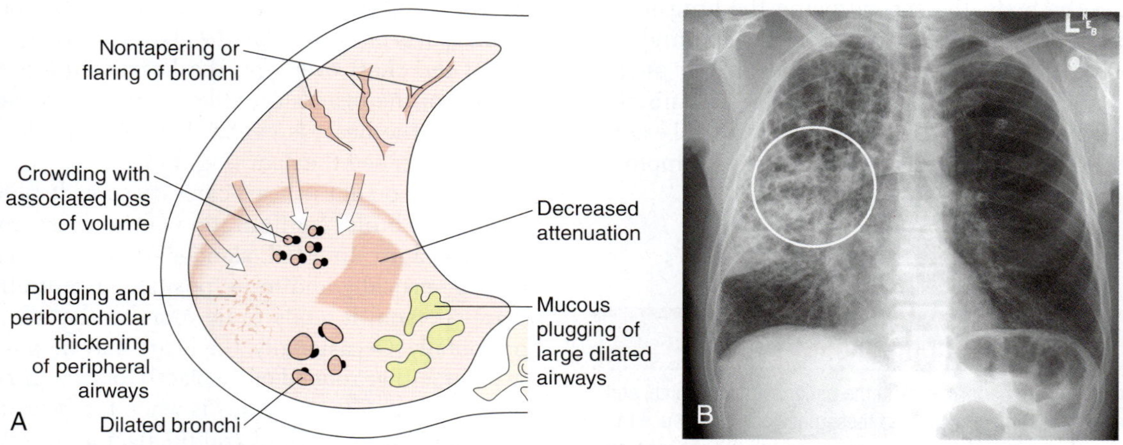

FIG. 14.40 (A) Bronchiectasis. (B) Patient with tuberculosis with multiple cystic structures *(white circle).* (A, From Spiro, S. G., Silvestri, G. A., & Agustí, A. (2012). *Clinical respiratory medicine* (4th ed.). Elsevier; B, from Herring, W. (2020). *Learning radiology* (4th ed.). Philadelphia: Elsevier.)

Chronic Bronchitis

Large airway inflammation, usually a result of chronic irritant exposure, most often smoking; more commonly a problem for patients older than 40

PATHOPHYSIOLOGY

- Large airways are chronically inflamed, leading to mucus production
- Smoking is prominent in the history, with many of these patients being emphysematous
- Recurrent bacterial infections are common

PATIENT DATA

Subjective Data

- Dyspnea may be present, although not severe
- Cough and sputum production are impressive

Objective Data

- Wheezing and crackles
- Hyperinflation with decreased breath sounds and a flattened diaphragm
- Severe chronic bronchitis may result in right ventricular failure with dependent edema

CHAPTER

15 Heart

The main heart function is to circulate blood through the body and lungs in two separate circulations (one circuit being the body, the second being the lungs). The heart lies in the mediastinum, to the left of the midline, just above the diaphragm, cradled between the medial and lower borders of the lungs. The cardiac examination is performed as part of the comprehensive physical examination or when a patient presents with signs or symptoms of cardiac or vascular disease.

Physical Examination Components

The following steps are performed with the patient sitting, supine, and in the left lateral recumbent positions; these positions are all used to compare findings or enhance the assessment. Having the patient lean forward while in the seated position can bring the heart closer to the chest wall and accentuate findings.

1. Inspect the precordium for:
   - Apical impulse
   - Pulsations
   - Heaves or lifts
2. Palpate the precordium to detect:
   - Apical impulse
   - Thrills, heaves, or lifts
3. Percuss to estimate the heart size (optional)
4. Systematically auscultate in each of five areas while the patient is breathing regularly and holding breath for:
   - Rate
   - Rhythm
   - S_1
   - S_2
   - Splitting
   - S_3 and/or S_4
   - Extra heart sounds (snaps, clicks, friction rubs, or murmurs)
5. Assess the characteristics of murmurs:
   - Timing and duration
   - Pitch
   - Intensity
   - Pattern
   - Quality
   - Location
   - Radiation
   - Variation with respiratory phase

ANATOMY AND PHYSIOLOGY

The heart is positioned behind the sternum and the contiguous parts of the third to the sixth costal cartilages. The area of the chest overlying the heart is the precordium. Because of the heart's conelike shape, the broader upper portion of the heart is called the *base,* and the narrower lower tip is called the *apex* (Fig. 15.1).

The position of the heart can vary considerably depending on body build, configuration of the chest, and level of the diaphragm. In a tall, slender person, the heart tends to hang vertically and to be positioned centrally. With a shorter person, it tends to lie more to the left and more horizontally. Occasionally, the heart may be positioned to the right, either rotated or displaced, or as a mirror image (dextrocardia). Situs inversus is when the heart and stomach are placed to the right and the liver to the left.

Structure

The pericardium is a tough, double-walled, fibrous sac encasing and protecting the heart. Several milliliters of fluid are present between the inner and outer layers of the pericardium, providing for low-friction movement (Fig. 15.2).

The epicardium, the thin outermost muscle layer, covers the surface of the heart and extends onto the great vessels. The myocardium, the thick muscular middle layer, is responsible for the pumping action of the heart. The endocardium, the innermost layer, lines the chambers of the heart and covers the heart valves and the small muscles associated with the opening and closing of these valves (Fig. 15.3).

The heart is divided into four chambers. The two upper chambers are the right and left atria (each atria has an ear-shaped projection, called an *auricle*), and the bottom chambers are the right and left ventricles. The left atrium and left ventricle together are referred to as the *left heart;* the right atrium and right ventricle together are referred to as the *right heart.* The left heart and right heart are divided by a blood-tight partition called the *interventricular septum* (see Fig. 15.1). On the anterior external surface of the heart, the coronary sulcus separates the atria from the ventricles (Fig. 15.4).

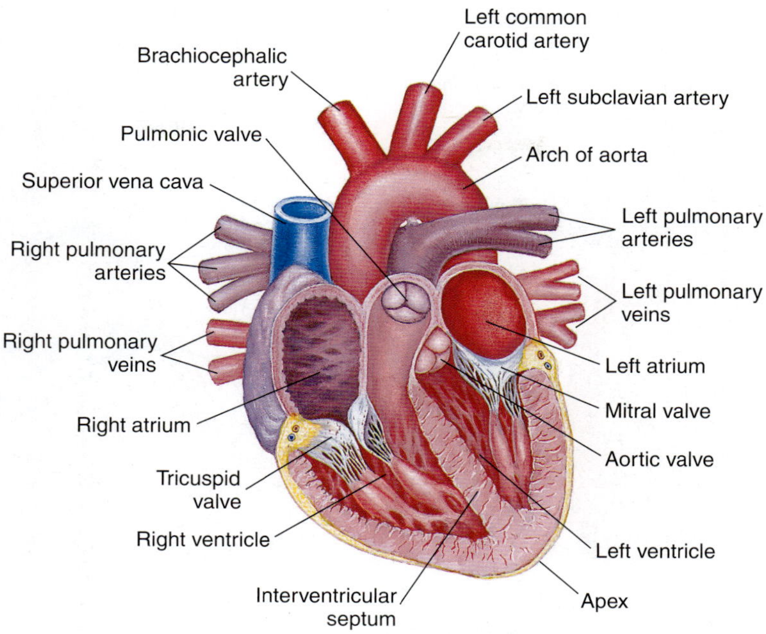

FIG. 15.1 Frontal section of the heart.

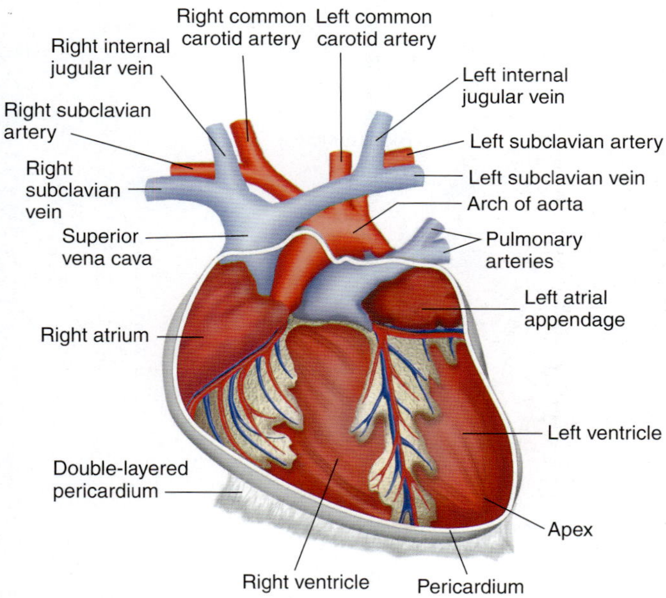

FIG. 15.2 Heart within the pericardium.

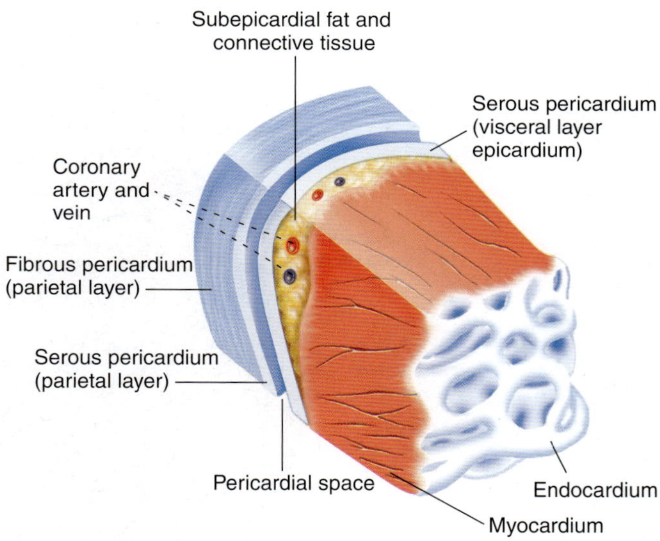

FIG. 15.3 Cross section of the cardiac muscle.

The atria are small, thin-walled structures acting primarily as reservoirs for blood returning to the heart from the veins throughout the body. The ventricles are large, thick-walled chambers that pump blood to the lungs and throughout the body. The right and left ventricles together form the primary muscle mass of the heart. In the adult heart, the left ventricle mass is greater than that of the right ventricle because the higher pressure in the systemic circulation requires a greater contractile force (and more muscle mass) for blood to be successfully pumped throughout the body. The adult heart is about 12 cm long, 8 cm wide at the widest point, and 6 cm in its anteroposterior diameter.

Most of the anterior surface of the heart is formed by the right ventricle. The left ventricle is positioned behind the right but extends anteriorly, forming the left border of the heart (see Fig. 15.4). The left atrium is above the left ventricle, forming the more posterior aspect of the heart. The heart is, in effect, turned ventrally on its axis, with its right side more anterior. The left ventricle's contraction and resulting thrust are usually felt as the apical impulse in the fifth left intercostal space at the midclavicular line. The right atrium lies above and slightly to the right of the right ventricle and is part of the right border of the heart.

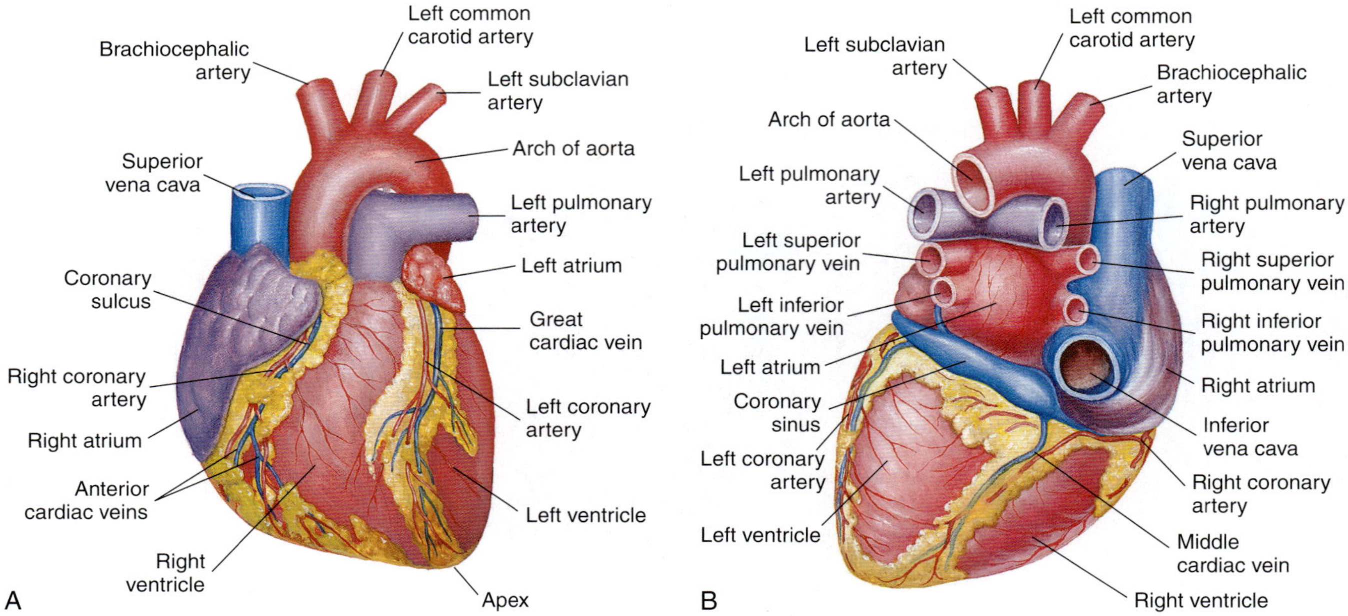

FIG. 15.4 Views of the heart. (A) Anterior. (B) Posterior.

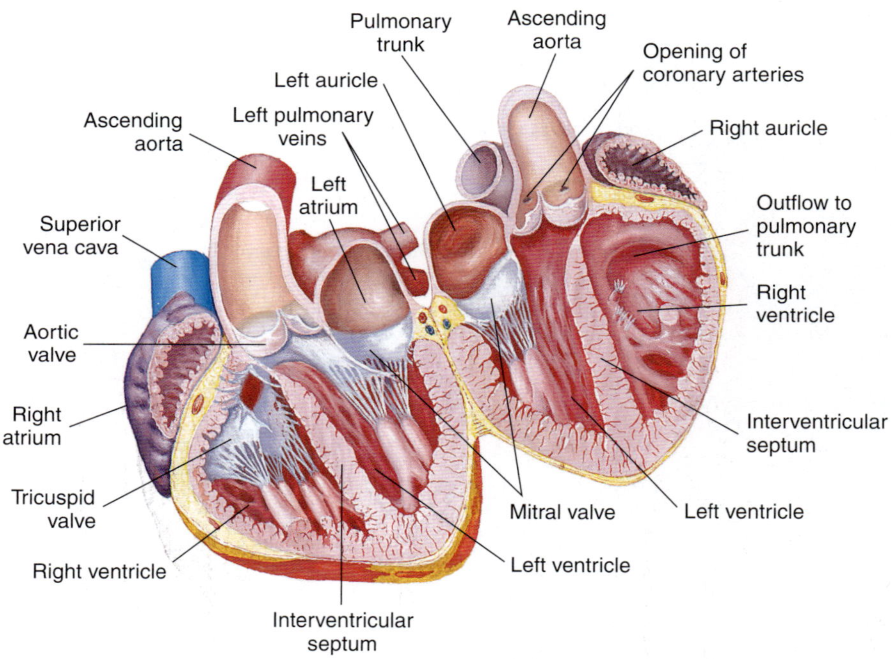

FIG. 15.5 Anterior cross section showing the valves and chambers of the heart.

The four chambers of the heart are connected by two sets of valves: the atrioventricular (AV) and semilunar valves. In a fully formed heart that is free of defect, these are the only intracardiac pathways and permit the flow of blood in only one direction (Fig. 15.5).

The AV valves, situated between the atria and the ventricles, include the tricuspid and mitral valves. The tricuspid valve, which has three cusps (or leaflets), separates the right atrium from the right ventricle. The mitral valve, which has two cusps, separates the left atrium from the left ventricle. When the atria contract (diastole), the AV valves open, allowing blood to flow into the ventricles. When the ventricles contract (systole), these valves snap shut, preventing blood from flowing back into the atria (Fig. 15.6). See Clinical Pearl, "Order of Valves."

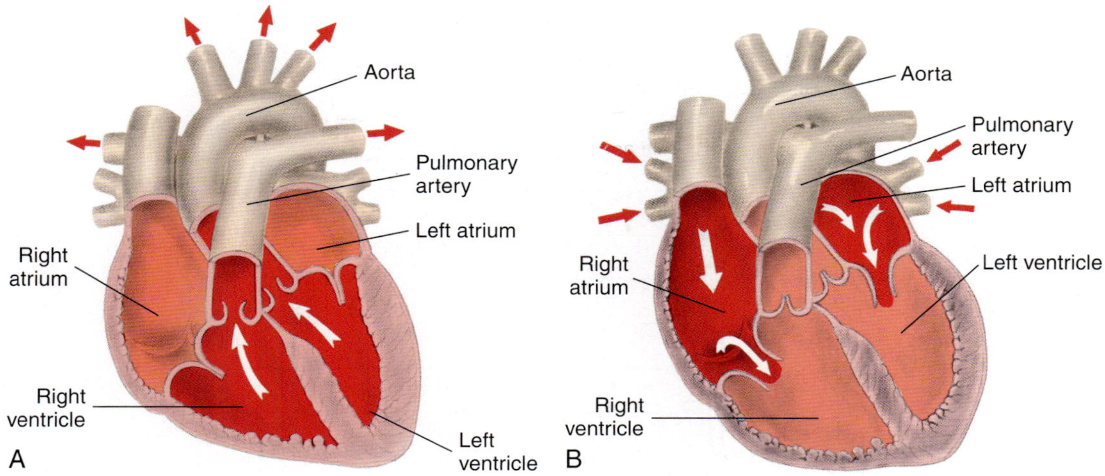

FIG. 15.6 Blood flow through the heart. (A) Systole. (B) Diastole. (From Canobbio, M. M. (1990). *Cardiovascular disorders.* St. Louis: Mosby.)

CLINICAL PEARL

Order of Valves

The order of blood flow through the cardiac valves can be remembered by using the sentence "Try Pulling My Arm" for **t**ricuspid, **p**ulmonic, **m**itral, and **a**ortic.

The two semilunar valves each have three cusps. The pulmonic valve separates the right ventricle from the pulmonary artery. The aortic valve lies between the left ventricle and the aorta. Contraction of the ventricles (systole) opens the semilunar valves, causing blood to rush into the pulmonary artery and aorta. When the ventricles relax (diastole), the valves close, shutting off backward blood flow into the ventricles (see Fig. 15.6).

Cardiac Cycle

The heart contracts and relaxes rhythmically, creating a two-phase cardiac cycle. During systole, the ventricles contract, ejecting blood from the left ventricle into the aorta and simultaneously from the right ventricle into the pulmonary artery. During diastole, the ventricles dilate, drawing blood into the ventricles as the atria contract, moving blood from the atria to the ventricles (see Fig. 15.6). The volume of blood and the pressure under which it is returned to the heart vary with the degree of physical and/or metabolic activity (e.g., with exercise or fever).

As systole begins, ventricular contraction raises the pressure in the ventricles and forces the mitral and tricuspid valves closed, preventing backflow. This valve closure produces the first heart sound (S_1), the characteristic "lub." The intraventricular pressure rises until it exceeds that in the aorta and pulmonary artery. Then the aortic and pulmonic valves are forced open, and ejection of blood into the arteries begins. Valve opening is usually a silent event (Fig. 15.7).

When the ventricles are almost empty, the pressure in them falls below that in the aorta and pulmonary artery, allowing the aortic and pulmonic valves to close. Closure of these valves causes the second heart sound (S_2), the "dub." The second heart sound has two components: A_2 is produced by aortic valve closure, and P_2 is produced by pulmonic valve closure. As ventricular pressure falls below atrial pressure, the mitral and tricuspid valves open to allow the blood collected in the atria to refill the relaxed ventricles. Diastole is a relatively passive interval until ventricular filling is almost complete. This filling sometimes produces a third heart sound (S_3). The S_3 is caused by blood quickly filling the ventricles, causing fluid waves to bounce off the walls and create low-frequency vibrations. It typically occurs about a third of the way into diastole at peak ventricular filling. Then the atria contract to ensure the ejection of any remaining blood. This can sometimes be heard as a fourth heart sound (S_4) in late diastole. An S_4 is caused by the forceful contraction of the left atrium against a stiff left ventricle, causing ventricular distension; see Clinical Pearl, "S_3 and S_4" and Risk Factors, "S_4 Heart Sound." The cycle begins anew, with ventricular contraction and atrial refilling occurring at about the same time. The cardiac cycle continues without resting and constantly adjusts to the variable demands of work, rest, digestion, and illness.

CLINICAL PEARL

S_3 and S_4 Heart Sounds

An S_3 sound is normal in children, young adults, and pregnant persons. An S_4 is hardly ever normal.

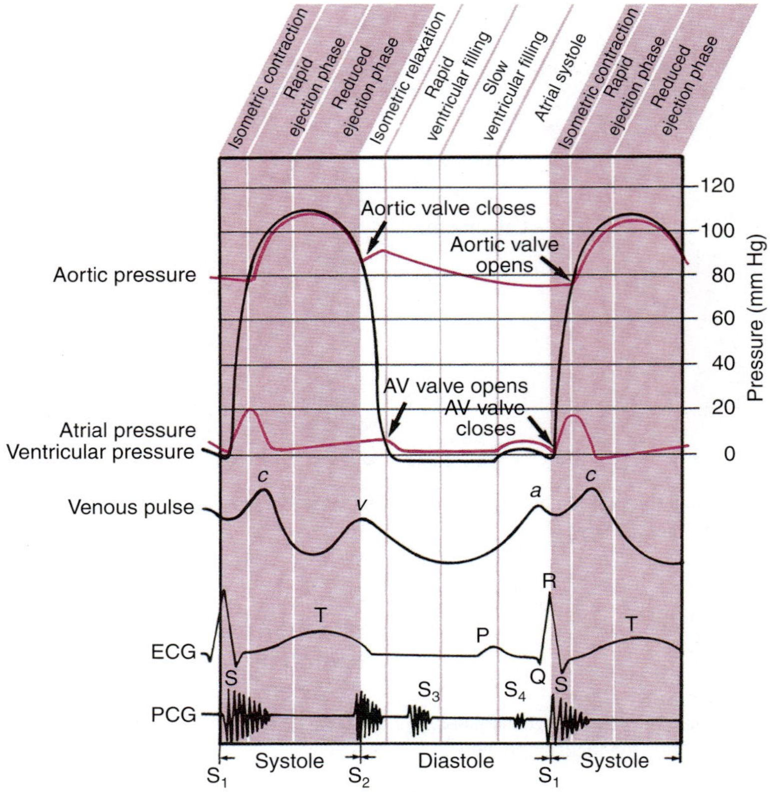

FIG. 15.7 Events of the cardiac cycle, showing venous pressure waves, electrocardiogram (ECG; the graphic representing the electrical activity during the cardiac cycle), and heart sounds in systole and diastole. *PCG,* Phonocardiogram. (Modified from Guzzetta, C. D., & Dossey, B. M. (1992). *Cardiovascular nursing: Holistic practice.* St. Louis: Mosby.)

Risk Factors

An S_4 heart sound is caused by diastolic overload and is associated with the following:

- Stiff left ventricle
- Elevated left ventricular end-diastolic pressure
- Elevated brain natriuretic peptide level
- Chronic hypertension
- Left ventricular cardiomyopathy
- Pulmonary hypertension
- Left ventricular outflow obstruction (e.g., hypertrophic cardiomyopathy)
- Ischemic heart disease

The events of the cardiac cycle are not exactly identical on both sides of the heart. In fact, pressures in the right ventricle, right atrium, and pulmonary artery are lower than in the left side of the heart, and the same events occur slightly later on the right side compared with the left side. The effect is that heart sounds sometimes have two distinct components, the first produced by the left side and the second by the right side. For example, the aortic valve closes slightly before the pulmonic, so that S_2 is often heard as two distinct components, referred to as a *split* S_2 (A_2, then P_2).

Closure of the heart valves during the cardiac cycle produces heart sounds in rapid succession. Although the valves are anatomically close to each other, their sounds are best heard in an area away from the anatomic site because the sound is transmitted in the direction of blood flow (see Fig. 15.15).

Electrical Activity

An intrinsic electrical conduction system enables the heart to contract and coordinates the sequence of muscular contractions taking place during the cardiac cycle. An electrical impulse stimulates each myocardial contraction. The impulse originates in and is paced by the sinoatrial (SA) node, located in the wall of the right atrium. The impulse then travels through both atria to the AV node, located in the atrial septum. In the AV node, the impulse is delayed but then passes down the bundle of His to the Purkinje fibers (heart muscle cells specialized for electrical conduction), located in the ventricular myocardium. Ventricular contraction is initiated at the apex and proceeds toward the base of the heart (Fig. 15.8).

An electrocardiogram (ECG) is a graphic recording of electrical activity during the cardiac cycle. The ECG records electrical current generated by the movement of ions into and out of the myocardial cell membranes.

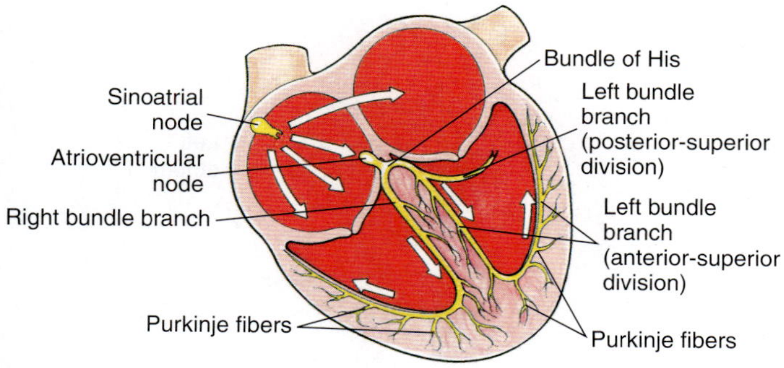

FIG. 15.8 **Cardiac conduction.** (From Canobbio, M. M. (1990). *Cardiovascular disorders.* St. Louis: Mosby.)

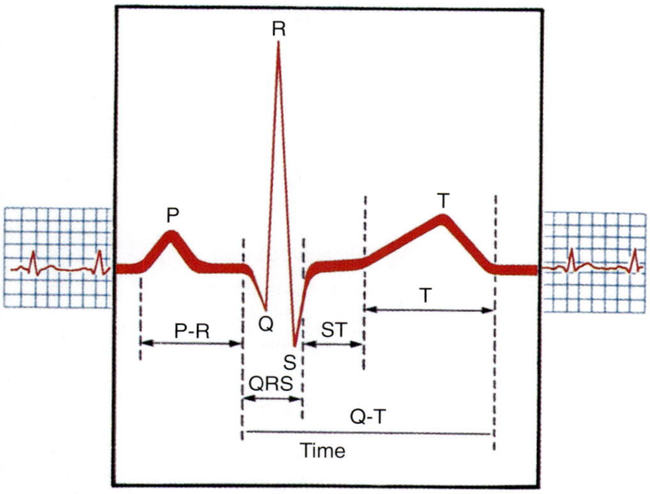

FIG. 15.9 **Usual electrocardiogram waveform.** (From Canobbio, M. M. (1990). *Cardiovascular disorders.* St. Louis: Mosby.)

The ECG records two basic events: depolarization, which is the spread of a stimulus through the heart muscle, and repolarization, which is the return of the stimulated heart muscle to a resting state. The ECG records electrical activity as specific waves (Fig. 15.9):

- P wave—the spread of a stimulus through the atria (atrial depolarization).
- PR interval—the time from initial stimulation of the atria to initial stimulation of the ventricles, usually 0.12 to 0.20 second.
- QRS complex—the spread of a stimulus through the ventricles (ventricular depolarization); normal is less than 0.12 second.
- ST segment and T wave—the return of stimulated ventricular muscle to a resting state (ventricular repolarization).
- U wave—a small deflection rarely seen just after the T wave, thought to be related to repolarization of the Purkinje fibers. This is commonly seen with bradycardia. This is also seen sometimes with electrolyte abnormalities, hypothermia, and hypothyroidism.
- QT interval—the time elapsed from the onset of ventricular depolarization until the completion of ventricular repolarization. The interval varies with the cardiac rate.

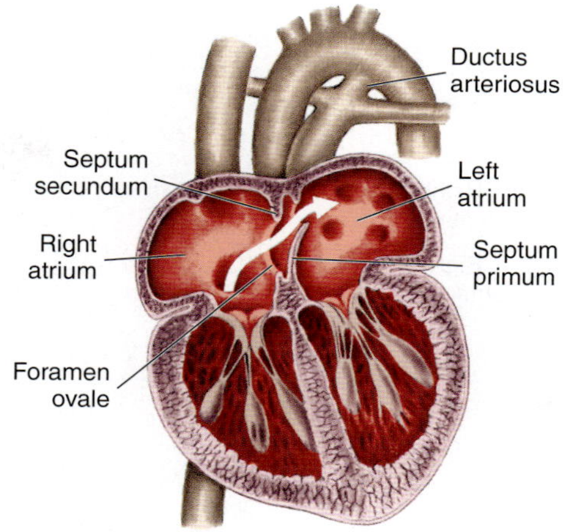

FIG. 15.10 **Anatomy of the fetal heart.** (From Thompson, J. M., et al. (1997). *Mosby's clinical nursing* (4th ed.). St. Louis: Mosby.)

Because the electrical stimulus starts the cycle, it precedes the mechanical response by a brief moment. The sequence of myocardial depolarization results in the events on the left side of the heart to occur slightly before those on the right. When the heart is beating at a rate of 68 to 72 beats/min, ventricular systole is shorter than diastole. As the rate increases to about 120 beats/min, because of stress or pathologic factors, the two phases of the cardiac cycle tend to approximate each other in length.

Infants and Children

Fetal circulation, which includes the umbilical vessels, compensates for the nonfunctional fetal lungs. Blood flows from the right atrium into the left atrium via the foramen ovale (Fig. 15.10). The right ventricle pumps blood through the patent ductus arteriosus rather than into the lungs. The right and left ventricles are equal in weight and muscle mass because they both pump blood into the systemic circulation, unlike the adult heart (Fig. 15.11; see also Fig. 15.10).

The changes at birth include closure of the ductus arteriosus, usually within 24 to 48 hours, and the functional closure of the interatrial foramen ovale as pressure rises in the left atrium. The mass of the left ventricle increases after birth in response to the left ventricle assuming responsibility for systemic circulation. By 1 year of age, the relative sizes of the left and right ventricles approximate the adult ratio of 2:1.

The heart lies more horizontally in the chest in infants and young children compared with adults. As a result, the apex of the heart rides higher, sometimes well into the fourth left intercostal space. In most cases, the adult heart position is reached by age 7 years.

Pregnant Patients

The pregnant patient's blood volume increases 40% to 50% over prepregnancy level. The rise is mainly due to an increase in plasma volume, which begins in the first trimester and reaches a maximum after the 30th week.

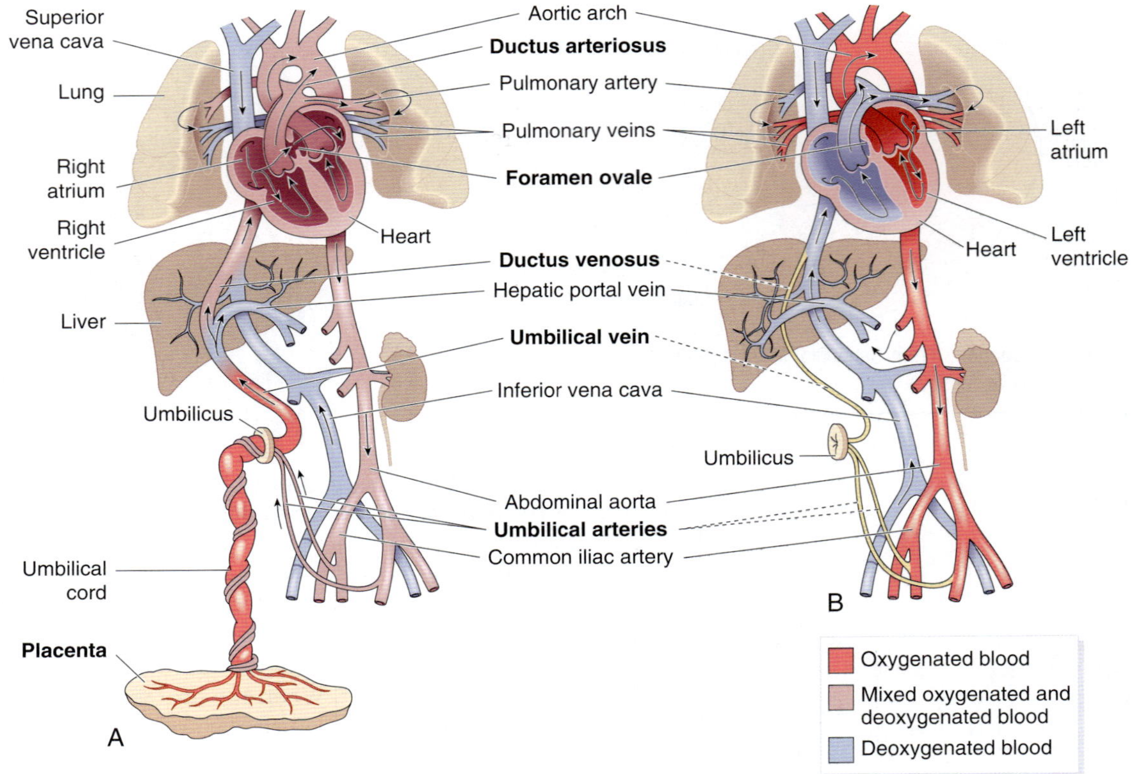

FIG. 15.11 Fetal circulation. (A) In utero. (B) After delivery. (From Waugh, A., & Grant, A. (2011). *Ross and Wilson anatomy and physiology in health and illness* (11th ed.). Elsevier.)

TABLE 15.1 Hemodynamic Changes During Pregnancy

	STAGE				
HEMODYNAMIC VARIABLE	FIRST TRIMESTER	SECOND TRIMESTER	THIRD TRIMESTER	LABOR AND DELIVERY	POSTPARTUM PERIOD
Heart rate	Increased	Peaks at 28th week	Slightly decreased	Increased; bradycardia at delivery	Prepregnancy level within 2–6 weeks
Blood pressure	Prepregnancy level	Slightly decreased	Prepregnancy level	Prepregnancy level	Prepregnancy level
Blood volume	Increased	Peaks at 20th week	Gradually decreased	Rises sharply	Prepregnancy level within 2–6 weeks
Stroke volume	Increased	Peaks at 28th week	Gradually decreased	Decreased	Prepregnancy level within 2–6 weeks
Cardiac output	Increased	Peaks at 20th week	Slightly decreased	Increased	Prepregnancy level within 2–6 weeks
Systemic vascular resistance	Decreased	Decreased	Decreased	Sharply decreased at delivery	Prepregnancy level within 2–6 weeks

On average, plasma volume increases 50% with a single pregnancy and as much as 70% with a twin pregnancy. The heart works harder to accommodate the increased heart rate and stroke volume required for the expanded blood volume. The left ventricle increases in both wall thickness and mass. The blood volume returns to prepregnancy levels within 3 to 4 weeks after delivery (Table 15.1).

The cardiac output increases approximately 30% to 40% over that of the nonpregnant state and reaches its highest level by about 25 to 32 weeks of gestation. This level is maintained until term. Cardiac output returns to prepregnancy levels about 2 weeks after delivery. As the uterus enlarges and the diaphragm moves upward in pregnancy, the position of the heart is shifted toward a horizontal position, with slight axis rotation.

Older Adults

Heart size may decrease with age unless hypertension or heart disease causes enlargement. The left ventricular wall thickens, and the valves tend to fibrose and calcify.

Stroke volume decreases, and cardiac output during exercise declines by 30% to 40%. The endocardium thickens. The myocardium becomes less elastic and more rigid so that recovery of myocardial contractility is delayed. The response to stress and increased oxygen demand is less efficient. Tachycardia is poorly tolerated, and after any type of stress, the return to an expected heart rate takes longer. Despite age-associated changes in heart architecture and contractile properties, the heart continues to function reasonably well at rest. Long-standing hypertensive disease, infarcts, and/or other insults, as well as loss of physical conditioning, may lead to severe compromise of the heart and to significant decline in cardiac output.

Cardiac function can be further compromised by fibrosis and sclerosis in the region of the SA node and in the heart valves (particularly the mitral valve and aortic cusps) and by increased vagal tone. ECG changes occur secondary to cellular alteration, to fibrosis within the conduction system, and to neurogenic changes.

REVIEW OF RELATED HISTORY

For each of the symptoms or conditions discussed in this section, particular topics to include in the history of the present illness are listed. Responses to questions about these topics provide clues for individualizing the physical examination and the development of a diagnostic evaluation for the patient. Questions regarding medication use (prescription and over-the-counter preparations), as well as complementary, alternative, and integrative therapies, are relevant for each area.

History of Present Illness

Chest Pain

See Boxes 15.1 and 15.2.

- Onset and duration: sudden, gradual, or vague onset, length of episode; cyclic nature; relation to physical exertion, rest, emotional experience, eating, coughing, cold temperatures, trauma; awakens from sleep
- Character: aching, sharp, tingling, burning, pressure, stabbing, crushing, or clenched fist (Levine) sign
- Location: radiating down arms, to neck, jaws, teeth, scapula; relief with rest or position change
- Severity: interference with activity, need to stop all activity until it subsides, disrupts sleep, severity on a scale of 0 to 10
- Associated symptoms: anxiety; dyspnea (shortness of breath); diaphoresis (sweating); dizziness; nausea or vomiting; faintness; cold, clammy skin; cyanosis; pallor; swelling or edema (noted anywhere, constant or at certain times during the day)

BOX 15.1 Chest Pain

The presence of chest pain suggests heart disease, and it has many causes. *Angina pectoris* is traditionally described as a pressure or choking sensation, either substernal or into the neck. The discomfort, which can be intense, may radiate to the jaw and down the left (and sometimes the right) arm. It often begins during strenuous physical activity, eating, exposure to intense cold, windy weather, or exposure to emotional stress. Relief may occur in minutes if the activity can be stopped. Signs of angina pectoris may vary in location, intensity, and radiation and often arise from sources other than the heart. In females, it may vary from the classic signs in males. The *precordial catch,* for example, is a sudden, sharp, relatively brief pain that does not radiate; occurs most often at rest; is unrelated to exertion; and may not have a discoverable cause.

Some Possible Causes of Chest Pain

Cardiac
Angina
Acute myocardial infarction
Coronary insufficiency
Myocardial infarction
Nonobstructive, nonspastic angina
Mitral valve prolapse

Aortic
Dissection of the aorta

Pleuropericardial Pain
Pericarditis
Pleurisy
Pneumothorax
Mediastinal emphysema

Gastrointestinal Disease
Hiatus hernia
Reflux esophagitis
Esophageal rupture
Esophageal spasm
Cholecystitis
Peptic ulcer disease
Pancreatitis

Pulmonary Disease
Pulmonary hypertension
Pneumonia
Pulmonary embolus
Bronchial hyperreactivity
Tension pneumothorax

Musculoskeletal
Cervical radiculopathy
Shoulder disorder or dysfunction (e.g., arthritis, bursitis, rotator cuff injury, biceps tendonitis)
Costochondral disorder
Xiphodynia

Psychoneurotic
Illicit drug use (e.g., cocaine)
Herpes zoster: when lesions occur in thoracic region

Unlike in adults, chest pain in children and adolescents is seldom due to a cardiac problem. It is often difficult to find a cause, but trauma, exercise-induced asthma, and, even in a somewhat younger child, the use of cocaine should be among the considerations.

BOX 15.2 Characteristics of Chest Pain

TYPE	CHARACTERISTICS
Cardiac	Substernal; provoked by effort, emotion, eating; relieved by rest and/or nitroglycerin; often accompanied by diaphoresis, occasionally by nausea
Pleural	Precipitated by breathing or coughing; usually described as sharp; present during respiration; absent when breath held
Esophageal	Burning, substernal, occasional radiation to the shoulder; nocturnal occurrence, usually when lying flat; relief with food, antacids, sometimes nitroglycerin
From a peptic ulcer	Almost always infradiaphragmatic and epigastric; nocturnal occurrence and daytime attacks relieved by food; unrelated to activity
Biliary	Usually under right scapula, prolonged in duration; often occurring after eating; will trigger angina more often than mimic it
Arthritis/bursitis	Usually lasts for hours; local tenderness and/or pain with movement
Cervical	Associated with injury; provoked by activity, persists after activity; painful on palpation and/or movement
Musculoskeletal (chest)	Intensified or provoked by movement, particularly twisting or costochondral bending; long-lasting; often associated with focal tenderness
Psychoneurotic	Associated with/after anxiety; poorly described; located in intramammary region

- Treatment: rest, position change, exercise, nitroglycerin
- Medications: digoxin, diuretics, aspirin, H2 blockers, proton pump inhibitors, beta-blockers, angiotensin-converting enzyme (ACE) inhibitors, calcium channel blockers, ranolazine, statins, nonsteroidal antiinflammatory drugs, nitrates, thrombolytics, or antihypertensive medications

Past Medical History

- Cardiac surgery or hospitalization for cardiac evaluation or disorder
- Congenital heart disease
- Rhythm disorder
- Acute rheumatic fever, characterized by unexplained fever, swollen joints, Sydenham chorea (St. Vitus dance), abdominal pain, skin rash (erythema marginatum), or nodules
- Kawasaki disease (see Chapter 16)
- Chronic illness: hypertension, bleeding disorder, hyperlipidemia, diabetes, thyroid dysfunction, coronary artery disease, obesity
- Viral-induced cardiomyopathy: coxsackie, parvovirus B19, adenovirus, echovirus, influenza, cytomegalovirus, SARS-CoV-2, Epstein-Barr virus, herpes simplex virus, human immunodeficiency virus, measles

Family History

- Long QT syndrome, Brugada syndrome, or Wolff-Parkinson-White syndrome
- Marfan syndrome (a genetic disorder of the connective tissue associated with mitral valve prolapse/regurgitation, aortic regurgitation, aortic dilatation, aneurysms, and

DIFFERENTIAL DIAGNOSIS

Comparison of Some Origins of Chest Pain

CARDIAC	MUSCULOSKELETAL	GASTROINTESTINAL
Presence of cardiac risk factors	History of trauma	History of indigestion
Specifically noted time of onset	Vague onset	Vague onset
Related to physical effort or emotional	Related to physical effort	Related to food consumption or psychosocial stress
Disappears if stimulating cause can be terminated	Continues after cessation of effort	May go on for several hours; unrelated to effort
Commonly forces patients to stop effort	Patients often can continue activity	Patients often can continue activity
Patient may awaken from sleep	Delays falling asleep	Patient may awaken from sleep, particularly during early morning
Relief at times with nitroglycerin	Relief at times with heat, nonsteroidal antiinflammatory drugs, or rest	Relief at times with antacids
Pain often in early morning or after washing and eating	Worse in evening after a day of physical effort	No particular relationship to time of day; related to food, tension
Greater likelihood in cold weather	Greater likelihood in cold, damp weather	Anytime

dissection) or Loeys-Dietz syndrome (a genetic disorder that affects connective tissue and can cause aneurysms, particularly of the aortic root)
- Diabetes
- Familial cardiac amyloidosis
- Heart disease
- Hypertrophic cardiomyopathy, dilated cardiomyopathy, or arrhythmogenic cardiomyopathy
- Dyslipidemia
- Hypertension
- Obesity
- Congenital heart disease: once it occurs in a family, the likelihood of its recurring increases
- Family members with risk factor: morbidity, mortality related to cardiovascular system; ages at time of illness or death; sudden death, particularly in young and middle-aged relatives

Risk Factors

Cardiac Disease

- Sex (males more at risk than females; female risk is increased in the postmenopausal years and with oral contraceptive use)
- Hyperlipidemia
- Hypertension
- Elevated homocysteine, C-reactive protein, or lipoprotein (a) level
- Tobacco use
- Family history of cardiovascular disease, diabetes, hyperlipidemia, hypertension, or sudden death in young adults
- Diabetes mellitus
- Alcohol use disorder
- Obesity: dietary habits, including an excessively fatty diet
- Obstructive sleep apnea
- Sedentary lifestyle without exercise
- Symptoms associated with cardiac disease
- Fatigue: unusual or persistent, inability to keep up with contemporaries, inability to maintain usual activities, earlier bedtime
- Associated symptoms: dyspnea on exertion, chest pain, palpitations, orthopnea (shortness of breath [dyspnea] when lying flat), paroxysmal nocturnal dyspnea (dyspnea that awakens the patient from sleep), anorexia, nausea, vomiting
- Cough:
  - Onset and duration
  - Character: dry, wet, nighttime, aggravated by lying down
  - Medications: ACE inhibitors
- Difficulty breathing (dyspnea, orthopnea)
- Worsening or remaining stable
- At rest or aggravated by exertion (How much?; Box 15.3); on level ground, climbing stairs
- Position: lying down or eased by resting on pillows (How many? or Sleep in a recliner?)
- Paroxysmal nocturnal dyspnea (recurring attacks of shortness of breath that wake the patient up at night gasping for air, coughing, wheezing, and feeling like they are suffocating)
- Loss of consciousness (transient syncope)
- Associated symptoms: palpitation, dysrhythmia
- When occurs: unusual exertion, sudden turning of neck (carotid sinus effect), looking upward (vertebral artery occlusion), change in posture

BOX 15.3 Physical Activity Recommendations and Exercise Intensity

Recommendations for Adults

- 150 minutes of moderate exercise or 75 minutes of vigorous exercise every week
  - Increase amount and intensity of physical activity gradually over time
  - Even more benefit is gained by being active 300 minutes (5 hours) every week
- Moderate- to high-intensity muscle strengthening (resistance or weights) twice weekly
- Spend less time sitting; high-intensity activity can offset some of the risks of being sedentary

Recommendations for Children

- Children 3 to 5 years old should be physically active and have opportunities to move throughout the day
- Children 6 to 17 years old should get at least 60 minutes of moderate to vigorous exercise daily
  - Exercise should be vigorous at least 3 days per week
  - Increase amount and intensity of physical activity gradually over time
- Muscle and bone strengthening (weight-bearing) activity should be at least 3 days per week

Exercise Intensity

Light: walking 10 to 15 steps, preparing a simple meal for one, retrieving a newspaper from just outside the door, pulling down a bedspread, brushing teeth

Moderate: making the bed, dusting and sweeping, walking a level short block, office filing, walking 2.5 miles per hour, biking slower than 10 miles per hour

Moderately vigorous: climbing one or two flights of stairs, lifting full cartons, long walks, sexual intercourse

Vigorous: jogging, vigorous athletics of any kind, cleaning the entire house in less than a day, raking a large number of leaves, mowing a large lawn with a hand mower, shoveling deep snow, biking more than 10 miles per hour

Adapted from U.S. Department of Health and Human Services. (2008). *Physical activity guidelines for Americans.* http://www.health.gov/paguidelines/default.aspx; American Heart Association (2024). *American Heart Association recommendations for physical activity in adults and kids,* https://www.heart.org/en/healthy-living/fitness/fitness-basics/aha-recs-for-physical-activity-in-adults

Personal and Social History

- Employment: physical demands; environmental hazards such as heat, chemicals, dust; sources of emotional stress
- Tobacco use: type (cigarettes, e-cigarettes, cigars, pipe, chewing tobacco), duration of use, amount, age started and stopped; pack-years (number of years smoking times number of packs per day)
- Nutritional status
- Usual diet: proportion of fat, use of salt, food preferences, history of dieting, caffeine intake
- Weight: loss or gain, amount and rate
- Alcohol consumption: amount, frequency, duration of current intake
- Known hypercholesterolemia and/or elevated triglycerides (see Risk Factors, “Cardiac Disease”)
- Relaxation/hobbies

- Exercise: type, amount, frequency, intensity (see Box 15.3)
- Substance use disorder: amyl nitrate, cocaine, injection drug use

Infants

- Tiring easily and/or sweating with feeding
- Breathing changes: more heavily or more rapidly than expected during feeding or defecation
- Cyanosis: perioral during eating, more widespread and more persistent, related to crying
- Excessive weight gain compared with caloric intake or poor growth
- Maternal health during pregnancy: medications taken, gestational diabetes, unexplained fever, illicit drug use

Children and Adolescents

- Tiring during play: amount of time before tiring, activities that are tiring, inability to keep up with other children
- Naps: longer than expected
- Knee-chest position or squatting after shortness of breath
- Headaches
- Nosebleeds
- Unexplained joint pain
- Height and weight gain (and any substantiating records)
- Change in physical and cognitive development (and any substantiating records)
- Palpitations
- Fatigue
- History of surgical repair of congenital heart disease

Pregnant Patients

- History of cardiac disease or surgery
- Dizziness or syncope or near-syncope on standing
- Indications of heart disease during pregnancy, including progressive or severe dyspnea, progressive orthopnea, paroxysmal nocturnal dyspnea, hemoptysis, syncope with exertion, and chest pain related to effort or emotion

Older Adults

- Common symptoms of cardiovascular disorders: confusion, dizziness, blackouts, syncope, palpitations, coughs and wheezes, hemoptysis, shortness of breath, chest pains or chest tightness, erectile dysfunction, fatigue, leg edema: pattern, frequency, time of day most pronounced
- If heart disease has been diagnosed: drug reactions; potassium excess (weakness, bradycardia, hypotension, confusion); potassium depletion (weakness, fatigue, muscle cramps, dysrhythmias); digitalis toxicity (anorexia, nausea, vomiting, diarrhea, headache, confusion, dysrhythmias, halo, yellow vision); interference with activities of daily living; ability of the patient and family to cope with the condition, perceived and actual; orthostatic hypotension

Think About It

Autonomic Failure Versus Hypovolemia

Transitioning from sitting to standing causes a decrease in venous return to the heart leading to decreased blood pressure. Normally this leads to a compensatory reflex, the baroreceptor reflex, resulting in a small decrease in systolic blood pressure, increase in diastolic blood pressure, and increase in heart rate. Orthostatic hypotension (reduction in blood pressure with standing) is common in older persons in part due to an impaired baroreceptor reflex. The absence of the reflex-induced increased heart rate as blood pressure falls is a physical examination sign indicating autonomic failure. This is in contrast with hypovolemia in which there is a compensatory increase in heart rate as blood pressure falls.

Patient Safety

Importance of a Healthy Lifestyle

Elevated serum cholesterol is a potent risk factor for myocardial infarction. Hyperlipidemia is one of the most common metabolic diseases because of the increasing obesity epidemic. The Centers for Disease Control and Prevention (CDC) recommends that children have their cholesterol checked between ages 9 and 11 years and again between 17 and 21 years (https://www.cdc.gov/cholesterol/testing/index.html).

- Adults 21 years or older with low-density lipoprotein (LDL) 190 mg/dL or greater or with known atherosclerotic cardiovascular disease (ASCVD) should be treated with high-intensity statin therapy unless contraindicated.
- Individuals with LDL 190 mg/dL or greater or triglycerides 500 mg/dL or greater should be evaluated for secondary causes of hyperlipidemia.
- Adults with an LDL 70 to 189 mg/dL and adults aged 40 to 75 years with diabetes or a 10-year ASCVD risk greater than 7.5% should be treated with moderate- to high-intensity statin therapy.

Use some of the time during the cardiac examination to remind the patient of the importance of healthy lifestyle in maintaining good cardiac health:

- Enjoy a diet that emphasizes vegetables, fruits, nuts, whole grains, lean vegetable or animal protein, and fish and also minimizes the intake of trans fats, red meat and processed red meats, refined carbohydrates, and sweetened beverages. If indicated, consider referral to a nutritionist.
- Exercise regularly with a goal of 150 minutes/week of moderate-intensity or 75 minutes/week of vigorous-intensity physical activity. Include resistance exercise in the plan.
- Cease smoking and avoid secondhand smoke. Various behavioral programs and medications can assist.
- Monitor blood pressure, blood glucose, inflammatory markers, and lipids annually.

Adapted from Arnett, D. K., Blumenthal, R. S., Albert, M. A., et al. (2019). 2019 ACC/AHA guideline on the primary prevention of cardiovascular disease: A report of the American College of Cardiology/American Heart Association Task Force on Clinical Practice Guidelines. *Circulation*, 2019;140, e596–e646.

EXAMINATION AND FINDINGS

Equipment

- Stethoscope
- Marking pencil
- Centimeter ruler

The examination of the heart includes the following: inspection, palpation, and percussion of the chest and then auscultation of the heart. Performing a successful examination requires a competence of each procedure and an ability to integrate and interpret the findings in relation to the cardiac events they reflect.

Findings from examinations of other body systems have a significant impact on judgments made about the cardiovascular system. For example, crackles auscultated in the lungs, palpation of an enlarged liver, and observation of peripheral edema are signs of heart failure. Examples of other influencing factors may include the following:

- Effect of a barrel chest or pectus deformity
- Xanthelasma (yellowish deposit of fat underneath the skin)
- Funduscopic changes of hypertension
- Ascites, pitting edema, or elevated jugular venous pulse
- Abdominal arterial bruit

In assessing cardiac function, it is a common error to auscultate the heart first. It is important to follow the proper sequence, beginning with inspection and proceeding to palpation, percussion, and performing auscultation last. Use a tangential light source to inspect the chest, allowing shadows to accent the surface flicker of any underlying cardiac movement. The room should be quiet because subtle, low-pitched sounds are hard to hear. Stand to the patient's right, at least at the start. A thorough examination of the heart requires the patient to assume a variety of positions: sitting erect and leaning forward, lying supine, and left lateral recumbent position. These changes in position mandate a comfortable examining table on which movement is easy. Large breasts can make examination difficult. Either the examiner or the patient can move the left breast up and to the left.

Inspection

In most adults the apical impulse is visible at about the midclavicular line in the fifth left intercostal space, but it is easily obscured by obesity, large breasts, or muscularity. In some patients it may be visible in the fourth left intercostal space. It should be seen in only one intercostal space if the heart is healthy. In some adults the apical impulse may become visible only when the patient sits up, bringing the heart closer to the anterior wall.

Examination findings are affected by the shape and thickness of the chest wall and the amount of tissue, air, and fluid through which the impulses are transmitted. For example, a readily visible and palpable impulse when the patient is supine suggests an intensity that may be the result of a problem. The absence of an apical impulse in addition to faint heart sounds, particularly when the patient is in the left lateral recumbent position, suggests some intervening extracardiac problem, such as pleural or pericardial fluid.

Inspection of other organs may reflect important information about the cardiac status. For example, inspecting the skin for cyanosis or venous distention and inspecting the nail bed for cyanosis and capillary refill time provide valuable clues to the cardiac evaluation.

Palpation

With warmed hands and the patient supine, palpate the precordium. Use the proximal halves of the four fingers held gently together or use the whole hand. Touch lightly and let the cardiac movements rise to your hand because sensation decreases as you increase pressure.

As always, be methodical. One suggested sequence is to begin at the apex, move to the inferior left sternal border, then move up the sternum to the base and down the right sternal border and into the epigastrium or axillae if the circumstance dictates (Fig. 15.12).

Feel for the apical impulse and identify its location by the intercostal space and the distance from the midsternal line. The point at which the apical impulse is most readily seen or felt should be described as the point of maximal impulse (PMI). The PMI is typically noted at the left fifth intercostal space, midclavicular line in adults, and fourth intercostal space medial to the nipple in children. Determine the diameter of the area in which it is felt. Usually it is palpable within a small diameter—no more than 1 cm. The impulse is usually gentle and brief, not lasting as long as systole. In some adults, the apical impulse is not felt because of the thickness of the chest wall (Fig. 15.13).

If the apical impulse is more vigorous than expected, characterize it as a "heave" or "lift." An apical impulse that is more forceful and widely distributed, fills systole, or is displaced laterally and downward may indicate increased cardiac output or left ventricular hypertrophy. A lift along the left sternal border may be caused by right ventricular hypertrophy. A loss of thrust may be related to overlying fluid or air or to displacement beneath the sternum. Displacement of the apical impulse to the right without a loss or gain in thrust suggests dextrocardia, diaphragmatic hernia, distended stomach, or a pulmonary abnormality.

Feel for a thrill—a fine, palpable, rushing vibration—a palpable murmur—often, but not always, over the base of the heart in the area of the right or left second intercostal space. It generally indicates turbulence or a disruption of the expected blood flow related to some defect in the closure of the aortic or pulmonic valve (generally aortic or pulmonic stenosis), pulmonary hypertension, or atrial septal defect (Box 15.4). Locate each sensation in terms of its intercostal space and relationship to the midsternal, midclavicular, or axillary lines. Chapter 14 describes the method for counting ribs and intercostal spaces.

While palpating the precordium, use your other hand to palpate the carotid artery so that you can describe the finding in relation to the cardiac cycle. The carotid pulse and S_1 are practically synchronous. The carotid pulse is located just medial to and below the angle of the jaw (Fig. 15.14).

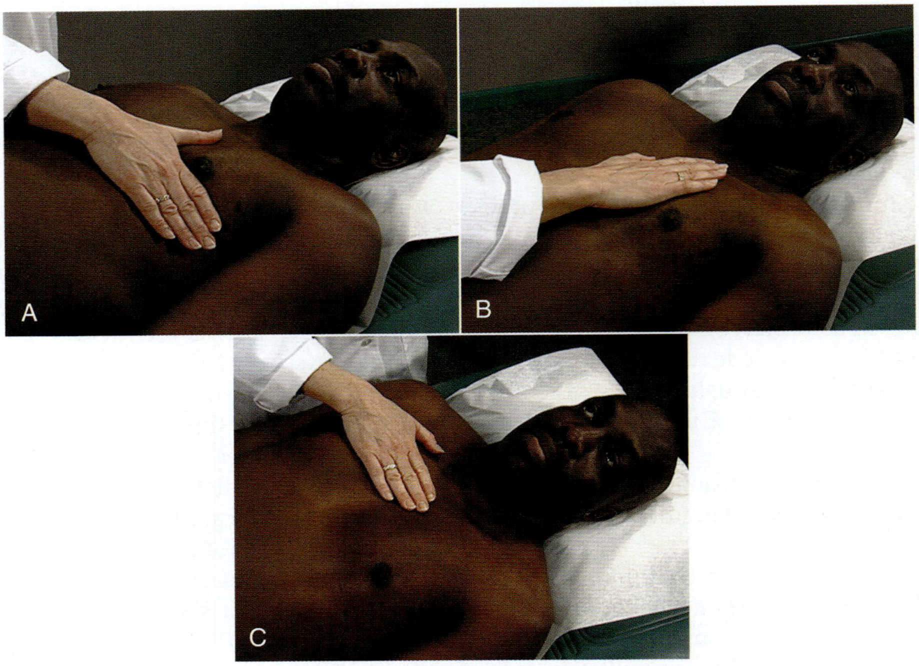

FIG. 15.12 **Sequence for palpation of the precordium.** (A) Apex. (B) Left sternal border. (C) Base.

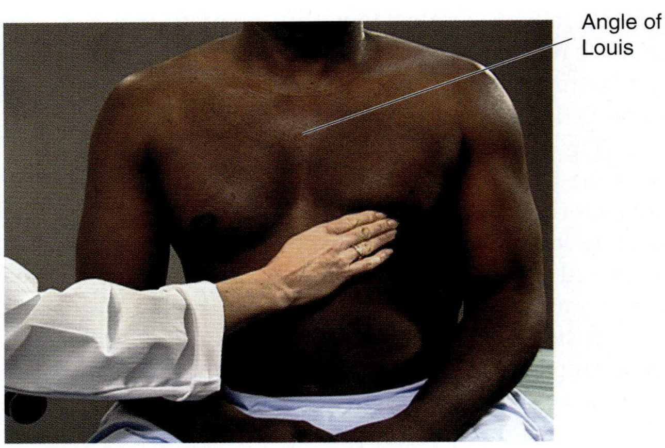

FIG. 15.13 **Palpation of the apical pulse.**

Percussion

Percussion is of limited value in defining the borders of the heart or determining its size because the shape of the chest is relatively rigid and can make the more malleable heart conform. Left ventricular size is better judged by the location of the apical impulse. The right ventricle tends to enlarge in the anteroposterior diameter rather than laterally, thus diminishing the value of percussion of the right heart border. Obesity, unusual muscular development, and some pathologic conditions (e.g., presence of air or fluids) can also easily distort the findings. A chest radiograph is far more useful in defining the heart borders.

If radiographic facilities are unavailable, percussion can be used to estimate the size of the heart. Begin tapping at the anterior axillary line, moving medially along the intercostal spaces toward the sternal border. The change from a resonant to a dull note marks the cardiac border. Note these points with a marking pen, and the outline of the heart is visually defined. On the left, the loss of resonance will generally be close to the PMI at the apex of the heart. Measure this point from the midsternal line at each intercostal space and record that distance. When percussing the right cardiac border, a change in resonance is usually

BOX 15.4 The Thrill of Heart Examination

A murmur at the grade IV level or more can be felt (see Tables 15.4 and 15.5). This palpable sensation is called a *thrill.* It may be appreciated in systole or diastole. The following are common.

TIMING	LOCATION	PROBABLE CAUSE
Systole	Suprasternal notch and/or second and third right intercostal space	Aortic stenosis
	Suprasternal notch and/or second and third left intercostal space	Pulmonic stenosis
	Fourth left intercostal space	Ventricular septal defect
	Apex	Mitral regurgitation
	Left lower sternal border	Tetralogy of Fallot
	Left upper sternal border, often with extensive radiation	Patent ductus arteriosus
Diastole	Right sternal border	Aortic regurgitation
		Aneurysm of ascending aorta
	Apex	Mitral stenosis

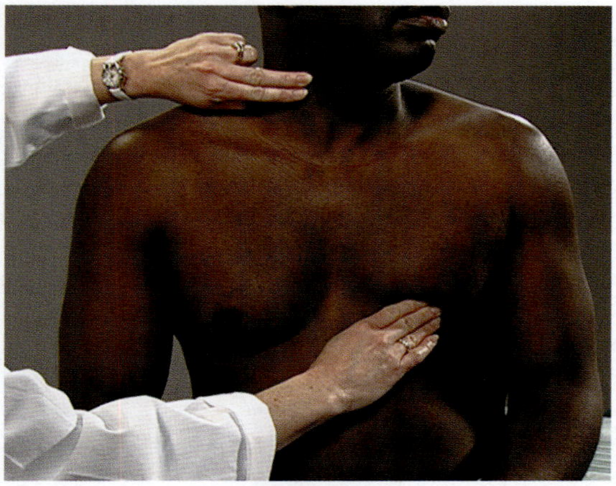

FIG. 15.14 Palpation of the carotid artery to time events felt over the precordium.

noted when the right sternal border is encountered. The right heart border is only found if it extends beyond the sternal border.

Auscultation

Because all heart sounds are of relatively low frequency in a range somewhat difficult for the human ear to detect, you must ensure a quiet environment. Because shivering and movement increase adventitious sound and because comfort is important, make certain the patient is warm and relaxed before beginning. Always place a comfortably warm stethoscope on the unclothed chest. You must also learn to appreciate the differences in findings when the chest is thin and nonmuscular (i.e., sounds are louder, closer), muscular, or obese (i.e., sounds are dimmer, more distant).

Because sound is transmitted in the direction of blood flow, specific heart sounds are best heard in areas where the blood flows after it passes through a valve (see Clinical Pearl, "Heart Sounds"). Approach each of the precordial areas systematically in a sequence that is comfortable for you, working your way from base to apex or apex to base (Box 15.5). Because the site of the apex of the heart may be changed by elevation of the diaphragm from pregnancy, ascites, or another intra-abdominal condition, many health care providers prefer to begin their examination at the base of the heart.

CLINICAL PEARL

Heart Sounds

It is a common error to try to hear all of the sounds in the cardiac cycle at once. Take the time to isolate each sound and each pause in the cardiac cycle, listening separately and selectively for as many beats as necessary to evaluate the sounds. It takes time to tune in; do not rush. Avoid jumping the stethoscope from one site to another; instead, inch the endpiece along the route. This maneuver helps prevent missing important sounds, such as more widely transmitted abnormal sounds. It also allows you to track a sound from its loudest point to its farthest reach (e.g., into the axilla or the back).

Auscultation should be performed in, but not be limited to, each of the five cardiac areas, using first the diaphragm and then the bell of the stethoscope. Use firm pressure with the diaphragm (best for higher-frequency sounds) and light pressure with the bell (best with low-frequency sounds). The five traditional auscultatory areas are located as follows (Fig. 15.15):

- Aortic valve area: second right intercostal space at the right sternal border
- Pulmonic valve area: second left intercostal space at the left sternal border
- Second pulmonic area: third left intercostal space at the left sternal border

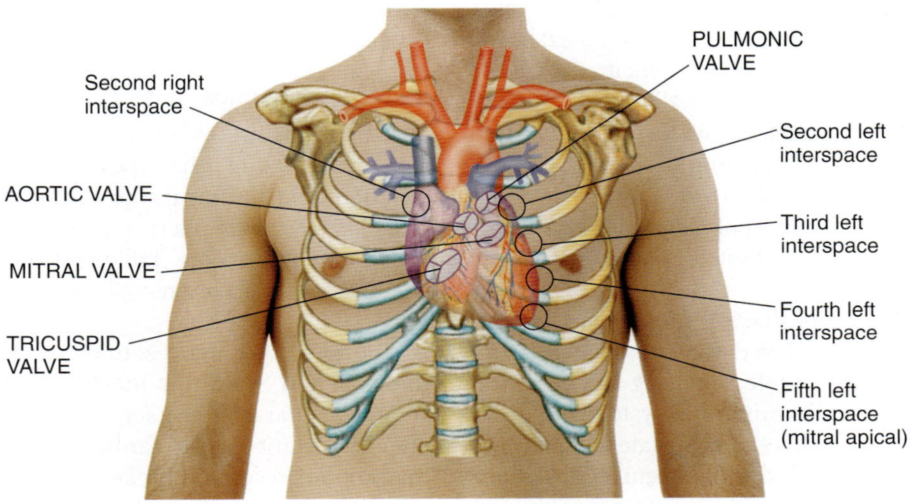

FIG. 15.15 Areas for auscultation of the heart.

HEART

BOX 15.5 Procedure for Auscultating the Heart

Adopt a routine for the various positions the patient is asked to assume for auscultating the heart; however, be prepared to alter the sequence if the patient's condition requires it. Instruct the patient when to breathe comfortably and when to hold the breath in expiration and inspiration. Listen carefully for each heart sound, isolating each component of the cardiac cycle, especially while the respirations are momentarily suspended. The following sequence is suggested:

Patient sitting up and leaning slightly forward and, preferably, in expiration: listen in all five areas (Fig. 15.16A). This is the best position to hear relatively high-pitched murmurs with the stethoscope diaphragm.

Patient supine: listen in all five areas (see Fig. 15.16B).

Patient left lateral recumbent: listen in all five areas. This is the best position to hear the low-pitched filling sounds in diastole with the stethoscope bell (see Fig. 15.16C).

Other positions depend on your findings. Having the patient in the right lateral recumbent position is the best for evaluating a right rotated heart of dextrocardia. Listen in all five areas.

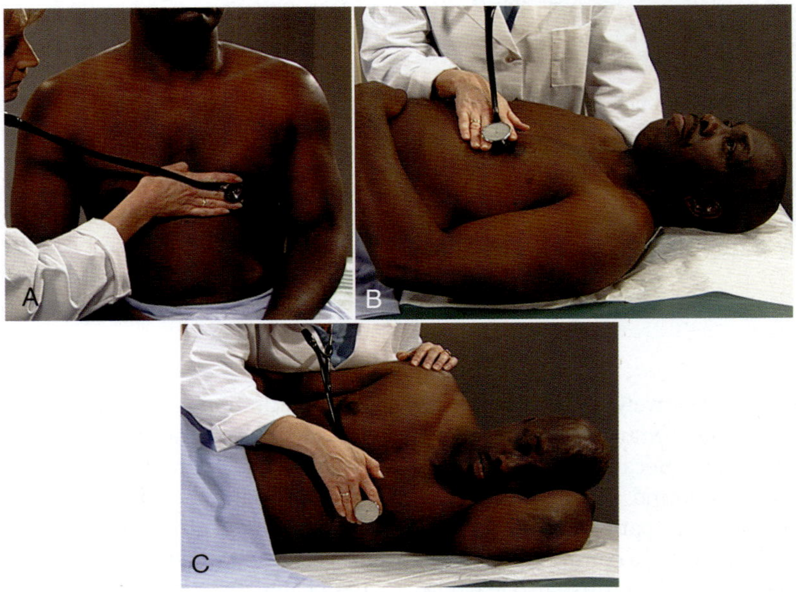

FIG. 15.16 Auscultation positions.

- Tricuspid area: fourth left intercostal space along the lower left sternal border
- Mitral (or apical) area: at the apex of the heart in the fifth left intercostal space at the midclavicular line

Assess the rate and rhythm of the heart at one auscultatory site where the tones are easily heard. Note that site. If the cardiac rhythm is irregular, compare the apical heart rate with the radial pulse rate. Note any deficit.

Instruct the patient to breathe normally and then hold the breath in expiration. Listen for S_1 while you palpate the carotid pulse. S_1 marks the beginning of systole. It coincides with the rise (upswing) of the carotid pulse. Note the intensity, any variations, the effect of respirations, and any splitting of S_1. Concentrate on systole, listening for any extra sounds or murmurs.

S_2 marks the initiation of diastole and closure of the aortic and pulmonic valves. Concentrate on diastole, usually a longer interval than systole, listening for any extra sounds or murmurs. Keep in mind that systole and diastole are equal in duration when the heart rate is rapid.

Instruct the patient to inhale deeply, listening closely for S_2 to become two components (split S_2) during inspiration. Split S_2 is best heard in the pulmonic auscultatory area.

Areas for inspection, palpation, and auscultation change if the heart is not located in its expected place in the left mediastinum. In situs inversus and dextrocardia, the heart is rotated to the right. In such a circumstance, adjust to the anatomic alteration by thinking of the examination sites as they would be in a mirror image of the expected location.

Basic Heart Sounds

Heart sounds are characterized in much the same way as respiratory and other body sounds: by pitch, intensity, duration, and timing in the cardiac cycle. Heart sounds are relatively low in pitch except in the presence of significant pathologic events. Table 15.2 summarizes their relative differences in intensity by auscultatory area (also see Fig. 15.19).

The four basic heart sounds are S_1, S_2, S_3, and S_4. Of these, S_1 and S_2 are the most distinct heart sounds and should be characterized separately because variations can offer important clues to cardiac function. S_3 and S_4 may or may not be present. Their absence is not an unusual finding. Thus evaluate S_3 and S_4 in relation to other sounds and events in the cardiac cycle.

TABLE 15.2 Intensity of Heart Sounds According to Auscultatory Area

	AORTIC	PUL-MONIC	SECOND PULMONIC	MITRAL	TRI-CUSPID
Pitch	$S_1 < S_2$	$S_1 < S_2$	$S_1 < S_2$	$S_1 > S_2$	$S_1 = S_2$
Loudness	$S_1 < S_2$	$S_1 < S_2$	$S_1 < S_2$[a]	$S_1 > S_2$[b]	$S_1 > S_2$
Duration	$S_1 > S_2$	$S_1 > S_2$	$S_1 > S_2$	$S_1 > S_2$	$S_1 > S_2$
S_2 split	Increased with inhalation in all auscultatory areas; the S_2 split may not be audible in the mitral area if P_2 is inaudible				
	Decreased with exhalation in all auscultatory areas				
A_2	Loudest	Loud	Decreased		
P_2	Decreased	Louder	Loudest		

[a]S_1 is relatively louder in the second pulmonic area than in the aortic area.
[b]S_1 may be louder in the mitral area than in the tricuspid area.

BOX 15.6 S_1 Intensity: Diagnostic Clues

When systole begins with the mitral valve open, the valve snaps shut more vigorously, producing a louder S_1. This occurs in the following situations:

- Blood velocity is increased (e.g., with anemia, fever, hyperthyroidism, anxiety, and during exercise).
- The mitral valve is stenotic.

If the mitral valve is not completely open, ventricular contraction forces it shut. The loudness produced by valve closure depends on the degree of opening:

- S_1 intensity is increased in the following situations:
  - Complete heart block is present.
  - Gross disruption of rhythm occurs, such as during fibrillation.
- The intensity of S_1 is decreased in the following situations:
  - Increased overlying tissue, fat, or fluid (e.g., as in emphysema, obesity, or pericardial fluid) obscures sounds.
  - Systemic or pulmonary hypertension is present, which contributes to more forceful atrial contraction. If the ventricle is noncompliant, the contraction may be delayed or diminished, especially if the valve is partially closed when contraction begins.
  - Fibrosis and calcification of a diseased mitral valve can result from rheumatic heart disease. Calcification diminishes valve flexibility so that it closes with less force.

S_1 and S_2. S_1, which results from closure of the mitral and tricuspid (AV) valves, indicates the beginning of systole. It is best heard toward the apex, where it is usually louder than S_2 (Box 15.6). At the base, S_1 is louder on the left than on the right but softer than S_2 in both areas. It is lower in pitch and a bit longer than S_2, and it occurs immediately after diastole (Fig. 15.17).

Although there is some asynchrony between closure of the mitral and tricuspid valves, S_1 is usually heard as one sound. If the asynchrony is more marked than usual, the sound may be split and is best heard in the tricuspid area. Other variations in S_1 depend on the competence of the pulmonary and systemic circulations, the structure of the heart valves, their position when ventricular contraction begins, and the force of the contraction.

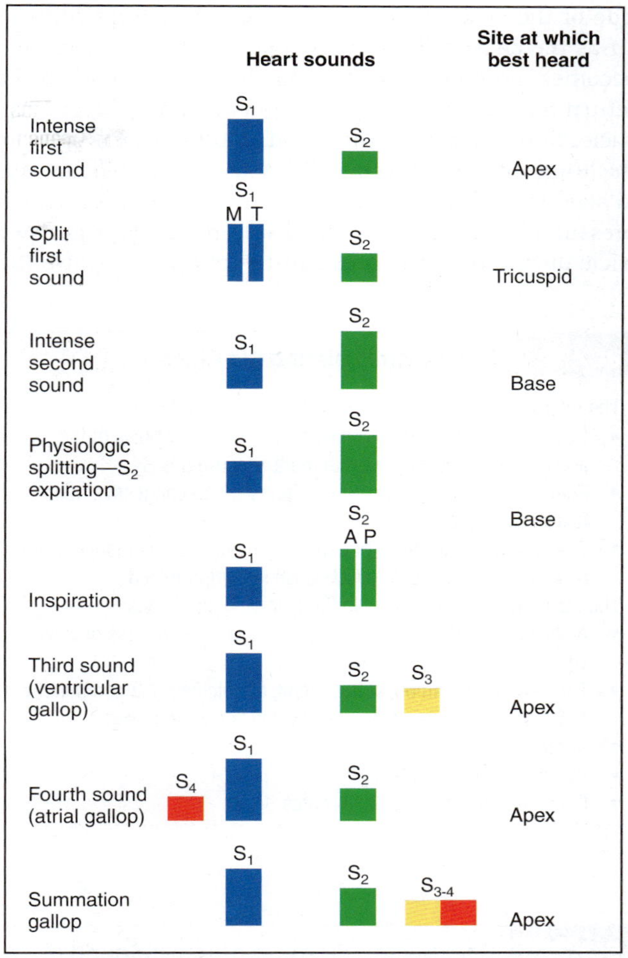

FIG. 15.17 **Heart sounds.** (Modified from Guzzetta, C. D., & Dossey, B. M. (1992). *Cardiovascular nursing: Holistic practice.* St. Louis: Mosby.)

S_2, the result of closure of the aortic and pulmonic (semilunar) valves, indicates the end of systole and is best heard in the aortic and pulmonic areas. It is of higher pitch and shorter duration than S_1. S_2 is louder than S_1 at the base of the heart; still, it is usually softer than S_1 at the apex (Box 15.7).

Splitting. *Splitting* occurs when the mitral and tricuspid valves or the pulmonic and aortic valves do not close simultaneously. Splitting of S_1 is not usually heard because the sound of the tricuspid valve closing is too faint to hear. Rarely, however, it may be audible in the tricuspid area, particularly on deep inspiration.

S_2 is generally two sounds that merge during expiration. The closure of the aortic valve (A_2) contributes most of the sound of S_2 when it is heard in the aortic or pulmonic areas. A_2 tends to mask the sound of pulmonic valve closure (P_2). During inspiration, P_2 occurs slightly later, giving S_2 two distinct components; this is a split S_2. Splitting is more often heard and easier to detect in the young; it is not well heard in older adults. This may be because of the tendency of the anteroposterior diameter of the chest to increase with age.

Splitting of S_2 is an expected event because pressures are higher and depolarization occurs earlier on the left side of the heart. During inspiration, the lungs fill with air as the chest wall expands. The intrathoracic pressure becomes more negative, and this increases venous blood return from the body into the right atrium and right ventricle. Simultaneously, the blood volume returning from the lungs into the left ventricle is reduced (the blood wants to stay in the lungs because of the negative intrathoracic pressure). The increased blood volume in the right ventricle during inspiration causes the pulmonary valve (P_2) to stay open longer during systole, whereas the aortic valve (A_2) closes slightly earlier due to reduced blood volume in the left ventricle (see Fig. 15.17). Ejection times tend to equalize when the breath is held in expiration, so this maneuver also tends to eliminate the split. The respiratory cycle is not always the dominant factor in splitting; the interval between the components may remain easily discernible throughout the respiratory cycle (Box 15.8).

BOX 15.7 S_2 Intensity: Diagnostic Clues

The intensity of S_2 increases in the following conditions:

- Systemic hypertension (S_2 may ring or boom), syphilis of the aortic valve, exercise, or excitement accentuates S_2.
- Pulmonary hypertension, mitral stenosis, and congestive heart failure accentuate P_2.
- The valves are diseased but still fully mobile; the component of S_2 affected depends on which valve is compromised.

The intensity of S_2 decreases in the following conditions:

- A shocklike state with arterial hypotension causes loss of valvular vigor.
- The valves are immobile, thickened, or calcified; the component of S_2 affected depends on which valve is compromised.
- Aortic stenosis affects A_2.
- Pulmonic stenosis affects P_2.
- Overlying tissue, fat, or fluid mutes S_2.

S_3 and S_4. During diastole, the ventricles fill in two steps: the early, passive flow of blood from the atria is followed by a more vigorous atrial ejection. The passive phase occurs relatively early in diastole, distending the ventricular walls and causing vibration. The resulting S_3 sound is quiet, low pitched, and often difficult to hear (see Fig. 15.17). In the second phase of ventricular filling, vibration in the valves, papillae, and ventricular walls produces S_4 (see Fig. 15.17). Because it occurs so late in diastole (presystole), S_4 may be confused with a split S_1.

S_3 and S_4 should be quiet and therefore somewhat difficult to hear. Increasing venous return (by asking the patient to raise a leg or inhale) or arterial pressure (by asking the patient to grip your hand tightly and repeatedly) may make these sounds easier to hear (see Fig. 15.19). When S_3 becomes intense and easy to hear, the resulting sequence of sounds simulates a gallop; this is the early diastolic gallop rhythm. It may be best heard when

BOX 15.8 Unexpected Splitting of Heart Sounds

Wide Splitting

The split becomes wider when delayed activation of contraction or right ventricle emptying slows pulmonic closure. This occurs, for example, in right bundle branch block, which splits both S_1 and S_2. Wide splitting of S_2 also occurs when stenosis delays closure of the pulmonic valve, when pulmonary hypertension delays ventricular emptying, or when mitral regurgitation or ventricular septal defect induces early closure of the aortic valve. The split becomes narrower and is even eliminated or paradoxical when closure of the aortic valve is delayed, such as in left bundle branch block, hypertrophic cardiomyopathy, and ventricular pacemakers.

Fixed Splitting

Splitting is said to be fixed when it is unaffected by respiration. This occurs with delayed closure of the pulmonic valve when output of the right ventricle is greater than that of the left. This can occur with large atrial septal defects.

Paradoxical (Reversed) Splitting

Paradoxical splitting occurs when closure of the aortic valve is delayed (e.g., as in left bundle branch block) so that P_2 occurs first, followed by A_2. In this case the interval between P_2 and A_1 is heard during expiration and disappears during inspiration.

See Fig. 15.18 for a visual depiction of variations in splitting of S_2 heart sounds.

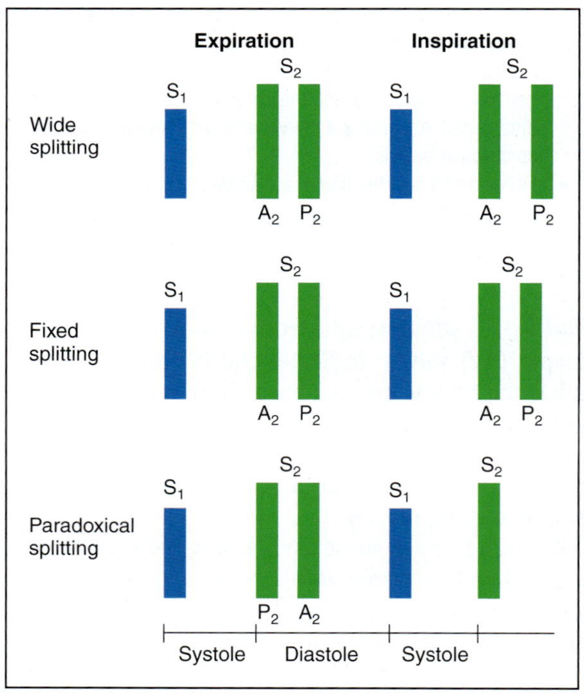

FIG. 15.18 Variations in splitting of S_2. (From Canobbio, M. M. (1990). *Cardiovascular disorders*. St. Louis: Mosby.)

the patient is in the left lateral decubitus (recumbent) position. S_4 may also become more intense, producing a readily discernible presystolic gallop rhythm. S_4 is most commonly heard in older patients, but it may be heard at any age when there is increased resistance to filling because the ventricular walls have lost compliance (e.g., in hypertensive disease and coronary artery disease) or with the increased stroke volume of high-output states (e.g., in profound anemia, pregnancy, and thyrotoxicosis). The rhythm of the heart sound when an S_3 is heard resembles the rhythm of pronouncing the word *Ken-TUCK-y*. When an S_4 is heard, it resembles the rhythm of pronouncing the word *TEN-nes-see*. A loud S_4 always suggests pathology and deserves additional evaluation.

The cardiac valves generally open noiselessly unless thickened, roughened, or otherwise altered as a result of disease. Valvular stenosis may produce an opening snap (mitral valve), ejection clicks (semilunar valves), or mid-to-late nonejection systolic clicks (mitral prolapse). The pulmonary ejection click is best heard on expiration in the second left intercostal space and is seldom heard on inspiration; aortic ejection clicks are less sharp, are less involved with S_1, and may be heard in the second right intercostal space. Extra heart sounds often accompany murmurs and should always be considered indicative of a pathologic process.

Extra Heart Sounds

A pericardial friction rub can be easily mistaken for cardiac-generated sounds. Inflammation of the pericardial sac causes a roughening of the parietal and visceral surfaces, which produces a rubbing machinelike sound audible on auscultation. It occupies both systole and diastole and overlies the intracardiac sounds. A pericardial friction rub may have three components that are associated in sequence with the atrial component of systole, ventricular systole, and ventricular diastole. It is usually heard widely but is more distinct toward the apex. A three-component

Heart sounds	First heart sound [$S_1(M_1T_1)$]	Second heart sound [$S_2(A_2P_2)$]	Third heart sound (S_3, ventricular gallop)	Fourth heart sound (S_4, atrial gallop)
	S_1 S_2 S_1 S_2	S_1 S_2 S_1 S_2	S_1 S_2 S_3 S_1 S_2 S_3	S_4 S_1 S_2 S_4 S_1 S_2
Anatomic reference	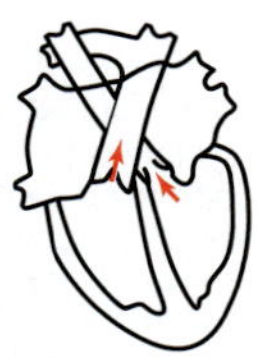	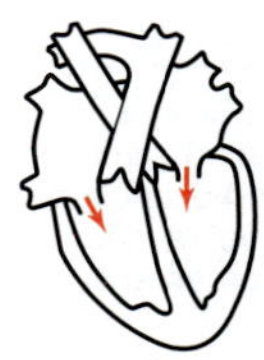	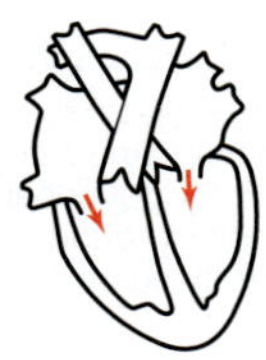	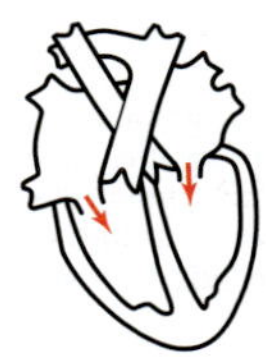
Preferable position of patient	Any position	Sitting or supine	Supine or left lateral	Supine or left semilateral
Area for auscultation	Entire precordium (apex)	A_2 at 2nd RICS P_2 at 2nd LICS	Apex	Apex
Endpiece	Diaphragm	Diaphragm	Bell	Bell
Pitch	High	High	Low	Low
Effects of respiration	Softer on inspiration	Fusion of A_2P_2 on expiration; physiologic split on inspiration	Increased on inspiration	Increased on inspiration
External influences	Increased with excitement, exercise, amyl nitrate, epinephrine, and atropine	Increased with thin chest walls and with exercise	Increased with exercise, fast heart rate, elevation of legs, and increased venous return	Increased with exercise, fast heart rate, elevation of legs, and increased venous return
Cause	Closure of tricuspid and mitral valves	Closure of pulmonic and aortic valves	Rapid ventricular filling	Forceful atrial ejection into distended ventricle

FIG. 15.19 Assessment of heart sounds. *LICS,* Left intercostal space; *RICS,* right intercostal space.

Continued

Quadruple rhythm	Summation gallop (triple gallop)	Ejection sounds	Systolic click	Opening snap
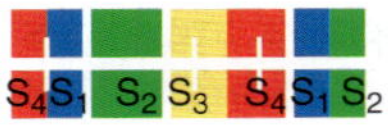	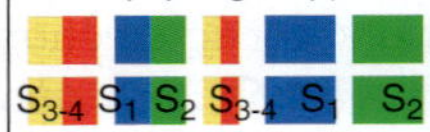	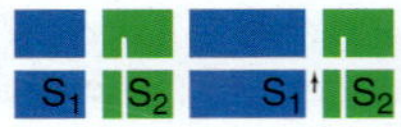	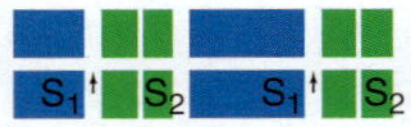	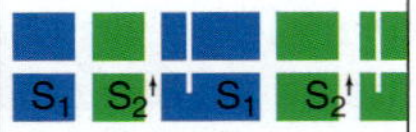
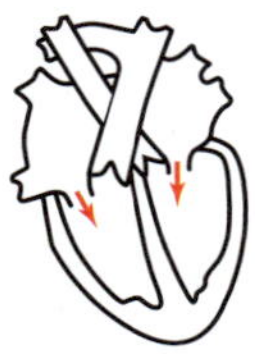	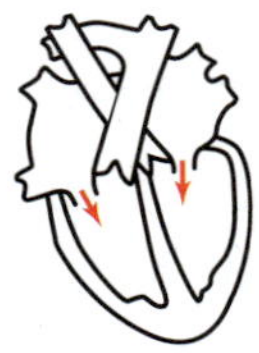	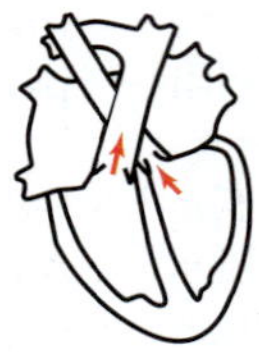	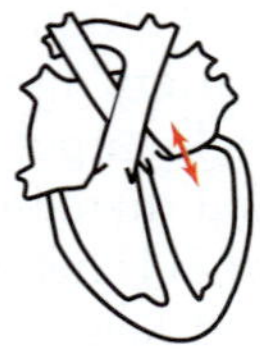	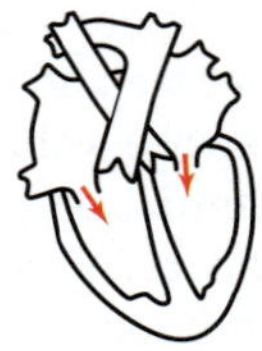
Supine or left lateral	Supine or left lateral	Sitting or supine	Sitting or supine	Any position
Apex	Apex	2nd RICS, 2nd LICS, or apex	Apex	Apex
Bell	Bell	Diaphragm	Diaphragm	Diaphragm
Low	Low	High	High	High
Increased on inspiration	Increased on inspiration	Increased on expiration with pulmonary stenosis	Increased on inspiration	Uninfluenced by inspiration
Aortic ejection sound same as S_1 and S_2; pulmonary ejection sound increased on expiration	Aortic ejection sound same as S_1 and S_2; pulmonary ejection sound increased on expiration	Aortic ejection sound same as S_1 and S_2; pulmonary ejection sound increased on expiration	Occurs later in systole with increased venous return (e.g., with elevated legs or supine position)	May be confused with S_3
S_1, S_2, S_3, and S_4, all heard separately	S_3 and S_4 fuse with fast heart rates	Opening of deformed semilunar valves	Prolapse of mitral valve leaflet	Abrupt recoil of stenotic mitral or tricuspid valve

FIG. 15.19, cont'd

friction rub may be intense enough to obscure the heart sounds. If there are only one or two components, the sound may not be intense or machinelike and may then be more difficult to distinguish from an intracardiac murmur. The detection of extra heart sounds is detailed in Table 15.3, along with associated causes (Fig. 15.19). See Clinical Pearl, "Heart Sounds After Surgical Procedures."

CLINICAL PEARL

Heart Sounds After Surgical Procedures

You should always know, based on history and chest inspection, whether a patient has had a cardiac surgical procedure. If this involves placement of a prosthetic mitral valve, listen for a distinct click early in diastole, loudest at the apex, and transmitted precordially. A prosthetic aortic valve causes a sound in early systole. The intensity of these sounds depends on the type of material used for the prosthesis. Animal tissue is the quietest and may even be silent. Pacemakers do not cause a sound.

Heart Murmurs

Heart murmurs are relatively prolonged extra sounds heard during systole or diastole. They often indicate a problem in adults. Murmurs are caused by some disruption in the flow of blood into, through, or out of the heart. The characteristics of a murmur depend on the adequacy of valve function, the size of the opening, the rate of blood flow, the vigor of the myocardium, and the thickness and consistency of the overlying tissues through which the murmur must be heard.

Diseased valves, a common cause of murmurs, either do not open or do not close well. When the leaflets are thickened and the passage narrowed, forward blood flow is restricted (stenosis). When valve leaflets, which are intended to fit together snugly, lose competency and leak, blood flows backward (regurgitation). Table 15.4 summarizes the characteristics of the heart murmurs. Murmurs are described in many ways (e.g., harsh, blowing, musical). Such descriptions may or may not be consistent with the

TABLE 15.3 Extra Heart Sounds

SOUNDS	DETECTION	TIMING AND DESCRIPTION
Increased S_3	Bell at apex; patient in left lateral recumbent position	Early diastole, low pitch
Increased S_4	Bell at apex; patient supine or in left lateral recumbent position	Late diastole or early systole, low pitch
Gallops	Bell at apex; patient supine or in left lateral recumbent position	Presystole, intense, easily heard
Mitral valve opening snap	Diaphragm medial to apex, may radiate to base; any position, second left intercostal space	Early diastole briefly, before S_3; high pitch, sharp snap, or click; not affected by respiration; easily confused with S_2
Aortic valve ejection click	Apex, base in second right intercostal space; patient sitting or supine	Early systole, intense, high pitch; radiates; not affected by respirations
Pulmonary valve ejection click	Second left intercostal space at sternal border; patient sitting or supine	Early systole, less intense than aortic click; intensifies on expiration, decreases on inspiration
Pericardial friction rub	Widely heard, sound clearest toward apex	May occupy all of systole and diastole; intense, grating, machinelike; may have three components and obliterate heart sounds; if only one or two components, may sound like murmur

TABLE 15.4 Characterization of Heart Murmurs

	CLASSIFICATION	DESCRIPTION
Timing and duration[a]	Early systolic	Begins with S_1, decrescendos, ends well before S_2
	Midsystolic (ejection)	Begins after S_1, ends before S_2; crescendo-decrescendo quality sometimes difficult to discern
	Late systolic	Begins mid-to-late systole, crescendos, ends at S_2; often introduced by mid-to-late systolic clicks
	Early diastolic	Begins with S_2
	Mid-diastolic	Begins at clear interval after S_2
	Late diastolic (presystolic)	Begins immediately before S_1
	Holosystolic (pansystolic)	Begins with S_1, occupies all of systole, ends at S_2
	Holodiastolic (pandiastolic)	Begins with S_2, occupies all of diastole, ends at S_1
	Continuous	Starts in systole, continues without interruption through S_2 into all or part of diastole; does not necessarily persist throughout entire cardiac cycle
Pitch	High, medium, low	Depends on pressure and rate of blood flow; low pitch is heard best with the bell
Intensity[b]	Grade I	Barely audible in quiet room
	Grade II	Quiet but clearly audible
	Grade III	Moderately loud
	Grade IV	Loud, associated with thrill
	Grade V	Very loud, thrill easily palpable
	Grade VI	Very loud, audible with stethoscope not in contact with chest, thrill palpable and visible
Pattern	Crescendo	Increasing intensity caused by increased blood velocity
	Decrescendo	Decreasing intensity caused by decreased blood velocity
	Square or plateau	Constant intensity
Quality	Harsh, raspy, machinelike, vibratory, musical, blowing	Quality depends on several factors, including degree of valve compromise, force of contractions, blood volume
Location	Anatomic landmarks (e.g., second left intercostal space on sternal border)	Area of greatest intensity, usually area to which valve sounds are normally transmitted
Radiation	Anatomic landmarks (e.g., to axilla or carotid arteries)	Site farthest from location of greatest intensity at which sound is still heard; sound usually transmitted in direction of blood flow
Respiratory phase	Intensity, quality, and timing may vary	Variations associated with venous return increase on inspiration or decrease on expiration

[a]Systolic murmurs are best described according to time of onset and termination; diastolic murmurs are best classified according to time of onset only.
[b]Discrimination among the six grades is more difficult for the diastolic murmur than for the systolic.

way you hear the sounds. Do not hesitate to use words that best suit your interpretation.

The most common source of significant murmurs is anatomic disorders of the heart valves (Fig. 15.20 and Table 15.5).

The discovery of a heart murmur requires careful assessment and diagnosis. Although some murmurs are benign (Box 15.9), others represent a pathologic process. Often additional testing is mandatory before a murmur is dismissed as functional.

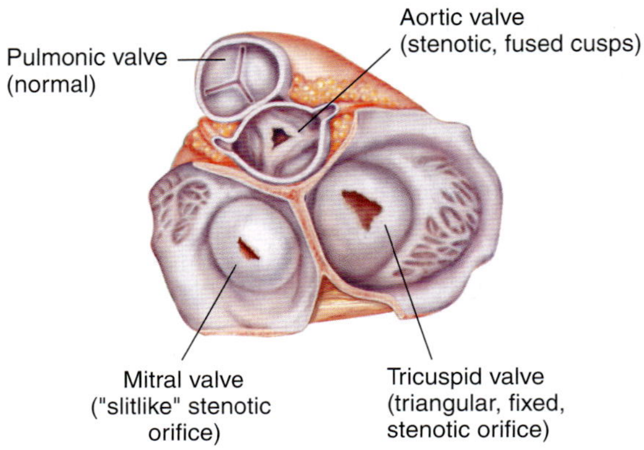

FIG. 15.20 Valvular heart disease. (Modified from Canobbio, M. M. (1990). *Cardiovascular disorders.* St. Louis: Mosby.)

Not all murmurs, however, are the result of valvular defects. Other causes include the following:

- High output demands that increase speed of blood flow (e.g., fever, thyrotoxicosis, anemia, pregnancy)
- Structural defects, either congenital or acquired, that allow blood to flow through inappropriate pathways (e.g., atrial or ventricular septal defects)
- Diminished strength of myocardial contraction
- Altered blood flow in the major vessels near the heart
- Transmitted murmurs resulting from valvular aortic stenosis, ruptured chordae tendineae of the mitral valve, or severe aortic regurgitation
- Vigorous left ventricular ejection (more common in children than in adults)
- Persistence of fetal circulation (e.g., patent ductus arteriosus)

It is not always possible on physical examination to identify with consistency the cause of a systolic murmur.

TABLE 15.5 Heart Murmurs

TYPE AND DETECTION	FINDINGS ON EXAMINATION	DESCRIPTION	
Mitral Stenosis			
Heard with bell at apex, patient in left lateral decubitus position	Low-frequency diastolic rumble, more intense in early and late diastole, does not radiate; systole usually quiet; palpable thrill at apex in late diastole common; S_1 increased and often palpable at left sternal border; S_2 split, often with accented P_2; opening snap follows P_2 closely Visible lift in right parasternal area if right ventricle hypertrophied Arterial pulse amplitude decreased	Narrowed valve restricts forward flow; forceful ejection into ventricle Often occurs with mitral regurgitation Caused by rheumatic fever or cardiac infection	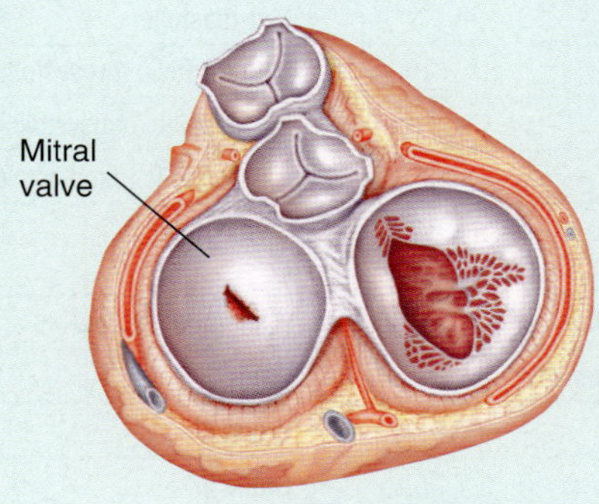 Mitral valve stenosis
Aortic Stenosis			
Heard over aortic area; ejection sound at second right intercostal border	Midsystolic (ejection) murmur, medium pitch, coarse, diamond-shaped,[a] crescendo-decrescendo; radiates along left sternal border (sometimes to apex) and to carotid with palpable thrill; S_1 often heard best at apex, disappearing when stenosis is severe, often followed by ejection click; S_2 soft or absent and may not be split; S_4 palpable; ejection sound muted in calcified valves; the more severe the stenosis, the later the peak of the murmur in systole Apical thrust shifts down and left and is prolonged if left ventricular hypertrophy is also present	Calcification of valve cusps restricts forward flow; forceful ejection from ventricle into systemic circulation Caused by congenital bicuspid (rather than the usual tricuspid) valve, rheumatic heart disease, atherosclerosis May be the cause of sudden death, particularly in children and adolescents, either at rest or during exercise; risk apparently related to degree of stenosis	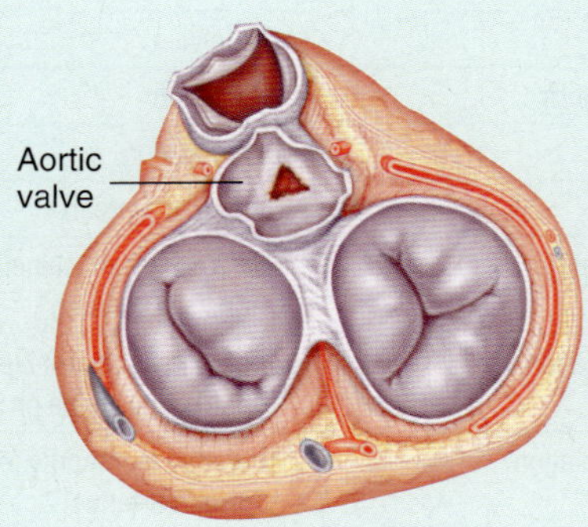 Aortic valve stenosis

TABLE 15.5 Heart Murmurs—cont'd

TYPE AND DETECTION	FINDINGS ON EXAMINATION	DESCRIPTION
Subaortic Stenosis Heard at apex and along left sternal border	Murmur fills systole, diamond-shaped, medium pitch, coarse; thrill often palpable during systole at apex and right sternal border; multiple waves in apical impulses; S_2 usually split; S_3 and S_4 often present Arterial pulse brisk, double wave in carotid common; jugular venous pulse prominent	Fibrous ring, usually 1–4 mm below aortic valve; most pronounced on ventricular septal side; may become progressively severe with time; difficult to distinguish from aortic stenosis on clinical grounds alone 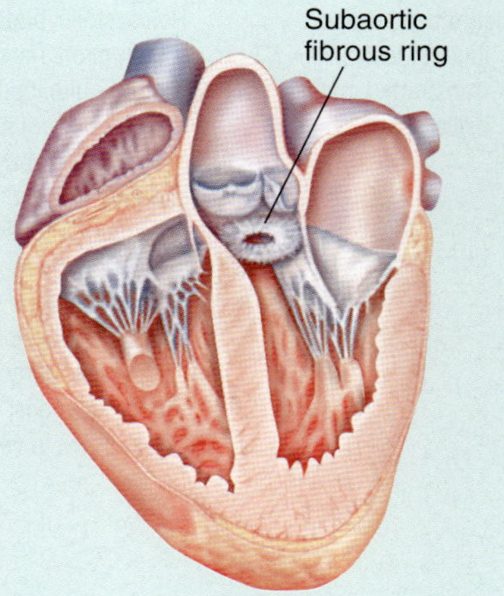 Subaortic stenosis
Pulmonic Stenosis Heard over pulmonic area radiating to left and into neck; thrill in second and third left intercostal spaces	Systolic (ejection) murmur, diamond-shaped, medium pitch, coarse; usually with thrill; S_1 often followed quickly by ejection click; S_2 often diminished, usually wide split; P_2 soft or absent; S_4 common in right ventricular hypertrophy; murmur may be prolonged and confused with that of a ventricular septal defect	Valve restricts forward flow; forceful ejection from ventricle into pulmonary circulation Cause is almost always congenital 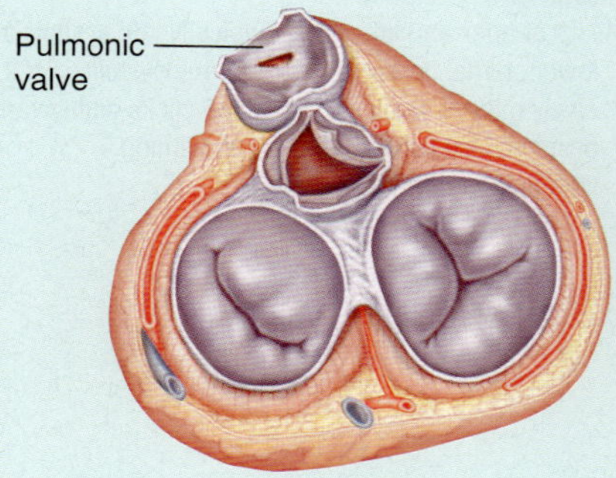 Pulmonic valve stenosis
Tricuspid Stenosis Heard with bell over tricuspid area	Diastolic rumble accentuated early and late in diastole, resembling mitral stenosis but louder on inspiration; diastolic thrill palpable over right ventricle; S_2 may be split during inspiration Arterial pulse amplitude decreased; jugular venous pulse prominent, especially A wave; slow fall of V wave (see Chapter 16)	Calcification of valve cusps restricts forward flow; forceful ejection into ventricles Usually seen with mitral stenosis; rarely occurs alone Caused by rheumatic heart disease, congenital defect, endocardial fibroelastosis, right atrial myxoma 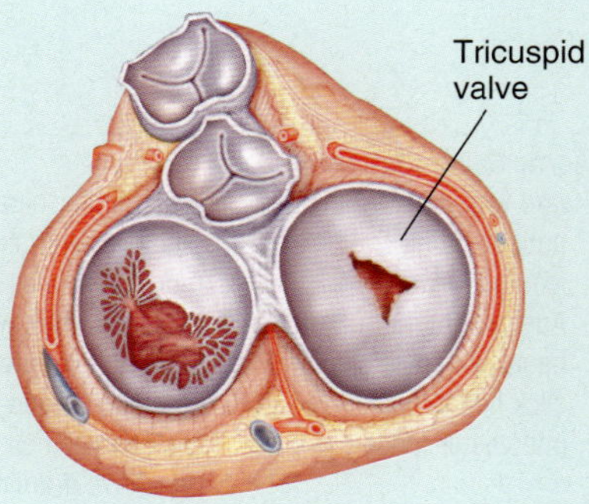 Tricuspid valve stenosis

Continued

TABLE 15.5 Heart Murmurs—cont'd

TYPE AND DETECTION	FINDINGS ON EXAMINATION	DESCRIPTION
Mitral Regurgitation Heard best at apex; loudest there, transmitted into left axilla	Holosystolic, plateau-shaped intensity, high pitch, harsh blowing quality, often quite loud and may obliterate S_2; radiates from apex to base or to left axilla; thrill may be palpable at apex during systole; S_1 intensity diminished; S_2 more intense with P_2 often accented; S_3 often present; S_3–S_4 gallop common in late disease If mild, late systolic murmur crescendos; if severe, early systolic intensity decrescendos; apical thrust more to left and down in ventricular hypertrophy	Valve incompetence allows backflow from ventricle to atrium Caused by rheumatic fever, myocardial infarction, myxoma, rupture of chordae 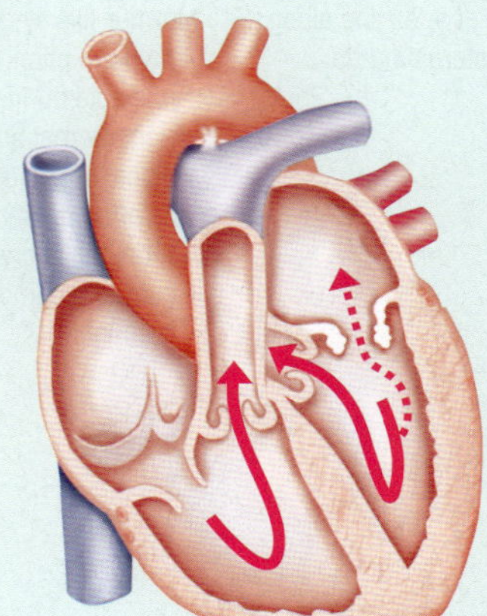 Mitral regurgitation (heart in systole)
Mitral Valve Prolapse Heard at apex and left lower sternal border; easily missed in supine position; also listen with patient upright	Typically late systolic murmur preceded by midsystolic clicks, but both murmur and clicks highly variable in intensity and timing	Valve is competent early in systole but prolapses into atrium later in systole; may become progressively severe, resulting in a holosystolic murmur; often concurrent with pectus excavatum 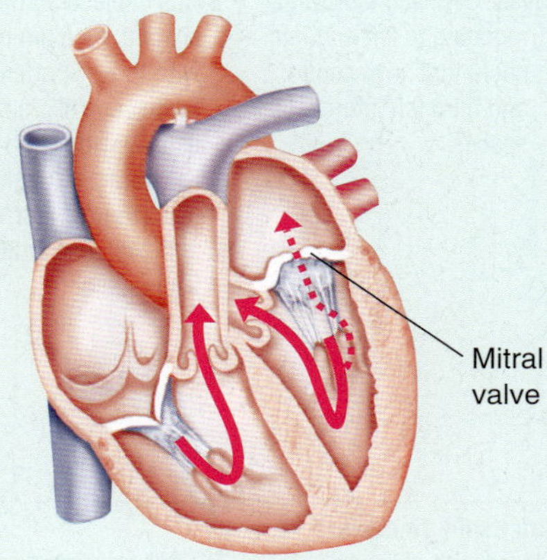 Mitral valve prolapse (heart in systole)
Aortic Regurgitation Heard with diaphragm, patient sitting and leaning forward; Austin-Flint murmur heard with bell; ejection click heard in second intercostal space	Early diastolic, high pitch, blowing, often with diamond-shaped midsystolic murmur, sounds often not prominent; duration varies with blood pressure; low-pitched, rumbling murmur at apex common (Austin-Flint); early ejection click sometimes present; S_1 soft; S_2 split may have drumlike quality; mitral (M_1) and A_2 often intensified, S_3–S_4 gallop common In left ventricular hypertrophy, prominent prolonged apical impulse down and to left Pulse pressure wide; water-hammer or Corrigan pulse common in carotid, brachial, and femoral arteries (see Chapter 16)	Valve incompetence allows backflow from aorta to ventricle Caused by rheumatic heart disease, endocarditis, aortic diseases (Marfan syndrome, medial necrosis), syphilis, ankylosing spondylitis, dissection, cardiac trauma 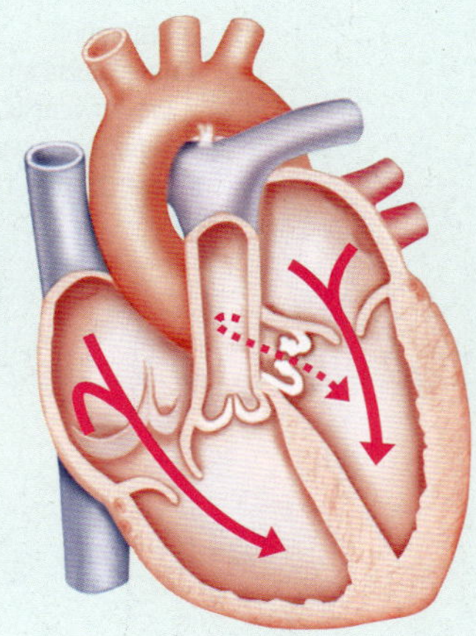 Aortic regurgitation (heart in diastole)

TABLE 15.5 Heart Murmurs—cont'd

TYPE AND DETECTION	FINDINGS ON EXAMINATION	DESCRIPTION	
Pulmonic Regurgitation			
	Difficult to distinguish from aortic regurgitation on physical examination	Valve incompetence allows backflow from pulmonary artery to ventricle Secondary to pulmonary hypertension or bacterial endocarditis	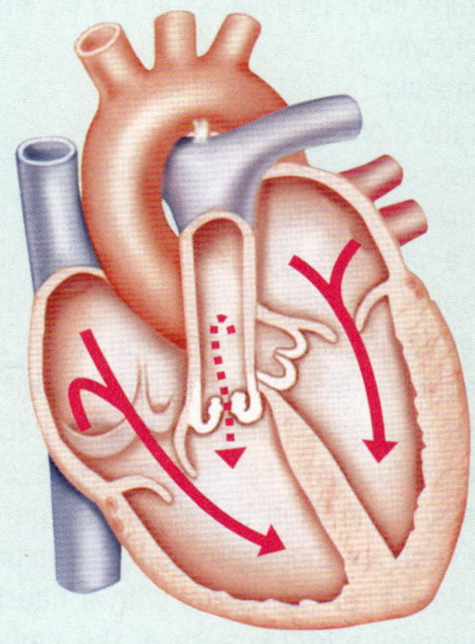 Pulmonic regurgitation (heart in diastole)
Tricuspid Regurgitation			
Heard at left lower sternum, occasionally radiating a few centimeters to the left	Holosystolic murmur over right ventricle, blowing, increased on inspiration; S_3 and thrill over tricuspid area common In pulmonary hypertension, pulmonary artery impulse palpable over second left intercostal space and P_2 accented; in right ventricular hypertrophy, visible lift to right of sternum Jugular venous pulse has large V waves (see Chapter 16)	Valve incompetence allows backflow from ventricle to atrium Caused by congenital defects, bacterial endocarditis (especially in intravenous drug abusers), pulmonary hypertension, cardiac trauma	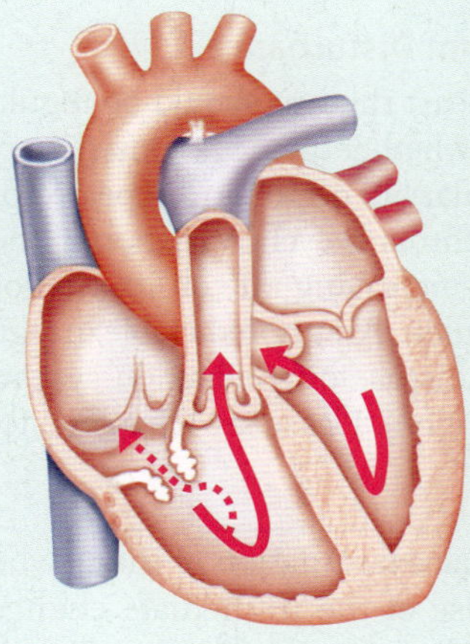 Tricuspid regurgitation (heart in systole)

[a]Diamond-shaped murmur is named for its recorded shape on phonocardiogram (a crescendo-decrescendo sound).

BOX 15.9 Are Some Murmurs Innocent?

Many murmurs—particularly in children, adolescents, and especially in young athletes—have no apparent cause and are called *Still murmers* (named after the physician who first described them). They are presumably a result of vigorous myocardial contraction, the consequent stronger blood flow in early systole or midsystole, and the rush of blood from the larger chamber of the heart into the smaller bore of a blood vessel. The thinner chests of the young make these sounds easier to hear, particularly with a lightly held bell. They are usually grade I or II, usually midsystolic, without radiation, medium pitch, blowing, brief, and often accompanied by splitting of S_2. They are often located in the second left intercostal space near the left sternal border. Such murmurs heard in a recumbent position may disappear when the patient sits or stands because of the tendency of the blood to pool. Do not confuse an "innocent" murmur with one that is "benign"—the result of a structural anomaly that is not severe enough to cause a clinical problem.

Evidence-Based Practice in Physical Examination

Cardiac Murmurs in Children

Structural heart disease is more likely when the murmur is:

- Holosystolic
- Diastolic
- Grade 3 or higher
- Associated with a systolic click
- Increased in intensity with standing
- Of a harsh quality

Chest radiography and electrocardiography rarely assist in the diagnosis of heart murmurs in children. The only clue available to the clinician that a critical congenital heart defect (CCHD) is present may be a mild decrease in the percutaneous oxygen saturation. For this reason, every infant should have pulse oximetry performed before discharge from the newborn nursery. Order echocardiography and consider referral to a pediatric cardiologist for newborns with a heart murmur, even if the child is asymptomatic, because of the higher prevalence of structural heart lesions in this population.

Risk Factors

Children at High Risk for an Underlying Structural Heart Defect

A SAFER approach—history taking to identify high-risk children—includes the following:

- **Syndromic features:** Heart defects are more common in infants with syndromes or chromosomal anomalies.
- **Age:** Murmurs in infants are more likely to be pathologic.
- **Family history:** Congenital heart defects have multifactorial inheritance and carry a slightly increased risk (3% to 5%) in the offspring.
- **Evaluation of feeding and growth:** A murmur in a child who presents with faltering growth, feeding difficulties, sweating during feeds, tachypnea, and/or cyanosis. Sometimes probing a bit further; for example, how long it takes for the infant to finish a bottle or whether the infant takes frequent breaks during feeds will help to identify heart failure earlier.
- **Rheumatic fever or other significant previous medical history:** History of rheumatic fever and Kawasaki disease in the past, especially in older children.

From Mikrou, P., & Ramesh, P. (2017). General paediatric evaluation of heart murmurs. *Paediatrics & Child Health, 27*(2), 90–92.

Rhythm Disturbance

The heart rhythm should be regular. If it is irregular, determine whether there is a consistent pattern. A heart rate that is irregular but occurs in a repeated pattern may indicate sinus arrhythmia, a cyclic variation of the heart rate characterized by an increasing rate on inspiration and decreasing rate on expiration. An unpredictable, irregular rhythm may indicate heart disease or conduction system impairment (e.g., atrial fibrillation). Please see Chapter 6 for expected heart rates.

Infants

Cardiac examination of the newborn presents a challenge because of the immediate change from fetal to systemic and pulmonary circulation. Examine the heart within the first 24 hours of life and again at about 2 to 3 days of age. Newborns in the nursery should have CCDH screening by pulse oximetry ideally after 24 hours of age or shortly before discharge if this occurs before 24 hours.

Complete evaluation of heart function includes examination of the skin, lungs, and liver. Infants with right-sided congestive heart failure have large, firm livers with the inferior edge as much as 5 to 6 cm below the right costal margin. Unlike adults, this finding may precede that of pulmonary crackles.

Inspect the color of the skin and mucous membranes. The well newborn should be reassuringly pink. A purplish plethora is associated with polycythemia (increased red cell mass); an ashen white color indicates shock; and central cyanosis (i.e., cyanosis of the skin and mucous membranes of the face and upper body) suggests congenital heart disease. Note the distribution and intensity of discoloration as well as the extent of change after vigorous exertion (e.g., crying or feeding). Acrocyanosis, cyanosis of the hands and feet without central cyanosis, does not signify pathology; it usually disappears within a few days, or even a few hours, after birth.

DIFFERENTIAL DIAGNOSIS

Comparison of Systolic Murmurs

ORIGIN	MANEUVER	EFFECT OF INTENSITY
Right-sided chambers	Inspiration	Increase
	Expiration	Decrease
Hypertrophic	Valsalva	Increase
Cardiomyopathy	Squatting to standing	Increase
	Standing to squatting	Decrease
	Passive leg elevation to 45 degrees, patient supine	Decrease
Mitral regurgitation[a]	Handgrip	Increase
Ventricular septal defect[a]	Transient arterial occlusion (sphygmomanometer placed on each of the patient's upper arms and simultaneously inflated to 20–40 mm Hg greater than patient's previously recorded blood pressures; intensity noted after 20 seconds)	Increase
Aortic stenosis	No maneuver distinguishes this murmur; the diagnosis can be made by exclusion	

[a]Handgrip, or transient arterial occlusion, will distinguish mitral regurgitation and ventricular septal defect from other causes of systolic murmurs; more than just auscultation is needed to make further distinction.

Cyanosis is a characteristic of congenital heart defects that allows a mixture of arterial and venous blood or prevents blood flow to the lungs. Severe cyanosis evident at birth or shortly thereafter suggests transposition of the great vessels, tetralogy of Fallot, tricuspid atresia, a severe septal defect, or severe pulmonic stenosis. Cyanosis that does not appear until after the neonatal period suggests pulmonic stenosis, Eisenmenger complex (heart defect that can lead to a right-to-left shunt), tetralogy of Fallot, or large septal defects.

Expect to see and palpate the apical impulse in the newborn at the fourth to fifth left intercostal space just medial to the midclavicular line. The smaller the baby or the thinner the chest, the more obvious it will be. It may be somewhat farther to the right in the first few hours of life, sometimes even substernal.

Note any enlargement of the heart. It is especially important to note the position of the heart if a baby is having trouble breathing. A pneumothorax (lung collapse) shifts the apical impulse away from the area of the pneumothorax. A diaphragmatic hernia, more commonly found on the left, shifts the heart to the right. Dextrocardia results in an apical impulse on the right.

The right ventricle is relatively more vigorous than the left in a well, full-term newborn. If the baby is thin, you might even be able to feel the closure of the pulmonary valve in the second left intercostal space.

S_2 in infants is somewhat higher in pitch and more discrete than S_1. The vigor and quality of the heart sounds of the newborn (and throughout infancy and early childhood) are major indicators of heart function. Diminished vigor may be the only apparent change when an infant is already in heart failure. Splitting of the heart sounds is common. S_2 is usually heard without a split at birth and then often splits within a few hours. See Clinical Pearl, "The Infant Heart and Liver."

CLINICAL PEARL

The Infant Heart and Liver

If you push up on the liver, thereby increasing right atrial pressure, the murmur of a left-to-right shunt through a septal opening or patent ductus will disappear briefly, whereas the murmur of a right-to-left shunt will intensify.

S_3 and S_4 are commonly heard in pediatric patients. Increased intensity of either sound may be indicative of an abnormality.

Murmurs are relatively common in the newborn until about 48 hours of age. Most are not pathologic but caused by the transition from fetal to pulmonic circulation rather than by a significant congenital abnormality. These murmurs are usually of grade I or II intensity, systolic, and unaccompanied by other signs and symptoms; they usually disappear within 2 to 3 days. Paradoxically, a significant congenital abnormality may be unaccompanied by a murmur.

If you cannot tell a murmur from respiration, listen while the baby is feeding, or time the sound with the carotid pulsation. Because of the rapid heart rate in infants, the heart sounds are more difficult to evaluate. A murmur heard immediately at birth is apt to be less significant than one continuously noted after the first few hours of life. If a murmur persists beyond the second or third day of life, is intense, fills systole, occupies diastole to any extent, or radiates widely, it must be investigated.

Murmurs that extend beyond S_2 and occupy diastole are said to have a machinelike quality; they may be associated with a patent ductus arteriosus. The murmur should disappear when the patent ductus closes in the first 2 or 3 days of life. Diastolic murmurs may be transient and possibly related to early closure of the ductus arteriosus or a mild, brief pulmonary insufficiency.

Children

The precordium of a child tends to bulge over an enlarged heart if the enlargement is longstanding. A child's thoracic cage, being more cartilaginous and yielding than that of an adult, responds more to the thrust of cardiac enlargement.

Sinus arrhythmia is a physiologic event during childhood. The heart rate varies in a cyclic pattern, usually faster on inspiration and slower on expiration. Most often, other dysrhythmias in children are ectopic in origin (e.g., supraventricular and ventricular ectopic beats). These and a variety of other seeming irregularities require extensive investigation only occasionally. Heart rates in children are discussed in Chapter 6.

Murmurs in infants and children may be the result of congenital heart disease; however, Kawasaki disease accounts for most acquired murmurs (see Chapter 16).

Some murmurs are innocent. A Still murmur—so named after George Frederic Still, the physician who first described it—occurs in active, healthy children between the ages of 3 and 7 years. Caused by the vigorous expulsion of blood from the left ventricle into the aorta, it increases in intensity with activity and diminishes when the child is quiet. It is often described as musical (see Box 15.9).

When examining a child with known heart disease, take careful note of weight gain (or loss), developmental delay, cyanosis, and clubbing of fingers and toes. Cyanosis is a major clue to congenital heart defects that impede oxygenation of blood.

Pregnant Patients

The heart position shifts during pregnancy, but the position varies with the size and position of the uterus. The apical impulse is upward and more lateral by 1 to 1.5 cm. Expect some changes in auscultated heart sounds because of the increased blood volume and extra effort of the heart. More audible splitting of S_1 and S_2 and S_3 may be readily heard after 20 weeks of gestation. A fourth heart sound is abnormal. In addition, systolic ejection murmurs may be heard over the pulmonic area in 90% of pregnant patients. The murmur is intensified during inspiration or expiration but should not be louder than grade II (see Table 15.4). There is no significant change in the ECG.

The presence of cyanosis, clubbing, or persistent neck vein distention or the development of a diastolic murmur suggests an abnormality.

Older Adults

You may need to slow the pace of your examination when asking an older patient to assume positions that may be uncomfortable or perhaps too difficult. Some older patients may not be able to lie flat, and some may not be able to control their breathing pattern at your request. The cardiac response to even minimal demand may be slowed or insufficient. An abrupt position change may cause a transient lightheadedness because of a drop in arterial pressure.

Frailty syndrome is characterized by signs and symptoms of being frail: weakness, slowing, decreased energy, lower activity, and, when severe, unintended weight loss. It is linked to comorbid conditions and carries an elevated risk of catastrophic declines in health and function, including disability, hospitalization, falls, fracture, and death. There is a lack of resilience and decreased ability to adapt to physical stressors. It is most common in adults older than 75 years and is increasingly common after age 85 (Walsh et al., 2023). Screening for frailty and early intervention may help minimize the risks of adverse outcomes. A simple screening scale is provided in Box 15.10.

BOX 15.10 The FRAIL Scale

A useful screening tool to help identify persons at risk for frailty is the FRAIL scale, which consists of five domains (Abellan van Kan et al., 2008):

- **F**atigue
- **R**esistance (ability to climb one flight of stairs)
- **A**mbulation (ability to walk one block)
- **I**llnesses (>5)
- **L**oss of weight (>5%)

The apical impulse may be harder to find in many persons because of the increased anteroposterior diameter of the chest. In obese older adults, the diaphragm is raised and the heart is more transverse.

Older adults who exercise regularly may reverse or avoid some of the age-associated changes.

S_4 is more common in older adults and may indicate decreased left ventricular compliance. Early, soft physiologic murmurs may be heard, caused by aortic lengthening, tortuosity, and sclerotic changes.

Common ECG changes in older patients include first-degree AV block, bundle branch blocks, ST-T wave abnormalities, premature systole (atrial and ventricular), left anterior hemiblock, left ventricular hypertrophy, and atrial fibrillation. Occasional ectopic beats are fairly common and may or may not be significant.

ABNORMALITIES

Heart

General Heart Abnormalities

Angina

Pain caused by myocardial ischemia

PATHOPHYSIOLOGY

- Occurs when myocardial oxygen demand exceeds supply
- Can be recurrent or present as initial incidence

PATIENT DATA

Subjective Data

- Substernal pain or intense pressure radiating to the neck, jaws, and arms, particularly the left
- Often accompanied by shortness of breath, fatigue, diaphoresis, faintness, and syncope

Objective Data

- No definitive examination findings suggest angina
- Tachycardia, tachypnea, hypertension, and/or diaphoresis
- Ischemia may lead to presence of crackles due to pulmonary edema or a reduction in S_1 intensity or an S_4
- Physical examination may suggest other comorbidities that place the patient at higher risk for angina symptoms, such as chronic obstructive pulmonary disease, xanthelasma, hypertension, evidence of peripheral arterial disease, abnormal pulsations on palpation over precordium, murmurs, or arrhythmias

Bacterial Endocarditis

Bacterial infection of the endothelial layer of the heart and valves

PATHOPHYSIOLOGY

- Individuals with congenital or acquired valve defects and those with a history of previous endocarditis or who use intravenous drugs are particularly susceptible (Fig. 15.21)

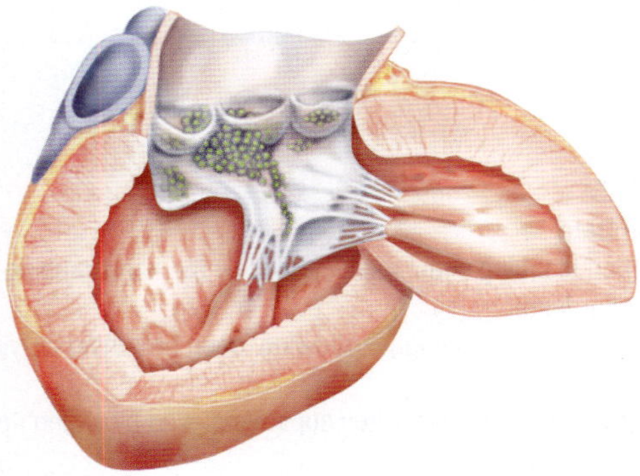

FIG. 15.21 Bacterial endocarditis. (Modified from Canobbio, M. M. (1990). *Cardiovascular disorders.* St. Louis: Mosby.)

PATIENT DATA

Subjective Data

- Fever, fatigue
- Sudden onset of congestive heart failure (e.g., shortness of breath, ankle edema)

Objective Data

- Murmur
- Signs of neurologic dysfunction
- Janeway lesions (small erythematous or hemorrhagic macules appearing on the palms and soles)
- Osler nodes (painful, red, raised lesions that appear on the tips of fingers or toes and are caused by septic emboli)

Congestive Heart Failure: Left-Sided

Heart fails to propel blood forward with its usual force, resulting in congestion in the pulmonary circulation

PATHOPHYSIOLOGY

Many causes:

- Left ventricular hypertrophy (high blood pressure leading to thickening of the left heart muscle)
- Cardiomyopathy (weakened heart muscle)
- Damaged aortic or mitral heart valves
- Ischemic cardiomyopathy (from coronary artery disease)
- Nonischemic cardiomyopathy
- Toxic exposures, such as alcohol or cocaine
- Viruses, such as coxsackie

Left-sided congestive heart failure (CHF) is characterized as systolic or diastolic:

- Systolic CHF is due to impaired contraction of the left ventricle
- Diastolic CHF is the result of advanced glycation cross-linking collagen and creating a stiff ventricle unable to dilate actively (impaired relaxation)
- Diastolic CHF occurs in older adults with diabetes mellitus whose tissue is exposed to glucose for a longer period

PATIENT DATA

Subjective Data

- Fatigue
- Breathing difficulty, shortness of breath
- Orthopnea
- Exercise intolerance

Objective Data

- Sudden with acute pulmonary edema or gradual symptom onset
- Crackles on pulmonary examination
- Systolic CHF has a narrow pulse pressure
- Diastolic CHF has a wide pulse pressure

Congestive Heart Failure: Right-Sided

Heart fails to propel blood forward with its usual force, resulting in congestion in the systemic circulation

PATHOPHYSIOLOGY

- Decreased cardiac output causes decreased blood flow to the tissues
- Many causes (see "Left-Sided")

PATIENT DATA

Subjective Data

- Peripheral edema, particularly at the end of the day or after prolonged sitting
- Weight gain

Objective Data

- Pitting edema in lower extremities
- Jugular venous distention
- Ascites
- Hepatomegaly

Evidence-Based Practice in Physical Examination

Can the Clinical Examination Diagnose Heart Failure in Adults?

The most helpful physical examination findings in the diagnosis of heart failure include displaced apex beat, irregular pulse, rales, pulse rate, heart murmur suggestive of mitral regurgitation, and elevated jugular venous pressure.

From Kelder, J. C., Cramer, M. J., van Wijngaarden, J., et al. (2011). The diagnostic value of physical examination and additional testing in primary care patients with suspected heart failure. *Circulation, 124*(25), 2865–2873. doi:10.1161/CIRCULATIONAHA.111.019216

Pericarditis

Inflammation of the pericardium

PATHOPHYSIOLOGY

- Often the result of a viral infection such as echovirus or coxsackievirus
- May be seen in:
  - Cancer (including leukemia)
  - HIV infection
  - Hypothyroidism
  - Kidney failure
  - Rheumatic fever
  - Tuberculosis
  - Kawasaki disease
- Other causes include:
  - Heart attack
  - Heart surgery or trauma to the chest, esophagus, or heart
  - Certain medications, such as procainamide, hydralazine, phenytoin, isoniazid
  - Radiation therapy to the chest
  - May cause a pericardial effusion and may increase and result in cardiac tamponade (Fig. 15.22)

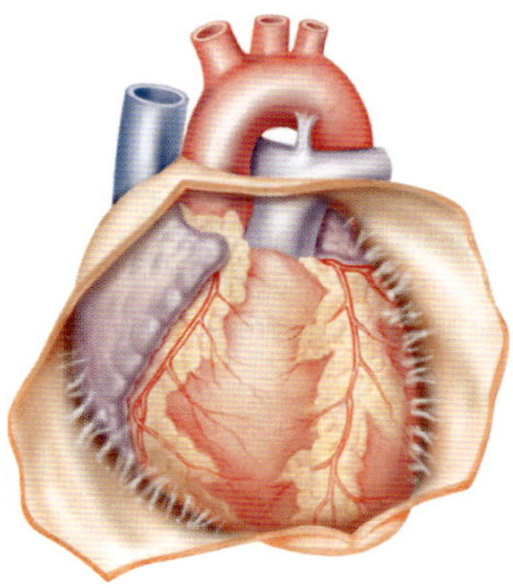

FIG. 15.22 Pericarditis. (Modified from Canobbio, M. M. (1990). *Cardiovascular disorders.* St. Louis: Mosby.)

PATIENT DATA

Subjective Data

- Sharp and stabbing chest pain (caused by the heart rubbing against the pericardium)
- Pain worse with coughing, swallowing, deep breathing or lying flat, or movement
- Pain may be most severe when supine, relieved by sitting up and leaning forward
- Pain in the back, neck, or left shoulder
- Difficulty breathing when lying down
- Dry cough
- Anxiety or fatigue

Objective Data

- Scratchy, grating, triphasic friction rub on auscultation, comprises ventricular systole, early diastolic ventricular filling, and late diastolic atrial systole
- Friction rub easily heard just left of the sternum in third and fourth intercostal spaces

Cardiac Tamponade

Excessive accumulation of effused fluids or blood between the pericardium and the heart (Fig. 15.23)

PATHOPHYSIOLOGY

- Seriously constrains cardiac relaxation, impairing blood return to the right heart
- Common causes: pericarditis, malignancy, aortic dissection, and trauma

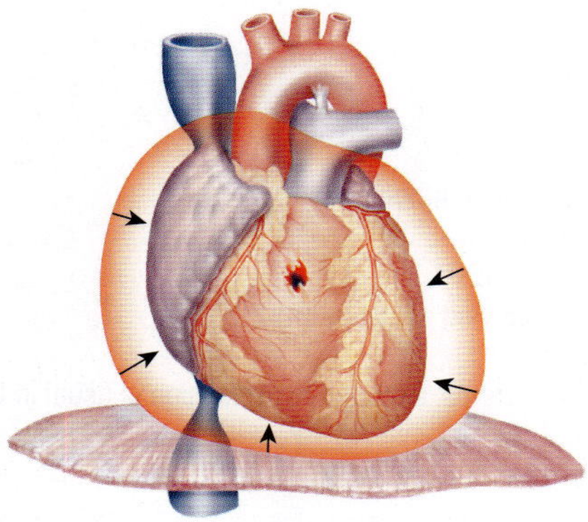

FIG. 15.23 Hemopericardium and cardiac tamponade. (Modified from Canobbio, M. M. (1990). *Cardiovascular disorders.* St. Louis: Mosby.)

PATIENT DATA

Subjective Data

- Anxiety, restlessness
- Chest pain
- Difficulty breathing
- Discomfort, sometimes relieved by sitting upright or leaning forward
- Syncope, lightheadedness
- Pale, gray, or blue skin
- Palpitations
- Rapid breathing
- Swelling of the abdomen or arms or neck veins

Objective Data

- Beck triad (jugular venous distention, hypotension, and muffled heart sounds)
- Chronically and severely involved pericardium may also scar and constrict, limiting cardiac filling; heart sounds are muffled, blood pressure drops, the pulse becomes weakened and rapid, and paradoxical pulse (see Chapter 16) becomes exaggerated

Cor Pulmonale

Enlargement of the right ventricle secondary to chronic lung disease (Fig. 15.24)

PATHOPHYSIOLOGY

- Usually chronic, occasionally acute
- In acute phase, the right side of the heart is dilated and fails
- Acute causes: massive pulmonary embolism and acute respiratory distress syndrome (ARDS)
- In chronic cor pulmonale, gradual hypertrophy of the right ventricle progresses until ultimate heart failure
- Results from chronic obstructive pulmonary disease (COPD) and pulmonary arterial hypertension

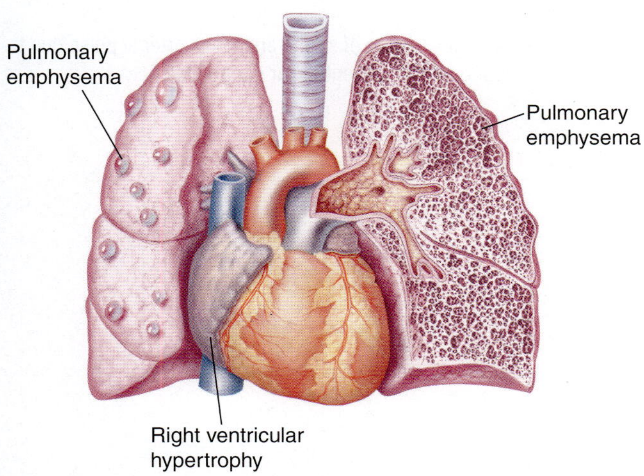

FIG. 15.24 Cor pulmonale. Notice extensive pulmonary emphysema and right ventricular hypertrophy. (Modified from Wilson, S. F., & Thompson, J. M. (1990). *Respiratory disorders.* St. Louis: Mosby.)

PATIENT DATA

Subjective Data

- Fatigue
- Tachypnea
- Exertional dyspnea
- Cough
- Hemoptysis
- Lightheadedness
- Syncope

Objective Data

- Evidence of pulmonary disease
- Wheezes and crackles on auscultation
- Increase in chest diameter
- Labored respiratory efforts with chest wall retractions
- Evidence of right heart failure and hypertrophy
- Distended neck veins with prominent A or V waves (see Chapter 16)
- Cyanosis
- Left parasternal systolic heave
- Loud S_2 exaggerated in the pulmonic region
- Lower extremity edema

Myocardial Infarction

Ischemic myocardial necrosis caused by abrupt decrease in coronary blood flow to a segment of the myocardium

PATHOPHYSIOLOGY

- Most commonly affects left ventricle
- Results from atherosclerosis of the coronary blood vessels
- Atherosclerotic plaques rupture, and thrombosis (a clot) forms, rapidly causing a sudden obstruction of blood flow

PATIENT DATA

Subjective Data

- Deep substernal or visceral pain that often radiates to the jaw, neck, and left arm (see Box 15.1)
- Discomfort may be mild, especially in older adults or patients with diabetes mellitus
- Nausea
- Fatigue
- Shortness of breath

Objective Data

- Dysrhythmias are common
- S_4 is usually present
- Distant heart sounds
- Soft, systolic, blowing apical murmur
- Thready pulse
- Blood pressure varies, although hypertension is usual in the early phases
- New ST elevation in two contiguous leads

Myocarditis

Focal or diffuse inflammation of the myocardium

PATHOPHYSIOLOGY

- Inflammation can occur from direct cytotoxic effect of secondary immune response
- Causes:
  - Viral—enterovirus, coxsackievirus, adenovirus, influenza, cytomegalovirus, SARS-CoV-2
  - Bacterial—tuberculosis, streptococci
  - Spirochetal—syphilis, Lyme disease
  - Fungal—candidiasis, aspergillosis, cryptococcosis, histoplasmosis
  - Protozoal—Chagas disease, toxoplasmosis, malaria
  - Helminthic—trichinosis, schistosomiasis
  - Bites/stings—scorpion venom, snake venom, black widow spider venom
  - Chemotherapeutic medications
  - Amphetamines, cocaine, catecholamines
  - Physical agents
  - Systemic inflammatory disease—giant cell myocarditis, sarcoidosis, Kawasaki disease, Crohn disease, systemic lupus erythematosus
  - Peripartum cardiomyopathy

PATIENT DATA

Subjective Data

- Initial symptoms vague
- Fatigue
- Dyspnea
- Fever
- Palpitations
- History of recent (within 1–2 weeks) flulike syndrome of fevers, arthralgias, and malaise or pharyngitis, tonsillitis, or upper respiratory tract infection

Objective Data

- Cardiac enlargement
- Murmurs
- Gallop rhythms
- Tachycardia
- Dysrhythmias
- Pulsus alternans (fluctuation of strong and weak arterial pulse due to alternating strong and weak ventricular contractions)

HEART RATE AND RHYTHM

Conduction Disturbances

Conduction disturbances either proximal to the bundle of His or diffusely throughout the conduction system

PATHOPHYSIOLOGY

- May result from a variety of causes: ischemic, infiltrative, or, rarely, neoplastic
- Antidepressant medications, digitalis, quinidine, and many other medications can be a precipitating factor

PATIENT DATA

Subjective Data

- Transient weakness
- Syncope may occur acutely without warning, sometimes as a "grayout" instead of a "blackout"; may precede the event
- Strokelike episodes
- Palpitations

Objective Data

- Rapid or irregular heartbeat
- Rhythm disturbances (Table 15.6)

TABLE 15.6 Abnormalities in Rates and Rhythms

TYPE AND DETECTION	FINDINGS ON EXAMINATION	DESCRIPTION
Atrial (Auricular) Flutter		
	Atrial rate far in excess of ventricular rate; heart sounds not necessarily weak	Regular uniform atrial contractions occur in excess of 200 beats/min, but the ventricular response is limited as a result of physiologic heart block. The conduction system cannot respond to the rapidity of the atrial rate, causing variance from the ventricular rate. The ECG may look like a sawtooth cog.
Atrial flutter with a constant 4:1 conduction ratio		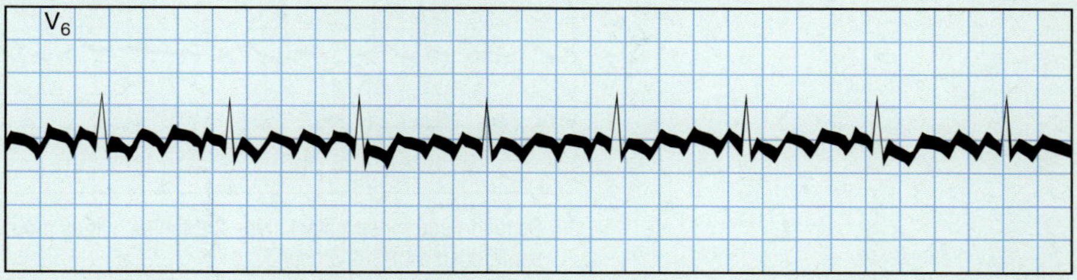
Sinus Bradycardia		
	Slow rate below 50 or 60/min	No disruption in conduction is not necessarily suggestive of a problem.
Sinus bradycardia		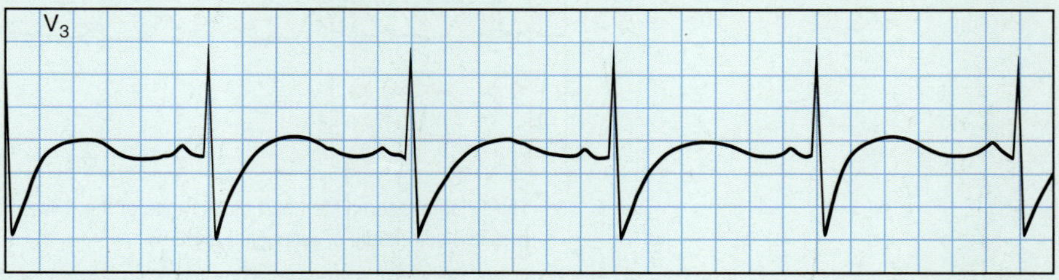
Atrial Fibrillation		
	Dysrhythmic contraction of the atria gives way to a rapid series of irregular spasms of the muscle wall; no discernible regularity in rhythm or pattern	The conduction system is malfunctioning and is in an anarchic state. Any contraction of the atria that is best described as "irregularly" irregular.
Atrial fibrillation with rapid ventricular response		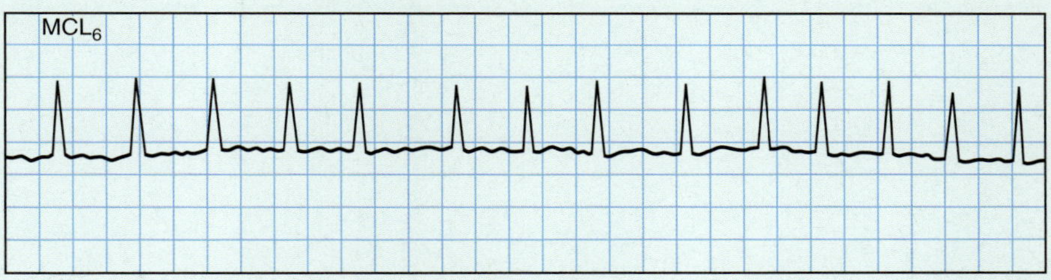

Continued

TABLE 15.6 Abnormalities in Rates and Rhythms—cont'd

TYPE AND DETECTION	FINDINGS ON EXAMINATION	DESCRIPTION
Heart Block	Heart rate slower than expected; incomplete heart block rate is often 25–45/min at rest	Conduction from atria to ventricles partially or completely disrupted. Conduction either occurs: 1. All the time (but taking a little longer than usual): first-degree heart block 2. Some of the time: second-degree heart block i. Type 1: Wenckebach/Mobitz 1 ii. Type 2: Mobitz 2 3. None of the time: third-degree or complete heart block
		ECG is necessary to determine the nature of heart block in conduction. 1. First-degree heart block: PR interval longer than 0.20 second 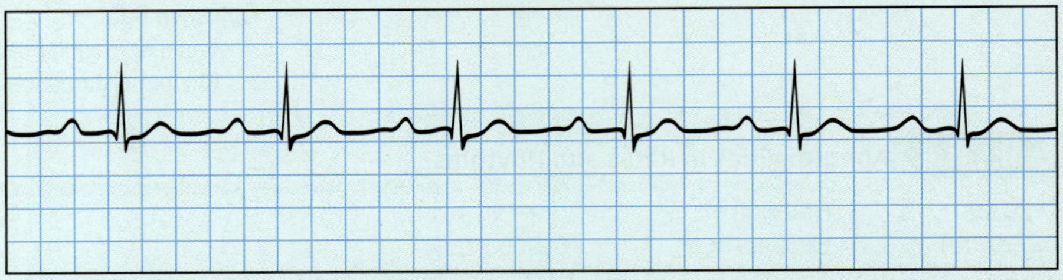
		2i. Second-degree heart block, type 1 (Wenckebach/Mobitz 1): benign, PR interval increases each beat until a QRS is dropped. 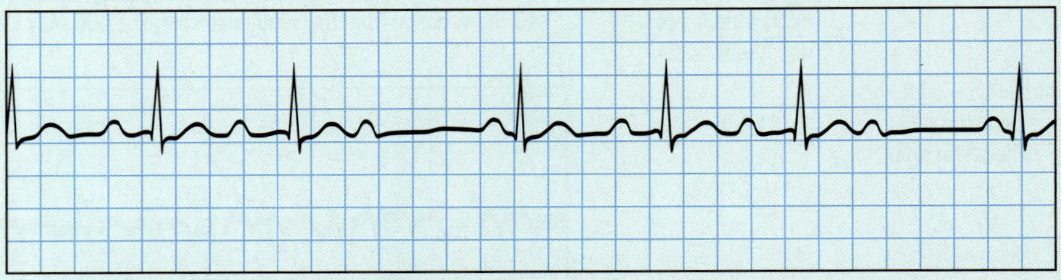
		2ii. Second-degree heart block, type 2 (Mobitz 2): may progress to compete heart block; PR interval stays the same, then a QRS is dropped. 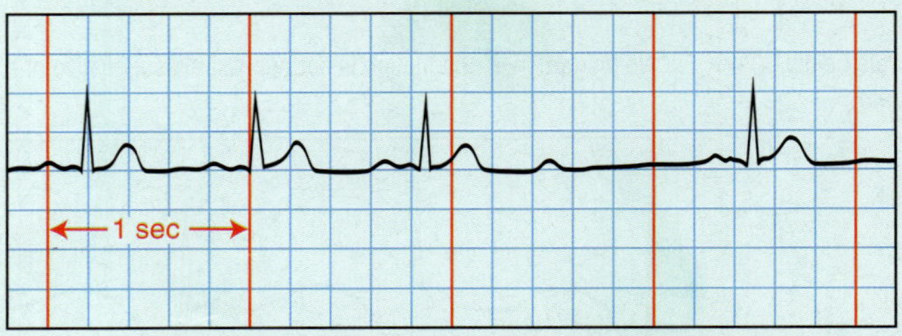 3. Third-degree, complete heart block: none of the P waves are conducted to the AV node; AV node generates a rate by itself (nodal or junctional rhythm) 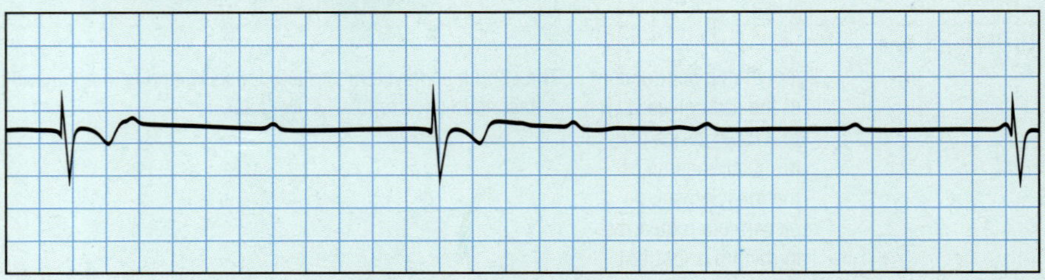

TABLE 15.6 Abnormalities in Rates and Rhythms—cont'd

TYPE AND DETECTION	FINDINGS ON EXAMINATION	DESCRIPTION
Supraventricular Tachycardia (SVT)		
	Rapid, regular heart rate and narrow QRS complex	Rapid heart rhythm originating at or above the atrioventricular node. The rate will occasionally decrease with vagal stimulation, holding a deep breath, or gentle massage of a carotid sinus. (Massage must always be done with care; see Chapter 16.)
Paroxysmal atrial tachycardia (PAT)		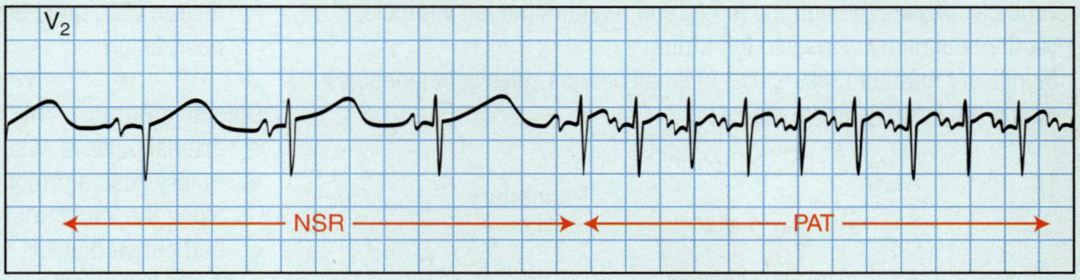
Ventricular Tachycardia		
	Rapid, relatively regular heartbeat (often nearly 200/min) without loss in apparent strength	The electrical source of the beat is an unusual focus somewhere in the ventricles. This usually arises in serious heart disease and is a grave prognostic sign.
Ventricular tachycardia		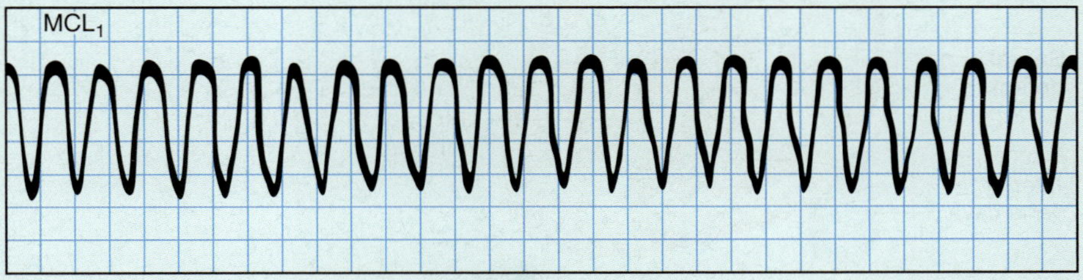
Ventricular Fibrillation		
	Complete loss of regular heart rhythm with expected conduction pattern absent if weakened and rapid, ventricular contraction is irregular	The ventricle has lost the rhythm of its expected response, and all evidence of vigorous contraction is gone. It calls for immediate action and may immediately precede sudden death.
Ventricular fibrillation		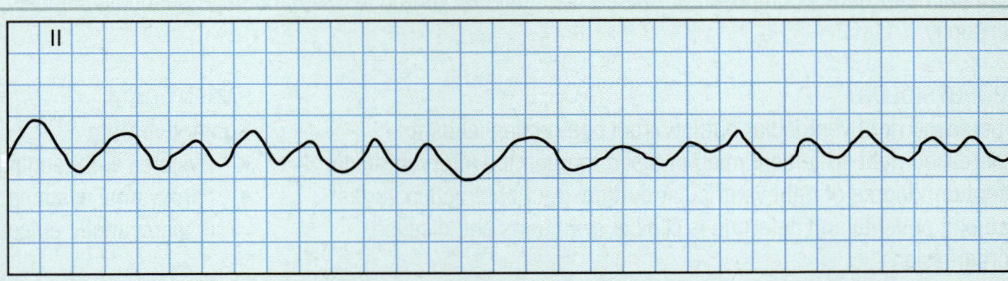

Sick Sinus Syndrome

Arrhythmias caused by a malfunction of the sinus node

PATHOPHYSIOLOGY

- Occurs secondary to hypertension, arteriosclerotic heart disease, or rheumatic heart, or without known cause (idiopathic)

PATIENT DATA

Subjective Data

- Fainting, transient dizzy spells, lightheadedness, seizures, palpitations, and angina

Objective Data

- Dysrhythmias
- Signs of congestive heart failure

Infants and Children

Ventricular Septal Defect

Opening between the left and right ventricles

PATHOPHYSIOLOGY

- During ventricular contraction, some blood from the left ventricle passes through the ventricular septal defect (VSD) into the right ventricle, passes through the lungs, and reenters the left ventricle via the pulmonary veins and left atrium
- Significant number (30%–50%) of small defects close spontaneously during the first 2 years of life

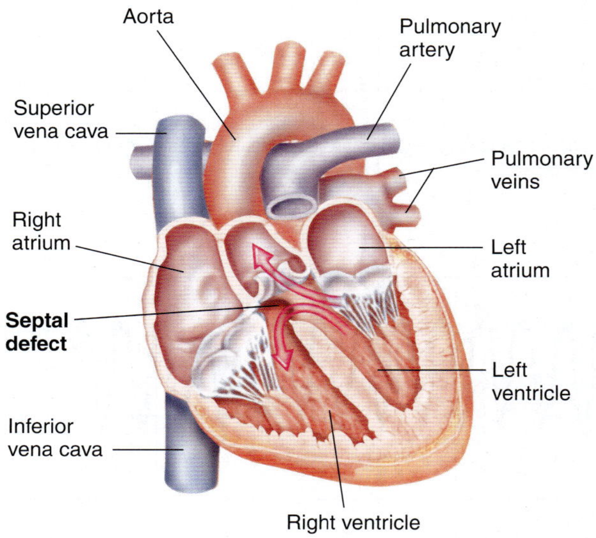

FIG. 15.25 **Tetralogy of Fallot.** (Modified from Canobbio, M. M. (1990). *Cardiovascular disorders.* St. Louis: Mosby.)

PATIENT DATA

Subjective Data

- Recurrent respiratory infections
- If large VSD, rapid breathing, poor growth, symptoms of congestive heart failure

Objective Data

- Arterial pulse is small, and jugular venous pulse is unaffected
- Holosystolic murmur, often loud, coarse, high-pitched, and best heard along the left sternal border in the third to fifth intercostal spaces
- Left peristernal lift
- A smaller defect causes a louder murmur and a more easily felt thrill than a large one (Fig. 15.25; see Table 15.5)

Tetralogy of Fallot

Congenital heart defect composed of four cardiac defects: ventricular septal defect, pulmonic stenosis, dextroposition of the aorta, and right ventricular hypertrophy

PATHOPHYSIOLOGY

- Increased right ventricular outflow tract obstruction leads to increased right-to-left shunting of blood through the interventricular septum; degree of right ventricular outflow tract obstruction varies among patients and determines clinical symptoms and disease progression
- Results in cyanosis during hypercontractile episodes, associated with agitation/crying

PATIENT DATA

Subjective Data

- Dyspnea with feeding, poor growth, exercise intolerance
- Paroxysmal dyspnea with loss of consciousness and central cyanosis (hypercyanotic episode or tetralogy spell)

Objective Data

- Parasternal heave and precordial prominence, systolic ejection murmur over the third intercostal space, sometimes radiating to the left side of the neck; a single S_2 is heard (Fig. 15.26)
- Older children develop clubbing of fingers and toes
- May develop heart failure if not surgically corrected

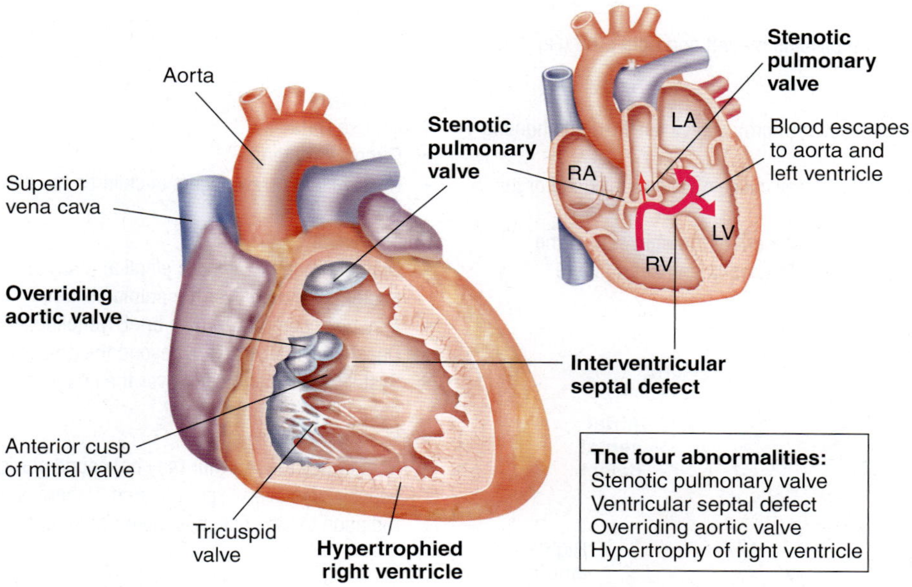

FIG. 15.26 Ventricular septal defect. (Modified from Canobbio, M. M. (1990). *Cardiovascular disorders.* St. Louis: Mosby.)

Patent Ductus Arteriosus

Failure of the ductus arteriosus to close after birth (Fig. 15.27)

PATHOPHYSIOLOGY

- Blood flows from the aorta through the ductus to the pulmonary artery during systole and diastole, increasing pressure in the pulmonary circulation and consequently the workload of the right ventricle

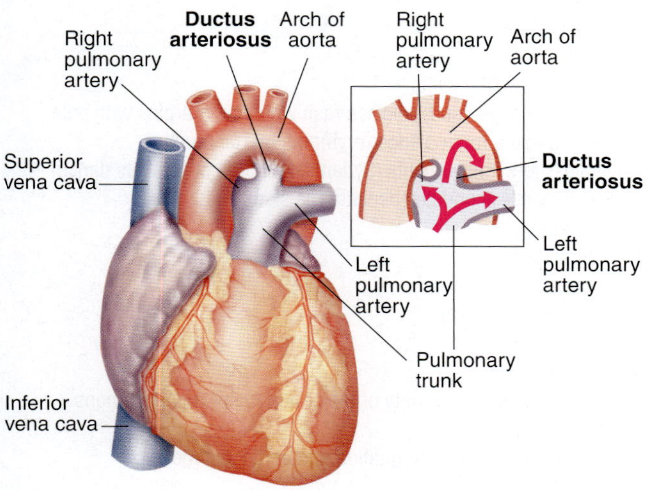

FIG. 15.27 Patent ductus arteriosus. (Modified from Canobbio, M. M. (1990). *Cardiovascular disorders.* St. Louis: Mosby.)

PATIENT DATA

Subjective Data

- Small shunt can be asymptomatic; a larger one causes dyspnea on exertion

Objective Data

- Dilated and pulsatile neck vessels
- Wide pulse pressure
- Harsh, loud, continuous murmur heard at the first to third intercostal spaces and the lower sternal border with a machinelike quality
- Murmur usually unaltered by postural change

Atrial Septal Defect

Congenital defect in the septum dividing the left and right atria (Fig. 15.28)

PATHOPHYSIOLOGY

- Large atrial septal defect (ASD; >9 mm), allows left-to-right shunting of blood
- Extra blood from the left atrium may cause a volume overload of the right atrium and the ventricle
- Untreated ASD can result in enlargement of the right side of the heart and shunt reversal (right-to-left shunt) and heart failure

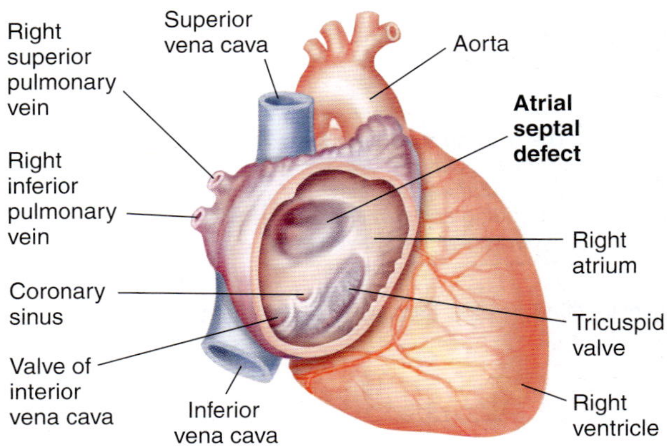

FIG. 15.28 Atrial septal defect.

PATIENT DATA

Subjective Data

- Often asymptomatic
- Heart failure rarely occurs in children but can often occur in adults

Objective Data

- Diamond-shaped systolic ejection murmur often loud, high-pitched, and harsh; heard over the pulmonic area
- May be accompanied by a brief, rumbling, early diastolic murmur
- Does not usually radiate beyond the precordium
- Systolic thrill may be felt over the area of the murmur, along with a palpable parasternal thrust
- S_2 may be widely split
- Sometimes the murmur may not sound particularly impressive, especially in overweight children; if there is a palpable thrust and radiation to the back, it is more apt to be significant

Acute Rheumatic Fever

Systemic connective tissue disease occurring after group A streptococcal pharyngitis or skin infection

PATHOPHYSIOLOGY

- Characterized by a variety of major and minor manifestations (Box 15.11)
- May result in serious cardiac valvular involvement of mitral or aortic valve; tricuspid and pulmonic are not often affected
- Affected valve becomes stenotic and regurgitant
- Children between 5 and 15 years of age are most commonly affected
- Prevention—adequate treatment for streptococcal pharyngitis or skin infections—is the best therapy
- The incidence of acute rheumatic fever is negligible in the United States but still occurs elsewhere and is most common in low-resource, low-income countries (Subhrajit & Sanyahumbi, 2021)

PATIENT DATA

Subjective Data

- Fever
- Inflamed swollen joints
- Flat or slightly raised, painless rash with pink margins with pale centers and a ragged edge (erythema marginatum)
- Aimless jerky movements (Sydenham chorea or St. Vitus dance)
- Small, painless nodules beneath the skin
- Chest pain
- Palpitations
- Fatigue
- Shortness of breath

Objective Data

- Characterized by a variety of major and minor manifestations (see Box 15.11)
- Murmurs of mitral regurgitation and aortic insufficiency
- Cardiomegaly
- Friction rub of pericarditis
- Signs of congestive heart failure

BOX 15.11 Jones Criteria for Diagnosis of Rheumatic Fever

MAJOR MANIFESTATIONS	MINOR MANIFESTATIONS
Carditis (echocardiography should be used to confirm the presence of carditis)	Clinical
Polyarthritis (can be monoarthritis in high-risk populations[a])	Previous rheumatic fever or rheumatic heart disease
Chorea	Polyarthralgia (can be monoarthralgia in high-risk populations[a])
Erythema marginatum	Fever
Subcutaneous nodules	Laboratory
	Acute phase reactions: erythrocyte sedimentation rate, C-reactive protein, leukocytosis
	Prolonged PR interval on electrocardiogram

Supporting Evidence of Streptococcal Infection

- Increased titer of antistreptolysin antibodies (antistreptolysin O in particular)
- Positive throat culture for group A streptococci
- Recent scarlet fever

The presence of two major or one major and two minor manifestations suggests a high probability of acute rheumatic fever if supported by evidence of a preceding group A streptococcal infection. Do not make the diagnosis on the basis of laboratory findings and two minor manifestations alone.[a]

[a]Acute rheumatic fever incidence >2 per 100,000 school-age children or all-age rheumatic heart disease prevalence of >1 per 1000 population per year.

From Gewitz, M. H., Baltimore, R. S., Tani, L. Y., et al. (2015). On behalf of the American Heart Association Committee on Rheumatic Fever, Endocarditis, and Kawasaki Disease of the Council on Cardiovascular Disease in the Young: Revision of the Jones criteria for the diagnosis of acute rheumatic fever in the era of Doppler echocardiography: A scientific statement from the American Heart Association. *Circulation, 131*, 1806–1818.

Older Adults

Atherosclerotic Heart Disease (Atherosclerosis, Coronary Heart Disease)

Narrowing of the small blood vessels that supply blood and oxygen to the heart

PATHOPHYSIOLOGY

- Caused by deposition of cholesterol or other lipids or by a complex inflammatory process
- Leads to vascular wall thickening and narrowing of the lumen

PATIENT DATA

Subjective Data

- May be asymptomatic
- Angina pectoris, shortness of breath, palpitations
- Family history of close relatives with atherosclerotic disease, early death, or dyslipidemia

Objective Data

- Dyslipidemia
- Dysrhythmias and signs of congestive heart failure

Senile Cardiac Amyloidosis

Deposition of amyloid, a fibrillary protein produced by chronic inflammation or neoplastic disease, in the heart

PATHOPHYSIOLOGY

- Heart contractility may be reduced
- Causes heart failure

PATIENT DATA

Subjective Data

- Palpitations, lower extremity edema, fatigue, reduced activity tolerance

Objective Data

- Pleural effusion
- Arrhythmia
- Lower extremity edema
- Dilated neck veins
- Hepatomegaly or ascites
- Electrocardiography or echocardiography shows small, thickened left ventricle; right ventricle may also be thickened

CHAPTER

16 Blood Vessels

The physical examination of the venous and arterial structures of the vascular system is a critical component of a patient's evaluation. You can gain great insight into their overall cardiovascular status, specifically the detection of peripheral artery disease (PAD) of the lower extremities, which is associated with an increased risk of stroke and cardiovascular events.

Physical Examination Components

Blood Vessels

1. Palpate the arterial pulses in distal extremities, comparing characteristics bilaterally for:
   - Rate
   - Rhythm
   - Contour
   - Amplitude
2. Auscultate the carotid; abdominal aorta; and renal, iliac, and femoral arteries for bruits.
3. With the patient reclining at a 45-degree angle, inspect for jugular venous pulsations and distention; differentiate jugular and carotid pulse waves, and evaluate jugular venous pressure.
4. Inspect the extremities for sufficiency of arteries and veins for:
   - Color, skin texture, and nail changes
   - Presence of hair
   - Muscular atrophy
   - Edema or swelling
   - Nonhealing ulcerations
   - Varicosities
5. Palpate the extremities for:
   - Warmth
   - Pulse quality
   - Tenderness along any superficial vein
   - Pitting edema

ANATOMY AND PHYSIOLOGY

The great vessels, the arteries leading from and the veins leading to the heart, are located in close proximity at the base of the heart. They include the aorta, superior and inferior venae cavae, pulmonary arteries, and pulmonary veins (Fig. 16.1). The aorta carries oxygenated blood from the left ventricle to the body. The pulmonary artery, which leaves the right ventricle and divides into right and left branches, carries deoxygenated blood to the lungs. The superior and inferior venae cavae carry deoxygenated blood from the upper and lower body, respectively, to the right atrium. The pulmonary veins return oxygenated blood from the lungs to the left atrium.

Blood Circulation

Once it leaves the heart, blood flows through two circulatory systems: the pulmonary and the systemic (Fig. 16.2). The pulmonary circulation routes blood through the lungs, where it is oxygenated before returning to the left atrium and ventricle of the heart. Venous blood arrives at the right atrium via the superior and inferior venae cavae and moves through the tricuspid valve to the right ventricle. During systole, deoxygenated blood is ejected through the pulmonic valve into the pulmonary artery; it then travels through the pulmonary arteries, arterioles, and capillaries until it reaches the alveoli, where gas exchange occurs.

Oxygenated blood of the systemic circulation returns to the heart and enters the systemic circulation through the pulmonary veins into the left atrium and then through the mitral valve into the left ventricle. The left ventricle contracts, forcing a volume of blood (stroke volume) with each beat through the aortic valve into the aorta, where it is distributed systemically through the arteries and capillaries. In the capillary bed, oxygen is provided to the tissues of the body; the now deoxygenated blood is rich in carbon dioxide. It passes into the venous system and returns to the heart via the superior and inferior venae cavae and into the right atrium (Fig. 16.3).

The structure of the arteries and veins reflects their function. The arteries are thicker, with a greater smooth muscle layer and less ability to stretch and expand (distention) from internal pressure. They are subjected to much more pressure than the veins. The veins are more distensible than the arteries (Fig. 16.4). Venous return occurs at a lower pressure than blood flow through the arteries, and veins contain valves to keep blood flowing in one direction. If circulatory volume increases significantly, the veins can expand and act as a repository for the extra volume.

Arterial Pulse and Pressure

The palpable and sometimes visible arterial pulses are the result of ventricular systole, which produces a pressure

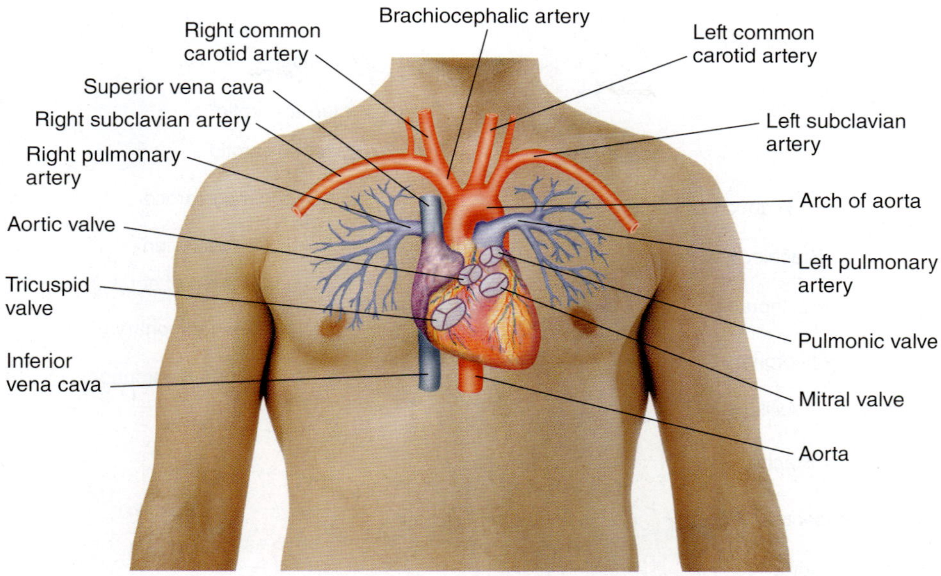

FIG. 16.1 Anatomic location of the great vessels and their relationship to the heart valves.

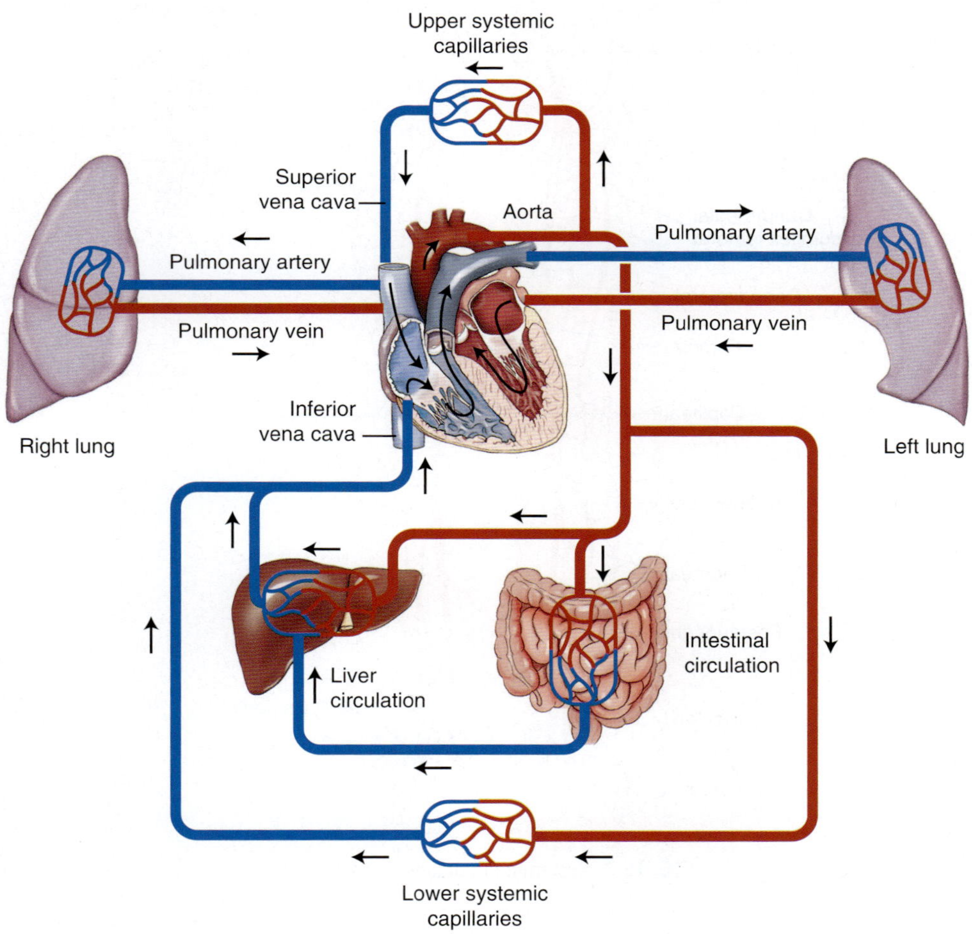

FIG. 16.2 Circulatory system.

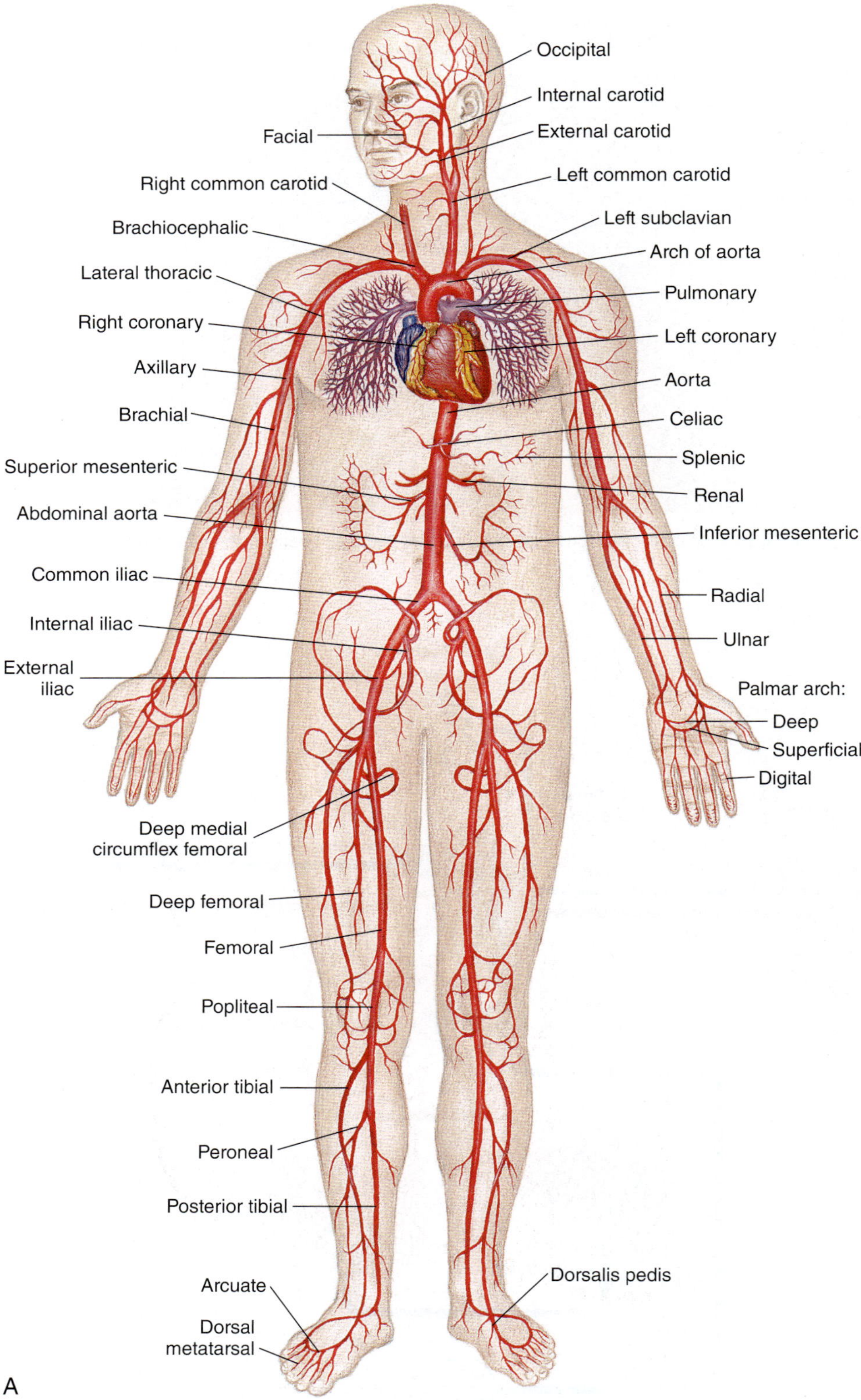

FIG. 16.3 Systemic circulation. (A) Arteries.

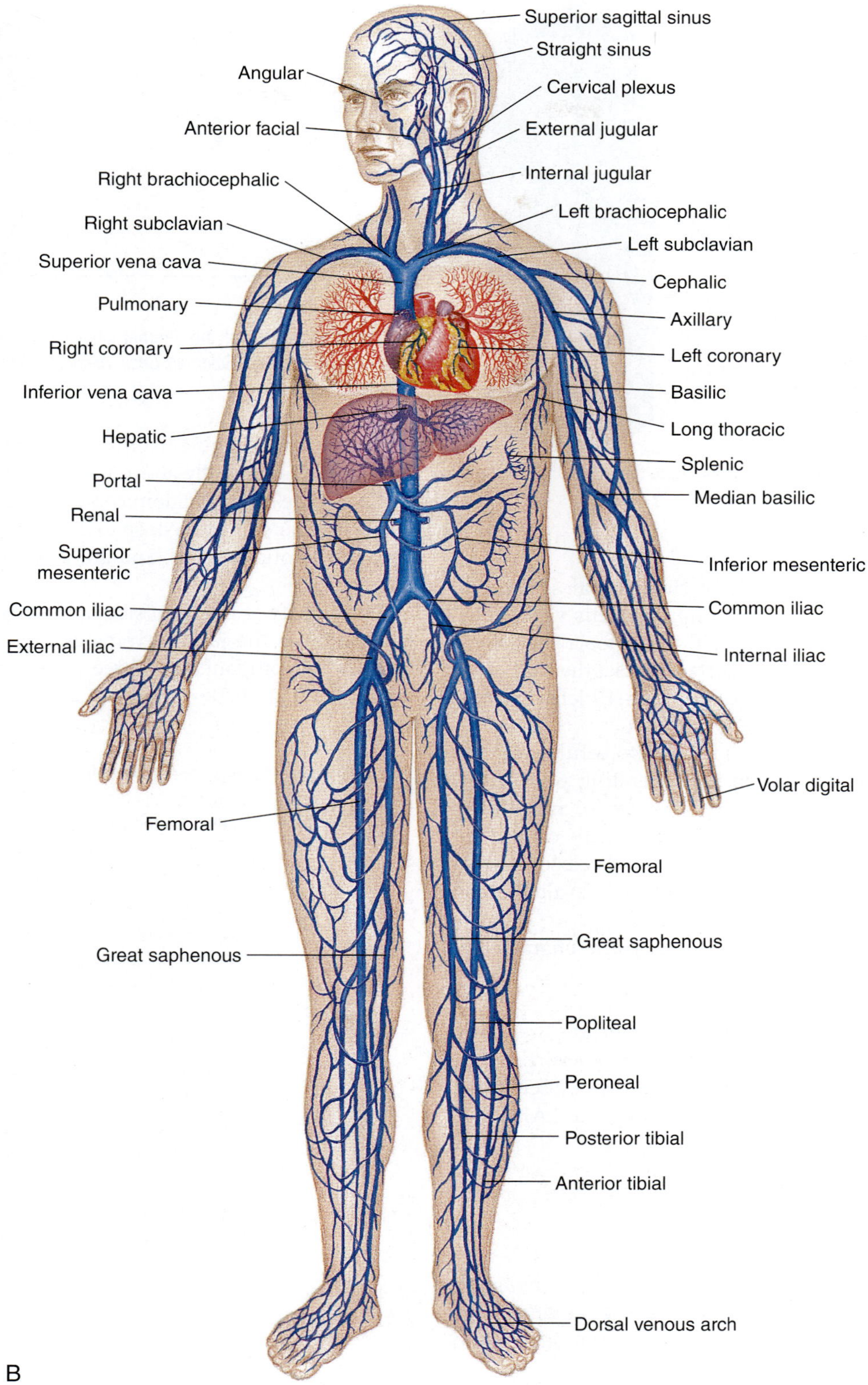

FIG. 16.3, cont'd (B) Veins.

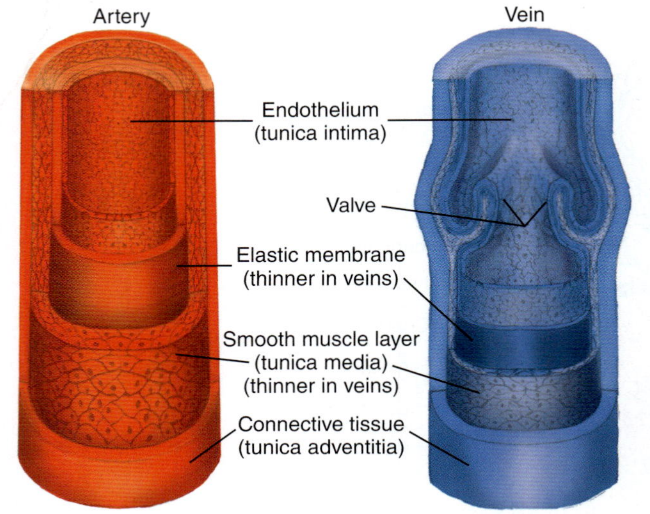

FIG. 16.4 **Structure of arteries and veins.** Note the relative thickness of the arterial wall.

wave (arterial pulse) throughout the arterial system. It takes barely 0.2 second for the impact of this wave to be felt in the dorsalis pedis artery within the foot. The arterial blood pressure is the force exerted against the wall of an artery as the bolus of blood exits the heart's left ventricle with each contraction.

The normal arterial pulse is felt as a forceful wave that is smooth and more rapid on the ascending part of the wave, whereas it becomes domed, less steep, and slower on the descending part (Fig. 16.5). Because the carotid arteries are the most accessible of the arteries closest to the heart, they have the most definitive pulse for evaluation of cardiac function.

The following variables contribute to the characteristics of the pulses:

- Volume of blood ejected (stroke volume)
- Distensibility of the aorta and large arteries
- Obstruction of blood flow (e.g., narrowing of aortic valve [stenosis] or aorta [coarctation or dissection], vasculitis—blood vessel inflammation with narrowing—or PAD)
- Peripheral artery resistance
- Viscosity of the blood

Jugular Venous Pulse and Pressure

The jugular veins, which empty directly into the superior vena cava, reflect the activity of the right side of the heart and offer clues to its competency. The level at which the jugular venous pulse is visible gives an indication of right atrial pressure.

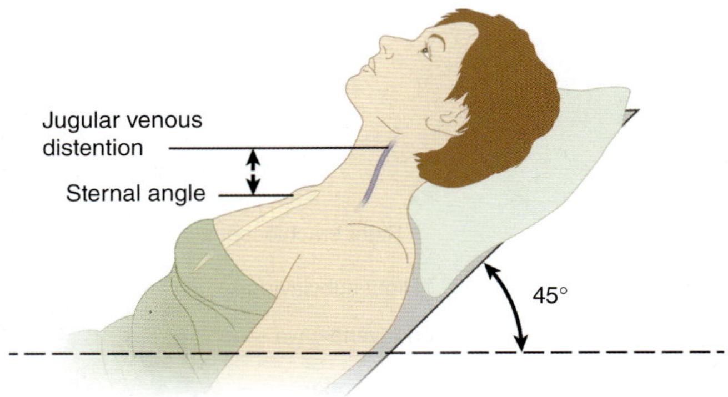

FIG. 16.6 Distention of the internal jugular vein. (From Goldman, L., & Schafer, A. I. (2016). *Goldman-Cecil medicine* (25th ed.). Philadelphia: Saunders.)

The external jugular veins are more superficial and more visible bilaterally above the clavicle, close to the insertion of the sternocleidomastoid muscles. The larger internal jugular veins run deep to the sternocleidomastoids, near the carotid arteries, and are less accessible to visual inspection (Fig. 16.6).

The activity of the right side of the heart is transmitted back through the jugular veins as a pulse[a] that has five identifiable components—three peaks and two descending slopes (Fig. 16.7):[a]

a wave	The upward a wave, the first and most prominent component, is the result of a brief backflow of blood to the vena cava during right atrial contraction. This peaks slightly before the first heart sound (S_1).
c wave	The upward c wave is a transmitted impulse from the vigorous backward push produced by closure of the tricuspid valve during right ventricular systole.
v wave	The upward v wave is caused by the increasing volume and concomitant increasing pressure in the right atrium. It occurs after the c wave, late in ventricular systole.
x slope	The downward x slope is caused by passive atrial filling. This ends with the initiation of the v wave.
y slope	The y slope following the v wave reflects the open tricuspid valve and the rapid filling of the right ventricle.

[a]Although often referred to as a pulse, this is not the same as an arterial pulse because it is reflected back from the right heart rather than pushed forward by the left heart. Unlike arterial pulses, it cannot be palpated, only visualized.

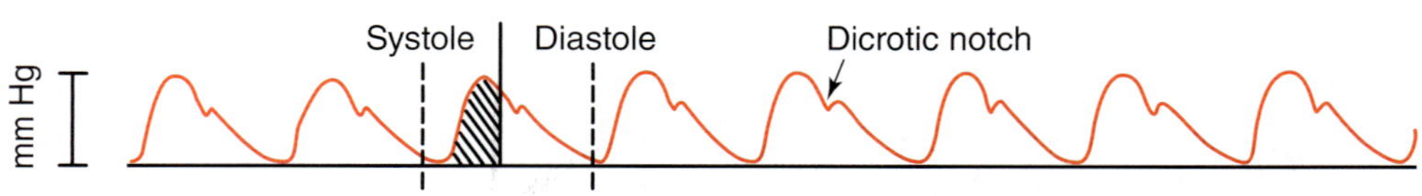

FIG. 16.5 Diagram of usual pulse.

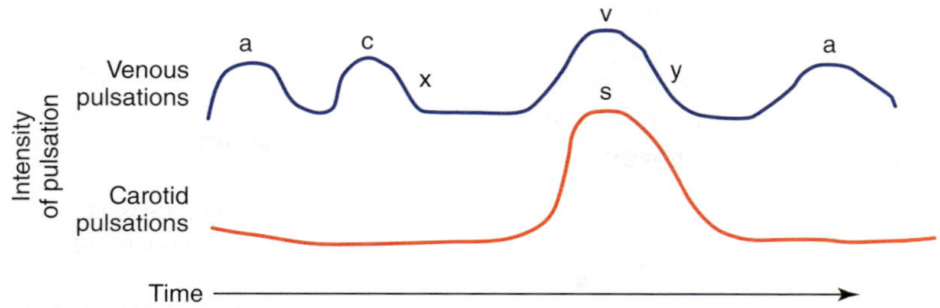

FIG. 16.7 Expected venous pulsations.

Infants and Children

At birth, the cutting of the umbilical cord, through which oxygen has been provided in utero, requires the infant to begin breathing. The onset of respiration expands the lungs and carries air to the alveoli. Pulmonary vascular resistance drops, allowing blood to flow more freely to the lungs. Systemic vascular resistance increases. In most full-term infants the ductus arteriosus closes, usually within the first 12 to 14 hours of life. Once pulmonary vascular resistance is lower than systemic resistance, blood flows into the pulmonary arteries rather than across the interatrial foramen ovale. The interatrial foramen ovale is functionally closed by the shifting pressures between the right and left sides of the heart.

Pregnant Patients

During pregnancy, the systemic vascular resistance decreases and peripheral vasodilation occurs, often resulting in palmar erythema and spider telangiectasias. The systolic blood pressure decreases slightly. There is a greater decrease in the diastolic pressure. The lowest levels occur in the second trimester and then rise but still remain below blood pressure readings before pregnancy. Maternal position affects blood pressure. Lower blood pressure can be noted when the patient is supine during the third trimester. This lower pressure is secondary to venous compression of the vena cava and impaired venous return. Blood in the lower extremities tends to pool in later pregnancy—except when the patient is in the lateral recumbent position—as a result of compression of the pelvic veins and inferior vena cava by the enlarged uterus. The compression may result in an increase in dependent edema, varicosities of the legs and vulva, and hemorrhoids.

Older Adults

Calcification and plaque buildup in the walls of the arteries can cause stiffness as well as dilation of the aorta, aortic branches, and carotid arteries. The arterial walls lose elasticity and vasomotor tone and are less distensible. The resulting increased peripheral vascular resistance may lead to elevated blood pressure, especially systolic.

REVIEW OF RELATED HISTORY

For each of the symptoms or conditions discussed in this section, targeted topics to include in the history of the present illness are listed. Responses to questions about these topics will provide clues for focusing on the physical examination and the development of an appropriate diagnostic evaluation. Questions regarding medication use (prescription and over-the-counter preparations) as well as complementary, alternative, and integrative therapies are relevant for each.

History of Present Illness

Leg Pain or Cramps

- Onset and duration: with activity or rest, recent injury or immobilization
- Character (e.g., sharp, dull, aching, throbbing)
- Continuous burning in toes, pain in thighs or buttocks, pain over specific location, induced by activity
- Skin changes: cold skin, pallor, sores, redness or warmth over vein, visible veins, darkened or ischemic skin
- Swelling of the leg
- Cramping: pain in buttock or calf with walking (claudication)
- Waking at night with leg or foot pain (rest pain)

Swollen Ankles

- Onset and duration: present in the morning, appearing as the day progresses, sudden onset, insidious onset
- Related circumstances: recent and long travel, postoperative immobilization, recent travel to high elevations, pregnancy, increased salt intake
- Associated symptoms: onset of nocturia, increased frequency of urination, increasing shortness of breath
- Treatment attempted (including rest, ice, massage, heat, elevation, use of compression stockings)
- Medications: heparin, warfarin, diuretics, antihypertensive medications

Past Medical History

- Cardiac surgery, or hospitalization for cardiac evaluation, congenital heart defect, vascular surgery or percutaneous interventions

- Chronic illness: hypertension and studies to define its cause, bleeding or clotting disorder, hyperlipidemia, diabetes, chronic kidney disease, thyroid dysfunction, stroke, vasculitis, thrombosis, transient ischemic attacks, coronary artery disease, atrial fibrillation or other type of dysrhythmia

Family History

Family members with risk factors, morbidity, and mortality related to the cardiovascular system; hypertension, dyslipidemia, diabetes, heart disease, thrombosis, varicose veins, venous insufficiency, peripheral vascular disease, abdominal aortic aneurysms, ages at time of illness or death

Personal and Social History

- Employment: physical demands; environmental hazards such as heat, chemicals, dust; sources of emotional stress
- Tobacco: type (cigarettes, cigars, pipe, chewing tobacco, marijuana, vaping, snuff); duration of use; amount; efforts to quit and methods used; age started and, perhaps, stopped; pack-years (Number of years smoking × Number of packs per day)
- Nutritional status
- Usual diet: proportion of fat, food preferences, salt intake, history of dieting
- Weight: loss or gain, amount and rate, expected or unexpected
- Exercise: type, amount, frequency, intensity
- Use of alcohol: amount consumed, frequency, duration of current intake
- Substance use: intravenous drug use, cocaine

Infants and Children

- Hemophilia
- Sickle cell disease
- Renal disease
- Coarctation of the aorta
- Leg cramps during exercise

Pregnant Patients

- Blood pressure: prepregnancy levels, elevation during pregnancy; evidence of preeclampsia with associated symptoms and signs such as headaches, visual changes, nausea and vomiting, epigastric pain, right upper quadrant pain, oliguria, rapid onset of edema (facial, abdominal, or peripheral), hyperreflexia, proteinuria, unusual bruising or bleeding. See Risk Factors, "Preeclampsia."
- Legs: edema, varicosities, pain or discomfort. See Risk Factors, "Varicose Veins."

Risk Factors

Preeclampsia

Age older than 40 years
First pregnancy
Preexisting chronic hypertension
Renal disease or diabetes mellitus
Multifetal gestation
Family history of preeclampsia or gestational hypertension
Previous preeclampsia or gestational hypertension
Obesity

Older Adults

- Leg edema: pattern, frequency, time of day most pronounced
- Interference with activities of daily living
- Ability of the patient and family to cope with the condition
- Claudication: area involved, unilateral or bilateral, distance one can walk before its onset, sensation, length of time required for relief
- Medications used for relief; efficacy of specific drugs

Risk Factors

Varicose Veins

Gender: four times more common in females than in males (during pregnancy in particular, increased hormonal levels weaken the walls of the vein and result in failure of the valves)
Genetic predisposition (children of parents with varicosities)
Tobacco use, sedentary lifestyle (habitual inactivity allows blood to pool in the veins, resulting in edema), occupations requiring prolonged standing, increased body mass index
Age: the veins of older adults are less elastic and more likely to be varicose
History of lower extremity trauma or venous thrombosis

EXAMINATION AND FINDINGS

Equipment

- Marking pencil
- Two separate centimeter rulers at least 15 cm long
- Stethoscope with bell and diaphragm

Palpation

The pulses are best palpated over arteries that are close to the surface of the body and lie over bones. These include the carotid, brachial, radial, femoral, popliteal, dorsalis pedis, and posterior tibial arteries (Fig. 16.8).

An arterial pulsation is essentially a bounding wave of blood that diminishes with increasing distance from the heart. The carotid pulses are most easily accessible and

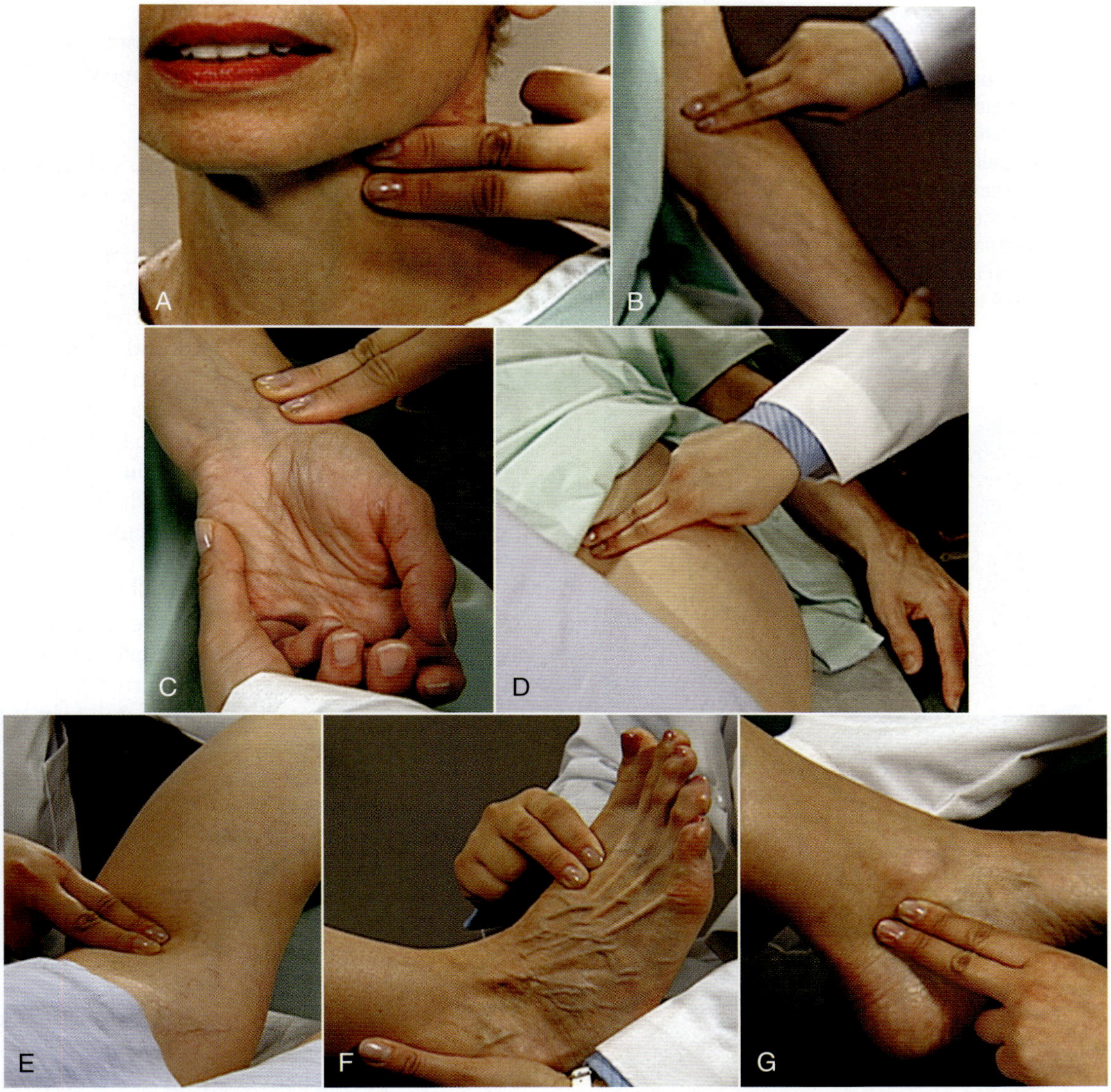

FIG. 16.8 Palpation of arterial pulses. (A) Carotid. (B) Brachial. (C) Radial. (D) Femoral. (E) Popliteal. (F) Dorsalis pedis. (G) Posterior tibial.

closest to the cardiac source, making them most useful in evaluating heart function. Examine the arterial pulses in the extremities to determine the sufficiency of the entire arterial circulation. Palpate at least one pulse point in each extremity, usually at the most distal point (see Clinical Pearl, "Carotid Palpation").

CLINICAL PEARL

Carotid Palpation

When palpating the carotid arteries, never palpate both sides simultaneously. Excessive carotid sinus massage can cause slowing of the pulse and a drop in blood pressure and compromise blood flow to the brain, leading to syncope. If you have difficulty feeling the pulse, rotate the patient's head to the side being examined to relax the sternocleidomastoid muscle.

Palpate the arterial pulses (most often the radial) to assess the heart rate and rhythm, pulse contour (waveform), amplitude (force), symmetry, and sometimes obstructions to blood flow. Palpate firmly but not so hard as to occlude the artery. The exception to this is when doing the Allen test to ensure ulnar artery patency before radial artery puncture (Box 16.1). Variations from the expected findings are described in Fig. 16.9.

The contour of the pulse wave is pliable. Healthy arteries have a smooth, rounded, or dome shape. Pay attention to the ascending portion, the peak, and the descending portion. Compare each wave crest with the next to detect cyclic differences.

BOX 16.1 The Allen Test

This test assesses the patency of the ulnar artery. Perform this test before radial artery puncture for arterial blood gas sampling or the insertion of a radial arterial catheter.

1. With the patient's palm facing upward, compress the radial and ulnar artery with your fingers (A).
2. Have the patient close and open the fist five times and then leave the blanched palm open.
3. Release pressure on the ulnar artery alone and watch for palmar reperfusion within 4 to 5 seconds.
4. If palmar reperfusion does not occur, suspect ulnar artery insufficiency and do not puncture the radial artery (B).

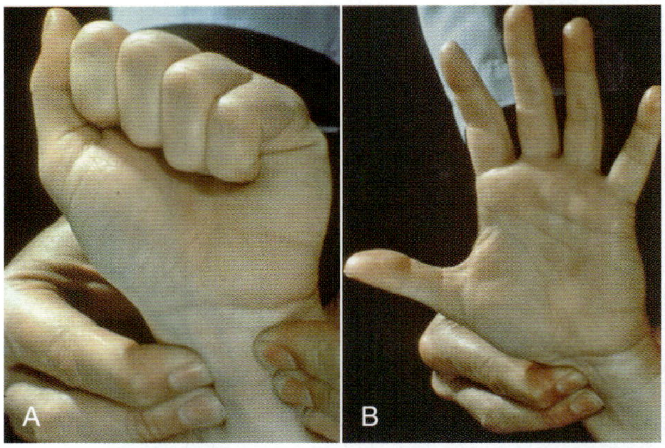

From Skirven, T. M., & Ostermen, A. L. (2011). *Rehabilitation of the hand and upper extremity* (6th ed.). Elsevier.

The amplitude of the pulse is described on a scale of 0 to 4:

4	Bounding, aneurysmal
3	Full, increased
2	Expected
1	Diminished, barely palpable
0	Absent, not palpable

Determine the regularity of the pulse. If it is irregular, determine whether there is a consistent pattern. An irregular heart rate that occurs in a repeated pattern may indicate sinus arrhythmia, a cyclic variation of the heart rate characterized by an increasing rate on inspiration and decreasing rate on expiration. A patternless, unpredictable, irregular rate may indicate heart disease or an impaired conduction system such as atrial fibrillation. If you note an irregular rate, record the beats per minute and compare it with the rate heard when auscultating the heart (see Chapter 15). Note the strength of the pulse.

Lack of symmetry (in pulse contour or strength) between the left and right extremities suggests impaired circulation. Compare the strength of the upper extremity pulses with those of the lower extremities and the left with the right. Ordinarily, the femoral is as strong as or stronger than the radial pulse. If the femoral pulsation is absent or diminished, proximal obstruction should be suspected, which may be due to such conditions as coarctation of the aorta, atherosclerotic peripheral arterial disease, or large vessel vasculitis.

Auscultation

Auscultate over an artery for a bruit (i.e., a murmur or unexpected sound) if you are following the radiation of murmurs first noted during the cardiac examination or looking for evidence of local obstruction. These sounds are usually low pitched and relatively hard to hear. Place the bell of the stethoscope directly over the artery. Sites to auscultate for a bruit are over the carotid, subclavian, abdominal aortic, renal, iliac, and femoral arteries. See Chapter 18 for auscultation of abdominal bruits. When listening over the carotid vessels, ask the patient to hold their breath for a few heartbeats so that respiratory sounds will not interfere with auscultation (Fig. 16.10). Sounds heard over the neck include venous hums and carotid bruits (Box 16.2).

Assessment for Peripheral Arterial Disease

Arteries in any location can become narrowed, leading to decreased blood flow. The first symptom is often pain that results from muscle ischemia, referred to as *claudication*. This pain can be characterized as a dull ache with accompanying muscle fatigue and cramps. It usually appears during sustained exercise, such as walking a distance or climbing several flights of stairs. Just a few minutes of rest will ordinarily relieve it. It recurs again with the same amount of activity. Continued activity causes worsening pain.

The site of pain is distal to the narrowing. After determining the distinguishing characteristics of the pain, note the following:

- Pulses (strong, weak, or possibly absent)
- Possible systolic bruits over the arteries that may extend through diastole
- Loss of expected body warmth in the affected area
- Localized pallor and cyanosis
- Collapsed superficial veins, with delay in venous filling
- Thin, atrophied skin; muscle atrophy (particularly with chronic insufficiency)

To judge the degree of narrowing and the potential severity of the arterial insufficiency, perform the following steps:

- Have the patient lie supine.
- Elevate the extremity.
- Note the degree of blanching.
- Have the patient sit on the edge of the bed or examining table to lower the extremity.
- Note the time for maximal return of color once the elevated extremity is lowered. Slight pallor on elevation and a return to full color as soon as the leg becomes dependent are the expected findings. A delay of many seconds or even minutes before the extremity regains full color indicates arterial insufficiency. When returning to full color takes as long as 2 minutes, the problem is severe.

A measurement of the capillary refill time provides another method of assessing severity (Box 16.3).

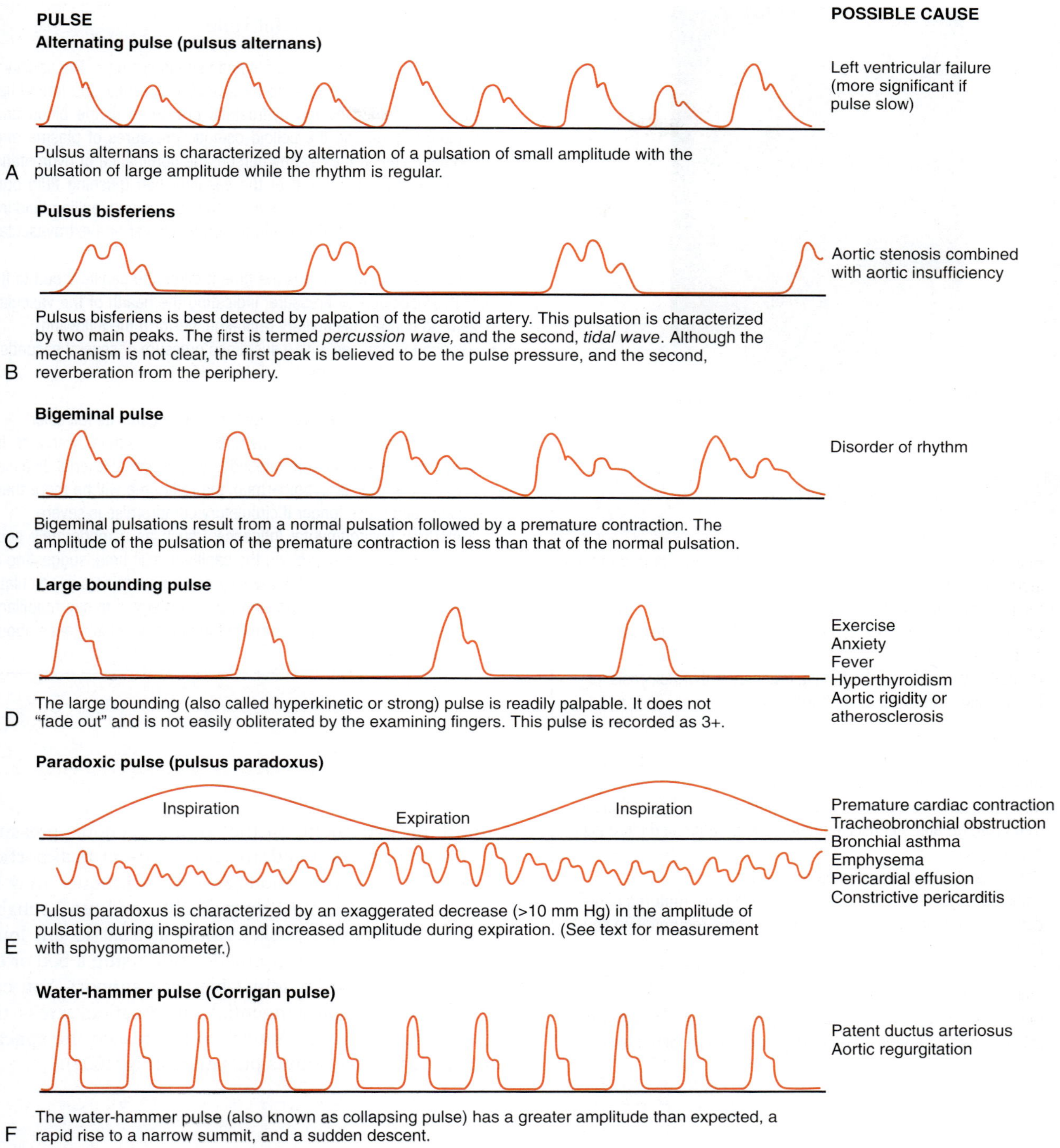

FIG. 16.9 Pulse abnormalities.

The following list provides a general guideline for assessment of possible causes of pain:

PAIN LOCATION	PROBABLE OBSTRUCTED ARTERY
Calf muscles	Superficial femoral artery
Thigh	Common femoral artery or external iliac artery
Buttock	Common iliac artery or distal aorta (erectile dysfunction may accompany stenosis of distal aorta)

If the pain is constant, the narrowing is likely critical; if it is excruciating, a major artery has probably been severely compromised acutely. Patients who present with acute limb ischemia (ALI) often demonstrate pain, pulselessness, paresthesias, paralysis, pallor, and poikilothermia. Determining the stage of ALI will help to dictate management. The following list provides a general guideline for assessment of these patients.

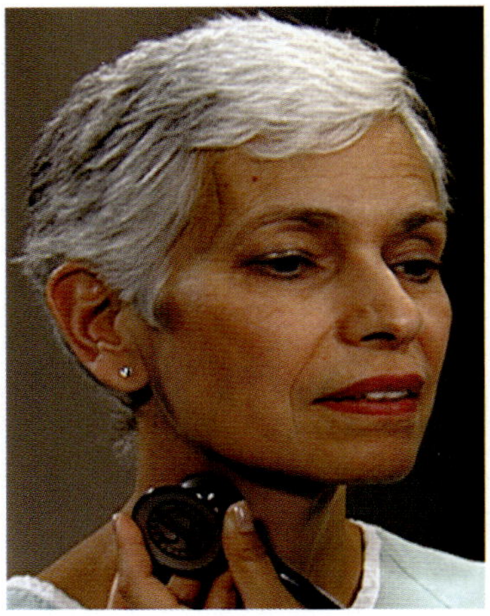

FIG. 16.10 Auscultation for bruits in the carotid artery.

BOX 16.2 Listening to the Neck

Venous Hum

- Heard at the medial end of the clavicle and anterior border of the sternocleidomastoid muscle
- Usually of no clinical significance
- Can be confused with carotid bruit, patent ductus arteriosus, and aortic regurgitation
- In adults, may occur with anemia, pregnancy, thyrotoxicosis, or intracranial arteriovenous malformation

Carotid Artery Bruits

- Heard at just above the medial end of the clavicle and anterior margin of the sternocleidomastoid muscle
- Mild obstruction produces a short, not particularly intense, localized bruit; greater stenosis lengthens the duration and increases the pitch
- Complete stenosis may eliminate the bruit
- Transmitted murmurs of valvular aortic stenosis, ruptured chordae tendineae of mitral valve, or severe aortic regurgitation can radiate to the carotid
- Can be heard with vigorous left ventricular ejection (more commonly in children than in adults)
- Occurs with arterial narrowing in cervical arteries (e.g., atherosclerotic carotid arteries, fibromuscular dysplasia, and arteritis)

STAGE	SENSORY IMPAIRMENT	MOTOR IMPAIRMENT	ARTERIAL DOPPLER SIGNAL	VENOUS DOPPLER SIGNAL
I (Viable)	No	No	Audible	Audible
IIa (Marginally Threatened)	Minimal	No	Often inaudible	Audible
IIb (Immediately Threatened)	Rest pain	Mild to moderate	Inaudible	Audible
III (Irreversible)	Anesthetic	Paralytic/ rigor	Inaudible	Inaudible

BOX 16.3 Capillary Refill Time

The capillary bed joins the arterial and venous systems. The capillary structure allows fluid exchange between the vascular and interstitial spaces, determined by the hydrostatic pressures of the blood and interstitial tissues and the colloid osmotic pressures of plasma and interstitial fluids. In the healthy person, the dominance of hydrostatic pressure at the arterial end of the capillary bed (pushing fluid out) and of the colloid osmotic pressure at the venous end (pulling fluid in) maintains the balance of fluids in the intravascular and extravascular spaces.

The capillary refill time is the time it takes the capillary bed to fill after it is occluded by pressure, indicating the health of the vascular system. To gauge the capillary refill time, perform the following:

- Blanch the nail bed with a sustained pressure of several seconds on a fingernail or toenail.
- Release the pressure.
- Observe the time elapsed before the nail regains its full color.

If the vascular system is intact, the refill time is less than 2 seconds. If, however, the system is compromised (e.g., peripheral arterial disease, hypovolemic shock, or hypothermia), the refill time will be more than 2 seconds and much longer if circulatory compromise is severe.

CAUTION: Environmental influences, such as a moderately cool room temperature, may prolong the capillary refill time, suggesting a problem that may not exist. Variability among examiners in calculating the time may also be a problem. One strategy is to say "capillary refill" as you release the pressure on the nail bed, which takes about 2 seconds, as a guide.

Peripheral Veins

Jugular Venous Pressure

Careful measurement of the jugular venous pressure (JVP) is an important and, in some cases, critical portion of the physical examination. Several techniques may be used. The simplest, most reproducible, and most reliable method requires two pocket rulers at least 15 cm long. Place the patient in the supine position using a bed or examining table with an adjustable back support. You can use a light to supply tangential illumination across the right side of the patient's neck to accentuate the appearance of the jugular venous pulsations (Fig. 16.11).

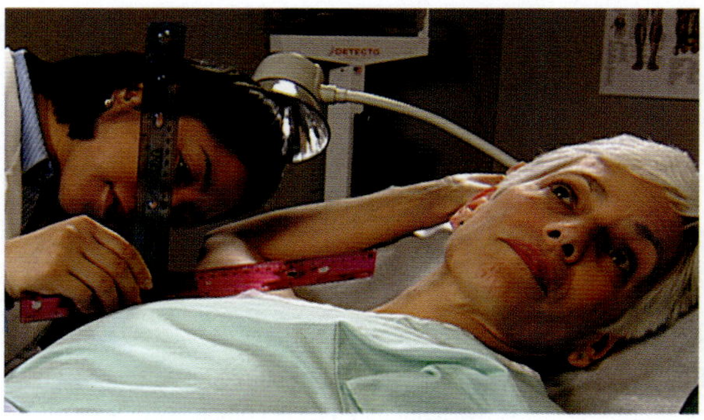

FIG. 16.11 Measuring jugular venous pressure.

When the supine patient is initially placed flat, note the engorgement of the jugular veins. Gradually raise the head of the bed until the jugular venous pulsations become evident between the angle of the jaw and the clavicle (see Fig. 16.6). Palpating the carotid pulse helps identify the venous pulsations and distinguish them from the carotid pulsations. Table 16.1 provides instructions on differentiating between jugular and carotid pulses. The jugular pulse can only be visualized; it cannot be palpated.

Several conditions may make the JVP examination more difficult: (1) severe right heart failure, tricuspid insufficiency, constrictive pericarditis, and cardiac tamponade may each cause extreme elevation of the JVP so that it is not apparent until the patient is sitting upright; (2) severe volume depletion makes the JVP difficult to detect even when the patient is flat; and (3) in extreme obesity, overlying adipose tissue obscures the jugular venous pulsations.

Place a ruler with its tip at the midaxillary line (the position of the heart within the chest) at the level of the nipple and extended vertically. Place the second ruler at the level of the meniscus of the JVP, extended horizontally to where it intersects the vertical ruler. The vertical distance above the level of the heart is noted as the mean JVP in centimeters of water (see Fig. 16.11). A value of less than 9 cm H_2O is the expected value.

Maneuvers useful for confirming the JVP measurement include hepatojugular reflux and the evaluation of the venous engorgement of the hands at various levels of elevation above the heart.

Hepatojugular Reflux

The hepatojugular reflux is exaggerated when right heart failure is present, and its measurement is used to evaluate that condition. To assess the hepatojugular reflux maneuver, use your hand to apply firm pressure for 10 seconds to the abdomen in the midepigastric region and instruct the patient to breathe regularly. Observe the neck for an elevation of at least 3 to 4 cm in JVP that lasts beyond a few seconds. The JVP equilibrates to its true level after removal of the abdominal hand pressure.

If the JVP is not obvious with this maneuver, the pressure is either much higher or much lower. Repeat the maneuver with the patient more supine if you suspect the pressure to be lower. Position the patient more upright if you suspect the JVP to be higher.

Evaluation of Hand Veins. The veins of the hand can be used as an "auxiliary manometer" of the right heart pressure when the patient does not have thrombosis or arteriovenous fistula in that arm or superior vena cava syndrome. With the patient semirecumbent, place their hand on the examination table or mattress. Palpate the hand veins, which should be engorged, to make sure they are compressible. Slowly raise the hand until the veins collapse (Fig. 16.12). Use a ruler to note the vertical distance between the midaxillary line at the nipple level (level of the heart) and the level of collapse of the hand veins. Confirm this level by lowering the hand slowly until the veins distend again and raise it back until they once again collapse. This distance should be identical to the mean JVP.

The hand vein measurement is particularly helpful to evaluate severe right heart failure when the pressure may be 20 to 30 cm H_2O (i.e., JVP is not evident with the patient sitting upright) or with volume depletion (i.e., JVP not visible with the patient supine).

Assessment for Venous Obstruction and Insufficiency. Obstruction of the venous system and a consequent insufficiency result in signs and symptoms that vary depending on how rapidly the obstruction develops and on the degree of localization. An acute obstruction may result from injury, external compression, or thrombosis. In the affected area, constant pain occurs simultaneously with the following:

- Swelling and tenderness over the muscles
- Engorgement of superficial veins
- Erythema and/or cyanosis

Inspect the extremities for signs of venous insufficiency (e.g., varicose veins, spider veins, hyperpigmentation, or edema). Examine the patient in both the standing and supine positions, particularly when you suspect chronic

TABLE 16.1 Comparison of the Jugular and Carotid Pulse Waves

ASSESSMENT	JUGULAR	CAROTID
Quality and character	Three positive waves in normal sinus rhythm	One wave
Palpate the carotid artery on one side of the neck and look at the jugular vein on the other side to tell the difference.	More undulating	More brisk
Effect of respiration	Level of pulse wave decreased on inspiration and increased on expiration	No effect
Venous compression	Easily eliminates pulse wave	No effect
Apply gentle pressure over vein at base of neck above clavicle.		
Abdominal pressure	May cause some increased prominence even in well persons; with right-sided heart failure, jugular vein may be more visible	No effect
Place the palm with moderate firmness over the right upper quadrant of the abdomen for 30 seconds.		

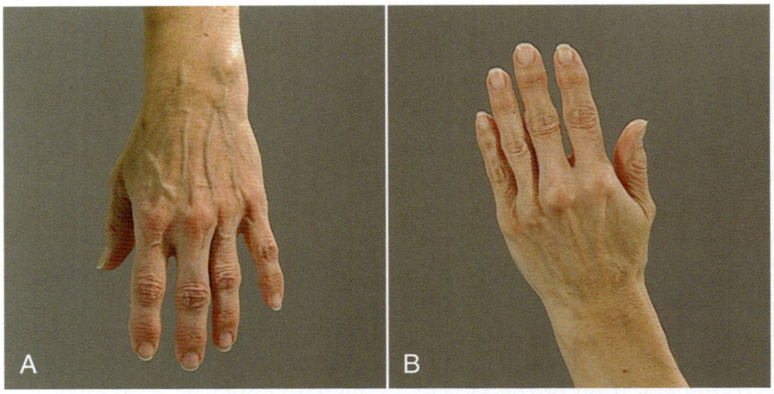

FIG. 16.12 Evaluation of hand veins. (A) Engorged veins in dependent hand. (B) Collapsed veins in elevated hand.

venous occlusion. Ultrasound studies can confirm the presence of venous occlusion and insufficiency.

Thrombosis. Note any redness, thickening, and tenderness along a superficial vein, suggesting thrombophlebitis of a superficial vein. Suspect a deep vein thrombosis if significant swelling, pain, and tenderness occur in an extremity over a deep vein. This cannot be confirmed on physical examination alone and requires diagnostic imaging.

Edema. Inspect the extremities for edema, manifested as a change in the usual contour of the leg. Press your index finger over the bony prominence of the tibia or medial malleolus for several seconds. A depression that does not rapidly refill and resume its original contour indicates orthostatic (pitting) edema. Usually this finding is not accompanied by thickening or pigmentation of the overlying skin. Right-sided heart failure leads to an increased fluid volume, which in turn elevates the hydrostatic pressure in the vascular space, causing edema in dependent parts of the body.

The severity of edema may be characterized by grading 1+ through 4+ (Fig. 16.13). Any concomitant pitting can be mild or severe, as evidenced by the following:

- 1+ Slight pitting, no visible distortion, disappears rapidly
- 2+ A somewhat deeper pit than in 1+, but again no readily detectable distortion; disappears in 10–15 seconds
- 3+ Noticeably deep pit that may last more than a minute; dependent extremity looks fuller and swollen
- 4+ Very deep pit that lasts as long as 2–5 minutes; dependent extremity is grossly distorted

Edema accompanied by some thickening and ulceration of the skin is frequently associated with deep venous obstruction or venous valvular incompetence. Edema that is related to valvular incompetence or an obstruction of a deep vein (usually in the legs) is caused by the mechanical pressure of increased blood volume in the area served by the affected vein. Circulatory disorders that cause edema so tense that it does not pit must be distinguished from lymphedema (see Chapter 10).

Varicose Veins. Varicose veins are dilated and engorged, with a diminished rate of blood flow and an increased intravenous pressure. These characteristics may result from incompetence of the vessel wall or venous valves or an obstruction in a more proximal vein.

Inspect the legs for superficial varicosities when the patient is standing. With varicosities, the veins appear dilated and often tortuous. If varicose veins are suspected, have the patient stand on their toes 10 times in succession. Palpate the legs to feel for the venous distention. When the venous system is competent, the distention of the veins disappears in a few seconds. If the distention of the veins is sustained for a longer time, you should suspect venous insufficiency.

To evaluate the direction of blood flow and the competency of the valves in the venous system, distend visible veins by putting the limb in a dependent position. Compress the vein with the finger or thumb of one hand and strip the vein of blood by compressing the vein and moving the fingers of the second hand proximally. If the compressed vessel fills before either compressing finger

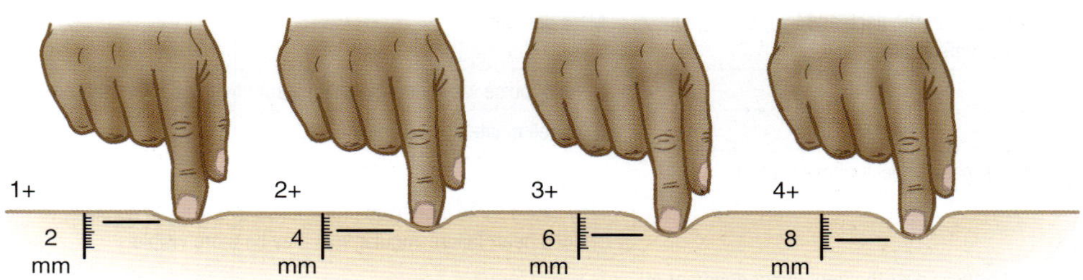

FIG. 16.13 Assessing for pitting edema.

is released, collateral circulation exists. If the compressing finger nearest the heart is released, the vessel should fill backward to the first valve only. If the entire venous column fills, the valves in that vessel are incompetent.

Infants

The brachial, radial, and femoral pulses of the newborn can easily be palpated. When the pulse is weaker than expected, cardiac output may be diminished or peripheral vasoconstriction may be present. A bounding pulse is associated with a large left-to-right shunt produced by a patent ductus arteriosus. In coarctation of the aorta, a difference is noted in pulse amplitude between the upper extremities or between the femoral and radial pulses, or the femoral pulses are weak or absent.

Capillary refill times in infants and children younger than 2 years of age are rapid, less than 1 second. A prolonged capillary refill time—longer than 2 seconds—indicates dehydration or hypovolemic shock.

Children

A venous hum, common in children, usually has no pathologic significance (see Box 16.2). It is caused by the turbulence of blood flow in the internal jugular veins. To detect a venous hum, ask the child to sit with the head turned away from you and tilted slightly upward. Auscultate over the supraclavicular space at the medial end of the clavicle and along the anterior border of the sternocleidomastoid muscle (Fig. 16.14). The intensity of the hum is increased when the patient is sitting with the head turned away from the area of auscultation, and it is diminished with a Valsalva maneuver. When present, the hum is a continuous, low-pitched sound that is louder during diastole. It may be interrupted by gentle pressure over the vein in the space between the trachea and the sternocleidomastoid muscle at about the level of the thyroid cartilage. The venous hum can be confused with patent ductus arteriosus, aortic regurgitation, and the murmur of valvular aortic stenosis transmitted into the carotid arteries.

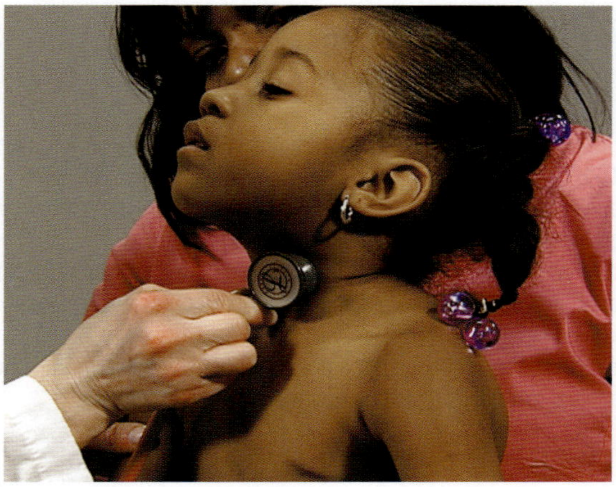

FIG. 16.14 Auscultation for venous hum.

Venous thrombosis occurs less commonly in children than in adults and is most often associated with placement of venous access devices. They can occur in any peripheral vessel and may cause swollen, painful extremities.

Pregnant Patients

With increasing cardiac output beginning in the first trimester, the pulse may be more easily palpated, with an abrupt rise and rapid fall. With increasing blood volume in the second trimester, jugular a and v waves may be easier to see. JVP should remain normal. Peripheral edema is a common finding as the pregnancy progresses. Varicose veins can develop during pregnancy and in the postpartum period.

Older Adults

The dorsalis pedis and posterior tibial pulses may be more difficult to find, and the superficial vessels are more apt to appear tortuous and distended.

ABNORMALITIES

VESSEL DISORDERS

Temporal Arteritis (Giant Cell Arteritis)

An inflammatory disease of the branches of the aortic arch, including the temporal arteries

PATHOPHYSIOLOGY

- Etiology unknown
- Inflammatory infiltrates develop in the thoracic aorta and neighboring arteries of the head and neck
- Arterial wall thickening and thrombosis can lead to reduced blood supply and ischemia of structures such as the masseter muscle, tongue, or optic nerve

PATIENT DATA

Subjective Data

- Usually affects persons older than 50 years of age
- Flulike symptoms (e.g., low-grade fever, malaise, anorexia) may be accompanied by polymyalgia rheumatica involving the hips, neck, and shoulders
- Headache in the temporal region on one or both sides, although the headache can occur in other regions
- Ocular symptoms, including loss of vision, are common
- Ischemia can also cause tongue pain and jaw claudication

Objective Data

- Area over the temporal artery may be red, swollen, tender, and nodular
- Temporal pulse may be strong, weak, or absent
- Biopsy required for definitive diagnosis

Arterial Aneurysm

A localized dilation, which is generally defined as 1.5 times the diameter of the normal artery, caused by a weakness in the arterial wall (Fig. 16.15)

PATHOPHYSIOLOGY

- Usually the result of atherosclerosis, with family history, tobacco use, and hypertension playing important roles
- Other causes include infection, iatrogenic injury, or traumatic injury
- Abdominal aneurysms are four times more common in males than in females
- Occurs most commonly in the aorta, although renal, femoral, and popliteal arteries are also common sites

PATIENT DATA

Subjective Data

- Generally asymptomatic until they rupture, dissect, or compress an adjacent structure
- With dissection, the patient may describe a severe, ripping pain

Objective Data

- Pulsatile swelling along the course of an artery
- A thrill or bruit may be evident over the aneurysm

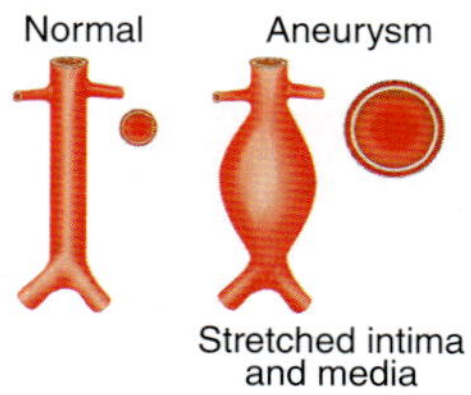

FIG. 16.15 Aortic aneurysm.

Arteriovenous Fistula

A pathologic communication between an artery and a vein

PATHOPHYSIOLOGY

- May be congenital or acquired
- Damage to vessels caused by catheterization is the most commonly acquired etiology
- If the fistula is large, there may be significant arterial-to-venous shunting of blood
- May result in an aneurysmal dilation

PATIENT DATA

Subjective Data

- Patients may present with lower extremity edema, varicose veins, or claudication due to ischemia

Objective Data

- A continuous bruit or thrill over the area of the fistula suggests its presence
- Edema or ischemia may develop in the involved extremity

Peripheral Arterial Disease

Stenosis of the blood supply to the extremities by atherosclerotic plaques

PATHOPHYSIOLOGY

- Most common cause is peripheral atherosclerosis
- Risk factors include diabetes, hypertension, dyslipidemia, and tobacco use
- Can also be a result of vascular trauma, radiation therapy, or vasculitis

PATIENT DATA

Subjective Data

- Pain in muscle after exercise that disappears with rest
- Amount of exercise needed to cause discomfort is predictable (e.g., occurring each time the same distance is walked)

Objective Data

- In claudication, the limb appears healthy, but pulses are weak or absent
- Progressive stenosis results in severe ischemia, in which the foot or leg is painful at rest, is cold and numb, and has skin changes (e.g., dry and scaling, with poor hair and nail growth)
- Edema seldom accompanies this disorder, but ulceration is common in severe disease, and the muscles may atrophy

Raynaud Phenomenon

An exaggerated spasm of the digital arterioles (occasionally in the nose and ears) usually in response to cold exposure (Fig. 16.16)

PATHOPHYSIOLOGY

- Primary Raynaud phenomenon occurs most commonly in young, otherwise healthy individuals, most commonly females, present with no evidence of underlying cause
- Secondary Raynaud phenomenon is associated with an underlying connective tissue disease such as scleroderma or systemic lupus erythematosus

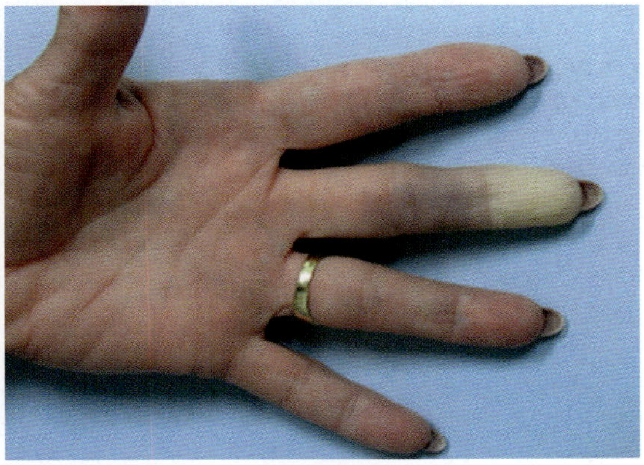

FIG. 16.16 Raynaud phenomenon. (From Klatt, E. C. (2020). *Robbins & Cotran atlas of pathology* (4th ed.). Elsevier Inc.)

PATIENT DATA

Subjective Data

- Involved areas feel cold and achy, improve on rewarming
- In secondary Raynaud, there can be intense pain from digital ischemia

Objective Data

- In primary Raynaud, there is a triphasic demarcated skin pallor (white), cyanosis (blue), and reperfusion (red) in the extremities
- The vasospasm may last from minutes to less than an hour
- In secondary Raynaud, ulcers may appear on the tips of the digits, and eventually the skin over the digits can appear smooth, shiny, and tight from loss of subcutaneous tissue

Arterial Embolic Disease

Emboli that are dispersed throughout the arterial system (Fig. 16.17)

PATHOPHYSIOLOGY

Emboli can be caused by:

- Thrombus
- Atherosclerotic plaques
- Infectious material from fungal and bacterial endocarditis
- Atrial myxomas (a mass of connective tissue)

PATIENT DATA

Subjective Data

- Pain is the most common symptom
- Paresthesias may also develop

Objective Data

- Occlusion of small arteries and necrosis of the tissue supplied by that vessel (e.g., blue toe syndrome)
- With endocarditis, splinter hemorrhages are seen in the nail beds

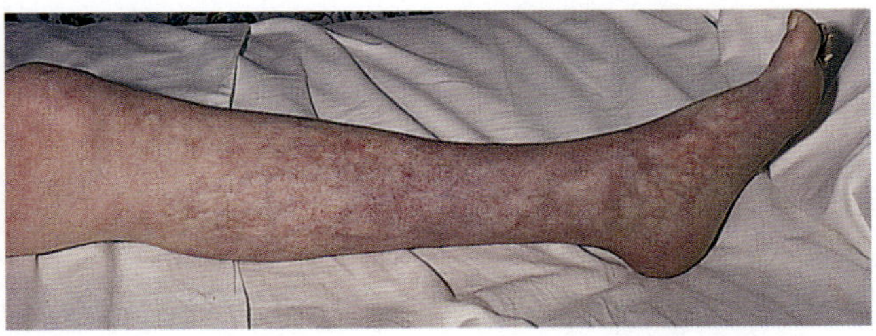

FIG. 16.17 Embolic phenomenon. (From Goldman, L., & Schafer, A. I. (2016). *Goldman-Cecil medicine* (25th ed.). Philadelphia: Saunders.)

Venous Thrombosis

Thrombosis can occur suddenly or gradually and with varying severity of symptoms; can be the result of trauma, a hypercoagulable state, or prolonged immobilization

PATHOPHYSIOLOGY

- Risk factors for venous thrombosis include prolonged immobilization (e.g., bed rest, recent surgery, long airplane flight); malignancy; trauma; use of contraceptive medication; and family or personal history of previous thrombosis

PATIENT DATA

Subjective Data

- Tenderness in area of thrombus, such as along the iliac vessels or the femoral canal, in the popliteal space, or over the deep calf veins
- Deep vein thrombosis in the femoral and pelvic circulations may be asymptomatic
- Pulmonary embolism may occur without warning

Objective Data

- Swelling may be distinguished only by measuring and comparing the circumference of the upper and lower legs bilaterally
- Minimal ankle edema, low-grade fever, and tachycardia

JUGULAR VENOUS PRESSURE DISORDER

Tricuspid Regurgitation

The backflow of blood into the right atrium during systole; a mild degree of tricuspid regurgitation can be seen in up to 75% of the normal adult population

PATHOPHYSIOLOGY

- Most commonly due to conditions that lead to dilation of the right ventricle (e.g., hypertension, pulmonary thrombosis)
- Less frequently, this can also result from primary valvular disease

PATIENT DATA

Subjective Data

- With mild to moderate tricuspid regurgitation, there are typically no symptoms
- With severe disease, you may see symptoms of right-sided heart failure such as ascites or peripheral edema

Objective Data

- The v wave is much more prominent and occurs earlier, often merging with the c wave (Fig. 16.18; for expected normal venous pulsations, see Fig. 16.7)
- A holosystolic murmur in the tricuspid region, a pulsatile liver, and peripheral edema

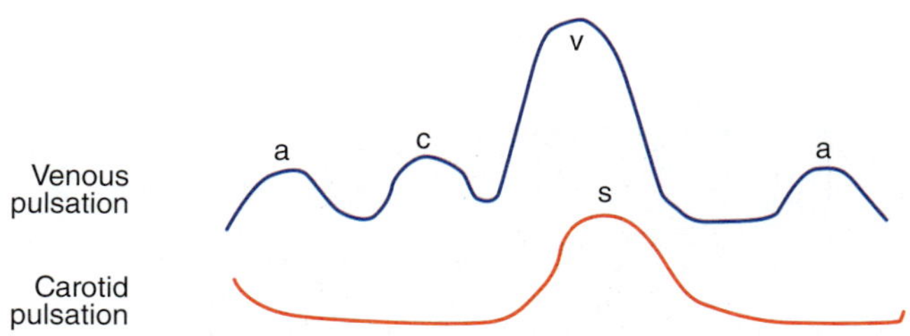

FIG. 16.18 Diagram of pulsation in tricuspid regurgitation.

Children

Coarctation of the Aorta

A stenosis seen most commonly in the descending aortic arch near the origin of the left subclavian artery and ligamentum arteriosum (Fig. 16.19)

PATHOPHYSIOLOGY

- Frequently due to congenital defect of the underlying vascular wall
- May also be acquired as a result of inflammatory aortic disease or severe atherosclerosis
- May occur with other left-sided heart defects
- More common in young males
- About 12% of young girls born with coarctation have Turner syndrome

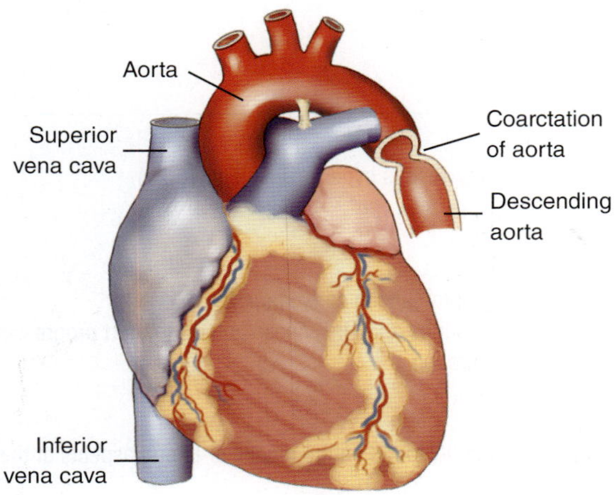

FIG. 16.19 Coarctation of the aorta.

PATIENT DATA

Subjective Data

- May be asymptomatic with mild narrowing
- In severe cases, hypertension or vascular insufficiency develops
- If symptomatic, the child may have symptoms of heart failure (e.g., difficulty feeding, poor appetite, and failure to thrive in an infant) or vascular insufficiency of an involved upper extremity with activity

Objective Data

- Differences in systolic blood pressure readings between the arm and leg readings
- Femoral pulses are weaker than radial pulses, or femoral pulses are absent

Kawasaki Disease

An acute small vessel vasculitis that may result in the development of coronary artery aneurysms

PATHOPHYSIOLOGY

- Cause of the vasculitis is unknown
- More common in young males than in young females
- Immune-mediated blood vessel damage can result in both vascular stenosis and aneurysm formation

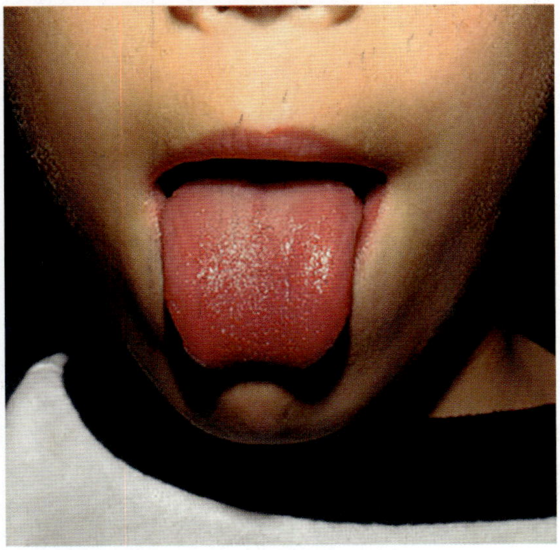

FIG. 16.20 Strawberry tongue. (From Fitzpatrick, J., & High, W. (2018). *Urgent care dermatology*. Philadelphia: Elsevier.)

PATIENT DATA

Subjective Data

- Symptoms are diffuse and typified by fever lasting 5 days or more
- Effects of a systemic vasculitis include weight loss, fatigue, and myalgias as well as arthritis

Objective Data

- Findings may include fever, conjunctival injection, strawberry tongue, and edema of the hands and feet
- Lymphadenopathy and polymorphous, nonvesicular rashes (Fig. 16.20)

Pregnant Patients

Preeclampsia-Eclampsia

A syndrome specific to pregnancy with hypertension that occurs after the 20th week of pregnancy and the presence of proteinuria; eclampsia is preeclampsia with seizures when no other cause for the seizures can be found

PATHOPHYSIOLOGY

- Theorized to result from a combination of vascular and immunologic abnormalities within the uteroplacental circulation

PATIENT DATA

Subjective Data

- May be diagnosed without proteinuria if other systemic symptoms are present (e.g., visual changes, headache, abdominal pain, pulmonary edema)

Objective Data

- Sustained elevation of the blood pressure (systolic >160 mm Hg, diastolic >110 mm Hg)

Older Adults

Venous Ulcers

Results from chronic venous insufficiency in which the lack of venous flow leads to lower extremity venous hypertension (Fig. 16.21)

PATHOPHYSIOLOGY

- Obstruction of venous flow may result from incompetent valves, obstruction of blood flow, or loss of the pumping effect of the leg muscles

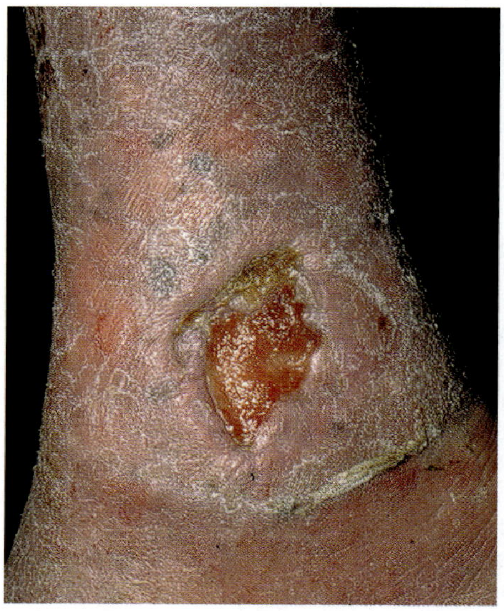

FIG. 16.21 Venous stasis ulcer. (From Ferri, F. F. (2020). *Ferri's clinical advisor 2021*. Philadelphia: Elsevier Inc.)

PATIENT DATA

Subjective Data

- Frequently asymptomatic in early stages
- Patients may describe a leg heaviness and discomfort progressing to edema and ulceration

Objective Data

- Ulcers are generally found on the medial or lateral aspects of the lower limbs
- Induration, edema, and hyperpigmentation are common associated findings

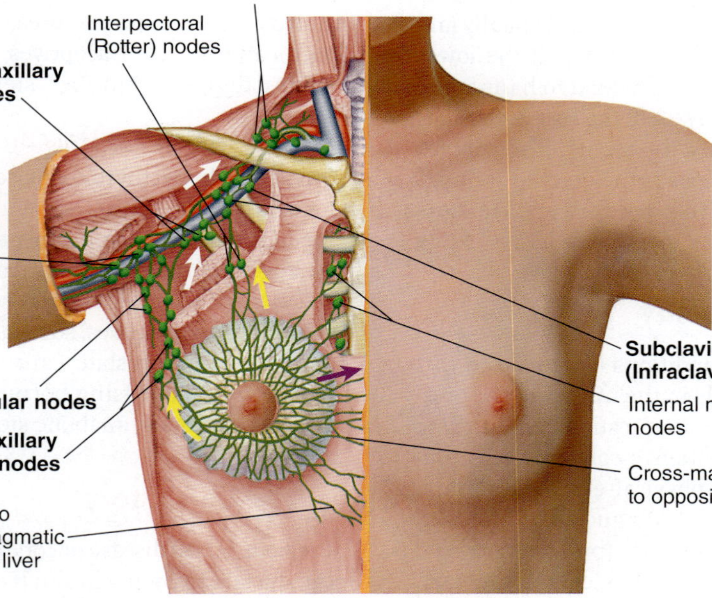

FIG. 17.3 **Lymphatic drainage of the breast.** Nodes in bold notation are accessible to palpation.

The complex of lymph nodes, their locations, and direction of drainage are illustrated in Fig. 17.3. The axillary nodes are more superficial and are accessible to palpation when enlarged. The anterior axillary (pectoral) nodes are located along the lower border of the pectoralis major, inside the lateral axillary fold. The midaxillary (central) nodes are high in the axilla close to the ribs. The posterior axillary (subscapular) nodes lie along the lateral border of the scapula and deep in the posterior axillary fold, whereas the lateral axillary (brachial) nodes can be felt along the upper humerus.

Children and Adolescents

The breast evolves in structure and function throughout life. Childhood and preadolescence represent a latent phase of breast development. Thelarche (breast development) represents the first sign of puberty in females. Breast development is classified using the five Tanner stages, also known as *sexual maturation rating,* as discussed in Chapter 8.

In using the Tanner system to stage breast development, it is important to note temporal relationships. It is unusual for the onset of menses to occur before stage 3. About 25% of females begin menstruation at stage 3. Approximately 75% are menstruating at stage 4 and are beginning to establish a regular menstrual cycle. About 10% do not begin to menstruate until stage 5. The average interval from the appearance of the breast bud (stage 2) to menarche is 2 years. Breasts develop at different rates in the individual, which can result in temporary asymmetry. Reassurance is often necessary. Delay in puberty for nonbinary, transgender, or intersex children through pubertal blockers limits or stops breast development and stops menstruation.

Pregnant Patients

Striking changes occur in the breasts during pregnancy. In response to luteal and placental hormones, the lactiferous ducts proliferate and the alveoli increase extensively in size and number, which may cause the breasts to enlarge two to three times their prepregnancy size. The increase in glandular tissue displaces connective tissue, and the breasts become softer and looser. Toward the end of pregnancy, as epithelial secretory activity increases, colostrum is produced and accumulates in the acinar cells (alveoli).

The areolae become more deeply pigmented and their diameter increases. The nipples become more prominent, darker, and more erectile. Montgomery tubercles often develop as sebaceous glands hypertrophy.

Mammary vascularization increases, causing veins to engorge and become visible as a blue network beneath the surface of the skin.

Lactating Patients

In the first few days after delivery, small amounts of colostrum are secreted from the breasts. Colostrum contains more protein and minerals than does mature milk as well as antibodies and other host resistance factors. Milk production replaces colostrum 2 to 4 days after delivery in response to surging prolactin levels, declining estrogen levels, and the stimulation of sucking. As the alveoli and lactiferous ducts fill, the breasts may become full and tense. This, combined with tissue edema and a delay in effective ejection reflexes, can produce breast engorgement.

At the termination of lactation, involution occurs over a period of about 3 months. Breast size decreases without loss of lobular and alveolar components; the breasts rarely return to their prelactation size.

Older Adults

After menopause, glandular tissue atrophies gradually and is replaced by fat. The inframammary ridge at the lower edge of the breast thickens. The breasts tend to hang more loosely from the chest wall as a result of the tissue changes and relaxation of the suspensory ligaments. The nipples become smaller and flatter and lose some erectile ability.

The skin may take on a relatively dry, thin texture. Loss of axillary hair may also occur.

REVIEW OF RELATED HISTORY

For each of the symptoms or conditions discussed in this section, targeted topics to include in the history of the present illness are listed. Responses to questions about these topics help to fully assess the patient's condition and provide clues for focusing on the physical examination and the development of an appropriate diagnostic evaluation. Questions regarding medication use (prescription and over-the-counter preparations) as well as complementary, alternative, and integrative therapies are relevant for each.

History of Present Illness

Breast Discomfort/Pain

- Temporal sequence: onset gradual or sudden; duration; persistent or intermittent
- Relationship to menses: timing, severity
- Character: stinging, pulling, burning, drawing, stabbing, aching, throbbing; unilateral or bilateral; localization; radiation
- Associated symptoms: lump or mass, discharge from nipple
- Contributory factors: skin irritation under breasts from tissue-to-tissue contact or from rubbing of undergarments; strenuous activity; recent injury to breast; use of breast binders
- Medications: hormones or bioidentical hormones; oral contraceptives

Breast Mass or Lump

- Temporal sequence: length of time since lump first noted; persistent or intermittent; relationship to menses
- Symptoms: tenderness or pain (characterize as described previously); dimpling or change in contour
- Changes in lump: size, character, relationship to menses (timing or severity)
- Associated symptoms: nipple discharge or retraction, tender lymph nodes
- Medications: hormones or bioidentical hormones

Nipple Discharge

- Character: spontaneous or provoked; unilateral or bilateral; onset gradual or sudden; duration, color, consistency, odor, amount
- Associated symptoms: nipple retraction; breast lump or discomfort
- Associated factors: relationship to menses or other activity; recent injury to breast
- Medications: contraceptives, hormones, phenothiazines, digitalis, diuretics, steroids

Breast Enlargement in Male Breasts (Gynecomastia)

- History of hyperthyroidism, testicular cancer, Klinefelter syndrome
- Medications: cimetidine, omeprazole, spironolactone, antiandrogens (finasteride), human immunodeficiency virus (HIV) medications (efavirenz), some chemotherapy agents, some antihypertensives, some antipsychotics, estrogen
- Treatment for prostate cancer with antiandrogens or gonadotropin-releasing hormone analogs
- Use of hormones, anabolic steroids, cannabis

Past Medical History

- Previous breast disease or conditions such as invasive cancer, ductal carcinoma in situ (DCIS), lobular carcinoma in situ (LCIS), ductal or lobular hyperplasia with or without atypia, papilloma fibroadenomas, fibrocystic changes
- Known *BRCA1, BRCA2, PALB2, CHEK2, CDH1, PTEN, STK11, TP53, ATM,* or other genetic mutation; known hereditary cancer syndrome (hereditary nonpolyposis colorectal cancer [HNPCC], Li-Fraumeni syndrome, or Cowden syndrome)
- Gender identity: female, male, nonbinary, transgender woman, transgender man, sex assignment at birth
- Previous other related cancers: ovarian, colorectal, endometrial
- Surgeries: breast biopsies, aspirations, implants, reductions, mastectomies, reconstructions, oophorectomy
- Risk factors for breast cancer (see Risk Factors box "Breast Cancer")
- Mammogram and other breast imaging history: frequency, date of last imaging, results
- Menstrual history: first day of last menstrual period; age at menarche and menopause; cycle length, duration, amount of flow, and regularity; associated breast symptoms (nipple discharge; pain or discomfort)
- Pregnancy: age at each pregnancy, length of each pregnancy, date of delivery or termination
- Lactation: number of children breastfed; duration of time for breastfeeding; date of termination of last breastfeeding; medications used to suppress lactation
- Menopause: onset, course, associated problems, residual problems
- Use of hormonal medications: name and dosage; reason for use (contraception, menstrual control, menopausal symptom relief; gender-affirming treatment); length of time on hormones; date of termination
- Other medications: nonprescription or prescription; hormones (estrogen, progesterone), selective estrogen receptor modulators (SERMs; tamoxifen, raloxifene), aromatase inhibitors (e.g., anastrozole, letrozole, exemestane); silicone injections

Risk Factors

Breast Cancer

Nonmodifiable Factors

Age: Risk increases with aging.

Gender: Higher incidence in female breasts. Transgender men who have not had bilateral mastectomies remain at risk for developing breast cancer.

Genetic risk factors: Patients with female breasts with an inherited *BRCA1* or *BRCA2* mutation have a 45% to 80% chance of developing breast cancer during their lifetime compared with the average risk of about 12%. Other inherited mutations can increase risk, but to a lesser degree.

Personal history of breast cancer: Cancer in one breast increases risk of developing a new cancer in the other breast.

Family history of breast cancer: One first-degree relative (parent, sibling, child) with breast cancer approximately doubles the risk; two first-degree relatives increase the risk threefold.

Certain benign breast conditions: Atypical hyperplasia with atypia or LCIS substantially increases breast cancer risk. Proliferative lesions without atypia may increase risk slightly. Lesions without proliferative changes (e.g., fibroadenoma, fibrocysts, papilloma) do not affect breast cancer risk.

Race: White persons are at higher risk than other racial/ethnic groups.

Previous breast radiation: Radiation therapy to the chest area as treatment for another cancer (such as Hodgkin disease or non-Hodgkin lymphoma) as a young adult significantly increases risk for breast cancer.

Menstrual periods: Menarche before age 12 or menopause after age 55 slightly increases risk.

Breast density: Breast tissue may be dense or fatty; older females whose mammograms show more dense tissue are at 1.2 to 2 times the risk.

Diethylstilbestrol (DES) therapy: Patients who received DES in the 1940s through the 1960s during their pregnancies have a slightly increased risk. Patients with female breasts who were exposed to DES in utero may have a slightly increased risk of breast cancer after age 40.

Modifiable/Lifestyle Factors

Childbirth: Nulliparity or late age at birth of first child (after age 30) is associated with an increased risk.

Hormone therapy: Use of combined estrogen and progesterone hormone replacement therapy (HRT) after menopause (more than 4 years of use) increases risk. The risk for transgender women taking estrogen hormones for at least 5 to 10 years is uncertain.

Alcohol: Risk increases by approximately 10% for each 10 g of daily alcohol intake (less than one standard drink, which is 14 g or 0.6 fluid ounces of alcohol)

Obesity and high-fat diets: Obesity is associated with an increased risk, especially after menopause. Having more fat tissue can increase estrogen levels and increase the likelihood of developing breast cancer.

Lack of physical activity: Patients with female breasts who are physically inactive throughout life may have an increased risk of breast cancer.

From American Cancer Society (2021, 2022); Deutsch (2016); and National Cancer Institute (2024).

Think About It

A solitary breast mass that is hard, fixed, and accompanied by other physical symptoms such as tethering, retraction, flattening, or peau d'orange is cancer until proven otherwise. The patient's assessed risk for breast cancer in the presence of those findings is irrelevant. Most breast cancers occur in females without additional risk factors or a family history.

Family History

- Breast cancer: primary relatives, secondary relatives; type of cancer; age at time of occurrence; treatment and results; known *BRCA1, BRCA2,* or other mutation
- Other cancers: ovarian, colorectal, known hereditary cancer syndromes (breast–ovarian cancer syndrome, HNPCC, Li-Fraumeni syndrome, or Cowden syndrome)
- Other breast disease in relatives: type of disease; age at time of occurrence; treatment and results

Personal and Social History

- Age
- Breast support used with strenuous exercise or sports activities
- Amount of caffeine intake and breast tissue response (pain, fibrocystic changes)
- Breast self-awareness: frequency, at what time in the menstrual cycle
- Use of alcohol, daily amounts
- Use of anabolic steroids or cannabis

Pregnant Patients

- Sensations: fullness, tingling, tenderness
- Presence of colostrum and knowledge about how to care for breasts and nipples during pregnancy
- Use of supportive bra
- Knowledge and information about breastfeeding
- Plans to breastfeed, experience, expectations, concerns

Lactating Patients

- Cleaning procedures for breasts: use of soap products that can remove natural lubricants, frequency of use; nipple preparations
- Use of breastfeeding bra
- Nipples: tenderness, pain, cracking, bleeding; retracted; related problems with feeding; exposure to air
- Associated problems: engorgement, leaking breasts, plugged duct (localized tenderness and lump), fever, infection; treatment and results; infant with oral candidal infection
- Breastfeeding routine: length of feeding, frequency, rotation of breasts, position(s)
- Breast milk pumping devices used, frequency
- Cultural beliefs about breastfeeding
- Food and environmental agents that can affect breast milk (e.g., caffeine, alcohol, pesticides)

- Medications that can cross the milk-blood barrier (e.g., cimetidine, clemastine, thiouracil); all medications—prescription and nonprescription—should be evaluated for potential side effects in the newborn

Older Adults

- Skin irritation under pendulous breasts from tissue-to-tissue contact or from rubbing of undergarments, treatment
- Hormone therapy during or since menopause: name and dosage of medication; duration of therapy

EXAMINATION AND FINDINGS

Equipment

- Small pillow or folded towel
- Ruler
- Flashlight with transilluminator
- Glass slide and cytologic fixative if nipple discharge is present

Adequate lighting is essential for revealing shadows and subtle variations in skin color and texture. Adequate exposure is also essential, requiring that the patient be disrobed to the waist. Simultaneous observation of both breasts is necessary to detect minor differences between them that may be significant. Stay attentive to modesty concerns and convey the need for full exposure. The presence of a chaperone may ease discomfort and protect both the patient and the examining clinician and should be used with adolescent patients.

Inspection

Breasts

As the patient sits with arms hanging loosely at the sides, inspect each breast and compare it with the other for size, symmetry, contour, skin color and texture, venous patterns, and lesions. Perform this portion of the examination for all patients. With patients assigned female at birth, transgender men with intact breasts, and transgender women with breast tissue, lift the breasts with your fingertips, inspecting the inferior and lateral aspects to determine changes in the color or texture of the skin.

Some transgender men bind the chest to create a masculine appearance and may be hesitant to remove the binder for a physical examination. Inspect for skin breakdown or skin lesions that may occur as a result of prolonged binding.

Breasts of patients assigned female at birth or transgender men with intact breasts vary in shape, from convex to pendulous or conical; often one breast is somewhat smaller than the other (Fig. 17.4). Breasts of patients assigned male at birth or transgender women not taking hormones or without surgical augmentation are generally even with the chest wall, although some, particularly in those who are overweight, have a convex shape. The amount of breast tissue in transgender women depends on the amount and duration of estrogen therapy. Breasts that have been surgically augmented vary in size and shape. Implants that have ruptured, contracted, or moved may distort the size and shape of the breast.

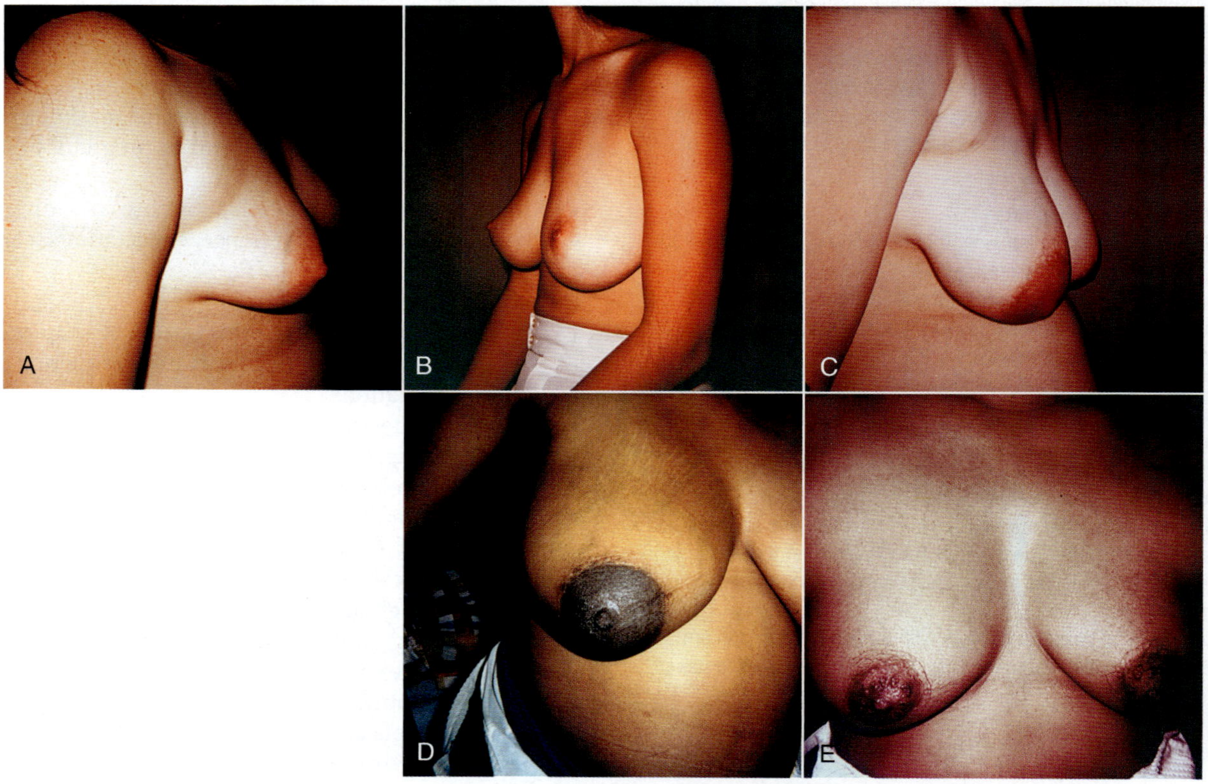

FIG. 17.4 Variations in breast size and contour. (A) Conical. (B) Convex. (C) Pendulous. (D) Large pendulous. (E) Right larger than left.

The skin texture should appear smooth, and the contour should be uninterrupted. Alterations in contour are best seen on bilateral comparison of one breast with the other. Retractions and dimpling signify the contraction of fibrotic tissue that may occur with carcinoma. A peau d'orange (orange skin) appearance of the skin indicates edema of the breast caused by blocked lymph drainage in advanced or inflammatory breast cancer (Fig. 17.5). The skin appears thickened with enlarged pores and accentuated skin markings. Healthy skin may look similar if the pores of the skin are large.

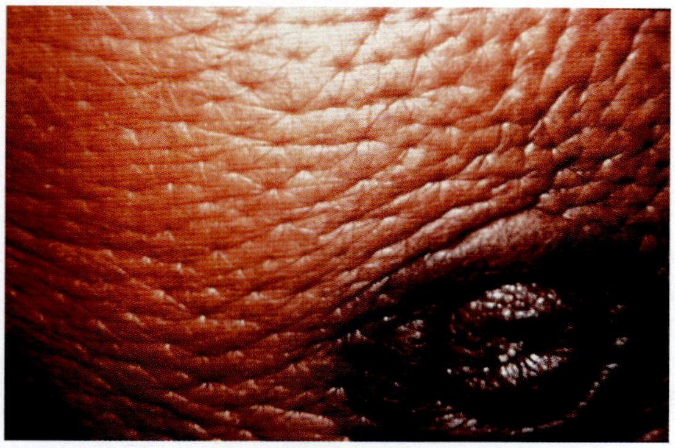

FIG. 17.5 Peau d'orange appearance from edema. (From: wartz, M. H. (2025). *Swartz textbook of physical diagnosis: History and examination* (9th ed.). Elsevier.)

Venous networks may be visible, although they are usually pronounced only in the breasts of pregnant or obese patients. Venous patterns should be symmetric. Unilateral venous patterns can occur as a result of increased blood flow to a malignancy. This finding requires further investigation.

Other markings and nevi that are long-standing, unchanging, or nontender are usually of little concern. Changes in or the recent appearance of any lesions always signal the need for closer investigation.

Nipples and Areolae

Inspect the areolae and nipples in all patients. The areola should be round or oval and bilaterally symmetric or nearly so. Areola color varies from light pink to very dark brown or black (Fig. 17.6).

Color tends to be lighter in light-skinned patients and darker in dark-skinned patients. A peppering of nontender, nonsuppurative Montgomery tubercles is a common and expected finding (Fig. 17.7). The surface should be otherwise smooth. Inflammation of the sebaceous glands in the areola can result in retention cysts that are tender and suppurative. The peau d'orange skin associated with cancer is often seen first in the areola.

Most nipples are everted (Fig. 17.8), but one or both may be inverted, with the nipple tucked inward. In these instanc-

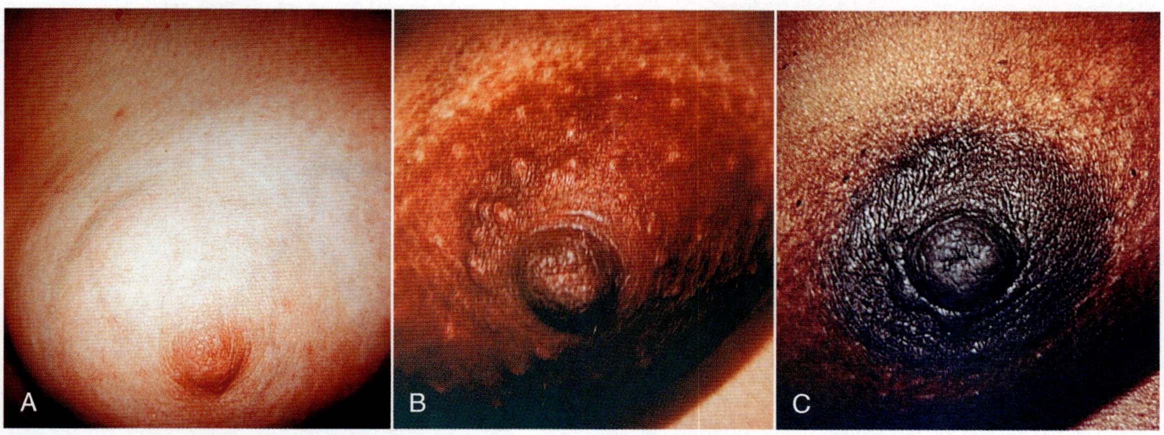

FIG. 17.6 Variations in color of areola. (A) Pink. (B) Brown. (C) Black.

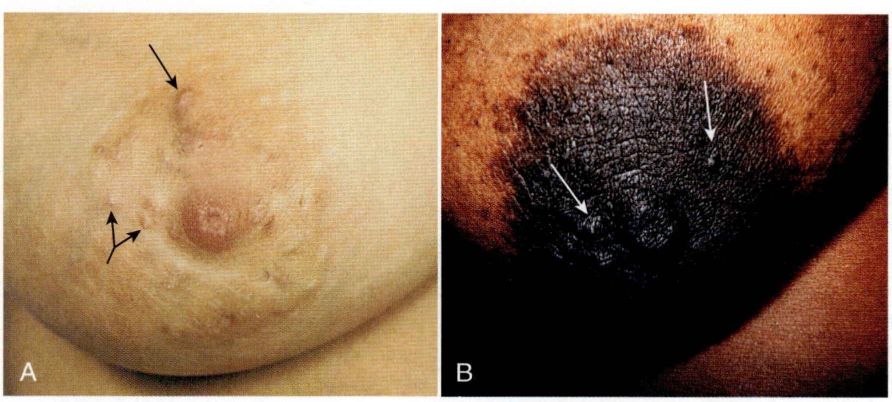

FIG. 17.7 Montgomery tubercles. (A) Light-skinned female. (B) Dark-skinned female. (A, From Mansel, R. E., & Bundred, N. J. (1995). *Color atlas of breast diseases.* St. Louis: Mosby.)

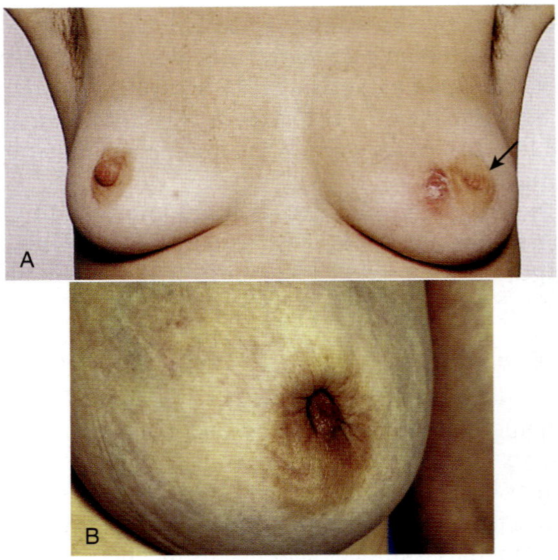

FIG. 17.8 (A) Left nipple inverted; right nipple everted. (B) Close-up of nipple inversion. A) Close-up view of woman body chest shows nipple turned inward with a brown patch, indicated by an arrow, on the left breast. B) Close-up view of breast shows nipple turned inward. (A, From Mansel R, Bundred N. (1995). *Color atlas of breast disease*, St Louis, Mosby; B, from Garden JO, Bradbury AW, et al. (2012). *Principles and practice of surgery*, (6th ed.). Philadelphia, Elsevier.)

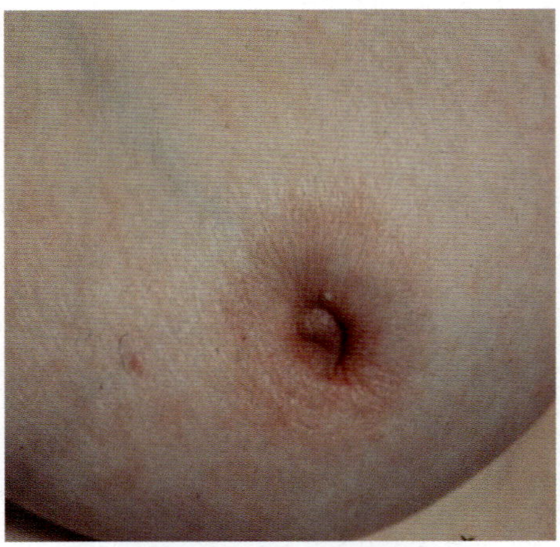

FIG. 17.9 Malignant retraction of the nipple. (From Dixon, J. M., & Barber, M. D. (Eds.). (2018). *Breast surgery* (6th ed.). Elsevier.)

es, ask whether there is a lifetime history of inversion. Recent unilateral inversion of a previously everted nipple suggests malignancy.

Simultaneous bilateral inspection is necessary to detect nipple retraction or deviation. Retraction is seen as a flattening or pulling back of the nipple and areola, which indicates inward pulling by inflammatory or malignant tissue (Fig. 17.9; see also Fig. 17.19). The fibrotic tissue of carcinoma can also change the axis of the nipple, causing it to point in a direction different from that of the other nipple.

The nipples should be a homogeneous color and match that of the areolae. Their surface may be either smooth or wrinkled but should be free of crusting, cracking, or

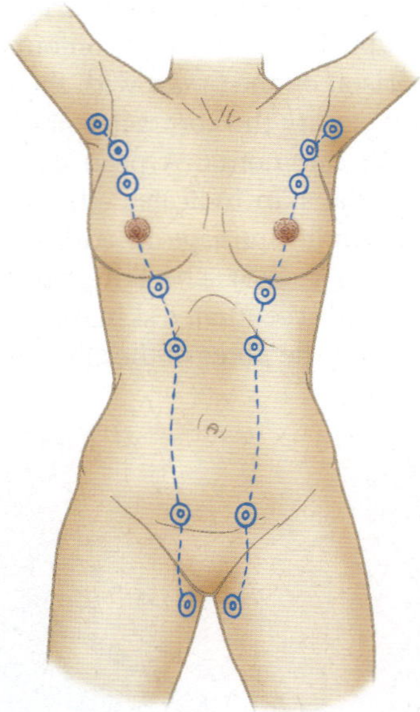

FIG. 17.10 Supernumerary nipples and tissue may arise along the "milk line," an embryonic ridge. (From Thompson, J. M., et al. (1997). *Mosby's clinical nursing* (4th ed.). St. Louis: Mosby.)

discharge. Supernumerary nipples, which are more common in Black patients than in White patients, appear as one or more extra nipples located along the embryonic mammary ridge (the "milk line"; Fig. 17.10). These nipples and areolae may be pink or brown, are usually small, and are commonly mistaken for moles (Fig. 17.11). Infrequently, some glandular tissue may accompany these nipples. In some cases, supernumerary nipples may be associated with congenital renal or cardiac anomalies, particularly in White patients.

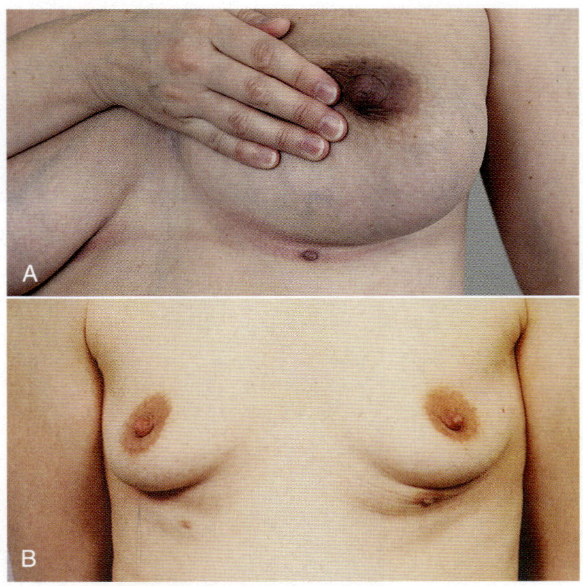

FIG. 17.11 (A) Supernumerary nipple without glandular tissue. (B) Supernumerary breast and nipple on left side and supernumerary nipple alone on right side. (B, From Mansel, R. E., & Bundred, N. J. (1995). *Color atlas of breast diseases.* St. Louis: Mosby.)

Evidence-Based Practice in Physical Examination

What Is the Evidence for Breast Cancer Screening Recommendations?

Breast cancer screening recommendations for females at average risk vary by authority; these recommendations also apply to transgender men with intact breasts (Deutsch, 2016). Issues regarding screening recommendations are the ages at which to start and stop screening; the screening interval (annual vs. biennial); and the screening modality (clinical breast examination [CBE], mammography, and tomosynthesis [creates a three-dimensional view], alone or in combination).

Evidence from the systematic reviews performed by the U.S. Preventive Services Task Force and the American Cancer Society reveal the following:

- Breast cancer mortality is reduced with mammography screening (although estimates are of borderline statistical significance); the magnitudes of effect are small for younger ages, and results vary depending on how cases were accrued in trials. Females at average risk should start screening at age 40 years. There are insufficient data to assess the benefits and harms of screening after age 75. Females should continue screening as long as they are in good health and have a life expectancy of at least 10 years.
- No head-to-head trials of different screening intervals have been conducted, and data from existing trials are insufficient to determine the specific effects of screening intervals. Recommendations on the screening interval (annual vs. biennial) vary.
- No direct evidence of any association between CBE alone (or in addition to mammography) with breast cancer mortality currently exists. No study addresses the comparative effectiveness of the modality on cancer-specific or all-cause mortality. Observational studies indicate that tomosynthesis with mammography reduces recalls but increases biopsies and cancer detection.

Authorities agree that breast cancer screening involves a trade-off of benefits and potential harms, and screening decisions should be made in the context of informed, shared decision making.

From American Cancer Society. (2023). *American Cancer Society recommendations for the early detection of breast cancer.* Accessed March 15, 2025, from https://www.cancer.org/cancer/types/breast-cancer/screening-tests-and-early-detection/american-cancer-society-recommendations-for-the-early-detection-of-breast-cancer.html; Deutsch, M. B. (Ed.). (2016). *Guidelines for the primary care of transgender and gender nonbinary people* (2nd ed.). UCSF Center of Excellence for Transgender Health; https://transcare.ucsf.edu/guidelines; Henderson, J. T., Webber, E. M., Weyrich, M. S., Miller, M., & Melnikow, J. (2024). Screening for breast cancer: Evidence report and systematic review for the U.S. Preventive Services Task Force. *JAMA, 331*(22), 1931–1946; and U.S. Preventive Services Task Force (2014). Accessed October 1, 2024, from https://www.uspreventiveservicestaskforce.org/uspstf/recommendation/breast-cancer-screening.

Reinspection in Varied Positions

Reinspect the breasts with the patient in the following positions:

- Seated with arms over the head or flexed behind the neck. This adds tension to the suspensory ligaments, accentuates dimpling, and may reveal variations in contour and symmetry (Fig. 17.12A).
- Seated with hands pressed against hips with shoulders rolled forward (or, alternatively, have the patient push her palms together). This contracts the pectoral muscles, which can reveal deviations in contour and symmetry (see Fig. 17.12B and C).
- Seated and leaning forward from the waist. This also causes tension in the suspensory ligaments; the breasts should hang equally. This maneuver can be particularly helpful in assessing the contour and symmetry of large breasts because the breasts fall away from the chest wall and hang freely. As the patient leans forward, support her by the hands (see Fig. 17.12D).

For all patient positions, the breasts should appear bilaterally symmetric with an even contour and absence of dimpling, retraction, or deviation.

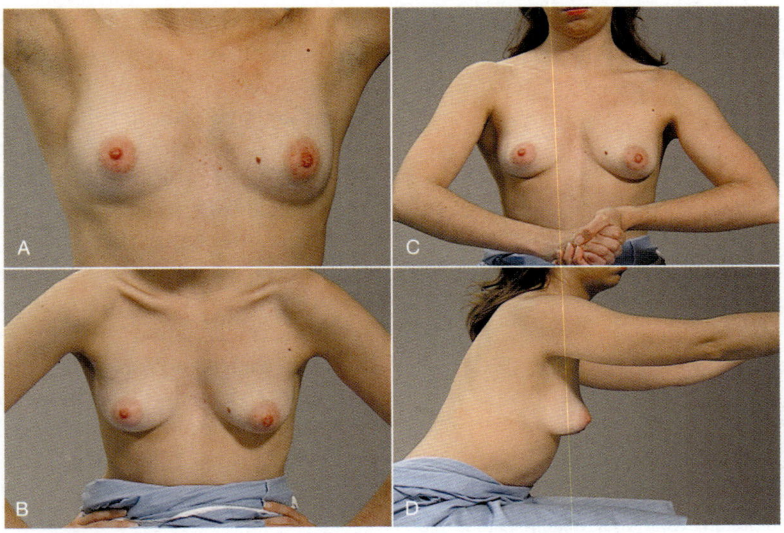

FIG. 17.12 Inspect the breasts in the following positions. (A) Arms extended overhead. (B) Hands pressed against hips. (C) Pressing hands together (an alternative way to flex the pectoral muscles). (D) Leaning forward from the waist.

Palpation

After a thorough inspection, systematically palpate the breasts, axillae, and supraclavicular and infraclavicular regions. Palpation of male breast tissue should not be omitted.

Patient in Seated Position

Chest Wall Sweep

Have the patient sit with arms hanging freely at the sides. Place the palm of your right hand at the patient's right clavicle at the sternum. Sweep downward from the clavicle to the nipple, feeling for superficial lumps. Repeat the sweep until you have covered the entire right chest wall. Repeat the procedure using your left hand for the left chest wall (Fig. 17.13).

Bimanual Digital Palpation

Place one hand, palmar surface facing up, under the patient's right breast. Position your hand so that it acts as a flat surface against which to compress the breast tissue. With the fingers of the other hand, walk across the breast tissue, feeling for lumps as you compress the tissue between your fingers and your flat hand. Repeat the procedure for the other breast (Fig. 17.14).

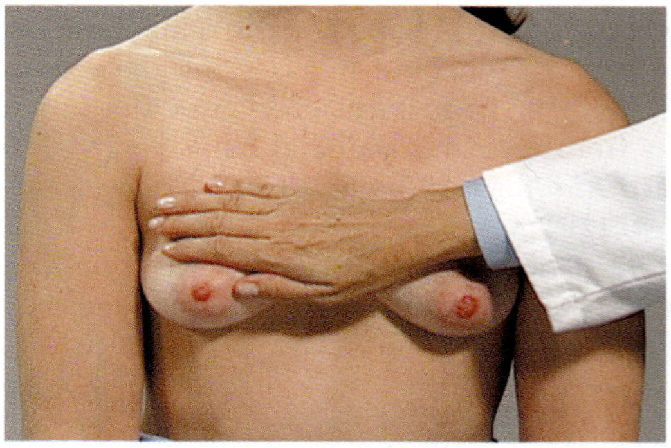

FIG. 17.13 Chest wall sweep. With the palm of your hand, sweep from the clavicle to the nipple, covering the area from the sternum to the midaxillary line.

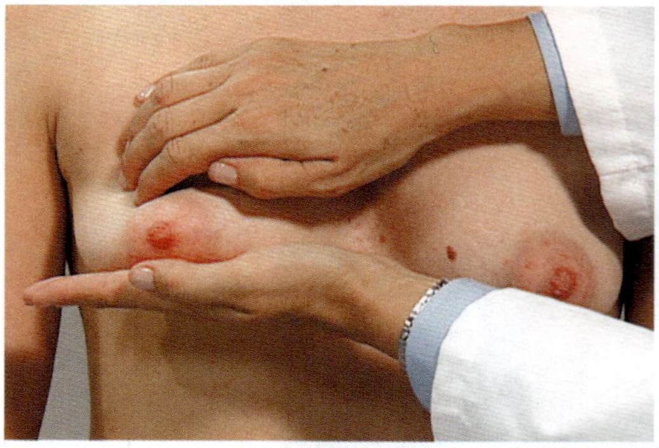

FIG. 17.14 Bimanual digital palpation. Walk your fingers across the breast tissue, compressing it between your fingers and the palmar surface of your other hand.

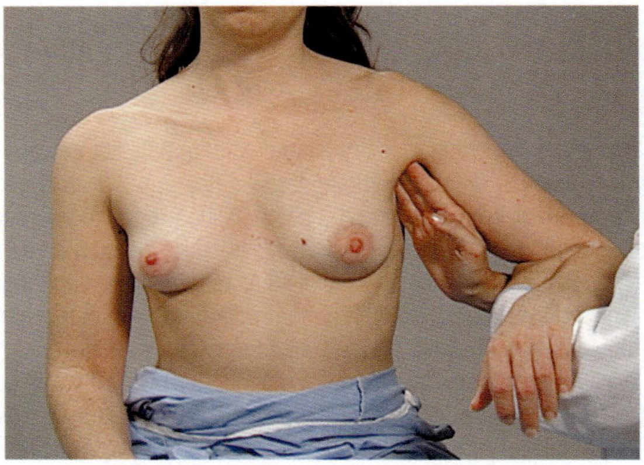

FIG. 17.15 Palpation of the axilla for lymph nodes.

Lymph Node Palpation

Palpate for lymph nodes in all patients. To palpate each axilla separately, have the patient seated with arms flexed at the elbow. For the left side, support the patient's left lower arm with your left hand while examining the left axilla with your right hand, as shown in Fig. 17.15. With the palmar surface of your fingers, reach deeply into the axillary hollow, pushing firmly so that you are gently rolling the soft tissue against the chest wall and muscles of the axilla. From the apex, palpate downward to the bra line and along the inner aspect of the upper arm down to the elbow. Reposition your fingers to palpate the medial aspect along the rib cage and into the anterior wall along the pectoral muscles. Reposition again to palpate the posterior wall along the border of the scapula. Repeat the mirror image of this maneuver for the right axilla.

Palpate the supraclavicular and infraclavicular areas for the presence of enlarged nodes. Hook your fingers over the clavicle and rotate them over the entire supraclavicular fossa. Have the patient turn their head toward the side being palpated and raise the same shoulder, allowing your fingers to reach more deeply into the fossa. Have the patient bend the head forward to relax the sternocleidomastoid muscle. These nodes are sentinel nodes (Virchow nodes), so any enlargement is highly significant. Palpable sentinel nodes are indicators for invasion of the lymphatics by cancer. Move your fingers to the infraclavicular area and palpate along the clavicle using a rotary motion with your fingers.

Lymph nodes in these areas are not usually palpable in the healthy adult. Palpable nodes may be the result of an inflammatory or malignant process. Move your fingers to the infraclavicular area and palpate along the clavicle using a rotary motion with your fingers. Nodes that are detected should be described according to location, size, shape, consistency, tenderness, fixation, and delineation of borders (see Chapter 10).

Patient in Supine Position

Have the patient raise one arm behind the head, then place a small pillow or folded towel under that shoulder to spread the breast tissue more evenly over the chest wall (Fig. 17.16). The ideal position for examination is to have the nipple pointing toward the ceiling. Patients with large breasts may need to roll slightly to achieve this position. Palpate each breast separately.

Palpate all areas of breast tissue, feeling for lumps or nodules (Box 17.1). Remember that the breast tissue extends from the second or third rib to the sixth or seventh rib and from the sternal margin to the midaxillary line. It is essential to include the tail of Spence in palpation. Recall that the greatest amount of glandular tissue lies in the upper outer quadrant of the breast, with tissue extending from this quadrant into the axilla to form the tail of Spence.

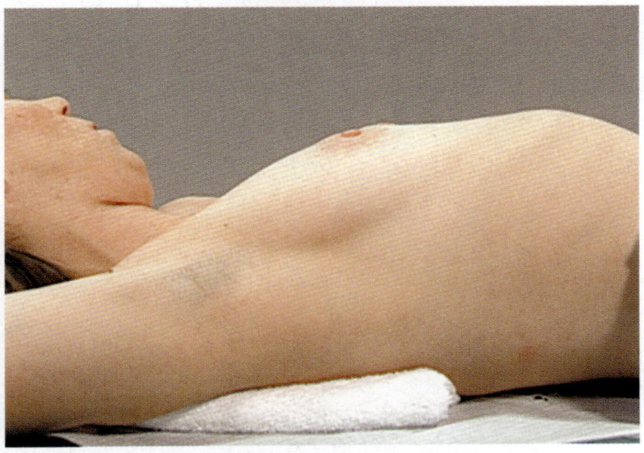

FIG. 17.16 Supine position for palpation.

In breasts that have been surgically augmented, palpate as usual. In some patients with surgical augmentation, capsular contraction may cause the breasts to feel hard.

Palpate using your finger pads because they are more sensitive than your fingertips. Palpate systematically, pushing gently but firmly, toward the chest wall as you rotate your fingers in a clockwise or counterclockwise pattern. At each point, as you rotate your fingers, press inward, using three depths of palpation: light, then medium, then deep. The exact sequence you select for palpation is not critical, but a systematic approach will help ensure that all portions of the breast are examined. Fig. 17.17 illustrates three methods that are commonly used. In the vertical strip technique, begin at the top of the breast and palpate, first downward, then upward, working your way over the entire breast. In the concentric circle technique,

BOX 17.1 Documenting Breast Masses

If a breast mass is felt, characterize it by its location, size, shape, consistency, tenderness, mobility, delineation of borders, and retraction (see Fig. 17.23). Ultrasound can be used to confirm the presence of fluid in certain masses. These characteristics are not diagnostic by themselves, but in conjunction with a thorough history, they provide a great deal of clinical information for correlation with findings from diagnostic testing.

Describe any breast mass or lump that you encounter using the following characteristics:

- Location: clock positions and distance from nipple
- Size (in centimeters): length, width, thickness
- Shape: round, discoid, lobular, stellate, regular or irregular
- Consistency: firm, soft, hard
- Tenderness
- Mobility: movable (in what directions) or fixed to overlying skin or subjacent fascia
- Borders: discrete or poorly defined
- Retraction: presence or absence of dimpling; altered contour

All new solitary or dominant masses must be investigated with further diagnostic testing.

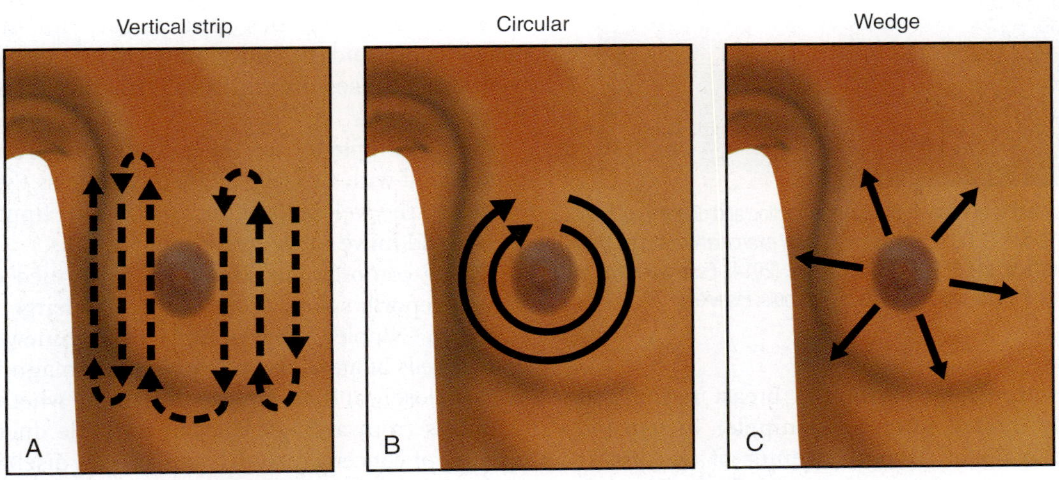

FIG. 17.17 **Various methods for palpation of the breast.** (A) Palpate from top to bottom in vertical strips. (B) Palpate in concentric circles. (C) Palpate out from the center in wedge sections.

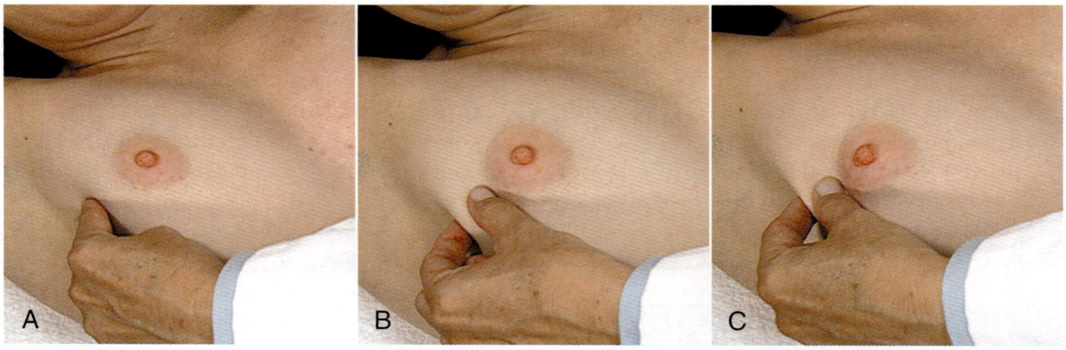

FIG. 17.18 (A) Palpating for consistency of a breast lesion. (B) Palpating for delineation of the borders of a breast mass. (C) Palpating for mobility of breast mass.

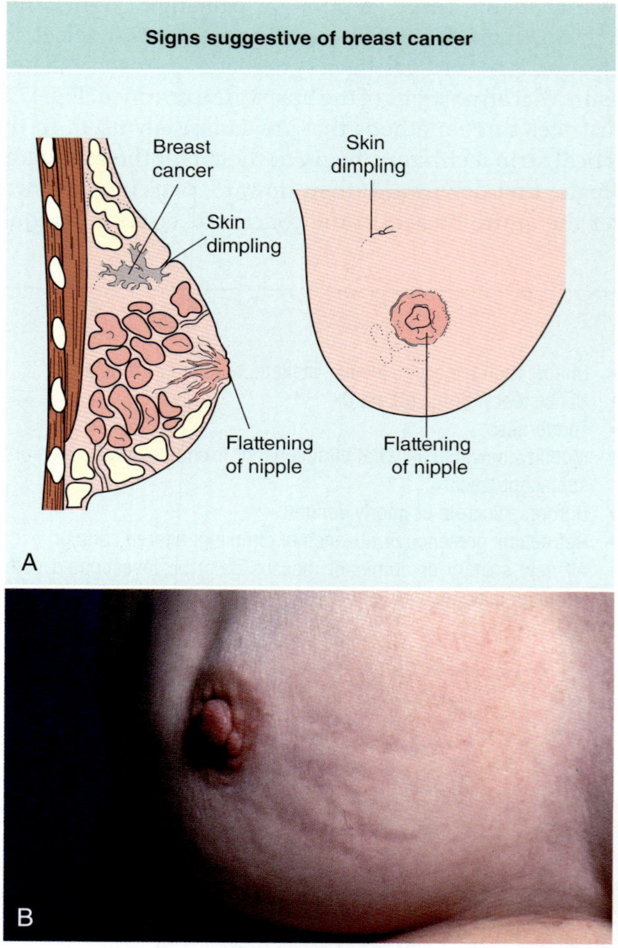

FIG. 17.19 (A) Clinical signs of cancer. (B) Nipple retraction and dimpling of skin. (A, From Epstein, O., Perkin, G. D., et al. (2008). *Clinical examination* (4th ed.). St. Louis: Elsevier; B, from Quick, C. R. G., Reed, J. B., et al. (2014). *Essential surgery: Problems, diagnosis and management* (5th ed.). St. Louis: Elsevier.)

begin at the outermost edge of the breast tissue and spiral your way inward toward the nipple. To use the wedge method, palpate from the center of the breast in radial fashion, returning to the areola to begin each spoke. Regardless of the method, glide your fingers from

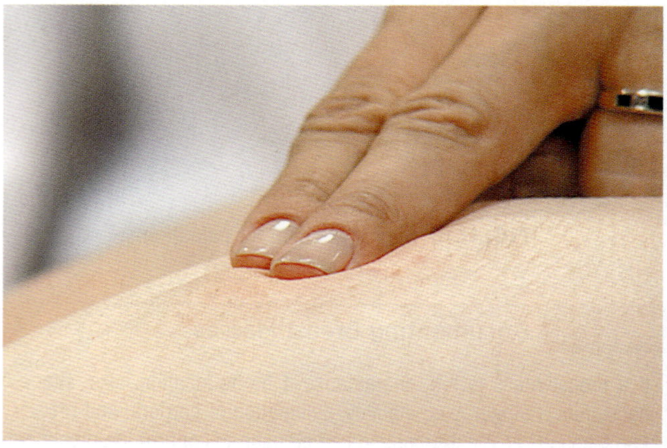

FIG. 17.20 Depressing the nipple inward into well behind the areola.

one point to the next. Avoid lifting your fingers off the breast tissue because doing so makes it easy to miss tissue.

Early lesions can be tiny and may be detected only through meticulous technique. If a breast mass is felt, note its characteristics and palpate its dimensions, consistency, and mobility (Fig. 17.18) and determine whether it causes dimpling or retraction (Fig. 17.19; see Box 17.1).

At the completion of the examination, return to the nipple, and with two fingers, gently depress the tissue inward into the well behind the areola. Your fingers and tissue should move easily inward (Fig. 17.20).

Nipple compression should be performed only if the patient reports spontaneous nipple discharge (see Clinical Pearl, "Nipple Compression"). Determine whether the discharge is bilateral or unilateral. Use a magnifying glass to look closely at the nipple to determine whether the discharge is from a single duct or multiple ducts. Characteristics of concern include spontaneous discharge that is unilateral and from a single duct. Fig. 17.21 shows various types of nipple discharge.

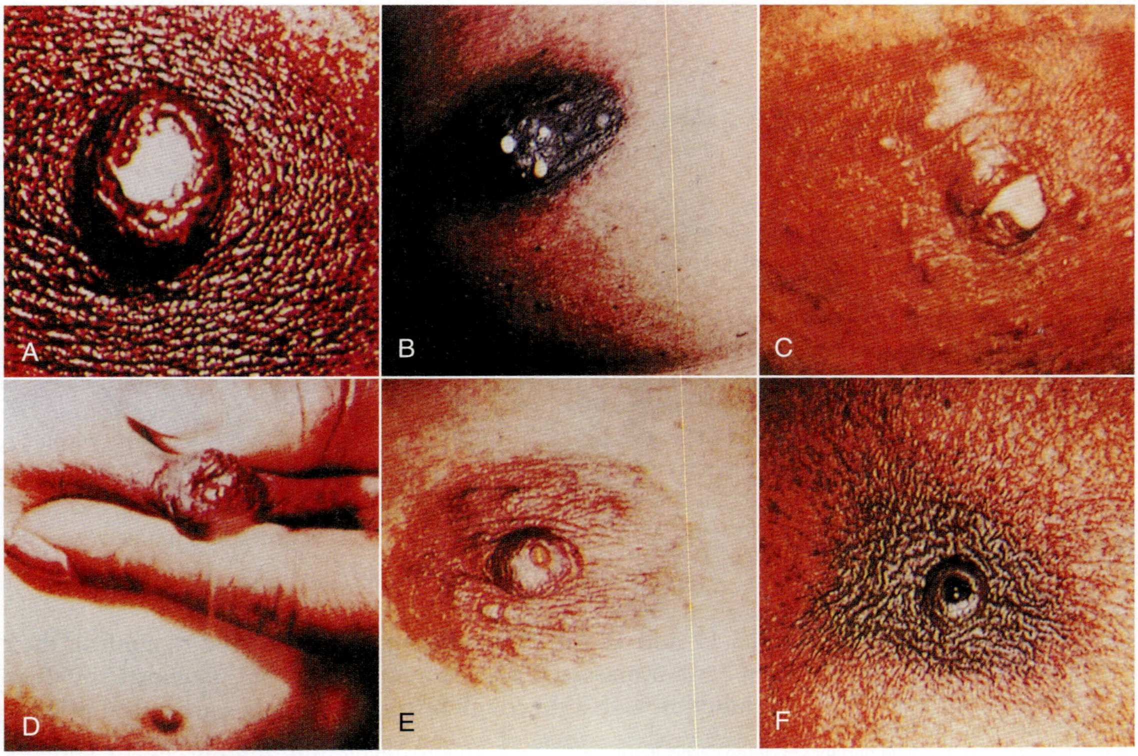

FIG. 17.21 Types of nipple discharge. (A) Milky discharge. (B) Multicolored, sticky discharge. (C) Purulent discharge. (D) Watery discharge. (E) Serous discharge. (F) Serosanguineous discharge. (From Gallager, H. S., et al. (1978). *The breast.* St. Louis: Mosby.)

Evidence-Based Practice: Palpation in Clinical Breast Examination

Reviews (McDonald et al., 2004; Saslow et al., 2004) reflect the recommendation for a vertical stripe search pattern, demonstrated as more thorough and superior in a study by Saunders et al. (1986) and in a systematic review by Barton et al. (1999). Although a study by Laufer et al. (2017) did not find evidence to support that recommendation, the authors did identify that the motion used by the clinician was an important determinant of accuracy. A rubbing motion, defined as repetitive movements in a circular motion or pushing the fingers in back and forth or right to left, was significantly associated with assessment accuracy. In an earlier study, Laufer et al. (2015) reported that increasing the amount of pressure in palpation improved the probability that the examiner would identify a deep-tissue breast lesion.

The universal recommendation is to engage in training with feedback and practice and use a standardized approach to clinical breast examination.

Barton, M., Harris, R., & Fletcher, S. W. (1999). Does this patient have breast cancer? The screening clinical breast examination: Should it be done? How? *JAMA, 282*(13), 1270–1280; Laufer, S., Cohen, E. R., Kwan, C., et al. (2015). Sensor technology in assessments of clinical skill. *New England Journal of Medicine, 372*(8), 784–786; Laufer, S., D'Angelo, A. D., Kwan, C., et al. (2017). Rescuing the clinical breast examination: Advances in classifying technique and assessing physician competency. *Annals of Surgery, 266*(6), 1069–1074.; McDonald, S., Saslow, D., & Alciati, M. H. (2004). Performance and reporting of clinical breast examination: A review of the literature. *CA: A Cancer Journal for Clinicians, 54,* 345–361; Saunders, K. J., Pilgrim, C. A., & Pennypacker, H. S. (1986). Increased proficiency of search in breast self-examination. *Cancer, 58,* 2531–2537; Saslow, D., Hannan, J., Osuch, J., et al. (2004). Clinical breast examination: Practical recommendations for optimizing performance and reporting. *CA: A Cancer Journal for Clinicians, 54*(6), 327–344.

CLINICAL PEARL

Nipple Compression

Nipple compression to provoke discharge is no longer performed as part of routine clinical breast examination. Many benign circumstances, including prior breastfeeding and nipple stimulation as a part of sexual activity, can result in nipple discharge when the nipple is compressed.

Findings in Patients With Female Breasts

The breast tissue of adults will feel dense, firm, and elastic. Expected variations include the lobular feel of glandular tissue (soft, nondiscrete bumps diffusely dispersed throughout the breast tissue) and the fine, granular feel of breast tissue in older adults. A firm transverse ridge of compressed tissue (the inframammary ridge) may be felt along the lower edge of the breast. It is easy to mistake this for a breast mass. A cyclical pattern of breast enlargement, increased nodularity, and tenderness is a common response to hormonal changes during the menstrual cycle. Be aware of where the patient is in the menstrual cycle because these changes are most likely to occur premenstrually and during menses. They are least noticeable during the week after menses. The procedure for examining the patient who has had a mastectomy is described in Box 17.2.

Patient Safety

Harms of Breast Cancer Screening

Although breast cancer screening is beneficial in reducing mortality, it also carries potential harms, so decisions about screening involve weighing the potential benefit against the potential harm. Potential harms include false-positive and false-negative results, additional testing, biopsies, overdiagnosis (diagnosis of lesions that would not become clinically significant) and subsequent treatment, pain from testing, and adverse psychological responses. As metrics for harm assessment are heterogeneous and estimates of harm are uncertain, the risk-benefit assessment is one that needs to be made by the individual patient in concert with the health care clinician.

From Myers, E. R., Moorman, P., Gierisch, J. M., et al. (2015). Benefits and harms of breast cancer screening: A systematic review. *JAMA, 314*(15), 1615–1634.

BOX 17.2 Examining the Patient Who Has Had a Mastectomy

- In the patient who has had a unilateral mastectomy, examine the unaffected breast in the usual manner.
- Inspect the mastectomy site(s) and axilla(e) for any visible signs of swelling, lumps, thickening, redness, color change, rash, or irritation to the scar. Note muscle loss or lymphedema that may be present, depending on the type and extent of the surgical procedure. If the mastectomy was performed for cancer treatment, pay particular attention to the scar. If malignancy recurs, it may be at the scar site.
- Palpate the surgical scar with two fingers, using small, circular motions to assess for swelling, lumps, thickening, or tenderness. Then palpate the chest wall, using three or four fingers in a sweeping motion across the area, being sure not to miss any spots. Intercostal residual breast tissue may exist. Position your fingers on either side of each rib, and run your fingers along the anterior ribs, using a stripping motion. Remember to use your finger pads and not your fingertips. Finally, palpate for lymph nodes in the axillary and supraclavicular and infraclavicular areas.
- If the patient has had breast reconstruction, augmentation, or a lumpectomy, perform breast examination in the usual manner with particular attention to any scars and new tissue.

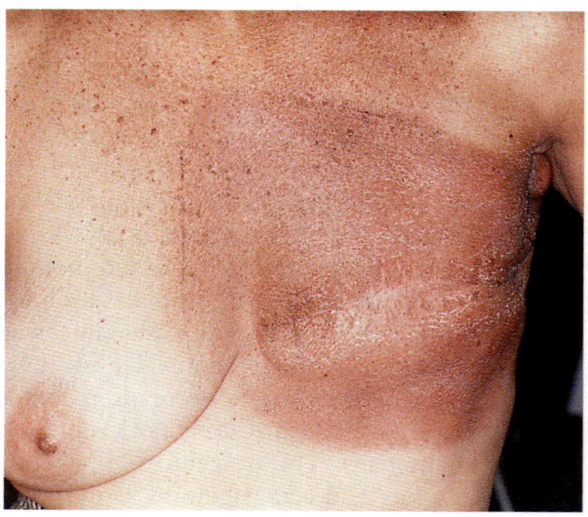

Findings in Patients With Male Breasts

In most patients, expect to feel a thin layer of fatty tissue overlying muscle. Obese patients may have a somewhat thicker fatty layer, giving the appearance of breast enlargement. A firm disk of glandular tissue can be felt in some patients. Transgender women taking hormones may have breast tissue and/or breast implants.

Infants

The breasts of many newborns are enlarged for a relatively brief time as a result of passively transferred maternal estrogen. The enlargement is rarely more than 1 to 1.5 cm in diameter and can be easily palpated behind the nipple. It usually disappears within 2 weeks and rarely lasts beyond 3 months of age. A small amount of clear or milky white fluid, commonly called *witch's milk,* also a result of maternal estrogen, is sometimes spontaneously expressed from the breast bud.

Children and Adolescents

The right and left breasts of the adolescent with female breasts may not develop at the same rate. Provide reassurance that asymmetry is common and that the breasts are developing appropriately. Chapter 8 describes the stages of breast development. Breast tissue of the adolescent feels homogeneous, dense, firm, and elastic. Although malignancy in this age group is rare, routine examination provides an excellent opportunity for reassurance and education for the patient and the parent.

Many male breasts at puberty have transient unilateral or bilateral subareolar masses. These are firm, sometimes tender, and are often a source of great concern to the patient and the parents. Reassure them that these breast buds will most likely disappear, usually within a year. They seldom enlarge to a point of cosmetic difficulty.

Occasionally, pubescent male breasts may enlarge, a condition called *gynecomastia,* which is usually benign and resolves spontaneously. It is typically caused by excess of estrogen relative to testosterone. If the enlargement is extreme and causes emotional distress, it can be corrected surgically for psychological or cosmetic reasons. In rare instances, biopsy is required to rule out the presence of cancer. Gynecomastia can be associated with the use of either prescription drugs or other substances, particularly cannabis and alcohol. Symptoms resolve after the drugs are discontinued.

Pregnant Patients

Pregnancy causes many breast changes, most becoming obvious during the first trimester. The patient may experience a sensation of fullness with tingling, tenderness, and a bilateral increase in size. Adequate support for the breasts may require alteration in the size and style of the bra worn.

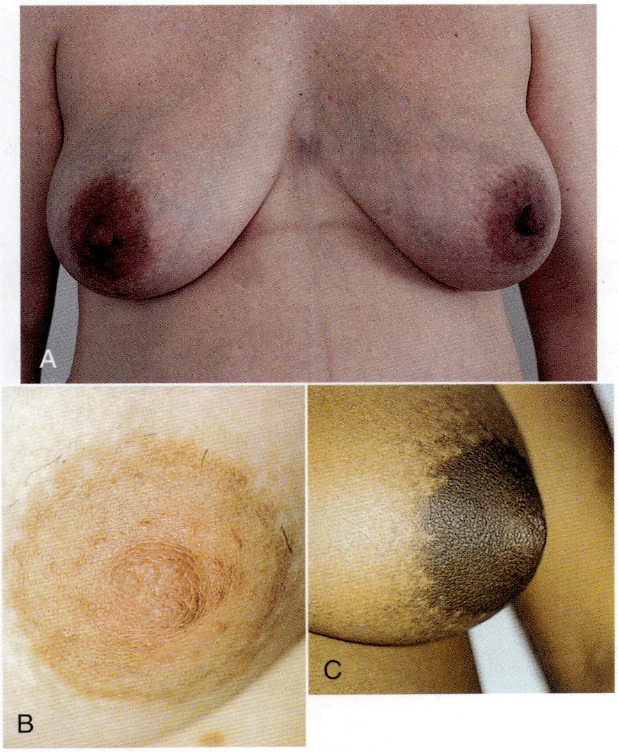

FIG. 17.22 Breast changes in pregnancy. (A) Note venous network, darkened areolae and nipples, and vascular spider. (B) Increased pigmentation and the development of raised sebaceous glands known as Montgomery tubercles. (C) Marked pigmentation in female with dark skin. (B and C, From Symonds, E. M., & Macpherson, M. B. A. (1994). *Color atlas of obstetrics and gynecology*. St. Louis: Mosby.)

Generally, the nipples enlarge and are more erectile. As the pregnancy progresses, the nipples sometimes become flattened or inverted. A crust caused by dried colostrum can be evident on the nipple. Inspect the breasts and expect to see areolae that are broader and darker. Montgomery tubercles are common (Fig. 17.22).

Palpation reveals a generalized coarse nodularity, and the breasts feel lobular because of hypertrophy of the mammary alveoli. Dilated subcutaneous veins may create a network of blue tracing across the breasts.

During the second trimester, telangiectasias (called *spider angiomas* or *vascular spiders*) may develop on the upper chest, arms, neck, and face as a result of elevated levels of circulating estrogen. The spiders are bluish in color and do not blanch with pressure. Striae may be evident as a result of stretching as the breasts increase in size.

Lactating Patients

During lactation, it is important to assess whether the breasts are adequately supported with a properly fitting bra. Palpate the breasts to determine the degree of softness. Full breasts, which are firm, dense, and slightly enlarged, may become engorged. Engorged breasts feel hard and warm and are enlarged, shiny, and painful. Engorgement is not an unusual condition in the first 24 to 48 hours after the breasts fill with milk; however, its later development may signal the onset of mastitis.

Clogged milk ducts are a relatively common occurrence in lactating patients. A clogged duct may result from either inadequate emptying of the breast or a bra that is too tight. The clogged duct will create a tender spot on the breast that may feel lumpy and hot. Frequent breastfeeding and/or expression of the milk, along with local application of heat, will help open the duct. A clogged duct left unattended may result in the development of mastitis.

Examine the nipples for signs of irritation (redness and tenderness) as well as for blisters or petechiae, which are precursors of overt cracking. Cracked nipples will be sore and may be bleeding. Lighter-colored nipples are no more prone to damage from breastfeeding than are darker nipples. Nipple damage from breastfeeding is associated with placement of the nipple in the infant's mouth.

After pregnancy and lactation, most of these changes regress. The areolae and nipples tend to retain their darker color, and the breasts become less firm than in their prepregnant state.

Older Adults

The breasts in postmenopausal females and transgender men with intact breasts may appear flattened, elongated, and suspended more loosely from the chest wall as the result of glandular tissue atrophy and relaxation of the suspensory ligaments. A finer granular feel on palpation replaces the lobular feel of glandular tissue. The inframammary ridge thickens and can be felt more easily. The nipples become smaller and flatter.

ABNORMALITIES

BREASTS

Breast Lumps

See the Differential Diagnosis table for characteristic differences between fibrocystic changes, fibroadenomas, and breast cancer. The differential signs and symptoms will help guide the next steps for diagnosis.

DIFFERENTIAL DIAGNOSIS

Signs and Symptoms of Breast Masses

CHARACTERISTIC	FIBROCYSTIC CHANGES	FIBROADENOMA	CANCER
Age range (yr)	20–49	15–55	30–80
Occurrence	Usually bilateral	Usually bilateral	Usually unilateral
Number	Multiple or single	Single; may be multiple	Single
Shape	Round	Round or discoid	Irregular or stellate
Consistency	Soft to firm; tense	Firm, rubbery	Hard, stonelike
Mobility	Mobile	Mobile	Fixed
Retraction signs	Absent	Absent	Often present
Tenderness	Usually tender	Usually nontender	Usually nontender
Borders	Well delineated	Well delineated	Poorly delineated; irregular
Variation with menses	Yes	No	No

Fibrocystic Changes

Benign fluid-filled cyst formation caused by ductal enlargement.

PATHOPHYSIOLOGY

- Usually bilateral and multiple
- Most common ages 30–55 years in female breasts
- Associated with a long follicular or luteal phase of the menstrual cycle

PATIENT DATA

Subjective Data

- Tender and painful breasts and/or palpable lumps that fluctuate with menses
- Usually worse premenstrually

Objective Data

- Round, soft-to-firm, tense, mobile masses with well-delineated borders
- Usually tender
- Usually bilateral
- Multiple or single

Fibroadenoma

Benign tumors composed of stromal and epithelial elements that represent a hyperplastic or proliferative process in a single terminal ductal unit.

PATHOPHYSIOLOGY

- May occur at any age during the reproductive years
- After menopause, the tumors often regress

PATIENT DATA

Subjective Data

- Painless lumps that do not fluctuate with the menstrual cycle
- May be asymptomatic with discovery on clinical breast examination or breast imaging

Objective Data

- Round or discoid, firm, rubbery, mobile masses with well-delineated borders
- Usually nontender
- Usually bilateral
- Single; may be multiple
- Biopsy often performed to rule out carcinoma

Malignant Breast Tumors

Ductal carcinoma arises from the epithelial lining of ducts, whereas lobular carcinoma originates in the glandular tissue of the lobules.

PATHOPHYSIOLOGY

- Mutations to normal cells result in uncontrolled cell division and tumor formation; as the tumor grows and invades surrounding tissue, metastases occur through the lymph and vascular systems
- Peak incidence between ages 40 and 75 years, with most malignant breast tumors occurring after age 50 years in female breasts

PATIENT DATA

Subjective Data

- Painless lump; change in size, shape, or contour of breast
- Axilla may be tender if lymph nodes involved
- May be asymptomatic with discovery on clinical breast examination or breast imaging

Objective Data

- May have palpable mass that is usually single; unilateral, irregular, or stellate in shape; poorly delineated borders; fixed; hard or stonelike; nontender
- Breast may have dimpling, retraction, prominent vasculature
- Skin may have peau d'orange or thickened appearance
- Nipple may be newly inverted or deviate in position (Fig. 17.23)

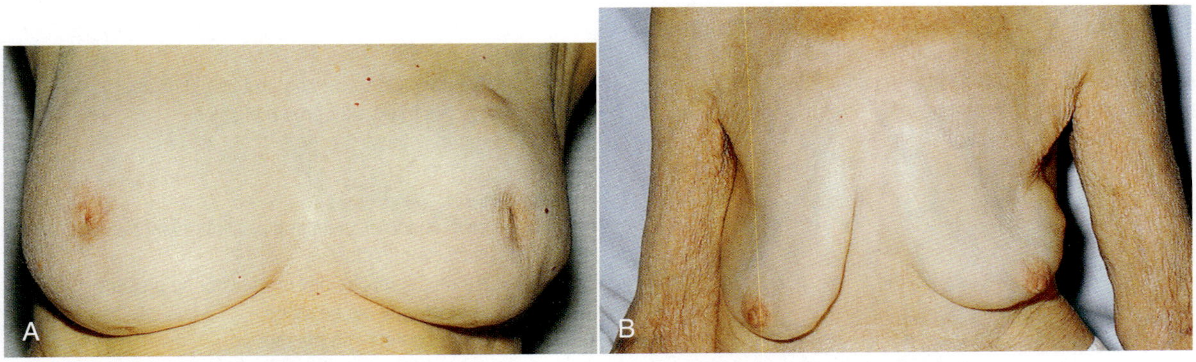

FIG. 17.23 (A) Patient with a lump and nipple retraction in the left breast. (B) Patient with altered nipple height resulting from breast cancer in the left breast. (From Mansel, R. E., & Bundred, N. J. (1995). *Color atlas of breast diseases*. St. Louis: Mosby.)

Fat Necrosis

Benign breast lump that occurs as inflammatory response to local injury.

PATHOPHYSIOLOGY

- Necrotic fat and cellular debris become fibrotic and may contract into a scar

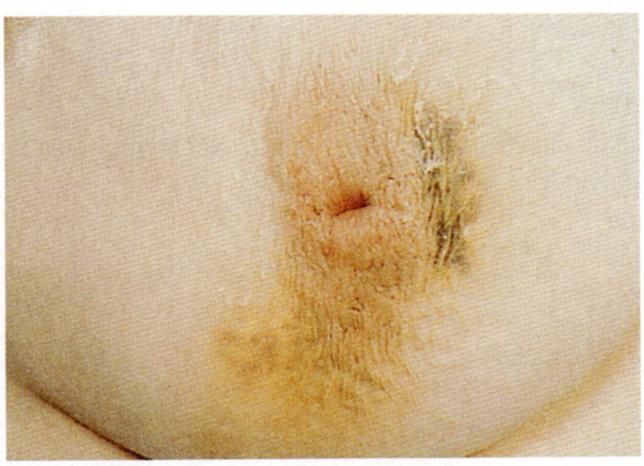

FIG. 17.24 Fat necrosis presenting as a hard mass in the breast after an episode of trauma sufficient to cause bruising. (From Mansel, R. E., & Bundred, N. J. (1995). *Color atlas of breast diseases*. St. Louis: Mosby.)

PATIENT DATA

Subjective Data

- History of trauma to the breast (including surgery)
- Painless lump

Objective Data

- Firm, irregular mass, often appearing as an area of discoloration (Fig. 17.24)
- May mimic breast malignancy on clinical examination or breast imaging, requiring biopsy for diagnosis

NIPPLES AND AREOLAE

Intraductal Papillomas and Papillomatosis

Benign tumors of the subareolar ducts that produce nipple discharge.

PATHOPHYSIOLOGY

- Epithelial hyperplasia produces a wartlike tumor in a lactiferous duct
- 2–3 cm in diameter
- May occur singly or in multiples

PATIENT DATA

Subjective Data

- Spontaneous nipple discharge
- Usually unilateral
- Usually serous or bloody

Objective Data

- Single-duct unilateral nipple discharge provoked on physical examination
- Mass behind the nipple may or may not be present
- May need excisional biopsy to rule out malignancy

Duct Ectasia

Benign condition of the subareolar ducts that produces nipple discharge.

PATHOPHYSIOLOGY

- Subareolar ducts become dilated and blocked with desquamating secretory epithelium, necrotic debris, and chronic inflammatory cells
- Occurs most commonly in menopause

PATIENT DATA

Subjective Data

- Spontaneous unilateral or bilateral nipple discharge
- Discharge often green or brown in color
- Discharge may be sticky

Objective Data

- Single or multiductal, unilateral or bilateral nipple discharge provoked on physical examination
- Mass behind the nipple may or may not be present
- Breast may or may not be tender
- Nipple retraction may be present

Galactorrhea

Lactation not associated with childbearing.

PATHOPHYSIOLOGY

- Elevated levels of prolactin, resulting in milk production, occur as a result of disruption of the communication between the pituitary and hypothalamus glands
- Common causes include pituitary-secreting tumors, hypothalamic-pituitary disorders, systemic diseases, numerous medications and herbs, physiologic conditions, or local factors

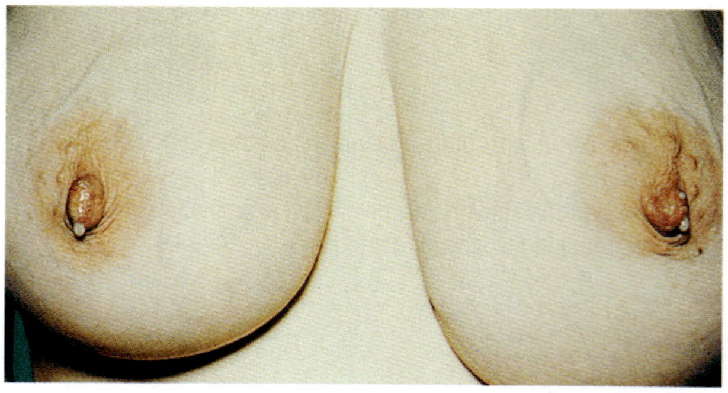

FIG. 17.25 **Galactorrhea produced by a prolactin-secreting pituitary tumor.** (From Mansel R, Bundred N. (1995). *Color atlas of breast disease*, St Louis, Mosby.)

PATIENT DATA

Subjective Data

- Spontaneous nipple discharge, usually bilateral; usually serous or milky
- Possible related medical history: amenorrhea, pregnancy, post abortion, hypothyroidism, Cushing syndrome, chronic renal failure
- Possible medication history: phenothiazines, tricyclic antidepressants, some antihypertensive agents, estrogens, H2 receptor blockers, cannabis, amphetamines, opiates
- Possible physiologic history: suckling, stress, dehydration, exercise, nipple stimulation

Objective Data

- Multiductal nipple discharge may or may not be provoked on physical examination (Fig. 17.25)
- No mass

Paget Disease

Surface manifestation of underlying ductal carcinoma.

PATHOPHYSIOLOGY

- Migration of malignant epithelial cells from the underlying intraductal carcinoma via the lactiferous sinuses into nipple skin
- Tumor cells disrupt the epithelial barrier, allowing extracellular fluid to seep out onto the nipple surface

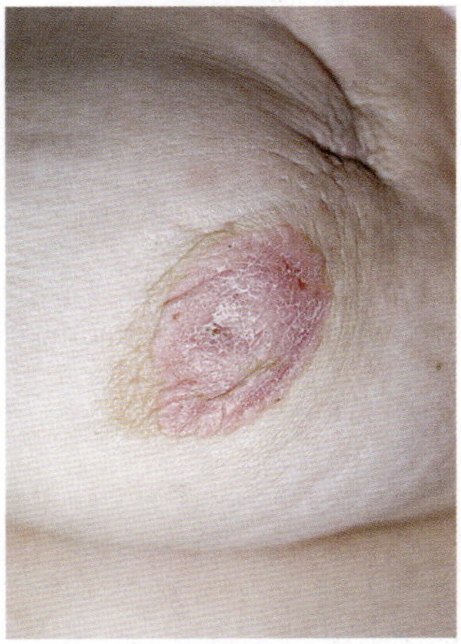

FIG. 17.26 Paget disease. (From Callen, J. P., et al. (2000). *Color atlas of dermatology* (2nd ed.). Philadelphia: Saunders.)

PATIENT DATA

Subjective Data

- Crustiness of the nipple, areola, and surrounding skin
- Pruritus of the nipple common

Objective Data

- Red, scaling, crusty patch on the nipple, areola, and surrounding skin (Fig. 17.26)
- May be unilateral or bilateral
- Appears eczematous but, unlike eczema, does not respond to steroids

Mastitis

Inflammation and infection of the breast tissue.

PATHOPHYSIOLOGY

- Most infections are staphylococcal, often *Staphylococcus aureus*
- Most common in lactating patients after milk is established, usually the second to third week after delivery; however, it may occur at any time
- Can occur in newborns, but uncommon
- Abscess formation can result

PATIENT DATA

Subjective Data

- Characterized by sudden onset of swelling, tenderness, redness, and heat in the breast
- Usually accompanied by chills, fever

Objective Data

- Tender, hard breast mass, with an area of fluctuation, erythema, and heat
- May have discharge of pus (suppuration)
- Underlying pus-filled abscess may impart a bluish tinge to the skin (Fig. 17.27)

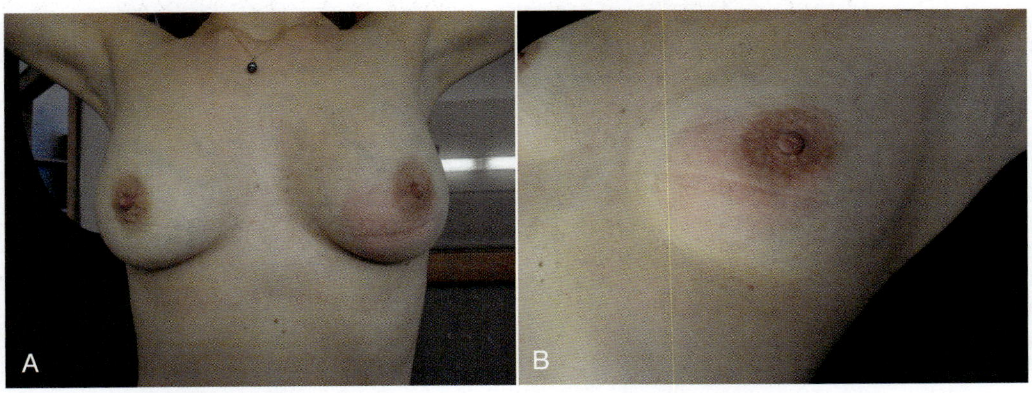

FIG. 17.27 Mastitis. (A) Seated position. (B) Supine. Note the area of erythema. (From Boutet, G. (2012). Breast inflammation: Clinical examination, aetiological pointers. *Diagnostic and Interventional Imaging*, *93*(2), 74–85.)

Gynecomastia

Breast enlargement in male breasts.

PATHOPHYSIOLOGY

- Result of increased body fat; hormone imbalance from puberty or aging; by testicular, pituitary, or hormone-secreting tumors; by liver failure; or by a variety of medications including anabolic steroids, cannabis, some antihypertensives, some antipsychotics, or those containing estrogens or antiandrogens
- When testosterone levels are low relative to estrogen, breasts grow larger and are more noticeable
- Increased body fat, which in turn produces more estrogen, can also cause breast enlargement

PATIENT DATA

Subjective Data

- Breast enlargement (Figs. 17.28 and 17.29)
- Relevant medication history (estrogens, antiandrogens, anabolic steroids, tricyclic antidepressants, spironolactone, 5-α reductase inhibitors, ketoconazole, cimetidine, substance use, and especially cannabis)

Objective Data

- Smooth, firm, mobile, tender disk of breast tissue located behind the areola
- Usually nontender
- May be unilateral or bilateral
- Amount of breast tissue varies; can be small overgrowth of breast tissue around the areola and nipple to larger, more "female-looking" breasts

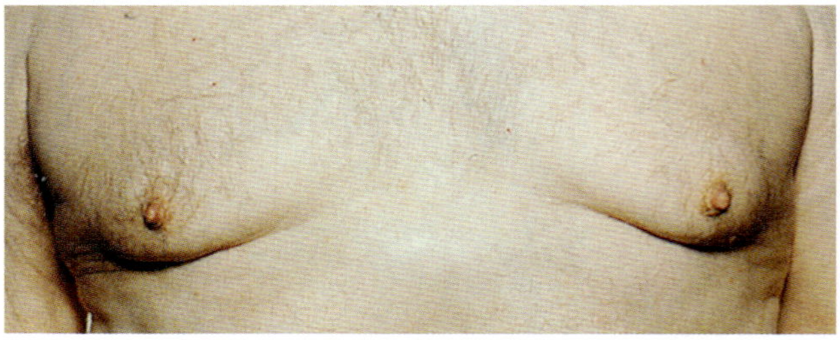

FIG. 17.28 Adult gynecomastia. (From Mansel, R. E., & Bundred, N. J. (1995). *Color atlas of breast diseases*. St. Louis: Mosby.)

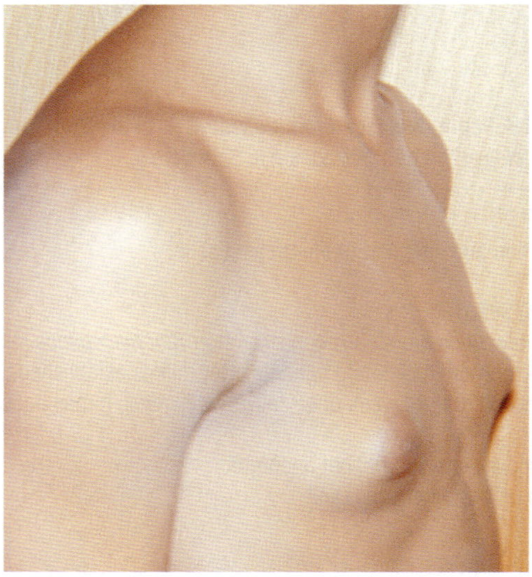

FIG. 17.29 Prepubertal gynecomastia, small and subareolar. (Courtesy Wellington Hung, MD, Children's National Medical Center, Washington, DC.)

Children

Premature Thelarche

Breast enlargement in children assigned female at birth younger than 8 years of age.

PATHOPHYSIOLOGY

- Cause is unknown; however, increased sensitivity of breast tissue to estradiol (E2), transient E2 secretion from ovarian cysts, dietary estrogen intake, and transient activation of the hypothalamus-pituitary-gonadal (HPG) axis have been proposed as possible mechanisms (Uçar et al., 2012)
- Most cases have an onset in young females under age 2 years
- In most cases, breasts continue to enlarge slowly throughout childhood until full development is reached during adolescence

PATIENT DATA

Subjective Data

- Breast enlargement

Objective Data

- Degree of enlargement varies from very slight to fully developed breasts
- Usually occurs bilaterally
- Other signs of sexual maturation may be absent

CHAPTER 18

Abdomen

The abdominal examination is performed as part of the comprehensive physical examination or when a patient presents with signs or symptoms suggestive of an abdominal disease process. It involves the core examination skills in a particular sequence: inspection, auscultation, percussion, and palpation. Additional procedures are used to detect serious abdominal pathology. During the abdominal examination, pay careful attention to the patient's comfort level or degree of distress.

Physical Examination Components

1. Inspect the abdomen for:
   - Skin characteristics
   - Venous return patterns
   - Symmetry
   - Surface motion
2. Inspect abdominal muscles as patient raises the head to detect the presence of:
   - Masses
   - Hernia
   - Separation of muscles
3. Auscultate with stethoscope diaphragm for bowel sounds.
4. Auscultate with stethoscope bell for bruits over aortic, renal, iliac, and femoral arteries.
5. Percuss the abdomen for:
   - Tone in all four quadrants (or nine regions)
   - Liver borders to estimate span
   - Splenic dullness in left midaxillary line
   - Gastric air bubble
6. Lightly palpate in all quadrants or regions for:
   - Muscular resistance
   - Tenderness
   - Masses
7. Deeply palpate for:
   - Bulges and masses around the umbilicus and umbilical ring
   - Liver border in right costal margin
   - Gallbladder below liver margin at lateral border of the rectus muscle
   - Spleen in left costal margin
   - Right and left kidneys
   - Aortic pulsation in midline
   - Other masses
8. With the patient sitting, percuss the left and right costovertebral angles for tenderness.

ANATOMY AND PHYSIOLOGY

The abdominal cavity contains several of the body's vital organs (Fig. 18.1). The peritoneum—a serous membrane—lines the cavity and forms a protective cover for many of the abdominal organs. Double folds of the peritoneum around the stomach constitute the greater and lesser omentum. The mesentery—a fan-shaped fold of the peritoneum—covers most of the small intestine and anchors it to the posterior abdominal wall.

Musculature and Connective Tissues

The rectus abdominis muscles anteriorly and the internal and external oblique muscles laterally form and protect the abdominal cavity (see Fig. 18.1A). The linea alba—a tendinous band—is located in the midline of the abdomen between the rectus abdominis muscles. It extends from the xiphoid process to the symphysis pubis and contains the umbilicus. The inguinal ligament (Poupart ligament) extends from the anterior-superior spine of the ilium on each side to the pubis.

Alimentary Tract

The alimentary tract—a tube approximately 27 feet long—runs from the mouth to the anus and includes the esophagus, stomach, small intestine, and large intestine. It functions to ingest and digest food; absorb nutrients, electrolytes, and water; and excrete waste products. Food and digestive products are moved along the length of the alimentary tract by peristalsis under autonomic (involuntary) nervous system control.

The esophagus—a collapsible tube about 10 inches long—connects the pharynx to the stomach. Just posterior to the trachea, the esophagus descends through the mediastinal cavity and diaphragm, entering the stomach at the cardiac orifice.

The stomach lies transversely in the upper abdominal cavity, just below the diaphragm. It consists of three sections: the fundus, lying above and to the left of the cardiac orifice; the middle two-thirds, or body; and the pylorus, the most distal portion that narrows and terminates in the pyloric orifice. The stomach secretes hydrochloric acid and digestive enzymes that break down fats and proteins.

Pepsin acts to digest proteins, whereas gastric lipase acts on emulsified fats. Little absorption takes place in the stomach.

The small intestine—about 21 feet long—begins at the pylorus. Coiled in the abdominal cavity, it joins the large intestine at the ileocecal valve. The first 12 inches of the small intestine—the duodenum—form a C-shaped curve around the head of the pancreas. The common bile duct and pancreatic duct open into the duodenum at the duodenal papilla, about 3 inches below the pylorus of the stomach. The next 8 feet of intestine, the jejunum, gradually become larger and thicker. The ileum makes up the remaining 12 feet of the small intestine. The ileocecal valve between the ileum and large intestine prevents backward flow of fecal material.

The small intestine completes digestion through the action of pancreatic enzymes, bile, and several other enzymes. Nutrients are absorbed through the mucosa of the small intestine. The functional surface area of the small intestine is increased by its circular folds and villi.

The large intestine begins at the cecum, a blind pouch about 2 to 3 inches long (see Fig. 18.1B). The ileal contents empty into the cecum through the ileocecal valve, and the vermiform appendix extends from the base of the cecum. The ascending colon rises from the cecum along the right posterior abdominal wall to the undersurface of the liver. The ascending colon turns toward the midline at the hepatic flexure and becomes the transverse colon. The transverse colon crosses the abdominal cavity toward the spleen and turns downward at the splenic flexure. The descending

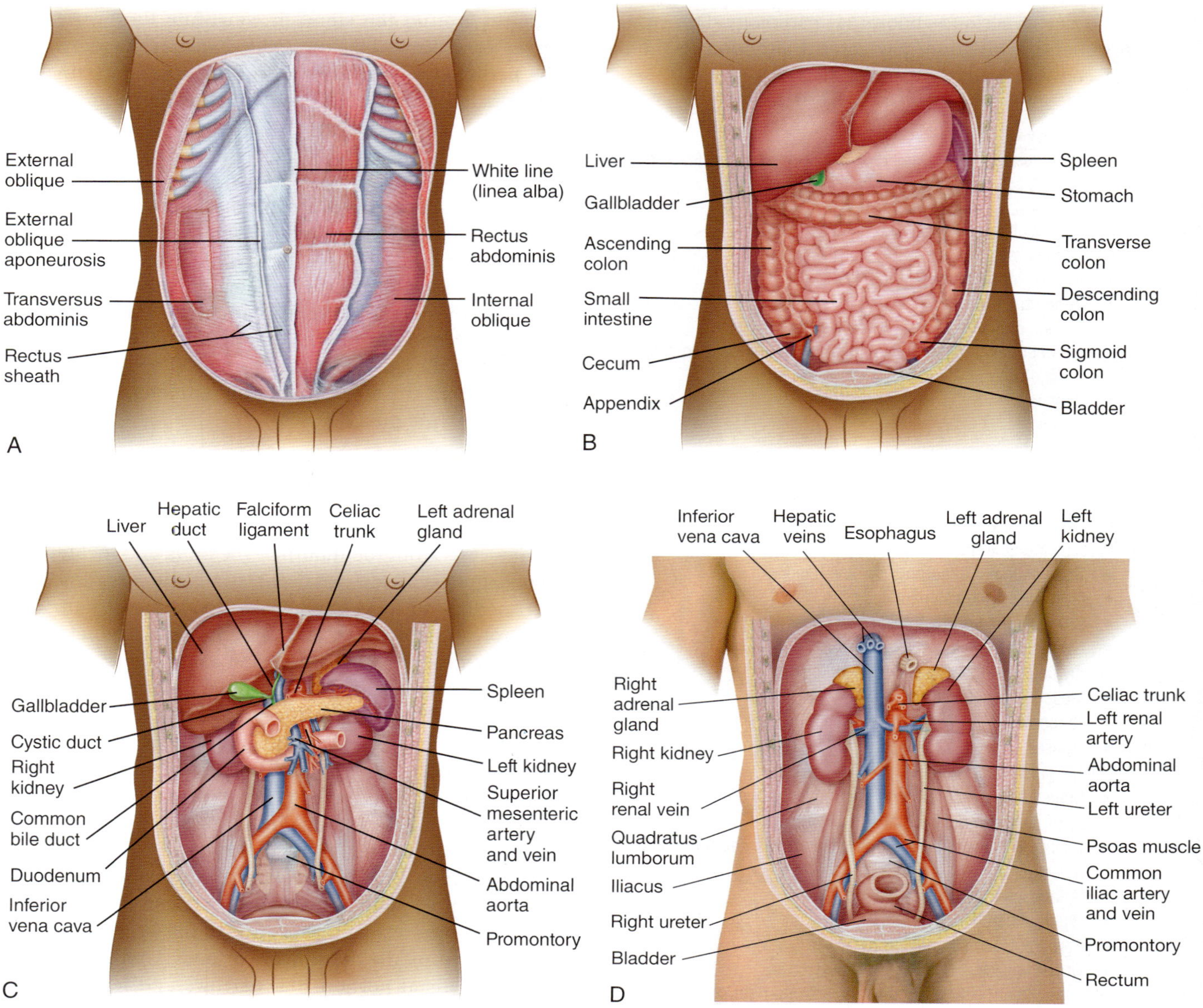

FIG. 18.1 Anatomic structures of the abdominal cavity.

colon continues along the left abdominal wall to the rim of the pelvis, where it turns medially and inferiorly to form the S-shaped sigmoid colon. The rectum extends from the sigmoid colon to the muscles of the pelvic floor. It continues as the anal canal and terminates at the anus.

The large intestine is about 4.5 to 5 feet long, with a diameter of 2.5 inches. Its main functions are to absorb water and transport waste. Mucous glands secrete large quantities of alkaline mucus that lubricate the intestinal contents and neutralize acids formed by intestinal bacteria. Live bacteria decompose undigested food residue, unabsorbed amino acids, cell debris, and dead bacteria through a process of putrefaction and fermentation.

Liver

The liver lies in the right upper quadrant of the abdomen (see Fig. 18.1C), just below the diaphragm and above the gallbladder, right kidney, and hepatic flexure of the colon. The heaviest organ in the body, the liver, weighs about 3 pounds. It is composed of four lobes containing lobules—the functional units. Each lobule is made up of liver cells radiating around a central vein. Branches of the portal vein, hepatic artery, and bile duct penetrate to the periphery of the lobules. Bile secreted by the liver cells drains from the bile ducts into the hepatic duct, which joins the cystic duct from the gallbladder to form the common bile duct.

The hepatic artery transports blood to the liver directly from the aorta, and the portal vein carries blood from the digestive tract and spleen to the liver. Repeated branching of both vessels makes the liver a highly vascular organ. Three hepatic veins carry blood from the liver and empty into the inferior vena cava (see Fig. 18.1D).

The liver plays an important role in the metabolism of carbohydrates, fats, and proteins. Glucose is converted and stored as glycogen until—in response to varying levels of insulin and regulatory hormones—it is reconverted and released again as glucose. The liver also can convert amino acids to glucose (gluconeogenesis). Fats, arriving at the liver in the form of fatty acids, are oxidized to two-carbon components in preparation for entry into the tricarboxylic acid cycle. Cholesterol is used by the liver to form bile salts. Synthesis of fats from carbohydrates and proteins also occurs in the liver. Proteins are broken down to amino acids through hydrolysis, and their waste products are converted to urea for excretion by the kidneys.

Other functions of the liver include storage of several vitamins and iron; detoxification of potentially harmful substances; production of antibodies; conjugation and excretion of steroid hormones; and the production of prothrombin, fibrinogen, and other substances for blood coagulation. The liver is responsible for the production of the majority of proteins circulating in the plasma. It serves as an excretory organ through the synthesis of bile, the secretion of organic wastes into bile, and the conversion of fat-soluble wastes to water-soluble material for renal excretion.

Gallbladder

The gallbladder is a saclike, pear-shaped organ about 4 inches long, lying recessed in the inferior surface of the liver (see Fig. 18.1C). It concentrates and stores bile from the liver. In response to cholecystokinin—a hormone produced in the duodenum—the gallbladder releases bile into the cystic duct. The cystic duct and hepatic duct join to form the common bile duct. Contraction of the gallbladder propels bile along the common duct and into the duodenum at the duodenal papilla. Composed of cholesterol, bile salts, and pigments, bile serves to maintain the alkaline pH of the small intestine, permitting emulsification of fats so that absorption of lipids can be accomplished.

Pancreas

The pancreas lies behind and beneath the stomach, with its head resting in the curve of the duodenum and tip extending across the abdominal cavity to almost touch the spleen (see Fig. 18.1C). As an exocrine gland, the acinar cells of the pancreas produce digestive juices containing inactive enzymes for breaking down proteins, fats, and carbohydrates. Collecting ducts empty into the pancreatic duct (duct of Wirsung), which runs the length of the organ. The pancreatic duct empties into the duodenum at the duodenal papilla alongside the common bile duct. Once introduced into the duodenum, the digestive enzymes are activated. As an endocrine gland, islet cells scattered throughout the pancreas produce the hormones insulin and glucagon.

Spleen

The spleen is in the left upper quadrant, lying above the left kidney and just below the diaphragm. White pulp (lymphoid tissue) constitutes most of the organ and functions as part of the reticuloendothelial system to filter blood and manufacture lymphocytes and monocytes. The red pulp of the spleen contains a capillary network and venous sinus system that allow for storage and release of blood, permitting the spleen to accommodate up to several hundred milliliters.

Kidneys, Ureters, and Bladder

The two kidneys are located in the retroperitoneal space of the upper abdomen (see Fig. 18.1D). Each extends from about the vertebral level of T12 to L3. The right kidney is usually slightly lower than the left, presumably because of the large, heavy liver just above it. Both kidneys are embedded in fat and fascia, which anchor and protect these organs. Each contains more than 1 million nephrons—the structural and functional units of the kidneys. The nephrons are composed of a tuft of capillaries, the glomerulus, a proximal convoluted tubule, the loop of Henle, and a distal convoluted tubule. The distal tubule empties into a collecting duct.

Each kidney receives about one-eighth of the cardiac output through the renal artery. The glomerular filtration rate (GFR)—used to measure kidney function—is typically 90 mL/min/1.73 m^2 or higher in healthy individuals. Most of the filtered material, including electrolytes, glucose, water, and small proteins, is actively reabsorbed in the proximal tubule. Some organic acids are also actively secreted in the distal tubule. Urinary volume is carefully controlled by antidiuretic hormone (ADH) to maintain a constant total body fluid volume. Urine passes into the renal pelvis via the collecting tubules and then into the ureters. Peristaltic waves move urine to the urinary bladder, which has a capacity of about 400 to 600 milliliters.

The kidney also serves as an endocrine gland responsible for the production of renin, which controls aldosterone secretion to regulate blood pressure. It is the primary source of erythropoietin production, thus influencing the body's red cell mass. In addition to synthesizing several prostaglandins, the kidney produces the biologically active form of vitamin D.

Vasculature

The abdominal portion of the descending aorta travels from the diaphragm through the abdominal cavity, just to the left of the midline (see Fig. 18.1D). At about the level of the umbilicus, the aorta branches into the two common iliac arteries. The splenic and renal arteries, which supply their respective organs, also branch off within the abdomen.

Fetal Development and Infancy

The pancreatic buds, liver, and gallbladder all begin to form during week 4 of gestation, by which time the intestine already exists as a single tube. The motility of the gastrointestinal tract develops in a cephalocaudal direction, permitting amniotic fluid to be swallowed by 17 weeks of gestation. Production of meconium—an end product of fetal metabolism—begins shortly thereafter. By 36 to 38 weeks of gestation, the gastrointestinal tract is capable of adapting to extrauterine life. However, the elasticity, musculature, and control mechanisms of the gastrointestinal tract continue to develop, reaching adult function at 2 to 3 years of age.

During gestation, the liver begins to form blood cells at about week 6, synthesize glycogen by week 9, and produce bile by week 12. The liver's role as a metabolic and glycogen storage organ accounts for its large size at birth. The liver remains the heaviest organ in the body.

Pancreatic islet cells are developed by 12 weeks of gestation and begin producing insulin. The spleen is active in blood formation during fetal development and the first year of life. Afterward, the spleen aids in the destruction of blood cells and functions as a lymphatic organ for immunologic response.

Nephrogenesis begins during the second month of gestation. By 12 weeks, the kidney is able to produce urine, and the bladder expands as a sac. Development of new nephrons ceases by 36 weeks of gestation. After birth, the kidney increases in size because of enlargement of the existing nephrons and adjoining tubules. The GFR is approximately 0.5 mL/min before 34 weeks of gestation and gradually increases in a linear fashion to the adulthood rate.

Pregnant Patients

As the uterus enlarges, the muscles of the abdominal wall stretch and lose tone. During the third trimester, the rectus abdominis muscles may separate, allowing abdominal contents to protrude at the midline (diastasis recti).

The umbilicus flattens or protrudes. Striae may form as the skin is stretched. A line of pigmentation at the midline (linea nigra) often develops from melanocyte-stimulating hormone produced by the placenta (Fig. 18.2). Abdominal muscles have less tone and are less active. The abdominal contour changes when lightening, or dropping, occurs (about 2 weeks before term in a nulliparous patient), and the fetal presenting part descends into the true pelvis. After pregnancy, the muscles gradually regain tone, though diastasis recti may persist.

During the second trimester, lower esophageal sphincter pressure decreases. Peristaltic wave velocity in the distal esophagus also decreases. Gastric emptying appears to be normal; however, gastrointestinal transit time is prolonged, at times leading to constipation. Incompetence of the pyloric sphincter may result in alkaline reflux of duodenal contents into the stomach. Because of relaxation of the lower esophageal sphincter, heartburn (gastroesophageal reflux) often occurs.

The gallbladder may become distended, accompanied by decreased emptying time and change in tone. The combination of gallbladder stasis and secretion of lithogenic bile increases formation of cholesterol crystals and the development of gallstones. Gallstones are more common in the second and third trimesters.

The kidneys enlarge by about 1 cm in length during pregnancy. The renal pelvis and ureters dilate from the effects of hormones and pressure from the enlarging

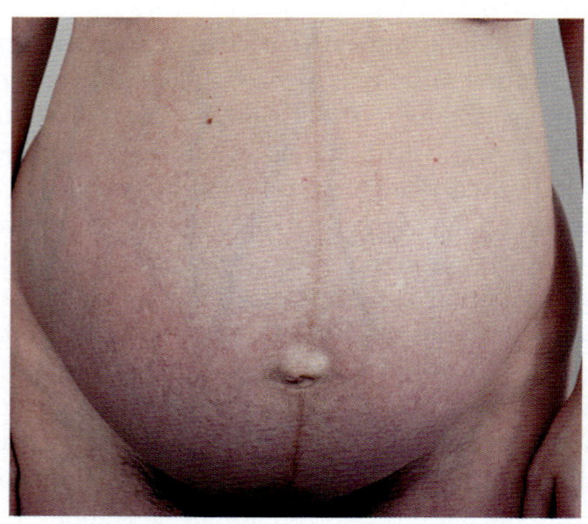

FIG. 18.2 Linea nigra in the third trimester of pregnancy.

uterus. Dilation of the ureter is greater on the right side than on the left, probably because it is affected by displacement of the uterus to the right by an enlarged right ovarian vein. The ureters also elongate and form single and double curves of varying sizes and angulation. These changes can lead to urinary stasis, which increases the risk of pyelonephritis in pregnant patients with asymptomatic bacteriuria. Renal function is most efficient if the individual lies in the lateral recumbent position, which helps prevent compression of the vena cava and aorta. These changes can last up to 3 or 4 months postpartum.

The bladder has increased sensitivity and compression during pregnancy, leading to urinary frequency and urgency during the first and third trimesters. After the fourth month, the increase in uterine size, hyperemia of all pelvic organs, and hyperplasia of muscle and connective tissue elevate the bladder trigone and cause thickening of the posterior margin. This process produces a marked deepening and widening of the trigone by the end of the pregnancy and may result in microhematuria. During the third trimester, compression may also result from the descent of the fetus into the pelvis; this, in turn, causes a sense of urgency and/or incontinence, even with a small amount of urine in the bladder.

The colon is displaced laterally upward and posteriorly, peristaltic activity may decrease, and water absorption is increased. As a result, bowel sounds are diminished, and constipation and flatus are more common. The appendix is displaced upward and laterally, away from the McBurney point, an anatomic landmark one-third of the distance from the anterior-superior iliac spine to the umbilicus.

In the postpartum period, the uterus involutes rapidly. Immediately after delivery, the uterus is approximately the size of a 20-week pregnancy (palpable at the level of the umbilicus). By the end of the first week, it is about the size of a 12-week pregnancy, palpable at the symphysis pubis. The muscles of the pelvic floor and the pelvic supports gradually regain tone during the postpartum period and may require 6 to 7 weeks to recover. Stretching of the abdominal wall during pregnancy may result in persistent striae.

Older Adults

The process of aging results in changes in the functional abilities of the gastrointestinal tract. Motility of the intestine is the most severely affected; secretion and absorption are affected to a lesser degree. Altered motility may be caused by age-related changes in neurons of the central nervous system and by changes in collagen properties that increase the resistance of the intestinal wall to stretching. Reduced circulation to the intestine often follows other systemic changes associated with hypoxia and hypovolemia.

As a result of epithelial atrophy, the secretion of both digestive enzymes and protective mucus decreases in the intestinal tract. Particular elements of the mucosal cells show a lesser degree of differentiation and are associated with reduction in secretory ability. These cells are also more susceptible to both physical and chemical agents, including ingested carcinogens. Bacterial flora of the intestine can undergo both qualitative and quantitative changes and become less biologically active. These changes may impair digestive ability and thereby cause food intolerances in the older adult.

Liver size decreases after 50 years of age, which parallels the decrease in lean body mass. Hepatic blood flow decreases as a result of a decline in cardiac output associated with aging. The liver loses some ability to metabolize certain drugs. Increasing obesity and the development of type 2 diabetes mellitus also put the liver at risk for the development of nonalcoholic fatty liver disease (NAFLD).

The size of the pancreas is unaffected by aging, although the main pancreatic duct and branches widen. With aging, there is an increase in fibrous tissue and fatty deposition with acinar cell atrophy; however, the large reserve of the organ results in no significant physiologic changes.

There may be an increase of biliary lipids—specifically the phospholipids and cholesterol—resulting in the formation of gallstones.

REVIEW OF RELATED HISTORY

For each of the symptoms or conditions discussed in this section, targeted topics to include in the history of the present illness are listed. Questions regarding these topics will help focus the physical examination and develop an appropriate diagnostic evaluation. Questions regarding medication use (prescription and over-the-counter) as well as complementary, alternative, and integrative therapies are relevant for each area.

History of Present Illness

Abdominal Pain

- Onset and duration: sudden or gradual; persistent, recurrent, intermittent
- Character: dull, sharp, burning, gnawing, stabbing, cramping, aching
- Location: at time of onset, change over time, radiation to another area, superficial or deep
- Associated symptoms: vomiting, diarrhea, constipation, passage of flatus, belching, jaundice, change in abdominal girth, weight loss or weight gain
- Relationship to: menstrual cycle, change in menses, intercourse, urination, defecation, inspiration, change in body position, food or alcohol intake, stress, time of day, trauma
- Recent stool characteristics: color, consistency, odor, frequency
- Urinary characteristics: frequency, color, volume congruent with fluid intake, force of stream, ease of starting stream, ability to empty bladder
- Medications: high doses of aspirin, steroids, nonsteroidal antiinflammatory drugs (NSAIDs)

Indigestion (Dyspepsia)

- Character: feeling of fullness, heartburn, discomfort, excessive belching, flatulence, loss of appetite, severe pain
- Location: localized or general, radiating to back, arms, or shoulders
- Relationship to: amount, type, and timing of food intake; menses
- Onset of symptoms: time of day or night, sudden or gradual
- Symptom relieved by antacids, change in diet, rest, activity
- Medications: antacids (calcium carbonate, H2 blockers, proton pump inhibitors)

Nausea and Vomiting

- Associated with vomiting; particular stimular (odors, activities, time of day, food intake)
- Occurs with particular stimuli (odors, activities, time of day, food intake)
- Character: nature (color, bright red blood or coffee grounds, bilious, undigested food particles), quantity, duration, frequency, ability to keep down liquids or food
- Associated symptoms: constipation, diarrhea, fever, chills, headache, weight loss, abdominal pain or cramping, heartburn, dizziness
- Relationship to: previous meal, change in appetite, medications, menses

Diarrhea

- Character: watery, copious, explosive; color; presence of blood, mucus, undigested food, oil, or fat; odor; frequency, duration; change in pattern
- Associated symptoms: fever, chills, thirst, weight loss, abdominal pain or cramping, constipation alternating with diarrhea, fecal incontinence
- Relationship to: amount, type, and timing of food intake; stressful life events or daily stressors
- Travel history and/or ill contacts
- Medications: laxatives or stool softeners; antidiarrheals

Constipation

- Character: presence of bright red blood, black or tarry appearance of stool; diarrhea alternating with constipation; accompanied by abdominal pain or discomfort; frequency, duration
- Pattern: last bowel movement, pain with defecation, change in consistency or size of stool
- Diet: recent change in diet, intake of high-fiber foods, change in fluid intake
- Medications: laxatives, stool softeners, iron, diuretics, glucagon-like peptide-1 (GLP-1) use, opioids, NSAIDs

Fecal Incontinence

- Character: stool characteristics, timing in relation to meals, number of episodes per day; occurring with or without warning sensation
- Associated with: use of laxatives, presence of underlying disease (cancer, inflammatory bowel disease, diverticulitis, colitis, proctitis, diabetic neuropathy, spinal cord injury)
- Relationship to: fluid and dietary intake, immobilization
- Medications: laxatives, stool softeners, diuretics

Jaundice

- Onset and duration
- Color of stools or urine
- Associated with abdominal pain, chills, fever, fatigue, lethargy
- Exposure to hepatitis, substance use, high-risk sexual activity, excessive alcohol use, ingestion of contaminated food or water
- Medications: high doses of acetaminophen; antipsychotics, antiepileptics, antibiotics

Dysuria

- Character: location (suprapubic, distal urethra), pain or burning, frequency or volume changes
- Associated fever or other systemic signs of illness: bacterial infection, tuberculosis, fungal or viral infection, parasitic infection
- Increased frequency of sexual intercourse or high-risk sexual activity
- Amount of daily fluid intake

Urinary Frequency

- Change in usual pattern and/or volume
- Associated with dysuria or other urinary characteristics: urgency, hematuria, incontinence, nocturia; increased thirst, weight loss
- Change in urinary stream; dribbling
- Medications: diuretics, caffeine intake

Urinary Incontinence

- Character: amount and frequency, constant or intermittent, dribbling versus frank incontinence
- Associated with: urgency, previous surgery, coughing, sneezing, lifting, laughing, standing up from sitting or lying, nocturia, menopause
- Medications: diuretics

Hematuria

- Character: color (bright red, rusty brown, cola-colored); present at beginning, end, or throughout voiding
- Associated symptoms: flank or costovertebral pain, passage of wormlike clots, pain on voiding
- Alternative possibilities: ingestion of foods containing red vegetable dyes (may cause red urinary pigment) like beets, blackberries, and fava beans; ingestion of laxatives containing phenolphthalein
- Medications: aspirin, NSAIDs, anticoagulants, diuretics, antibiotics

Risk Factors

Persons at Risk for Viral Hepatitis

RISK FACTOR	HEPATITIS A	HEPATITIS B	HEPATITIS C
Sexual contact with an infected individual		√	√
People experiencing homelessness	√		
Men who have sex with men	√	√	
International travelers to countries with intermediate or high prevalence	√	√	
Close person-to-person contact with an infected individual	√		
Infants born to infected mothers		√	√
People with human immunodeficiency virus (HIV) infection		√	√
People with clotting factor disorders	√		
People who received clotting factor concentrates made before 1987			√
People who received blood transfusions or solid organ transplants before July 1992			√
People with end-stage renal disease, including hemodialysis patients		√	√
People with chronic liver disease		√	
People sharing contaminated needles, syringes, or other injection drug equipment		√	√
People who use injection or noninjection drugs	√	√	
Health care and public safety workers at risk for occupational exposure to blood or blood-contaminated body fluids		√	√
People receiving immunosuppressive therapy		√	
People who are incarcerated		√	√
People who received tattoos from unregulated vendors			√

Modified from Centers for Disease Control and Prevention. (2020). *The ABCs of hepatitis—for health professionals.* https://www.cdc.gov/hepatitis/resources/professionals/pdfs/abctable.pdf

Past Medical History

- Gastrointestinal disorder: peptic ulcer, polyps, inflammatory bowel disease, irritable bowel syndrome, intestinal obstruction, pancreatitis, hyperlipidemia
- Hepatitis or cirrhosis of the liver
- Abdominal or urinary tract surgery or injury
- Urinary tract infection: number of episodes, treatment
- Major illness: cancer, arthritis (steroids, NSAIDs, or aspirin use), kidney disease, cardiac disease
- Blood transfusions
- Immunization status (hepatitis A and hepatitis B)
- Colorectal cancer or related cancers—breast, ovarian, endometrial
- Sexually transmitted infections

Family History

- Colorectal cancer and familial colorectal cancer syndromes—familial adenomatous polyposis, hereditary nonpolyposis colorectal cancer (Lynch syndrome)
- Gallbladder disease
- Kidney disease: renal stone, polycystic disease, renal tubular acidosis, renal or bladder carcinoma
- Malabsorption syndrome: cystic fibrosis, celiac disease
- Hirschsprung disease (congenital aganglionic megacolon)
- Familial Mediterranean fever (periodic peritonitis)

Personal and Social History

- Nutrition: 24-hour dietary recall; food preferences and dislikes; ethnic foods, religious food restrictions, food intolerances, lifestyle effects on food intake, use of probiotics or dietary supplements; voluntary and involuntary weight gain or loss
- First day of last menstrual period
- Alcohol intake: frequency, type, and usual amounts
- Stressful life events or chronic daily stressors: physical, social, and psychological changes
- Exposure to infectious diseases: hepatitis, influenza; travel history; occupational or environmental exposures

- Trauma: through type of work, physical activity, physical or emotional abuse, intimate partner violence, community or neighborhood violence
- Substance use (cocaine, marijuana)
- Tobacco use: smoking cigarettes or e-cigarettes frequency, amount, duration, pack-years

Infants

- Gestational age and birth weight (preterm and less than 1500 g at higher risk for necrotizing enterocolitis)
- Passage of first meconium stool within 24 hours, constipation
- Jaundice: in newborn period; exchange transfusions, prolonged use of total parenteral nutrition, phototherapy; exclusively breastfed infant; appearance later in first month of life
- Vomiting: increasing in amount or frequency, forceful or projectile (pyloric stenosis), blood in emesis, back arching (gastroesophageal reflux); associated with intermittent abdominal pain or drawing up of the legs (intussusception)
- Diarrhea, fussiness, failure to gain weight, weight loss, steatorrhea (malabsorption)
- Abdominal distention (with or without pain)

Children

- Constipation: toilet training methods; soiling; diarrhea; abdominal distention; stool size, shape, consistency (types 1 and 2 on Bristol Stool Chart; Fig. 18.3), typical frequency, and time of last stool; rectal bleeding; painful passage of stool
- Dietary habits: lack of fiber in diet, change in appetite, daily fluid intake; pica (eating non-nutritive substances like ice or soil)
- Abdominal pain: splinting of abdominal movement, resists movement, keeps knees flexed
- Psychosocial stressors: home, school, neighborhood, and peers

Bristol Stool Chart

Type 1	Separate hard lumps, like nuts (hard to pass)
Type 2	Sausage-shaped but lumpy
Type 3	Like a sausage but with cracks on the surface
Type 4	Like a sausage or snake, smooth and soft
Type 5	Soft blobs with clear-cut edges
Type 6	Fluffy pieces with ragged edges, a mushy stool
Type 7	Watery, no solid pieces. Entirely liquid

FIG. 18.3 Bristol Stool Chart.

Pregnant Patients

- Urinary symptoms: frequency, urgency, nocturia (common in early and late pregnancy); burning, dysuria, odor (signs of infection)
- Abdominal pain: weeks of gestation (pregnancy can alter the usual location of pain)
- Fetal movement
- Contractions: onset, frequency, duration, intensity; accompanying symptoms; lower back pain; leakage of fluid, vaginal bleeding

Older Adults

- Urinary symptoms: nocturia, change in stream, dribbling, incontinence
- Change in bowel patterns, constipation, diarrhea, fecal incontinence
- Dietary habits: inclusion of fiber in diet, change in ability to tolerate certain foods, change in appetite, daily fluid intake

EXAMINATION AND FINDINGS

Equipment

- Stethoscope
- Centimeter measuring tape
- Marking pen

Preparation

To perform the abdominal examination, you will need a good light source; full exposure of the abdomen; warm hands with short fingernails; and, ideally, a comfortable, relaxed patient. Have patients empty their bladder before the examination begins; a full bladder interferes with accurate examination of nearby organs and makes the examination uncomfortable. Place the patient in a supine position with arms at the sides. Approach the patient from the right side. The patient's abdominal musculature should be relaxed to allow access to the underlying structures. It may be helpful to place a small pillow under the patient's head and another under slightly flexed knees. Drape a sheet over the patient's chest for warmth and privacy. Make your approach slow and gentle, avoiding sudden movements. Ask the patient to point to any tender areas and examine those last.

Risk Factors

Colon Cancer

- Age older than 50 years
- Family history of colorectal cancer or adenomatous polyps in one or more first-degree relatives (higher risk if relative was diagnosed before 50 years or more than one relative affected)
- Family history of syndromic colon cancer, including hereditary nonpolyposis colorectal cancer (HNPCC) or Lynch syndrome from a mutation in the *MLH1, MSH2, MSH6, PMS2,* or *EPCAM* genes; familial adenomatous polyposis (FAP) from mutations in the *APC* gene, which includes attenuated FAP or AFAP (fewer than 100 polyps and occurs in patients in their 40s and 50s); Turcot syndrome (associated with medulloblastoma); and Gardner syndrome (associated with noncancer tumors of skin, soft tissue, and bones)
- Family history of Peutz-Jeghers syndrome caused by mutations in *STK11 (LKB1)* gene (affected individuals often have freckles around the mouth and hamartomas in the digestive tract) and *MUTYH*-associated polyposis (MAP) caused by mutations in the *MUTYH* gene (associated with other cancers including gastrointestinal, breast, ovary, and thyroid)
- Cystic fibrosis (CF) caused by mutations in the *CFTR* gene (colon cancer may occur earlier than those without CF, and risk is higher in patients who had an organ transplant)
- Personal history of colon cancer, adenomatous polyps, inflammatory bowel disease (Crohn disease, ulcerative colitis)
- Native American, Alaska Native, or African American race
- Jews of Eastern European descent (Ashkenazi Jews)
- Diet: low-fiber, high in red meat, processed meats, and foods fried, broiled, grilled increases risk; diet high in fruits and vegetable decreases risk
- Overweight and obesity
- Long-term diet high in red meats and processed meats
- Tobacco use
- Physical inactivity
- Moderate to severe alcohol use
- Type 2 diabetes (independent of overweight/obesity)

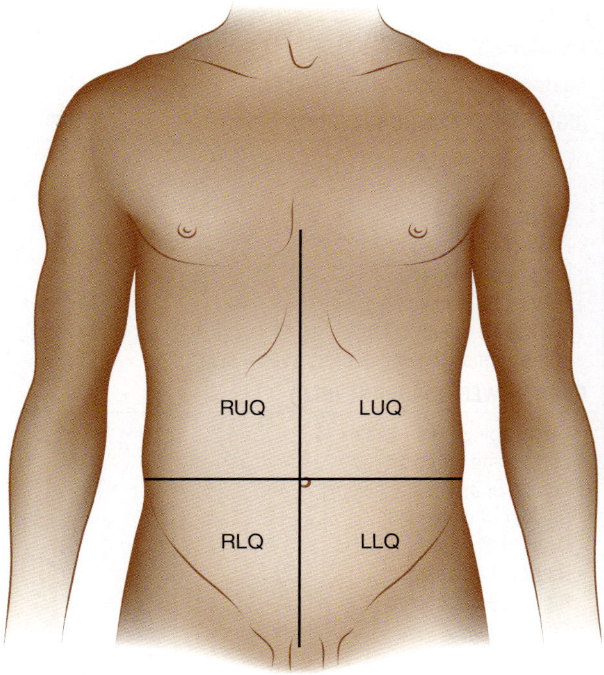

FIG 18.4 Four quadrants of the abdomen. (From Wilson, S. F., & Giddens, J. F. (2009). *Health assessment for nursing practice* (4th ed.). St. Louis: Mosby.)

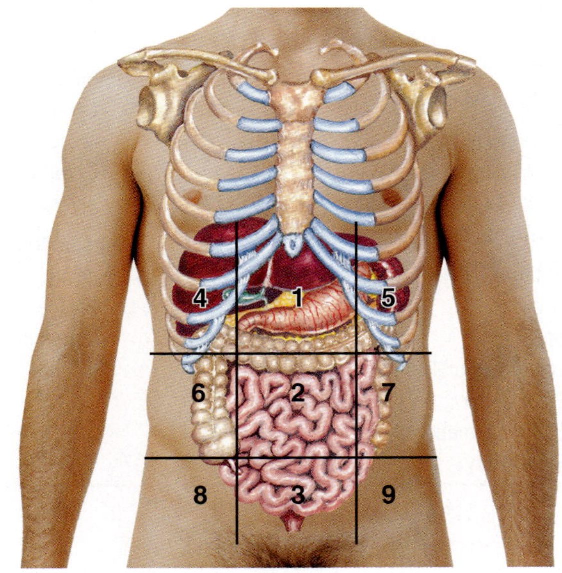

FIG. 18.5 Nine regions of the abdomen. *1,* Epigastric; *2,* umbilical; *3,* hypogastric; *4* and *5,* right and left hypochondriac; *6* and *7,* right and left lumbar; *8* and *9,* right and left inguinal. (Modified from Wilson, S. F., & Giddens, J. F. (2009). *Health assessment for nursing practice* (4th ed.). St. Louis: Mosby.)

For the purposes of examination, the abdomen is commonly divided into four quadrants, first by drawing an imaginary line from the sternum to the pubis through the umbilicus. Draw a second imaginary line perpendicular to the first, horizontally across the abdomen through the umbilicus (Fig. 18.4). Alternatively, the abdomen is divided into nine regions using the following imaginary lines: two horizontal lines, one across the lowest edge of the costal margin and the other across the edge of the iliac crest, and two vertical lines running bilaterally from the midclavicular line to the middle of the Poupart ligament, approximating the lateral borders of the rectus abdominis muscles (Fig. 18.5). Choose one of these mapping methods and use it consistently. Box 18.1 lists the contents of the abdomen in each of the quadrants and regions. Mentally visualize the underlying organs and structures in each of the zones as you proceed with the examination. Certain anatomic landmarks are useful in describing the location of pain, tenderness, and other findings. These landmarks are illustrated in Fig. 18.6.

BOX 18.1 Landmarks for Abdominal Examination

Anatomic Correlates of the Four Quadrants of the Abdomen

RIGHT UPPER QUADRANT (RUQ)	LEFT UPPER QUADRANT (LUQ)
Liver and gallbladder	Left lobe of liver
Pylorus	Spleen
Duodenum	Stomach
Head of pancreas	Body of pancreas
Right adrenal gland	Left adrenal gland
Portion of right kidney	Portion of left kidney
Hepatic flexure of colon	Splenic flexure of colon
Portions of ascending and transverse colon	Portions of transverse and descending colon
RIGHT LOWER QUADRANT (RLQ)	**LEFT LOWER QUADRANT (LLQ)**
Lower pole of right kidney	Lower pole of left kidney
Cecum and appendix	Sigmoid colon
Portion of ascending colon	Portion of descending colon
Bladder (if distended)	Bladder (if distended)
Ovary and salpinx	Ovary and salpinx
Uterus (if enlarged)	Uterus (if enlarged)
Right spermatic cord	Left spermatic cord
Right ureter	Left ureter

Anatomic Correlates of the Nine Regions of the Abdomen

Right Hypochondriac
- Right lobe of liver
- Gallbladder
- Portion of duodenum
- Hepatic flexure of colon
- Portion of right kidney
- Right adrenal gland

Right Lumbar
- Ascending colon
- Lower half of right kidney
- Portion of duodenum and jejunum

Right Inguinal
- Cecum
- Appendix
- Lower end of ileum
- Right ureter
- Right spermatic cord
- Right ovary

Epigastric
- Pylorus
- Duodenum
- Pancreas
- Portion of liver

Umbilical
- Omentum
- Mesentery
- Lower part of duodenum
- Jejunum and ileum

Hypogastric (Pubic)
- Ileum
- Bladder
- Uterus (if enlarged)

Left Hypochondriac
- Stomach
- Spleen
- Tail of pancreas
- Splenic flexure of colon
- Upper pole of left kidney
- Left adrenal gland

Left Lumbar
- Descending colon
- Lower half of left kidney
- Portions of jejunum and ileum

Left Inguinal
- Sigmoid colon
- Left ureter
- Left spermatic cord
- Left ovary

Inspection

Surface Characteristics

Begin by inspecting the abdomen from a seated position at the patient's right side. This position allows a tangential view that enhances shadows and contouring. Observe the skin color and surface characteristics. The skin of the abdomen should have the same expected variations in color and surface characteristics as the rest of the body. The skin may be somewhat paler if not exposed to the sun. A fine venous network is often visible. Above the umbilicus, venous return should be toward the head; below the umbilicus, it should be toward the feet (Fig. 18.7A). When abdominal vessels appear distended or more pronounced, use the following procedure to determine the direction of venous return. Place the index fingers of both hands side by side perpendicularly over a vein. Press and separate the fingers, milking to empty a section of vein. Release one finger and time the refill. Release the other finger and time the refill. The flow of venous blood is in the direction of the faster filling. Flow patterns are altered in some disease states (see Fig. 18.7B and C).

Unexpected skin findings include generalized color changes such as jaundice or cyanosis. A glistening, taut appearance suggests ascites (fluid accumulation in the abdomen). Inspect for bruises and localized discoloration. Areas of redness may indicate inflammation. A bluish periumbilical discoloration (Cullen sign) suggests

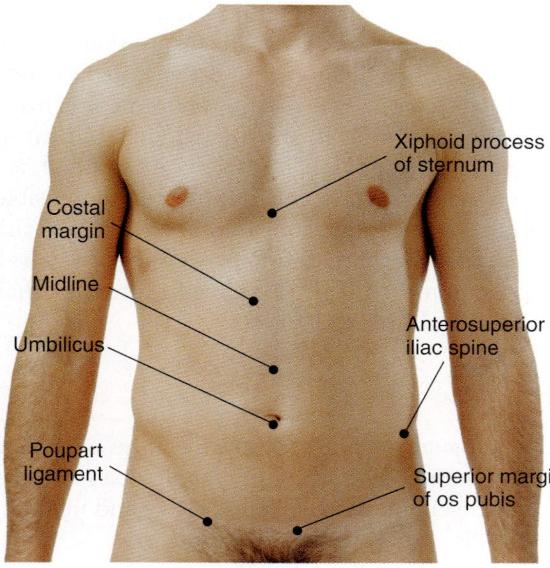

FIG. 18.6 Landmarks of the abdomen. (From Wilson, S. F., & Giddens, J. F. (2009). *Health assessment for nursing practice* (4th ed.). St. Louis: Mosby.)

intra-abdominal bleeding. Striae often result from pregnancy or weight gain. Striae of recent origin are pink or blue in color but turn silvery white over time. Abdominal tumors or ascites can produce striae. The striae of Cushing syndrome remain purplish.

Inspect for any lesions, particularly nodules. Lesions are of particular importance because gastrointestinal diseases often produce secondary skin changes. A pearl-like, enlarged, and sometimes painful umbilical nodule from cancer metastasis, known as a *Sister Mary Joseph nodule,* may be the first sign of an intra-abdominal malignancy (Ben Kridis et al., 2023). Skin and gastrointestinal lesions may arise from the same cause or may occur without relationship to one another. See Clinical Pearl, "Scars."

CLINICAL PEARL

Scars

Note any scars and describe their location, configuration, and relative size in the electronic medical record (EMR). Many EMRs include tools for illustrating skin findings. If the cause of a scar was not explained during the history, now is a good time to pursue that information. The presence of scarring should alert you to the possibility of intra-abdominal adhesions.

Contour

Contour is the abdominal profile from the rib margin to the pubis, viewed on the horizontal plane. The expected contours can be described as flat, rounded, or scaphoid. A flat contour is common in athletic adults. The rounded or convex contour is characteristic of young children, but in adults it is the result of subcutaneous fat or poor muscle tone. The abdomen should be evenly rounded with the maximum height of convexity at the umbilicus. The scaphoid or concave contour is seen in thin adults. Inspect the abdomen for contour, symmetry, and surface motion, using tangential lighting to illuminate contour and visible peristalsis.

Note the location and contour of the umbilicus. It should be centrally located without displacement upward, downward, or laterally. The umbilicus may be inverted or protrude slightly, but it should be free of inflammation, swelling, or bulge that may indicate a hernia.

Inspect for symmetry from a seated position at the patient's side, then move to a standing position behind the patient's head, if possible. Contralateral areas of the abdomen should be symmetric in appearance and contour. Look for any distention or bulges.

Generalized symmetric distention may occur as a result of obesity, enlarged organs, and fluid or gas. Distention from the umbilicus to the symphysis can be caused by pregnancy, uterine fibroids, a distended bladder, or an

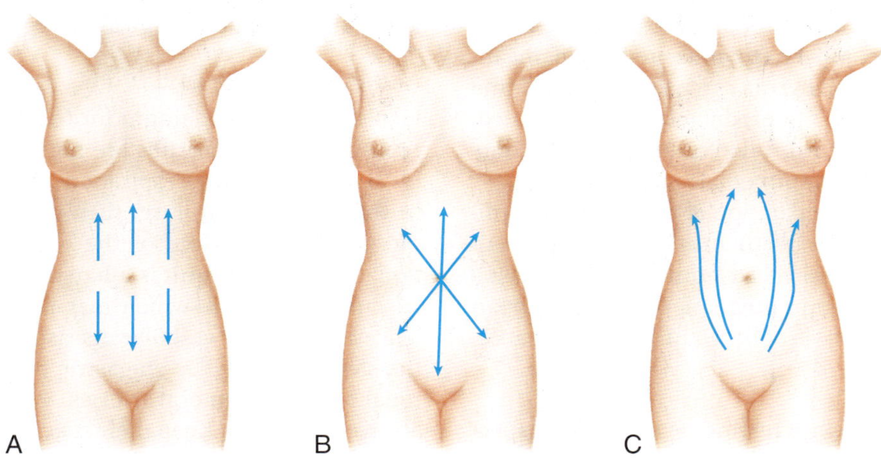

FIG. 18.7 Abdominal venous patterns. (A) Expected. (B) Portal hypertension. (C) Inferior vena cava obstruction.

ovarian tumor. Distention of the upper half, above the umbilicus, can be due to gastric dilation, a pancreatic cyst, or tumor. Asymmetric distention or protrusion may indicate hernia, tumor, cysts, bowel obstruction, muscle or soft tissue hematoma, or enlargement of abdominal organs. See Clinical Pearl, "Abdominal Distention."

CLINICAL PEARL

Abdominal Distention

You are examining a patient with a significantly distended abdomen and whose bowel sounds are hypoactive or even absent. There is no particular pain, and you feel no masses. The deep tendon reflexes are diminished. The patient is on diuretics for treatment of hypertension. Think of hypokalemia as a cause of a paralytic ileus (intestinal pseudo-obstruction): diuretics/distention/deficiency of potassium. Use of opioids and hypothyroidism are two other common causes of paralytic ileus.

Ask the patient to take a deep breath and hold it. The contour should remain smooth and symmetric. This maneuver lowers the diaphragm and compresses the organs of the abdominal cavity, which may cause previously unseen bulges or masses to appear. Next, ask the patient to raise their head from the table. This contracts the rectus abdominis muscles, which produces muscle prominence in thin or athletic adults. Superficial abdominal wall masses may become visible. If a hernia is present, the increased abdominal pressure may cause it to protrude.

An incisional hernia is caused by a defect in the abdominal musculature that develops after a surgical incision, resulting in a protrusion in the area of the surgical scar. Protrusion of the navel indicates an umbilical hernia. An umbilical hernia may develop during pregnancy, in long-standing ascites, or when intrathoracic pressure is repeatedly increased, as occurs in chronic respiratory disease. Hernias may also occur in the midline of the epigastrium due to small fascial defects in the linea alba. This type of hernia contains a bit of fat and may be felt as a small, tender nodule. Most hernias are reducible, meaning that the contents of the hernia can be pushed back into place. If not, the hernia is nonreducible or incarcerated, where blood supply to the protruded contents may become obstructed, which requires immediate surgery.

In addition to hernias, separation of the rectus abdominis muscles (i.e., diastasis recti) may become apparent when the patient raises their head from the table. Diastasis recti occurs more often in pregnancy and the postpartum period. The condition is of little clinical significance.

Movement

With the patient's head again resting on the table, inspect the abdomen for movement. Smooth, even movement should occur with respiration. Individuals with a greater inclination of the ribs show mostly costal movement, whereas others exhibit abdominal movement. Limited abdominal motion associated with respiration may indicate peritonitis in an ill-appearing patient. Surface motion from peristalsis, seen as a rippling movement across the abdomen, may be seen in thin individuals but can also be a sign of intestinal obstruction. Abdominal aortic pulsations seen in the upper midline are often visible in thin adults. Marked pulsations may occur as the result of increased pulse pressure (difference between systolic and diastolic blood pressure often seen with valve insufficiency) or abdominal aortic aneurysm.

Auscultation

Unlike the usual sequence, always perform auscultation of the abdomen before percussion and palpation because these maneuvers may alter the frequency and intensity of bowel sounds.

Bowel Sounds

Lightly place the diaphragm of a warmed stethoscope on the abdomen. Some clinicians say they prefer to use the bell; in reality, they tend to pull the skin taut with the bell and, in effect, make a diaphragm. A cold stethoscope, like cold hands, may initiate contraction of the abdominal muscles. Listen for bowel sounds and note frequency and character. They are usually heard as clicks and gurgles that occur irregularly and range from 5 to 35 per minute. Bowel sounds are generalized, so most often they can be assessed adequately by listening in one place. Loud prolonged gurgles are called *borborygmi* (stomach growling). Increased (hyperactive) bowel sounds may occur with gastroenteritis, early intestinal obstruction, or hunger. High-pitched tinkling sounds suggest intestinal fluid and air under pressure, as in early obstruction. Decreased (hypoactive) bowel sounds occur with peritonitis and paralytic ileus. Auscultate in all four quadrants if you have a concern. Absent bowel sounds, referring to an inability to hear any bowel sounds after 3 to 5 minutes of continuous listening, may be associated with abdominal pain and rigidity and indicate a surgical emergency.

Additional Sounds and Bruits

Listen with the diaphragm for friction rubs over the liver and spleen. Friction rubs are high pitched and are heard in association with respiration. Although friction rubs in the abdomen are rare, they indicate inflammation of the peritoneal surface of the organ from tumor, infection, or infarct. A bruit is a harsh or musical intermittent auscultatory sound, which may reflect blood flow turbulence and indicate vascular disease. Listen with the bell of the stethoscope in the epigastric region and in the aortic, renal, iliac, and femoral arteries. Vascular sounds are usually well localized. Keep their specific locations in mind as you listen at those sites (Fig. 18.8). Auscultate with the bell of the stethoscope in the epigastric region and around the umbilicus for a venous hum, which is soft, low pitched,

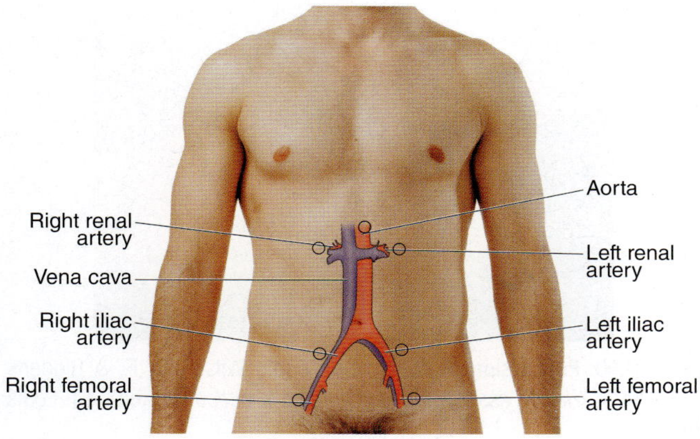

FIG. 18.8 Sites to auscultate for bruits: renal arteries, iliac arteries, aorta, and femoral arteries. (Modified from Wilson, S. F., & Giddens, J. F. (2009). *Health assessment for nursing practice* (4th ed.). St. Louis: Mosby.)

and continuous. A venous hum occurs with increased collateral circulation between the portal and systemic venous systems.

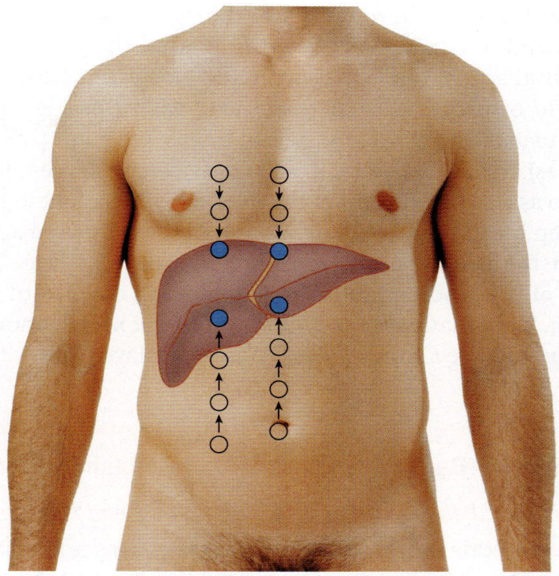

FIG. 18.9 Liver percussion routes along midclavicular and midsternal lines. (Modified from Wilson, S. F., & Giddens, J. F. (2009). *Health assessment for nursing practice* (4th ed.). St. Louis: Mosby.)

Percussion

Percussion is used to assess the size and density of the organs in the abdomen and to detect the presence of fluid, air, and fluid-filled or solid masses. Percussion is used either independently or concurrently with palpation of specific organs and can validate palpatory findings. For simplicity, percussion and palpation are discussed separately.

First, percuss all quadrants or regions of the abdomen for a sense of overall tympany and dullness (Table 18.1). Tympany is the predominant sound because air is present in the stomach and intestines. Dullness is heard over organs and solid masses. A distended bladder produces dullness in the suprapubic area. Develop a systematic route for percussion.

Liver Span

Now, go back and percuss individually the liver, spleen, and stomach. Begin liver percussion at the right midclavicular line over an area of tympany. Always begin with an area of tympany and proceed to an area of dullness because that sound change is easiest to detect. Percuss upward along the midclavicular line, as shown in Fig. 18.9, to determine the lower border of the liver. The area of liver dullness is usually heard at the costal margin or slightly below it. Mark the border with a marking pen. A lower liver border that is more than 2 to 3 cm (0.75 to 1 inch) below the costal margin may indicate organ enlargement or downward displacement of the diaphragm because of chronic obstructive pulmonary disease.

To determine the upper border of the liver, begin percussion on the right midclavicular line at an area of lung resonance around the third intercostal space. Continue downward until the percussion tone changes to one of dullness; this marks the upper border of the liver. Mark the location with the pen. The upper border is usually in the fifth intercostal space. An upper border below this may indicate downward displacement or liver atrophy. Dullness extending above the fifth intercostal space suggests upward displacement from abdominal fluid or a mass.

Measure the distance between the marks to estimate the vertical span of the liver. The usual span is approximately 6 to 12 cm (2.5 to 4.5 inches). A span greater than this may indicate liver enlargement, whereas a lesser span suggests atrophy. Age and gender influence liver size. Liver span is usually greater in males and in tall individuals.

Percussion provides a gross estimate of liver size. Errors in estimating liver span can occur when the dullness of a pleural effusion or lung consolidation obscures the upper liver border. Similarly, gas in the colon may produce tympany in the right upper quadrant and obscure the dullness of the lower liver border.

If liver enlargement is suspected, additional percussion maneuvers can provide further information. Percuss

TABLE 18.1 Percussion Notes of the Abdomen

NOTE	DESCRIPTION	LOCATION
Tympany	Musical note of higher pitch than resonance	Over air-filled viscera
Hyperresonance	Pitch lies between tympany and resonance	Base of left lung
Resonance	Sustained note of moderate pitch	Over lung tissue and sometimes over the abdomen
Dullness	Short, high-pitched note with little resonance	Over solid organs adjacent to air-filled structures

upward and then downward over the right midaxillary line. Liver dullness is usually detected around the seventh intercostal space. You can also percuss along the midsternal line to estimate the midsternal liver span (see Fig. 18.9). The usual span at the midsternal line is 4 to 8 cm (1.5 to 3 inches). Spans exceeding 8 cm suggest liver enlargement.

To assess the descent of the liver, ask the patient to take a deep breath and hold it while you percuss upward again from the abdomen at the right midclavicular line. The area of lower border dullness should move downward 2 to 3 cm. This maneuver will guide subsequent palpation of the organ. See Clinical Pearl, "Assessing Liver Size."

Evidence-Based Practice in Physical Examination

Liver Size: Percussion Correlates With Ultrasound Findings

In a prospective study of adults with liver disease, liver size measured by physical examination (percussion along the midclavicular line) correlated with the gold standard of ultrasound (transaxial measurement). Of the 101 patients examined, the mean liver span by percussion was 8.9 cm ± 1.13 and mean liver span by ultrasound was 14.3 cm ± 1.6. With a correction factor of 1.6, transaxial liver span can be accurately predicted by measurement using liver percussion. This finding can be particularly helpful in resource-limited settings.

From Loloi, J., Patel, N., McDevitt, P., et al. (2019). How strongly do physical examination estimates and ultrasound measurements of liver size correlate? A prospective study. *American Journal of Medicine, 132*(1), 103–108. https://www.sciencedirect.com/science/article/pii/S0002934318308799.

CLINICAL PEARL

Assessing Liver Size

It is best to report the size of the liver in two ways: liver span as determined from percussing the upper and lower borders and the extent of liver projection below the costal margin. When the size of a patient's liver is important in assessing the clinical condition, projection below the costal margin alone will not provide enough comparative information. Be sure to specify which landmarks were used for future measurement comparison (e.g., midclavicular line).

Spleen

Percuss the spleen just posterior to the midaxillary line on the left side as shown in Fig. 18.10. Percuss in several directions beginning at areas of lung resonance. You may hear a small area of splenic dullness from the sixth to the ninth rib. The Traube space is a semilunar region defined by the sixth rib superiorly, the midaxillary line laterally, and the left costal margin inferiorly. This area is typically tympanitic because it overlies the fundus of the stomach. With splenic enlargement, tympany changes to dullness as the spleen is brought forward and downward with inspiration (splenic percussion sign). However, a full stomach, feces-filled intestine, or left-sided pleural effusion may also produce dullness. The inability to detect the spleen with palpation and/or percussion does not rule out splenomegaly. If dullness is appreciated in the Traube space, palpation should follow as described later. If clinical suspicion is high and splenomegaly is not appreciated on examination, an abdominal ultrasound may be helpful (Aldulaimi & Mendez, 2021).

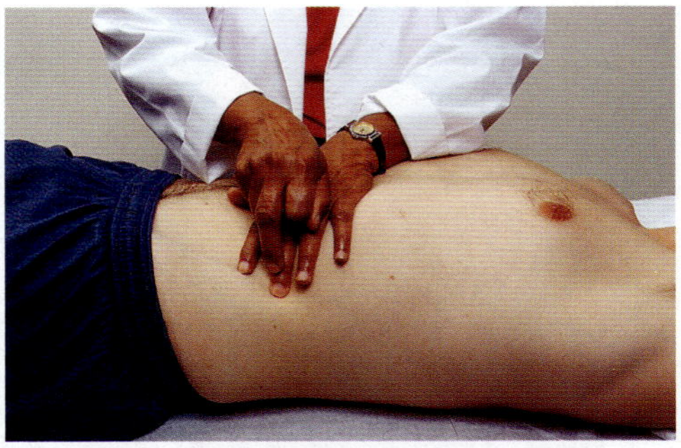

FIG. 18.10 **Percussion of the spleen.** (From Wilson, S. F., & Giddens, J. F. (2009). *Health assessment for nursing practice* (4th ed.). St. Louis: Mosby.)

Gastric Bubble

Percuss for the gastric air bubble in the area of the left lower anterior rib cage and left epigastric region. The tympany produced by the gastric bubble is lower in pitch than the tympany of the intestine.

Kidneys

To assess each kidney for tenderness, ask the patient to assume a sitting position. Place the palm of your hand over the right costovertebral angle and strike your hand with the ulnar surface of the fist of your other hand (Fig. 18.11A). Repeat the maneuver over the left costovertebral angle. Direct percussion with the fist over each costovertebral angle may also be used (see Fig. 18.11B). The patient should perceive a thud, but it should not cause pain unless there is underlying renal pathology. For efficiency of time and motion, this maneuver is performed while examining the back rather than the abdomen.

Palpation

Use palpation to assess the organs of the abdominal cavity and to detect muscle spasms, masses, fluid, and areas of tenderness. Evaluate the abdominal organs for size, shape, mobility, and consistency. Stand at the patient's right side with the patient in the supine position. Attempt to make the patient as comfortable and relaxed as possible. Use warm hands and bend the patient's knees to help relax the abdominal muscles. Ticklishness may be a challenge (Box 18.2).

Light Palpation

Begin with a light, systematic palpation of all four quadrants—or nine regions—initially avoiding any areas

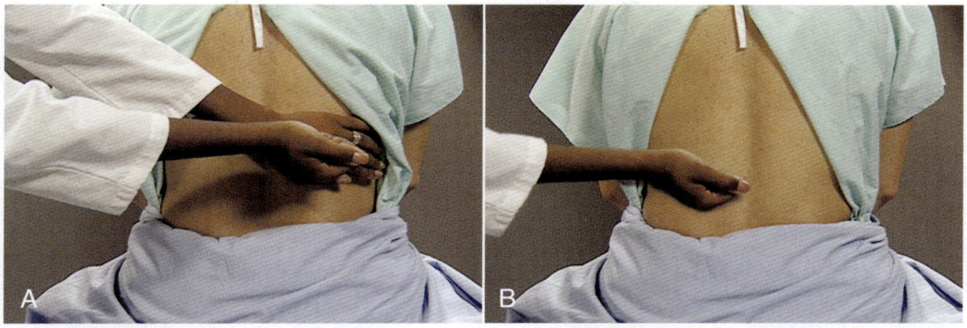

FIG. 18.11 Fist percussion of the costovertebral angle for kidney tenderness. (A) Indirect percussion. (B) Direct percussion.

BOX 18.2 Examining the Abdomen in a Ticklish Patient

The ticklishness of a patient can sometimes make it difficult to palpate the abdomen satisfactorily; however, there are ways to overcome this problem. Ask the patient to perform self-palpation, and place your hands over the patient's fingers, not quite touching the abdomen itself. After a time, let your fingers drift slowly onto the abdomen while still resting primarily on the patient's fingers. You can still learn a good deal, and ticklishness might be less of a problem. You might also use the diaphragm of the stethoscope (making sure it is warm enough) as a palpating instrument. This serves as a starting point, and again your fingers can drift over the edge of the diaphragm and palpate without eliciting an excessively ticklish response. Applying a stimulus to another, less sensitive part of the body with your nonpalpating hand can also decrease a ticklish response. In some instances, a patient's ticklishness cannot be overcome, and you just have to palpate as best you can.

the patient had identified as painful. Lay the palm of your hand lightly on the abdomen, with the fingers extended and held together (Fig. 18.12). With the palmar surface of your fingers, depress the abdominal wall no more than 1 cm, using a light and even pressing circular motion. Avoid short, quick jabs. The abdomen should feel smooth, with a consistent softness. The patient's abdomen may tense if you press too deeply, your hands are cold, the patient is ticklish, or intra-abdominal inflammation is present. Guarding—tensing of the abdominal musculature to protect inflamed organs—should alert you to move cautiously through the remainder of the examination.

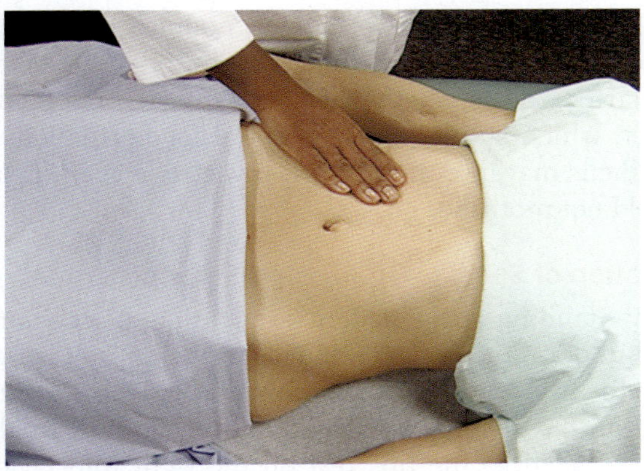

FIG. 18.12 Light palpation of the abdomen. With fingers extended and approximated, press in no more than 1 cm.

Light palpation is useful in identifying muscular resistance and areas of tenderness. A large mass or distended structure may be appreciated on light palpation as a sense of resistance. If resistance is present, determine whether it is voluntary or involuntary by placing a pillow under the patient's knees and asking the patient to breathe slowly through the mouth as you feel for relaxation of the rectus abdominis muscles on expiration. If the tenseness remains, it is probably an involuntary response to localized or generalized rigidity. Rigidity is a boardlike hardness of the abdominal wall overlying areas of peritoneal irritation.

Moderate Palpation

Continue palpation with the same hand position and technique used for light palpation, exerting moderate pressure as an intermediate step to gradually approach deep palpation. Tenderness not elicited on light palpation may become evident with deeper pressure. An additional maneuver of moderate palpation is performed with the side of your hand (Fig. 18.13). This maneuver is useful in assessing organs that move with respiration, specifically the liver and spleen. Palpate during the entire respiratory cycle. As the patient inspires, the organ is displaced downward, and you may be able to feel it as it bumps gently against your hand.

Deep Palpation

Deep palpation is necessary to thoroughly delineate abdominal organs and to detect less obvious masses. Use the palmar surface of your extended fingers, pressing deeply and evenly into the abdominal wall (Fig. 18.14). Palpate all four quadrants or nine regions, moving the fingers back and forth over the abdominal contents. Often, you are able to feel the borders of the rectus abdominis muscles, the aorta, and portions of the colon. Tenderness not elicited with light or moderate palpation may become evident. Deep pressure may also evoke tenderness in the

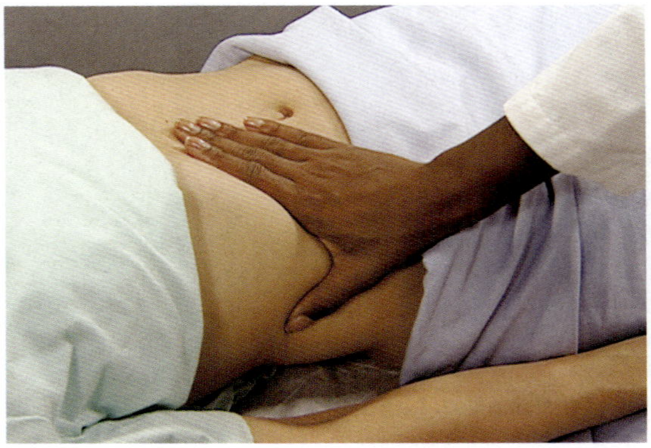

FIG. 18.13 Moderate palpation using the side of the hand.

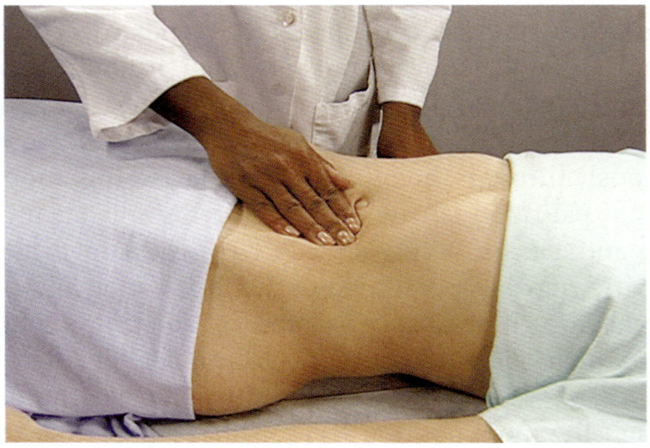

FIG. 18.14 Deep palpation of the abdomen. Press deeply and evenly with the palmar surface of extended fingers.

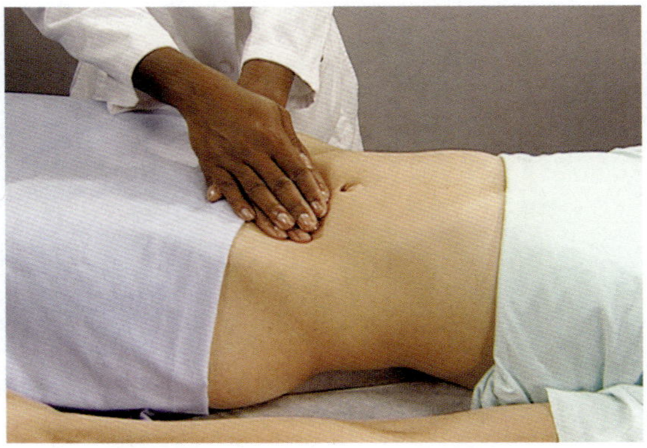

FIG. 18.15 Deep bimanual palpation.

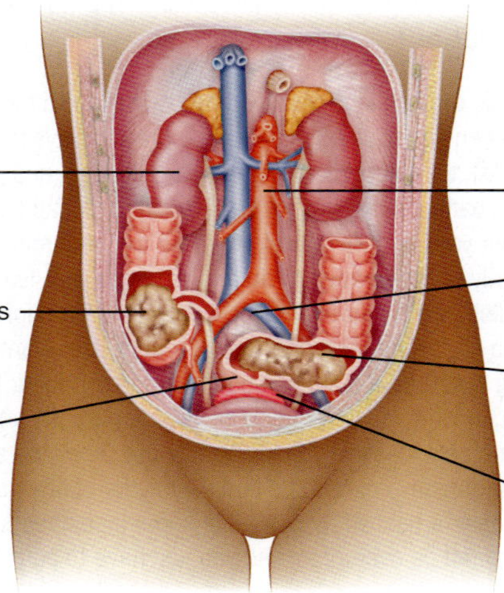

FIG. 18.16 Abdominal structures commonly felt as masses.

healthy person over the cecum, sigmoid colon, and aorta and in the midline near the xiphoid process. If deep palpation is difficult because of obesity or muscular resistance, you can use a bimanual technique with one hand atop the other, as shown in Fig. 18.15. Exert pressure with the top hand while concentrating on sensation with the other hand. Some clinicians prefer to use the bimanual technique for all patients.

Masses

Identify any masses and note the following characteristics: location, size, shape, consistency, tenderness, pulsation, mobility, and movement with respiration. To determine whether a mass is superficial (i.e., located in the abdominal wall) or intra-abdominal, have the patient lift their head from the examining table, thus contracting the abdominal muscles. Masses in the abdominal wall will continue to be palpable, but those located in the abdominal cavity will be more difficult to feel because they are obscured by abdominal musculature. The presence of feces in the colon, sometimes mistaken for an abdominal mass, may be felt as a soft, rounded, boggy mass in the cecum and in the ascending, descending, or sigmoid colon. Other structures that could be mistaken for masses are the lateral borders of the rectus abdominis muscles, uterus, aorta, sacral promontory, and common iliac artery (Fig. 18.16). By mentally visualizing the location of the abdominal structures, you can distinguish between what ought to be there and an unexpected finding.

Umbilical Ring

Palpate the umbilical ring and around the umbilicus. The area should be free of bulges, nodules, and granulation. The umbilical ring should be round and free of irregularities. Note whether it is incomplete or soft in the center, which suggests the potential for herniation. The umbilicus may be either slightly inverted or everted, but it should not protrude.

Palpation of Specific Organs and Structures

Liver. Standing at the patient's right side, place your left hand under the 11th and 12th ribs, pressing upward to elevate the liver toward the abdominal wall. Place your right hand on the abdomen, fingers pointing toward the head and extended so the tips rest on the right midclavicular line below the level of liver dullness, as shown in Fig. 18.17A. Alternatively, you can place your right hand

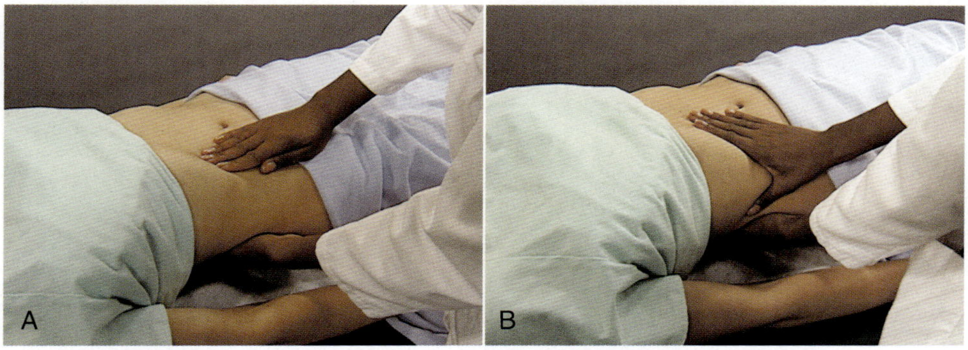

FIG. 18.17 Palpating the liver. (A) Fingers are extended, with tips on right midclavicular line below the level of liver dullness and pointing toward the head. (B) Alternative method for liver palpation with the fingers parallel to the costal margin.

parallel to the right costal margin, as shown in Fig. 18.17B. In either case, press your right hand gently but deeply, in and up. Have the patient breathe regularly a few times and then take a deep breath. Try to feel the liver edge as the diaphragm pushes it down to meet your fingertips. Ordinarily, the liver is not palpable, although it may be felt in some thin persons without pathologic conditions. If the liver edge is felt, it should be firm, smooth, even, and nontender. Feel for nodules, tenderness, and irregularity. If the liver is palpable, repeat the maneuver medially and laterally to the costal margin to assess the liver contour and surface.

Liver: Alternative Techniques. An alternative technique is to hook your fingers over the right costal margin below the border of liver dullness, as shown in Fig. 18.18. Stand on the patient's right side facing their feet. Press in and up toward the costal margin with your fingers and ask the patient to take a deep breath. Try to feel the liver edge as it descends to meet your fingers.

If the abdomen is distended or the abdominal muscles tense, the usual techniques for determining the lower liver border may be challenging, and the scratch test may be useful (Fig. 18.19). This technique uses auscultation to detect the differences in sound transmission over solid and hollow organs. Place the diaphragm of the stethoscope over the liver and with the finger of your other hand scratch the abdominal surface lightly, moving toward the liver border. When you encounter the liver, the sound should intensify.

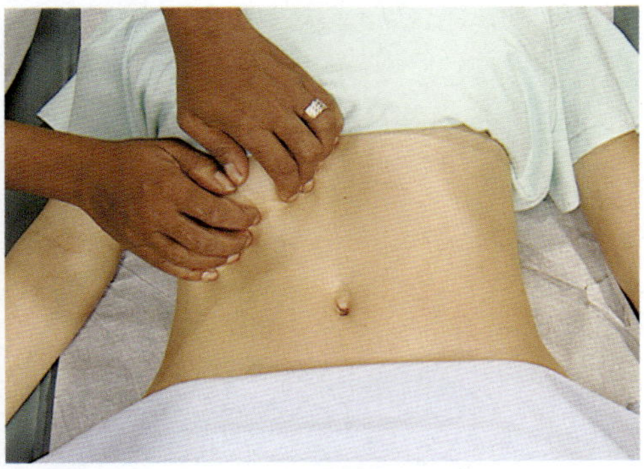

FIG. 18.18 Palpating the liver with fingers hooked over the costal margin.

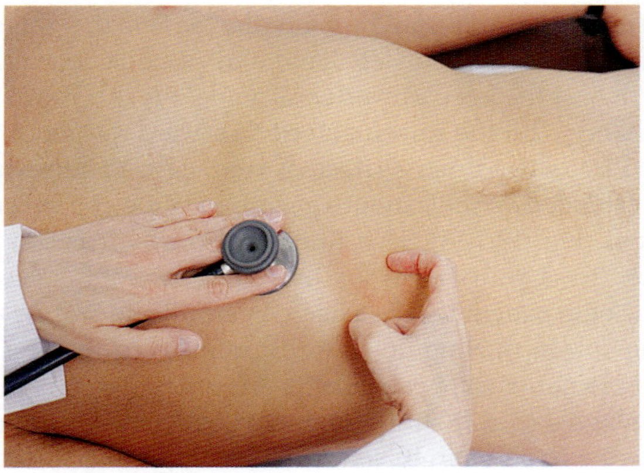

FIG. 18.19 Scratch technique for auscultating the liver. With the stethoscope over the liver, lightly scratch the abdominal surface, moving toward the liver. The sound will be intensified over the liver.

Consider using indirect fist percussion to check for liver tenderness when the liver is not palpable and there is clinical suspicion for hepatobiliary infection. Place the palmar surface of one hand over the lower right rib cage, and then strike your hand with the ulnar surface of the fist of your other hand. The healthy liver is not tender to percussion.

Gallbladder. Palpate below the liver margin at the lateral border of the rectus abdominis muscle for the gallbladder. A healthy gallbladder will not be palpable. A palpable, tender gallbladder indicates cholecystitis, whereas nontender enlargement suggests common bile duct obstruction. If you suspect cholecystitis, have the patient take a deep breath during deep palpation. As the inflamed gallbladder comes in contact with the examining fingers, the patient will experience pain and abruptly halt inspiration (Murphy sign).

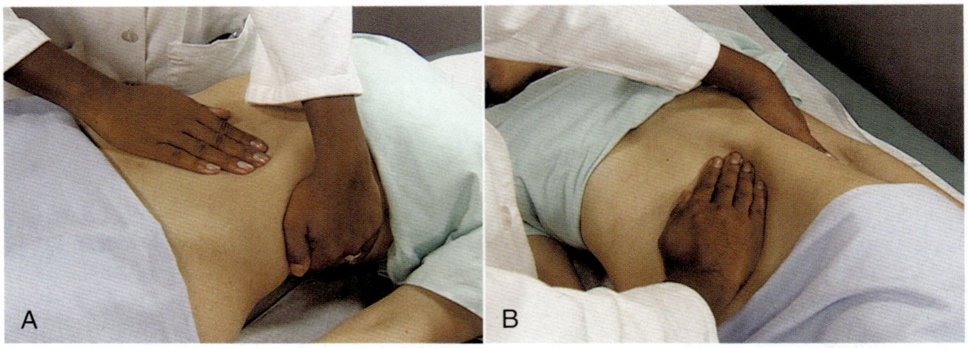

FIG. 18.20 **Palpating the spleen.** (A) Press upward with the left hand at the patient's left costovertebral angle. Feel for the spleen with the right hand below the left costal margin. (B) Palpating the spleen with the patient lying on the side. Press inward with the left hand and tips of the right fingers.

Spleen. While still standing on the patient's right side, reach across with your left hand and place it beneath the patient over the left costovertebral angle. Press upward with that hand to lift the spleen anteriorly toward the abdominal wall. Place the palmar surface of your right hand with fingers extended on the patient's abdomen below the left costal margin (Fig. 18.20A). Use findings from percussion as a guide. Press your fingertips inward toward the spleen as you ask the patient to take a deep breath. Try to feel the edge of the spleen moving downward toward your fingers. The spleen is not usually palpable; if you can feel it, it is probably enlarged (Box 18.3). Be sure to palpate with your fingers below the costal margin so that you will not miss the lower edge of an enlarged spleen. Be gentle in palpation. In patients with splenomegaly from infectious mononucleosis, the spleen can be three to four times its normal size and there is a small risk for splenic rupture (Bartlett et al., 2016).

Repeat the palpation while the patient is lying on the right side with hips and knees flexed (see Fig. 18.20B). Still standing on the right side, press inward with your left hand to assist gravity in bringing the spleen forward. Press inward with the fingertips of your right hand and feel for the edge of the spleen. Again, you will not usually feel it; if you can, it is probably enlarged.

Left Kidney. Standing on the patient's right side, reach across with your left hand as you did in spleen palpation and place your hand over the left flank. Place your right hand at the patient's left costal margin. Have the patient take a deep breath and then elevate the left flank with your left hand and palpate deeply (because of the retroperitoneal position of the kidney) with your right hand (Fig. 18.21). Try to feel the lower pole (bottom part) of the kidney with your fingertips as the patient inhales. The left kidney is ordinarily not palpable.

Another approach is to capture the kidney. Move to the patient's left side and position your hands as before, with the left hand over the patient's left flank and the right hand at the left costal margin. Ask the patient to take a deep breath. At the height of inspiration, press the fingers of your two hands together to capture the kidney between the fingers. Ask the patient to breathe out and hold the exhalation while you slowly release your fingers (Fig. 18.22). If you have captured the kidney, you may feel it slip beneath your fingers as it moves back into place. Although the patient may feel the capture and release, the maneuver should not be painful. Again, a left kidney is seldom palpable.

BOX 18.3 An Enlarged Spleen or an Enlarged Left Kidney?

When an organ is palpable below the left costal margin, it may be difficult to differentiate an enlarged spleen from an enlarged left kidney. Percussion should help distinguish between the organs. The percussion note over an enlarged spleen is dull because the spleen displaces the bowel. The usual area of splenic dullness will be increased downward and toward the midline. The percussion note over an enlarged kidney is resonant because the kidney is deeply situated behind the bowel. In addition, the edge of the spleen is sharper than that of the kidney. A palpable notch along the medial border suggests an enlarged spleen rather than an enlarged kidney.

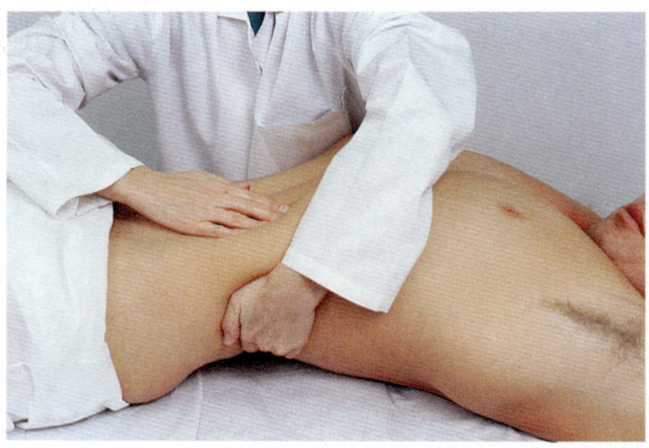

FIG. 18.21 **Palpating the left kidney.** Elevate the left flank with the left hand. Palpate deeply with the right hand.

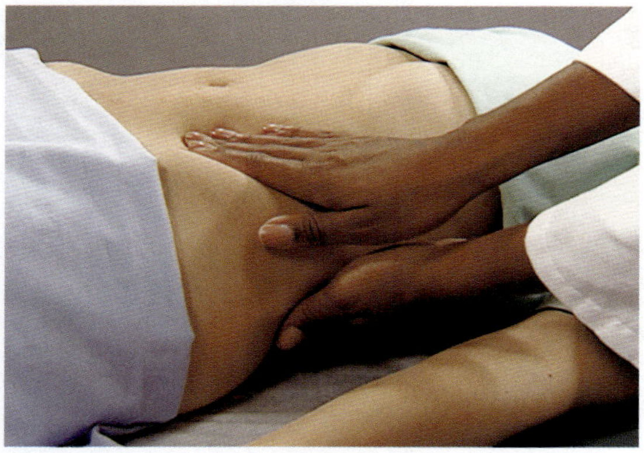

FIG. 18.22 Capture technique for palpating the kidney (left kidney palpation shown). As the patient takes a deep breath, press the fingers of both hands together. As the patient exhales, slowly release the pressure and feel for the kidney to slip between the fingers.

Evidence-Based Practice in Physical Examination

Detecting Abdominal Aortic Aneurysms

Although clinicians can detect asymptomatic abdominal aortic aneurysms (AAAs) by palpation, the overall sensitivity is somewhat low. A negative examination does not rule out the diagnosis, especially in patients with obesity and in those who are unable to relax their abdominal musculature during the examination. In general, palpation has a moderate sensitivity for detecting aneurysms large enough to be referred for surgery. The U.S. Preventive Services Task Force currently recommends a one-time screening ultrasound for AAA in males 65 to 75 years of age who have ever smoked.

From U.S. Preventive Services Task Force. (2019). *Final recommendation statement: Abdominal aortic aneurysm screening.* Rockville, MD: U.S. Department of Health and Human Services, Agency for Healthcare Research and Quality.

Right Kidney. Stand on the patient's right side, placing one hand under the patient's right flank and the other hand at the right costal margin. Perform the same maneuvers as you did for the left kidney. Because of the anatomic position of the right kidney (slightly lower than the left), it is more commonly palpable than the left kidney. If it is palpable, it should be smooth, firm, and nontender. It may be difficult to distinguish the kidney from the liver edge. The liver edge tends to be sharp, whereas the kidney is more rounded. The liver also extends more medially and laterally and cannot be captured.

Aorta. Palpate deeply slightly to the left of the midline and feel for the aortic pulsation. If the pulsation is prominent, try to determine the direction of pulsation. A prominent lateral pulsation suggests an aortic aneurysm. If you are unable to feel the pulse on deep palpation, an alternative technique may help. Place the palmar surface of your hands with fingers extended on the midline. Press the fingers deeply inward on each side of the aorta and feel for the pulsation. In thin individuals, you can use one hand, placing the thumb on one side of the aorta and the fingers on the other side (Fig. 18.23).

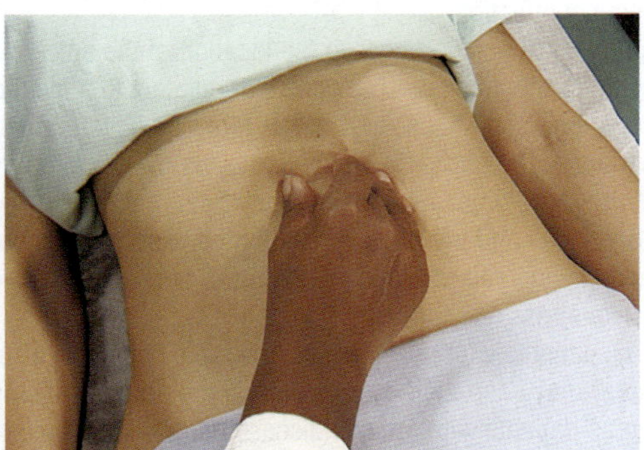

FIG. 18.23 Palpating the aorta. Place the thumb on one side of the aorta and the fingers on the other side.

Urinary Bladder. The urinary bladder is not palpable in a healthy patient unless the bladder is distended with urine, at which time you will feel it as a smooth, round, tense mass. You can determine the distended bladder outline with percussion; a distended bladder will elicit a lower percussion note than the surrounding air-filled intestines.

Advanced Skills

Ascites Assessment

Ascites—a pathologic increase in fluid in the peritoneal cavity—may be suspected in the patient with risk factors (e.g., hepatitis, congestive heart failure) who has a protuberant abdomen or bulging flank when lying supine. Percuss for areas of dullness and resonance with the patient supine. Because ascites fluid settles with gravity, expect to hear dullness in the dependent parts of the abdomen and tympany in the upper parts where the relatively lighter bowel has risen. Mark the borders between tympany and dullness. Several physical examination maneuvers are used to detect the presence of ascites.

Shifting Dullness

After identifying the borders between tympany and dullness, have the patient lie on one side and again percuss for tympany and dullness and mark the borders. In the patient without ascites, the borders will remain relatively constant. With ascites, the border of dullness shifts to the dependent side (approaches the midline) as the fluid resettles with gravity (Fig. 18.24).

Fluid Wave

This procedure requires assistance from the patient or another examiner (Fig. 18.25). With the patient supine, ask them or another person to press the edge of the hand and forearm firmly along the vertical midline of the abdomen. This positioning helps stop the transmission of

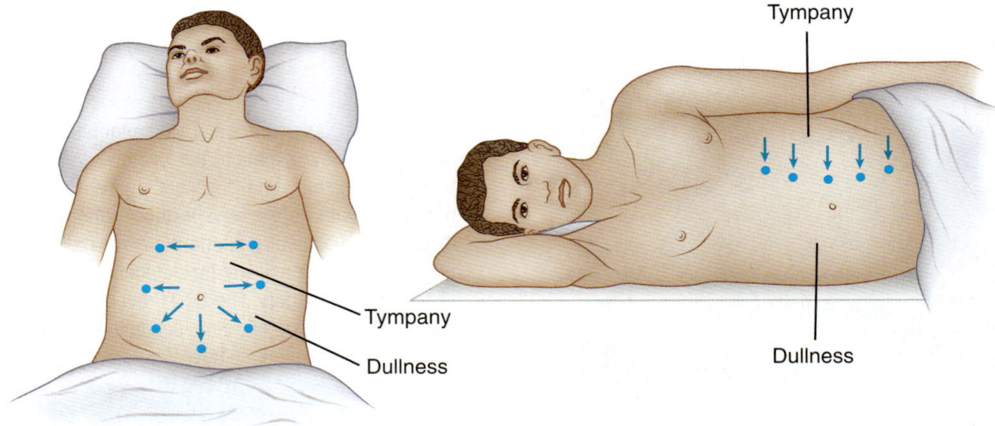

FIG. 18.24 Testing for shifting dullness. Dullness shifts to the dependent side.

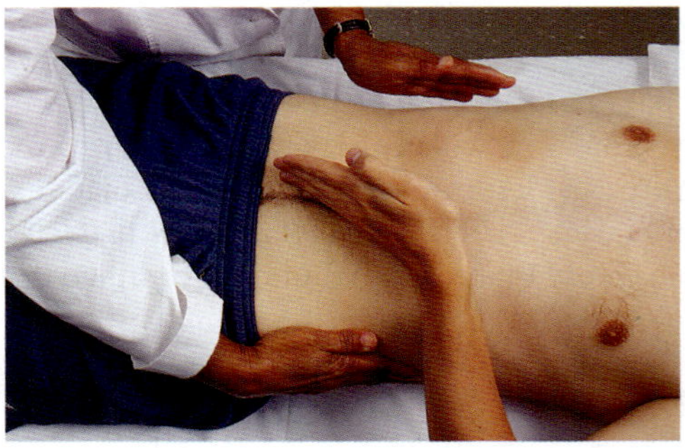

FIG. 18.25 Testing for fluid wave. Strike one side of the abdomen sharply with the fingertips. Feel for the impulse of a fluid wave with the other hand. (From Wilson, S. F., & Giddens, J. F. (2009). *Health assessment for nursing practice* (4th ed.). St. Louis: Mosby.)

a wave through adipose tissue. Place your hands on each side of the abdomen and strike one side sharply with your fingertips. Feel for the impulse of a fluid wave with the fingertips of your other hand. An easily detected fluid wave suggests ascites. However, a fluid wave can sometimes be felt in people without ascites and, conversely, may not occur in people with early ascites.

Evidence-Based Practice in Physical Examination

Detecting Ascites

The most sensitive maneuvers for detecting ascites are flank dullness (84%) and the presence of bulging flanks (81%), both of which have a specificity of 59%. The most specific test is the presence of a fluid wave (90%), although its sensitivity is fair (62%). Because these maneuvers may miss smaller amounts of peritoneal fluid, abdominal ultrasound may be necessary.

From Simel, D. L. (2009). Update: Ascites. In D. L. Simel & D. Rennie (Eds.), *The rational clinical examination evidence-based clinical diagnosis.* New York: McGraw Hill.

Pain Assessment

Abdominal pain is a common symptom but sometimes challenging to evaluate. Pain that is severe enough to make the patient unwilling to move, accompanied by nausea and vomiting, and marked by areas of localized tenderness generally suggests underlying pathology. While examining the abdomen, keep your eyes on the patient's face. The facial response is as important in your evaluation as the patient's verbal response to questions about the quality and degree of pain (Box 18.4). Ask the patient to

BOX 18.4 Clues in Diagnosing Abdominal Pain

There are all types of rules for identifying whether pain in the abdomen has significance. The following are a few of them:

Patients may give a "touch-me-not" warning—that is, not to touch in a particular area; however, these patients may not actually have pain if their face seems relaxed and unconcerned, even smiling. When you touch, they might recoil, but the unconcerned face persists. (This sign is helpful in other areas of the body as well as the abdomen.)

Patients with an organic cause for abdominal pain are generally not hungry. A negative response to the question, "Do you want something to eat?" is likely, particularly with appendicitis or intra-abdominal infection.

Ask the patient to point a finger to the location of the pain. If it is not directed to the umbilicus but goes immediately to a fixed point, there is a greater likelihood that this has significant pathologic importance. The farther from the umbilicus the pain, the more likely it will be organic in origin (Apley rule). If the finger goes to the umbilicus and the patient seems otherwise well to you, you should expand your differential diagnosis to include other etiologies like stress and trauma.

In general, patients with nonspecific abdominal pain from a functional disorder may keep their eyes closed during abdominal palpation, whereas patients with organic disease usually keep their eyes open. Similarly, pain that is elicited with manual palpation—but not with pressing the stethoscope during auscultation—may not have an organic disorder.

cough or take a deep breath. Assess the patient's willingness to stand up, walk, or jump. Is the pain exacerbated by movement?

Common causes of abdominal pain are described in Tables 18.2 and 18.3. Careful assessment of the quality (Table 18.4) and location (Box 18.5) of pain can usually narrow the possible causes, allowing you to select additional diagnostic studies with greater efficiency.

Findings associated with peritoneal irritation are summarized in Box 18.6. Appendicitis is the most common indication for emergency abdominal surgery. An accurate diagnosis based on history and physical examination can facilitate immediate surgical evaluation and definitive treatment and prevent unnecessary use of imaging studies. Historical symptoms that increase the likelihood of appendicitis are right lower quadrant (RLQ) pain, initial periumbilical pain with migration to the RLQ, and the presence of pain before vomiting. The presence of rigidity, a positive psoas sign (see "Iliopsoas Muscle Test"), fever, and/or rebound tenderness are physical examination findings that increase the likelihood of appendicitis. On physical examination, the lack of RLQ pain, rigidity, or guarding makes appendicitis less likely. Clinicians rarely rely on a single symptom or sign to make a diagnosis; however, the precision and accuracy of combinations of these findings have not been reported. No single finding effectively rules out appendicitis. The Evidence-Based Practice box describes the use of clinical prediction rules to help with diagnosing appendicitis.

TABLE 18.2 Conditions Producing Acute Abdominal Pain

CONDITION	USUAL PAIN CHARACTERISTICS	POSSIBLE ASSOCIATED SIGNS AND SYMPTOMS
Appendicitis	Initially periumbilical or epigastric; colicky; later becomes localized to RLQ, often at McBurney point	Guarding, tenderness; + iliopsoas and + obturator signs, RLQ skin hyperesthesia; anorexia, nausea, or vomiting after onset of pain; low-grade fever; + Aaron, Rovsing, Markle, and McBurney signs[a]
Peritonitis	Onset sudden or gradual; pain generalized or localized, dull or severe, and unrelenting; guarding; pain on deep inspiration	Shallow respiration; + Blumberg, Markle, and Ballance signs; reduced or absent bowel sounds, nausea and vomiting; + obturator + iliopsoas signs
Cholecystitis	Severe, unrelenting RUQ or epigastric pain; may be referred to right subscapular area	RUQ tenderness and rigidity; + Murphy sign, palpable gallbladder, anorexia, vomiting, fever, possible jaundice
Pancreatitis	Dramatic, sudden, excruciating LUQ, epigastric, or umbilical pain; may be present in one or both flanks; may be referred to left shoulder and penetrates to back	Epigastric tenderness, vomiting, fever, shock; + Grey Turner sign; + Cullen sign: both signs occur 2–3 days after onset
Salpingitis	Lower quadrant, worse on left	Nausea, vomiting, fever, suprapubic tenderness, rigid abdomen, pain on pelvic examination
Pelvic inflammatory disease	Lower quadrant, increases with activity	Tender adnexa and cervix, cervical discharge, dyspareunia
Diverticulitis	Epigastric, radiating down left side of abdomen especially after eating; may be referred to back	Flatulence, borborygmus, diarrhea, dysuria, tenderness on palpation
Perforated gastric or duodenal ulcer	Abrupt RUQ; may be referred to shoulders	Abdominal free air and distention with increased resonance over liver; tenderness in epigastrium or RUQ; rigid abdominal wall, rebound tenderness
Intestinal obstruction	Abrupt, severe, colicky, spasmodic; referred to epigastrium, umbilicus	Distention, minimal rebound tenderness, vomiting, localized tenderness, visible peristalsis; bowel sounds absent (with paralytic obstruction) or hyperactive high pitched (with mechanical obstruction)
Volvulus	Referred to hypogastrium and umbilicus	Distention, nausea, vomiting, guarding; sigmoid loop volvulus may be palpable
Leaking abdominal aneurysm	Steady throbbing midline over aneurysm; may penetrate to back, flank	Nausea, vomiting, abdominal mass, bruit
Biliary stones, colic	Episodic, severe, RUQ, or epigastrium lasting 15 minutes to several hours; may be lower	RUQ tenderness, soft abdominal wall, anorexia, vomiting, jaundice, subnormal temperature
Renal calculi	Intense; flank, extending to groin and genitals; may be episodic	Fever, hematuria; + Kehr sign
Ectopic pregnancy	Lower quadrant; referred to shoulder; with rupture is agonizing	Hypogastric tenderness, symptoms of pregnancy, spotting, irregular menses, soft abdominal wall, mass on bimanual pelvic examination; ruptured: shock, rigid abdominal wall, distention; + Kehr and Cullen signs
Ruptured ovarian cyst	Lower quadrant, steady, increases with cough or motion	Vomiting, low-grade fever, anorexia, tenderness on pelvic examination
Splenic rupture	Intense; LUQ, radiating to left shoulder; may worsen with foot of bed elevated	Shock, pallor, lowered temperature

LUQ, Left upper quadrant; *RLQ,* right lower quadrant; *RUQ,* right upper quadrant.
[a]See Table 18.5 for explanation of signs.

TABLE 18.3 Conditions Producing Chronic Abdominal Pain

CONDITION	USUAL PAIN CHARACTERISTICS	POSSIBLE ASSOCIATED SIGNS AND SYMPTOMS
Irritable bowel syndrome	Hypogastric pain; crampy, variable, infrequent; associated with bowel function	Unremarkable physical examination Pain associated with gas, bloating, distention; relief with passage of flatus, feces
Lactose intolerance	Crampy pain after drinking milk or eating milk products	Associated diarrhea; unremarkable physical examination
Diverticular disease	Localized pain	Abdominal tenderness, fever
Constipation	Colicky or dull and steady pain that does not progress and worsen	Fecal mass palpable, stool in rectum
Uterine fibroids	Pain related to menses, intercourse	Palpable myoma(s)
Hernia	Localized pain that increases with exertion or lifting	Hernia on physical examination
Esophagitis/gastroesophageal reflux disease	Burning or gnawing pain in midepigastrium, worsens with recumbency and certain foods	Unremarkable physical examination
Peptic ulcer	Burning or gnawing pain	May have epigastric tenderness on palpation
Gastritis	Constant burning pain in epigastrium	May be accompanied by nausea, vomiting, diarrhea, or fever Unremarkable physical examination

Modified from Dains, J. E., Baumann, L. C., & Scheibel, P. (2007). *Health assessment and clinical diagnosis in primary care* (3rd ed.). St Louis: Mosby.

TABLE 18.4 Quality and Onset of Abdominal Pain

CHARACTERISTIC	POSSIBLE RELATED CONDITIONS
Burning	Peptic ulcer
Cramping	Biliary colic, gastroenteritis
Colicky	Appendicitis with impacted feces; renal stone
Aching	Appendiceal irritation
Knifelike	Pancreatitis
Ripping, tearing	Aortic dissection
Gradual onset	Infection
Sudden onset	Duodenal ulcer, acute pancreatitis, obstruction, perforation

BOX 18.5 Some Causes of Pain Perceived in Anatomic Regions

RIGHT UPPER QUADRANT		LEFT UPPER QUADRANT
Duodenal ulcer Hepatitis Hepatomegaly Lower lobe pneumonia Cholecystitis		Ruptured spleen Gastric ulcer Aortic aneurysm Perforated colon Lower lobe pneumonia
RIGHT LOWER QUADRANT	**PERIUMBILICAL**	**LEFT LOWER QUADRANT**
Appendicitis Salpingitis Ovarian cyst Ruptured ectopic pregnancy Tubo-ovarian abscess Renal/ureteral stone Strangulated hernia Meckel diverticulitis Regional ileitis Perforated cecum	Intestinal obstruction Acute pancreatitis Early appendicitis Mesenteric thrombosis Aortic aneurysm Diverticulitis	Sigmoid diverticulitis Salpingitis Ovarian cyst Ruptured ectopic pregnancy Tubo-ovarian abscess Renal/ureteral stone Strangulated hernia Perforated colon Regional ileitis Ulcerative colitis

BOX 18.6 Findings in Peritoneal Irritation

- Involuntary rigidity of abdominal muscles
- Tenderness and guarding
- Absent bowel sounds
- Positive obturator test
- Positive iliopsoas test
- Rebound tenderness (Blumberg sign and McBurney sign; see Table 18.5)
- Abdominal pain on walking
- Positive heel jar test (Markle sign; see Table 18.5)
- Right lower quadrant pain intensified by left lower quadrant abdominal palpation (Rovsing sign; see Table 18.5)

Evidence-Based Practice in Physical Examination

Diagnosing Appendicitis

Several clinical prediction rules (CPRs) have been developed based on history, physical examination, and laboratory values. The Alvarado score (also known as the MANTRELS [Migration of pain, Anorexia, Nausea/vomiting, Tenderness in the right lower quadrant, Rebound pain, Elevation of temperature, Leukocytosis, Shift to the left] score) has been validated in children and adults and remains the most widely accepted and simplest decision tool (Abdella Bahta et al., 2023). The Pediatric Appendicitis Score (PAS), which includes RLQ pain with cough, percussion or hopping, has also been used. The Ohmann score, which uses patient age, history, physical examination, and laboratory findings, is another tool to help identify patients at low, moderate, and high risk of having appendicitis. In a systematic literature review assessing 12 studies, the most valid CPR for diagnosing appendicitis in children are the Alvarado score and the PAS (Kulik et al., 2013). In another systematic review of 12 studies examining CPRs in adults, the appendicitis inflammatory response (AIR) score, which includes symptoms (fever, vomiting), physical exam (rebound tenderness), and laboratory findings, showed the highest sensitivity (92%) and specificity (63%) for diagnosing appendicitis (Kularatna et al., 2017).

CLINICAL PEARL

Ectopic Pregnancy

Unfortunately, ectopic pregnancy is often not diagnosed before rupture because symptoms are mild. In a pregnant patient, a dramatic change from mild, even vague, abdominal pain that is not particularly distressing to a sudden onset of severe abdominal tenderness in the hypogastric area—particularly on the involved side—is very worrisome. Rigidity and rebound may come on early or late. If a patient of childbearing age presents with vague abdominal symptoms, be sure to conduct a sexual health and menstrual history and strongly consider performing a urine pregnancy test. Do not disregard the mild tenderness that might be evoked. Instead, try to anticipate the emergency of a rupture.

Abdominal Signs

"Classic" abdominal pain signs have often been given the name of the person who first described them. Some of the most common and historical signs are included in Table 18.5.

Rebound Tenderness

Several maneuvers can be used to assess for peritoneal inflammation (see Box 18.6). Rebound tenderness is identified in the following manner. Holding your hand at a 90-degree angle to the abdomen with the fingers extended, press gently and deeply into a region remote from the area of abdominal discomfort. Rapidly withdraw your hand and fingers (Fig. 18.26). The return to position—or "rebound" of the structures that were compressed by your fingers—causes a sharp stabbing pain at the site of peritoneal inflammation (positive Blumberg sign). Rebound tenderness over the McBurney point in the RLQ suggests appendicitis (positive McBurney sign). The maneuver for rebound tenderness should be performed at the end of the examination because a positive response produces pain and muscle spasms that can interfere with any subsequent examination. Because light percussion produces a mild localized response in the presence of peritoneal inflammation, assessing for rebound tenderness is considered unnecessary by many clinicians. See Clinical Pearl, "Ectopic Pregnancy."

Iliopsoas Muscle Test

This test is performed when you suspect appendicitis because an inflamed appendix may cause irritation of the lateral iliopsoas muscle. Ask the patient to lie supine and then place your hand over the lower right thigh. Ask the patient to raise the right leg, flexing at the hip, while you push downward (Fig. 18.27A). An alternative technique is to position the patient on the left side and ask that the right leg be raised from the hip while you press downward against it. A third technique is to hyperextend the right leg by drawing it backward while the patient is lying on the left side (see Fig. 18.27B). Pain with any of these techniques is considered a positive psoas sign, indicating irritation of the iliopsoas muscle.

Obturator Muscle Test

This test can be performed when you suspect a ruptured appendix or a pelvic abscess caused by irritation of the obturator muscle. While the patient is in the supine position, ask them to flex the right leg at the hip and knee to 90 degrees. Hold the leg just above the knee, grasp the ankle, and rotate the leg laterally and medially (Fig. 18.28). Pain in the right hypogastric region is a positive sign, indicating irritation of the obturator muscle.

TABLE 18.5 Abdominal Signs Associated With Common Abdominal Conditions

SIGN	DESCRIPTION	ASSOCIATED CONDITIONS
Aaron	Pain or distress occurs in area of patient's heart or stomach on palpation of McBurney point	Appendicitis
Ballance	Fixed dullness to percussion in left flank and dullness in right flank that disappears on change of position	Peritoneal irritation
Blumberg	Rebound tenderness	Peritoneal irritation; appendicitis
Cullen	Ecchymosis around umbilicus	Hemoperitoneum; pancreatitis; ectopic pregnancy
Dance	Absence of bowel sounds in right lower quadrant	Intussusception
Gray Turner	Ecchymosis of flanks	Hemoperitoneum; pancreatitis
Howship-Romberg	Pain down the medial aspect of the thigh to the knees	Strangulated obturator hernia
Kehr	Abdominal pain radiating to left shoulder	Spleen rupture; renal calculi; ectopic pregnancy
Markle (heel jar)	Patient stands with straightened knees, then raises up on toes, relaxes, and allows heels to hit floor, thus jarring body; action will cause abdominal pain if positive	Peritoneal irritation; appendicitis
McBurney	Rebound tenderness and sharp pain when McBurney point is palpated	Appendicitis
Murphy	Abrupt cessation of inspiration on palpation of gallbladder	Cholecystitis
Rovsing	Right lower quadrant pain intensified by left lower quadrant abdominal palpation	Peritoneal irritation; appendicitis

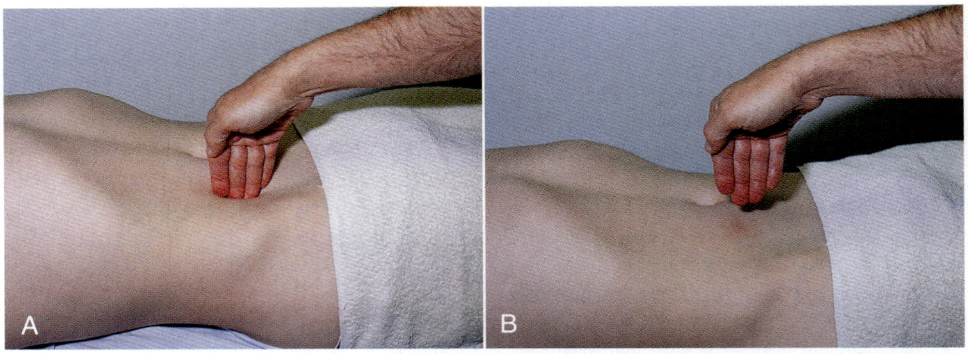

FIG. 18.26 Testing for rebound tenderness. (A) Press deeply and gently into the abdomen. (B) Then rapidly withdraw the hands and fingers.

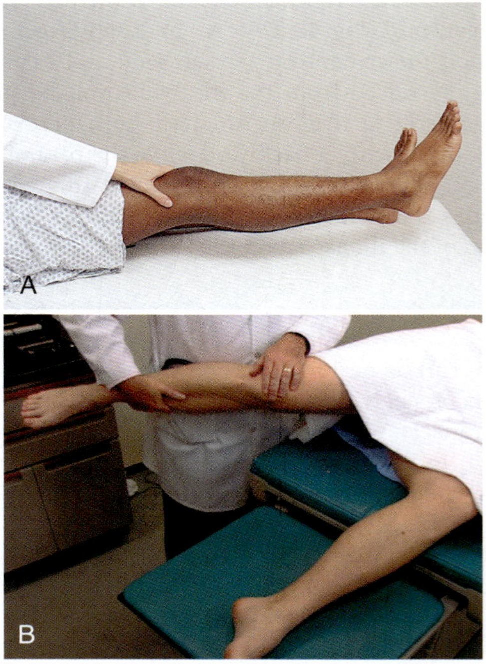

FIG. 18.27 Iliopsoas muscle test. (A) The patient raises the leg from the hip while the examiner pushes downward against it. (B) Alternative technique. The examiner hyperextends the right leg by drawing it backward while the patient lies on the left side. (B, From Swartz, M. H. (2006). Textbook of physical diagnosis (5th ed.). Philadelphia: Elsevier.)

Ballottement

Ballottement is a palpation technique used to assess an organ or a mass. To perform abdominal ballottement with one hand, place your extended fingers, hand, and forearm at a 90-degree angle to the abdomen. Push in toward the organ or mass with the fingertips (Fig. 18.29A). If the mass is freely movable, it will float upward and touch the fingertips as fluid and other structures are displaced by the maneuver. To perform bimanual ballottement, place one hand on the anterior abdominal wall and one hand against the flank. Push inward on the abdominal wall while palpating with the flank hand to determine the presence and size of the mass (see Fig. 18.29B).

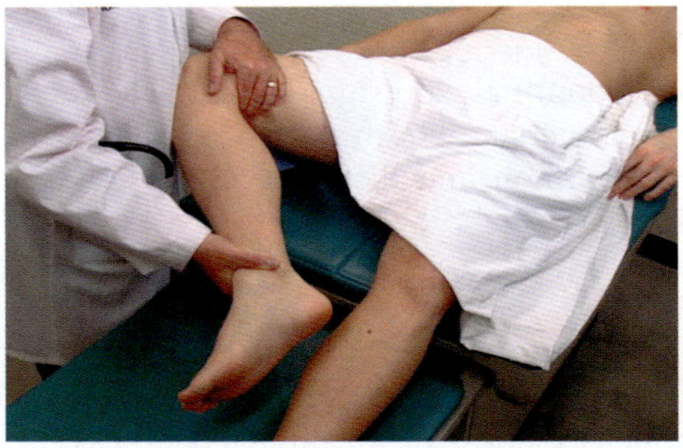

FIG. 18.28 Obturator muscle test. With the right leg flexed at the hip and knee, rotate the leg laterally and medially. (From Swartz, M. H. (2006). Textbook of physical diagnosis (5th ed.). Philadelphia: Elsevier.)

Infants and Children

If possible, the infant's abdomen should be examined during a time of relaxation and quiet. It is often best to do this at the start of the overall examination, especially before initiating any procedure that might cause distress (Fig. 18.30). Sucking on a pacifier may help relax the infant. The parent's lap often makes the best examining surface as the infant or toddler will feel most secure. Sit facing the parent and conduct the abdominal examination entirely on the parent's lap. This works well during the first several months—and often the first 2 to 3 years—of life (Fig. 18.31).

Inspection

Inspect the abdomen, noting its shape, contour, and movement with respiration. It should be rounded and dome shaped because the abdominal musculature has not fully developed. Note any localized fullness. Abdominal and chest movements should be synchronous, with a slight bulge of the abdomen at the beginning of respiration. Note whether the abdomen protrudes above the level of the chest or is scaphoid. A distended or protruding abdomen can result from feces, a mass, or organ enlargement. A scaphoid abdomen in a patient in respiratory distress suggests that the abdominal contents are displaced into

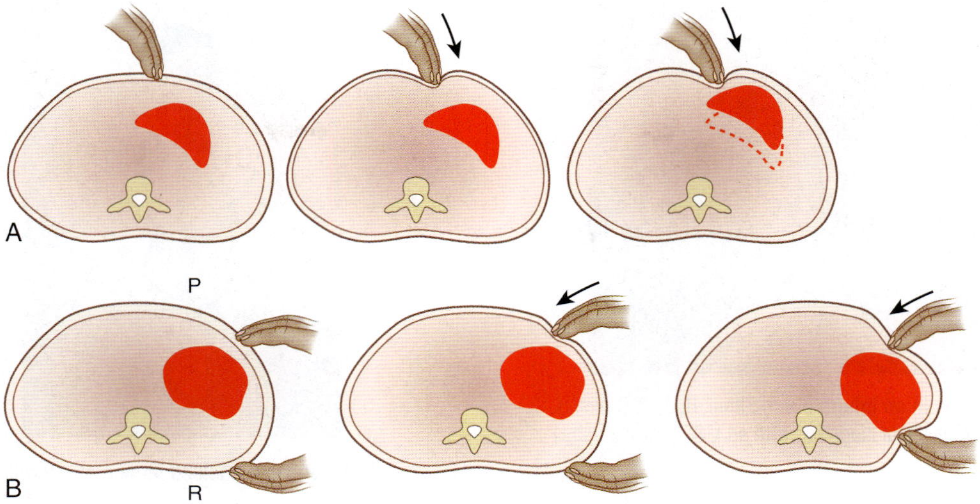

FIG. 18.29 **Ballottement technique.** (A) Single-handed ballottement. Push inward at a 90-degree angle. If the object is freely movable, it will float upward to touch the fingertips. (B) Bimanual ballottement. *P*, Pushing hand; *R*, receiving hand.

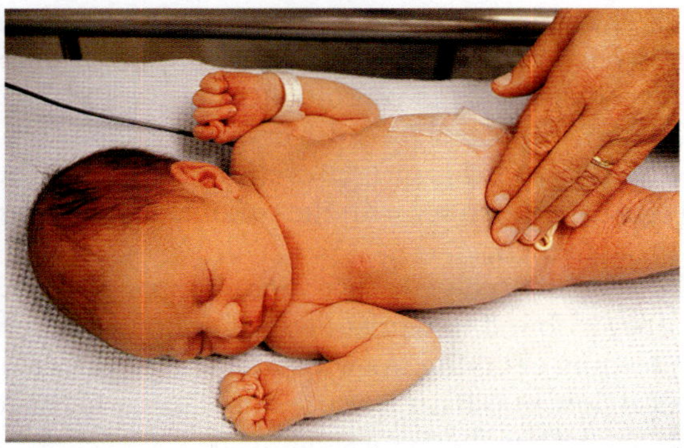

FIG. 18.30 **Positioning for examination of the infant's abdomen.**

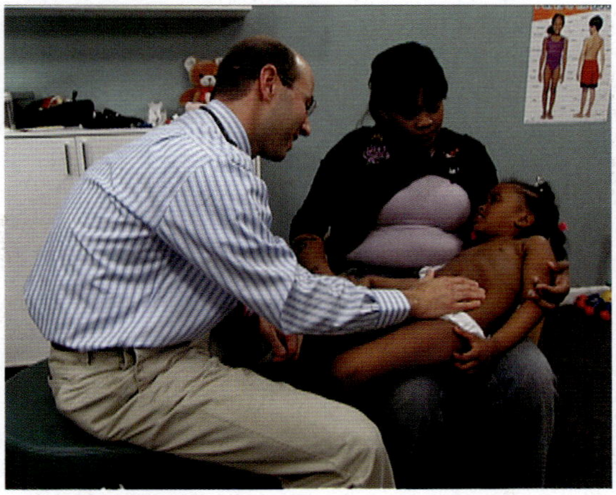

FIG. 18.31 **Positioning for examination of a toddler in a parent's lap.**

the thorax due to a congenital diaphragmatic hernia or diaphragm rupture from blunt trauma.

Note any pulsations over the abdomen. Pulsations in the epigastric area are common in newborns and infants. Superficial veins are usually visible in the thin infant; however, distended veins across the abdomen are an unexpected finding suggestive of vascular obstruction or abdominal distention or obstruction. Spider nevi may indicate liver disease.

If you are present at the time of delivery, inspect the umbilical cord of the newborn, counting the number of vessels. Two arteries and one vein should be present. A single umbilical artery should alert you to the possibility of congenital anomalies. Any intestinal structure present in the umbilical cord or protruding into the umbilical area and visible through a thick transparent membrane suggests an omphalocele (see Clinical Pearl, "Umbilical Cord").

When examining newborns in the office, the umbilical stump area should be dry and odorless. Inspect it for discharge, redness, induration, and skin warmth. Once the stump has separated, typically by 2 weeks of age, serous or serosanguineous discharge may indicate a granuloma when no other signs of infection are present. Inspect all folds of skin in the umbilicus for a nodule of granulomatous tissue. If drainage persists after cord separation, consider the possibility of a patent urachal cyst or remnant.

Note any protrusion through the umbilicus or rectus abdominis muscles when the infant strains. The umbilicus is usually inverted. A small umbilical hernia (i.e., the protrusion of omentum and intestine through the umbilical opening, forming a visible and palpable bulge) is a common finding in infants. Umbilical hernias can be large and impressive (Fig. 18.32). It is ordinarily easy to reduce them temporarily by pushing the contents back into the intra-abdominal position. Measure the diameter of the umbilical opening rather than the protruding contents to determine the size. The maximum size is generally reached by

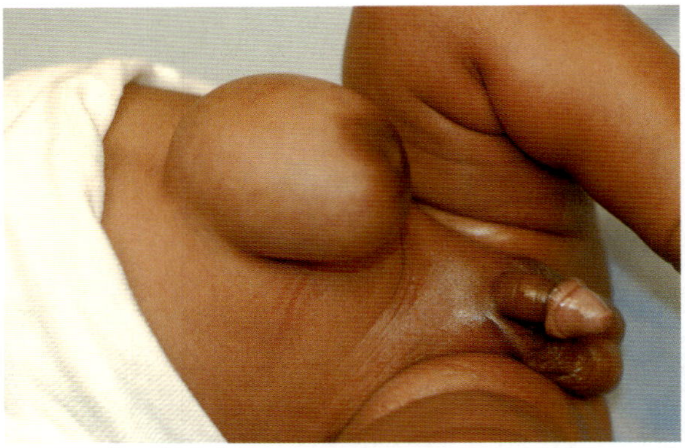

FIG. 18.32 Umbilical hernia in an infant. (From Zitelli, B. J., & Davis, H. W. (2012). Atlas of pediatric physical diagnosis (6th ed.). St. Louis: Mosby.)

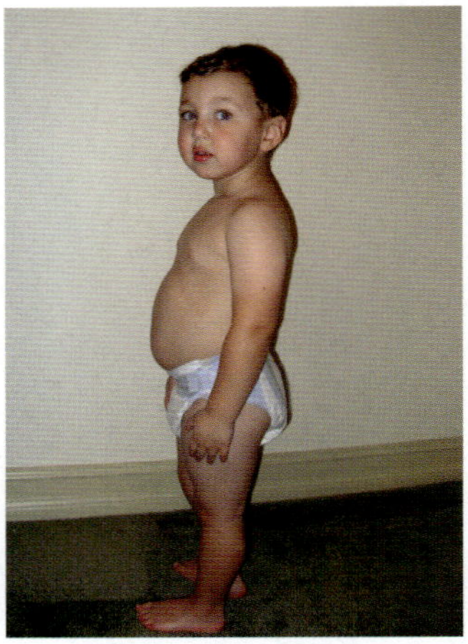

FIG. 18.33 Potbellied stance of a toddler.

1 month of age, and most small umbilical hernias will close spontaneously by 1 to 2 years of age.

Diastasis rectus abdominis, a separation 1 to 4 cm wide in the midline, usually between the xiphoid and the umbilicus, is a common finding when the rectus abdominis muscles do not approximate each other. Ordinarily, there is no need for surgical repair. Although rare, herniation through the rectus abdominis muscles can occur.

If the infant is vomiting frequently, use tangential lighting and observe the abdomen at eye level for peristaltic waves. Peristalsis is not usually visible. Peristaltic waves may sometimes be seen in thin, malnourished infants, but their presence usually suggests an intestinal obstruction such as pyloric stenosis.

The abdomen of the young child protrudes slightly, giving a potbellied appearance when the child is standing, sitting, and supine (Fig. 18.33). After age 5 years, the contour of the child's abdomen, when supine, may become convex and will not extend above an imaginary line drawn from the xiphoid process to the symphysis pubis. Respirations will continue to be abdominal until the child is 6 to 7 years old. Restricted abdominal respiration in young children can be caused by peritoneal irritation requiring urgent medical evaluation.

CLINICAL PEARL

Umbilical Cord

A thick umbilical cord suggests a well-nourished fetus; a thin cord suggests otherwise.

Auscultation and Percussion

The procedures of auscultation and percussion of the abdomen do not differ from those used for adults. Bowel sounds should be present within 1 to 2 hours after birth, and peristalsis is detected when a metallic tinkling sound is heard every 10 to 30 seconds. A scaphoid abdomen in a newborn with respiratory distress suggests a congenital diaphragmatic hernia. In this instance, bowel sounds may be appreciated in the chest. Bruits and venous hums should not be heard on abdominal auscultation.

Renal bruits are associated with renal artery stenosis and, rarely, with a renal arteriovenous fistula. The bruit of stenosis has a high frequency and is soft; the bruit of an arteriovenous fistula is continuous. Both are difficult to hear. When suspicious (because of hypertension), try first with the patient held upright or sitting, listening at the posterior flank; then try with the patient supine, listening over the abdomen.

The abdomen may produce more tympany on percussion than is found in adults because infants swallow air when feeding or crying. As with adults, tympany in a distended abdomen is usually the result of gas, whereas dullness may indicate fluid or a solid mass.

Palpation

Palpate the abdomen with the infant's feet slightly elevated and knees flexed to promote relaxation of the abdominal musculature (see Clinical Pearl, "Palpating an Infant's Abdomen"). Begin with superficial palpation to detect the spleen, liver, and masses close to the surface. The spleen is usually palpable 1 to 2 cm below the left costal margin during the first few weeks after birth. A detectable spleen tip at the left costal margin is a common finding in well infants and young children. An enlarged spleen may indicate congenital hemolytic disease or sepsis in an ill-appearing infant.

CLINICAL PEARL

Palpating an Infant's Abdomen

The abdomen of an infant can seem very tiny in relation to the size of your hand. Place your right hand gently on the abdomen with the thumb at the right upper quadrant and the index finger at the left upper quadrant. Press very gently at first, only gradually increasing pressure (never too vigorously) as you palpate over the entire abdomen.

CLINICAL PEARL

Enlarged Liver

An infant of a mother with diabetes may have an enlarged liver. Typically, these infants have macrosomia (birth weight over 4000 g). This history and/or findings should alert the clinician to check the infant for hypoglycemia, hyperbilirubinemia, and congenital anomalies like heart defects.

Liver Palpation

To assess the liver, superficially palpate at the right midclavicular line 3 to 4 cm below the costal margin. As the infant inspires, wait to feel a narrow mass tap your finger. Gradually move your fingers up the midclavicular line until the sensation is felt. The liver edge is usually palpable just below the right costal margin in the newborn. The liver edge may be palpable at 1 to 3 cm below the right costal margin in infants and toddlers. Estimation of true liver size can be accomplished only by percussing the upper border, as well as palpating the lower edge. The upper edge of the liver should be detected by percussion at the sixth intercostal space. Together, the techniques provide an estimate of liver span, rather than just a projection of size below the costal margin (see Clinical Pearl, "Enlarged Liver").

Hepatomegaly is present when the liver is more than 3 cm below the right costal margin, suggesting infection, cardiac failure, or liver disease. Before 2 years of age, females have a slightly larger liver span than males. The mean range of liver spans by percussion in infants and children is as follows:

AGE	LIVER SPAN (cm)
0–2 months	4.0–6.3
2–12 months	4.0–7.9
1–5 years	6.3–10.5
5–10 years	6.9–11.4
10–15 years	7.4–12.3

From Amatya, P., Shah, D., Gupta, N., & Bhatta, N. K. (2014). Clinical and ultrasonographic measurement of liver size in normal children. *Indian Journal of Pediatrics, 81*(5), 441–445.

Deep Palpation

Following light palpation, perform deep palpation in all quadrants or regions. Note the location, size, shape, tenderness, and consistency of any masses. More than half of all masses detected in newborns are genitourinary in origin; hydronephrosis and multicystic dysplastic kidney are the most common. In young children, Wilms tumor and neuroblastoma typically present as large abdominal masses. All masses should be investigated with imaging studies.

DIFFERENTIAL DIAGNOSIS

Abdominal Masses in Infants and Children

NEONATES	INFANTS AND CHILDREN
Hydronephrosis	Feces (constipation)
Multicystic dysplastic kidney	Pyloric stenosis
Polycystic kidney disease	Gastrointestinal duplication
Renal vein thrombosis	Intussusception
Wilms tumor	Meckel diverticulum
Ovarian cyst	Neuroblastoma
Hydrocolpos	Wilms tumor
Hydrometrocolpos	Lymphoma
Gastrointestinal duplication	Hepatoblastoma
	Ovarian cyst
	Teratoma

The olive-shaped mass of pyloric stenosis may be detected with deep palpation in the right upper quadrant immediately after the infant vomits. It can be helpful to sit the infant in your lap, folding the upper body gently against your palpating hand and bringing the pyloric mass into opposition with your hand. Almost all other palpable masses in the abdomen of the newborn are typically renal in origin. A sausage-shaped mass in the left or right upper quadrant may indicate intussusception in an ill-appearing or lethargic infant or toddler. A midline suprapubic mass suggests Hirschsprung disease in which feces fill the rectosigmoid colon. A soft mass in the left lower quadrant of a child of any age may indicate feces in the sigmoid colon associated with constipation.

In the infant and toddler, the bladder can usually be palpated and percussed in the suprapubic area. A distended bladder, felt as a firm, central, dome-shaped structure in the lower abdomen, may indicate urethral obstruction. Compared with newborns, abdominal tumors are more commonly palpated in infants and toddlers, the most common being neuroblastoma, Wilms tumor, and lymphoma. Palpation of the femoral arteries is performed during the abdominal examination as described in Chapter 16.

Tenderness or pain on palpation may be difficult to detect in the infant; however, pain and tenderness are assessed by such behaviors as change in the pitch of crying, facial grimacing, disinterest in sucking, and drawing the knees to the abdomen with palpation. Examine the infant on the parent's lap. If the infant continues to cry throughout the examination, seize the quiet moment in the respiratory cycle to palpate to distinguish between a firm and soft abdomen. The abdomen should be soft during inspiration. If the abdomen remains hard with a noticeable rigidity or resistance to pressure during both respiratory phases, peritoneal irritation may be present. It is often necessary to delay examination of a distressed infant, waiting for a quieter moment, unless there is reason for urgency. Causes of abdominal pain in pediatric patients vary by age.

DIFFERENTIAL DIAGNOSIS

Causes of Acute Abdominal Pain in Infants, Children, and Adolescents

DIAGNOSIS	INFANCY (<2 YEARS)	PRESCHOOL AGE (2–5 YEARS)	SCHOOL AGE (5–12 YEARS)	ADOLESCENCE (>12 YEARS)
Intra-abdominal Causes				
Appendicitis		√	√	√
Cholecystitis				√
Constipation	√	√	√	√
Functional			√	√
Gastritis				√
Gastroenteritis	√	√	√	√
Gastroesophageal reflux disease	√			√
Hepatitis				√
Incarcerated hernia	√			
Inflammatory bowel disease			√	√
Henoch-Schönlein purpura		√		
Intussusception	√	√		
Milk protein allergy	√			
Pancreatitis				√
Volvulus	√			
Extra-abdominal Causes				
Dysmenorrhea				√
Ectopic pregnancy				√
Epididymitis				√
Group A streptococcal pharyngitis			√	√
Nephrolithiasis				√
Ovarian torsion				√
Pelvic inflammatory disease				√
Pneumonia		√	√	√
Pregnancy			√	
Testicular torsion			√	√
Urinary tract infection		√	√	√

Diagnoses are included for age groups in which they are most commonly seen.
Modified from Marin, J. R., & Alpern, E. R. (2011). Abdominal pain in children. *Emergency Medicine Clinics of North America, 29*(2), 401–428, ix–x.

Palpate the abdomen of a child who is ticklish with a firm rather than soft touch. If this is unsuccessful, place the child's hand under the palm of your examining hand, leaving your fingers free to palpate. Localization of abdominal tenderness or pain may be difficult in the young child who cannot verbally describe the site or character of pain. Distract the child with a toy or question the child about a favorite activity as you begin palpating in the abdominal region believed most distant from the area of pain. Observe for changes in facial expression during palpation to identify the location of greatest pain. Check for rebound tenderness and make the same observations of the child's facial expression. As with adults, check for rebound tenderness cautiously. Once a child has experienced palpation that is too intense, a subsequent clinician has little chance for a successful abdominal examination.

Adolescents

The techniques of abdominal examination of the adolescent are the same as those used for adults. Do not overlook the possibility of pregnancy or ovarian torsion as a cause of abdominal pain or lower abdominal mass in young adolescent females.

Evidence-Based Practice in Physical Examination

Ovarian Torsion

In a study of 82 female children and adolescents found to have ovarian torsion, most reported severe intermittent pain for 24 hours' duration. More often, patients reported pain in the right lower quadrant compared with the left lower quadrant (61% vs. 34%). Most (91%) had abdominal tenderness, 27% had guarding, and 18% had rebound tenderness on examination.

From Rossi, B. V., Ference, E. H., Zurakowski, D., Scholz, S., Feins, N. R., Chow, J. S., & Laufer, M. R. (2012). The clinical presentation and surgical management of adnexal torsion in the pediatric and adolescent population. *Journal of Pediatric and Adolescent Gynecology, 25*(2), 109–113.

Pregnant Patients

Uterine changes that can be detected on pelvic examination are discussed in Chapter 19. Nausea and vomiting are common in the first trimester. Constipation is a common occurrence, and hemorrhoids often develop later in pregnancy. Bowel sounds will be diminished as a result of decreased peristaltic activity. Striae and a midline band of pigmentation (linea nigra) may be present (see Fig. 18.2). Assessment of the abdomen of pregnant patients includes uterine size estimation for gestational age, fetal growth, position of the fetus, monitoring of fetal well-being, and presence of uterine contractions (see Chapter 19).

Older Adults

The techniques of examination are the same as those used for younger adults. The abdominal wall of the older adult becomes thinner and less firm as a result of the loss of connective tissue and muscle mass that accompanies aging. Palpation therefore may be relatively easier and yield more accurate findings. A pulsating AAA may be more readily palpable than in younger patients. Deposition of fat over the abdominal area is common despite concurrent loss of fatty tissue over the extremities. The abdominal contour is often rounded as a result of loss of muscle tone.

Use judgment in determining whether a patient is able to assume a particular position. Rotation of joints, such as with the obturator muscle test, may cause discomfort in patients who have decreased muscle flexibility or increased joint tenderness.

Be aware that respiratory changes can produce corresponding findings in the abdominal examination. The liver in patients with hyperexpanded lungs from chronic obstructive pulmonary disease may be displaced downward but not necessarily enlarged. In this case, both the upper and lower borders of the liver may be detected 1 to 2 cm below the usual markers, but the liver span should still be between 6 and 12 cm. On the other hand, with the decrease in liver size after 50 years of age, you may find a smaller midclavicular liver span.

With decreased intestinal motility associated with aging, intestinal disorders are common in older adults, so be particularly sensitive to patient concerns and related findings. Constipation is a common symptom, and you are more likely to feel stool in the sigmoid colon. The sensation of bloating or increased gas may be reflected by increased tympany on percussion. Fecal impaction is a common finding in older adults with severe or chronic constipation. See Clinical Pearl, "Constipation With Diarrhea."

Obstruction may be a problem with older adults, occurring as a result of hypokalemia; myocardial infarction; and infections such as pneumonia, sepsis, peritonitis, and pancreatitis. Vomiting, distention, diarrhea, and constipation can signal obstruction.

The incidence of gastrointestinal cancer increases with age. Symptoms depend on the site of the tumor and include dysphagia, nausea, vomiting, anorexia, and hematemesis. Patients may also report changes in stool frequency, size, consistency, or color. See Chapter 21 for a discussion of the rectal digital examination, an important step in the detection of colon cancer.

Pain perception may be altered as part of the aging process, and older patients may exhibit atypical pain symptoms. These can include less severe or totally absent pain with disease states that characteristically produce pain in younger adults. Therefore evaluation of pain in the older adult must take into account concurrent symptoms and accompanying findings.

CLINICAL PEARL

Constipation With Diarrhea

Be aware that people with apparent diarrhea may still have constipation. Some may have loose stools around a major fecal impaction and develop overflow incontinence that leads to encopresis (soiling).

ABNORMALITIES

Alimentary Tract

Acute Diarrhea

Three or more watery or loose stools per day

PATHOPHYSIOLOGY

- Viral gastroenteritis is the most common cause and typically self-limited in those without signs or symptoms or other organ involvement
- International travelers may acquire foodborne infection (e.g., enterotoxigenic *Escherichia coli, Salmonella, Shigella,* or *Entamoeba histolytica*)
- Camping or well water exposes individuals to *Giardia* and *Campylobacter* through untreated water
- *Cryptosporidium* is a potential cause from contaminated water in urban areas of the United States
- *Salmonella* or *Campylobacter jejuni* from undercooked poultry
- Undercooked beef or unpasteurized milk may contain *E. coli* 0157:H7
- Raw shellfish is a potential source of Norwalk virus
- Consider food poisoning if diarrhea develops in two or more persons after ingestion of the same food

PATIENT DATA

Subjective Data

- Usually, abrupt onset and lasts less than 2 weeks
- Abdominal pain
- Nausea
- Vomiting
- Fever
- Tenesmus (feeling of incomplete defecation)
- Vomiting within several hours of ingesting a particular food suggests food poisoning
- Bloody diarrhea may occur with organisms such as *Campylobacter* and *Shigella*

Objective Data

- Diffuse abdominal tenderness
- Examination can mimic peritoneal inflammation with right lower quadrant (RLQ) pain or guarding
- If severe, may have findings consistent with moderate to severe dehydration, particularly in infants, children, and older adults (e.g., tachycardia, hypotension, and altered mental status)

Gastroesophageal Reflux Disease

Backward flow of gastric contents, which are typically acidic, into the esophagus

PATHOPHYSIOLOGY

- Caused by relaxation or incompetence of the lower esophageal sphincter
- Delayed gastric emptying is a predisposing factor
- More common among older adults and in pregnant patients

PATIENT DATA

Subjective Data

- Heartburn or acid indigestion (burning chest pain, localized behind the sternum that moves up toward the neck and throat)
- Bitter or sour taste of acid in the back of the throat
- Hoarseness
- Infants and toddlers may exhibit back arching, fussiness with feeding, or regurgitation and vomiting; can be severe enough to cause weight loss and failure to thrive
- Can precipitate an acute asthma exacerbation or cause chronic respiratory problems from aspiration and esophageal bleeding

Objective Data

- Generally, no physical examination findings
- With severe disease may have erythema of the posterior pharynx and edematous vocal cords

Irritable Bowel Syndrome

Functional chronic gastrointestinal disorder with symptoms of pain and change in stooling patterns

PATHOPHYSIOLOGY

- Cause unknown
- Most common disorder seen by gastroenterologists; estimated 10%–15% of U.S. adults affected, 5%–7% diagnosed
- Occurs more often in females
- Usually begins in late adolescence or early adult life and rarely appears for the first time after 45 years of age

PATIENT DATA

Subjective Data

- Commonly report a cluster of symptoms, consisting of abdominal pain, bloating, constipation; or abdominal pain, urgency, and diarrhea; or mixed constipation and diarrhea (see Table 18.3)

Objective Data

- Generally, unremarkable examination
- Diagnosis is typically made after excluding other potential causes
- Rome IV diagnostic criteria include abdominal pain, on average, at least 1 day a week in the past 3 months associated with two or more of the following:• Related to defecation
  - Associated with a change in frequency of stool
  - Associated with a change in form (consistency) of stool
  - Symptoms must have started at least 6 months ago (Drossman, 2016)

Patient Safety

Avoiding Foodborne Infection

Adults and children are susceptible to foodborne infection, both at home and while traveling. Prevention measures include the following:

- Cook all ground beef and poultry thoroughly. Send restaurant food back if it is not cooked well. Eat only food that has been cooked thoroughly and is still hot.
- Do not drink unpasteurized juices or milk.
- Refrigerate ground beef and perishable food right away after shopping.
- Wash hands and food utensils with hot, soapy water after handling meat and poultry.
- Avoid cooked food that has been kept at room temperature for several hours.

Travelers can minimize their risk for "traveler's diarrhea" by practicing the following effective preventive measures:

- Avoid eating foods or drinking beverages purchased from street vendors or restaurants where unhygienic conditions are present.
- Wash hands with soap when available.
- Avoid eating raw or undercooked meat and seafood.
- Avoid eating raw fruits (e.g., oranges, bananas, avocados) and vegetables unless the traveler peels them.
- Avoid ice unless it has been made from safe water.
- Avoid dishes containing raw or undercooked eggs.
- NOTE: Due to the emergence of antimicrobial resistance, prophylactic antibiotics are not recommended for most travelers.

Hiatal Hernia

Part of the stomach passes through the esophageal hiatus in the diaphragm into the chest cavity

PATHOPHYSIOLOGY

- About 95% are classified as sliding hernias where the gastroesophageal junction is displaced above the diaphragm; 5% of hernias are paraesophageal, typically occurring after surgical management of reflux
- Very common; occurs most often in females and older adults
- Associated with obesity, pregnancy, heavy lifting, hard coughing, and straining with bowel movements

PATIENT DATA

Subjective Data

- Most are asymptomatic and discovered incidentally
- May have symptoms of gastroesophageal reflux, like epigastric pain and/or heartburn, that worsens with lying down and is relieved by sitting up or antacids, water brash (mouth fills with fluid from the esophagus), or dysphagia
- Symptoms of incarcerated hernia include sudden onset of vomiting, pain, and complete dysphagia

Objective Data

- Generally, no physical examination findings

Stomach and Duodenal Ulcers (Peptic Ulcer Disease)

Chronic circumscribed break in the stomach or duodenal mucosa that scars with healing

PATHOPHYSIOLOGY

- Typically develops from infection with *Helicobacter pylori* resulting in increased gastrin production and acid secretion
- May be caused by Zollinger-Ellison syndrome, a rare disorder where one or more tumors (gastrinomas) secrete gastrin
- Occurs approximately twice as often in males as in females
- Long-term use of aspirin or NSAIDs can increase risk

PATIENT DATA

Subjective Data

- Localized epigastric pain that occurs when the stomach is empty and is relieved by food or antacids
- With upper gastrointestinal bleeding, symptoms include hematemesis and melena; significant blood loss may result in dizziness and syncope

Objective Data

- Anterior stomach wall ulcers may produce tenderness on palpation of the abdomen
- Ulcers occur on both the anterior and posterior walls of the duodenal bulb; anterior ulcers are more likely to perforate, whereas posterior ulcers are more likely to bleed
- Perforation of the duodenum presents with signs of an acute abdomen (abdominal distention, rebound, and guarding)
- With significant bleeding, may show hypotension and tachycardia

Crohn Disease

Chronic inflammatory disorder that can affect any part of the gastrointestinal tract that produces ulceration, fibrosis, and malabsorption; terminal ileum and colon are the most common sites

PATHOPHYSIOLOGY

- Cause is unknown but is thought to be immune related and occurs from an imbalance between proinflammatory and antiinflammatory mediators in genetically susceptible individuals
- Smokers are more likely to develop Crohn disease and the disease course is more complicated than nonsmokers (Veloso, 2016)

PATIENT DATA

Subjective Data

- Chronic diarrhea with compromised nutritional status
- Other systemic manifestations may include arthritis, iritis, and erythema nodosum
- Disease course characterized by unpredictable flares and remissions

Objective Data

- May have RLQ tenderness
- Abdominal mass may be palpated secondary to thickened or inflamed bowel
- Perianal skin tags, fistulae, and abscesses may be seen
- Extraintestinal examination findings include erythema nodosum and pyoderma gangrenosum as well as arthritis involving the large joints
- Colonoscopy and pathology show characteristic cobblestone appearance of the mucosa
- Fistula and abscess formation, sometimes extending to the skin, is common (Fig. 18.34) as well as perianal skin tags (Fig. 18.35).

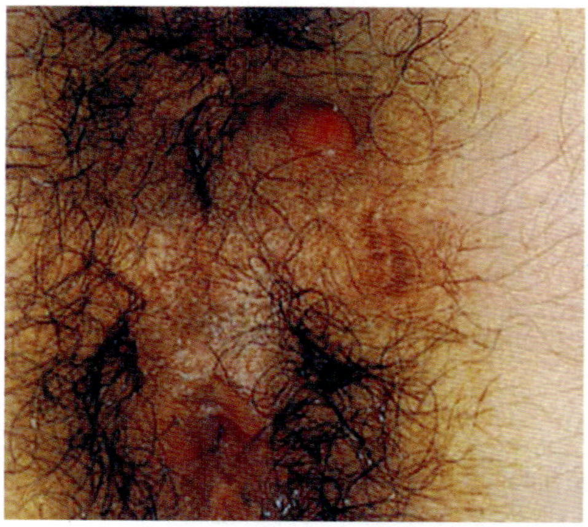

FIG. 18.34 Crohn disease showing a perianal abscess, a raised and erythematous lesion, above a small scar from a prior incision and drainage procedure. (From Zitelli, B. J., & Davis, H. W. (2012). Atlas of pediatric physical diagnosis (6th ed.). St. Louis: Mosby.)

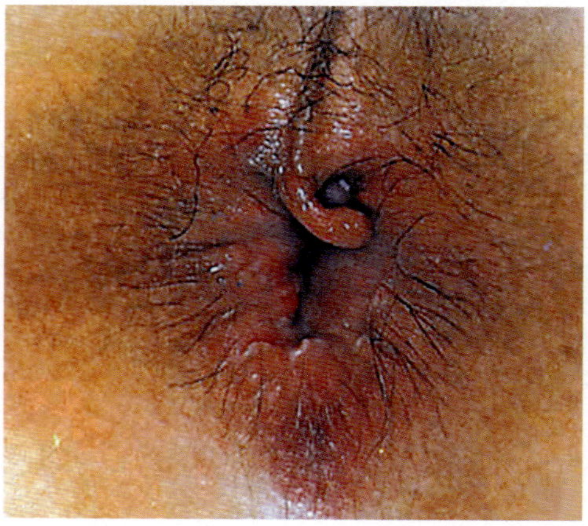

FIG. 18.35 Crohn disease. Note a scar from a previous incision and drainage. Perianal skin tags are common in Crohn disease and a good clue to diagnosis. (From Zitelli, B. J., & Davis, H. W. (2012). Atlas of pediatric physical diagnosis (6th ed.). St. Louis: Mosby.)

Ulcerative Colitis

Chronic inflammatory disorder of the colon and rectum that produces mucosal friability and areas of ulceration

PATHOPHYSIOLOGY

- Cause is unknown, but immunologic, environmental, and genetic factors have been implicated
- Active chronic ulcerative colitis predisposes an individual to developing colon cancer
- Males and females equally affected
- Typically develops between 15 and 30 years of age or after age 60
- Occurs more often in those with a family history of inflammatory bowel disease and those of Jewish descent

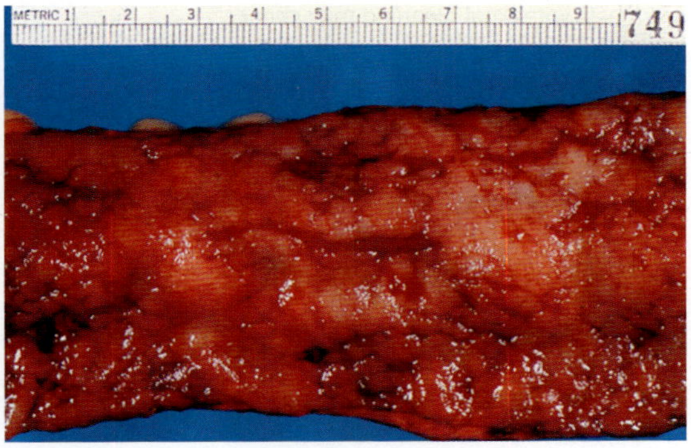

FIG. 18.36 Ulcerative colitis showing severe mucosal edema and inflammation with ulcerations and bleeding. (From Doughty, D. B., & Jackson, D. B. (1993). Gastrointestinal disorders. St. Louis: Mosby.)

PATIENT DATA

Subjective Data

- Bloody, frequent, watery diarrhea, with as many as 20–30 diarrheal stools per day
- May exhibit weight loss, fatigue, and general debilitation
- May range from mild to severe, depending on the degree of colon involvement
- May remain in remission for years after an acute phase of the illness
- Sclerosing cholangitis (inflammation, scarring, and destruction of bile ducts) may present with fatigue and jaundice

Objective Data

- Generally, do not have fistulae or perianal disease
- Contrast radiographs typically show loss of the normal mucosal pattern
- Sclerosing cholangitis may occur with a cholestatic pattern of elevated transaminase levels
- Endoscopic findings show mucosal edema with ulcerations and bleeding (Fig. 18.36)

Gastric Cancer

Malignancy that arises from epithelial cells of the mucous membrane

PATHOPHYSIOLOGY

- One of the most common malignancies worldwide
- Twice as common in males than in females
- *Helicobacter pylori* infection is a major risk factor
- Other modifiable risk factors include tobacco use, alcohol consumption, and poor diet
- Up to 10% of cases are familial
- Most commonly found in lower half of the stomach
- In early stages, the growth is confined to the mucosa and submucosa; as disease progresses, the muscular layer of the stomach becomes involved; metastases, local and distant, are common

PATIENT DATA

Subjective Data

- May have vague and nonspecific symptoms, including loss of appetite, feeling of fullness, weight loss, dysphagia, and persistent epigastric pain

Objective Data

- May have midepigastric tenderness, hepatomegaly, enlarged supraclavicular nodes, and ascites
- An epigastric mass may be palpable in the late stages of disease

Diverticular Disease

Small bulges or saclike outpouchings (diverticula) through colonic muscle in the intestine

PATHOPHYSIOLOGY

- May involve any part of the gastrointestinal tract; the sigmoid is the most commonly affected location (Fig. 18.37)
- Cause unknown but may be caused by colonic dysmotility, defective muscular structure, and defects in collagen and aging

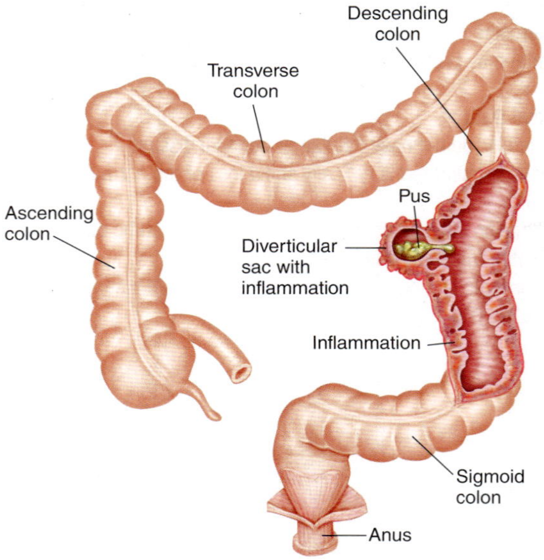

FIG. 18.37 Diverticulosis (diverticulitis). (From Doughty, D. B., & Jackson, D. B. (1993). Gastrointestinal disorders. St. Louis: Mosby.)

PATIENT DATA

Subjective Data

- Most patients are asymptomatic
- With diverticulitis (when diverticula become inflamed), may experience left lower quadrant pain, anorexia, nausea, vomiting, and altered bowel habits (usually constipation)
- Pain usually localizes to the site of inflammation

Objective Data

- May have abdominal distention with tympany to percussion with decreased bowel sounds and localized tenderness (see Table 18.2)
- Lower gastrointestinal bleeding may occur

Colon Cancer (Colorectal Cancer)

May involve the rectum, sigmoid, proximal, and descending colon

PATHOPHYSIOLOGY

- About 100,000 new cases of colon cancer and 40,000 new cases of rectal cancer are diagnosed each year in the United States
- Lifetime risk for males and females is about 4% (see Risk Factors box earlier in the chapter)

PATIENT DATA

Subjective Data

- Symptoms depend on cancer location, size, and presence of metastases
- May describe abdominal pain, blood in the stool, or a recent change in the frequency or character of stools
- Earliest sign may be occult blood in the stool, which can be detected by guaiac-based fecal occult blood testing (gFOBT)

Objective Data

- Few early examination findings
- If disease has progressed, may have palpable abdominal mass in right or left lower quadrant or show signs of anemia from occult blood loss (e.g., pallor and tachycardia)
- Rectal cancer may be palpable by digital rectal examination (see Chapter 21)
- Evidence-Based Practice in Physical Examination box highlights recent colon cancer screening test recommendations

Evidence-Based Practice in Physical Examination

Screening for Colorectal Cancer

Of cancers affecting females and males, colorectal cancer is the third leading cause of cancer-related deaths in the United States, accounting for about 52,000 deaths each year. Many of these deaths are preventable through appropriate screening. Colorectal cancer is most often diagnosed in individuals 65 to 74 years of age, though a rise in cancer diagnoses is occurring in adults 40 to 49 years of age. In 2021, the U.S. Preventive Services Task Force (USPSTF) updated its previous recommendations based on a review of the evidence assessing both benefits and harms of screening in adults 40 years of age or older. With high certainty of substantial net benefit, the USPSTF recommends colorectal cancer screening for adults 50 to 75 years of age. They also recommend screening adults 45 to 49 years of age with moderate certainty of moderate net benefit. For individuals 76 to 86 years of age who have been screened in the past, there was moderate certainty of a small net benefit. The recommendations apply to asymptomatic adults 45 years and older who are at average risk of colorectal cancer (i.e., no prior diagnosis of colorectal cancer, adenomatous polyps, or inflammatory bowel disease; no personal diagnosis or family history of known genetic disorders predisposing them to colorectal cancer). Colorectal screening tests fall into two categories: (1) stool-based tests to primarily identify colorectal cancer and (2) direct visualization tests to detect both cancer and premalignant adenomatous polyps.

The USPSTF discusses the following screening tests in their 2021 recommendation:

- Annual guaiac-based fecal occult blood test (gFOBT) with high test sensitivity
- Annual fecal immunochemical test (FIT) with high test sensitivity
- Multitarget stool DNA test (sDNA-FIT) with high sensitivity (testing interval 1 to 3 years per manufacturer)
- Colonoscopy every 10 years
- Computed tomography colonography every 5 years
- Flexible sigmoidoscopy (FSIG) every 5 years
- FSIG every 10 years with FIT every year

From U.S. Preventive Services Task Force. (2021). Screening for colorectal cancer: U.S. Preventive Services Task Force Recommendation Statement. *JAMA, 325*(19), 1965–1977.

HEPATOBILIARY SYSTEM

Hepatitis

Inflammatory process characterized by diffuse or patchy hepatocellular necrosis

PATHOPHYSIOLOGY

- Most commonly caused by viral infection, alcohol, drugs, or toxins
- Acute viral hepatitis is caused by at least five distinct agents; see Risk Factors box regarding hepatitis A, B, and C earlier in the chapter
- Hepatitis D occurs only in those infected with hepatitis B, either as a coinfection in acute hepatitis B or as a superinfection in chronic hepatitis B
- Hepatitis E is a self-limited type that may occur after a natural disaster because of fecal-contaminated water or food

PATIENT DATA

Subjective Data

- Some are asymptomatic; others report jaundice, anorexia, abdominal pain, clay-colored stools, tea-colored urine, and fatigue

Objective Data

- Liver function tests are abnormal
- Examination findings may include jaundice and hepatomegaly
- With severe or progressive disease, may develop cirrhosis with its associated examination findings

Cirrhosis

Late stage of liver disease characterized by fibrosis (scarring), alteration of normal hepatic architecture, and loss of function

PATHOPHYSIOLOGY

- Progression of liver disease to cirrhosis can happen over weeks to years
- Signs and symptoms occur as a result of decreased liver synthetic function, decreased detoxification capabilities, or portal hypertension
- Most common causes in the United States are hepatitis C and alcohol-associated liver disease
- Less common causes include autoimmune hepatitis, primary biliary cirrhosis, Wilson disease, hemochromatosis, α_1-antitrypsin deficiency, and sarcoidosis

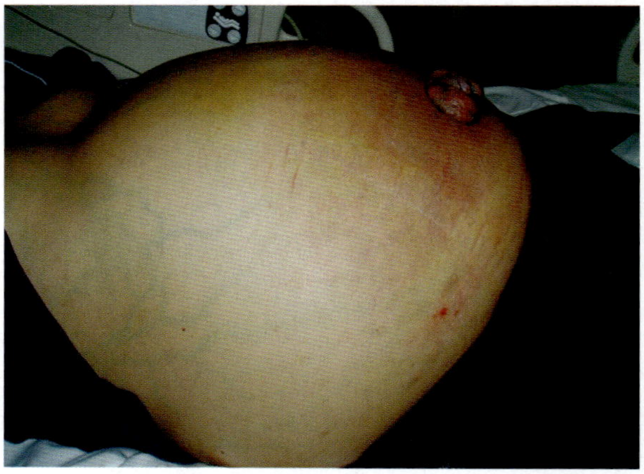

FIG. 18.38 Marked ascites and an umbilical hernia, which had ruptured a few days before the photograph, in a patient with cirrhosis and portal hypertension secondary to hepatitis C.

PATIENT DATA

Subjective Data

- May be asymptomatic; others report jaundice, anorexia, abdominal pain, clay-colored stools, tea-colored urine, and fatigue
- May describe prominent abdominal vasculature, cutaneous spider angiomas, hematemesis, and abdominal fullness

Objective Data

- On examination, the liver is initially enlarged with a firm, nontender border on palpation; as scarring progresses, liver size is reduced and generally cannot be palpated
- Neurologic examination abnormalities may be seen (e.g., hepatic encephalopathy)
- With progressive disease, portal hypertension and ascites may occur (Fig. 18.38)
- Muscle wasting and nutritional deficiencies may be evident in late-stage disease
- May have abnormal laboratory values (e.g., liver function tests and coagulopathy)

Hepatocellular Carcinoma

Primary tumor of the liver that usually occurs in patients with chronic liver disease

PATHOPHYSIOLOGY

- Most common type of liver cancer in the United States
- Risk factors include hepatitis C infection, hepatitis B infection, excessive alcohol intake, obesity, diabetes, nonalcoholic fatty liver disease (NAFLD), and tobacco use
- Median survival time from diagnosis is months (Petrick et al., 2016)
- Can metastasize to the lungs, portal vein, periportal nodes, bone, and brain
- Widespread vaccination for hepatitis A and B, routine screening for hepatitis B and C, and treatment of hepatitis C may reduce the incidence

PATIENT DATA

Subjective Data

- Symptoms may include jaundice, anorexia, fatigue, abdominal fullness, clay-colored stools, and tea-colored urine

Objective Data

- On examination, hepatomegaly with a hard, irregular liver border may be palpated
- Liver nodules may be present and palpable, and the liver may be tender or nontender
- Examination findings related to cirrhosis may be seen (see earlier)

Cholelithiasis

Stone formation in the gallbladder occurs when certain substances reach a high concentration in bile and produce crystals

PATHOPHYSIOLOGY

- Crystals mix with mucus and form gallbladder sludge; over time, the crystals enlarge, mix, and form stones
- Main substances involved in gallstone formation are cholesterol (>80%) and calcium bilirubinate
- Chronic disease can result in fibrosis and gallbladder dysfunction and predispose to gallbladder cancer

PATIENT DATA

Subjective Data

- Many patients are asymptomatic
- Symptoms may include indigestion, colic, and mild transient jaundice

Objective Data

- Condition commonly produces episodes of acute cholecystitis

Cholecystitis

Inflammatory process of the gallbladder most commonly due to obstruction of the cystic duct from cholelithiasis, which may be acute or chronic

PATHOPHYSIOLOGY

- With cystic duct obstruction, the gallbladder becomes distended and blood flow is compromised, leading to ischemia and inflammation
- Acute cholecystitis has associated stone formation (cholelithiasis) in 90% of cases, causing obstruction and inflammation
- Acute cholecystitis without stones (acalculous) results from any condition that affects the regular emptying and filling of the gallbladder, such as immobilization with major surgery, trauma, sepsis, or long-term total parenteral nutrition
- Chronic cholecystitis refers to repeated attacks of acute cholecystitis in a gallbladder that is scarred and contracted

PATIENT DATA

Subjective Data

- Primary symptom is right upper quadrant (RUQ) pain with radiation around the mid-torso to the right scapular region; pain is abrupt and severe and lasts for 2–4 hours
- May have associated symptoms including fever, jaundice, and anorexia
- With chronic cholecystitis may exhibit fat intolerance, flatulence, nausea, anorexia, and nonspecific abdominal pain

Objective Data

- In acute cholecystitis, classic examination finding is marked tenderness in the RUQ or epigastrium (see Table 18.2)
- Involuntary guarding or rebound tenderness may be present
- Some may have a full palpable gallbladder in the RUQ
- Some may have subtle examination findings, including diffuse abdominal pain; others may have an unremarkable examination
- In chronic cholecystitis, the gallbladder is typically not palpated due to fibrosis

Metabolic Dysfunction–Associated Steatotic Liver Disease

Steatotic liver disease in patients with at least one risk factor for cardiometabolic dysfunction and minimal or no alcohol consumption

PATHOPHYSIOLOGY

- Formerly known as *nonalcoholic fatty liver disease* (NAFLD), patients have at least one metabolic risk factor: obesity, hypertension, dyslipidemia, or type 2 diabetes mellitus
- Disease may progress to metabolic dysfunction–associated steatotic liver disease (MASLD) with metabolic dysfunction-associated steatohepatitis (MASH) where patients have evidence of hepatocellular injury (formerly known as nonalcoholic steatohepatitis [NASH])
- Pathogenesis is unclear, though likely due to inflammation and insulin resistance; genetic variants have been associated with disease progression
- Worldwide prevalence of 30%, with higher incidence in males compared with females (Le et al., 2023)

PATIENT DATA

Subjective Data

- Most patients are asymptomatic
- Some describe vague RUQ discomfort, fatigue, malaise, and jaundice

Objective Data

- Usually identified after discovering abnormal liver function tests; most have elevated transaminases with aspartate aminotransferase (AST) and alanine aminotransferase (ALT) being two to three times the upper limits of normal
- Other than an elevated body mass index (BMI; overweight or obese by criteria), usually no other clinical signs
- Some patients may have hepatomegaly
- In more severe disease, patients may have jaundice, splenomegaly, and ascites
- Liver steatosis seen on abdominal ultrasound, computed tomography (CT), or magnetic resonance imaging (MRI)
- Liver biopsy may be needed if diagnosis is uncertain despite laboratory and imaging findings

PANCREAS

Acute Pancreatitis

Acute inflammatory process in which release of pancreatic enzymes results in pancreatic glandular autodigestion

PATHOPHYSIOLOGY

- Although unclear what pathophysiologic mechanism initiates acute pancreatitis, there are a number of known causes, including biliary disease (cholelithiasis) and chronic alcohol use, accounting for approximately 80% of cases

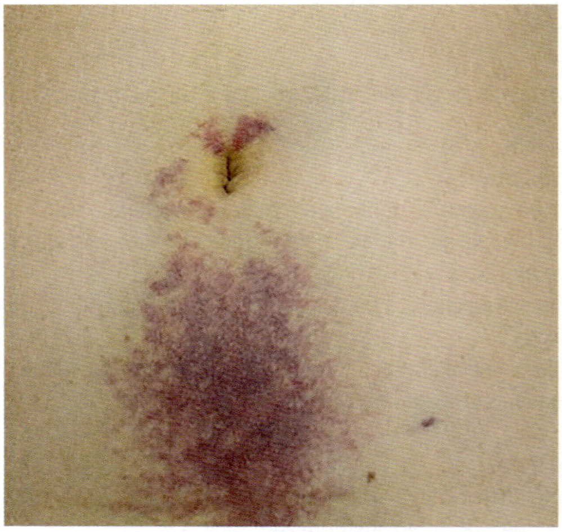

FIG. 18.39 Cullen sign seen in a patient with rectus sheath hematoma. (From Harris, S., & Naina, H. V. (2008). Cullen's sign revisited. *American Journal of Medicine*, *121*(8), 682–683.)

PATIENT DATA

Subjective Data

- Symptoms range from mild to severe sudden onset of persistent epigastric pain that may radiate to the back; pain is typically described as constant and dull
- Often associated with nausea, vomiting, abdominal distention, fever, and anorexia

Objective Data

- Most patients have diffuse abdominal tenderness to palpation; involuntary guarding and abdominal distention can occur (see Table 18.2)
- Decreased bowel sounds may be appreciated as a result of an ileus
- In severe necrotizing pancreatitis, Cullen and Grey Turner signs may be appreciated on examination (see Table 18.5 and Figs. 18.39 and 18.40)
- Some may present with fever and tachycardia
- Others may have dyspnea due to diaphragm irritation
- Pancreatic enzymes (amylase and lipase) are elevated

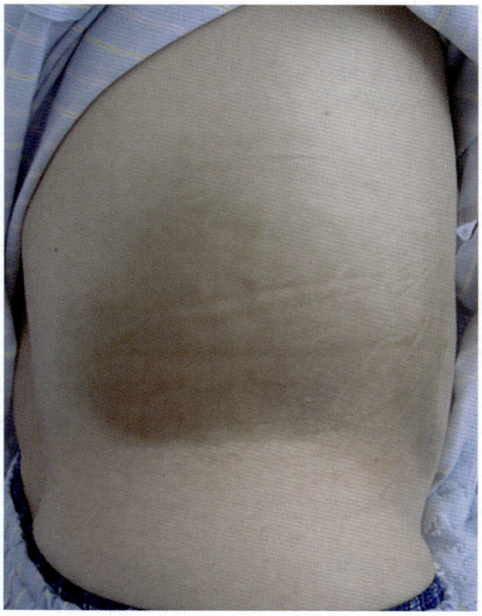

FIG. 18.40 Grey Turner sign. A dirty green ecchymosis developed in the right flank on the third day of hospitalization.

Chronic Pancreatitis

Chronic inflammatory process of the pancreas, characterized by irreversible morphologic changes resulting in atrophy, fibrosis, and pancreatic calcifications

PATHOPHYSIOLOGY

- Most common cause is chronic alcohol use; other causes include congenital structural abnormalities of the pancreas, hereditary pancreatitis, cystic fibrosis, medication-induced disease, and autoimmune pancreatitis

PATIENT DATA

Subjective Data

- Symptoms may include constant, unremitting abdominal pain; weight loss; and steatorrhea

Objective Data

- Examination findings are similar to those in acute pancreatitis; however, with chronic disease, there is a greater likelihood of pseudocyst formation
- With advanced disease, some may exhibit signs of malnutrition with decreased subcutaneous fat and temporal wasting
- Pancreatic enzyme levels (amylase and lipase) are elevated, and glucose intolerance may be seen

SPLEEN

Spleen Laceration/Rupture

PATHOPHYSIOLOGY

- Most commonly injured organ in abdominal trauma because of its anatomic location
- Mechanism of injury can be either blunt or penetrating but is more often blunt (e.g., from motor vehicle crashes)

PATIENT DATA

Subjective Data

- Symptoms include pain in the left upper quadrant with radiation to the left shoulder (positive Kehr sign); see Table 18.5
- Depending on degree of blood loss, may have symptoms of hypovolemia (e.g., lightheadedness, tachycardia, syncope)
- See Chapter 26

Objective Data

- Examination is remarkable for left upper quadrant pain with palpation; signs of peritoneal irritation may be seen (involuntary guarding or rebound tenderness; see Table 18.2)
- Diagnosis is made by paracentesis or CT
- Depending on the degree of blood loss, patients may present with hypotension and a decreasing hematocrit

KIDNEY

Acute Glomerulonephritis

Inflammation of the capillary loops of the renal glomeruli

PATHOPHYSIOLOGY

- Accounts for about 20% of chronic kidney disease
- Results from immune complex deposition or formation
- Many causes; most common include infection (poststreptococcal) and immune mediated (IgA nephropathy)

PATIENT DATA

Subjective Data

- Symptoms are usually nonspecific and include nausea and malaise; flank pain may be reported as well as headache secondary to hypertension
- Some patients report tea-colored urine or gross hematuria
- May be asymptomatic and identified with an elevated blood pressure reading

Objective Data

- May have an unremarkable examination and normal blood pressure
- Examination findings may include edema, hypertension, and oliguria
- About 85% of affected children develop peripheral and periorbital edema
- Microscopic hematuria occurs in all affected patients (red blood cell casts are seen on urine microscopy)

Hydronephrosis

Dilation of the renal pelvis and calyces due to an obstruction of urine flow anywhere from the urethral meatus to the kidneys

PATHOPHYSIOLOGY

- Increasing ureteral pressure from urine results in changes in glomerular filtration, tubular function, and renal blood flow

PATIENT DATA

Subjective Data

- With an acute obstruction, may have intermittent, severe pain (renal colic) with nausea and vomiting
- With secondary infection, may report abdominal pain, flank pain, hematuria, and fever

Objective Data

- Most will have an unremarkable physical examination
- In severe cases, the kidneys may be palpable during the abdominal examination; costovertebral angle tenderness may be present
- With lower urinary tract obstruction, a distended bladder may be palpable (e.g., posterior urethral valves in a newborn)
- Most are asymptomatic; hydronephrosis is found during radiologic screening (e.g., fetal ultrasound) or diagnostic imaging

Pyelonephritis

Infection of the kidney and renal pelvis

PATHOPHYSIOLOGY

- Gram-negative bacilli (*Escherichia coli* and *Klebsiella*) and *Enterococcus faecalis* are the most common pathogens
- Less common organisms occur in hospitalized patients and/or those with indwelling catheters
- Risk factors include indwelling catheters, diabetes mellitus, sexual activity, prior history of urinary tract infections (UTIs), vesicoureteral reflux (infants and children), and urinary incontinence (older adults)

PATIENT DATA

Subjective Data

- Typically present with fever, dysuria, and flank pain
- Other symptoms include rigors, polyuria, urinary frequency, urgency, and hematuria

Objective Data

- Most are generally ill appearing with significant pain or discomfort
- Fever and costovertebral angle (CVA) tenderness distinguish pyelonephritis from uncomplicated UTIs
- On laboratory evaluation, pyuria and bacteriuria are present and confirm the diagnosis

Renal Abscess

Localized infection in the medulla or cortex of the kidney

PATHOPHYSIOLOGY

- Abscesses in the renal cortex are often caused by gram-positive organisms (*Staphylococcus aureus* and *Enterococcus faecalis*)
- Medullary abscesses are commonly caused by gram-negative bacilli (*Escherichia coli* and *Klebsiella*)

PATIENT DATA

Subjective Data

- Symptoms of pyelonephritis (chills, fever, dysuria, and flank pain) persist beyond 72 hours of appropriate antibiotic therapy

Objective Data

- Similar to pyelonephritis, most are generally ill appearing with fever and significant pain or discomfort
- CVA tenderness is typically present on examination
- Urinalysis may show pyuria and bacteriuria if the abscess is in the renal medulla; pyuria may be the only laboratory finding if the abscess is located in the cortex
- Renal imaging: ultrasound, CT, or MRI are common diagnostic tools

Renal Calculi

Stones formed in the pelvis of the kidney associated with obstruction and infections in the urinary tract

PATHOPHYSIOLOGY

- Stones are composed of calcium, oxalate, uric acid, cystine, xanthine, and phosphate
- Situations leading to alkaline urine are conducive to calcium and phosphate stone formation; acidic urine (low PH) promotes cystine and uric acid stone formation; urine temperature, ionic strength, and concentration also affect stone formation
- About twice as prevalent in males compared with females

PATIENT DATA

Subjective Data

- Symptoms include fever, dysuria, hematuria, and flank pain
- Renal colic is marked by severe, cramping flank pain with nausea and vomiting; as the stone passes through the ureter, the pain typically moves from the flank to the groin and then to the scrotal or labial area (see Table 18.2)

Objective Data

- Most present to an emergency or urgent care facility with severe, cramping pain
- Examination findings may include CVA tenderness and/or abdominal tenderness with palpation
- Urinalysis may show microscopic hematuria; an elevated urinary calcium-to-creatinine ratio is suggestive

Infants

Intussusception

Prolapse, or telescoping, of one segment of intestine into another causes intestinal obstruction

PATHOPHYSIOLOGY

- Commonly occurs in infants between 3 and 12 months old and is the most common cause of bowel obstruction in infants and children 3 months to 6 years of age; four times as likely to occur in females as in males
- Some episodes may resolve spontaneously, but if untreated, most cases result in bowel infarction, perforation, and peritonitis
- Although the cause of most cases is unknown, lymph tissue hyperplasia is thought to lead to mucosal prolapse, with the most common site being the terminal ileum into the colon; in a small percentage of children, lead points are identified (Meckel diverticulum, polyp, lymphoma); lead points are more common in children older than 2 years
- In adults, about 1%–5% of bowel obstruction is from intussusception; usually there is a pathologic lead point (malignancy in more than half of cases; Marinis et al., 2009; Fig. 18.41)

PATIENT DATA

Subjective Data

- Symptoms include acute intermittent abdominal pain, abdominal distention, and vomiting
- Symptoms can be dramatic in onset; previously well child may start with paroxysms of crying and severe abdominal pain, sometimes awakening from sleep; intermittent bouts of lethargy may also occur
- Child is often inconsolable, sometimes with legs and knees flexed (doubled up) with pain
- Stool appears normal in the early stages; as ischemia progresses, subsequent stools may be mixed with blood and mucus with a red currant jelly appearance (Fig. 18.42)

Objective Data

- Sausage-shaped mass may be palpated in the right or left upper quadrant, whereas the right lower quadrant feels empty (positive Dance sign)
- As disease progresses, may display findings of bowel perforation (abdominal distention and guarding)
- Diagnosis and treatment most often carried out with the use of an air-contrast enema

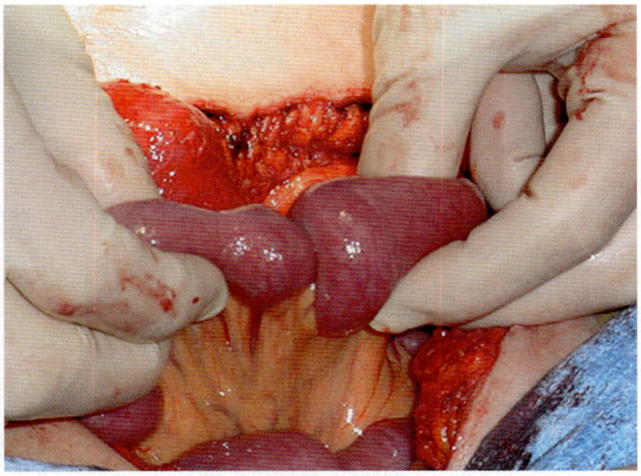

FIG. 18.41 Jejunojejunal intussusception in an adult patient.

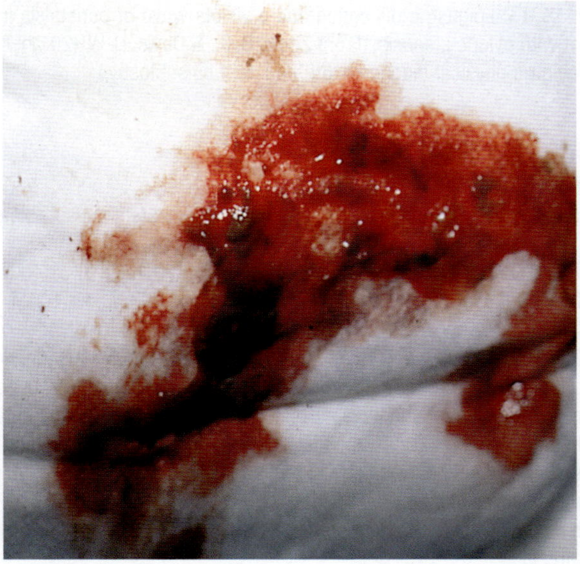

FIG 18.42 The intussusception—the invaginated portion of bowel—becomes congested and ischemic, leading to the passage of bloody stool mixed with mucus (currant jelly stool). (From Zitelli, B. J., & Davis, H. W. (2018). Zitelli and Davis' atlas of pediatric physical diagnosis (7th ed.). Philadelphia: Elsevier.)

Pyloric Stenosis

Hypertrophy of the circular muscle of the pylorus, leading to obstruction of the pyloric sphincter

PATHOPHYSIOLOGY

- Occurs in 1–3/1000 infants in the United States; males are affected about four times as often as females, and there is a strong familial tendency
- Cause is unknown; an association has been found with use of erythromycin

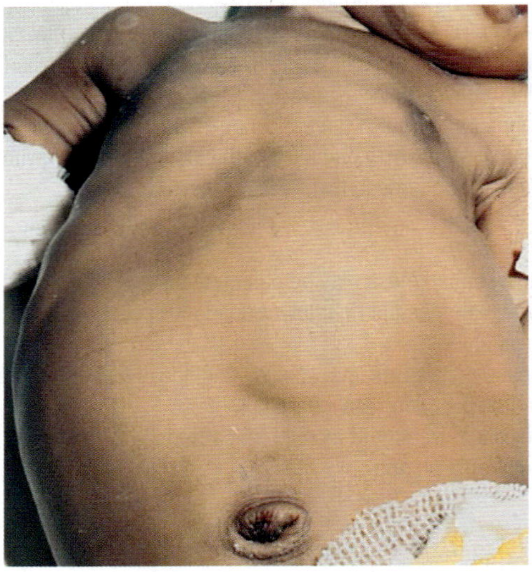

FIG. 18.43 Epigastric distention and a visible wave of peristalsis in an infant with pyloric stenosis. (From Zitelli, B. J., & Davis, H. W. (2012). Atlas of pediatric physical diagnosis (6th ed.). St. Louis: Mosby.)

PATIENT DATA

Subjective Data

- Symptoms typically develop after several weeks of age and include regurgitation progressing to projectile vomiting (i.e., vigorous, shoots out of the mouth, and carries a short distance); feeding eagerly (even after a vomiting episode); and failure to gain weight

Objective Data

- Epigastric distention from an obstructed stomach may be seen as well as a visible wave of peristalsis (left to right; Fig. 18.43)
- Small, rounded, olive-shaped mass sometimes palpable in the right upper quadrant, particularly after the infant vomits
- Ultrasound and/or surgical consult should be obtained with suspected cases

Meconium Ileus

Distal intestinal obstruction caused by thick, inspissated, impacted meconium in the lower intestine of a newborn

PATHOPHYSIOLOGY

- May be the first manifestation of cystic fibrosis (CF); about 10%–20% of newborns with CF have meconium ileus
- Pancreatic insufficiency or congenital pancreatic anomalies (pancreatic duct stenosis) are thought to be contributing factors; however, many affected infants have normal pancreatic function and structure
- In uncomplicated cases, the distal ileum narrows with proximal intestinal distention; up to one-half of cases are complicated (volvulus, atresia, or meconium peritonitis)
- If condition occurs in utero, fetal volvulus may cause intestinal atresia

PATIENT DATA

Subjective Data

- Most affected newborns present with failure to pass meconium in the first 24 hours after birth
- Symptoms related to distal intestinal obstruction develop (vomiting and abdominal distention)

Objective Data

- Newborns will present with abdominal distention
- In complicated cases (volvulus), infants can present with signs of shock (e.g., tachycardia and hypotension)
- Uncomplicated cases are treated with hyperosmolar enemas under fluoroscopic guidance; resolution occurs in more than half of affected infants

Biliary Atresia

Congenital obstruction or absence of some or all of the bile duct system, resulting in bile flow obstruction; most have complete absence of entire extra-hepatic biliary tree

PATHOPHYSIOLOGY

- Classified as postnatal onset (85%–90% of cases) or embryonic onset
- In postnatal onset, disease inflammation and necrosis of extrahepatic bile ducts are thought to result from a perinatal insult (e.g., viral infection)
- Embryonic onset is thought to result from gene mutations controlling bile duct formation and differentiation early in gestation; intrahepatic cholestasis and biliary tract fibrosis develop; this type is associated with other congenital anomalies (polysplenia syndrome)

PATIENT DATA

Subjective Data

- Symptoms of neonatal cholestasis develop in the first several weeks of life and include jaundice, light clay-colored stools, and dark urine (Fig. 18.44)
- Newborns may show failure to gain weight or have normal weight gain

Objective Data

- Most infants are full term and develop jaundice in the first 2 months of life; hepatomegaly may be firm to palpation
- Splenomegaly may occur and indicates progressive disease with portal hypertension (Fig. 18.45)
- In the embryonic type, infants may have heart murmurs, indicating associated congenital heart disease
- Abdominal ultrasound is diagnostic; without prompt surgical correction, secondary biliary cirrhosis occurs

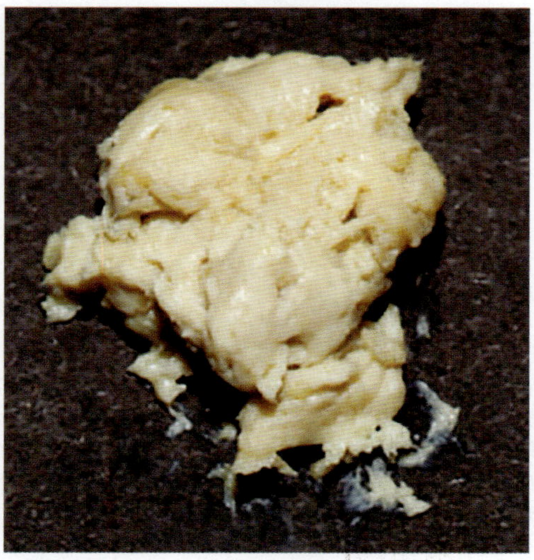

FIG. 18.44 Pale stool secondary to biliary atresia. (From Lissauer, T. & Will, C. (2017). Illustrated textbook of paediatrics (5th ed.). Philadelphia: Elsevier.)

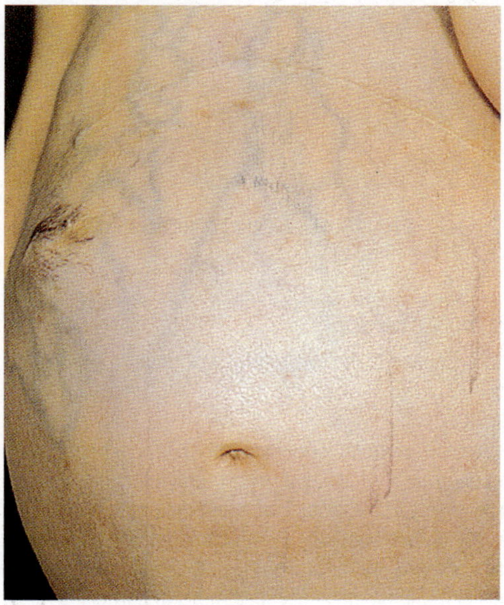

FIG. 18.45 Child with biliary atresia and cirrhosis with prominent abdominal veins. (From Zitelli, B. J., & Davis, H. W. (2012). Atlas of pediatric physical diagnosis (6th ed.). St. Louis: Mosby.)

Meckel Diverticulum

Outpouching of the ileum that varies in size from a small appendiceal process to a segment of bowel several inches long, often in the proximity of the ileocecal valve

PATHOPHYSIOLOGY

- Develops from incomplete obliteration of the vitelline duct resulting in a blind-ending pouch that contains all the mucosal layers in the ileum (Fig. 18.46)
- Most common congenital anomaly of the gastrointestinal tract, occurring in about 2% of the general population

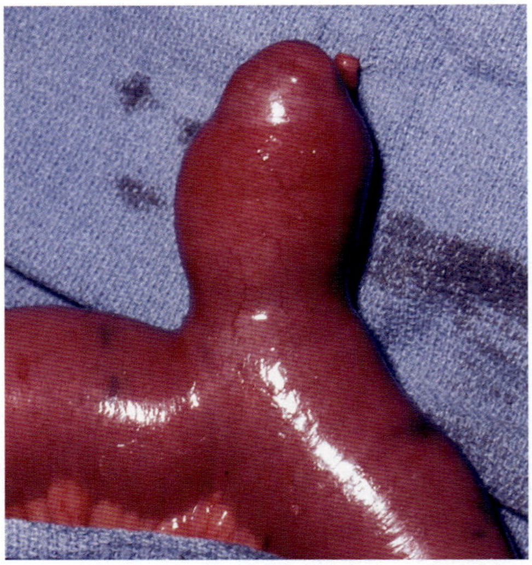

FIG. 18.46 Meckel diverticulum.

PATIENT DATA

Subjective Data

- Most are asymptomatic
- Often found as an incidental finding during a radiologic study or intra-abdominal surgery for other reasons
- In children, bright or dark red rectal bleeding with little, if any, abdominal pain is a common presenting concern
- Some present with abdominal pain that can be severe in character; others may present with signs of intestinal obstruction or diverticulitis, similar to acute appendicitis with bilious emesis

Objective Data

- Painless rectal bleeding is the most common presenting finding on examination
- Some patients present with intestinal obstruction (abdominal tenderness, involuntary guarding) and rebound tenderness); in severe cases, perforation can occur with peritoneal signs and hypovolemic shock (tachycardia and hypotension)

Necrotizing Enterocolitis

Inflammatory disease of the gastrointestinal mucosa associated with prematurity and gut immaturity

PATHOPHYSIOLOGY

- Most common gastrointestinal emergency in neonates
- Varying degrees of mucosal or transmural intestinal necrosis occur, most commonly in the distal ileum and proximal colon
- Cause is unknown but likely multifactorial; an infectious cause is thought to have a primary role in the development; coagulation necrosis is found on intestinal specimens at surgery
- Incidence is 1%–5% of infants in neonatal intensive care units; incidence and mortality are inversely related to gestational age

PATIENT DATA

Subjective Data

- Symptoms may be subtle, including inability to tolerate feedings (oral or nasogastric); may also present suddenly and progress quickly
- Abdominal distention, vomiting, and bloody stools often prompt an evaluation in at-risk neonates

Objective Data

- May display temperature instability and subtle signs of distress
- Examination signs may include lethargy, abdominal distention, apnea, and respiratory distress
- Plain abdominal radiograph may show pneumatosis intestinalis (air in the bowel wall)
- Often fatal due to complications of intestinal perforation and sepsis

Children

Neuroblastoma

Solid malignancy of embryonal origin in the peripheral sympathetic nervous system

PATHOPHYSIOLOGY

- Considered a spectrum of tumors of varying degrees of neural differentiation
- Although commonly arising from the adrenal medulla, may occur anywhere along the craniospinal axis
- Cause is unknown, but genetic and environmental factors are proposed; associations have been found with parental occupational chemical exposures, and familial cases have been reported

PATIENT DATA

Subjective Data

- Typically presents as an asymptomatic abdominal mass in a young child
- Symptoms may include malaise, loss of appetite, weight loss, and protrusion of one or both eyes

Objective Data

- Examination findings include a firm, fixed, nontender, irregular, and nodular abdominal mass that crosses the midline
- Metastases to the periorbital region result in proptosis and infraorbital ecchymoses
- Horner syndrome, ataxia, and opsomyoclonus ("dancing eyes and dancing feet") may be seen on physical examination
- Radiologic studies may show a calcified mass with hemorrhage into surrounding structures

Wilms Tumor (Nephroblastoma)

Most common intra-abdominal tumor of childhood; usually appears between 3 and 5 years of age

PATHOPHYSIOLOGY

- Most cases are sporadic; a small percentage have a family history
- Wilms tumor gene, *WT1,* is located on chromosome 11 and regulates normal kidney development; about 20% of affected children have mutations of this gene
- Associated with several syndromes; WAGR includes Wilms tumor, aniridia, genitourinary abnormalities, and intellectual disability

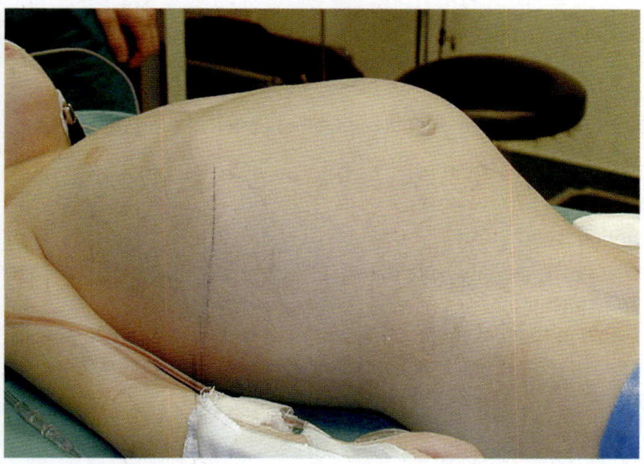

FIG. 18.47 Wilms tumor. Large left-sided flank mass seen on visual inspection.

PATIENT DATA

Subjective Data

- Most present with painless enlargement of the abdomen or an abdominal mass (often found while parents are bathing their young child)
- Some present with abdominal pain, vomiting, and hematuria
- Some are identified during screening due to associated congenital abnormalities

Objective Data

- May be felt on abdominal examination as a firm, nontender mass deep within the flank, only slightly movable, and not usually crossing the midline (Fig. 18.47); sometimes bilateral
- Hypertension may be present

Hirschsprung Disease (Congenital Aganglionic Megacolon)

Primary absence of parasympathetic ganglion cells in a segment of the colon, which interrupts intestinal motility

PATHOPHYSIOLOGY

- Abnormal intestinal innervation results in the absence of peristalsis, which leads to the accumulation of stool proximal to the defect and intestinal obstruction
- Most common cause of lower intestinal obstruction in newborns
- Three to four times as common in males as in females
- Genetic mutations have been identified in some patients

PATIENT DATA

Subjective Data

- Symptoms typically begin at birth with failure to pass meconium in the first 24–48 hours
- Other symptoms include failure to thrive, constipation, abdominal distention, and episodes of bilious vomiting and diarrhea
- Older infants and young children may present with severe constipation

Objective Data

- Examination findings consistent with severe constipation include abdominal distention and stool palpated in the left lower abdomen

Hemolytic Uremic Syndrome

Triad of microangiopathic hemolytic anemia, thrombocytopenia, and uremia

PATHOPHYSIOLOGY

- One of the most common causes of acute kidney injury in children, generally occurring in those younger than 4 years
- Most common cause of hemolytic uremic syndrome (HUS) in the United States is the Shiga-like toxin produced by *Escherichia coli* 0157:H7; other bacterial pathogens such as *Shigella* can cause HUS, as well as some viruses
- Risk factors include ingestion of undercooked meat or unpasteurized milk

PATIENT DATA

Subjective Data

- Most have a preceding upper respiratory infection or gastroenteritis with fever, abdominal pain, and vomiting; diarrhea often becomes bloody
- Gastrointestinal involvement may lead to symptoms of an acute abdomen, with occasional perforation
- Some present with a sudden onset of pallor, weakness, lethargy, and decreased urine output

Objective Data

- Typically present with dehydration, edema, petechiae, and hepatosplenomegaly
- With severe gastrointestinal disease, may display peritoneal signs (abdominal distention, involuntary guarding, rebound tenderness)

Older Adults

Fecal Incontinence

Inability to control bowel movements, leading to leakage of stool; associated with three major causes—fecal impaction, underlying disease, and neurogenic disorders

PATHOPHYSIOLOGY

- Fecal impaction (most common cause) is associated with immobilization and poor fluid and dietary intake; laxative overuse may also be a cause
- Local neurogenic disorders refer to any process that causes degeneration of the mesenteric plexus and lower bowel, resulting in a lax sphincter muscle, diminished sacral reflex, and decreased puborectal muscle tone
- Cognitive neurogenic disorders usually result from stroke or dementia

PATIENT DATA

Subjective Data

- Most have "overflow incontinence" (a soft stool that oozes around the impaction)
- Unable to recognize rectal fullness and with an inability to inhibit intrinsic rectal contractions; stools normally formed and occur in a set pattern, usually after a meal

Objective Data

- Diagnosed through digital rectal examination when assessing rectal tone or other abnormalities
- Radiologic and manometry studies are often helpful in determining the underlying cause such as cancer, inflammatory bowel disease, diverticulitis, colitis, proctitis, or diabetic neuropathy

CHAPTER 19

Female Genitalia

For ease of communication, in this textbook the term *female genitalia* refers to the following internal and external anatomic structures: mons pubis, labia, clitoris, vestibular glands, vagina, cervix, uterus, fallopian tubes, ovaries, and bony pelvis, regardless of the gender identity of the patient. Examination of the female genitalia is typically performed when a patient presents with a specific concern, as part of the newborn examination, for the sexually active adolescent, or as part of a routine health visit. Examination of the anus and rectum (see Chapter 21) is often performed at the same time.

Physical Examination Components

External Genitalia

1. Inspect the pubic hair characteristics and distribution.
2. Inspect and palpate the labia for:
   - Symmetry of color
   - Caking of discharge
   - Inflammation
   - Irritation or excoriation
   - Swelling
3. Inspect the urethral meatus and vaginal opening for:
   - Discharge
   - Lesions or caruncles
   - Polyps
   - Fistulas
4. Milk the Skene glands.
5. Palpate the Bartholin glands.
6. Inspect and palpate the perineum for:
   - Smoothness
   - Tenderness, inflammation
   - Fistulas
   - Lesions or growths
7. Inspect for prolapse and urinary incontinence as the patient bears down.
8. Inspect the perineal area and anus for:
   - Skin characteristics
   - Lesions
   - Fissures or excoriation
   - Inflammation

Internal Genitalia Speculum Examination

1. Insert the speculum along the path of least resistance.
2. Inspect the cervix for:
   - Color
   - Position
   - Size
   - Surface characteristics
   - Discharge
   - Size and shape of os
3. Collect necessary specimens.
4. Inspect vaginal walls for:
   - Color
   - Surface characteristics
   - Secretions

Bimanual Examination

1. Insert the index and middle fingers of one hand into the vagina and place the other hand on the abdominal midline.
2. Palpate the vaginal walls for:
   - Smoothness
   - Tenderness
   - Lesions (cysts, nodules, or masses)
3. Palpate the cervix for:
   - Size, shape, and length
   - Position
   - Mobility
4. Palpate the uterus for:
   - Location
   - Position
   - Size, shape, and contour
   - Mobility
   - Tenderness
5. Palpate the ovaries for:
   - Size
   - Shape
   - Consistency
   - Tenderness
6. Palpate adnexal areas for masses and tenderness.

Rectovaginal Examination

1. Insert the index finger into the vagina and the middle finger into the anus.
2. Assess sphincter tone.
3. Palpate the rectovaginal septum for:
   - Thickness
   - Tone
   - Nodules
4. Palpate the posterior aspect of the uterus.
5. Palpate the anterior and posterior rectal wall for:
   - Masses, polyps, or nodules
   - Strictures, other irregularities, or tenderness
6. Note characteristics of feces when the gloved finger is removed.

ANATOMY AND PHYSIOLOGY

External Genitalia

The vulva—or external female genital organs—includes the mons pubis, labia majora, labia minora, clitoris, vestibular glands, vaginal vestibule, vaginal orifice, and urethral opening (Fig. 19.1). The symphysis pubis is covered by a pad of adipose tissue called the *mons pubis* or *mons veneris,* which postpuberty is covered with coarse terminal hair. Extending downward and backward from the mons pubis are the labia majora—two folds of adipose tissue covered by skin. The labia majora vary in appearance depending on the amount of adipose tissue present. The outer surfaces of the labia majora are also covered with hair after puberty.

Lying inside and usually hidden by the labia majora are the labia minora—two hairless, flat, reddish folds. The labia minora meet at the anterior of the vulva, where each labium divides into two lamellae, with the lower pair fusing to form the frenulum of the clitoris and the upper pair forming the prepuce. Tucked between the frenulum and the prepuce is the clitoris, a small bud of erectile tissue, the homologue of the penis and a primary center of sexual excitement. Posteriorly, the labia minora meet as two ridges that fuse to form the fourchette.

The labia minora enclose the area designated as the vestibule, which contains six openings: the urethra, the vagina, two ducts of Bartholin glands, and two ducts of Skene glands. The lower two-thirds of the urethra lie immediately above the anterior vaginal wall and terminate in the urethral meatus at the midline of the vestibule just above the vaginal opening and below the clitoris. Skene ducts drain a group of urethral glands and open onto the vestibule on each side of the urethra. The ductal openings may be visible.

The vaginal opening occupies the posterior portion of the vestibule and varies in size and shape. Surrounding the vaginal opening is the hymen—a connective tissue membrane that may be circular, crescentic, or fimbriated. After the hymen tears and becomes permanently divided, the edges either disappear or form hymenal tags. Bartholin glands, located posteriorly on each side of the vaginal orifice, open onto the sides of the vestibule in the groove between the labia minora and the hymen. The ductal openings are not usually visible. During sexual excitement, Bartholin glands secrete mucus into the introitus for lubrication.

The pelvic floor consists of a group of muscles that form a supportive sling for the pelvic contents. The muscle fibers insert at various points on the bony pelvis and form functional sphincters for the vagina, rectum, and urethra (Fig. 19.2).

Internal Genitalia

The vagina is a musculomembranous tube that has transverse rugae (anatomic folds) during the reproductive phase of life. It inclines posteriorly at an angle of approximately 45 degrees with the vertical plane of the body (Fig. 19.3). The anterior wall of the vagina is separated from the bladder and urethra by connective tissue called the *vesicovaginal septum.* The posterior vaginal wall is separated from the rectum by the rectovaginal septum. The anterior and posterior walls of the vagina lie in close proximity, with only a small space between them. The upper end of the vagina is a blind vault into which the uterine cervix projects. The pocket formed around the cervix is divided into the anterior, posterior, and lateral fornices. These are of clinical importance, as the internal pelvic organs can be palpated through their thin walls. The vagina carries menstrual flow from the uterus, serves as the terminal portion of the birth canal, and is the receptive organ for the penis during sexual intercourse. The anatomy of a neovagina created in a transgender woman differs from that of a natal

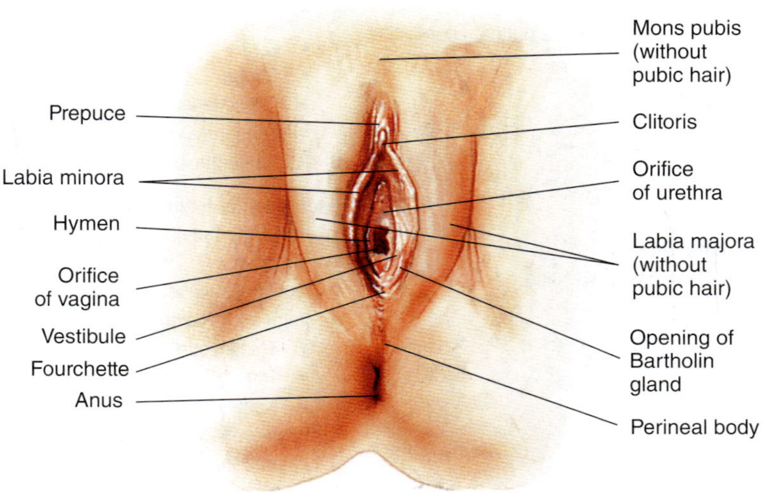

FIG. 19.1 External female genitalia. (Lowdermilk, D. L., & Perry, S. E. (2007). *Maternity and women's health care* (8th ed.). St. Louis: Mosby.)

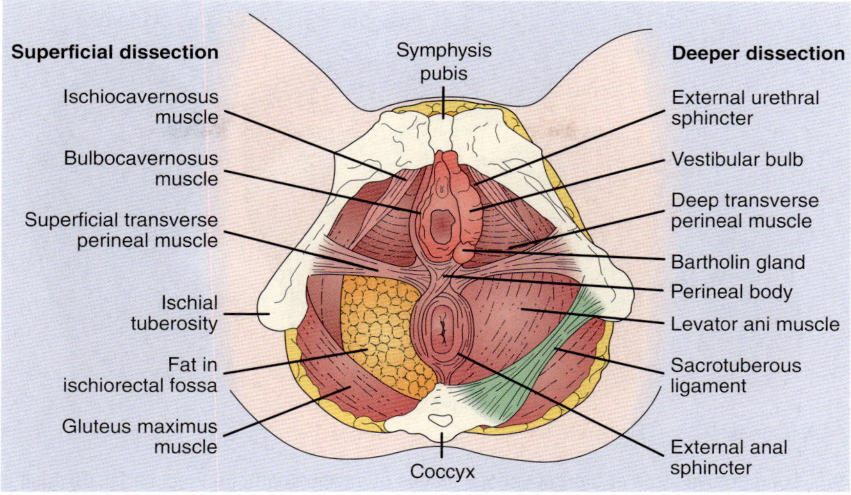

FIG. 19.2 **Musculature of the perineum.** (From Black, M., Ambros-Rudolph, C. M., et al. (2008). *Obstetric and gynecologic dermatology* (3rd ed.). Elsevier.)

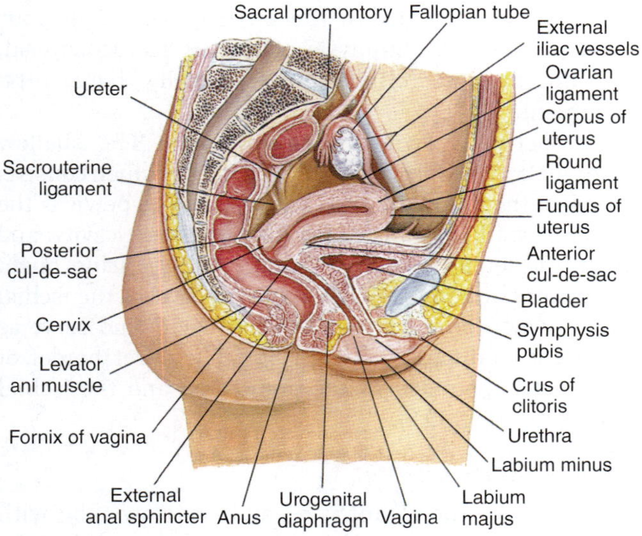

FIG. 19.3 **Midsagittal view of the female pelvic organs.**

vagina. It is a blind cuff, lacks a cervix and surrounding fornices, and may have a more posterior orientation.

The uterus sits in the pelvic cavity between the bladder and the rectum. It is an inverted, pear-shaped, muscular organ that is relatively mobile (Fig. 19.4). The uterus is covered by the peritoneum and lined by the endometrium, which is shed during menstruation. The rectouterine cul-de-sac (pouch of Douglas) is a deep recess formed by the peritoneum as it covers the lower posterior wall of the uterus and upper portion of the vagina, separating it from the rectum. The uterus is flattened anteroposteriorly and usually inclines forward at a 45-degree angle, although it may be anteverted, anteflexed, retroverted, or retroflexed. In nulliparous patients, the size is approximately 5.5 to 8 cm long, 3.5 to 4 cm wide, and 2 to 2.5 cm thick. The uterus of a parous patient may be larger by 2 to 3 cm in any of the dimensions. The uterus of a nulliparous patient weighs approximately 40 to 50 g (Fig. 19.5), and that of a multiparous patient is 20 to 30 g heavier.

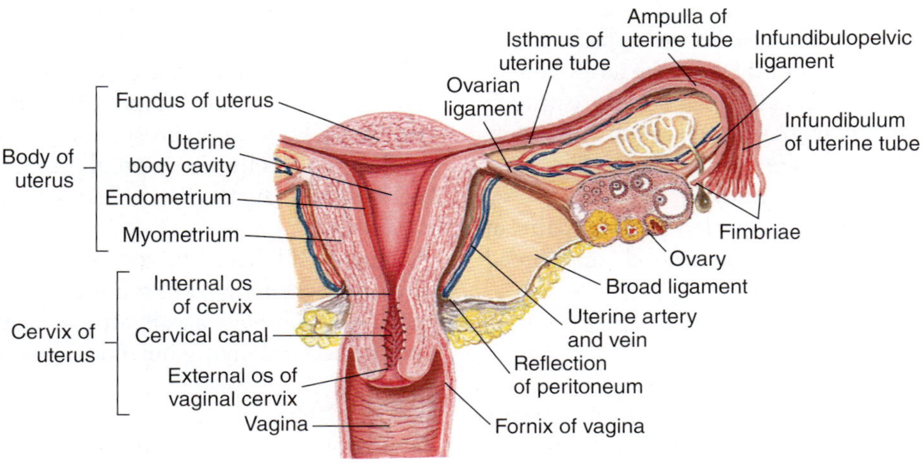

FIG. 19.4 **Cross-sectional view of internal female genitalia and pelvic contents.**

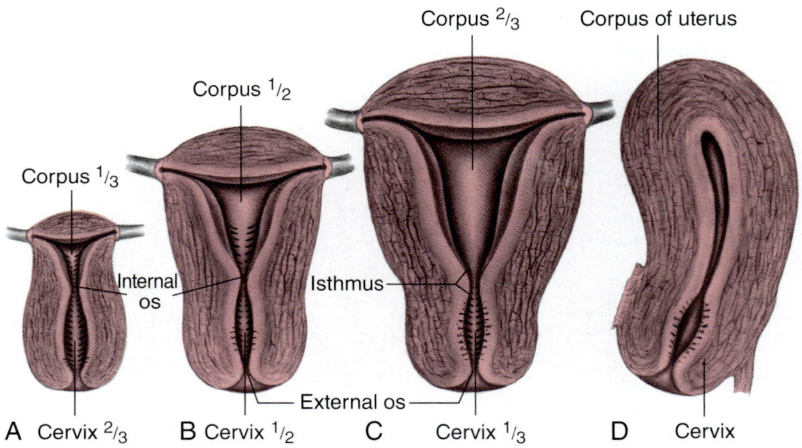

FIG. 19.5 **Comparative sizes of uteri at various stages of development.** (A) Prepubertal. (B) Adult nulliparous. (C) Adult multiparous. (D) Lateral view, adult multiparous. The fractions give the relative proportion of the size of the corpus and the cervix.

The uterus is divided anatomically into the corpus and cervix. The corpus consists of the fundus, which is the convex upper portion between the points of insertion of the fallopian tubes; the main portion or body; and the isthmus, which is the constricted lower portion adjacent to the cervix. The cervix extends from the isthmus into the vagina. The uterus opens into the vagina via the external cervical os.

The fallopian tubes and ovaries comprise the adnexa of the uterus. The fallopian tubes insert into the upper portion of the uterus and extend laterally to the ovaries. Each tube ranges from 8 to 14 cm long and is supported by a fold of the broad ligament called the *mesosalpinx*. The isthmus end of the fallopian tube opens into the uterine cavity. The fimbriated end opens into the pelvic cavity, with a projection that extends to the ovary and captures the ovum. Rhythmic contractions of the tubal musculature transport the ovum to the uterus.

The ovaries are a pair of oval organs resting in a slight depression on the lateral pelvic wall at the level of the anterosuperior iliac spine. The ovaries are approximately 3 cm long, 2 cm wide, and 1 cm thick in the adult patient during the reproductive years. Ovaries secrete estrogen and progesterone, hormones that have several functions, including controlling the menstrual cycle (Fig. 19.6; Table 19.1) and supporting pregnancy.

The internal genitalia are supported by four pairs of ligaments: the cardinal, uterosacral, round, and broad ligaments.

Bony Pelvis

The pelvis is formed from four bones: two innominate (each consisting of the ilium, ischium, and pubis); the sacrum; and the coccyx (Fig. 19.7). The bony pelvis is important in accommodating a growing fetus during pregnancy and in the birth process. The four pelvic joints—the symphysis pubis, the sacrococcygeal, and the two sacroiliac joints—usually have little movement.

The pelvis is divided into two parts. The shallow upper section is considered the false pelvis, which consists mainly of the flared-out iliac bones. The true pelvis is the lower curved bony canal, including the inlet, cavity, and outlet; the fetus must pass through these during birth. The upper border of the outlet is at the level of the ischial spines, which project into the pelvic cavity and serve as important landmarks during labor. The lower border of the outlet is bounded by the pubic arch and the ischial tuberosities (Fig. 19.8).

Infants and Children

The vagina of the infant is a small, narrow tube with fewer epithelial layers than those of the adult. The uterus is approximately 35 mm long, with the cervix constituting about two-thirds of the entire length of the organ. The ovaries are tiny and functionally immature. The labia minora are relatively avascular, thin, and pale. The labia majora are hairless and nonprominent. The hymen is a thin diaphragm just inside the introitus, usually with a crescent-shaped opening in the midline. The clitoris is small. External genitalia may be swollen at birth due to estrogen from the pregnant patient.

During childhood, the genitalia—except for the clitoris—grow incrementally at varying rates. Anatomic and functional development accelerate with the onset of puberty and the accompanying hormonal changes.

Adolescents

During puberty, the external genitalia increase in size and begin to assume adult proportions. The clitoris becomes more erectile and the labia minora more vascular. The labia majora and mons pubis become more prominent and begin to develop hair, often occurring simultaneously with breast development. Growth changes and secondary sex characteristic developments that occur during puberty are discussed in Chapter 8.

If the hymen is intact, the vaginal opening is about 1 cm. The vagina lengthens, and the epithelial layers thicken. The vaginal secretions become acidic.

The uterus, ovaries, and fallopian tubes increase in size and weight. The uterine musculature and vascular supply

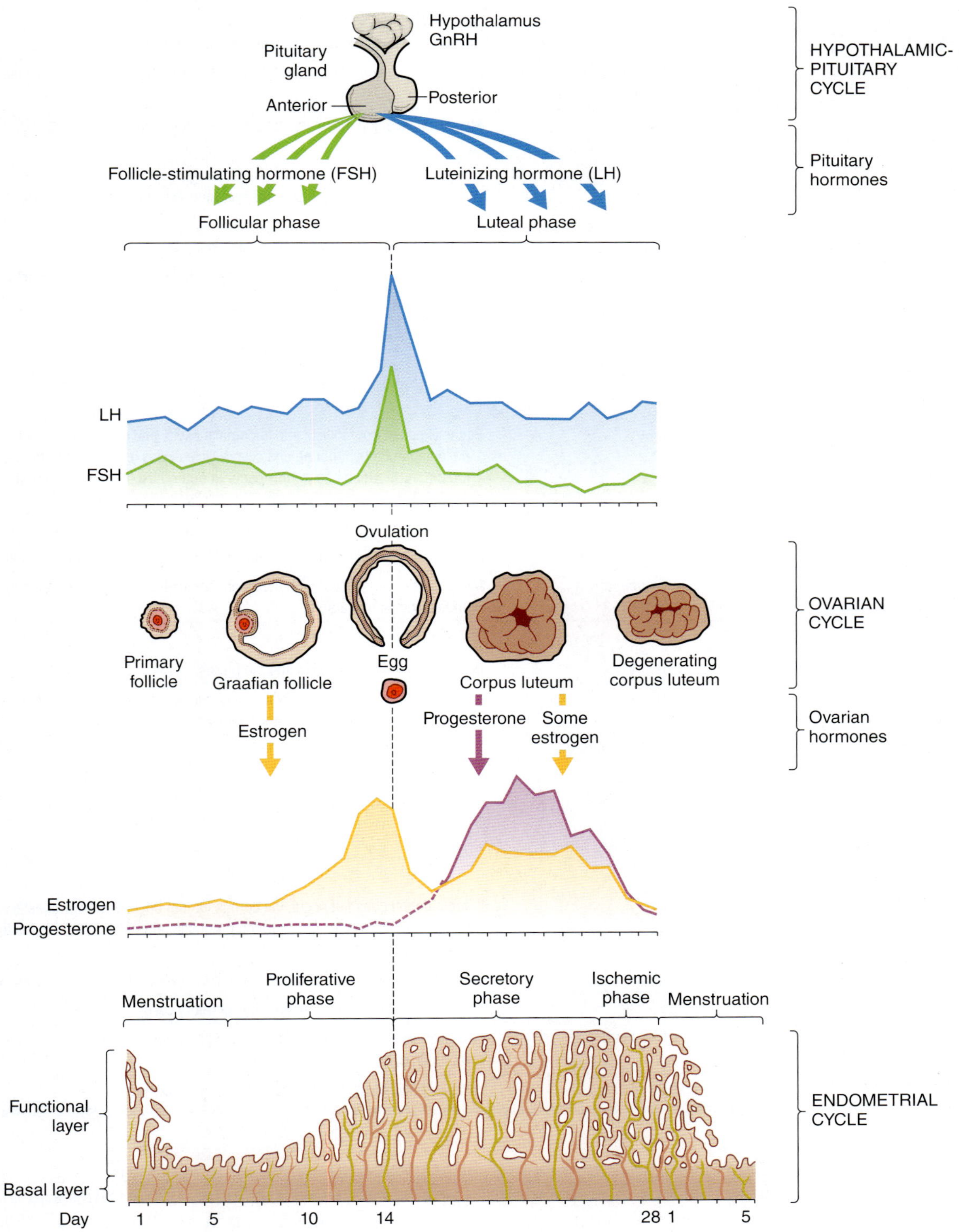

FIG. 19.6 Female menstrual cycle. Diagram shows the interrelationship of the cerebral, hypothalamic, pituitary, and uterine functions throughout a standard 28-day menstrual cycle. (From Lowdermilk, D. L., & Perry, S. E. (2007). *Maternity and women's health care* (8th ed.). St. Louis: Mosby.)

TABLE 19.1 The Menstrual Cycle

PHASE		DESCRIPTION
Menstrual Phase: Days 1–4		
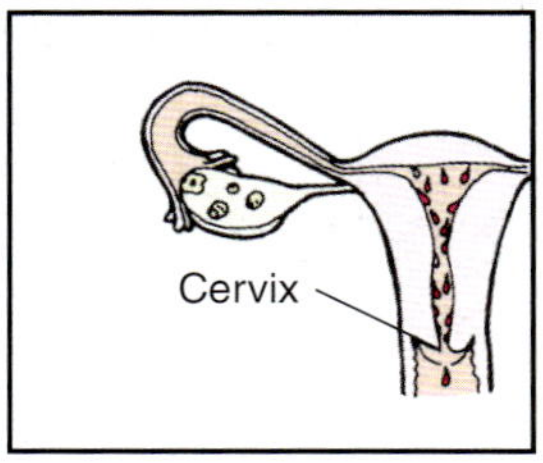	Ovary	Estrogen levels begin to rise, preparing follicle and egg for the next cycle.
	Uterus	Progesterone stimulates endometrial prostaglandins that cause vasoconstriction; upper layers of endometrium shed.
	Breast	Cellular activity in the alveoli decreases; breast ducts shrink.
	Central nervous system (CNS) hormones	Follicle-stimulating hormone (FSH) and luteinizing hormone (LH) levels decrease.
	Symptoms	Menstrual bleeding may vary, depending on hormones and prostaglandins.
Postmenstrual, Preovulatory Phase: Days 5–12		
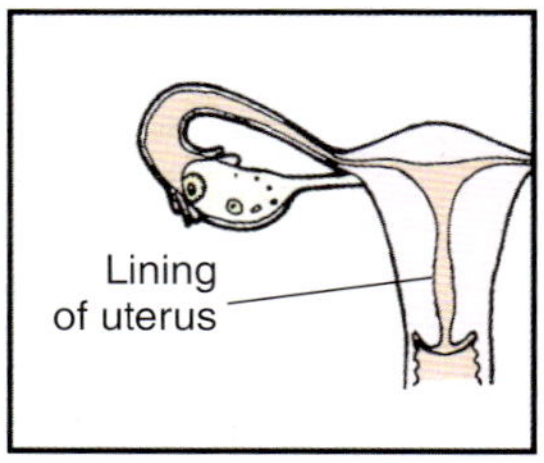	Ovary	Ovary and maturing follicle produce estrogen; follicular phase—egg develops within follicle.
	Uterus	Proliferative phase—uterine lining thickens.
	Breast	Parenchymal and proliferation (increased cellular activity) of breast ducts occurs.
	CNS hormones	FSH stimulates ovarian follicular growth.
Ovulation: Day 13 or 14		
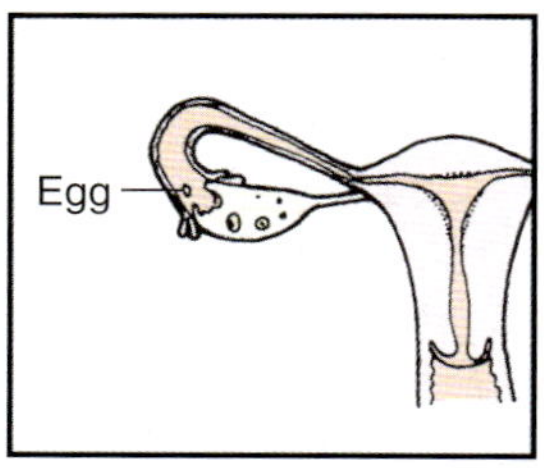	Ovary	Egg is expelled from follicle into abdominal cavity and drawn into the uterine (fallopian) tube by fimbriae and cilia; follicle closes and begins to form corpus luteum; fertilization of egg may occur in outer third of tube if sperm are unimpeded.
	Uterus	End of proliferative phase; progesterone causes further thickening of the uterine wall.
	CNS hormones	LH and estrogen levels increase rapidly; LH surge stimulates release of egg.
	Symptoms	Mittelschmerz may occur with ovulation; cervical mucus is increased and is stringy and elastic (spinnbarkeit).
Secretory Phase: Days 15–20		
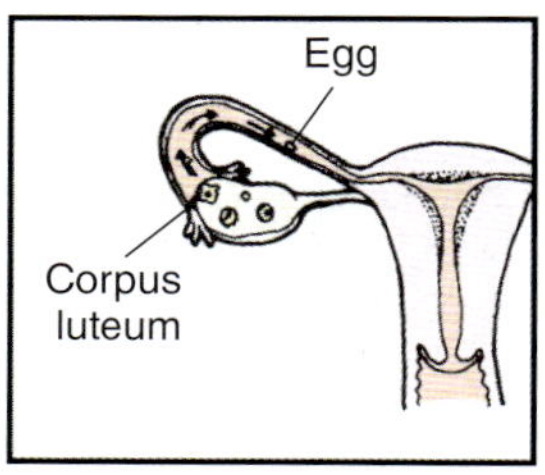	Ovary	Egg (ovum) is moved by cilia into the uterus.
	Uterus	After the egg is released, the follicle becomes a corpus luteum; secretion of progesterone increases and predominates.
	CNS hormones	LH and FSH levels decrease.
Premenstrual, Luteal Phase: Days 21–28		
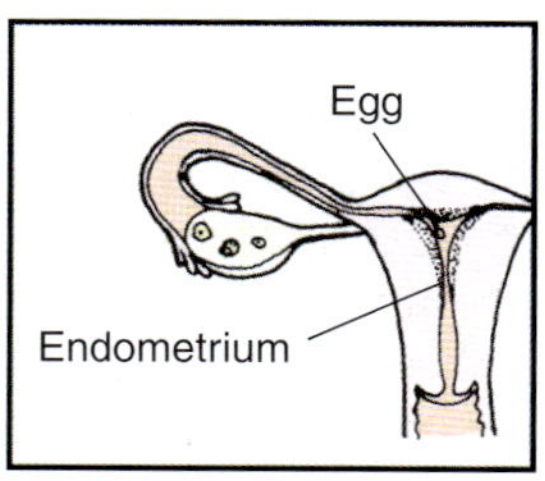	Ovary	If implantation does not occur, the corpus luteum degenerates; progesterone production decreases, and estrogen production drops and then begins to rise as a new follicle develops.
	Uterus	Menstruation starts around day 28, which begins day 1 of the menstrual cycle.
	Breast	Alveolar breast cells differentiate into secretory cells.
	CNS hormones	Increased levels of gonadotropin-releasing hormone (GnRH) cause increased secretion of FSH.
	Symptoms	Vascular engorgement and water retention may occur.

increase. The endometrial lining thickens in preparation for the onset of menstruation (menarche). Historically, average age at menarche in the United States has been between 12 and 13 years. There is evidence that the average age at menarche has been decreasing among younger generations, especially in racial minorities and those with lower socioeconomic statuses (Wang et al., 2024). Just before menarche, vaginal secretions increase.

Functional maturation of the reproductive organs is reached during puberty. Due to immaturity of the

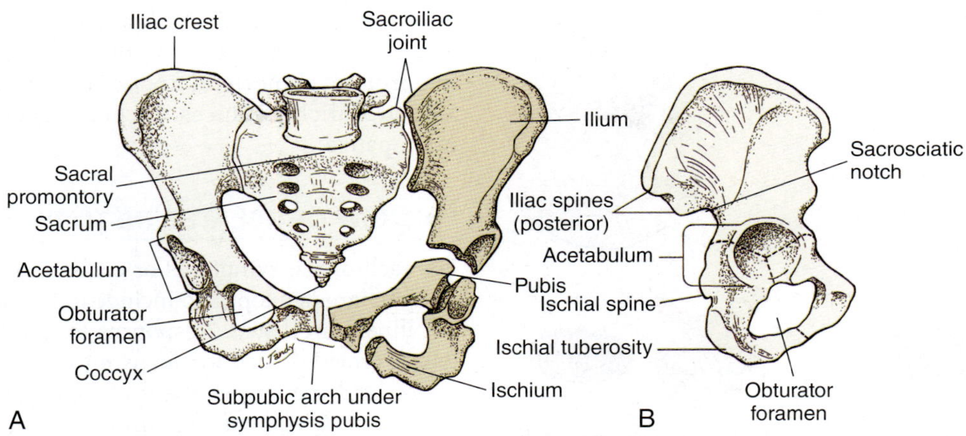

FIG. 19.7 **Adult female pelvis.**(A) Anterior view. The three embryonic parts of the left innominate bone are lightly shaded. (B) External view of right innominate bone (fused). (From Lowdermilk, D. L., & Perry, S. E. (2007). *Maternity and women's health care* (8th ed.). St. Louis: Mosby.)

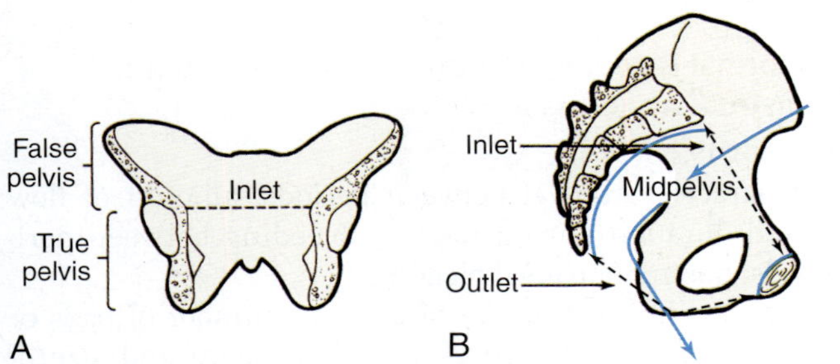

FIG. 19.8 **Female pelvis.** (A) Cavity of the false pelvis is a shallow basin above the inlet; the true pelvis is a deeper cavity below the inlet. (B) Cavity of the true pelvis is an irregularly curved canal (*arrows*). (From Lowdermilk, D. L., & Perry, S. E. (2007). *Maternity and women's health care*, (8th ed.). St. Louis: Mosby.)

hypothalamic-pituitary-ovarian axis, irregular menstrual cycles are common during the early years after menarche as a result of anovulation.

Pregnant Patients

The high levels of estrogen and progesterone that are necessary to support pregnancy are responsible for uterine enlargement during the first trimester. After the third month, uterine enlargement is primarily the result of mechanical pressure of the growing fetus. As the uterus enlarges, the muscular walls strengthen and become more elastic. As the uterus becomes larger and more ovoid, it rises out of the pelvis; by 12 weeks of gestation, it reaches into the abdominal cavity. During the first months, the walls become thicker but then gradually thin to about 1.5 cm or less at term. Uterine weight at term, excluding the fetus and placenta, will usually have increased more than 10-fold and the capacity increases 500 to 1000 times that of the nonpregnant uterus. In the postpartum period the uterus involutes rapidly. Immediately after delivery the uterus is approximately the size of a 20-week pregnancy (at the level of the umbilicus). By the end of the first week, it is about the size of a 12-week pregnancy, palpable at the symphysis pubis.

Hormonal activity (relaxin and progesterone) is responsible for the softening of the pelvic cartilage and strengthening of the pelvic ligaments. Consequently, the pelvic joints separate slightly, allowing some mobility; this results in the characteristic "waddle" gait. The symphysis pubis relaxes and increases in width, with marked mobility of the pelvis at term. The symphysis pubis returns to the pre-pregnancy state within 3 to 5 months postpartum. Protrusion of the abdomen as the uterus grows causes the pelvis to tilt forward, placing additional strain on the back and sacroiliac joints.

During pregnancy, an increase in uterine blood flow and lymph causes pelvic congestion and edema. As a result, the uterus, cervix, and isthmus soften (Goodell sign), and the cervix takes on a bluish color (Chadwick sign). The cervical canal is obstructed by thick mucus soon after conception, protecting the infant from infection. When this plug dislodges at the beginning of labor, it produces a sign of labor called *bloody show*. The glands near the external os proliferate with eversion of the columnar endocervical glands. The softness and compressibility of the isthmus result in exaggerated uterine anteflexion during the first 3 months of pregnancy, causing the fundus to press on the urinary bladder.

Both the mucosa of the vaginal walls and the connective tissue thicken, and smooth muscle cells hypertrophy. These changes result in an increased length of the vaginal walls, so that at times they can be seen protruding from the vulvar opening. The papillae of the mucosa have a hobnailed appearance. The vaginal secretions increase and have an acidic pH due to an increase in lactic acid production by the vaginal epithelium. The increase in pH helps keep bacteria from multiplying in the vagina but also can support *Candida* infection. Fig. 19.9 compares the changes that

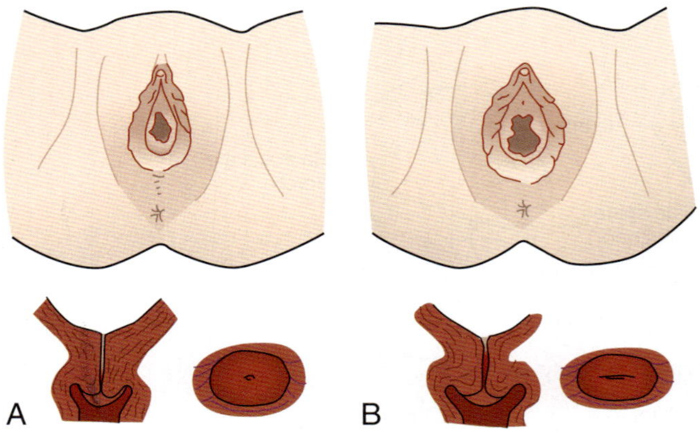

FIG. 19.9 Comparison of vulva and cervix in a nullipara patient (A) and a multipara patient (B) at the same stage of pregnancy. (From Lowdermilk, D. L., & Perry, S. E. (2007). *Maternity and women's health care* (8th ed.). St. Louis: Mosby.)

occur in a patient experiencing the first pregnancy with those in a patient who has experienced more than one pregnancy.

Older Adults

Concurrent with endocrine changes, ovarian function diminishes during a patient's 40s, and menstrual periods begin to cease, although fertility may continue. The median age of menopause in the United States is 51 years (range 41 to 59 years). Menopause is defined as 1 year with no menses (amenorrhea). Just as menarche in the adolescent is one aspect of puberty, similarly, cessation of menses is one aspect of this transitional phase of the life cycle. During this time, estrogen levels decrease, causing the labia and clitoris to become smaller. The labia majora also become flatter as body fat is lost. Pubic hair turns gray and is usually sparser. Both adrenal androgens and ovarian testosterone levels markedly decrease after menopause, which may account in part for decreases in libido and in muscle mass and strength.

The vaginal introitus gradually constricts. The vagina narrows, shortens, and loses its rugae, and the mucosa becomes thin, pale, and dry, which may result in pain during sexual intercourse (dyspareunia). The cervix becomes smaller and paler. The uterus decreases in size, and the endometrium thins.

The ovaries also decrease to approximately 1 to 2 cm. Follicles gradually disappear, and the surface of the ovary convolutes. Ovulation usually ceases about 1 to 2 years before menopause.

The ligaments and connective tissue of the pelvis sometimes lose their elasticity and tone, thus weakening the supportive sling for the pelvic contents. The vaginal walls may lose some of their structural integrity.

Menopause has systemic effects, which include an increase in body fat and intra-abdominal deposition of body fat (tendency toward male pattern of body fat distribution). Levels of total and low-density lipoprotein cholesterol increase. Thermoregulation is altered, which produces the hot flashes associated with menopause.

REVIEW OF RELATED HISTORY

For each of the symptoms or conditions discussed in this section, targeted topics to include in the history of the present illness are listed. Responses to questions about these topics provide clues for focusing on the physical examination and the development of an appropriate diagnostic evaluation. Questions regarding medication use (prescription and over-the-counter preparations) as well as complementary, alternative, and integrative therapies are relevant for each.

History of Present Illness

Abnormal Bleeding (Postmenopausal Bleeding, Menstrual Abnormalities)

See Box 19.1.

- Character: interval between periods, amount of flow and duration during menses, bleeding between periods; postmenopausal bleeding
- Change in flow: nature of change, number of pads or tampons saturated in 24 hours, presence and size of clots

BOX 19.1 Abnormal Uterine Bleeding: Parameters

Abnormal uterine bleeding (AUB) is a broad term that describes irregularities in the menstrual cycle involving frequency, regularity, duration, and volume of flow outside of pregnancy. AUB also includes intermenstrual bleeding.

PARAMETER	DESCRIPTION
Frequency	Absent (no bleeding) = amenorrhea Infrequent (>38 days) Normal (24 to ≤38 days) Frequent (<24 days)
Duration	Normal (≤8 days) Prolonged (>8 days)
Regularity	Normal or "regular" (shortest to longest cycle variation: ≤7–9 days) Irregular (shortest to longest cycle variation: ≥8–10 days)
Flow volume (patient determined)	Light Normal Heavy
Intermenstrual bleeding	Bleeding between cyclically regular onset of menses Random or cyclical: early, mid, or late cycle

From Munro, M. G., Critchley, H. O. D., Fraser, I. S., for the FIGO Menstrual Disorders Committee (2018).

- Temporal sequence: onset, duration, precipitating factors, course since onset
- Associated symptoms: pain, cramping, abdominal distention, pelvic fullness, change in bowel habits, weight loss or gain
- Medications: oral contraceptives; hormones; tamoxifen

Pain

- Temporal sequence: date and time of onset, sudden versus gradual onset, course since onset, duration, recurrence
- Character: specific location, type, and intensity of pain
- Associated symptoms: vaginal discharge or bleeding, gastrointestinal symptoms, abdominal distention or tenderness, pelvic fullness
- Association with menstrual cycle: timing, location, duration, changes
- Relationship to body functions and activities: voiding, eating, defecation, flatus, exercise, walking up stairs, bending, stretching, sexual activity
- Aggravating or relieving factors
- Previous medical care for this problem
- Efforts to treat
- Medications: analgesics

Vaginal Discharge

- Character: amount, color, odor, consistency, changes in characteristics
- Occurrence: acute or chronic
- Douching habits
- Clothing habits: use of underwear with noncotton crotch, tight pants or jeans
- Sexual history—see “Personal and Social History”
- Presence of discharge or symptoms in sexual partner
- Use of spermicide or latex condoms
- Associated symptoms: itching; tender, inflamed, or bleeding external tissues; dyspareunia; dysuria or burning on urination; abdominal pain or cramping; pelvic fullness
- Efforts to treat: vaginal cream
- Medications: oral contraceptives, antibiotics, aromatase inhibitors, hormones

Premenstrual Symptoms

- Symptoms: headaches, weight gain, edema, breast tenderness, irritability, or mood changes
- Frequency
- Interference with activities of daily living
- Relief measures
- Aggravating factors
- Medications: analgesics, diuretics

Menopausal Symptoms

- Age at menopause or currently experiencing
- Symptoms: menstrual changes, mood changes, tension, hot flashes, sleep disruption
- Postmenopausal uterine bleeding
- General feelings about menopause: self-image, effect on intimate relationships
- Mother’s or sibling’s experience with menopause
- Birth control measures during menopause
- Medications: hormones—dose and duration; serum estrogen receptor modulators
- Use of complementary or alternative therapy: soy, other natural estrogen products; black cohosh (used as an alternative to hormonal treatment for menopause)

Infertility

- Length of time attempting pregnancy, sexual activity practices, knowledge of fertile period in menstrual cycle, length of cycle
- Abnormalities of vagina, cervix, uterus, fallopian tubes, ovaries
- Contributing factors: stress, nutrition, chemical substances
- Partner factors (see Chapter 20)
- Diagnostic evaluation to date

Urinary Symptoms (Dysuria, Burning on Urination, Frequency, Urgency)

- Character: acute or chronic; frequency of occurrence; last episode; onset; course since onset; feel like bladder is empty or not after voiding; pain at start, throughout, or at cessation of urination
- Description of urine: color, presence of blood or particles, clear or cloudy
- Associated symptoms: vaginal discharge or bleeding, abdominal pain or cramping, abdominal distention, pelvic fullness or pressure, flank pain
- Medications: urinary tract analgesics, antispasmodics

Past Medical History

- Gender identity: female, male, nonbinary; transgender man; transgender woman; sex assignment at birth
- Organ inventory: clitoris (natal or surgically constructed), vagina (natal or surgically constructed), cervix, uterus, fallopian tubes, ovaries, prostate gland, penis (natal or surgically constructed), scrotum and testicles (natal or surgically constructed)
- Menstrual history
    - Age at menarche and/or menopause
    - Date of last normal menstrual period: first day of last cycle
    - Number of days in cycle and regularity of cycle
    - Character of flow: amount (number of pads or tampons used in 24 hours on heaviest days), duration, presence and size of clots
    - Dysmenorrhea: characteristics, duration, frequency, relief measures

- Intermenstrual bleeding or spotting: amount, duration, frequency, timing in relation to phase of cycle
- Intermenstrual pain: severity, duration, timing; association with ovulation
- Premenstrual symptoms: see "History of Present Illness"
- Obstetric history
  - **G:** Gravidity (total number of pregnancies)
  - **T:** number of term pregnancies
  - **P:** number of preterm pregnancies
  - **A:** number of abortions, spontaneous or induced
  - **L:** number of living children
  - Complications of pregnancy, delivery, abortion, or with fetus or neonate
- Menopause history: see "History of Present Illness"
- Gynecologic history
  - Date of last pelvic examination
  - Prior Papanicolaou (Pap) smears, human papillomavirus (HPV) testing and results
  - Prior abnormal Pap smears or HPV test—when, how treated, follow-up
  - Sexually transmitted infections (STIs)
  - Pelvic inflammatory disease
  - Vaginal infections
  - Recent and past gynecologic/genitourinary procedures or surgery, including tubal ligation, hysterectomy, oophorectomy, laparoscopy, cryosurgery, conization, colposcopy, hysterectomy, vaginectomy, oophorectomy, orchiectomy, feminizing vaginoplasty, masculinizing phalloplasty, scrotoplasty, erectile implants, metoidioplasty (clitoral release/enlargement, which may include urethral lengthening)
  - Chronic diseases: diabetes, cancer of reproductive organs or related cancers (breast, colorectal)

Risk Factors

Cervical Cancer

HPV infection: HPV infection is common, and only a small percentage of those infected with untreated HPV will develop cervical cancer. The "high-risk" types include HPV 16, 18, 31, 33, and 45 as well as some others.

HPV vaccination: protective factor; decreases risk of cervical cancer

Pap smear history: lack of regular screening for cervical cancer; transgender men are less likely to be current on cervical cancer screening

High parity: patients with three or more full-term pregnancies have an increased risk of developing cervical cancer (likely related to HPV exposure or susceptibility).

Young age at parity: patients who were younger than 20 years when they had their first full-term pregnancy are more likely to develop cervical cancer later in life than those who were not pregnant until they were 25 years or older.

Cigarette smoking: doubles the risk; tobacco by-products have been found in the cervical mucus of patients who smoke.

HIV infection: increased susceptibility to HPV infections

Chlamydia infection: increases risk for cervical cancer

Diet: diets low in fruits and vegetables may increase risk for cervical cancer; overweight patients are more likely to develop this cancer.

DES exposure: increased risk in patients exposed in utero to diethylstilbestrol (DES; prescribed between 1940 and 1971 to pregnant patients at high risk of miscarriages)

Oral contraceptives (OCs): some evidence indicates that risk increases the longer OCs are used; the risk decreases with cessation of OCs.

Low socioeconomic status: likely related to access to health care services, including cervical cancer screening and treatment of precancerous cervical disease

From American Cancer Society. (2020). *Risk factors for cervical cancer.* https://www.cancer.org/cancer/types/cervical-cancer/causes-risks-prevention/risk-factors.html. Accessed September 24, 2024; and Deutsch, M. B. (Ed.). (2016).

Risk Factors

Ovarian Cancer

Age: risk increases with age. Most ovarian cancers develop after menopause.

Inherited genetic mutation or syndromes: increased risk with known inherited mutation of the *BRCA1* or *BRCA2* or *PTEN* gene. Increased risk of hereditary nonpolyposis colon cancer syndrome (HNPCC), Peutz-Jeghers syndrome, MUTYH-associated polyposis. Other genes linked to ovarian cancer include *ATM, BRIP1, RAD51C, RAD51D,* and *PALB2.*

Family history: one or more first-degree relatives (parent, sibling, child) with ovarian and/or breast cancer; strong family history of colon cancers; Ashkenazi Jewish descent; and a family history of breast and/or ovarian cancer

Obesity: patients with a body mass index of at least 30 have a higher risk of developing ovarian cancer.

Reproductive history: nulliparity or parity after age 35 years increases the risk.

Use of fertility drugs: increased risk in some studies, especially if pregnancy is not achieved

Personal history: increased risk with breast, endometrial, and/or colon cancers

Hormone replacement therapy: increased risk in postmenopausal patients. The risk seems to be higher in patients taking estrogen alone (without progesterone) for at least 5 or 10 years.

Use of OCs: protective use for 4 or more years is associated with an approximately 50% reduction in ovarian cancer risk in the general population.

Testosterone therapy: no evidence that transgender men taking testosterone have an increased risk

Diet: high-fat diet associated with higher rates of ovarian cancer in industrialized nations, but the link remains unproven

From American Cancer Society (2021); and Deutsch, M. B. (Ed.), (2016). *Guidelines for the primary care of transgender and gender nonbinary people* (2nd ed.). UCSF Center of Excellence for Transgender Health.

Risk Factors

Endometrial Cancer

Total number of menstrual cycles: increased risk with more menstrual cycles during a patient's lifetime (i.e., early menarche plus late menopause)

Infertility or nulliparity: during pregnancy, the hormonal balance shifts toward more progesterone. Therefore having many pregnancies reduces endometrial cancer risk, and nulliparity increases risk.

Obesity: having more fat tissue can increase a patient's estrogen levels and therefore increase the endometrial cancer risk.

Endometrial hyperplasia: atypical hyperplasia increases risk; can be caused by use of tamoxifen, an antiestrogen drug that acts like an estrogen in the uterus

Estrogen replacement therapy (ERT): estrogen alone (without progestins) in patients with a uterus increases risk.

Testosterone therapy: no evidence that transgender men taking testosterone have an increased risk

Ovarian diseases: polycystic ovaries and some ovarian tumors such as granulosa–theca cell tumors cause an increase in estrogen relative to progestin. Some of these conditions lead to hysterectomy and oophorectomy, ending the risk for endometrial cancer.

Diet: diet high in animal fat

Diabetes: endometrial cancer more common in patients with both type 1 and type 2 diabetes

Age: risk increases with age; 95% of endometrial cancers occur in patients 40 years of age or older.

Family history: history of endometrial, breast, ovarian, or colorectal cancers

Personal history: breast or ovarian cancer or hereditary nonpolyposis colorectal cancer syndrome (Lynch syndrome); known genetic mutation in *BRCA1* or *BRCA2*

Prior pelvic radiation therapy: radiation used to treat some other cancers can damage the DNA of cells, sometimes increasing the risk of developing a second type of cancer such as endometrial cancer.

From American Cancer Society (2019); and Deutsch, M. B. (Ed.), (2016). *Guidelines for the primary care of transgender and gender nonbinary people* (2nd ed.). UCSF Center of Excellence for Transgender Health, 2016.

Family History

- Diabetes
- Cancer of reproductive organs
- Pregnancies with multiple births (e.g., twins, triplets)
- Congenital anomalies

Personal and Social History

- Cleansing routines: use of sprays, powders, perfume, antiseptic soap, deodorants, or ointments
- Contraception history
  - Current method: length of time used, effectiveness, consistency of use, side effects, satisfaction with method
  - Previous methods: duration of use for each, side effects, and reasons for discontinuing each
  - Douching history: frequency—length of time since last douche; number of years douching, method, solution used, reason for douching
- Sexual history
  - Current sexual activity: number of current and previous partners; gender of partner(s)
  - Satisfaction with relationship(s), sexual pleasure achieved, frequency
  - Problems: pain on penetration (entry or deep); decreased lubrication, lack of orgasm of partner(s), sexual preference
  - STI history
  - Use of barrier protection for STIs
  - Partner testing for STIs
- Sexual assault or abuse
  - Screening for intimate partner violence (IPV), domestic violence, and sex trafficking: see Chapter 2.
- Performance of genital self-examination (see Patient Safety box "Self-Examination to Detect STIs")
- Substance use

Infants and Children

Routinely, no questions are required unless there is a specific concern from the parent, other adult, or child.

- Bleeding
  - Character: onset, duration, precipitating factor if known, course since onset
  - Age of mother at menarche
  - Signs of breast development and pubic hair (thelarche and adrenarche)
  - Suspicion about retained toilet tissue or insertion of foreign objects by child
  - Suspicion about possible sexual abuse
- Pain
  - Character: type of pain, onset, course since onset, duration
  - Specific location
  - Associated symptoms: vaginal discharge or bleeding, urinary symptoms, gastrointestinal symptoms, child fearful of parent or other adults
  - Contributory problems: use of bubble bath, irritating soaps, or detergents; suspicion about insertion of foreign objects by child or about possible sexual abuse
  - Recent trauma (straddle injury)
- Vaginal discharge
  - Relationship to diapers: use of powder or lotions, how frequently diapers are changed
  - Associated symptoms: pain, bleeding
  - Contributory problems: use of bubble bath, irritating soaps, or detergents; suspicion about insertion of foreign objects by child or about possible sexual abuse
- Masturbation (Box 19.2)

Adolescents

As the older child matures, ask the same questions that you ask adult patients. Do not assume that youthful age precludes sexual activity or any of the related concerns. While taking the history, it is necessary at some point to talk with the adolescent alone while the parent is out of the room to provide a confidential safe space for discussion of sensitive topics. When you set the agenda at the start of the visit, let the adolescent and parent know you provide this space for all adolescent patients. Your questions should be posed in a gentle, matter-of-fact, and nonjudgmental manner.

Patient Safety

Self-Examination to Detect STIs

Genital self-examination (GSE) is recommended for anyone who is at risk for contracting an STI. This includes sexually active persons who have had more than one sexual partner or whose partner has had other partners. The purpose of GSE is to detect any signs or symptoms that might indicate the presence of an STI. Many people who have an STI do not know that they have one, and some STIs can remain undetected for years. GSE should become a regular part of routine self–health care practices.

Explain and demonstrate the following procedure to your patient and give the opportunity to perform a GSE under your guidance. Emphasize hand washing before and afterward.

Instruct the patient to start by examining the area that the pubic hair covers. Patients may want to use a mirror and position it so that they can see their entire genital area. The pubic hair should then be spread apart with the fingers, and the patient should carefully look for any bumps, sores, or blisters on the skin. Bumps and blisters may be red or light-colored or resemble pimples. Also instruct the patient to look for warts, which may look similar to warts on other parts of the body. At first, they may be small, bumpy spots; left untreated, however, they could develop a fleshy, cauliflower-like appearance (see Fig. 19.47).

Next, instruct the patient to spread the outer vaginal lips and look closely at the hood of the clitoris. The patient should gently pull the hood up to see the clitoris and again look for any bumps, blisters, sores, or warts. Then both sides of the inner vaginal lips should be examined for the same signs.

Have the patient move on to examine the area around the urinary and vaginal openings, looking for any bumps, blisters, sores, or warts (see Figs. 19.48 through 19.51). Some signs of STIs may be out of view—in the vagina or near the cervix. Therefore if patients believe that they have come in contact with an STI, they should see their clinician even if no signs or symptoms are discovered during self-examination.

Also educate patients about other symptoms associated with STIs—specifically, pain or burning on urination, pain in the pelvic area, bleeding between menstrual periods, or an itchy rash around the vagina. Some STIs may cause a vaginal discharge. Patients should try to be aware of what their normal discharge looks like. Discharge caused by an STI will be different from the usual; it may be yellow and thicker and have an odor.

Instruct patients to see a clinician if they have any of the preceding signs or symptoms.

BOX 19.2 Evaluation of Masturbation in Children

Masturbation is a common, healthy, self-discovery activity in children. Parents sometimes express concern about their child's masturbation activity. The following guidelines can help you determine when such activity might be a cause for concern.

HEALTHY ACTIVITY	NEEDS FURTHER ASSESSMENT
Occasional	Frequent, compulsive excessive/obsessive
Discreet, private	No regard for privacy Age-inappropriate public masturbation
Not preferred over other activity or play	Often preferred over other activity or play Combined with other emotional and/or behavioral problems
No physical signs or symptoms	Produces genital discomfort, irritation, or physical signs
External stimulation of genitalia only	Involves penetration of the genital orifices; aggressive; includes bizarre practices or rituals

From Haka-Ikse, K., & Mian, M. (1993). Sexuality in children. *Pediatrics in Review, 14*(10), 401–407 and Mallants, C., & Casteels, K. (2008). Practical approach to childhood masturbation—a review. European *Journal of Pediatric Surgery, 167*(10), 1111–1117.

Pregnant Patients

- Expected date of delivery (EDD) or weeks of gestation
- Previous obstetric history:
  - **G:** gravidity (total number of pregnancies)
  - **T:** number of term pregnancies
  - **P:** number of preterm pregnancies
  - **A:** number of abortions, spontaneous or induced
  - **L:** number of living children
  - Prenatal complications, infertility treatment
- Previous birth history: length of gestation at birth, birth weight, fetal outcome, length of labor, fetal presentation, type of delivery, use of forceps, lacerations and/or episiotomy, complications (natal and postnatal)
- Previous menstrual history (see menstrual history under "Past Medical History")
- Surgical history: prior uterine surgery and type of scar
- Family history: diabetes mellitus, multiple births, preeclampsia, genetic disorder
- Involuntary passage of fluid, which may result from rupture of membranes (ROM): determine onset, duration, color, odor, amount, and if still leaking
- Bleeding
  - Character: onset, duration, precipitating factor if known (e.g., intercourse, trauma), course since onset, amount
  - Associated symptoms
- Pain: type (e.g., sharp or dull, intermittent or continuous), onset, location, duration
- Gastrointestinal symptoms: nausea, vomiting, heartburn

Older Adults

- Menopause history: see "History of Present Illness"
- Symptoms associated with age-related physiologic changes: itching, urinary symptoms, dyspareunia
- Changes in sexual desire or behavior in self or partner(s)

EXAMINATION AND FINDINGS

Equipment

- Lamp or light source
- Drapes
- Speculum
- Gloves
- Water-soluble lubricant
- Pap smear/HPV collection equipment
  - Collection device: (wooden or plastic spatula, cervical brush or broom)
  - Glass slides and cytologic fixative or fluid collection media
- Other specimen collection equipment as needed:
  - Cotton swabs
  - Culture plates or media
  - DNA tests for organisms

Preparation

Although most patients express lack of enthusiasm in anticipation of a pelvic examination, most do not experience anxiety (see Clinical Pearl, "Anxiety"). Explain in general terms what you are going to do. Maintain eye contact with the patient, both before and—as much as possible—during the examination. Be sensitive to cultural variations in behavior. Patients from some cultural or ethnic groups may not return eye contact as a show of respect. If the patient has not seen the equipment before, show it and explain its use.

The genital and pelvic examination may be anxiety producing for transgender patients. The use of a gender-affirming approach during the examination—for example, use of correct name and pronouns—demonstrates respect and can help reduce anxiety. Patients who have undergone gender-affirming surgeries may have varying physical examination findings depending on the procedures performed.

> **CLINICAL PEARL**
>
> **Anxiety**
>
> Marked anxiety before an examination may be a sign that something is not quite right. Before beginning, you should attempt to uncover the source of the anxiety. It could be a bad experience, either in a patient's personal life (e.g., child abuse, sexual assault) or during a previous pelvic examination. It could be the lack of familiarity with what to expect during the examination; it could be worry about possible findings or their meaning. Do not assume you know—use your skills and ask. It is your job to minimize the patient's apprehension and discomfort.

Assure the patient that you will explain what you are doing as the examination proceeds. Advise that you will be as gentle as possible and to inform you of any discomfort.

Have the patient empty the bladder before the examination. Bimanual examination is uncomfortable for the patient if the bladder is full. A full bladder also makes it difficult to palpate the pelvic organs.

Make sure that the room temperature is comfortable. Do what you can to ensure privacy. The door should be securely closed and should be opened only with permission of both the patient and examiner. The examination table is best positioned so that the patient faces away from the door during the examination. A drawn curtain can ensure that any door opening will not expose the patient. A chaperone, often required by practice or institutional policy, protects both the clinician and patient. Some patients may be reluctant to reveal confidential and sensitive information in the presence of an observer chaperone, but this should not supersede the need to have a chaperone present for the examination.

Positioning

Assist the patient into the lithotomy position on the examining table. (If a table with stirrups is not available or if the patient is unable to assume the lithotomy position, the examination can be performed in other positions.) Help the patient stabilize the feet in the stirrups and slide the buttocks down to the edge of the examining table. If the patient is not positioned correctly, you will have difficulty with the speculum examination.

Draping and Gloving

The patient can be draped in such a way that allows minimal exposure. A good method is to cover the knees and symphysis, depressing the drape between the knees. This allows you to see the patient's face (and the patient, yours) throughout the examination (Fig. 19.10).

Once the patient is positioned and draped, make sure that any equipment is nearby and in easy reach. Arrange

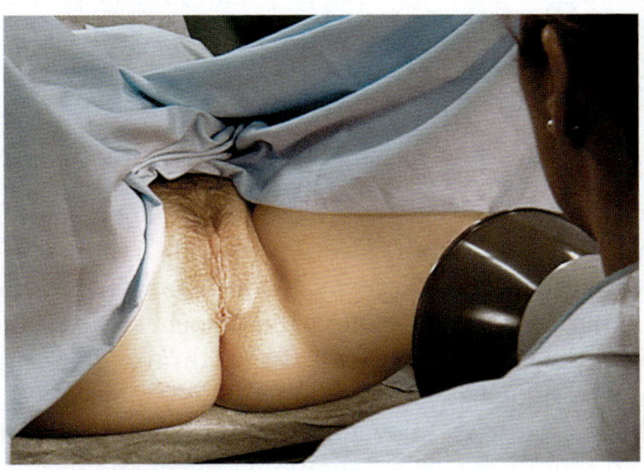

FIG. 19.10 Draped patient in dorsal lithotomy position.

the examining lamp so that the external genitalia are clearly visible. Wash or sanitize your hands and put gloves on both hands (see Clinical Pearl, "Gloving").

Ask the patient to drop open the knees. Never try to separate the legs forcibly or even gently. The pelvic examination is an intrusive procedure, and you may need to wait a moment until the patient is ready. Tell the patient that you are going to begin, then start with a neutral touch on the lower thigh, moving your examining hand along the thigh without breaking contact to the external genitalia.

CLINICAL PEARL

Gloving

Once you have touched any part of the patient's genital area, assume that your glove is contaminated. Do not touch any surfaces or instruments that will not be discarded or immediately disinfected until you remove or change your gloves. This includes lights, drawers, door handles, counter surfaces, examining table surfaces, fixative and specimen bottles and jars, computers or electronic devices, and patient forms. Change gloves as often as you need to. Some clinicians prefer to double or triple glove at the beginning of an examination and then remove a glove when a clean hand is needed.

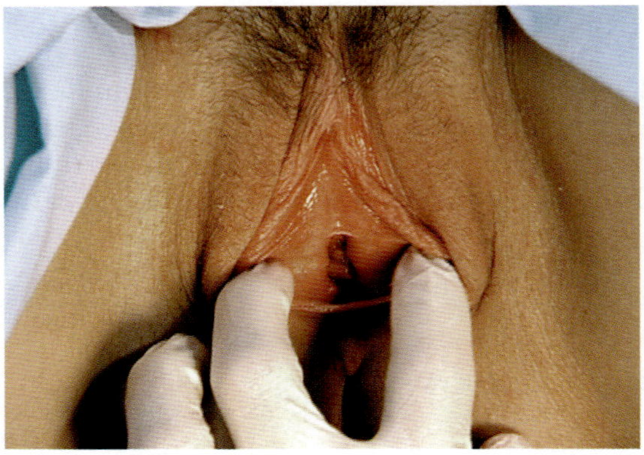

FIG. 19.11 Separation of the labia.

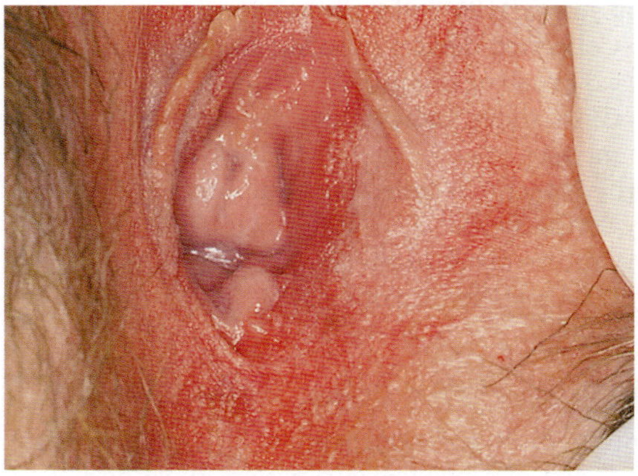

FIG. 19.12 **Normal vulva with finely textured, papular sebaceous glands on the inner labia majora and labia minora.** (From Morse, S. A., et al. (2003). *Atlas of sexually transmitted diseases and AIDS* (3rd ed.). St. Louis: Mosby.)

External Examination

Inspection and Palpation

Sit at the end of the examining table and inspect and palpate the external genitalia. Look at the hair distribution and notice the surface characteristics of the mons pubis and labia majora. The skin should be smooth and clean, and the hair should be free of nits or lice.

Labia Majora

The labia majora may be gaping or closed and may appear dry or moist. They are usually symmetric and may be either shriveled or full. The tissue should feel soft and homogeneous. Labial swelling, redness, or tenderness—particularly if unilateral—may be indicative of a Bartholin gland infection. Look for excoriation, rashes, or lesions, which suggest an infectious or inflammatory process. If any of these signs are present, ask if the patient has been scratching. Observe for discoloration, varicosities, obvious stretching, or signs of trauma or scarring.

Labia Minora

Separate the labia majora with the fingers of one hand and inspect the labia minora. Use your other hand to palpate the labia minora between your thumb and second finger; then separate the labia minora and inspect and palpate the inside of the labia minora, clitoris, urethral orifice, vaginal introitus, and perineum (Fig. 19.11).

The labia minora may appear symmetric or asymmetric, and the inner surface should be moist and dark pink. The tissue should feel soft, homogeneous, and without tenderness (Fig. 19.12). Look for inflammation, irritation, excoriation, or caking of discharge in the tissue folds, which suggests vaginal infection or poor hygiene. Discoloration or tenderness may be the result of traumatic bruising. Ulcers or vesicles may be signs of an STI. Palpate for irregularities or nodules.

Clitoris

Inspect the clitoris for size. Generally, the clitoris is about 2 cm or less in length and 0.5 cm in diameter. Enlargement may be a sign of a masculinizing condition. Observe also for atrophy, inflammation, or adhesions.

Urethral Orifice

The urethral orifice appears as an irregular opening or slit. It may be close to or slightly within the vaginal introitus and is usually in the midline. Inspect for discharge, polyps, caruncles, and fistulas. A caruncle is a bright red polypoid vascular growth that protrudes from the urethral meatus; most urethral caruncles cause no symptoms (Fig. 19.13).

Signs of irritation, inflammation, or dilation suggest repeated urinary tract infections or insertion of foreign objects. Ask questions about any findings at a later

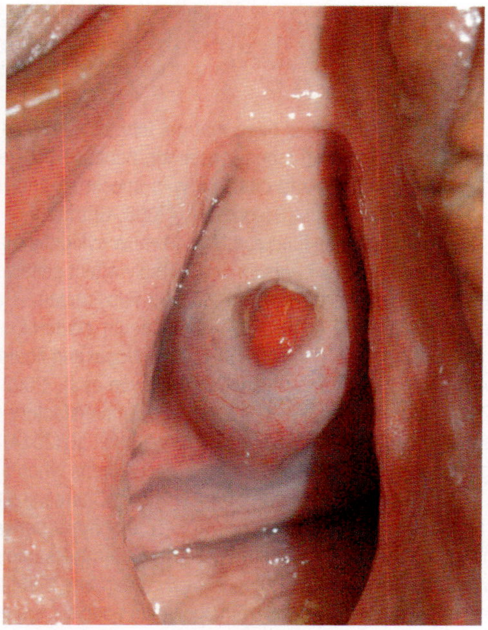

FIG. 19.13 Urethral caruncle, a red, fleshy lesion at the urethral meatus. (From Black, M., Ambros-Rudolph, C. M., et al. (2008). *Obstetric and gynecologic dermatology* (3rd ed.). Elsevier.)

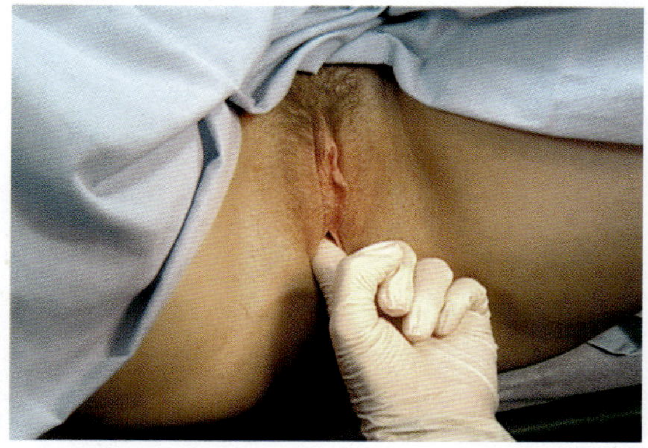

FIG. 19.14 Palpation of Skene glands.

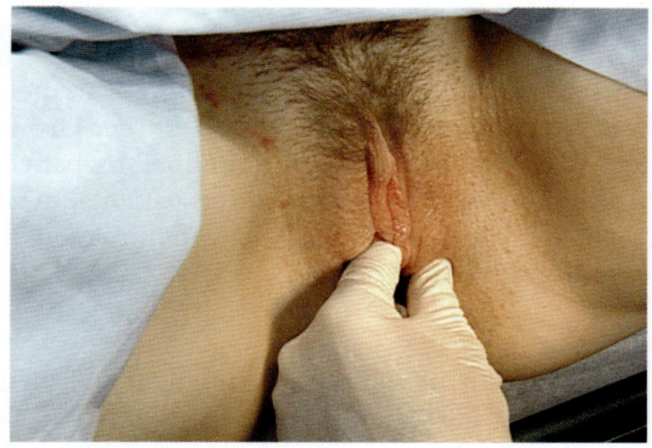

FIG. 19.15 Palpation of Bartholin glands.

time—not during the pelvic examination when the patient feels most vulnerable.

Vaginal Introitus

The vaginal introitus can be a thin vertical slit or a large orifice with irregular edges from hymenal remnants (myrtiform caruncles). The tissue should be moist. Look for swelling, discoloration, discharge, lesions, fistulas, or fissures.

Skene and Bartholin Glands

With the labia still separated, examine the Skene and Bartholin glands. Tell the patient you are going to insert one finger in the vagina and that they will feel you pressing forward with it. With your palm facing upward, insert the index finger of the examining hand into the vagina as far as the second joint of the finger. Exerting upward pressure, milk the Skene glands by moving the finger outward. Do this on both sides of the urethra, and then directly on the urethra (Fig. 19.14). Look for discharge and note any tenderness. If a discharge occurs, note its color, consistency, and odor, and obtain a culture. Discharge from the Skene glands or urethra usually indicates an infection—most commonly, but not necessarily, gonococcal.

With your finger still in place, you can then locate the cervix and note the direction in which it points. This may help you locate the cervix when you insert the speculum.

Maintaining labial separation and with your finger still in the vaginal opening, tell the patient to expect pressure around the entrance to the vagina. Palpate the lateral tissue between your index finger and thumb. Palpate the entire area, paying particular attention to the posterolateral portion of the labia majora where the Bartholin glands are located. Note any swelling, tenderness, masses, heat, or fluctuation. Observe for discharge from the opening of the Bartholin gland duct. Palpate and observe bilaterally because each gland is separate (Fig. 19.15). Note the color, consistency, and odor of any discharge, and obtain a specimen for laboratory evaluation. Swelling that is painful, hot to the touch, and fluctuant is indicative of infection of the Bartholin gland. The infection is usually gonococcal or staphylococcal in origin and is filled with pus. A nontender mass is indicative of a Bartholin cyst, which is the result of chronic inflammation of the gland.

Muscle Tone

Test muscle tone if the patient has delivered children or has told you about signs of weak muscle tone (e.g., urinary incontinence or the sensation of something “falling out”). To test, ask the patient to squeeze the vaginal opening around your finger, explaining that you are testing muscle tone. Then ask the patient to bear down as you watch for urinary incontinence and uterine prolapse. Uterine prolapse is marked by protrusion of the cervix or uterus on straining.

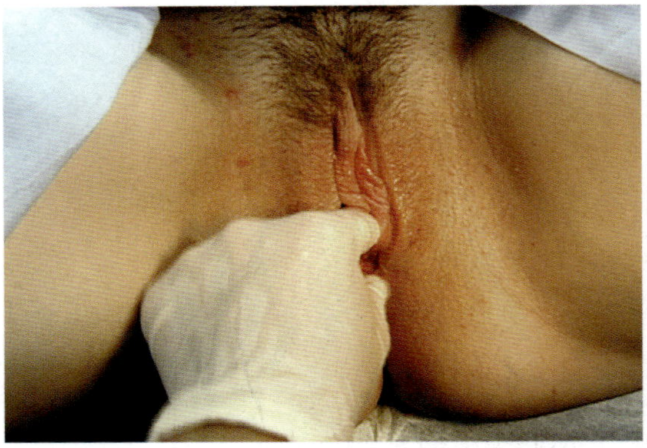

FIG. 19.16 Palpating the perineum.

Perineum

Inspect and palpate the perineum (Fig. 19.16). The perineal surface should be smooth; episiotomy scarring may be evident in patients who have borne children. The tissue will feel thick and smooth in the nulliparous patient. It will be thinner and rigid in multiparous patients. In either case, it should not be tender. Look for inflammation, fistulas, lesions, or growths.

Anus

The anal surface is more darkly pigmented, and the skin may appear coarse. It should be free of scarring, lesions, inflammation, fissures, lumps, skin tags, or excoriation. If you touch the anus or perianal skin, be sure to change your gloves so that you do not introduce bacteria into the vagina during the internal examination.

Internal Examination

Preparation

It is essential that you become familiar with how the speculum operates before you begin the examination so that you do not inadvertently hurt the patient through mishandling of the instrument. Chapter 3 describes the proper use of the speculum. Become familiar with both the reusable stainless steel and the disposable plastic specula because their mechanisms of action are somewhat different.

Lubricate the speculum (and the gloved fingers) with water or a water-soluble lubricant. Most clinicians routinely lubricate with water only. An added advantage of using water as a lubricant is that a cold speculum can be warmed by rinsing in warm (but not hot) water. A speculum can also be warmed by holding it in your hand (if it is warm) or under the lamp for a few minutes.

Select the appropriate-size speculum (see Chapter 3) and hold it in your hand with the index finger over the top of the proximal end of the anterior blade and the other fingers around the handle. This position controls the blades as the speculum is inserted into the vagina.

Evidence-Based Practice in Physical Examination

Lubricating the Speculum

The conventional wisdom has been that gel lubricants should not be used when collecting a Pap smear specimen because the gel could obscure cellular elements and interfere with specimen analysis and interpretation. Some studies (Gilson et al., 2006; Griffith et al., 2005; Harer et al., 2003) question this premise and show evidence that using a water-soluble gel lubricant does not adversely affect cellular analysis with either conventional or liquid-based Pap smears. However, another report (Zardawi et al., 2003) documents contamination by excess gel in some instances with both conventional and liquid-based Pap smears, and two other studies (Charoenkwan et al., 2008; Köşüş et al., 2012) document a higher proportion of unsatisfactory smears that were contaminated with gel. Additionally, Lin et al. (2014) reported a significantly higher rate of insufficient specimens when a water-soluble lubricant containing carbomers was used. Charoenkwan et al. (2008) also reported discordance in cytologic diagnosis between the gel-contaminated and uncontaminated smears from the same patient. Our advice: Until further studies conclusively determine that gel lubricant does not adversely interfere with specimen analysis, we continue to recommend lubrication with water. However, if gel lubricant is used, a thin layer on the external surface of the blades only will help avoid contamination of the specimen.

Insertion of Speculum

Tell the patient to expect your touch, and gently insert a finger of your other hand just inside the vaginal introitus and apply pressure downward. Ask the patient to breathe slowly and try to consciously relax the muscles or the muscles of the buttocks. Wait until you feel the relaxation (Fig. 19.17A). Use the fingers of that hand to separate the labia minora so that the vaginal opening becomes clearly visible. Then slowly insert the speculum along the path of least resistance, often slightly downward, avoiding trauma to the urethra and vaginal walls. Some clinicians insert the speculum blades at an oblique angle; others prefer to keep the blades horizontal. In either case, avoid touching the clitoris, catching pubic hair, or pinching labial skin (see Fig. 19.17B and C). Insert the speculum the length of the vaginal canal. While maintaining gentle downward pressure with the speculum, open it by pressing on the thumb piece. Sweep the speculum slowly upward until the cervix comes into view. Gently reposition the speculum, if necessary, to locate the cervix. Adjust the light source.

Once you visualize the cervix, manipulate the speculum to fully expose the cervix between the anterior and posterior blades. Lock the speculum blades into place to stabilize the distal spread of the blades and adjust the proximal spread as needed (see Fig. 19.17D).

Cervix

Inspect the cervix for color, position, size, surface characteristics, discharge, and size and shape of the os.

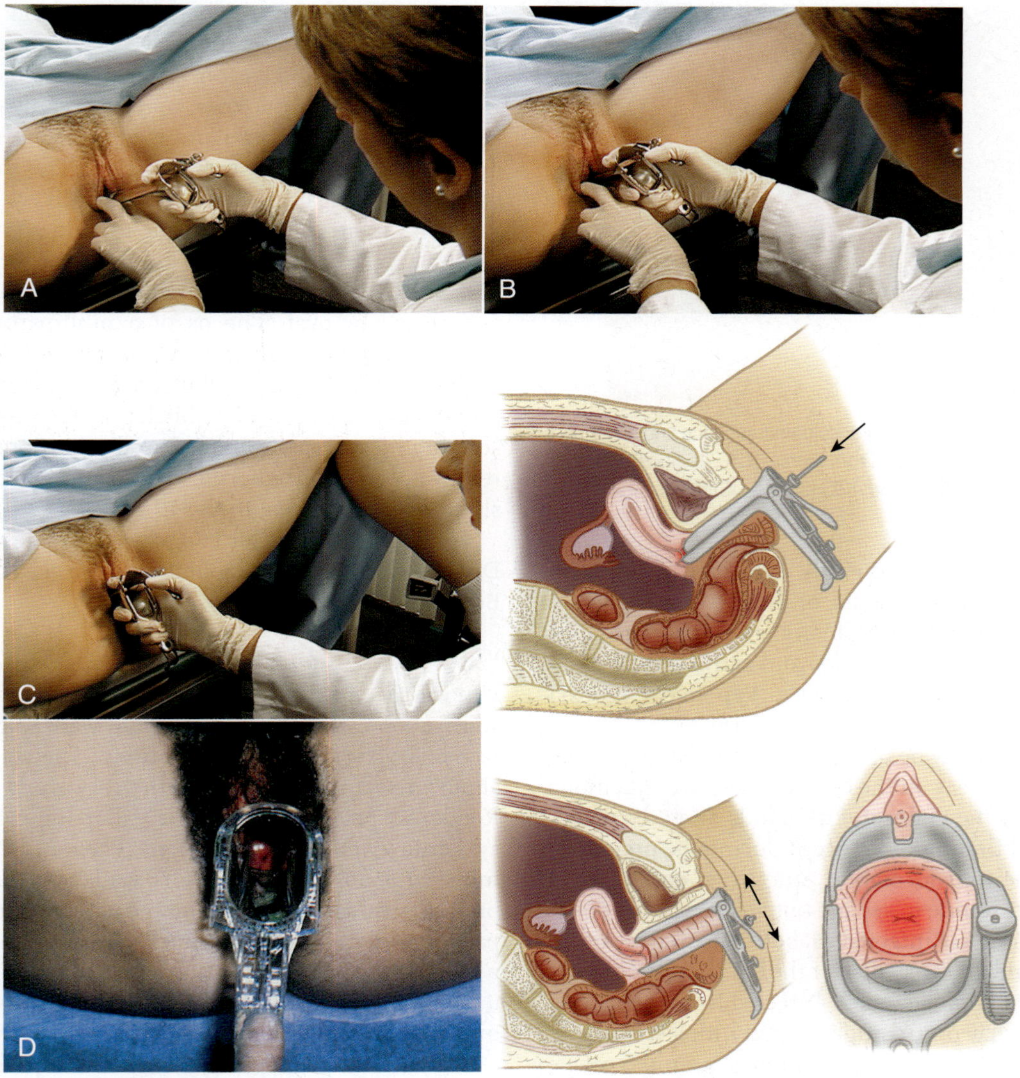

FIG. 19.17 Examination of the internal genitalia with a speculum. Begin by inserting a finger and applying downward pressure to relax the vaginal muscles. (A) Gently insert the closed speculum blades into the vagina. (B) Direct the speculum along the path of least resistance. (C) Insert the speculum the length of the vaginal canal. (D) Speculum is in place, locked, and stabilized. Note cervix in full view. (D, Photograph from Edge, V., & Miller, M. (1994). Women's health care. St. Louis: Mosby.)

Color. Expect the cervix to be pink, with the color evenly distributed. A bluish color indicates increased vascularity, which may be a sign of pregnancy. Symmetric circumscribed redness around the os is an expected finding that indicates exposed columnar epithelium from the cervical canal. However, beginning clinicians should consider any reddened areas an unexpected finding, especially if patchy or if the borders are irregular. A pale cervix is associated with anemia.

Position. The anteroposterior position of the cervix correlates with the position of the uterus. A cervix that is pointing anteriorly indicates a retroverted uterus; one pointing posteriorly indicates an anteverted uterus. A cervix in the horizontal position indicates a uterus in midposition. The cervix should be located in the midline. Deviation to the right or left may indicate a pelvic mass, uterine adhesions, or pregnancy. The cervix may protrude 1 to 3 cm into the vagina. Projection greater than 3 cm may indicate a pelvic or uterine mass. The cervix of a patient of childbearing age is usually 2 to 3 cm in diameter.

Surface Characteristics. The surface of the cervix should be smooth. Usually the transformation zone (the junction of squamous and columnar epithelium) is just barely visible inside the external os. Some squamocolumnar epithelium of the cervical canal may be visible as a symmetric reddened circle around the os (Fig. 19.18). Cervical ectropion occurs when eversion of the endocervix exposes columnar epithelium. The everted epithelium has a red, shiny appearance

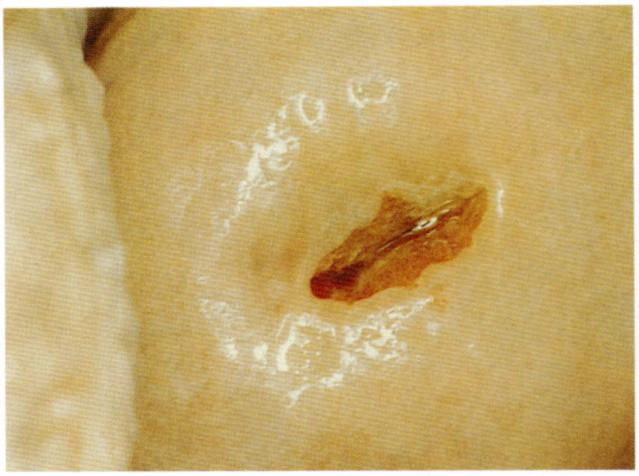

FIG. 19.18 Normal cervix. The squamocolumnar junction and lower part of the endocervical canal are seen. (From Morse, S. A., et al. (2003). *Atlas of sexually transmitted diseases and AIDS* (3rd ed.). St. Louis: Mosby.)

around the os and may bleed easily. Ectropion is common in adolescents, pregnant patients, or those taking estrogen-containing contraceptives. Ectropion is not an abnormality, but because it is indistinguishable from early cervical carcinoma, further diagnostic studies (e.g., Pap smear, biopsy) must be performed for differential diagnosis.

Nabothian cysts may be observed as small, white or yellow, raised, round areas on the cervix. These are mucinous retention cysts of the endocervical glands and are considered an expected finding. They occur during the process of metaplasia at the transformation zone when endocervical columnar cells continue to secrete but are covered by squamous epithelium. An infected Nabothian cyst becomes swollen with fluid and may distort the shape of the cervix, giving it an irregular appearance. Infected Nabothian cysts vary in size and may occur singly or in multiples.

Look for friable tissue, red patchy areas, granular areas, and white patches that could indicate cervicitis, infection, or carcinoma.

Note the presence of any cervical polyps, which are bright red, soft, and fragile. They usually arise from the endocervical canal (Fig. 19.19).

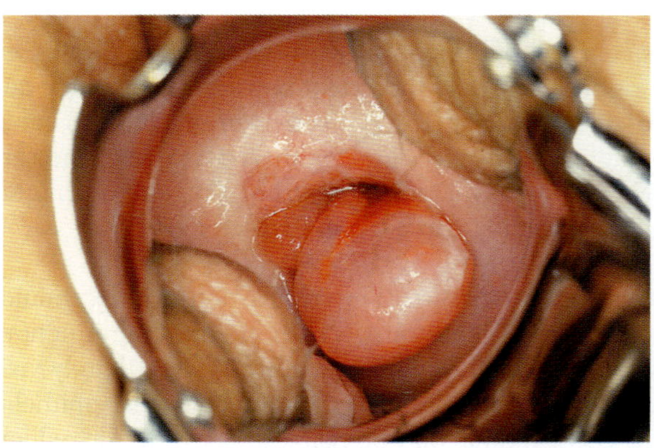

FIG. 19.19 Polyp protruding through the cervical os. (From Baggish, M. S. (2003). Colposcopy of the cervix, vagina, and vulva: A comprehensive textbook, Philadelphia: Mosby.)

Discharge. Note any discharge. Determine whether the discharge comes from the cervix itself or whether it is vaginal in origin and has only been deposited on the cervix. Usual discharge is odorless; may be creamy or clear; may be thick, thin, or stringy; and is often heavier at midcycle or immediately before menstruation. The discharge of a bacterial or fungal infection will more likely have an odor and will vary in color from white to yellow, green, or gray.

Size and Shape. The os of the nulliparous patient is small and round or oval. The os of a multiparous patient is usually a horizontal slit or may be irregular and stellate. Cervical lacerations caused by trauma from childbirth can produce lateral transverse, bilateral transverse, or stellate scarring. Trauma from induced abortion or difficult removal of an intrauterine device may also change the shape of the os to a slit (Fig. 19.20).

Obtain specimens for Pap smear, HPV testing, culture, DNA testing, or other laboratory analysis as indicated in Box 19.3.

Withdrawal of Speculum

Unlock the speculum and remove it slowly and carefully so that you can inspect the vaginal walls. Note color, surface characteristics, and secretions. The color should be about the same color pink as the cervix or a little lighter. Reddened patches, lesions, or pallor indicates a local or systemic pathologic condition. The surface should be moist and homogeneous. The walls will have rugae in premenopausal patients and be smooth in postmenopausal patients. Look for cracks, lesions, bleeding, nodules, and swelling. Secretions that may be expected are usually thin, clear or cloudy, and odorless. Secretions indicative of infection are often profuse; may be thick, curdy, or frothy; appear gray, green, or yellow; and may have a foul odor.

Look for the presence of a cystocele or rectocele. A cystocele is a hernial protrusion of the urinary bladder through the anterior wall of the vagina, sometimes even exiting the introitus (Fig. 19.24). The bulging can be seen and felt as the patient bears down. More severe degrees of cystocele are accompanied by urinary stress incontinence. Seen as a bulge on the posterior wall of the vagina, a rectocele (or proctocele) is a hernial protrusion of part of the rectum through the posterior vaginal wall (Fig. 19.25).

As you withdraw the speculum, the blades will tend to close themselves. Avoid pinching the cervix and vaginal walls. Maintain downward pressure of the speculum to avoid trauma to the urethra. Hook your index finger over the anterior blade as it is removed. Keep one thumb on the handle lever and control the closing of the speculum. Make sure that the speculum is fully closed when the blades pass through the hymenal ring. Note the odor of any vaginal discharge that has pooled in the posterior blade and obtain a specimen if you have not already done so. Deposit the speculum in the proper container.

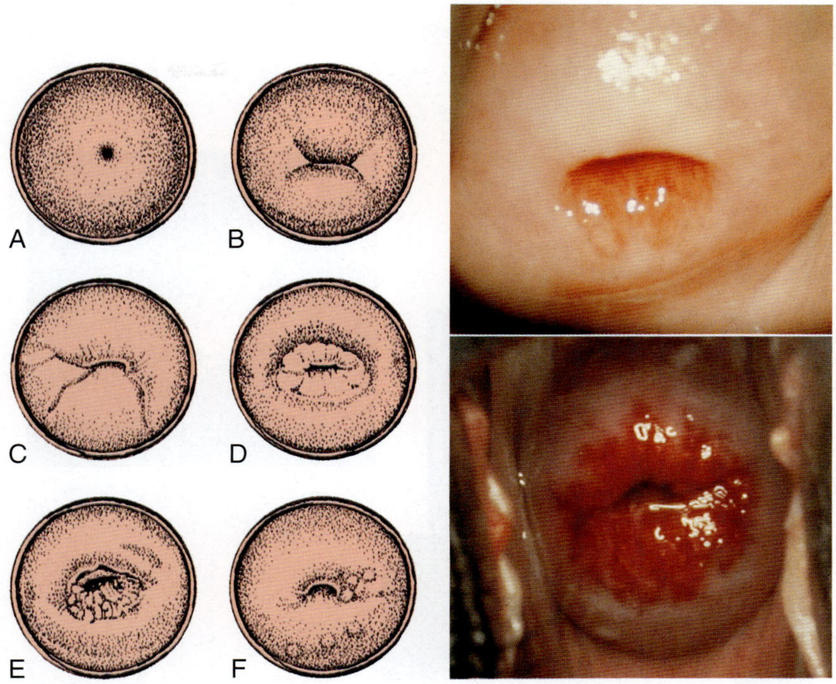

FIG. 19.20 **Common appearances of the cervix.** (A) Normal nulliparous cervix. The surface is covered with pink squamous epithelium that is uniform in consistency. The os is small and round. A small area of ectropion is visible inferior to the os. (B) Parous cervix. Note slit appearance of os. (C) Multiparous, lacerated. (D) Everted. Columnar mucosal cells usually found in the endocervical canal have extended out into the surface of the cervix, creating a circular, raised, erythematous appearance. Note the normal nonpurulent cervical mucus. This normal variant is not to be confused with cervicitis. (E) Eroded. (F) Nabothian cysts. (Photographs from Zitelli, B. J., & Davis, H. W. (1997). *Atlas of pediatric physical diagnosis* (3rd ed.). St. Louis: Mosby; A, courtesy C. Stevens, DO, Houston, TX; D, Courtesy E. Jerome, MD.)

BOX 19.3 Obtaining Vaginal Smears and Specimens

Vaginal specimens for smears and cultures are often obtained during the speculum examination. Vaginal specimens are obtained while the speculum is in place but after the cervix and its surrounding tissue have been inspected. Collect specimens as indicated for Pap smear, HPV testing, sexually transmitted infection screening, and wet mount. Be sure to follow Standard Precautions for the safe collection of human secretions. Label the specimen with the patient's name, date, and a description of the specimen (e.g., cervical smear, vaginal smear, culture). If the Pap smear cervical specimen is from a transgender man, it is essential to make clear to the laboratory that the sample is a cervical Pap smear (especially if the listed gender marker is "male") to avoid the sample being run incorrectly as an anal Pap or discarded. The use of testosterone or presence of amenorrhea should be indicated on the requisition.

Conventional Papanicolaou Smear

Brushes and brooms are now being used in conjunction with, or instead of, the conventional spatula to improve the quality of cells obtained. The cylindric-type brush collects endocervical cells only. First, collect a sample from the ectocervix with a spatula (Figs. 19.21 and 19.22A). Insert the longer projection of the spatula into the cervical os; rotate it 360 degrees, keeping it flush against the cervical tissue. Withdraw the spatula and spread the specimen on a glass slide. A single light stroke with each side of the spatula is sufficient to thin the specimen out over the slide. Immediately spray with cytologic fixative and label the slide as the ectocervical specimen. Then introduce the brush device into the vagina and insert it into the cervical os until only the bristles closest to the handle are exposed (see Fig. 19.22B and C). Slowly rotate one half-turn. Remove and prepare the endocervical smear by rolling and twisting the brush with moderate pressure across a glass slide. Fix the specimen with spray and label as the endocervical specimen.

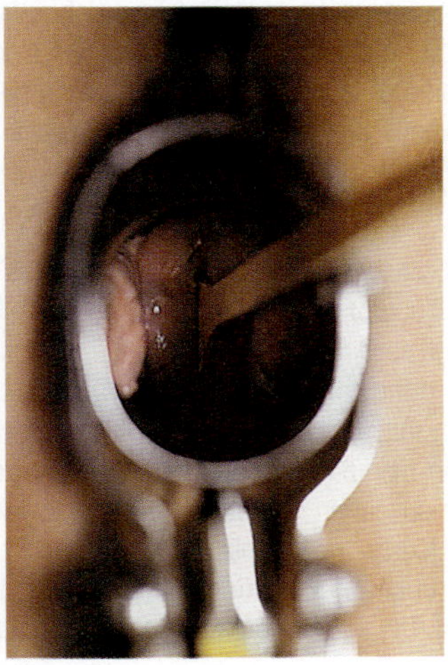

FIG. 19.21 **Scrape the cervix with the bifid end of the spatula to obtain a Pap smear.** (From Symonds, E. M., & Macpherson, M. B. A. (1994). Color atlas of obstetrics and gynecology. St. Louis: Mosby.)

Continued

BOX 19.3 Obtaining Vaginal Smears and Specimens—cont'd

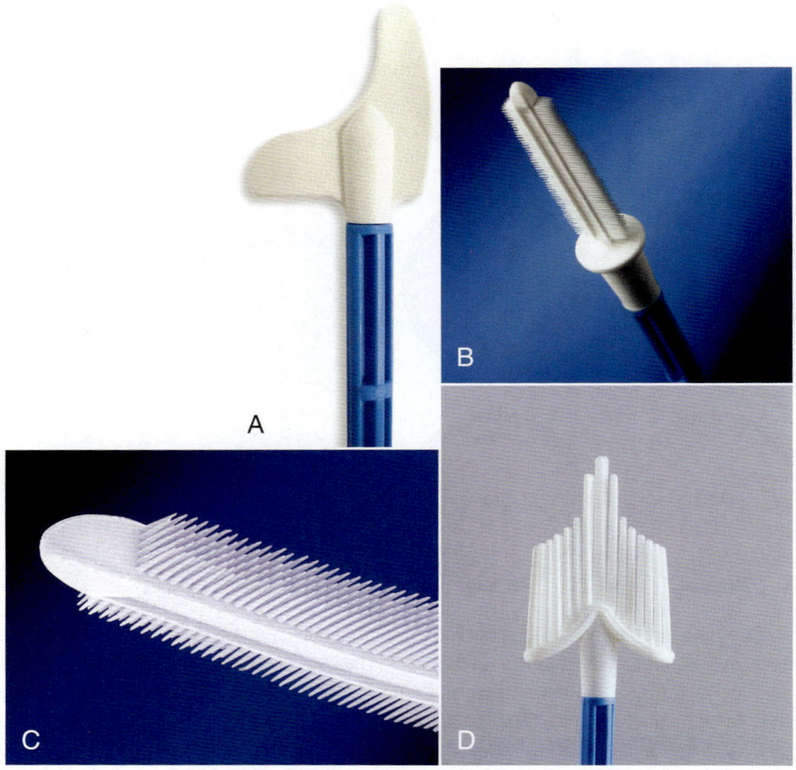

FIG. 19.22 Implements used to obtain a Pap smear. (A) Close-up of spatula. (B) Brush device. (C) Close-up of brush. (D) Broom device. (Courtesy Therapak Corporation, Irwindale, CA.)

The broom-type device is used for collecting both ectocervical and endocervical cells at the same time (see Fig. 19.22D). This broom uses flexible plastic bristles, which are reported to cause less blood spotting after the examination. Introduce the brush into the vagina and insert the central long bristles into the cervical os until the lateral bristles bend fully against the ectocervix. Maintain gentle pressure and rotate the brush by rolling the handle between the thumb and forefinger three to five times to the left and right. Withdraw the brush and transfer the sample to a glass slide with two single paint strokes: apply first one side of the bristle, turn the brush over, and paint the slide again in exactly the same area. Apply fixative and label as the ectocervical and endocervical specimen.

Liquid-Based Pap Testing

The liquid-based cytology replaces the use of a glass slide and fixative spray. Use a brush and/or the broom-type device to collect the specimen following the same collection steps as with the conventional Pap smear. Rinse the brush in the solution by swirling. Deposit the broom end of the device directly into the collection vial. With any collection device, be sure to follow the manufacturer and laboratory instructions to collect and preserve the specimen appropriately. Close the vial tightly to prevent leakage and loss of the sample during transport. Label with patient name, date, and origin of specimen (ectocervical only or ectocervical and endocervical). The liquid sample is also used to test for HPV.

Gonococcal Culture Specimen

Immediately after the Pap smear is obtained, introduce a sterile cotton swab into the vagina and insert it into the cervical os (Fig. 19.23); hold it in place for 10–30 seconds. Withdraw the swab and spread

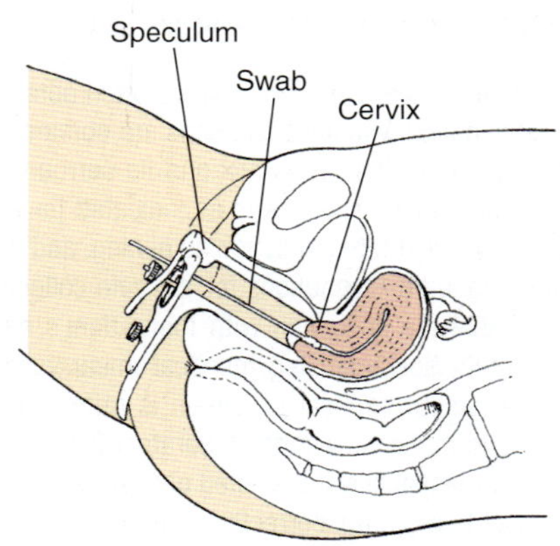

FIG. 19.23 Obtaining a cervical specimen by inserting a swab into the cervical os. (From Grimes, D. (1991). Infectious diseases. St. Louis: Mosby.)

the specimen in a large Z pattern over the culture medium, rotating the swab at the same time. Label the tube or plate and follow agency routine for transporting and maintaining appropriate temperature of the specimen. If indicated, an anal culture can be obtained after the vaginal speculum has been removed. Insert a fresh, sterile cotton swab about 2.5 cm into the rectum and rotate it full circle; hold it in place for 10 to 30 seconds. Withdraw the swab and prepare the specimen as described for the vaginal culture. Gonococcal cultures are now used less commonly than the combined DNA probe for chlamydia and gonorrhea.

BOX 19.3 Obtaining Vaginal Smears and Specimens—cont'd

DNA Testing for Organisms

These tests involve the construction of a nucleic acid sequence that will match to a sequence in the DNA or RNA of the target tissue; the results are rapid and sensitive. Use a Dacron swab (with plastic or wire shaft) when collecting your specimen, as wooden cotton-tipped applicators may interfere with the test results. Also be sure to check the expiration date so as not to use out-of-date materials. Insert the swab into the cervical os and rotate the swab in the endocervical canal for 30 seconds to ensure adequate sampling and absorption by the swab. Avoid contact with the vaginal mucous membranes, which would contaminate the specimen. Remove the swab and place it in the tube containing the specimen reagent. Single- or dual-organism tests are available for *Chlamydia trachomatis* and *Neisseria gonorrhoeae.* Multiorganism tests are available for *Trichomonas vaginalis, Gardnerella vaginalis, Candida* species, and *Mycoplasma genitalium.*

Wet Mount and Potassium Hydroxide (KOH) Procedures

In a patient with vaginal discharge, these microscope examinations can demonstrate the presence of *T. vaginalis,* bacterial vaginosis, or candidiasis. For the wet mount, obtain a specimen of vaginal discharge using a swab. Smear the sample on a glass slide and add a drop of normal saline. Place a coverslip on the slide, and view under the microscope. The presence of trichomonads indicates *T. vaginalis.* The presence of bacteria-filled epithelial cells (clue cells) indicates bacterial vaginosis. On a separate glass slide, place a specimen of vaginal discharge, apply a drop of aqueous 10% KOH, and put a coverslip in place. The presence of a fishy odor (the "whiff test") suggests bacterial vaginosis. The KOH dissolves epithelial cells and debris and facilitates visualization of the mycelia of a fungus. View under the microscope for the presence of mycelial fragments, hyphae, and budding yeast cells, which indicate candidiasis.

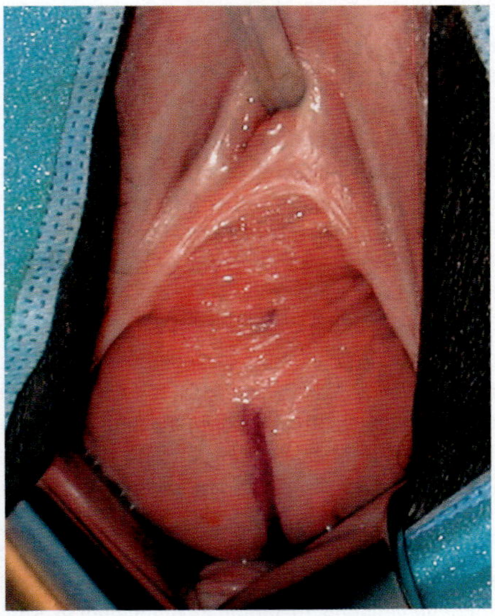

FIG. 19.24 **Cystocele.** (From Wein, A. J., Kavoussi, L. R., et al. (2016). *Campbell-Walsh Urology* (11th ed.). Philadelphia: Elsevier.)

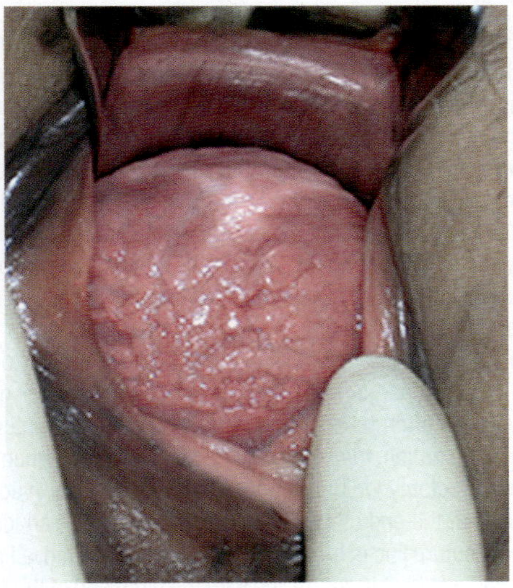

FIG. 19.25 **Rectocele.** (From Corton, M. M. (2009). Anatomy of pelvic floor dysfunction. *Obstetrics and Gynecology Clinics of North America,* 36(3), 401–419.)

Bimanual Examination

Inform the patient that you are going to examine internally with your fingers. Change your gloves or remove the outer glove and lubricate the index and middle fingers of your examining hand. Insert the tips of the gloved index and middle fingers into the vaginal opening and press downward, again waiting for the muscles to relax. Gradually and gently insert your fingers their full length into the vagina. Palpate the vaginal wall as you insert your fingers. It should be smooth, homogeneous, and nontender. Feel for cysts, nodules, masses, or growths.

Be careful where you place your thumb during the bimanual examination. You can tuck it into the palm of your hand, but that will cut down on the distance you can insert your fingers. Be aware of where the thumb is and keep it from touching the clitoris, which can produce discomfort (Fig. 19.26).

Box 19.4 describes the examination of a patient who has had a hysterectomy. Box 19.5 describes pelvic examination with transgender patients.

Evidence-Based Practice in Physical Examination

Cervical Cancer Screening After Hysterectomy?

Experts agree that patients who have had a hysterectomy for noncancer reasons, with the cervix removed, no evidence of malignancy, and no history of abnormal cancerous cell growth, can discontinue screening for cervical cancer. The yield of cytologic screening is very low after hysterectomy, and there is no evidence that continuing screening improves health outcomes.

From American Cancer Society (2021); and U.S. Preventive Services Task Force (2018).

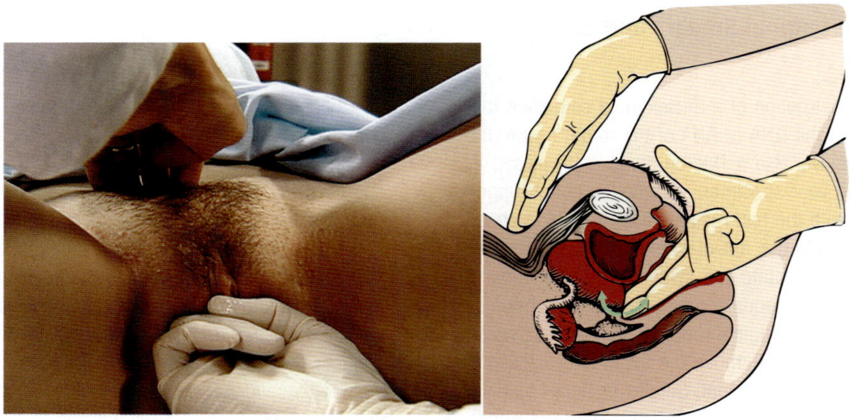

FIG. 19.26 Bimanual palpation of the uterus.

BOX 19.4 Examining the Patient Who Has Had a Hysterectomy

Examination of a patient who has had a hysterectomy is essentially no different from the usual procedure. The same examination steps and sequence are followed, with minor variation in what you are assessing. Getting an accurate history before the examination will assist you in knowing what to look for. Determine whether the surgical approach was vaginal or abdominal; whether the patient had a total hysterectomy, a supracervical hysterectomy (cervix left intact), or a partial hysterectomy (fallopian tubes and ovaries left intact); the reason for the hysterectomy; if there have been bladder or bowel changes since the surgery; and the presence of menopausal symptoms.

Examine the external genitalia for atrophy, skin changes, decreased resilience, and discharge. In these patients, specimens for gonococci or chlamydia are often taken at the vestibule rather than internally. On speculum examination, the cervix will be absent except when a supracervical hysterectomy was performed. The surgical scar (vaginal cuff) will be visible at the end of the vaginal canal and will be an identifiable white or pink suture line in the posterior fornix. If indicated, a Pap smear should be taken from this suture line with the blunt end of the spatula or blunt broom. Be sure to label the specimen as vaginal cells; otherwise, the report may be sent back as incomplete or unsatisfactory because of a lack of endocervical cell sample. Assess the walls, mucosa, and secretions as you ordinarily would. The vaginal canal of a patient who has had a total hysterectomy might show the same changes as those that occur with menopause (e.g., a decrease in rugae and secretions), especially if the patient is not receiving hormone therapy. Examine for a cystocele or rectocele. Stress incontinence may be a problem, so observe for this when having the patient bear down.

On bimanual examination, the uterus will obviously not be present; further findings will depend on whether the hysterectomy was total or partial. If partial, proceed with the examination as usual, assessing the ovaries and surrounding area. If the hysterectomy was total, assess the adnexal area for masses, adhesions, or tenderness. The bladder and bowel may feel more prominent than usual.

BOX 19.5 Pelvic Examination With Transgender Patients

Pelvic examination in transgender women who have had vaginoplasty—the creation of a neovagina—may be appropriate to screen for lesions, granulation tissue, or stenosis or to test for sexually transmitted infections (STIs). Be aware of defenses in the neovagina—it ends in a blind cuff, does not have a cervix or fornices, and may have a more posterior orientation. Select an appropriate sized speculum and allow the anatomy to guide the insertion of the speculum. The neovagina does not self-lubricate and requires the use of a lubricant.

Pelvic examination in transgender men who have an intact vagina and cervix may be appropriate for cancer screening or to test for STIs. When sending a specimen for Pap smear, it is essential to clearly identify the specimen as cervical, especially if the patient's listed gender is "male." Otherwise, the specimen may be discarded or incorrectly run as an anal Pap. The use of testosterone or presence of amenorrhea should be indicated.

Pelvic examination in transgender patients may produce anxiety and be perceived as traumatic because many transgender patients have experienced violence, including sexual violence. The provision of information, choices, decision-making ability, and a sense of control is important. In testing for STIs, some transgender patients may prefer to collect their own specimens. If a patient refuses a speculum examination, consider offering an external or bimanual examination as a beginning step. A positive experience can establish trust and comfort and may facilitate further examination in the future.

Cervix

Locate the cervix with the palmar surface of your fingers, feel its end, and run your fingers around its circumference to feel the fornices. Feel the size, length, and shape, which should correspond with your observations from the speculum examination. The consistency of the cervix in a nonpregnant patient will be firm, like the tip of the nose; during pregnancy, the cervix is softer. Feel for nodules, hardness, and roughness. Note the position of the cervix as discussed in the speculum examination. The cervix should be in the midline and may be pointing anteriorly or posteriorly.

Grasp the cervix gently between your fingers and move it from side to side. Observe the patient for any expression of pain or discomfort with movement (cervical motion tenderness). The cervix should move 1 to 2 cm in each direction with minimal or no discomfort. Painful cervical

Patient Safety

HPV and Cancer Prevention

HPV infection can cause cervical, vaginal, vulvar, penile, anal, and oropharyngeal cancers as well as genital warts. Vaccination against HPV before exposure to the virus through sexual activity is recommended for all 9- to 12-year-olds. The immune response is also more robust in preteen years. Because parents most often make the decision about this vaccine, the gynecologic examination presents an opportunity to educate about the vaccine and to discuss it in terms of cancer prevention rather than HPV as an STI. Catch-up HPV vaccination is recommended through age 26 years for everyone, if not vaccinated already. Shared clinical decision making is recommended for individuals aged 27 through 45 years who are not vaccinated.

The Centers for Disease Control and Prevention and American Academy of Pediatrics provide tools and resources for clinicians to successfully communicate with parents about HPV vaccination.

From American Academy of Pediatrics (2023); American Congress of Obstetricians and Gynecologists (2019); and Centers for Disease Control and Prevention (2024).

movement suggests a pelvic inflammatory process such as pelvic inflammatory disease or a ruptured tubal pregnancy.

Uterus

Position. Palpate the uterus. Place the palmar surface of your other hand on the abdominal midline, midway between the umbilicus and the symphysis pubis. Place the intravaginal fingers in the anterior fornix. Slowly slide the abdominal hand toward the pubis, pressing downward and forward with the flat surface of your fingers. At the same time, push inward and upward with the fingertips of the intravaginal hand while you push downward on the cervix with the backs of your fingers. Think of it as trying to bring your two hands together as you press down on the cervix. If the uterus is anteverted or anteflexed (the most common position), you will feel the fundus between the fingers of your two hands at the level of the pubis (Fig. 19.27A and B).

If you do not feel the uterus with the previous maneuver, place the intravaginal fingers together in the posterior fornix with the abdominal hand immediately above the symphysis pubis. Press firmly downward with the abdominal hand while you press against the cervix inward with the other hand. A retroverted or retroflexed uterus should be felt with this maneuver (see Fig. 19.27C and D).

If you still cannot feel the uterus, move the intravaginal fingers to each side of the cervix. Keeping contact with the cervix, press inward and feel as far as you can. Then slide your fingers so that one is on top of the cervix and one is underneath. Continue pressing inward while moving your fingers to feel as much of the uterus as you can. When the uterus is in the midposition, you will not be able to feel the fundus with the abdominal hand (see Fig. 19.27E).

Confirm the location and position of the uterus by comparing your inspection findings with your palpation findings. The uterus should be located in the midline regardless of its position. Deviation to the right or left is indicative of possible adhesions, pelvic masses, or pregnancy. Knowing the position of the uterus is essential before performing any intrauterine procedure, including insertion of an intrauterine contraceptive device.

Size, Shape, and Contour. Palpate the uterus for size, shape, and contour. It should be pear shaped and 5.5 to 8 cm long, although it is larger in all dimensions in multiparous patients. A uterus larger than expected in a patient of childbearing age is indicative of pregnancy, fibroid, or tumor. The contour should be rounded, and the walls should feel firm and smooth in the nonpregnant patient. The contour smoothness will be interrupted by pregnancy or tumor.

Mobility. Gently move the uterus between the intravaginal hand and abdominal hand to assess for mobility and tenderness. The uterus should be mobile in the anteroposterior plane. A fixed uterus indicates adhesions. Tenderness on movement suggests a pelvic inflammatory process or ruptured tubal pregnancy.

Adnexa and Ovaries

Palpate the adnexal areas and ovaries. Place the fingers of your abdominal hand on the right lower quadrant. With the intravaginal hand facing upward, place both fingers in the right lateral fornix. Press the intravaginal fingers deeply inward and upward toward the abdominal hand while sweeping the flat surface of the fingers of the abdominal hand deeply inward and obliquely downward toward the symphysis pubis. Palpate the entire area by firmly pressing the abdominal hand and intravaginal fingers together. Repeat the maneuver on the left side (Fig. 19.28).

The ovaries—if palpable—should feel firm, smooth, ovoid, and approximately 3 by 2 by 1 cm in size. The healthy ovary is slightly to moderately tender on palpation. Marked tenderness, enlargement, and nodularity are unexpected. Usually, no other structures are palpable except for round ligaments. Fallopian tubes are usually not palpable, so a problem may exist if they are felt. You are also palpating for adnexal masses—and if any are found, they should be characterized by size, shape, location, consistency, and tenderness.

The adnexa are often difficult to palpate because of their location and position and the presence of excess adipose tissue in some patients. If you are unable to feel anything in the adnexal areas with thorough palpation, you can assume that no abnormality is present, provided no clinical symptoms exist (see Clinical Pearl, "Mittelschmerz and Adnexal Tenderness").

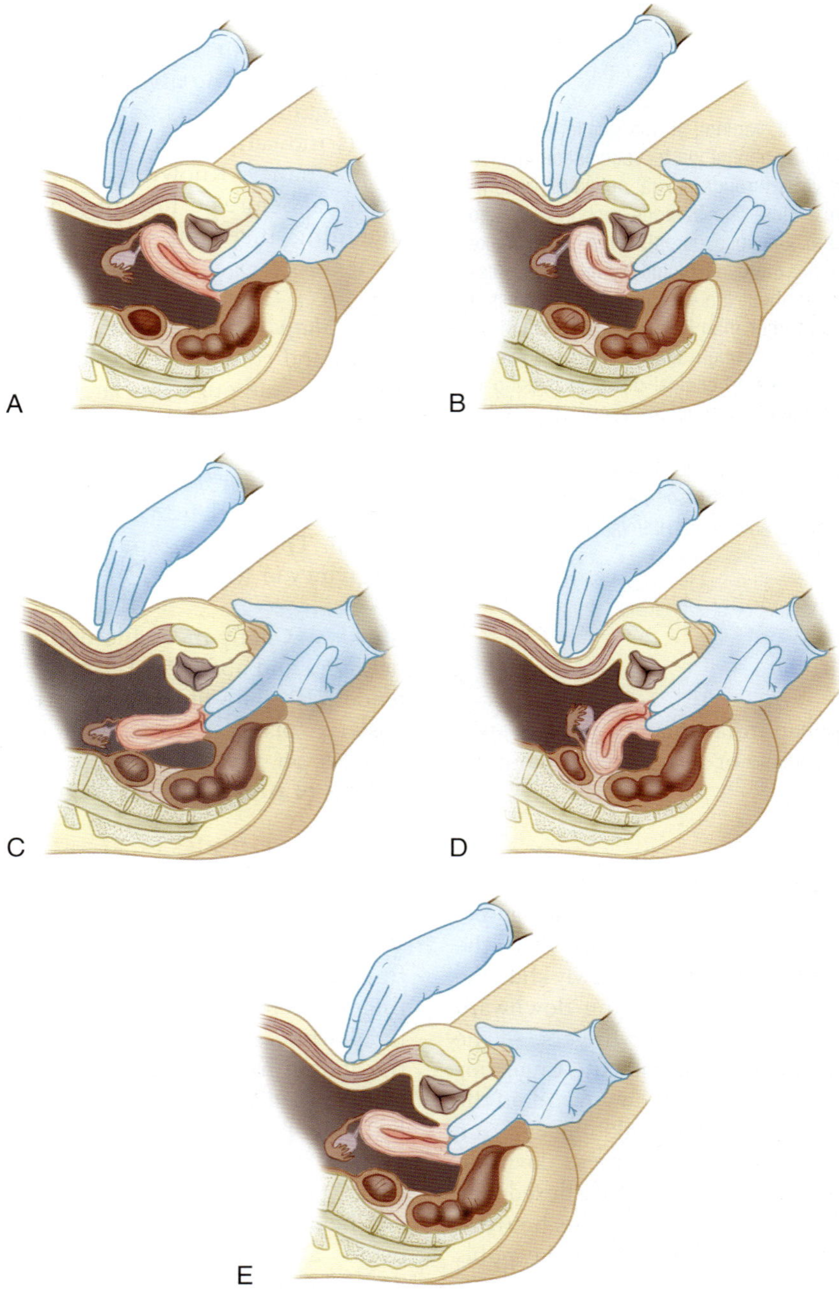

FIG. 19.27 **Varying positions of uteri.** (A) Anteverted. (B) Anteflexed. (C) Retroverted. (D) Retroflexed. (E) Midposition.

> **CLINICAL PEARL**
>
> **Mittelschmerz and Adnexal Tenderness**
>
> Mittelschmerz—lower abdominal pain associated with ovulation—may be accompanied by tenderness on the side in which ovulation took place that month. The timing is, of course, essential in the history. The onset of pain is usually sudden, and remission is spontaneous. On pelvic examination, you may discover a bit of adnexal tenderness, but the examination will otherwise be reassuringly negative.

Rectovaginal Examination

Preparation

The rectovaginal examination is an important part of the total pelvic examination. It allows you to reach almost 2.5 cm (1 inch) higher into the pelvis, which enables you to better evaluate the pelvic organs and structures. It is an uncomfortable examination for patients, however, and they may ask you to omit it. Nevertheless, it is important to perform, and you should explain why it is necessary.

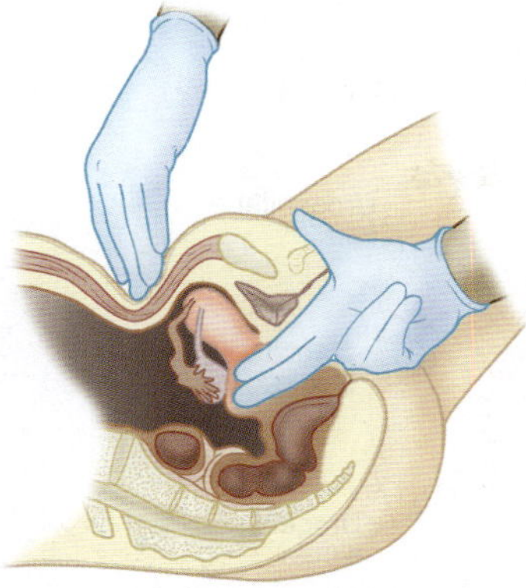

FIG. 19.28 Bimanual palpation of adnexa. Sweep abdominal fingers downward to capture the ovary.

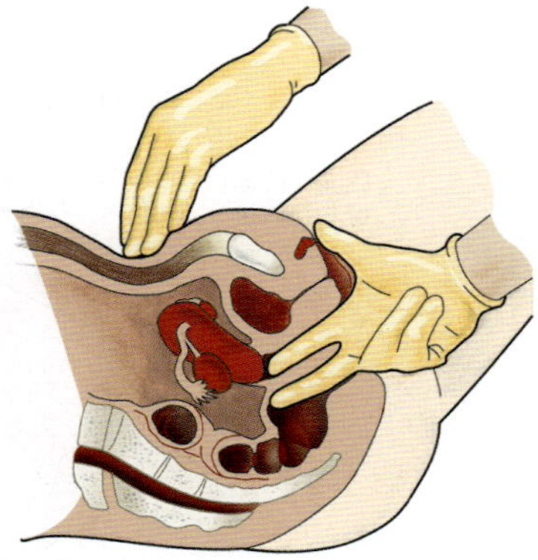

FIG. 19.29 Rectovaginal palpation. (From Lowdermilk, D. L., & Perry, S. E. (2007). *Maternity and women's health care* (8th ed.). St. Louis: Mosby.)

As you complete the bimanual examination, withdraw your examining fingers, change gloves, and lubricate the fingers. Tell the patient that the feeling of urgency of a bowel movement is common but reassure that it will not occur. Have the patient breathe slowly and consciously try to relax the sphincter, rectum, and buttocks because tightening the muscles makes the examination more uncomfortable.

Anal Sphincter

Assess the anal sphincter if there are concerns. Place your index finger in the vagina, and then press your middle finger against the anus and ask the patient to bear down while slipping the tip of the finger into the rectum just past the sphincter. Palpate the area of the anorectal junction and just above it. Ask the patient to tighten and relax the anal sphincter. Observe sphincter tone. An extremely tight sphincter may be the result of anxiety about the examination, may be caused by scarring, or may indicate spasticity caused by fissures, lesions, or inflammation. A lax sphincter suggests neurologic deficit, whereas an absent sphincter may result from improper repair of a third-degree perineal laceration after childbirth or trauma.

Rectal Walls and Rectovaginal Septum

Slide both your vaginal and rectal fingers in as far as they will go and then ask the patient to bear down. This will bring an additional centimeter within reach of your fingers. Rotate the rectal finger to explore the anterior rectal wall for masses, polyps, nodules, strictures, irregularities, and tenderness. The wall should feel smooth and uninterrupted. Palpate the rectovaginal septum along the anterior wall for thickness, tone, and nodules. You may feel the uterine body and occasionally the uterine fundus in a retroflexed uterus.

Uterus

Press firmly and deeply downward with the abdominal hand just above the symphysis pubis while you position the vaginal finger in the posterior vaginal fornix and press strongly upward against the posterior side of the cervix. Palpate as much of the posterior side of the uterus as possible, confirming your findings from the vaginal examination regarding location, position, size, shape, contour, consistency, and tenderness of the uterus. This maneuver is particularly useful in evaluating a retroverted uterus (Fig. 19.29).

Adnexa

If you were unable to palpate the adnexal areas on bimanual examination or if the findings were questionable, repeat the adnexal examination using the same maneuvers described in the bimanual examination.

Stool

As you withdraw your fingers, rotate the rectal finger to evaluate the posterior rectal wall just as you did earlier for the anterior wall. Gently remove your examining fingers and observe for secretions and stool. Note the color and presence of any blood. Prepare a specimen for occult blood testing, if indicated. Unless the patient is unable to do so, provide a wipe for removal of the lubricating gel. The patient can do a more thorough and comfortable job. Be sure to provide an appropriate disposal receptacle.

Completion

Assist the patient into a sitting position and give the opportunity to regain equilibrium and composure. Provide a sanitary pad if the patient is menstruating. Share findings and ask the patient to voice feelings about the examination. This conversation may be brief, but it should never be avoided. Some clinicians prefer to leave the room and give the patient the opportunity to dress before discussing findings.

Infants

The appearance of the external genitalia can help in the assessment of gestational age in the newborn. Examination is conducted with the infant's legs held in a frog position. The labia majora appear widely separated, and the clitoris is prominent up to 36 weeks of gestation, but by full term, the labia majora completely cover the labia minora and clitoris.

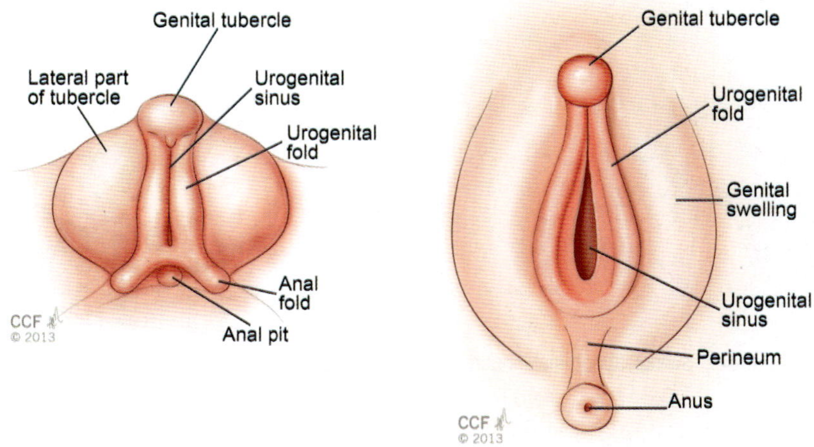

FIG. 19.30 Normal appearance of the female genitalia. (A) Genitalia of a newborn girl. The labia majora are full, and the thickened labia minora protrude between them. (B) Genitalia of a 2-year-old girl. The labia majora are flattened, and the labia minora and hymen are thin and flat. (From Walters, M. D., & Karram, M. M. (2015). *Urogynecology and reconstructive pelvic surgery* (4th ed.). Elsevier.)

The newborn's genitalia reflect the influence of maternal hormones. The labia majora and minora may be swollen, with the labia minora often more prominent. The hymen is often protruding, thick, and vascular, and it may simulate an extruding mass. These are all transient phenomena and will disappear in a few weeks (Fig. 19.30).

The clitoris may appear relatively large; this usually has no significance. True hypertrophy is not common; however, in newborns, an enlarged clitoris must alert the clinician to the possibility of congenital adrenal hyperplasia.

The central opening of the hymen is usually about 0.5 cm in diameter. It is important to determine the presence of an opening; however, make no effort to stretch the hymen. An imperforate hymen is rare but can cause difficulty later, including hydrocolpos in the child and hematocolpos in the adolescent.

Malformations in the external genitalia are often difficult to discern. If the baby was a breech delivery, the genitalia may be swollen and bruised for many days after delivery. Any ambiguous appearance or unusual orifice in the vulvar vault or perineum must be expeditiously explored before gender assignment occurs.

A mucoid, whitish vaginal discharge is commonly seen during the newborn period and sometimes as late as 4 weeks after birth. The discharge is occasionally mixed with blood. This is the result of passive hormonal transfer from the pregnant patient and is an expected finding. Parental reassurance is often necessary.

Thin but difficult-to-separate adhesions between the labia minora are often seen during the first few months or even years of life. Sometimes they completely cover the vulvar vestibule. There may be just the smallest of openings through which urine can escape. These may require separation, using the gentlest of teasing or the application of estrogen creams.

Vaginal discharge in infants and young children may occur as the result of irritation from the diaper or powder. The discharge is usually mucoid.

Children

Indications for Examination. The extent of the gynecologic examination depends on the child's age and concerns or parental concerns. For the well child, the examination includes only inspection and palpation of the external genitalia. The internal vaginal examination is performed on a young child only when there is a specific problem, such as bleeding, discharge, trauma, or suspected sexual abuse. Bubble bath vaginitis is common in young children and does not require an internal examination. Speculum examination on a young child requires special equipment and an experienced and knowledgeable gynecologist or pediatrician.

The young child usually cooperates with examination of the external genitalia if your approach is very matter of fact. The very young child might prefer to lie in the parent's lap, with legs held in a frog position by the parent. The preschool child can be placed on the examining table, lying back against the head of the table, which should be raised about 30 degrees. The parent can help the child hold the legs up in a frog position.

A school-age child may not like the examination but is likely to cooperate if you take the time to reassure that you will only look at and touch the outside. However, you must realize that a child in this circumstance, lying down, underpants off, will most often feel quite vulnerable. You might have the child help by taking the hand and first having the child touch the genitalia. The child should be positioned on the table on the back with the knees flexed and drawn up. The examination should be approached with the same degree of respect, explanation, and caution as with the adult patient.

It is always necessary to have a chaperone during examination of the genitalia.

Inspection and Palpation

Inspect the perineum, all the structures of the vulvar vestibule, and the urethral and vaginal orifices by separating the labia with the thumb and forefinger of one hand.

Adequate visualization of the interior of the vagina and the hymenal opening can be difficult in prepubertal patients. A technique that can be helpful is that of anterior labial traction. Firmly grasp both labia majora (not the minora) with the thumb and index finger of each hand, then gently but firmly pull the labia forward and slightly to the side. Gentle but firm traction will not cause discomfort. A previously obscured hymenal opening almost always becomes visible with this technique, as does the interior of the vagina, nearly to the cervix. Most foreign bodies are visible with this method. With the help of an assistant, a swab is easily inserted through the hymenal opening to obtain cultures if needed.

Bartholin and Skene glands are usually not palpable; if they are, enlargement exists. This indicates infection, which is most often (but not always) gonococcal. If there is concern about an imperforate hymen, ask the patient to cough, and observe the hymen. An imperforate hymen will bulge, whereas one with an opening will not.

Discharge

Vaginal discharge often irritates the perineal tissues, causing redness and perhaps excoriation. Other sources of perineal irritation include bubble baths, soaps, detergents, and urinary tract infections. Carefully question the parent for a history of hematuria, dysuria, or other symptoms that would indicate urinary tract infection. A foul odor is more likely indicative of a foreign body (particularly in preschool children), especially if a secondary infection is present. Vaginal discharge may also result from trichomonal, gonococcal, or candidal infection. When considering these diagnoses, an evaluation by a clinician with expertise in sexual abuse evaluation is warranted.

Injuries

Swelling of vulvar tissues, particularly if accompanied by bruising or foul-smelling discharge, should alert you to the possibility of sexual abuse (Box 19.6). It must always be suspected if a young child has an STI or if there is injury to the external genitalia. Injuries to the softer structure

BOX 19.6 Red Flags for Sexual Abuse

The following signs and symptoms in children or adolescents should raise your suspicion for sexual abuse. Remember, however, that any sign or symptom by itself is of limited significance; it may be related to sexual abuse, or it may be from another cause altogether. Also, the physical examination is often normal. This is an area in which good clinical judgment is imperative. Each sign or symptom must be considered in context with the particular child's health status, stage of growth and development, and entire history.

Medical Concerns and Findings

- Evidence of general physical abuse or neglect
- Evidence of trauma and/or scarring in genital, anal, and perianal areas
- Unusual changes in skin color or pigmentation in genital or anal area
- Presence of sexually transmitted infection (oral, anal, genital)
- Anorectal problems such as itching, bleeding, pain, fecal incontinence, poor anal sphincter tone, bowel habit dysfunction
- Genitourinary problems such as rash or sores in genital area, vaginal odor or discharge, pain (including abdominal pain), itching, bleeding, discharge, dysuria, hematuria, urinary tract infections, enuresis

Examples of Nonspecific Behavioral Manifestations

- Problems with school
- Dramatic weight changes or eating disturbances
- Depression
- Anxiety
- Sleep problems or nightmares
- Sudden change in personality or behavior
- Increased aggression and impulsivity, sudden avoidance of certain people or places

Examples of Sexual Behaviors That Are Concerning

- Use of sexually provocative mannerisms
- Excessive masturbation or sexual behavior that cannot be redirected
- Age-inappropriate sexual knowledge or experience
- Repeated object insertion into vagina and/or anus
- Child asking to be touched or kissed in genital area
- Sex play between children with 4 years or more age difference
- Sex play that involves the use of force, threats, or bribes

Modified from Hornor, G. (2004); Jenny, C., & Crawford-Jakubiak, J. E., & Committee on Child Abuse and Neglect, & American Academy of Pediatrics (2013); Kellogg, N. D. (2010); Koop, C. E. (1988); and McClain, N., et al. (2000).

of the external genitalia are not caused by bicycle seats. A straddle injury from a bicycle seat is generally evident over the symphysis pubis where the structures are more fixed. The injuries resulting from sexual abuse are generally more posterior and may involve the perineum grossly. The examination does not require the use of instruments in most cases. Separation of the labia and gentle labial traction while the child is supine with the knees bent and hips abducted (frog-leg position) will adequately expose the genital structures. Speculum examinations are contraindicated in prepubertal children in the office setting. If intravaginal trauma is suspected, vaginoscopy should be performed under anesthesia. Consider referral to a specialized clinic or child advocacy center where children are seen, such that an experienced clinician can perform the examination and collect appropriate forensic specimens. Additionally, psychologists and other mental health counselors are typically in these centers. Careful questioning of the parent or guardian is mandatory, as well as a report to the appropriate social service agencies for further investigation. In most cases of sexual abuse, the physical examination is normal. A normal examination does not rule out sexual abuse if there is suspicion.

Bleeding

Vaginal bleeding in children is often the result of unintentional injury, experimentation with a foreign body (e.g., toy), or sexual abuse. Rarely, there may be an ovarian tumor or carcinoma of the cervix. Remember, too, that some children may have precocious puberty and begin menstruation well before the expected time (Box 19.7). If this occurs, further evaluation is necessary.

Rectal Examination

On occasion, a rectal examination may be indicated to determine the presence or absence of the uterus, the presence of a foreign body in the vagina, or concerns about GI bleeding. The parent or guardian can assist and offer reassurance to the child during the examination. The rectal examination may be performed with the patient lying on the back, feet held together, and knees bent up on the abdomen. Steady the child by placing one hand on the knees and slip the gloved examining finger into the rectum. Most examiners prefer the index finger, but this is not mandatory. Once your finger is introduced, you may release the legs and use your free hand to simultaneously palpate the abdomen. If old enough to cooperate, have the child pant like a puppy to relax the muscles. A foreign body may be palpable, as well as the cervix. The ovaries are not usually felt. There may be bleeding and even a transient mild rectal prolapse after the examination, so be sure to warn the parent of this.

BOX 19.7 Causes of Genital Bleeding in Children

Vaginal bleeding during childhood is always clinically important and requires further evaluation. Common causes in children include the following:

- Genital lesions
- Vaginitis
- Foreign body
- Trauma
- Tumors
- Endocrine changes
- Estrogen ingestion
- Precocious puberty
- Hormone-producing ovarian tumor

Adolescents

The adolescent requires the same examination and positioning as the adult. Ask whether this is the young patient's first gynecologic examination. The first examination sets the stage for future examinations. Take time to explain what you will be doing. Use models or illustrations to show what will happen and what you will look for. Techniques such as deep breathing throughout the procedure, alternating tightening and relaxation of the perineal muscles, or progressive muscle relaxation may help the adolescent stay relaxed during the examination. An adolescent should be allowed the privacy of having the examination without a parent or guardian present, but a chaperone is always necessary. An interview without the parent is necessary to obtain an accurate sexual history, including sexual abuse, sex trafficking, and IPV, and to discuss sexual play (see Chapter 2). This is typically conducted before the pelvic examination.

Choose the appropriate size speculum. A pediatric speculum with blades that are 1 to 1.5 cm wide can be used and should cause minimal discomfort. If the adolescent is sexually active, a small adult speculum may be used.

As the patient goes through puberty, you will see the maturational changes of sexual development (see Chapter 8). Just before menarche, there is a physiologic increase in vaginal secretions. The hymen may or may not be stretched across the vaginal opening. By menarche, the opening should be at least 1 cm wide. As the adolescent matures, the findings are the same as those for the adult.

Pregnant Patients

The gynecologic examination for the pregnant patient follows the same procedure as that for the nonpregnant adult patient. Assessment of pregnant patients includes gestational age estimation, uterine size and contour, pelvic size estimates, and cervical dilation and length. Examination also includes fetal assessment: growth, position, and well-being. During labor, fetal station and head position are also assessed.

Gestational Age

Calculation is performed to determine the EDD. The Naegele rule is often used to calculate EDD: Add 1 year to the first day of the last normal menstrual period, subtract 3 months, and add 7 days.

The average duration of pregnancy is considered to be 280 days, or 40 weeks. The pregnancy is then divided into trimesters, each of which is slightly more than 13 weeks, or 3 calendar months. The clinically appropriate unit of measure, however, is weeks of gestation completed. Weeks of gestation completed can be easily calculated by using an obstetric wheel or an electronic pregnancy calculator.

Uterus Size and Contour

Estimate uterine size by manual measurement of fundal height. This technique provides an estimate for the length of the pregnancy, fetal growth, and gestational age. Have the patient empty the bladder before the procedure. Ask the patient to lie supine. Early uterine enlargement may not be symmetric, and you may feel deviation of the uterus to one side and an irregularity in its contour at the site of implantation. This uterine irregularity occurs around weeks 8 to 10 (Piskacek sign).

There is a lack of consensus about the accuracy of estimates of the size of the uterus at the various weeks; however, some estimate should be made. The size of various fruits is a common, although not reliable, means for describing the size of the uterus in early pregnancy. Centimeters are more accurate units of measurement and should be used as soon as possible.

With a nonstretchable tape measure, measure from the upper part of the symphysis pubis to the superior fundus uterus (Fig. 19.31). Record the measurement in centimeters. The same person should perform the measurement each time to decrease chances of individual variation.

This measurement is most accurate between 20 and 32 weeks of gestation when the fundal height in centimeters correlates well with the gestational age in weeks, ±2 cm. A 1-cm increase per week in fundal height is an expected pattern. Suspect twin pregnancy or other conditions that enlarge the uterus if during the second trimester the uterine size is larger than expected based on the EDD. A variation of more than 2 cm may indicate the need for further evaluation with ultrasound. If the uterine size is smaller than expected, consider the possibility of intrauterine growth restriction. The accuracy of fundal height as a screening tool for intrauterine growth restriction is poor but can provide clinical suspicion indicating a need for sonography. Customized charts based on maternal height, weight, parity, and ethnicity are more accurate. Factors that can affect the accuracy of fundal height measurement are obesity, amount of amniotic fluid, myomata, multiple gestation, fetal size, and position of the uterus.

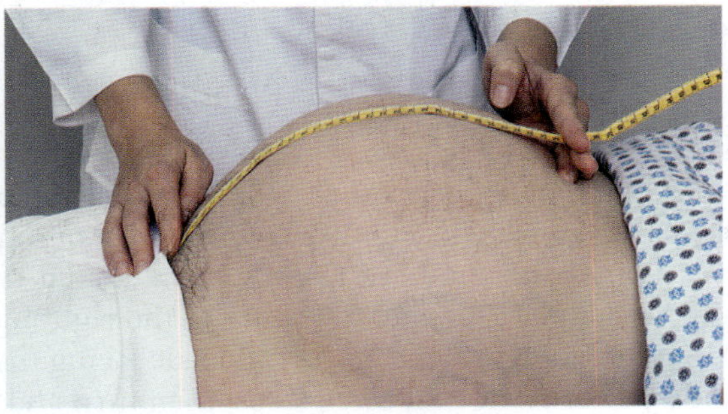

FIG. 19.31 Measurement of fundal height from the symphysis pubis to the superior fundus uterus.

Changes in fundal height at the various weeks of gestation are shown in Fig. 19.32, along with some changes that are detectable on examination.

Pelvic Examination

In early pregnancy you can feel a softening of the isthmus, whereas the cervix is still firm. In the second month of pregnancy, the cervix, vagina, and vulva acquire their bluish color from increased vascularity. The cervix itself softens and will feel more like lips than like the firmness of the nose tip. The fundus flexes easily on the cervix. There is slight fullness and softening of the fundus near the site of implantation. These findings are summarized in Box 19.8. You will notice increased vaginal secretions as a result of increased vascularity. None of these findings

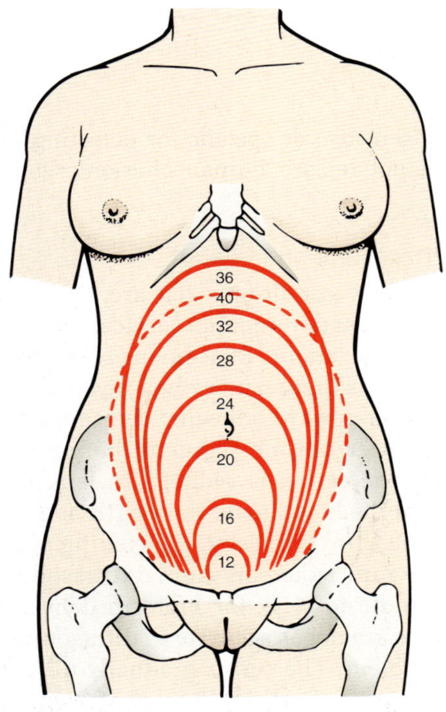

FIG. 19.32 **Changes in fundal height with pregnancy.** Weeks 10 to 12: Uterus within pelvis; fetal heartbeat can be detected with Doppler. Week 12: Uterus palpable just above symphysis pubis. Week 16: Uterus palpable halfway between symphysis and umbilicus; ballottement of fetus is possible by abdominal and vaginal examination. Week 20: Uterine fundus at lower border of umbilicus; fetal heartbeat can be auscultated with a fetoscope. Weeks 24 to 26: Uterus changes from globular to ovoid shape; fetus palpable. Week 28: Uterus approximately halfway between umbilicus and xiphoid; fetus easily palpable. Week 34: Uterine fundus just below xiphoid. Week 40: Fundal height drops as fetus begins to engage in pelvis.

BOX 19.8 Early Signs of Pregnancy

The following are physical signs that occur early in pregnancy. These signs—along with internal ballottement, palpation of fetal parts, and positive test results for urine or serum human chorionic gonadotropin—are probable indicators of pregnancy. They are considered probable because clinical conditions other than pregnancy can cause any one of them. Their occurrence together, however, creates a strong case for the presence of a pregnancy.

SIGN	FINDING	APPROXIMATE WEEKS OF GESTATION
Goodell	Softening of the cervix	4–6
Hegar	Softening of the uterine isthmus	6–8
McDonald	Fundus flexes easily on the cervix	7–8
Braun von Fernwald	Fullness and softening of the fundus near the site of implantation	7–8
Piskacek	Palpable lateral bulge or soft prominence of one uterine cornu	7–8
Chadwick	Bluish color of the cervix, vagina, and vulva	8–12

is perfectly sensitive or specific for detecting pregnancy and should not replace human chorionic gonadotropin testing.

Cervical Effacement and Dilation

Other pregnancy conditions that are assessed during the pelvic examination include cervical effacement and dilation and effacement. Effacement refers to the thinning of the cervix that results when myometrial activity pulls the cervix upward, allowing the cervix to become part of the lower uterine segment during prelabor or early labor. The cervix is reduced in length. Ultrasonographic methods estimate its length at 3 to 4 cm at the end of the third trimester. Shortening of the cervix (less than 29 mm) noted on vaginal ultrasound in midpregnancy indicates risk for preterm delivery. Digital examinations are not as accurate as ultrasound and may miss the problem. The cervix gradually thins to only a few millimeters (paper thin). Record effacement in centimeters. Effacement usually precedes cervical dilation in the primipara and often occurs with dilation in the multipara.

Dilation involves the opening of the cervical canal to allow for the passage of the fetus. The process is measured in centimeters and progresses from a closed os (internal) to 10 cm, which is full or complete dilation. During labor, the time may vary among patients for progression of cervical dilation related to parity, weeks of gestation (some dilation may be present late in pregnancy), and progress of labor.

Fetal Well-Being

Assessment of fetal well-being includes but is not limited to measurement of fetal heart rate (FHR) and fetal movement (FM). FHR is detected by Doppler by 11 to 12 weeks of gestation and heard by fetoscope at 19 to 20 weeks of gestation. Count the FHR or impulse for 1 minute and compare it with the pregnant patient's pulse during that time. Note the quality and rhythm of the heart tones. Documenting the results is sometimes done using a two-line figure in which the point of intersection is the umbilicus, and the four quadrants are the maternal abdomen. Use an X or FHR to record the location of the maximal impulse on the maternal abdomen (see example in the accompanying figure).

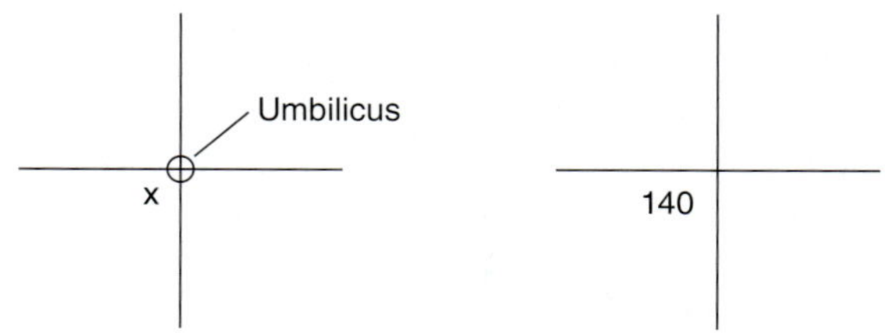

FM typically is appreciated by pregnant patients between 16 and 20 weeks of gestation. Maternal assessment of FM can be used as an indicator of fetal well-being. Instruct the patient to note the pattern of movement over a given time. If the pattern shows a decrease, or if movement ceases, the patient should notify their clinician immediately. One of the most used techniques is the Cardiff count-to-10 method, where the patient counts 10 movements, noting the length of time for them to occur. There are no universally accepted FM count criteria, but the standard ranges from 10 times in 1 hour to 10 times in 12 hours. If there are fewer than 10 movements in 12 hours, the patient should notify the health care professional. If no monitoring technique is used, the occurrence of three or fewer FMs in 2 hours for 2 consecutive days while the patient is at rest in the left lateral position signals the need for further evaluation of fetal well-being. If there are no identifiable risks of uteroplacental insufficiency, patients may be asked to start recording FM between 34 and 36 weeks of gestation. If there are risk factors, monitoring should start as early as 28 weeks.

Fetal Position

In the latter half of the third trimester, assessment of fetal position can be performed using the four steps of the Leopold maneuvers (Fig. 19.33). After positioning the patient supine with the head slightly elevated and knees slightly flexed, place a small towel under the right hip. If you are right-handed, stand at the right side facing the patient and perform the first three steps, then turn and face the feet for the last step; if you are left-handed, stand on the patient's left for the first three steps, then turn and

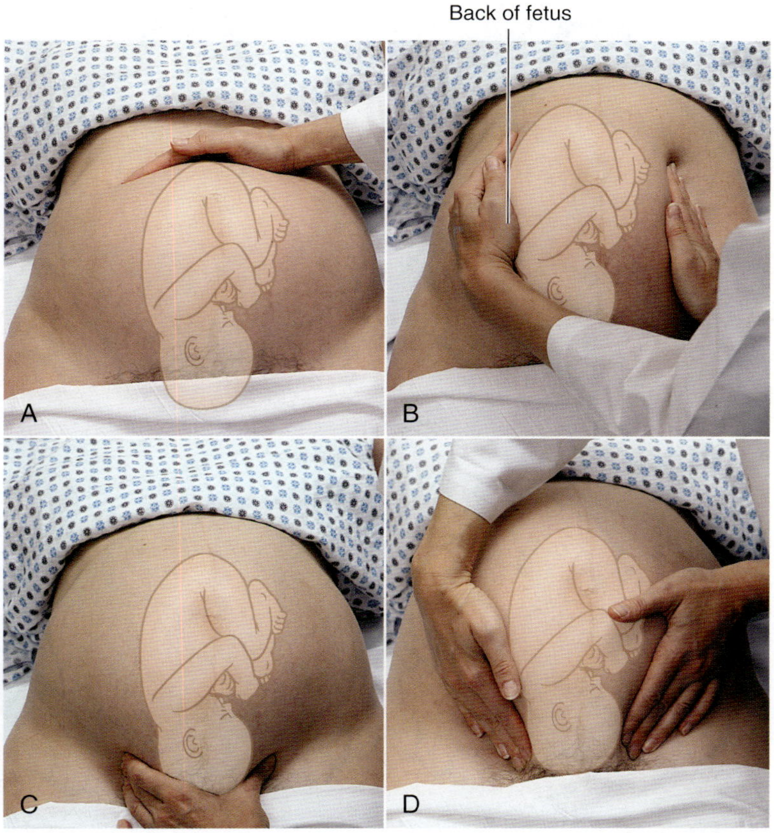

FIG. 19.33 Leopold maneuvers. (A) First maneuver. Place hand(s) over fundus and identify the fetal part. (B) Second maneuver. Use the palmar surface of one hand to locate the back of the fetus. Use the other hand to feel the irregularities, such as hands and feet. (C) Third maneuver. Use thumb and third finger to grasp presenting part over the symphysis pubis. (D) Fourth maneuver. Use both hands to outline the fetal head. With a head presenting deep in the pelvis, only a small portion may be felt.

face the feet for the last step. The maneuvers are performed as follows:

1. Place hands over the fundus and identify the fetal part (see Fig. 19.33A). The head feels round, firm, and freely movable and is detectable by ballottement. The buttocks feel softer and less mobile and regular.
2. With the palmar surface of your hand, locate the back of the fetus by applying gentle but deep pressure (see Fig. 19.33B). The back feels smooth and convex, whereas the small parts (the feet, hands, knees, and elbows) feel more irregular.
3. With the right hand (if you are right-handed) or with the left (if you are left-handed), using the thumb and third finger, gently grasp the presenting part over the symphysis pubis (see Fig. 19.33C). The head will feel firm and, if not engaged, will be movable from side to side and easily displaced upward. If the buttocks are present, they will feel softer. If the presenting part is not engaged, the fourth step is used.
4. Turn and face the patient's feet and use two hands to outline the fetal head (see Fig. 19.33D). If the head is presenting and is deep into the pelvis, only a small portion may be felt. Palpation of the cephalic prominence (the part of the fetus that prevents descent of the examiner's hand) on the same side as the small parts suggests that the head is flexed, and the vertex is present. This is the optimal position. Palpation of the cephalic prominence on the same side as the back suggests that the presenting part is extended.

When recording the information obtained from abdominal palpation, include the presenting part (i.e., vertex if the head, or breech if the buttocks); the lie (the relationship of the long axis of the fetus to the long axis of the pregnant patient) as longitudinal, transverse (perpendicular), or oblique; and the attitude of the fetal head if it is the presenting part (flexed or extended). With experience, you will also be able to estimate the weight of the fetus. A bedside ultrasound can confirm the position.

Twins or other multiple fetuses are a variation, often suspected when there is the presence of two or more fetal heart tones or on abdominal palpation when additional sets of fetal parts are detected. Diagnosis is made by ultrasound. The technique for abdominal palpation in twin pregnancy is depicted in Fig. 19.34.

The FHR can also be used to estimate the position of the fetus. The areas of maximal intensity of the FHR and the position of the fetus are depicted in Fig. 19.35.

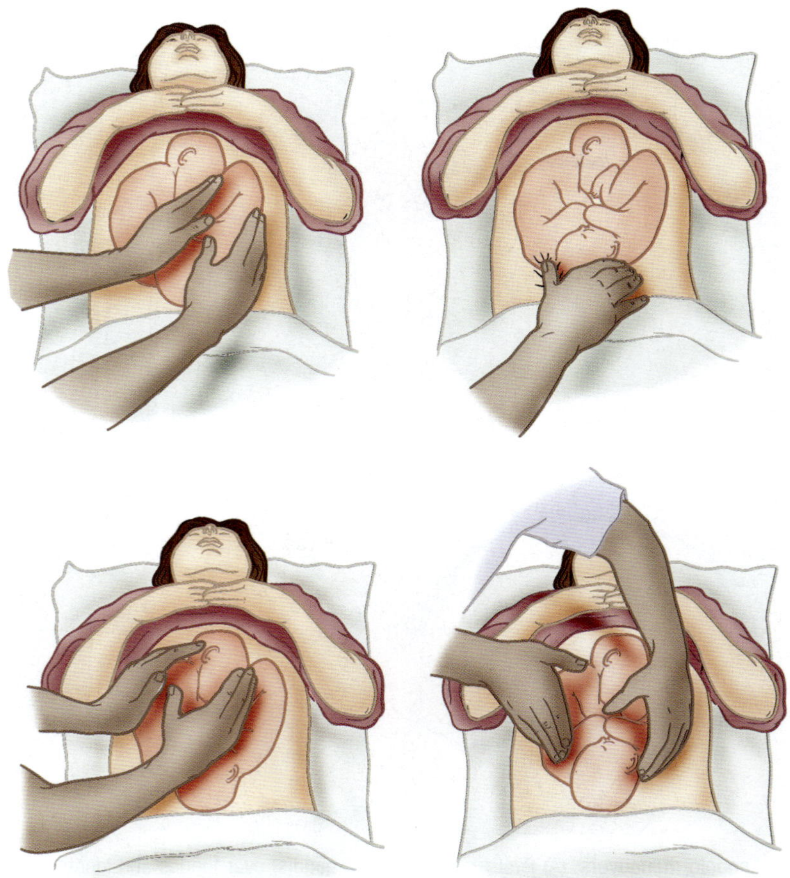

FIG. 19.34 Abdominal palpation of twin pregnancy.

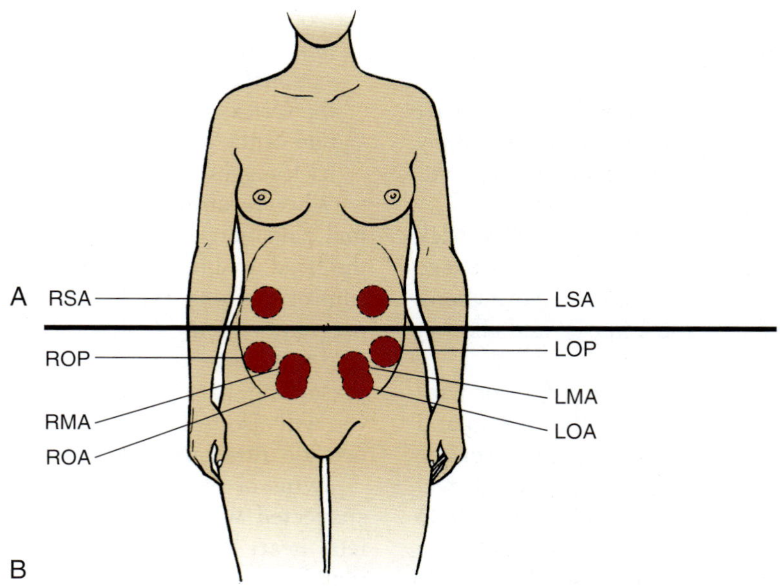

FIG. 19.35 Areas of maximal intensity of fetal heart rate (FHR) for differing positions. (A) Presentation is breech if FHR is heard above umbilicus. (B) Presentation is vertex if FHR is heard below umbilicus. *LMA,* Left mentum anterior; *LOA,* left occipitoanterior; *LOP,* left occipitoposterior; *LSA,* left sacrum anterior; *RMA,* right mentum anterior; *ROA,* right occipitoanterior; *ROP,* right occipitoposterior; *RSA,* right sacrum anterior. (From Lowdermilk, D. L., et al. (1997). *Maternity and women's health care* (6th ed.). St. Louis: Mosby.)

Station

Station is the relationship of the presenting part to the ischial spines of the pregnant patient's pelvis. Vaginal examination and palpation are performed during labor to estimate the descent of the presenting part. The measurement is determined by centimeters above and below the ischial spines and is recorded by plus and minus signs (Fig. 19.36). For example, the station at 1 cm below the spines is recorded as a +1, at the spines as a 0, and at 1 cm above the spines as a –1. Record (in centimeters) the routine cervical examination findings for dilation, cervical length, and station, in that order.

Contractions

Uterine contractions may begin as early as the third month of gestation and are called *Braxton-Hicks contractions*. They may go unnoticed by the patient but may become painful at times, especially as the pregnancy progresses and with increased gravidity. The regular occurrence of more than four to six uterine contractions per hour before 37 weeks of gestation requires evaluation.

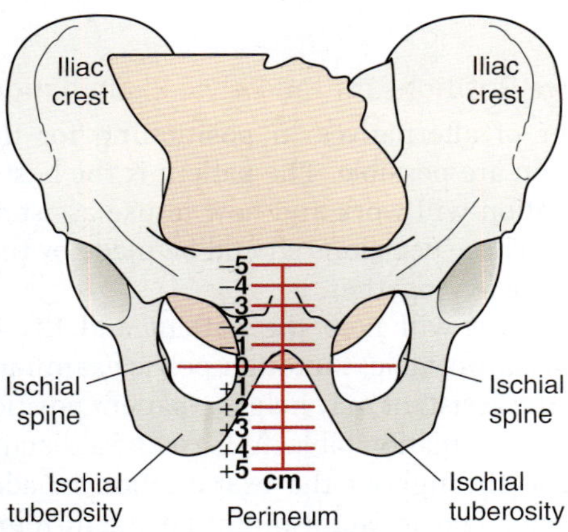

FIG. 19.36 Stations of presenting part (degree of descent). Silhouette shows head of infant at station 0. (Courtesy Ross Products Division, Abbott Laboratories Inc., Columbus, OH. From Lowdermilk, D. L., & Perry, S. E. (2007). *Maternity and women's health care* (8th ed.). St. Louis: Mosby.)

You can assess uterine contractions with abdominal palpation, but more accuracy is obtained using electronic monitoring equipment, either indirectly through the abdominal wall or directly with the placement of an intrauterine pressure catheter. Assessment through abdominal palpation is helpful when equipment is not available to determine the onset or course of labor, either preterm or term. Practice is needed to determine the difference between mild, moderate, and strong contractions. Place the fingertips on the abdomen so that you are able to detect the contraction and relaxation of the uterus and keep them there throughout the entire contraction, including the period of relaxation.

The strength of the contraction is classified as follows:

Mild: slightly tense fundus that is easy to indent with the fingertips

Moderate: firm fundus that is difficult to indent with the fingertips

Strong: rigid or hard, boardlike fundus or one that does not indent with the fingertips

The duration of the contraction is measured in seconds from the beginning until relaxation occurs. The frequency of contractions is measured from the beginning of one contraction to the beginning of the next. The frequency of contractions is assessed for regularity (at regular intervals, such as every 5 minutes, or at irregular or sporadic intervals). Each patient's experience of the discomfort created by the contracting uterus varies due to physiologic makeup, past experiences, cultural influences, expectations, prenatal education, support, and other factors. The patient's sense of the event should not be discounted based on physiologic and subjective measures.

Fetal Head Position

The position of the fetal head can be determined by vaginal examination once dilation has begun. Insert your fingers anteriorly into the posterior aspect of the vagina and then move your fingers upward over the fetal head as you turn them, locating the sagittal suture with the posterior and anterior fontanels at either end (Fig. 19.37A). The position

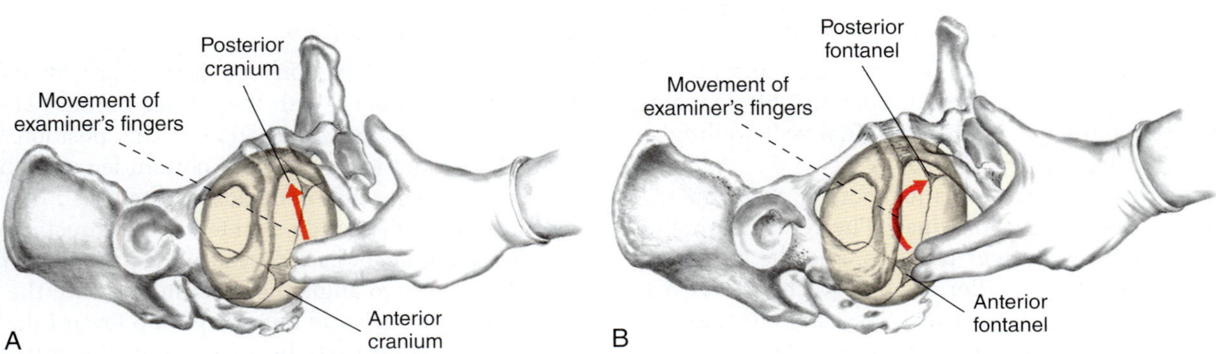

FIG. 19.37 (A) Locating the sagittal suture on vaginal examination. (B) Differentiating the fontanels on vaginal examination.

of the fontanels is determined by examining the anterior aspect of the sagittal suture and then using a circular motion to pass alongside the head until the other fontanel is felt and differentiated (see Fig. 19.37B). The position of the face and breech are easier to determine because the various parts are more distinguishable.

Other Pregnancy-Associated Changes

The uterus may become more anteflexed during the first 3 months from softening of the isthmus. As a result, the fundus may press on the urinary bladder, causing the patient to experience urinary frequency.

Vulvar varicosities occur commonly during pregnancy. The varicosities may involve both the vulva and the rectal area. Pressure from the pregnant uterus and possibly hereditary factors contribute to the formation of the varicosities.

Skin and breast changes that occur with pregnancy are discussed in Chapters 9 and 17.

Older Adults

The temptation with older adults is to defer the examination because of their age. This is often not appropriate. The examination procedure for the older patient is the same as that for the patient of childbearing age, with a few modifications for comfort. The older patient may require more time and assistance to assume the lithotomy position. The patient may need assistance from another individual to help hold the legs, as they may tire easily when the hip joints remain in abduction for an extended period. Patients with orthopnea will need to have their head and chest elevated during examination. You may need to use a smaller speculum, depending on the degree of introital constriction that occurs with aging.

Note that the labia appear flatter and smaller, corresponding with the degree of loss of subcutaneous fat elsewhere on the body. The skin is drier and shinier than that of a younger adult, and the pubic hair is gray and may be sparse. The clitoris is smaller than that of a younger adult.

The urinary meatus may appear as an irregular opening or slit. It may be located more posteriorly than in younger patients—very near or within the vaginal introitus—as a result of relaxed perineal musculature.

The vaginal introitus may be constricted and may admit only one finger. In some multiparous older patients, the introitus may gape, with the vaginal walls rolling toward the opening.

The vagina is narrower and shorter, and you will see and feel the absence of rugae. The cervix is smaller and paler than in younger patients, and the surrounding fornices may be smaller or absent. The cervix may seem less mobile if it protrudes less far into the vaginal canal. The os may be smaller but should still be palpable.

The uterus diminishes in size and may not be palpable, and the ovaries are rarely palpable because of atrophy. Ovaries that are palpable should be considered suspicious for tumor, and additional workup to exclude cancer is required.

The rectovaginal septum will feel thin, smooth, and pliable. Anal sphincter tone may be somewhat diminished. As the pelvic musculature relaxes, look particularly for stress incontinence and prolapse of the vaginal walls or uterus.

As with younger patients, as you inspect and palpate you are evaluating for signs of inflammation (older adults are particularly susceptible to atrophic vaginitis), infection, trauma, tenderness, masses, nodules, enlargement, irregularity, and changes in consistency.

Patients With Disabilities

Preparation

The clinician can do a number of things to promote a comfortable pelvic examination experience for a patient with disabilities. See Chapter 3 for a discussion of common approaches to patients with mobility or sensory impairments and patients with spinal cord injury or lesions.

Alternative Positions for the Pelvic Examination

A number of alternatives in positioning for the pelvic examination are possible. The patient is the best judge of which position will work and how to use assistants most effectively. These decisions should be made by the patient and the clinician together.

An assistant will help the patient and the clinician facilitate a comfortable, thorough pelvic examination. For example, the assistant may help the patient position themself on the examination table. At least one assistant should be available throughout the examination in addition to the clinician. The assistant might be a staff member, an attendant, or a friend of the patient.

Many patients cannot comfortably assume the traditional (lithotomy) pelvic examination position. A patient who experiences one or more conditions such as joint stiffness, pain, paralysis, or lack of muscle control may require the use of an alternative position.

Knee-Chest Position

In the knee-chest position, the patient lies on the side with both knees bent, with the top leg brought closer to the chest (Fig. 19.38). A variation of this position would allow the patient to lie with the bottom leg straightened while the top leg is still bent close to the chest. Insert the speculum with the handle pointed in the direction of the patient's abdomen or back. Because the patient is lying on the side, be sure to angle the speculum toward the small of the patient's back and not straight up toward the head. Once the speculum has been removed, the patient will need to roll onto the back.

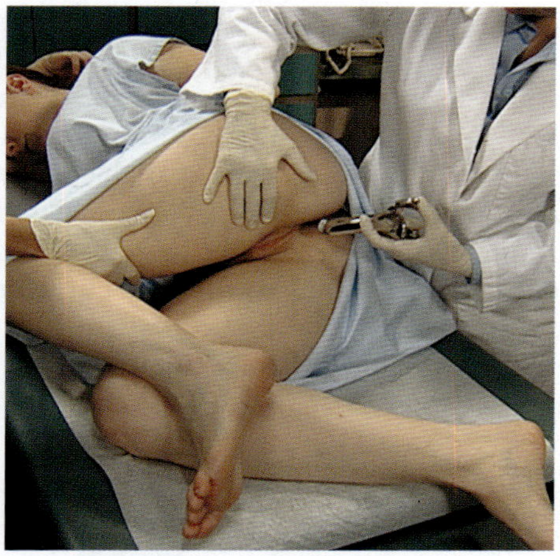

FIG. 19.38 The knee-chest position.

The assistant may provide support for the patient while on the examination table, help the patient straighten the bottom leg if the preferred variation of this position, or support the patient in rolling onto the back for the bimanual examination. If the patient cannot separate the legs, the assistant may help elevate one leg.

The knee-chest position does not require the use of stirrups. It is particularly good for a patient who feels most comfortable and balanced lying on a side.

Diamond-Shaped Position

In the diamond-shaped position, the patient lies on the back with knees bent so that both legs are spread flat and the heels meet at the foot of the table (Fig. 19.39). Insert the speculum with the handle up and perform the bimanual examination from the side or foot of the table.

The assistant may help the patient with self-support on the table and hold the feet together in alignment with the spine to maintain this position. A patient may be more comfortable using pillows or an assistant to elevate the thighs and/or using a pillow under the small of the back.

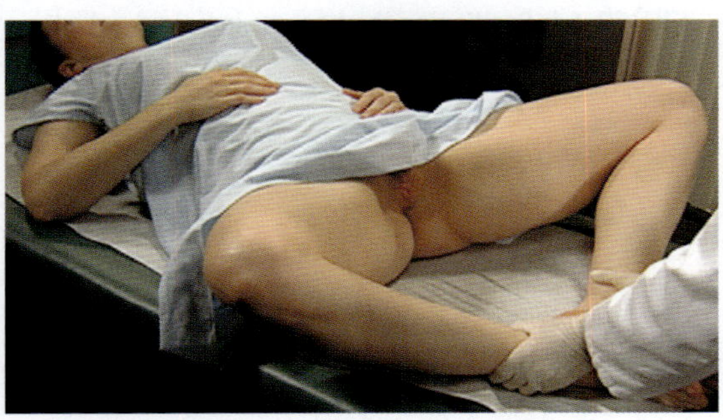

FIG. 19.39 The diamond-shaped position.

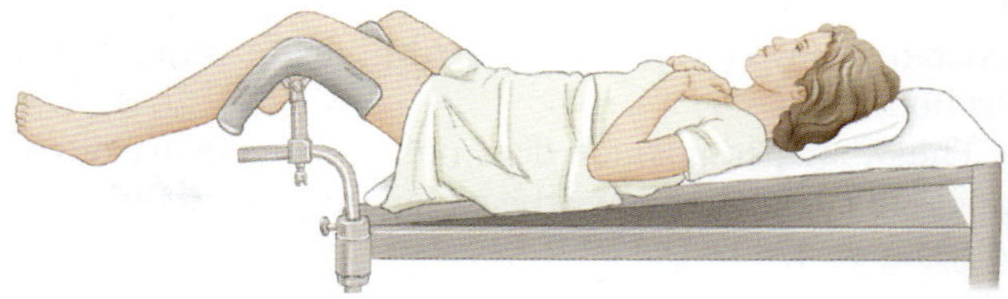

FIG. 19.40 The obstetric stirrups position.

The diamond-shaped position does not require the use of stirrups. A patient must be able to lie flat on the back to use this position.

Obstetric Stirrups Position

In the obstetric stirrups position, the patient lies on the back near the foot of the table with legs supported under the knee by obstetric stirrups (Fig. 19.40). Insert the speculum with the handle down and perform the bimanual examination from the foot of the table.

The patient may require assistance in putting the legs into the stirrups. The stirrups can be padded to increase comfort and reduce irritation. A strap can be attached to each stirrup to hold a patient's legs securely in place if the patient prefers this increased support.

Obstetric stirrups provide much more support than the traditionally used foot stirrups. This position allows a patient who has difficulty using the foot stirrups to assume the traditional pelvic examination position.

M-Shaped Position

In the M-shaped position, the patient lies supine, knees bent and apart, and feet resting on the examination table close to the buttocks (Fig. 19.41). Insert the speculum with the handle up and perform the bimanual examination from the foot of the table.

If the patient feels the legs are not completely stable on the examination table, an assistant may support the feet

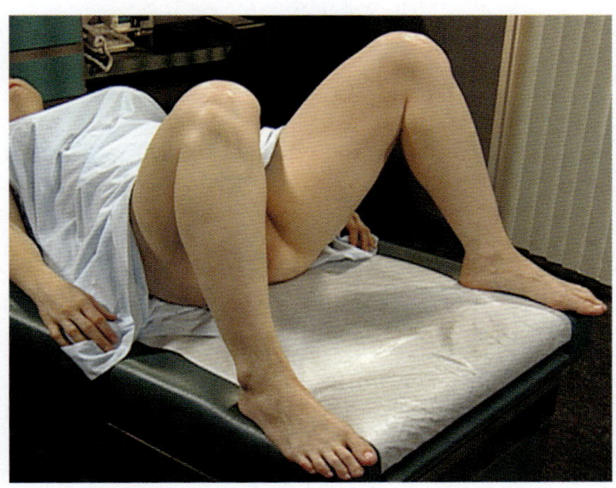

FIG. 19.41 The M-shaped position.

or knees. If a patient has had bilateral leg amputations, assistants may elevate the residual limbs to simulate this position.

The M-shaped position does not require the use of stirrups. This position allows the patient to lie with the entire body supported by the table.

V-Shaped Position

In the V-shaped position, the patient lies supine with straightened legs separated widely to either side of the table (Fig. 19.42). If a patient is able to put one foot in the stirrup, a variation of this position would allow the patient to hold one leg out straight and keep one foot in a stirrup. Insert the speculum with the handle up and perform the bimanual examination from the side or foot of the table.

At least one and possibly two assistants are needed to enable the patient to maintain this position. The assistants should support each straightened leg at the knee and ankle. The patient may be more comfortable if the legs are slightly elevated or if a pillow is used under the small of the back or tailbone.

The V-shaped position may or may not require stirrups. The patient must be able to lie comfortably on the back to use this position.

Patients With Sensory Impairment

A patient with visual or hearing impairment will probably want to utilize the usual foot-stirrup position for the pelvic examination (Figs. 19.43 and 19.44). Before the examination, you can ask if the patient would like to examine the speculum, swab, or other instruments that will be used during the examination. If three-dimensional genital models are available, they can be used to familiarize the patient with the examination process. You may elevate the head of the table for a patient with a hearing impairment so that the clinician and/or interpreter are visible. The drape that is used to cover the patient's body below the waist should be kept low between the legs.

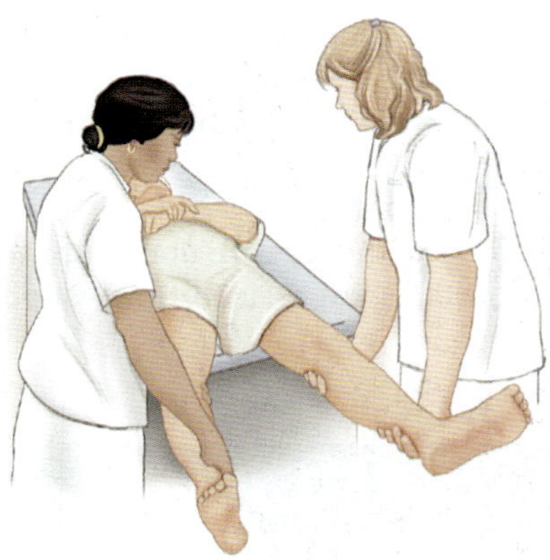

FIG. 19.42 The V-shaped position.

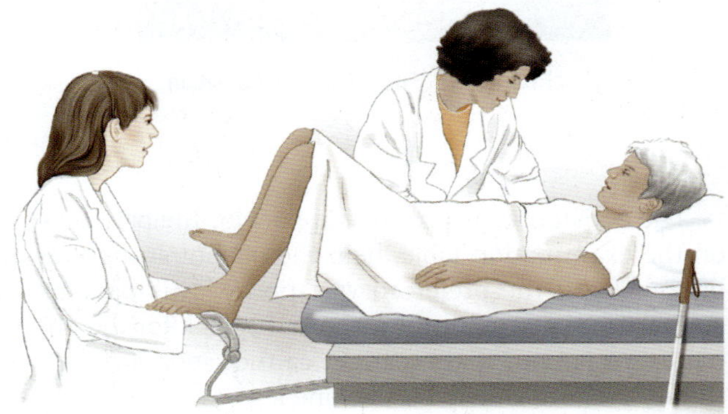

FIG. 19.43 Positioning the visually impaired patient.

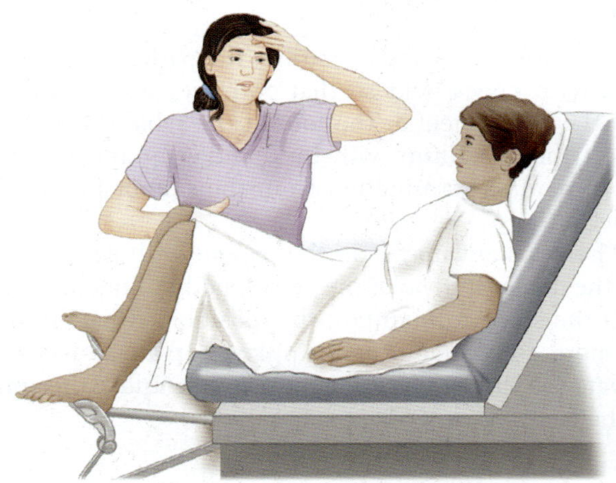

FIG. 19.44 Positioning the hearing-impaired patient.

ABNORMALITIES

Female Genitalia

Premenstrual Syndrome

A collection of physical, psychological, and mood symptoms related to a patient's menstrual cycle

PATHOPHYSIOLOGY

- Etiology unclear; likely causes include hormonal factors and responses to hormonal factors
- Usually begins in a patient's late 20s and increases in incidence and severity as menopause approaches

PATIENT DATA

Subjective Data

- Symptoms may include breast swelling and tenderness, acne, bloating and weight gain, headache or joint pain, food cravings, irritability, difficulty concentrating, mood swings, crying spells, and depression
- Symptoms occur 5–7 days before menses (luteal phase) and subside with onset of menses

Objective Data

- None
- Diagnosis based on symptoms and temporal relationship to menstrual cycle

Infertility

The inability to conceive over a period of 1 year of unprotected sexual intercourse

PATHOPHYSIOLOGY

- Many causes, including both male and female conditions
- Contributing factors in the patient include abnormalities of the vagina, cervix, uterus, fallopian tubes, and ovaries
- Male infertility can be caused by insufficient, nonmotile, or immature sperm; ductal obstruction of sperm; and transport-related factors
- Factors influencing fertility include stress, nutrition, chemical substances, chromosomal abnormalities, certain disease processes, sexual and relationship problems, and hematologic and immunologic disorders

PATIENT DATA

Subjective Data

- Unsuccessful attempts to become pregnant

Objective Data

- Varies with underlying cause
- Often no findings on physical examination

Endometriosis

The presence and growth of endometrial tissue outside the uterus (Figs. 19.45 and 19.46)

PATHOPHYSIOLOGY

- Pathogenesis not definitive
- Thought to be due to retrograde reflux of menstrual tissue from the fallopian tubes during menstruation

PATIENT DATA

Subjective Data

- Pelvic pain, dysmenorrhea, and heavy or prolonged menstrual flow

Objective Data

- No findings
- On bimanual examination, tender nodules may be palpable along the uterosacral ligaments
- Diagnosis confirmed by laparoscopy

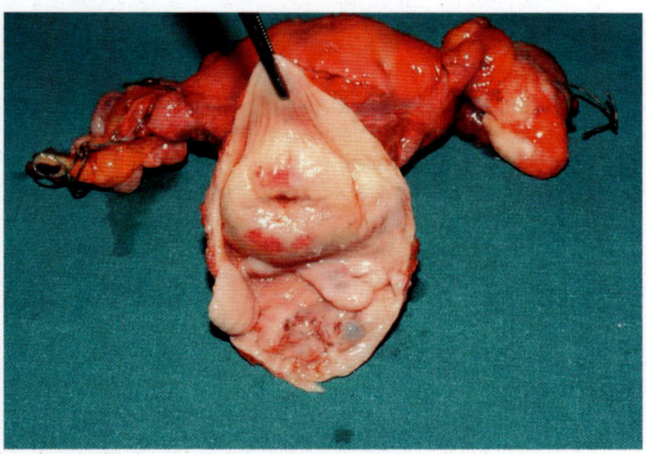

FIG. 19.45 Endometriosis. (From Fedele, L., et al. (2005). Tailoring radicality in demolitive surgery for deeply infiltrating endometriosis. *American Journal of Obstetrics & Gynecology*, 193, 114–117.)

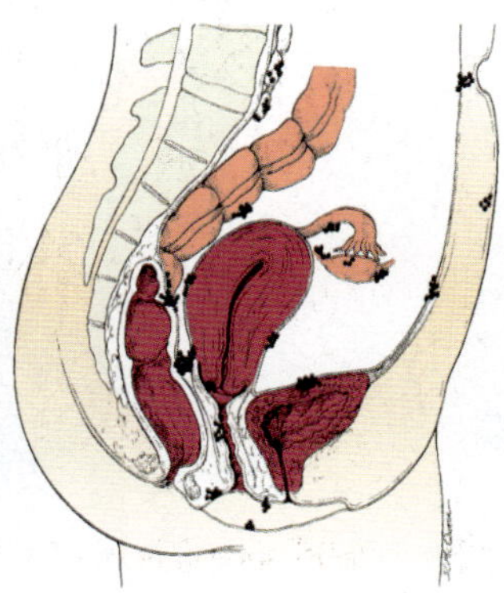

FIG. 19.46 Common sites of endometriosis. (From Stenchever, M., et al. (2001). *Comprehensive gynecology* (4th ed.). St. Louis: Mosby.)

LESIONS FROM SEXUALLY TRANSMITTED INFECTIONS

Condyloma Acuminatum (Genital Warts)

Warty lesions caused by STI with HPV

PATHOPHYSIOLOGY

- HPV invades the basal layer of the epidermis; virus penetrates through skin and causes mucosal microabrasions
- Latent viral phase begins with no signs or symptoms and can last from a month to several years
- After latency, viral DNA, capsids, and particles are produced; host cells become infected and develop the characteristic skin lesions
- Considered an STI

PATIENT DATA

Subjective Data

- Soft, painless, wartlike lesions
- History of sexual contact

Objective Data

- Flesh-colored, whitish pink to reddish brown, discrete, soft growths on labia, vestibule, or perianal area (Fig. 19.47)
- Lesions may occur singly or in clusters and may enlarge to form cauliflower-like masses

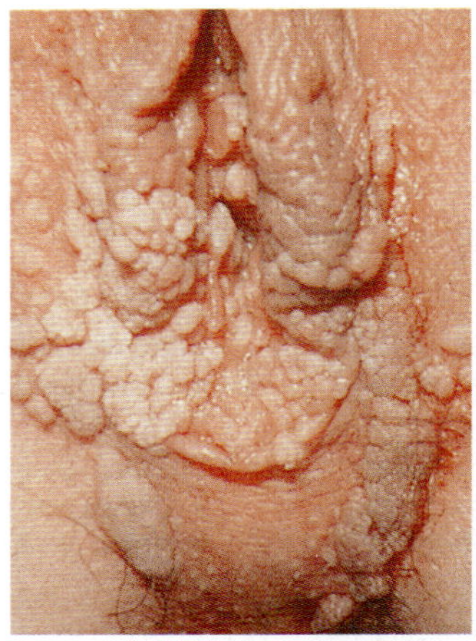

FIG. 19.47 **Condyloma acuminatum.** (From Morse, S. A., et al. (2003). *Atlas of sexually transmitted diseases and AIDS* (3rd ed.). St. Louis: Mosby.)

Molluscum Contagiosum

Viral infection of the skin and mucous membranes; considered an STI in adults, in contrast to the common nonsexually transmitted infection occurring in young children (Fig. 19.48)

PATHOPHYSIOLOGY

- Caused by a poxvirus; the virus enters the skin through small breaks of hair follicles
- Spreads through direct person-to-person contact and through contact with contaminated object
- After incubation period, growths appear
- Genital lesions are sexually transmitted

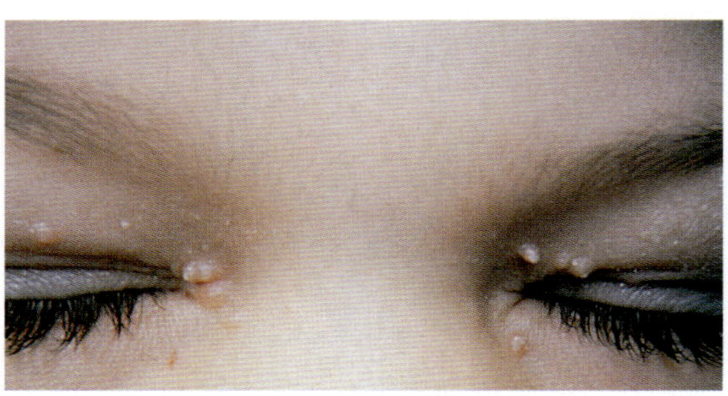

FIG. 19.48 **Molluscum contagiosum.** Note that these have occurred around the eyes. (Courtesy Walter Tunnesen, MD, Chapel Hill, NC.)

PATIENT DATA

Subjective Data

- Painless lesions in genital area
- Sexually active

Objective Data

- White or flesh-colored, dome-shaped papules that are round or oval
- Surface has a characteristic central umbilication from which a thick, creamy core can be expressed
- Lesions may last from several months to several years
- Diagnosis usually based on the clinical appearance of the lesions
- Direct microscopic examination of stained material from the core will reveal typical molluscum bodies within the epithelial cell

Syphilitic Chancre

Skin lesion associated with primary syphilis

PATHOPHYSIOLOGY

- Sexually transmitted infection caused by the bacterium *Treponema pallidum*
- Transmitted through direct contact with a syphilis sore
- Lesions of primary syphilis generally occur 2 weeks after exposure
- Chancre lasts 3–6 weeks, heals without treatment

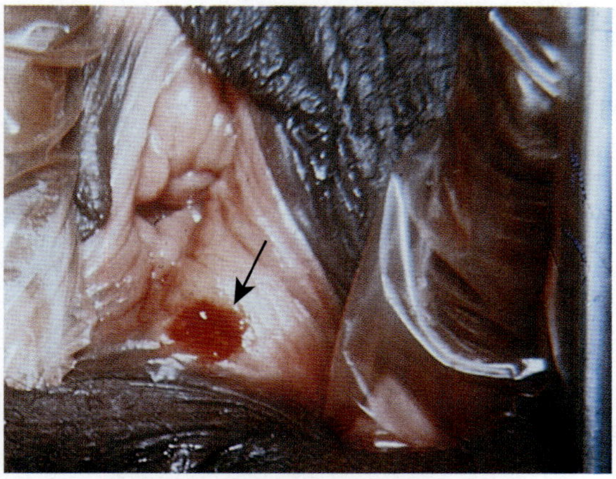

FIG. 19.49 **Primary syphilitic chancre in vagina.**

PATIENT DATA

Subjective Data

- Often no lesion noted, as may be internal (Fig. 19.49)
- Painless genital ulcer
- Sexually active

Objective Data

- Solitary lesion; firm, round, small, painless ulcer
- Lesion has indurated borders with a clear base
- Scrapings from the ulcer, examined microscopically, show spirochetes

Condyloma Latum

Lesions of secondary syphilis

PATHOPHYSIOLOGY

- Sexually transmitted infection caused by the bacterium *T. pallidum*
- Appear about 6–12 weeks after infection

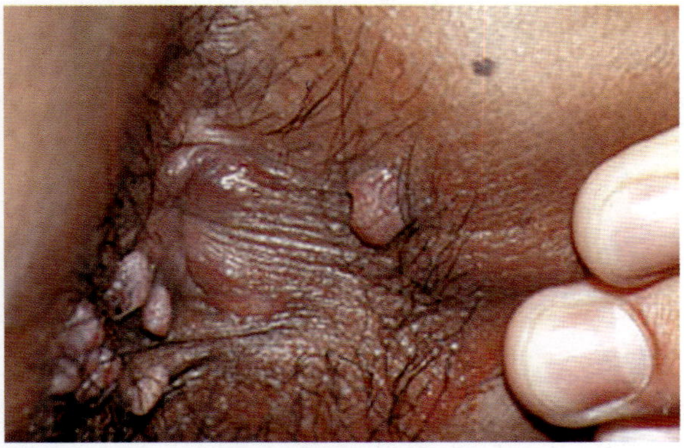

FIG. 19.50 **Condyloma latum.** (From Cohen, B. (2013). *Pediatric dermatology* (4th ed.). Elsevier.)

PATIENT DATA

Subjective Data

- Healed solitary genital lesion
- Sexually active

Objective Data

- Flat, round, or oval papules covered by a gray exudate (Fig. 19.50)

Genital Herpes

A sexually transmitted viral infection of the skin and mucosa

PATHOPHYSIOLOGY

- Caused by the herpes simplex virus (HSV)
- Most transmission of HSV occurs when individuals shed the virus in the absence of symptoms

PATIENT DATA

Subjective Data

- Painful lesions in genital area
- History of sexual contact
- May report burning or pain with urination

Objective Data

- Superficial vesicles in the genital area; internal or external (Figs. 19.51 and 19.52); may be eroded
- Initial infection is often extensive, whereas recurrent infection is usually confined to a small, localized patch on the vulva, perineum, vagina, or cervix

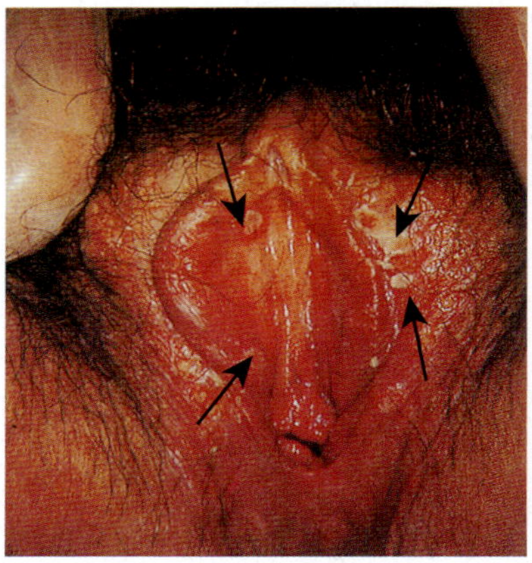

FIG. 19.51 Herpes lesions. Scattered erosions covered with exudate. (From Habif, T. P. (2004). *Clinical dermatology* (4th ed.). St. Louis: Mosby.)

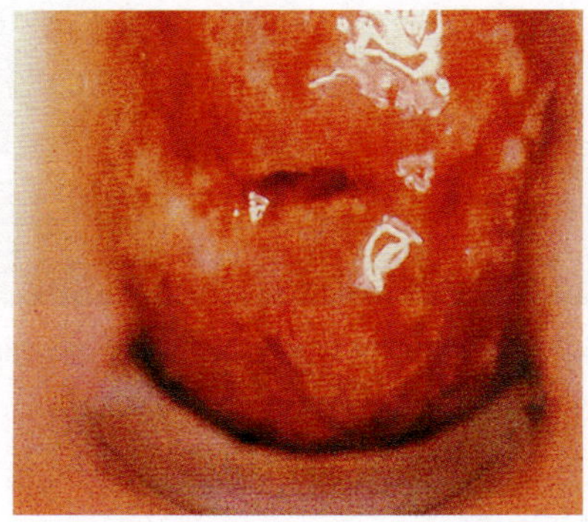

FIG. 19.52 Herpetic cervicitis. Erythema, purulent exudate, and erosions are present on the cervix. (From Morse, S. A., et al. (2003). *Atlas of sexually transmitted diseases and AIDS* (3rd ed.). St. Louis: Mosby.)

VULVA AND VAGINA

Inflammation of Bartholin Gland

PATHOPHYSIOLOGY

- Commonly, but not always, caused by *Neisseria gonorrhoeae*
- May be acute or chronic

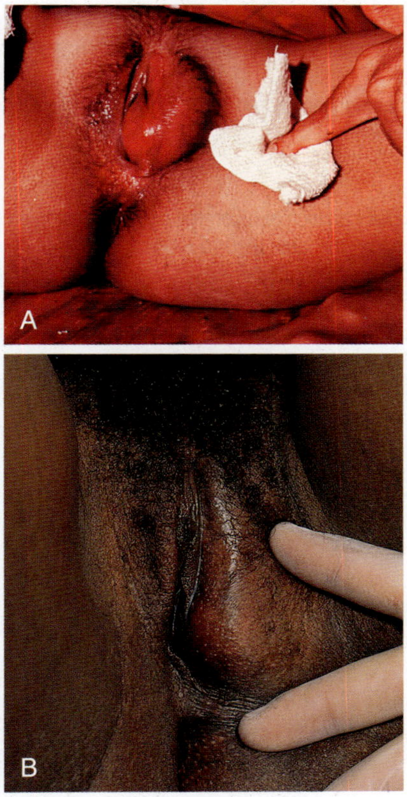

FIG. 19.53 Inflammation of Bartholin gland. (A, From Elsevier; B, from Swartz, M. H. (2006). *Textbook of physical diagnosis* (5th ed.). Philadelphia: Elsevier.)

PATIENT DATA

Subjective Data

- Pain and swelling in the groin

Objective Data

- Hot, red, tender, fluctuant swelling of the Bartholin gland that may drain pus (Fig. 19.53)
- Chronic inflammation results in a nontender cyst on the labium

Vaginal Carcinoma

Classified according to the type of tissue from which the cancer arises: squamous cell, adenocarcinoma, melanoma, and sarcoma

PATHOPHYSIOLOGY

- Squamous cell carcinoma begins in the epithelial lining of the vagina; may be caused by HPV; develops over a period of many years from precancerous changes called *vaginal intraepithelial neoplasia* (VAIN)
- Adenocarcinoma begins in the glandular tissue
- Malignant melanoma develops from pigment-producing cells called *melanocytes*
- Sarcomas form deep in the wall of the vagina, not on its surface epithelium

PATIENT DATA

Subjective Data

- Abnormal vaginal bleeding
- Difficult or painful urination
- Pain during sexual intercourse
- Pain in the pelvic area, back, or legs
- Edema in the legs
- Risk factor: patient exposed in utero to DES

Objective Data

- Vaginal discharge, lesions, and masses
- Melanoma tends to affect the lower or outer portion of the vagina
- Tumors vary greatly in size, color, and growth pattern
- Diagnosis is based on tissue biopsy

Vulvar Carcinoma

Classified according to the type of tissue from which the cancer arises: squamous cell, adenocarcinoma, melanoma, and basal cell

PATHOPHYSIOLOGY

- Squamous cell carcinoma arises from epithelial cells; most common form of vulvar cancer
- Adenocarcinoma starts in the Bartholin glands or vulvar sweat glands and accounts for a small percentage of vulvar cancer cases
- Melanoma accounts for about 2%–4% of vulvar cancer; patients with melanoma on other parts of their body have an increased risk of developing vulvar melanoma
- Basal cell carcinoma, common on sun-exposed areas, is a rare form of vulvar cancer

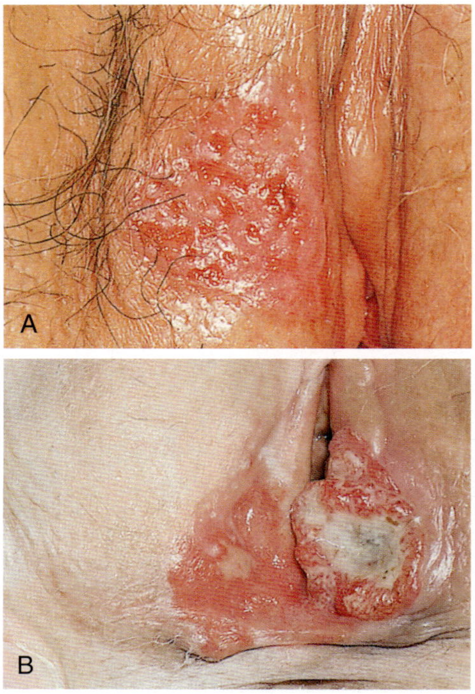

FIG. 19.54 (A) Ulcerative squamous cell carcinoma of the vulva. (B) Basal cell carcinoma of the vulva. (From Symonds, E. M., & Macpherson, M. B. A. (1994). Color atlas of obstetrics and gynecology. St. Louis: Mosby.)

PATIENT DATA

Subjective Data

- Lump or growth in or on the vulvar area or a patch of skin that is differently textured or colored
- Ulcer that persists for longer than 1 month
- Bleeding from vulvar area
- Change in the appearance of an existing mole (specific to vulvar melanoma)
- Persistent itching, pain, soreness, or burning in the vulvar area
- Painful urination

Objective Data

- Squamous cell carcinoma: ulcerated or raised lesion on the vulva; usually found on the labia (Fig. 19.54A)
- Adenocarcinoma: ulcerated or raised lesion usually found on the sides of the vaginal opening
- Melanoma: dark-colored lesion most often on the clitoris or the labia minora
- Basal cell: ulcerated lesion (see Fig. 19.54B)
- Diagnosis is based on tissue biopsy

Vaginal Infections

Vaginal infections often produce a discharge (Figs. 19.55 and 19.56); see the Differential Diagnosis table

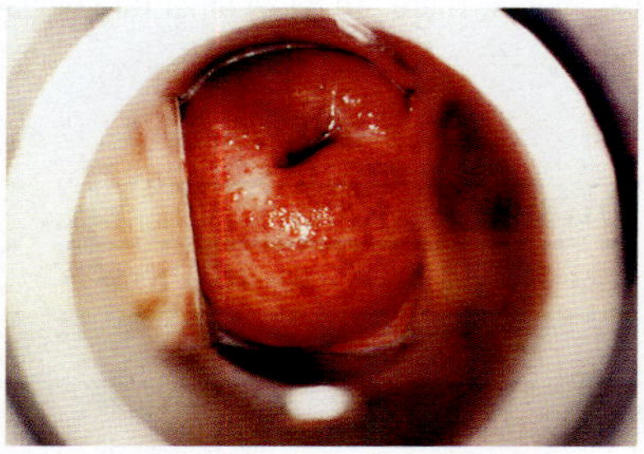

FIG. 19.55 **Trichomoniasis.** The vaginal mucosa is inflamed and often speckled with petechial lesions. In adolescents, petechial hemorrhages may also be found on the cervix, resulting in the so-called *strawberry cervix.* (From Rein, M. (Ed.). (1996). *Atlas of infectious diseases* (Vol. v). Sexually transmitted diseases. Philadelphia: Churchill Livingstone.)

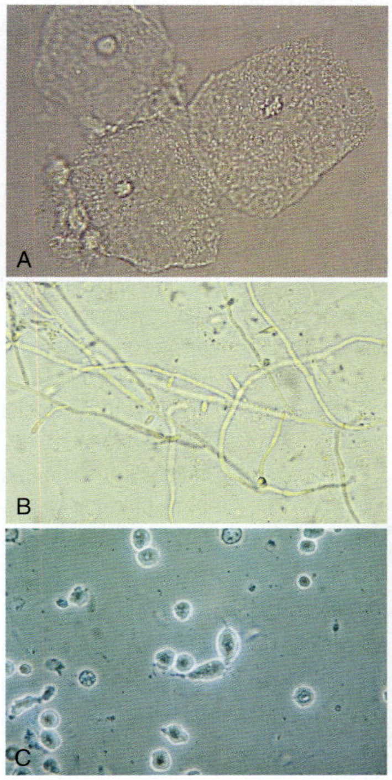

FIG. 19.56 Microscopic differentiation of vaginal infections. (A) Bacterial vaginosis: clue cells. (B) Candida vulvovaginitis: budding, branching hyphae. (C) Trichomoniasis: motile trichomonads. (A, From Klatt, E. C. (2015). *Robbins and Cotran atlas of pathology* (3rd ed.). Elsevier; B, from Zitelli, B. J., & Davis, H. W. (2018). *Zitelli and Davis' atlas of pediatric physical diagnosis* (7th ed.). Philadelphia: Elsevier; C, Bennett, J. E., Dolin, R., et al. (2015). *Mandell, Douglas, and Bennett's principles and practice of infectious diseases, updated edition* (8th ed.). Elsevier.)

DIFFERENTIAL DIAGNOSIS

Vaginal Discharges and Infections

CONDITION	HISTORY	PHYSICAL FINDINGS	DIAGNOSTIC TESTS
Physiologic vaginitis	Increase in discharge	Clear or mucoid discharge	Wet mount: up to 3–5 WBCs; epithelial cells
Bacterial vaginosis *(Gardnerella vaginalis)*	No foul odor, itching, or edema Foul-smelling discharge; complains of "fishy odor"	Homogeneous thin, white or gray discharge; pH >4.5	+KOH "whiff" test; wet mount: + clue cells (see Fig. 19.56A)
Candida vulvovaginitis *(Candida albicans)*	Pruritic discharge; itching of labia; itching may extend to thighs	White, curdy discharge; pH 4.0–5.0; cervix may be red; may have erythema of perineum and thighs	KOH prep: mycelia, budding, branching yeast, pseudohyphae (see Fig. 19.56B)
Trichomoniasis *(Trichomonas vaginalis)*	Watery discharge; foul odor; dysuria and dyspareunia with severe infection	Profuse, frothy, greenish discharge; pH 5.0–6.6; red, friable cervix with petechiae ("strawberry" cervix; see Fig. 19.55)	Wet mount: round or pear-shaped protozoa; motile "gyrating" flagella (see Fig. 19.56C)
Gonorrhea *(Neisseria gonorrhoeae)*	Partner with STI; often asymptomatic or may have symptoms of PID	Purulent discharge from cervix; Skene/Bartholin gland inflammation; cervix and vulva may be inflamed	Gram stain Culture DNA probe
Chlamydia *(Chlamydia trachomatis)*	Partner with nongonococcal urethritis; often asymptomatic; may complain of spotting after intercourse or urethritis	± Purulent discharge; cervix may or may not be red or friable	DNA probe
Atrophic vaginitis	Dyspareunia; vaginal dryness; perimenopausal or postmenopausal	Pale, thin vaginal mucosa; pH >4.5	Wet mount: folded, clumped epithelial cells
Allergic vaginitis	New bubble bath, soap, douche, or other hygiene products	Foul smell; erythema; pH may be altered	Wet mount: WBCs
Foreign body	Red and swollen vulva; vaginal discharge; history of use of tampon, condom, or diaphragm	Bloody or foul-smelling discharge	Wet mount: WBCs

KOH, Potassium hydroxide; *PID,* pelvic inflammatory disease; *STI,* sexually transmitted infection; *WBC,* white blood cell.

CERVIX

Cervical Cancer

Classified according to the type of tissue from which the cancer arises: squamous cell carcinoma and adenocarcinoma. There are a few other rare types of cervical cancer.

PATHOPHYSIOLOGY

- Typically originates from a dysplastic or premalignant lesion present at the active squamocolumnar junction
- Lesions gradually progress through recognizable stages before developing into invasive disease
- The transformation from mild dysplastic to invasive carcinoma generally occurs slowly over several years
- HPV is the most important causative agent in cervical carcinogenesis at the molecular level; vaccination against HPV before exposure is effective in reducing risk

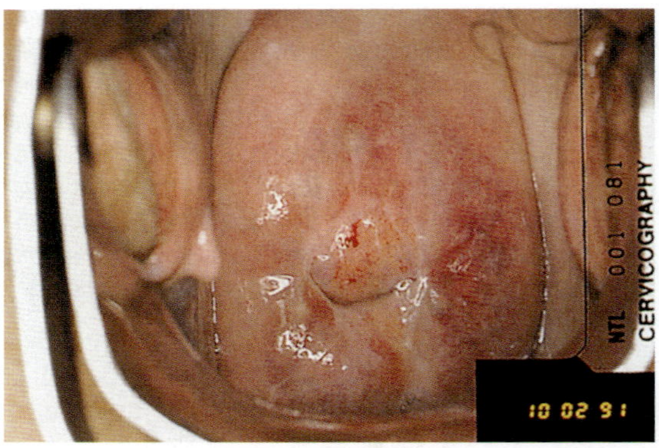

FIG. 19.57 The cervical cancer lesion is predominantly around the external os. (From Symonds, E. M., & Macpherson, M. B. A. (1994). Color atlas of obstetrics and gynecology. St. Louis: Mosby.)

PATIENT DATA

Subjective Data

- Usually asymptomatic
- May report unexpected vaginal bleeding or spotting

Objective Data

- Often no findings on physical examination
- A hard granular surface at or near the cervical os
- Lesion can evolve to form an extensive irregular cauliflower growth that bleeds easily (Fig. 19.57)
- Early lesions are indistinguishable from ectropion
- Ulcerated area
- Precancerous and early cancer changes are detected by Pap smear, not by physical examination

UTERUS

Uterine Prolapse

Descent or herniation of the uterus into or beyond the vagina

PATHOPHYSIOLOGY

- Result of weakening of the supporting structures of the pelvic floor, often occurring concurrently with a cystocele and rectocele
- Uterus becomes progressively retroverted and descends into the vaginal canal (Fig. 19.58)

PATIENT DATA

Subjective Data

- Sensation of pelvic heaviness and/or uterus falling out
- Tissue protruding from vagina
- Urine leakage or urge incontinence, difficulty having a bowel movement, or low back pain

Objective Data

- First-degree prolapse: the cervix remains within the vagina
- Second-degree prolapse: the cervix is at the introitus
- Third-degree prolapse: the cervix and vagina drop outside the introitus (Fig. 19.59)

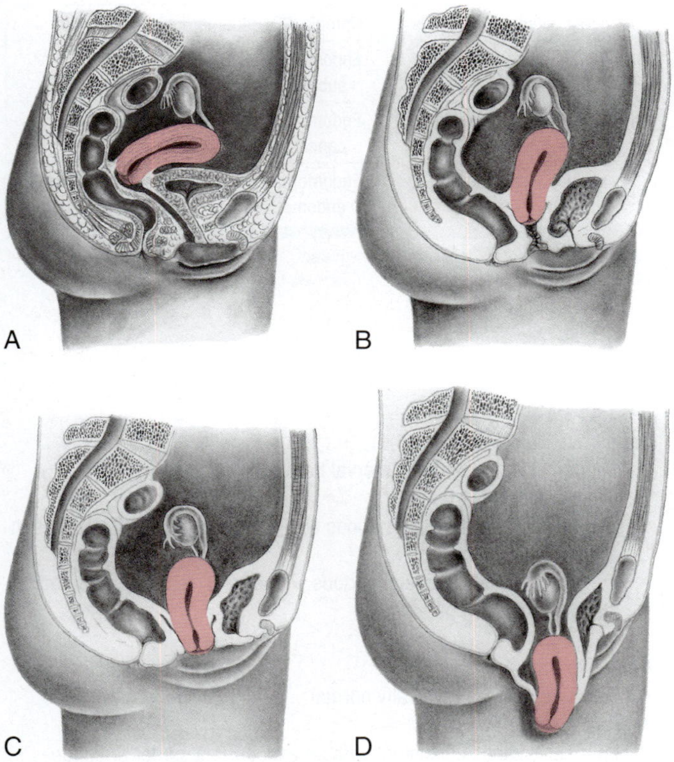

FIG. 19.58 Uterine prolapse. (A) Expected uterine position. (B) First-degree prolapse of the uterus. (C) Second-degree prolapse of the uterus. (D) Complete prolapse of the uterus.

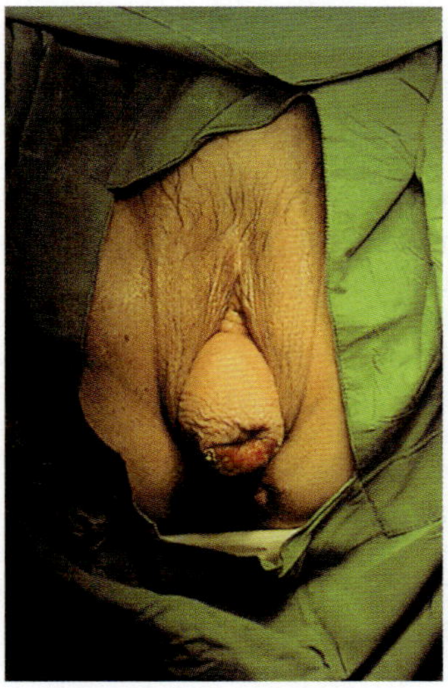

FIG. 19.59 Third-degree prolapse of the uterus and vaginal walls. (From Symonds, E. M., & Macpherson, M. B. A. (1994). Color atlas of obstetrics and gynecology. St. Louis: Mosby.)

Uterine Bleeding

Abnormality in menstrual bleeding and inappropriate uterine bleeding are common gynecologic problems (Table 19.2).

Think About It

In interpreting unexpected uterine bleeding, age is a primary consideration. In a prepubertal patient, the major considerations are early menarche, foreign body, and trauma (including sexual abuse). In a patient of childbearing age with a uterus, it is axiomatic that the patient is pregnant until proven otherwise. While careful history, accompanied by a thorough examination, will head you toward a diagnostic conclusion, pregnancy testing is an essential early step. In a postmenopausal patient with a uterus, any vaginal bleeding is a red flag for endometrial cancer regardless of history and examination findings.

TABLE 19.2 Types of Uterine Bleeding and Associated Causes

	COMMON CAUSES
Midcycle spotting	Midcycle estradiol fluctuation associated with ovulation
Delayed menstruation	Anovulation or threatened abortion with excessive bleeding
Frequent bleeding	Chronic PID, endometriosis, anovulation
Profuse menstrual bleeding	Endometrial polyps, adenomyosis, submucous bleeding leiomyomas, IUD
Intermenstrual or irregular bleeding	Endometrial polyps, uterine or cervical cancer, oral contraceptives
Postmenopausal bleeding	Endometrial hyperplasia, estrogen therapy, endometrial cancer

IUD, Intrauterine device; *PID*, pelvic inflammatory disease.
Modified from Thompson, J. M., et al. (1997). *Clinical nursing* (4th ed.). St. Louis: Mosby.

PATHOPHYSIOLOGY

Nonpregnant patients:

- Structural causes (PALM)
  - Polyp
  - Adenomyosis
  - Leiomyoma
  - Malignancy or hyperplasia of the endometrium
- Nonstructural causes (COEIN)
  - Coagulopathy
  - Ovulatory dysfunction: irregular or unpredictable release of progesterone by the ovary; primary ovarian abnormality such as polycystic ovarian syndrome (PCOS); or a systemic endocrinologic disorder that affects the hypothalamic-pituitary-ovarian axis
  - Endometrial: loss of the homeostatic control mechanisms that initiate and terminate uterine bleeding at the endometrial cellular level
  - Iatrogenic (e.g., from medications such as antibiotics, phenobarbital, rifampin, phenytoin, or carbamazepine)
  - Not otherwise classified (e.g., trauma, postsurgical, infection)

Pregnancy-related:

- Pregnancy implantation, placental abnormalities, threatened abortion and ectopic pregnancy

PATIENT DATA

Subjective Data (see Box 19.1)

- Shortened or lengthened interval between periods
- Absence of menstruation
- Normal intervals between periods with excessive flow and/or duration or decreased flow
- Irregular intervals between periods with excessive flow and duration
- Bleeding between periods

Objective Data

- Pelvic examination typically normal
- Palpable leiomyomas
- Physical findings consistent with an endocrine disorder or coagulopathy
- Findings consistent with stage of pregnancy

Myomas (Leiomyomas, Fibroids)

Common, benign uterine tumors (Fig. 19.60)

PATHOPHYSIOLOGY

- Arise from the overgrowth of smooth muscle and connective tissue in the uterus
- May occur singly or in multiples and vary greatly in size

PATIENT DATA

Subjective Data

- Fibroid symptoms are related to the number of tumors, as well as to their size and location. Symptoms may include the following:
  - Heavy menses
  - Abdominal cramping usually felt during menstruation
  - Urinary frequency, urgency, and/or incontinence from pressure on the bladder
  - Constipation, difficult defecation, or rectal pain from pressure on the colon
  - Abdominal cramping from pressure on the small bowel
  - Generalized pelvic and/or lower abdominal discomfort

Objective Data

- Firm, irregular nodules in the contour of the uterus on bimanual examination
- Uterus may be enlarged

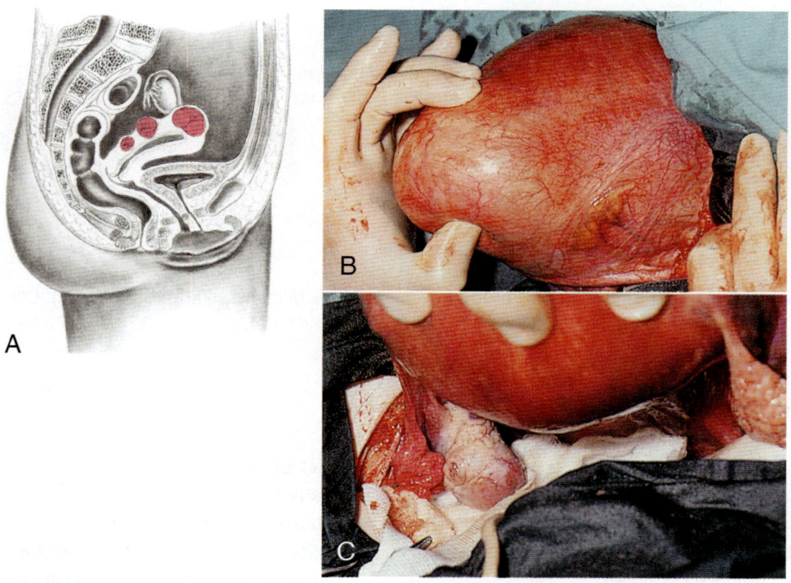

FIG. 19.60 Myomas of the uterus (fibroids). (A) Common location of myomas. (B) Multiple uterine fibroids. (C) Multiple uterine fibroids with enlarged ovaries resulting from multiple small cysts. (B and C, From Symonds, E. M., & Macpherson, M. B. A. (1994). Color atlas of obstetrics and gynecology. St. Louis: Mosby.)

Endometrial Cancer

Classified by histologic subtype, including endometrioid, serous , clear cell mixed , undifferentiated/dedifferentiated, carcinosarcoma, and other rare subtypes.

PATHOPHYSIOLOGY

- Occurs most often in postmenopausal patients
- Nearly all endometrial cancers are cancers of the glandular cells found in the lining of the uterus; most known risk factors for endometrial cancer are linked to the imbalance between estrogen and progesterone in the body
- Patients with a uterus taking tamoxifen are at increased risk

PATIENT DATA

Subjective Data

- Postmenopausal vaginal bleeding—red flag for endometrial cancer

Objective Data

- None; diagnosed by endometrial biopsy

ADNEXA

Ovarian Cysts

Fluid-filled sac in an ovary (Fig. 19.61)

PATHOPHYSIOLOGY

- Follicle undergoes varying rates of maturation, and cysts can occur as the result of hypothalamic-pituitary dysfunction or because of native anatomic defects in the reproductive system
- Can occur unilaterally or bilaterally
- Can be present from the neonatal period to postmenopause
- Most ovarian cysts occur during infancy and adolescence, which are hormonally active periods of development
- Most are functional in nature and resolve with minimal treatment

PATIENT DATA

Subjective Data

- Usually asymptomatic
- May report lower abdominal pain: sharp, intermittent, sudden, and severe
- Sudden onset of abdominal pain may suggest cyst rupture

Objective Data

- Pelvic mass may be palpated
- Cervical motion tenderness may be elicited
- Often an incidental finding during ultrasonography performed for other reasons

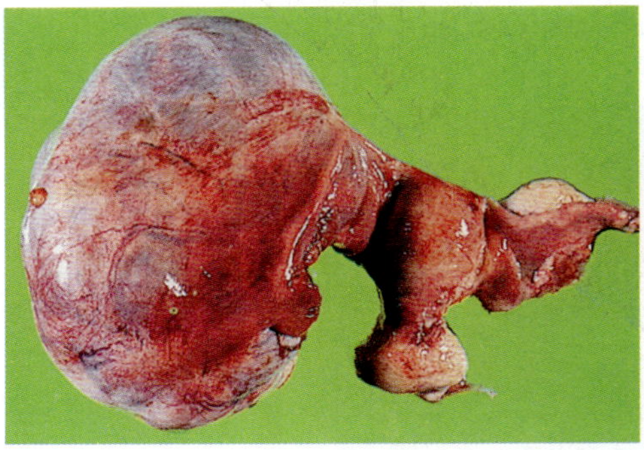

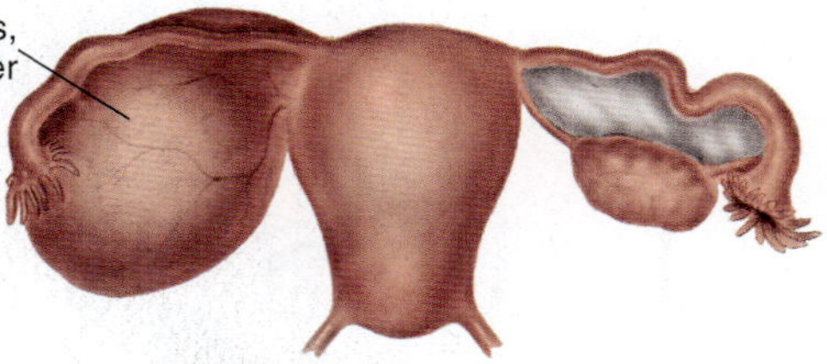

FIG. 19.61 Ovarian cyst. (Photograph from Symonds, E. M., & Macpherson, M. B. A. (1994). Color atlas of obstetrics and gynecology. St. Louis: Mosby.)

Ovarian Cancer

Classified by the cells from which the cancer arises: epithelial, stromal, or germ cell

PATHOPHYSIOLOGY

- Epithelial tumors: arise from a layer of germinal epithelium on the outside of the ovary; most common form of ovarian cancer
- Stromal tumors develop from connective tissue cells that help form the structure of the ovary and produce hormones
- Germ cell tumors arise from germ cells (cells that produce the egg); develop most often in young patients (including teenagers)

PATIENT DATA

Subjective Data

- Often asymptomatic at first
- Suspect ovarian cancer in a patient older than 40 years with persistent and unexplained vague gastrointestinal symptoms such as generalized abdominal discomfort and/or pain, gas, indigestion, pressure, swelling, bloating, cramps, or feeling of fullness even after a light meal

Objective Data

- May have no physical findings
- On bimanual examination, an ovary that is enlarged in a premenopausal patient or a palpable ovary in a postmenopausal patient should be considered suspicious for cancer
- Further diagnostic tests are required

Tubal (Ectopic) Pregnancy

Ectopic pregnancy occurring outside the uterus

PATHOPHYSIOLOGY

- Most common site is in one of the fallopian tubes but can occur in other areas
- Ectopic pregnancy usually caused by a condition that blocks or slows the movement of a fertilized egg through the fallopian tube to the uterus
- May be caused by a physical blockage in the tube; most cases from scarring caused by past ectopic pregnancy, past infection in the fallopian tubes, pelvic inflammatory disease, or surgery of the fallopian tubes

PATIENT DATA

Subjective Data

- Abnormal vaginal bleeding
- Low back pain
- Mild cramping on one side of the pelvis
- Pain in the lower abdomen or pelvic area
- If the area of the abnormal pregnancy ruptures and bleeds, symptoms may worsen
- Feeling lightheaded or syncope
- Pain that is felt in the shoulder area
- Severe, sharp, and sudden pain in the lower abdomen

Objective Data

- Marked pelvic tenderness, with tenderness and rigidity of the lower abdomen
- Cervical motion tenderness; a tender, unilateral adnexal mass may indicate the site of the pregnancy (Fig. 19.62)
- Tachycardia and hypotension reflect hemorrhage of a ruptured tubal pregnancy into the peritoneal cavity and impending cardiovascular collapse
- A ruptured tubal pregnancy is a surgical emergency

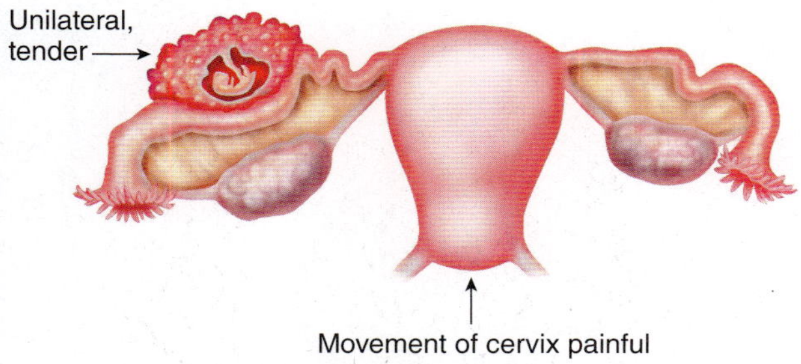

FIG. 19.62 **Ruptured tubal pregnancy.**

Pelvic Inflammatory Disease

Infection of the uterus, fallopian tubes, and other reproductive organs; a common and serious complication of some STIs (Fig. 19.63)

PATHOPHYSIOLOGY

- Often caused by *Neisseria gonorrhoeae* and *Chlamydia trachomatis*
- May be acute or chronic

PATIENT DATA

Subjective Data

- Symptoms may be mild or absent
- Unusual vaginal discharge that may have a foul odor
- Symptoms include painful intercourse, painful urination, irregular menstrual bleeding, and pain in the upper abdomen

Objective Data

- Acute PID produces very tender, bilateral adnexal areas; the patient guards and usually cannot tolerate bimanual examination
- Symptoms of chronic PID are bilateral, tender, irregular, and fairly fixed adnexal areas

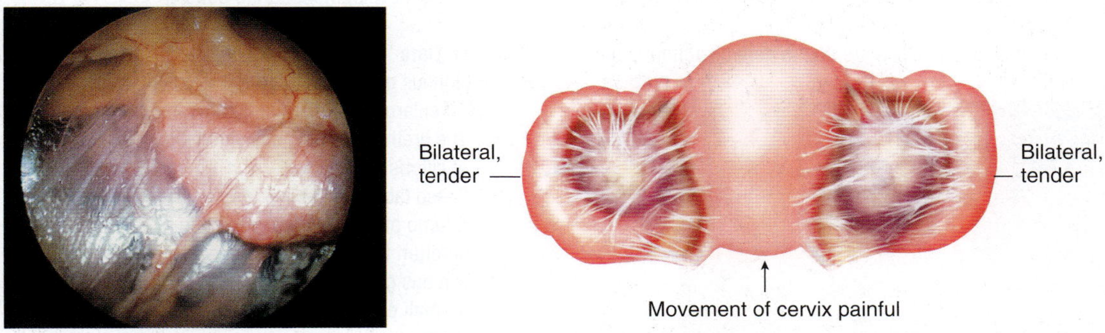

FIG. 19.63 **Pelvic inflammatory disease.** The photograph shows a sheet of fine adhesions covering the fallopian tubes and ovary, which is buried beneath the fallopian tubes. (Photograph from Symonds, E. M., & Macpherson, M. B. A. (1994). Color atlas of obstetrics and gynecology. St. Louis: Mosby.)

Salpingitis

Inflammation or infection of the fallopian tubes, often associated with PID; can be acute or chronic (Fig. 19.64)

PATHOPHYSIOLOGY

- Most cases of acute salpingitis occur in two stages: the first involves acquisition of a vaginal or cervical infection; the second involves ascent of the infection to the upper genital tract
- Organisms most commonly associated with acute salpingitis are *N. gonorrhoeae* and *C. trachomatis*

PATIENT DATA

Subjective Data

- Lower quadrant pain; constant and dull or cramping; pain may be accentuated by motion or sexual activity
- Coexisting purulent vaginal discharge
- Abnormal vaginal bleeding
- Nausea, vomiting, fever

Objective Data

- Cervical motion tenderness and/or adnexal tenderness on bimanual examination
- Mucopurulent cervical discharge

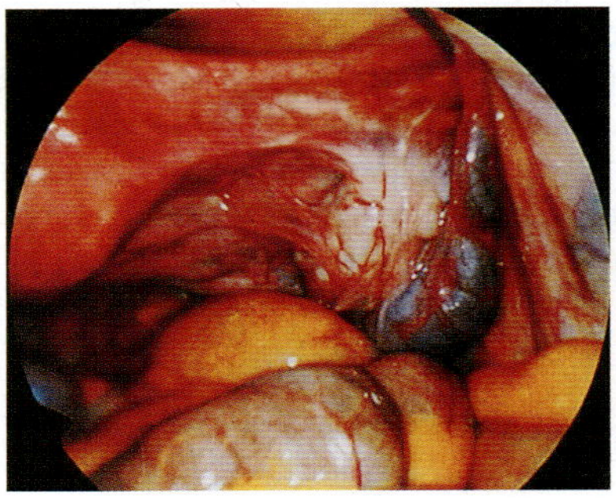

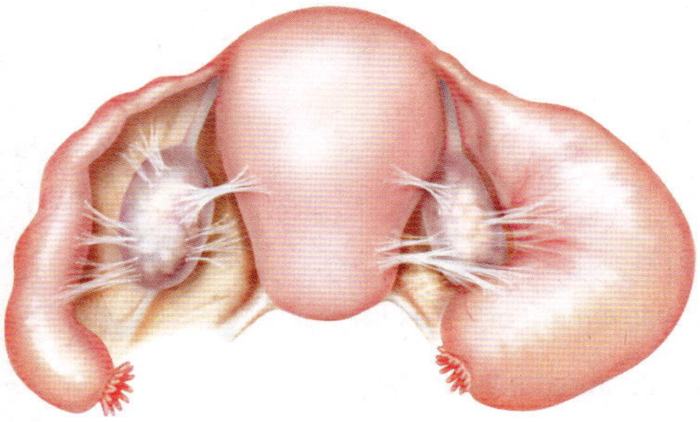

FIG. 19.64 Salpingitis. The photograph shows acute salpingitis with adhesions. Dye has been instilled into the grossly swollen fallopian tube on the right. Dense adhesions obscure the ovary. (Photograph from Morse, S. A., et al. (2003). *Atlas of sexually transmitted diseases and AIDS* (3rd ed.). St. Louis: Mosby.)

Infants and Children

Ambiguous Genitalia

The newborn's genitalia are not clearly either male or female (Fig. 19.65).

PATHOPHYSIOLOGY

- Presence or absence of male hormones controls the development of the sex organs during fetal development; male genitalia develop because of male hormones from the fetal testicles; in the female fetus, without the effects of male hormones, the genitalia develop as female
- A deficiency of male hormones in a genetic male fetus results in ambiguous genitalia; in a female fetus, the presence of male hormones during development results in ambiguous genitalia
- Most causes of ambiguous genitalia are due to genetic abnormalities

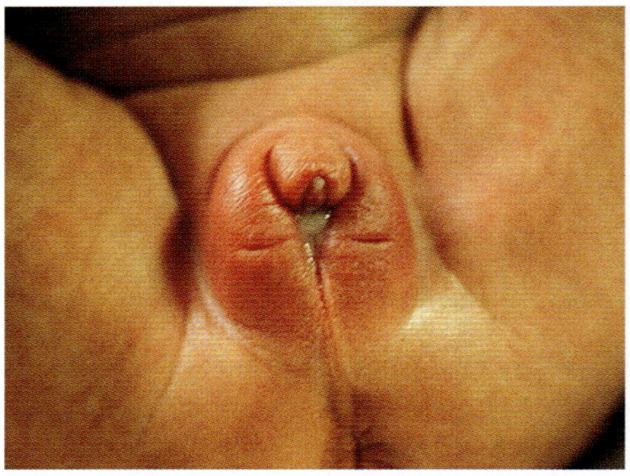

FIG. 19.65 Ambiguous genitalia. (Courtesy Patrick C. Walsh, MD, The Johns Hopkins School of Medicine, Baltimore, MD.)

PATIENT DATA

Subjective Data

Family history of:

- Genital abnormalities
- Known congenital adrenal hyperplasia
- Unexplained deaths in early infancy
- Infertility in close relatives
- Abnormal development during puberty

Objective Data

- Ambiguous genitalia in a genetic female:
  - An enlarged clitoris that has the appearance of a small penis
  - The urethral opening anywhere along, above, or below the surface of clitoris
  - Fused labia resembling a scrotum
  - A lump of tissue is felt within the fused labia, making it look like a scrotum with testicles
- Ambiguous genitalia in a genetic male:
  - A small penis that resembles an enlarged clitoris
  - Urethral opening anywhere along, above, or below the penis or as low as on the peritoneum, further making the infant appear to be female
  - Small scrotum with any degree of separation, resembling labia
  - Undescended testicles commonly accompany ambiguous genitalia
- Infant should have chromosomal studies performed

CLINICAL PEARL

Looks Can Be Deceiving

Looks can be deceiving. Do not jump to conclusions. The pictures accompanying prove the point. The patient is not a genetic male. The clitoris is enlarged; the labia are fused. Inspection must be very careful.

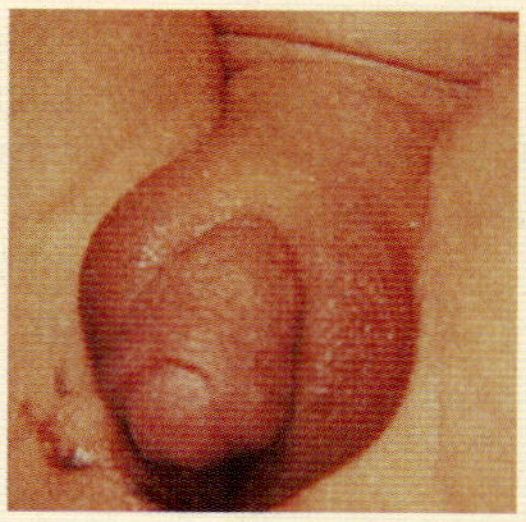

(Photograph from Biomedical Photography, Johns Hopkins University School of Medicine, Baltimore, MD.)

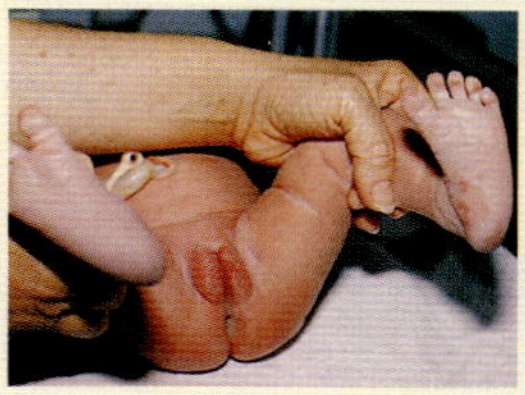

Standard infant female external genitalia. (From Lowdermilk, D. L., & Perry, S. E. (2007). *Maternity and women's health care* (8th ed.). St. Louis: Mosby.)

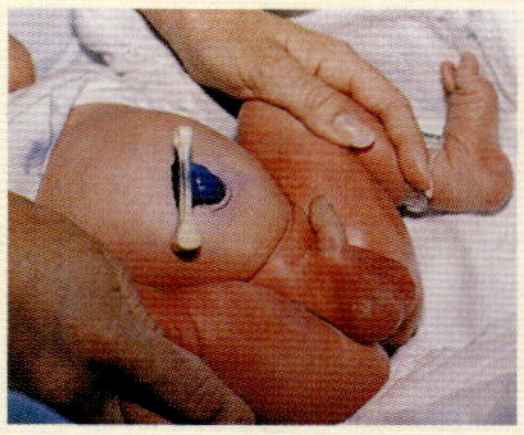

Standard infant male external genitalia. (From Lowdermilk, D. L., & Perry, S. E. (2007). *Maternity and women's health care* (8th ed.). St. Louis: Mosby.)

Hydrocolpos

Distention of the vagina caused by accumulation of fluid due to congenital vaginal obstruction

PATHOPHYSIOLOGY

- Obstruction usually caused by an imperforate hymen or, less commonly, a transverse vaginal septum

PATIENT DATA

Subjective Data

- None

Objective Data

- Small midline lower abdominal mass or a small cystic mass between the labia
- Condition may resolve spontaneously or may require surgical intervention
- Abdominal sonography is helpful in making the correct diagnosis, showing a large midline translucent mass displacing the bladder forward

Vulvovaginitis

Inflammation of the vulvar and vaginal tissues

PATHOPHYSIOLOGY

- Possible causes include sexual abuse; trichomonal, monilial, or gonococcal infection; secondary infection from a foreign body; nonspecific infection from bubble baths; diaper irritation; urethritis; injury; or pinworm infection
- Recent pharyngitis can lead to group A beta-hemolytic streptococcal (GABHS) vaginitis
- Asymptomatic vaginal discharge often occurs in the months before menarche and represents a physiologic response to increasing estrogen levels

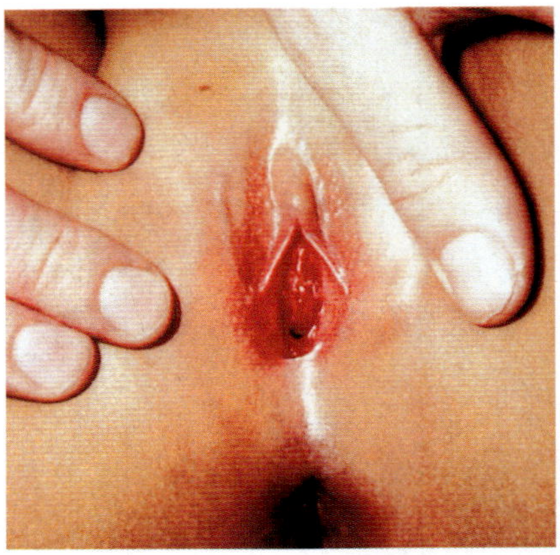

FIG. 19.66 **Nonspecific inflammation characteristic of chemical irritant vulvovaginitis.** (From Zitelli, B. J., & Davis, H. W. (2007). *Atlas of pediatric physical diagnosis* (5th ed.). St. Louis: Mosby.)

PATIENT DATA

Subjective Data

- Vaginal discharge
- Discomfort, pain, or pruritus
- Vulvar irritation
- Burning on urination
- With infants and young children, the parent may report a discharge on the diaper or panties, an abnormal vaginal odor, or redness of the vulva
- Wiping the anus from posterior to anterior, wearing tight-fitting synthetic undergarments, and using vaginal irritants such as bubble baths

Objective Data

- Warm, erythematous, and swollen vulvar tissues (Fig. 19.66)
- Vaginal pruritus, especially at night, suggests pinworm infection
- Itching, soreness, bleeding, and vaginal discharge; bloody and foul-smelling discharge may suggest a vaginal foreign body

Pregnant Patients

Premature Rupture of Membranes

The spontaneous premature rupture of the membranes (PROM) in a preterm pregnancy carries a high risk of perinatal morbidity and mortality, as well as maternal morbidity and mortality

PATHOPHYSIOLOGY

- Cause of PROM is not known; however, certain conditions such as infection and hydramnios have been implicated; some health care professionals also consider the rupture of membranes before the onset of labor in a term pregnancy to be premature rupture if labor does not begin within 12 hours

PATIENT DATA

Subjective Data

- During pregnancy before term, premature passage of fluid from the vagina

Objective Data

- PROM should be verified with a sterile speculum examination to collect fluid for testing with Nitrazine paper and microscopic examination
- Amniotic fluid has a pH of 7.15 and will turn Nitrazine paper blue-green
- Amniotic fluid placed on a slide and air-dried will have a "fern" pattern
- Ultrasound evaluation of fluid will reveal decreased or absent amniotic fluid

Vaginal Bleeding During Pregnancy

Vaginal bleeding that can occur early or late in pregnancy

PATHOPHYSIOLOGY

- In early pregnancy, may be due to unknown causes of little consequence or due to a potentially life-threatening condition, such as an ectopic pregnancy
- Late in pregnancy, causes of bleeding may range from benign conditions such as cervical changes to a potentially life-threatening abruptio placentae

PATIENT DATA

Subjective Data

- Vaginal bleeding
- May or may not be accompanied by pain

Objective Data

- Diagnosis based on the gestational age and the character of the bleeding (light or heavy, associated with pain or painless, intermittent or constant)
- Patients with vaginal bleeding in labor or who have a suspected placenta previa (prepare for emergency cesarean delivery before examination)
- Laboratory and imaging tests are used to confirm or revise the initial diagnosis

Older Adults

Atrophic Vaginitis

Inflammation of the vagina due to the thinning and shrinking of the tissues, as well as decreased lubrication

PATHOPHYSIOLOGY

- Caused by lack of estrogen during perimenopause and menopause

PATIENT DATA

Subjective Data

- Vaginal soreness or itching
- Discomfort or bleeding with sexual intercourse

Objective Data

- Vaginal mucosa is dry and pale, although it may become reddened and develop petechiae and superficial erosions
- Accompanying vaginal discharge may be white, gray, yellow, green, or blood tinged
- Can be thick or watery but, although it varies in amount, rarely profuse

Urinary Incontinence

See Chapter 18.

CHAPTER

20 Male Genitalia

For ease of communication, in this textbook the term *male genitalia* refers to the following anatomic structures: penis, testes (testicles), epididymides, scrotum, prostate gland, and seminal vesicles, regardless of the gender identity of the patient. Examination of the male genitalia is typically performed when a patient presents with a specific concern, as part of the newborn examination, or as part of a routine well child or adult health visit. In adults, examination of the anus, rectum, and prostate (see Chapter 21) is often performed at the same time.

Physical Examination Components

1. Inspect the pubic hair characteristics and distribution.
2. Retract the foreskin if the patient is uncircumcised (limited retraction in infants and young children).
3. Inspect the glans of the penis with the foreskin retracted, noting:
   - Color
   - Smegma
   - External meatus of urethra
   - Urethral discharge
   - Lesions
4. Palpate the penis for tenderness and induration.
5. Strip the urethra for discharge.
6. Inspect the scrotum and ventral surface of the penis for:
   - Color
   - Texture
   - Asymmetry
   - Lesions
   - Unusual thickening
   - Presence of hernia
7. Palpate the inguinal canal for a direct or indirect hernia.
8. Palpate the testes, epididymides, and vas deferens for:
   - Consistency
   - Size
   - Tenderness
   - Bleeding, masses, lumpiness, or nodules
9. Transilluminate masses in the scrotum.
10. Palpate for inguinal lymph nodes.
11. Elicit the cremasteric reflex bilaterally.

ANATOMY AND PHYSIOLOGY

The penis, testes, epididymides, scrotum, prostate gland, and seminal vesicles constitute the male genitalia (Fig. 20.1).

The penis serves as the final excretory organ for urine and, when erect, as the means of introducing semen into the vagina. The penis consists of the corpora cavernosa, which form the dorsum and sides, and the corpus spongiosum, which contains the urethra. The corpus spongiosum expands at its distal end to form the glans penis. The urethral orifice is a slitlike opening located approximately 2 mm ventral to the tip of the glans (Figs. 20.2 and 20.3). The skin of the penis is thin, redundant to permit erection, and free of subcutaneous fat. It is generally more darkly pigmented than body skin. Unless the patient has been circumcised, the prepuce (foreskin) covers the glans. In the uncircumcised penis, smegma is formed by the secretion of sebaceous material by the glans and the desquamation of epithelial cells from the prepuce. It appears as a cheesy white material on the glans and in the fornix of the foreskin.

The scrotum, like the penis, is generally more darkly pigmented than body skin. A septum divides the scrotum into two pendulous sacs, each containing a testis, epididymis, spermatic cord, and muscle layer termed the *cremasteric muscle* that allows the scrotum to relax or contract (Fig. 20.4). Testicular temperature is controlled by altering the distance of the testes from the body through muscular action. Spermatogenesis requires maintenance of temperatures lower than 37°C.

The testes are responsible for the production of both spermatozoa and testosterone. The adult testis is ovoid and measures approximately 4 × 3 × 2 cm. The epididymis is a soft, comma-shaped structure located on the posterolateral and upper aspect of the testis. It provides for storage, maturation, and transit of sperm. The vas deferens begins at the tail of the epididymis, ascends the spermatic cord, travels through the inguinal canal, and unites with the seminal vesicle to form the ejaculatory duct.

The prostate gland, which resembles a large chestnut and is approximately the size of a testis, surrounds the urethra at the bladder neck. It produces the major volume of ejaculatory fluid, which contains fibrinolysin. This enzyme liquefies the coagulated semen, a process that may be important for satisfactory sperm motility. The seminal vesicles extend from the prostate onto the posterior surface of the bladder.

Erection of the penis occurs when the two corpora cavernosa become engorged with blood, generally 20 to 50 mL. Arterial dilation and decreased venous outflow produce the increased blood supply; both processes are under the control of the autonomic nervous system

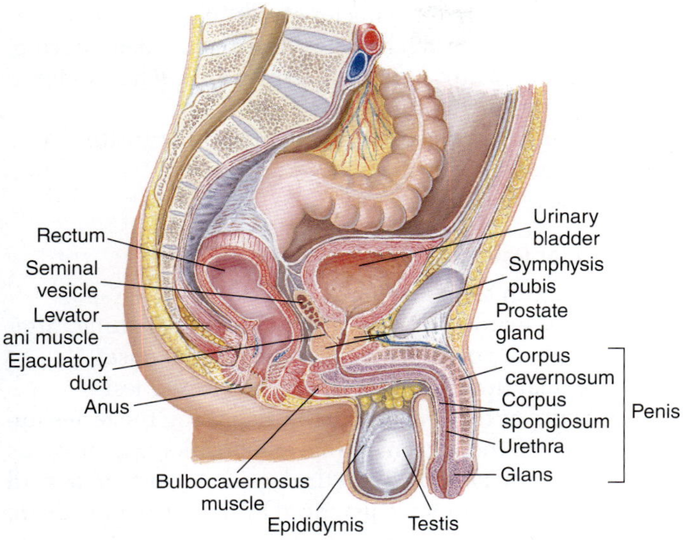

FIG. 20.1 Male pelvic organs.

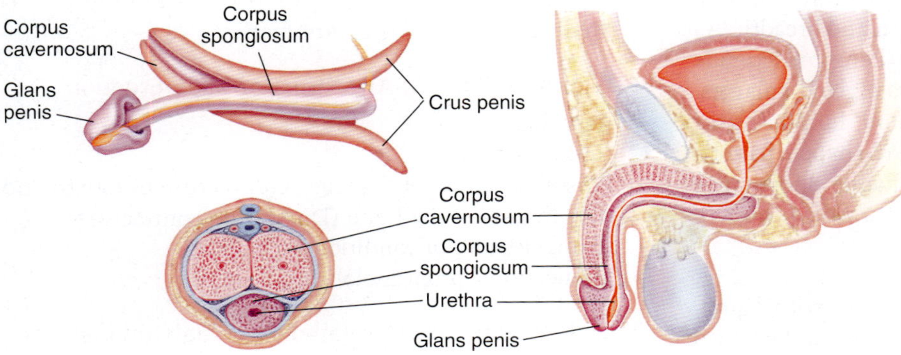

FIG. 20.2 Anatomy of the penis.

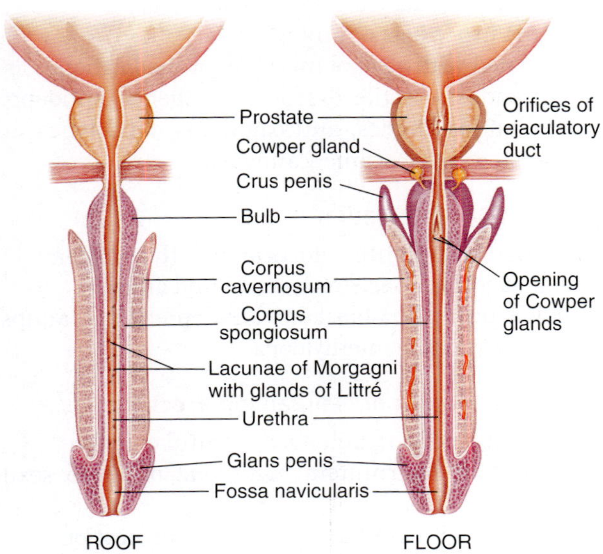

FIG. 20.3 **Anatomy of urethra and penis.** (From Lowdermilk, D. L., et al. (1997). *Maternity and women's health care* (6th ed.). St. Louis: Mosby.)

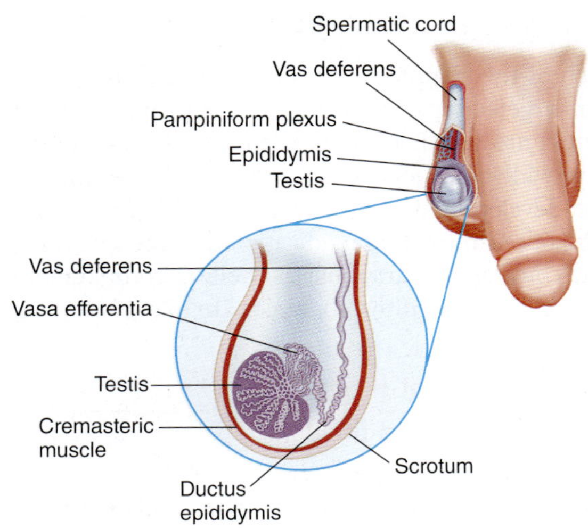

FIG. 20.4 Scrotum and its contents.

and occur because of the local synthesis of nitric oxide. Ejaculation during orgasm consists of the emission of secretions from the vas deferens, epididymides, prostate, and seminal vesicles. Orgasm is followed by constriction of the vessels supplying blood to the corpora cavernosa and gradual detumescence (subsidence of the erection).

Infants and Children

The external genitalia are sex undifferentiated at 8 weeks of gestation, but by 12 weeks of gestation, sex differentiation has occurred. Any fetal insult during 8 or 9 weeks of gestation may lead to major anomalies of the external genitalia. Minor morphologic abnormalities arise during later stages of gestation.

During the third trimester, the testes descend from the retroperitoneal space through the inguinal canal to the scrotum. At full term, one or both testes may still lie within the inguinal canal, with the final descent into the scrotum occurring in the early postnatal period. Descent of the testes may be arrested at any point, however, or they may follow an abnormal path.

Small separations between the glans and the inner preputial epithelium begin during the third trimester. Separation of the prepuce from the glans is usually incomplete at birth and often remains so until the age of 3 to 4 years in uncircumcised children.

Adolescents

With the onset of puberty, testicular growth begins and the scrotal skin reddens, thins, and becomes increasingly pendulous. Sparse, downy, straight hair appears at the base of the penis. The penis enlarges in length and breadth. As maturation continues, the pubic hair darkens and extends over the entire pubic area, and the prostate gland enlarges. By the completion of puberty, the pubic hair is curly, dense, and coarse and forms a diamond-shaped pattern from the umbilicus to the anus. (See Chapter 8 for stages of genital developmental and sexual maturation.)

Older Adults

Pubic hair becomes finer and less abundant with aging, and pubic alopecia may occur. The scrotum becomes more pendulous. An erection may develop more slowly, and orgasm may be less intense.

REVIEW OF RELATED HISTORY

For each of the symptoms or conditions discussed in this section, targeted topics to include in the history of the present illness are listed. Responses to questions about these topics provide clues for focusing the physical examination and the development of an appropriate diagnostic evaluation. Questions regarding medication use (prescription and over-the-counter preparations) as well as complementary, alternative, and integrative therapies are relevant for each.

History of Present Illness

Discharge or Lesion on the Penis

- Character of lumps, sores, rash
- Discharge: color, consistency, odor, tendency to stain underwear
- Symptoms: itching, burning, stinging
- Exposure to sexually transmitted infection (STI): multiple partners, infection in partners, failure to use condom or incorrect condom use, history of prior STI

Swelling in Inguinal Area

- Intermittent or constant, association with straining or lifting, duration, presence of pain
- Change in size or character of swelling
- Pain in the groin: character (tearing, sudden, searing, or cutting pain); associated activity (lifting heavy object, coughing, or straining at stool)
- Use of supportive undergarment or other treatment
- Frequent heavy lifting
- Medications: analgesics

Testicular Pain or Mass

- Change in testicular size
- Events surrounding onset: noted while bathing, after trauma, during a sporting event; sudden onset
- Irregular lumps, soreness, or heaviness of testes
- Practice of tucking: manually displacing the testes upward into the inguinal canal and positioning the penis and scrotal skin between the legs and rearward toward the anus. Commonly practiced by transgender women. Tight underwear, tape, or a special garment known as a *gaff* may be used to maintain this positioning.
- Medications: analgesics, antibiotics

Curvature of Penis in Any Direction With Erection

- Associated pain
- Injury to penis
- Personal history of diabetes, contracture of fourth and fifth fingers of the hand (Dupuytren contracture)
- Family history of condition
- Medications: propranolol

Persistent Erections Unrelated to Sexual Stimulation

- Current history of sickle cell disease, leukemia, multiple sclerosis, diabetes, spinal cord injury
- Trauma to genitals or groin
- Associated with alcohol ingestion or medication
- Medications: erectile dysfunction agents, antidepressants, antipsychotics, anticoagulants, anxiolytics, recreational drugs (cocaine, cannabis)

Difficulty With Ejaculation

- Painful or premature, efforts to treat the problem
- Ejaculate color, consistency, odor, and amount
- Medications: alpha-blockers, antidepressants, antipsychotics, clonidine, methyldopa

Difficulty Achieving or Maintaining Erection

- Pain with erection; prolonged, painful erection
- Constant or intermittent, with one or more sexual partners
- Associated with alcohol ingestion or medication
- Medications: diuretics, sedatives, antihypertensive agents, anxiolytics, estrogens, inhibitors of androgen synthesis, antidepressants, carbamazepine, erectile dysfunction agents

Infertility

- Lifestyle factors that may increase temperature of scrotum: tight clothing, briefs, hot baths, employment in high-temperature environment or requiring prolonged sitting

- Length of time attempting pregnancy, sexual activity pattern, knowledge of fertile period of partner's reproductive cycle
- History of varicocele, hydrocele, or undescended testes
- Diagnostic evaluation to date: semen analysis, physical examination, sperm antibody titers
- Medications: testosterone, glucocorticoids, hypothalamic-releasing hormone, marijuana

Past Medical History

- Gender identity: male, female, nonbinary, transgender woman, transgender man; sex assignment at birth
- Organ inventory: penis (natal or surgically constructed), scrotum and testes (natal or surgically constructed), prostate gland, clitoris (natal or surgically constructed), vagina (natal or surgically constructed), cervix, uterus, fallopian tubes, ovaries
- Congenital anomaly and/or surgery of genitourinary tract: undescended testes, hypospadias, epispadias, hydrocele, varicocele, hernia, prostate; vasectomy
- STIs: single or multiple infections; specific organism (gonorrhea, syphilis, herpes, human papillomavirus [HPV]), chlamydia); treatment; effectiveness; residual problems; vaccination for HPV (see Patient Safety: "HPV Immunization")
- Chronic illness: testicular or prostatic cancer, neurologic or vascular impairment, diabetes mellitus, cardiac disease
- Recent and past genitourinary/gynecologic procedures: masculinizing phalloplasty, scrotoplasty, erectile implants, vaginectomy, metoidioplasty (clitoral release/enlargement that may include urethral lengthening), hysterectomy, oophorectomy, orchiectomy, feminizing vaginoplasty

Patient Safety

HPV Immunization

HPV infection can cause cervical, vaginal, vulvar, penile, anal, and oropharyngeal cancers as well as genital warts. Vaccination against HPV before exposure to the virus through sexual activity is recommended for all 9- to 12-year-olds. The immune response is more robust in the preteen years. Because parents most often make the decision about this vaccine, the genital examination presents an opportunity to educate about the vaccine and to discuss it in terms of cancer prevention rather than HPV as a sexually transmitted infection. Catch-up HPV vaccination is recommended through age 26 for everyone, if not vaccinated already. Shared clinical decision making is recommended for individuals aged 27 through 45 years who are not vaccinated.

The Centers for Disease Control and Prevention and American Academy of Pediatrics provide tools and resources for clinicians to successfully communicate with parents about HPV vaccination.

From American Academy of Pediatrics. (2023). Human papilloma virus (HPV). Accessed August 9, 2025, from https://www.aap.org/en/news-room/campaigns-and-toolkits/human-papillomavirus-hpv/?srsltid=AfmBOoojENM_hTDlAuj3tlghh4Du6L511Gd3nw-gdiYeyP-pXByZcEYxt; 2023; and U.S. Centers for Disease Control and Prevention. (2024). Human papillomavirus (HPV). Accessed August 9, 2025, from http://www.cdc.gov.hpv/index,html

Family History

- Infertility in siblings
- History of prostate, testicular, penile, or breast cancer
- Hernias
- Peyronie disease (contracture of penis)

Personal and Social History

- Occupational risk of trauma to suprapubic region or genitalia, exposure to radiation or toxins
- Exercise: use of a protective device with contact sports or bicycle riding
- Concerns about genitalia: size, shape, surface characteristics, texture
- Testicular/genital self-examination practices (see Patient Safety, "Self-Examination for STIs")
- Concerns about sexual behaviors including sexual partners (single or multiple)
- Concerns about sexual orientation (heterosexual, homosexual, bisexual) or gender identity (transgender, cisgender, agender)
- Reproductive function: number of children, form of contraception used, frequency of ejaculation
- Alcohol, cannabis, cocaine, other recreational drug use: quantity and frequency

Infants and Children

- Maternal use of sex hormones or birth control pills during pregnancy
- Circumcised: complications from procedure
- Uncircumcised: hygiene measures, retractability of foreskin, interference with urinary stream
- Scrotal swelling with crying or bowel movement
- Congenital anomalies: hypospadias, epispadias, undescended testes, ambiguous genitalia
- Parental concerns with masturbation, sexual exploration
- Swelling, discoloration, or sores on the penis or scrotum; pain in the genitalia
- Concern for sexual abuse

Adolescents

- Knowledge of reproductive function, source of information about sexual activity and function
- Presence of nocturnal emissions, pubic hair, enlargement of genitalia, age at time of each occurrence and of first nocturnal emissions
- Concern of sexual abuse
- Sexual activity, protection used for contraception and STI prevention

Older Adults

- Change in frequency of sexual activity or desire: related to loss of spouse or other sexual partner; no sexual partner; sexually restrictive environment; depression; physical illness resulting in fatigue, weakness, or pain

- Change in sexual response: longer time required or inability to achieve full erection, less forceful ejaculation, more rapid detumescence, longer interval between erections, prostate surgery

Patient Safety

Self-Examination to Detect STIs

Genital self-examination (GSE) is recommended for anyone who is at risk for contracting a sexually transmitted infection (STI). This includes sexually active persons who have had more than one sexual partner or whose partner has had other partners. The purpose of the GSE is to detect any signs or symptoms that might indicate the presence of an STI. Many people who have an STI do not know they have one, and some STIs can remain undetected for years. GSE should become a part of routine self-examination health care practices. Explain and demonstrate the following procedure to your patients and give them the opportunity to perform a GSE with your guidance.

Instruct the patient to hold the penis in the hand and examine the head. If not circumcised, the patient should gently pull back the foreskin to expose the glans. Inspection and palpation of the entire head of the penis should be performed in a clockwise motion while the patient carefully looks for any bumps, sores, or blisters on the skin. Bumps and blisters may be red or light colored or may resemble pimples. Have the patient also look for genital warts, which may look like warts on other parts of the body. Examine the urethral meatus for any discharge.

Next, the patient will examine the entire shaft and look for the same signs. Instruct the patient to separate the pubic hair at the base of the penis and carefully examine the skin underneath. Be sure to include the underside of the shaft in the examination; a mirror may be helpful.

Instruct the patient to examine the scrotal skin and contents; hold each testicle gently and inspect and palpate the skin, including the underside of the scrotum, looking for any lesions, lumps, swelling, or soreness. Educate the patient about other symptoms associated with STIs, specifically pain or burning on urination or discharge from the penis. The discharge may vary in color, consistency, and amount.

Any of the preceding signs or symptoms require evaluation by a clinician.

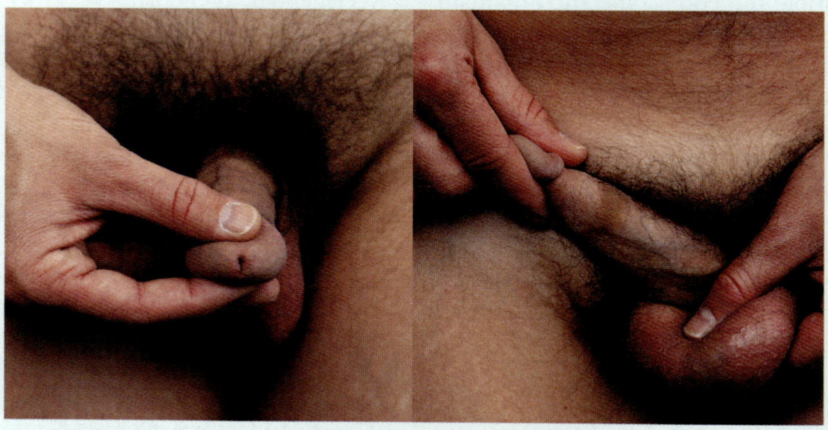

From American Cancer Society. (2018). *Risk factors for penile cancer.* Accessed September 30, 2024, from https://www.cancer.org/cancer/types/penile-cancer/causes-risks-prevention/risk-factors.html; American Cancer Society. (2024). *Risk factors for testicular cancer.* Accessed September 30, 2024, from https://www.cancer.org/cancer/types/testicular-cancer/causes-risks-prevention/risk-factors.html; and Deutsch, M. B. (Ed.). (2016). *Guidelines for the primary care of transgender and gender nonbinary people* (2nd ed.). UCSF Center of Excellence for Transgender Health. http://transhealth.ucsf.edu/trans?page=guidelines-home

Risk Factors

Cancer of the Male Genitalia

Penile

- Infection with high-risk types of HPV
- Lack of circumcision with failure to maintain good hygiene
- Phimosis
- Age: risk increases with age
- Smoking (smoking alone increases risk; smokers with HPV infection are at even higher risk)
- HIV infection
- Ultraviolet (UV) light treatment of psoriasis if genitalia exposed

Testicular

- Undescended testicle (cryptorchidism): risk elevated for both testicles
- Personal history of testicular cancer (the opposite testicle is at increased risk)
- Family history of testicular cancer
- HIV infection
- Age: about half of testicular cancer cases occur between the ages of 20 and 34 years; can occur at any age
- Race: White persons have a five times greater risk than Black persons and more than three times greater risk than Asian American and Native American persons
- Androgen suppression: likely decreases the risk in transgender women

EXAMINATION AND FINDINGS

Equipment

- Gloves
- Drapes
- Penlight for transillumination

Examination of the genitalia involves inspection, palpation, and transillumination of any mass found and requires that you are gloved. The patient may be anxious about examination of the genitalia, so it is important to examine the genitalia carefully and completely but also efficiently (Box 20.1). Patients who have undergone gender-affirming surgeries may have varying physical examination findings depending on the procedures performed. The patient may be lying or standing for this part of the examination. A chaperone, often required by policy, protects both the clinician and the patient. Some patients may be reluctant to reveal confidential and sensitive information in the presence of a chaperone, but this should not supersede the need to have a chaperone present for the examination.

Inspection and Palpation

Genital Hair Distribution

First inspect the genital hair distribution. Genital hair is coarser than scalp hair. It should be abundant in the pubic region and may continue in a narrowing midline pattern to the umbilicus (the biologic male escutcheon pattern). Depending on how the patient is positioned, it may be possible to note that the distribution continues around the scrotum to the anal orifice. The penis itself is not covered with hair, and the scrotum generally has a scant amount.

Penis

Examine the penis. The dorsal vein should be apparent on inspection. Note whether the patient is circumcised or uncircumcised (Fig. 20.5). If the patient is uncircumcised, retract the foreskin or ask the patient to do so. It should retract easily, and a bit of smegma (white, cheesy sebaceous matter that collects between the glans penis and the foreskin) may be seen over the glans. Occasionally the foreskin is tight and cannot be retracted. This condition is called *phimosis* (Fig. 20.6) and may occur during the first 6 years of life or as a result of recurrent balanitis (inflammation of the glans; Fig. 20.7) or balanoposthitis (inflammation of the glans penis and prepuce), which occur in

BOX 20.1 Minimizing the Patient's Anxiety

The physical examination is laden with anxiety-provoking elements for most people, but examination of the genitals is particularly likely to arouse anxiety. Patients are often fearful of having an erection during the examination. Patients may worry about whether their genitals are "normal," and misinformation on sexual matters can add to their concerns. For transgender patients, the use of a gender-affirming approach during the examination (e.g., use of correct name and pronouns and acceptance of gender-affirming treatments and procedures) can demonstrate respect and help reduce anxiety. Your attitude and ability to communicate can reassure the apprehensive patient. Some important elements to remember:

- Know the language. It is inappropriate to talk down to anyone, but you and the patient must understand each other. You may not be entirely comfortable with some of the common words and phrases you hear from the patients, but the common language may be appropriate in certain circumstances. Know the language and use it effectively, without apology, and in a nondemeaning fashion.
- Never make jokes. Light, casual talk or jokes about the genitalia or sexual function are always inappropriate, no matter how well you know the patient. Feelings about one's own sexuality run deep and are often well masked. Do not pull at the edges of a mask you may not suspect is there.
- Remember that your face is easily seen by the patient when you are examining the genitalia. An unexpected finding may cause a sudden change in your expression. You must guard against what you reveal by nonverbal communication.
- Remember that you are a professional, fulfilling the responsibility of a professional.

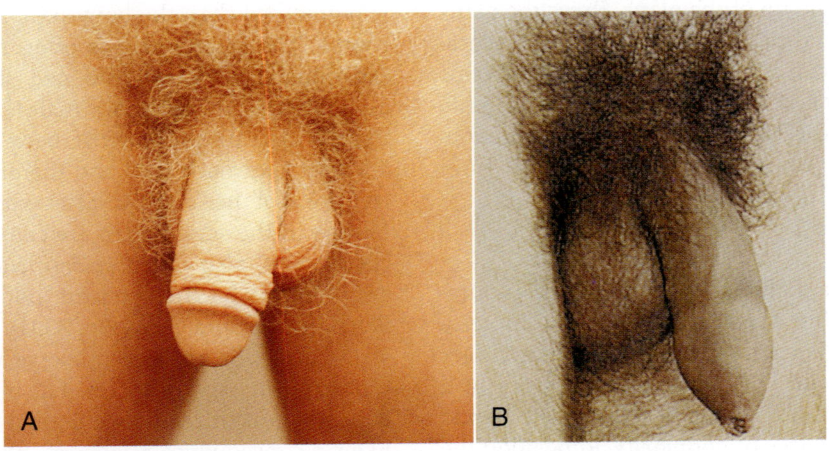

FIG. 20.5 Appearance of male genitalia. (A) Circumcised. (B) Uncircumcised.

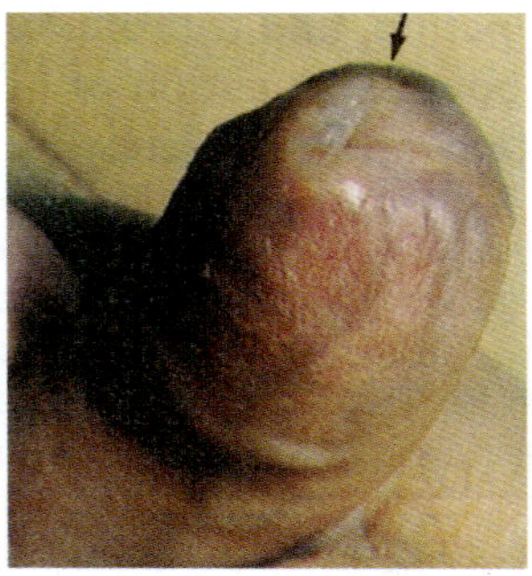

FIG. 20.6 **Phimosis.** (From Wolfe, J. (1984). 400 Self-assessment picture tests in clinical medicine. Chicago: Elsevier.)

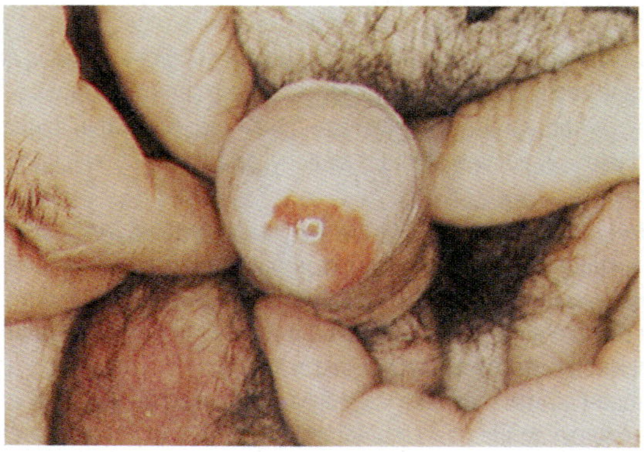

FIG. 20.7 **Balanitis.** (From Lloyd-Davies R. W., et al. (1994). *Color atlas of urology* (2nd ed.). London: Mosby.)

uncircumcised individuals and may be caused by either bacterial or fungal infections. It is most commonly seen in patients with poorly controlled diabetes mellitus. Phimosis may also be caused by previous unsuccessful efforts to retract the foreskin that have caused radial tearing of the preputial ring, resulting in adhesions of the foreskin to the glans.

If the patient is circumcised, the glans is exposed and appears erythematous and dry. No smegma will be present.

Urethral Meatus

Examine the external meatus of the urethra. The orifice should appear slitlike and be located on the ventral surface just millimeters from the tip of the glans. Press the glans between your thumb and forefinger to open the urethral orifice (Fig. 20.8). You can ask the patient to perform this procedure. The opening should be glistening and pink. Bright erythema or a discharge indicates inflammation, whereas a pinpoint or round opening may result from meatal stenosis.

Penile Shaft

Palpate the shaft of the penis for tenderness and induration. Strip the urethra for discharge by firmly compressing the base of the penis with your thumb and forefinger and moving them toward the glans. The presence of a discharge may indicate an STI. The texture of the flaccid penis should be soft and free of nodularity. Reposition the foreskin after performing these maneuvers.

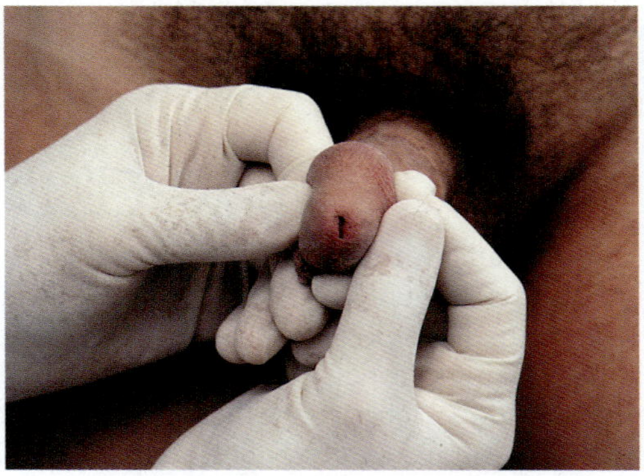

FIG. 20.8 **Examination of urethral orifice.**

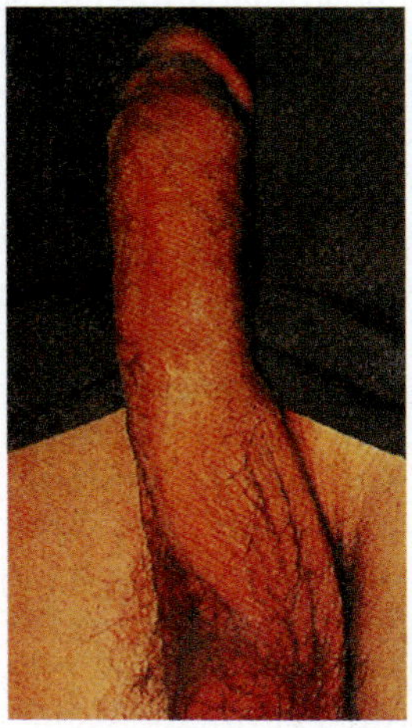

FIG. 20.9 **Priapism.** (From Lloyd-Davies R. W., et al. (1994). *Color atlas of urology* (2nd ed.). London: Mosby.)

Rarely, you may see a patient with a prolonged penile erection, called *priapism* (Fig. 20.9), which may be painful. Although in most cases the condition is idiopathic, it can occur in patients with leukemia or hemoglobinopathies such as sickle cell disease or as a result of medications for erectile dysfunction.

Scrotum

Inspect the scrotum (Fig. 20.10). It may appear more deeply pigmented than the body skin, and the surface may be coarse. The scrotal skin is often reddened in red-haired individuals; however, reddened skin in other individuals may indicate an inflammatory process. The scrotum usually appears asymmetric because the left testicle has a longer spermatic cord and therefore is often lower. The thickness of the scrotum varies with temperature and age. Lumps in the scrotal skin are commonly caused by sebaceous cysts, also called *epidermoid cysts*. They appear as small lumps on the scrotum, but they may enlarge and discharge oily material (Fig. 20.11).

Occasionally you may observe unusual thickening of the scrotum caused by edema, often with pitting. This does not generally imply a genital condition, but is more likely a consequence of general fluid retention associated with cardiac, renal, or hepatic disease.

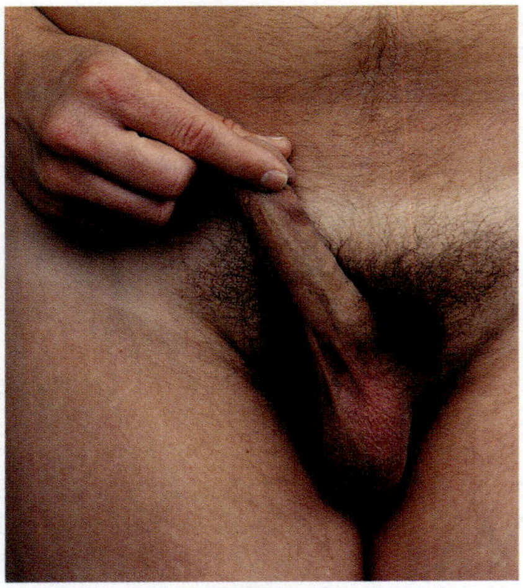

FIG. 20.10 Inspection of scrotum and ventral surface of penis as the patient positions the penis.

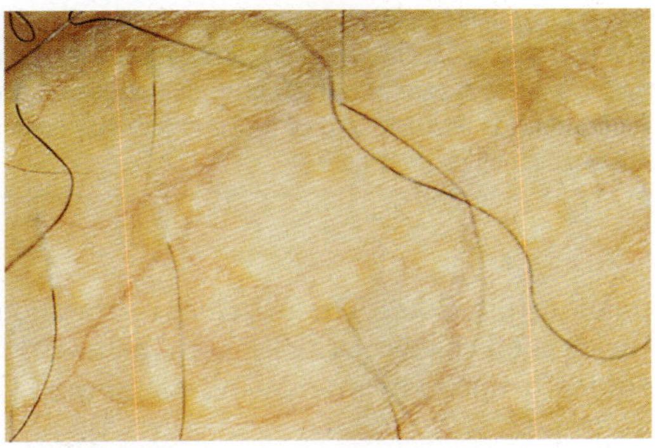

FIG. 20.11 Sebaceous glands on the scrotum. (From Morse, S.A., et al. (2003). *Atlas of sexually transmitted diseases and AIDS* (3rd ed.). St. Louis: Mosby.)

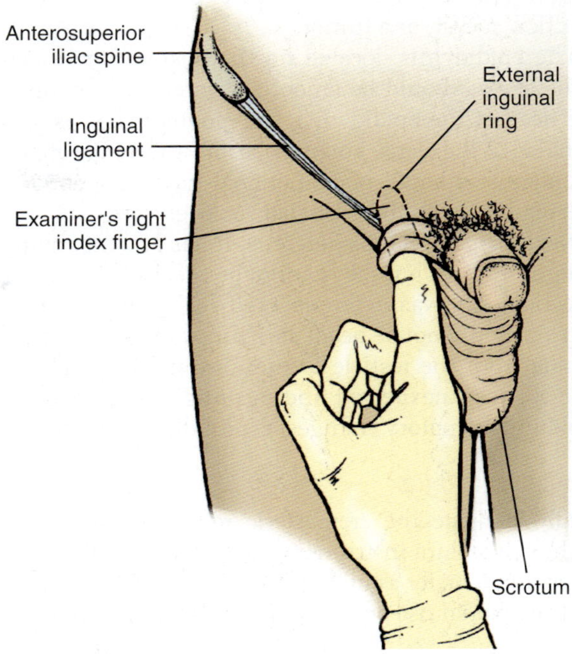

FIG. 20.12 Checking for inguinal hernia; gloved finger inserted through inguinal canal.

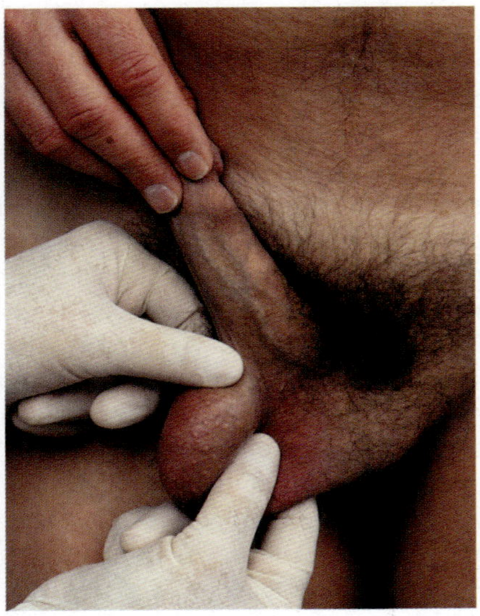

FIG. 20.13 Palpating contents of the scrotal sac.

Hernia

Examine for evidence of a hernia. Fig. 20.16, later in the chapter, shows the anatomy of the region and the three common types of hernias. With the patient standing, ask them to bear down as if having a bowel movement. During this maneuver inspect the area of the inguinal canal and the region of the fossa ovalis. After asking the patient to relax again, insert your examining finger into the lower part of the scrotum and carry it upward along the vas deferens into the inguinal canal (Fig. 20.12). You can auscultate for bowel sounds, which will be present in uncomplicated reducible hernias.

Which finger you use depends on the size of the patient. In the young child, the little finger is appropriate; in the adult, the index or middle finger is generally used. You should be able to feel the oval external ring. Ask the patient to cough. If an inguinal hernia is present, you should feel the sudden presence of a bulge against your finger. The hernia is described as indirect if it lies within the inguinal canal. It may also come through the external canal and even pass into the scrotum. Because an indirect hernia on one side strongly suggests the possibility of bilateral herniation, be sure to examine both sides thoroughly. If the bulge is felt medial to the external canal, it probably represents a direct inguinal hernia.

Testes

Palpate the testes using the thumb and first two fingers. The testes should be sensitive to gentle compression but not tender, and they should feel smooth and rubbery and be free of nodules (Fig. 20.13). Transgender women may have testicles that have decreased in size or are completely retracted. In some conditions (e.g., syphilis and diabetic neuropathy), a testis may be totally insensitive to painful stimuli. Irregularities in texture or size may indicate an infection, a cyst, or a tumor.

The epididymis, located on the posterolateral surface of the testis, should be smooth, discrete, and nontender. The head of the epididymis, the globus major, is located cephalad to the testis. You may be able to feel the appendix epididymis, a small nonfunctional tissue appendage, as an irregularity on the cephalad surface.

Next, palpate the vas deferens. It has accompanying arteries and veins, but they cannot be precisely identified by palpation. The vas deferens itself feels smooth and discrete; it should not be beaded or lumpy in its course as you palpate from the testicle to the inguinal ring. The presence of such unexpected findings might indicate diabetes or old inflammatory changes, especially tuberculosis.

Cremasteric Reflex

Finally, evaluate the cremasteric reflex. Stroke the inner thigh with a blunt instrument such as the handle of the reflex hammer or, for a child, with your finger. The testicle and scrotum should rise on the stroked side (see Chapter 23).

Prostate

Examination of the prostate is detailed in Chapter 21.

Infants

Examine the genitalia of the newborn for congenital anomalies, incomplete development, and sexual ambiguity. Inspect the penis for size, placement of the urethral meatus, and any anomalies. The nonerect length of the penis at birth is usually 2 to 3 cm. Transitory erection of the penis during infancy is common, and the penis should have a straight projection. An unusually small penis (micropenis), defined as less than 1.9 cm measured at stretched penile length, may be associated with conditions of abnormal testicular development (e.g., Klinefelter syndrome) and may not be appropriate for circumcision. The micropenis must also be differentiated from the unusually large clitoris (clitoromegaly) that may be seen at birth in congenital adrenal hyperplasia. A hooked, downward bowing of the penis suggests abnormal development of the penis (chordee), most evident on erection. Look for an accompanying hypospadias (location of the urethral meatus on the ventral surface of the penis). Hypospadias is a contraindication for circumcision.

Inspection and Palpation

Inspect the glans penis of the neonate. The foreskin in the uncircumcised infant is commonly tight, but should retract enough to permit a good urinary stream. Do not retract the foreskin more than necessary to see the urethra, especially if the neonate will not be circumcised. Mobility of the foreskin increases with time and usually is fully retractable by 3 or 4 years of age. The slitlike urethral meatus should be located near the tip. Inspect the glans of the circumcised infant for ulcerations, bleeding, and inflammation (Box 20.2). The urinary stream should be strong, with good caliber. Dribbling or a reduced force or caliber of the urinary stream may indicate stenosis of the urethral meatus.

BOX 20.2 Circumcision

There has been much discussion about the appropriateness of routine circumcision in neonates. In 2007 the American Academy of Pediatrics (AAP) convened a multidisciplinary workgroup to evaluate the evidence regarding circumcision. In 2012 the AAP released the following policy statement: "Evaluation of current evidence indicates that the health benefits of newborn male circumcision outweigh the risks; furthermore, the benefits of newborn male circumcision justify access to this procedure for families who choose it" (AAP, 2012).

Specific benefits from circumcision of the penis were identified for the prevention of urinary tract infections, acquisition of HIV, transmission of some sexually transmitted infections, and penile cancer. Circumcision did not appear to adversely affect penile sexual function/sensitivity or sexual satisfaction. Adequate training for both sterile techniques and effective pain management was imperative.

The AAP recognizes the sociocultural and ethical issues embedded in the circumcision decision and advises that parents should weigh the health benefits and risks in light of their own religious, cultural, and personal preferences, as the medical benefits alone may not outweigh these other considerations for individual families. Your role as a clinician is to provide factually correct, nonbiased information about circumcision and assist parents by explaining, in a nonbiased manner, the potential benefits and risks and by ensuring that they understand the elective nature of the procedure.

CLINICAL PEARL

Retraction of the Foreskin

It is important to carefully retract the foreskin because forced retraction may contribute to the formation of binding adhesions. Some adherence of the prepuce to the glans may continue until 6 years of age.

Inspect the scrotum for size, symmetry, shape, rugae, presence of testicles, and anomalies (Fig. 20.14). The scrotum of the premature infant may appear underdeveloped, without rugae and without testes, whereas the full-term neonate should have a loose, pendulous scrotum with

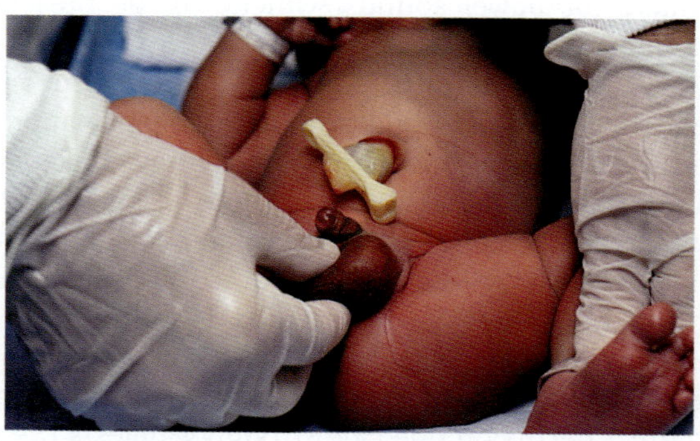

FIG. 20.14 Palpating the scrotum of an infant.

Condyloma Acuminata

"Genital warts" caused by HPV.

PATHOPHYSIOLOGY

- HPV invades the basal layer of the epidermis; virus penetrates through skin and causes mucosal microabrasions
- Latent viral phase begins with no signs or symptoms and can last from a month to several years
- Following latency, viral DNA, capsids, and particles are produced; host cells become infected and develop the characteristic skin lesions
- Considered an STI

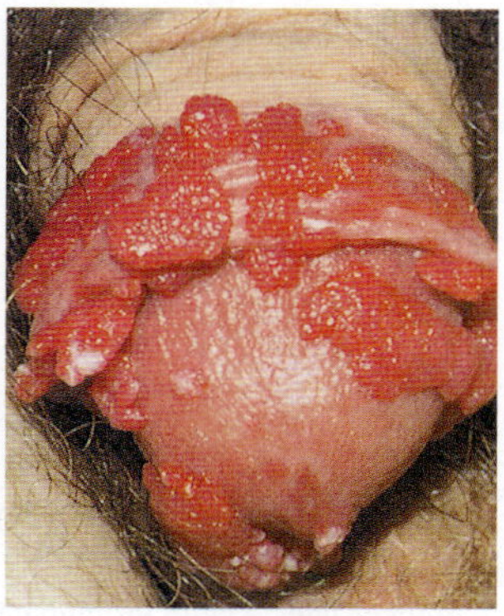

FIG. 20.21 **Condyloma acuminata (genital warts).** (From Wolfe, J. (1984). 400 Self-assessment picture tests in clinical medicine. Chicago: Elsevier.)

PATIENT DATA

Subjective Data

- Soft, painless, wartlike lesions on penis
- History of sexual contact

Objective Data

- Single or multiple papular lesions
- May be pearly, filiform, fungating (ulcerating and necrotic), cauliflower, or plaquelike (Figs. 20.21 and 20.22)
- Can be smooth, verrucous, or lobulated
- May be the same color as the skin or may be reddish or hyperpigmented
- Lesions are commonly present on the prepuce, glans penis, and penile shaft, but they may be present within the urethra as well

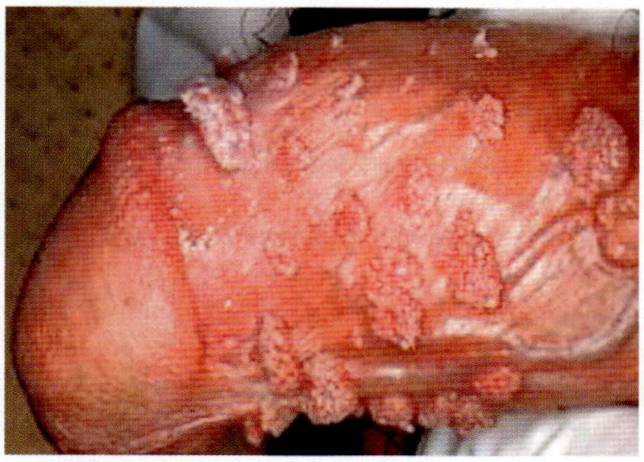

FIG. 20.22 **Condyloma acuminata (genital warts).** (From Monk, B. J., et al. (2007). The spectrum and clinical sequelae of human papillomavirus infection. *Gynecologic Oncology*, *107*(2), S6–S13.)

Lymphogranuloma Venereum

STI of the lymphatics.

PATHOPHYSIOLOGY

- Caused by *Chlamydia trachomatis*
- Organism enters through skin breaks and abrasions, or it crosses the epithelial cells of mucous membranes
- Initial lesion occurs at the site of entry
- Travels via lymphatics to regional lymph nodes, where organism replicates within macrophages
- Subsequently, local lymph nodes become involved; draining sinus tracts may form

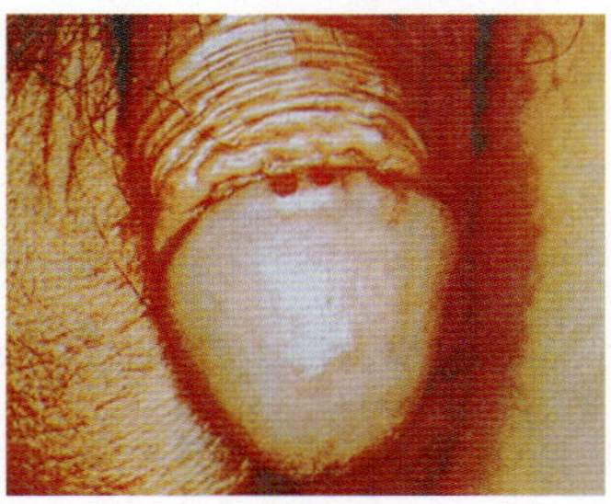

FIG. 20.23 **Lymphogranuloma venereum.** (From Meheus, A., & Ursi, J. P. (1982). Sexually transmitted diseases. Kalamazoo, MI: Upjohn.)

PATIENT DATA

Subjective Data

- Painless lesion on penis
- Symptoms may be systemic (fever, malaise)
- History of sexual contact

Objective Data

- Initial lesion is a painless erosion at or near the coronal sulcus (Fig. 20.23)
- Enlarged regional lymph nodes
- If lymphatic drainage is blocked, penile and scrotal lymphedema may ensue
- Draining sinus tract in untreated infection

Molluscum Contagiosum

Viral infection of the skin and mucous membranes; considered an STI in adults.

PATHOPHYSIOLOGY

- Caused by a poxvirus that infects only the skin
- Spread by skin-to-skin contact or by contact with an object that has touched infected skin
- Virus enters the skin through small breaks in the skin barrier
- After an incubation period, growths appear

PATIENT DATA

Subjective Data

- Painless lesions on penis
- Contact with an infected person

Objective Data

- Lesions are pearly gray, often umbilicated, smooth, dome-shaped, and with discrete margins (Fig. 20.24)
- Lesions most common on the glans penis

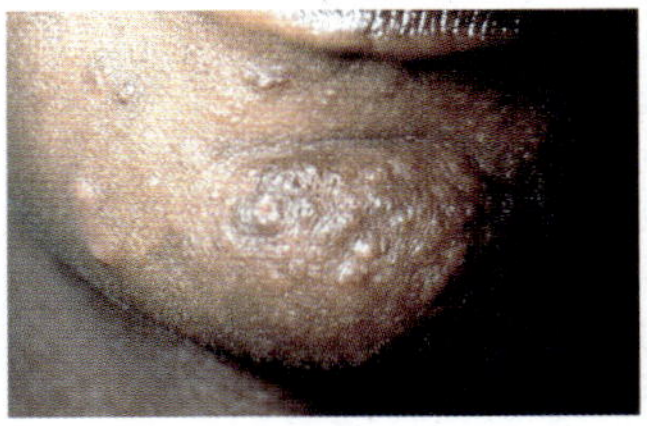

FIG. 20.24 Molluscum contagiosum. (From Procop, G. W., & Pritt, B. S. (2015). Pathology of infectious diseases. Elsevier.)

Peyronie Disease

Characterized by a fibrous band in the corpus cavernosum.

PATHOPHYSIOLOGY

- Dense, fibrous scar tissue (plaque) forms in the tunica albuginea (wall of the corpus cavernosum)
- Plaque focally interferes with expansion of the corpus cavernosum during erection
- Etiology unclear; may occur as the result of trauma, inflammation, or inherited disorder
- Acute phase: first 6–18 months with progression of penile deformity
- Chronic phase: plateau of symptoms for at least 3–6 months; the deformity remains stable

PATIENT DATA

Subjective Data

- Bending and/or indentation of the erection (Fig. 20.25)
- Loss of penile length on erection
- May have pain on erect or flaccid state (primarily in acute phase)
- Family history of the condition
- History of Dupuytren contracture (finger joint flexion contractures; most commonly fourth and fifth fingers of the hand)

Objective Data

- One or more palpable hardened areas
- Reduced elasticity of the flaccid penis
- Radiography or ultrasound can show plaque calcification

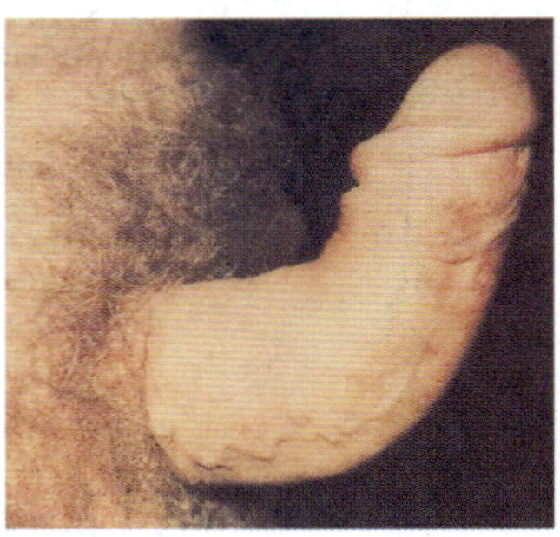

FIG. 20.25 Peyronie disease. (Courtesy Patrick C. Walsh, MD, The Johns Hopkins University School of Medicine, Baltimore, MD.)

Penile Cancer

Almost all cases are squamous cell carcinoma, usually originating in the glans or foreskin.

PATHOPHYSIOLOGY

- Associated with HPV types 16 and 18
- Patients who have been circumcised rarely develop penile cancer
- Lesions start as superficial neoplasms of the prepuce or glans penis and then progress to invade the corpora cavernosa and urethra, with subsequent development of metastases to the inguinal lymph nodes

PATIENT DATA

Subjective Data

- Painless ulceration that fails to heal
- Uncircumcised
- Poor penile hygiene

Objective Data

- Lesion, usually on glans, may present as a reddened area
- Papule or pustule
- Warty growth, shallow erosion, or a deep ulceration with rolled edges (Fig. 20.26)
- May have a phimosis that obscures the lesion

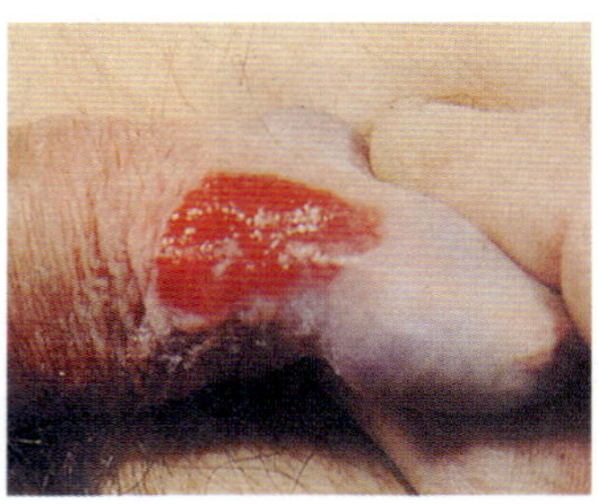

FIG. 20.26 Cancer of the penis. (Courtesy Patrick C. Walsh, MD, The Johns Hopkins University School of Medicine, Baltimore, MD.)

SCROTUM

Spermatocele

Benign cystic accumulation of sperm occurring on the epididymis.

PATHOPHYSIOLOGY

- Etiology and pathophysiology unknown

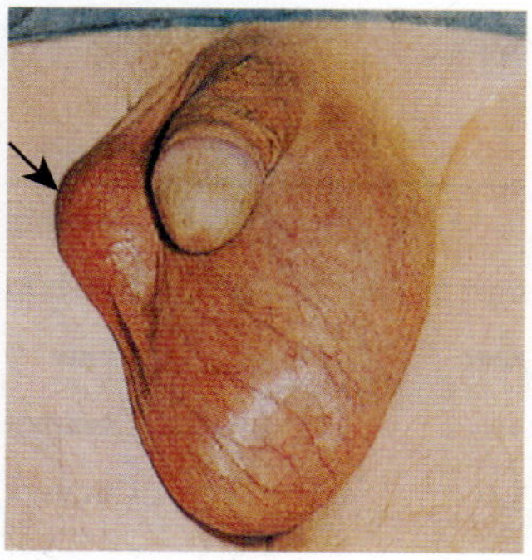

FIG. 20.27 **Spermatocele.** (From Lloyd-Davies, R. W., et al. (1994). *Color atlas of urology* (2nd ed.). London: Mosby.)

PATIENT DATA

Subjective Data

- Asymptomatic; incidental finding on physical examination or self-examination

Objective Data

- Smooth, spherical, nontender mass at epididymis (superior and posterior to the testis; Fig. 20.27)
- Usually smaller than 1 cm

Varicocele

Abnormal tortuosity and dilation of veins of the pampiniform plexus within the spermatic cord (Fig. 20.28).

PATHOPHYSIOLOGY

- More common in the left testicle than in the right because of several anatomic factors, including the angle at which the left testicular vein enters the left renal vein, the lack of effective antireflux valves at the juncture of the testicular vein and renal vein, and the increased renal vein pressure due to its compression between the superior mesenteric artery and the aorta
- May be associated with reduced fertility, probably from increased venous pressure and elevated testicular temperature

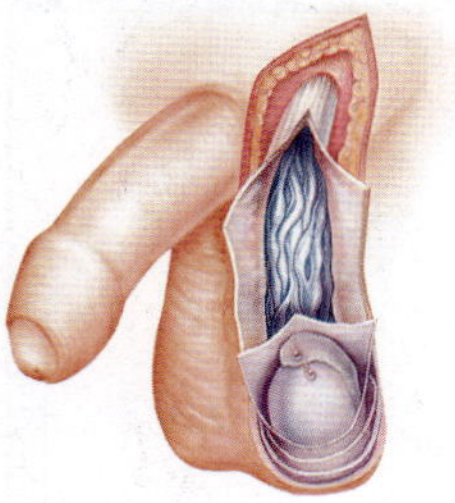

FIG. 20.28 Varicocele.

PATIENT DATA

Subjective Data

- Usually asymptomatic (and found in the course of an evaluation for infertility)
- May report scrotal pain or heaviness

Objective Data

- Often visible only when the patient is standing; is classically described as a "bag of worms"
- Graded as:
  - Small: palpated only during Valsalva maneuver
  - Moderate: easily palpated without Valsalva maneuver
  - Large: causing visible bulging of the scrotum

Orchitis

Acute inflammation of the testis secondary to infection.

PATHOPHYSIOLOGY

- Uncommon except as a complication of mumps in the adolescent or adult
- Is generally unilateral and results in testicular atrophy in 50% of cases
- In older adults may result from bacterial migration from a prostate infection

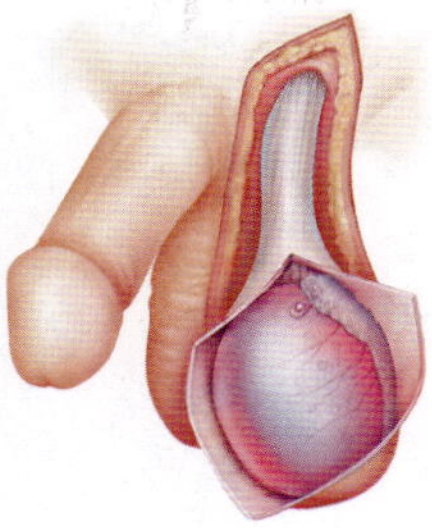

FIG. 20.29 Orchitis.

PATIENT DATA

Subjective Data

- Acute-onset testicular pain and swelling
- Pain ranges from mild discomfort to severe
- Associated systemic symptoms: fatigue, malaise, myalgias, fever
- Mumps orchitis follows the development of parotitis by 4–7 days

Objective Data

- Enlarged, tender testis (Fig. 20.29)
- Erythematous and edematous scrotal skin
- Enlarged epididymis associated with epididymo-orchitis

Epididymitis

Inflammation of the epididymis (a major consideration in the differential diagnosis is testicular torsion, which is a surgical emergency; see the Differential Diagnosis table, "Acute Testicular Swelling").

PATHOPHYSIOLOGY

- Often seen in association with a urinary tract infection
- May also occur as a result of an STI
- Occasionally, chronic epididymitis may occur as a consequence of tuberculosis

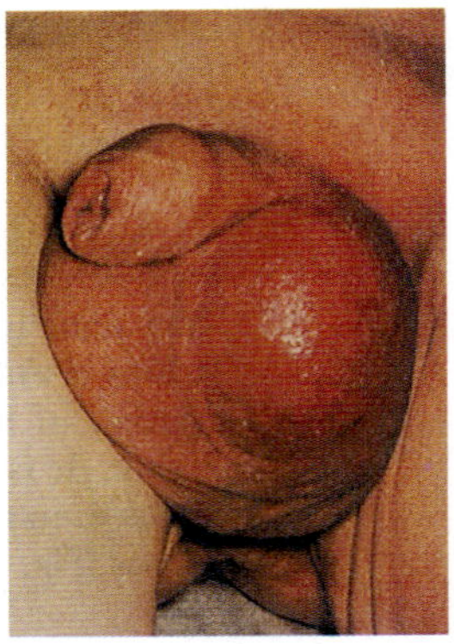

FIG. 20.30 **Epididymitis.** (From Lloyd-Davies, R. W., et al. (1994). *Color atlas of urology* (2nd ed.). London: Mosby.)

PATIENT DATA

Subjective Data

- Painful scrotum
- Urethral discharge
- Fever
- Pyuria
- Recent sexual activity

Objective Data

- Epididymis feels firm and lumpy; is tender (Fig. 20.30)
- Vasa deferentia may be beaded
- Overlying scrotum may be markedly erythematous

DIFFERENTIAL DIAGNOSIS

Acute Testicular Swelling

	TORSION	EPIDIDYMITIS
Cause	Twisting of testis on spermatic cord	Bacterial infection (STI or UTI)
Age	Newborn to adolescence	Adolescence to adulthood
Onset of pain	Acute	Gradual
Vomiting	Common	Uncommon
Anorexia	Common	Uncommon
Fever	Uncommon	Possible
Dysuria	Uncommon	Possible
Supporting findings	Absence of cremasteric reflex on side of acute swelling	Urethral discharge
	Scrotal discoloration	History of recent sexual activity
		Fever
		Pyuria
		Thickened or nodular epididymis

STI, Sexually transmitted infection; *UTI*, urinary tract infection.

Testicular Cancer

Classified by the cells from which the cancer arises.

PATHOPHYSIOLOGY

- Seminomas and nonseminomas arise from germ cells (sperm-producing cells)
- Non–germ cell tumors arise from supportive and hormone-producing tissue
- Most testicular cancers are germ cell cancers
- Germ cell tumors tend to occur in young males and are the most common tumor in males 15–30 years of age

PATIENT DATA

Subjective Data

- Presence of painless mass in testicle
- May report scrotal enlargement or swelling
- Sensation of heaviness in the scrotum
- Dull ache in the lower abdomen, back, or groin
- Sudden collection of fluid in the scrotum

Objective Data

- Irregular, nontender mass fixed on the testis (Fig. 20.31)
- Does not transilluminate
- May also have hydrocele (does transilluminate)
- May have associated inguinal lymphadenopathy

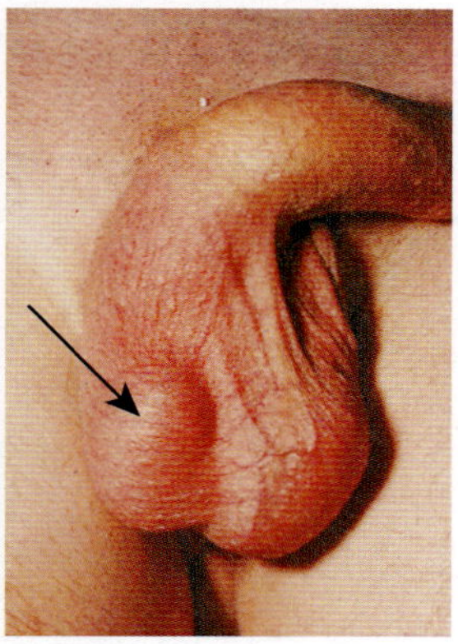

FIG. 20.31 Testicular tumor. (From Wolfe, J. (1984). 400 Self-assessment picture tests in clinical medicine. Chicago: Elsevier.)

INFERTILITY

See Chapter 19.

Infants

Ambiguous Genitalia

See Chapter 19.

Hypospadias

Congenital defect in which the urethral meatus is located on the ventral surface of the glans penile shaft or the base of the penis.

PATHOPHYSIOLOGY

- Congenital defect that is thought to occur embryologically during urethral development, from 8 to 20 weeks of gestation
- Several etiologies suggested, including genetic, endocrine, and environmental factors
- Presence of hypospadias puts the infant at greater risk of having undescended testicles

PATIENT DATA

Subjective Data

- Parent may note penile defect or may be discovered by a clinician in the nursery

Objective Data

- Diagnosis generally made on examination of the newborn infant
- Urethral meatus located on the ventral surface of the glans penile shaft or the base of the penis (Fig. 20.32)
- Dorsal hood of foreskin and glandular groove are evident, but prepuce is incomplete ventrally
- Penis may have ventral shortening and curvature, called *chordee,* with more proximal urethral defects

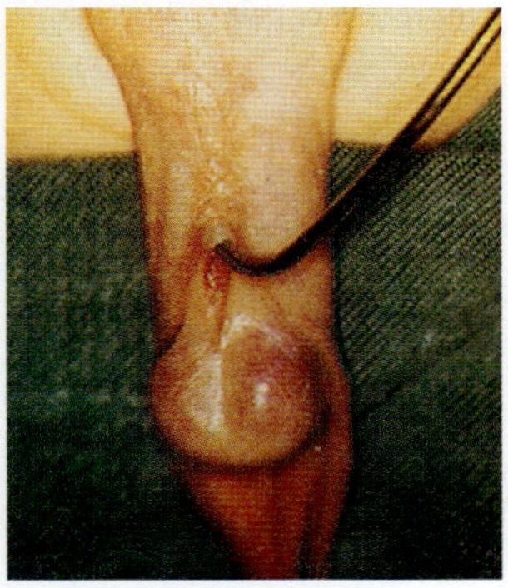

FIG. 20.32 Hypospadias. (From Wolfe, J. (1984). *400 Self-assessment picture tests in clinical medicine.* Chicago: Elsevier.)

Hydrocele

Fluid accumulation in the scrotum.

PATHOPHYSIOLOGY

- Fluid accumulates in the scrotum as a result of a defect in the tunica vaginalis; this condition is common in infancy; if the tunica vaginalis is not patent, the hydrocele will generally disappear spontaneously in the first 6 months of life

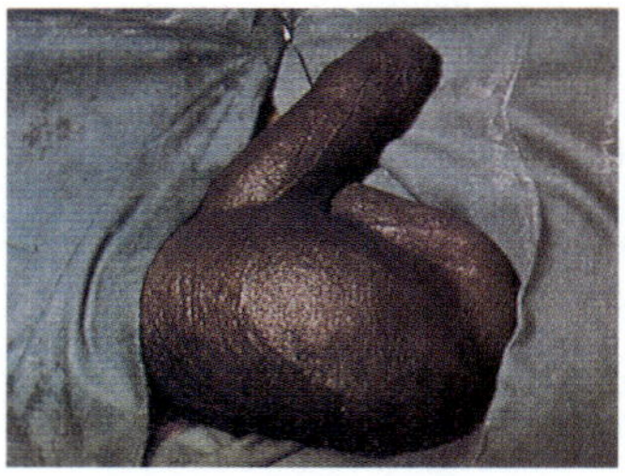

FIG. 20.33 Hydrocele. (From Lloyd-Davies, R. W., et al. (1994). *Color atlas of urology* (2nd ed.). London: Mosby.)

PATIENT DATA

Subjective Data

- Painless enlargement or swelling of the scrotum

Objective Data

- Nontender, smooth, firm mass superior and anterior to the testes (Fig. 20.33)
- Transilluminates
- Confined to the scrotum and does not enter the inguinal canal, unless it has been present for a long time and is very large and taut

Adolescents

Testicular Torsion

Twisting of testis around the spermatic cord; testicular torsion is a surgical emergency (see the Differential Diagnosis table, "Acute Testicular Swelling").

PATHOPHYSIOLOGY

- Twisting of the spermatic cord cuts off the blood supply to the testicle
- Occurs in newborns to adolescents; most common in adolescents

PATIENT DATA

Subjective Data

- Acute onset of scrotal pain, often accompanied by nausea and vomiting
- Absence of systemic symptoms such as fever and myalgia
- Risk factors: trauma and strenuous physical activity

Objective Data

- The testicle is exquisitely tender
- Testicle is elevated ("high riding") from a twisted or shortened cord
- Scrotal discoloration is often present
- Absence of cremasteric reflex on side of acute swelling

Think About It

Although the differential diagnosis for scrotal or testicular pain includes less urgent causes, such as epididymitis, hydrocele, referred pain, and inguinal hernia, the occurrence of testicular torsion creates a surgical emergency that requires prompt diagnosis and intervention. Doppler ultrasonography is the modality of choice for diagnosis; when not readily available or if inconclusive, direct surgical consult for high-risk patients should not be delayed. The Testicular Workup for Ischemia and Suspected Torsion (TWIST) score is a validated score for determining risk in pediatric populations. It uses urologic history and physical examination to assess risk of testis torsion. Parameters include testis swelling (2 points), hard testis (2), absent cremasteric reflex (1), nausea/vomiting (1), and high-riding testis (1). Patients with scores ≥6 are considered high risk.

Klinefelter Syndrome

Congenital anomaly associated with XXY chromosomal inheritance.

PATHOPHYSIOLOGY

- Caused by an extra X chromosome
- Infant with Klinefelter syndrome appears normal at birth; condition becomes apparent in puberty when secondary sexual characteristics fail to develop
- Symptoms depend on the number of XXY cells, the level of testosterone, and the age when the condition is diagnosed

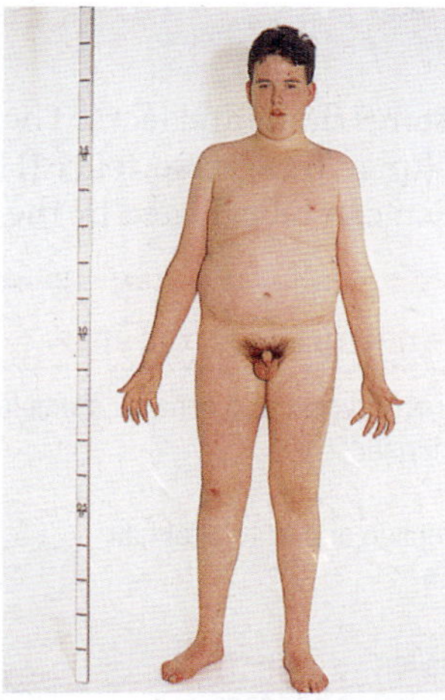

FIG. 20.34 **Klinefelter syndrome.** (From Patton, K. T., & Thibodeau, G. A. (2010). *Anatomy & physiology* (7th ed.). St. Louis: Mosby.)

PATIENT DATA

Subjective Data

- Differences in physical, language, and social development compared with others of the same age
- Concern over delayed pubertal development

Objective Data

- Hypogonadism, including a small scrotum
- Diminished pubic, axillary, and facial hair
- Enlarged breast tissue
- Tall stature, long legs, short trunk (Fig. 20.34)
- In mild cases, no abnormalities will be present; however, the individual will be infertile

CHAPTER

21 Anus, Rectum, and Prostate

Examination of the anus and rectum may be performed as part of a routine health visit. In patients with a prostate, examination may include the prostate. Examination of these structures is also performed when the patient has a specific concern.

ANATOMY AND PHYSIOLOGY

The rectum and anus form the terminal portions of the gastrointestinal (GI) tract (Fig. 21.1). The anal canal is approximately 2.5 to 4 cm long and opens onto the perineum. The tissue visible at the external margin of the anus is moist, hairless mucosa. Juncture with the perianal skin is characterized by increased pigmentation and, in the adult, the presence of hair.

The anal canal is normally kept securely closed by concentric rings of muscle, the internal and external sphincters. The internal ring of smooth muscle is under involuntary autonomic control. The urge to defecate occurs when the rectum fills with feces, which causes reflexive stimulation that relaxes the internal sphincter. Defecation is controlled by the striated external sphincter, which is under voluntary control. The lower half of the canal is supplied with somatic sensory nerves, making it sensitive to painful stimuli, whereas the upper half is under autonomic control and is relatively insensitive. Therefore conditions of the lower anus may cause pain, whereas those of the upper anus usually will not.

Internally, the anal canal is lined by columns of mucosal tissue (columns of Morgagni) that fuse to form the anorectal junction. The spaces between the columns are called *crypts,* into which anal glands empty. Inflammation of the crypts can result in fistula or fissure formation. Anastomosing veins cross the columns, forming a ring called the *zona hemorrhoidalis.* Internal hemorrhoids result from dilation of these veins. The lower segment of the anal canal contains a venous plexus that drains into the inferior rectal veins. Dilation of this plexus results in external hemorrhoids.

The rectum lies superior to the anus and is approximately 12 cm long. Its proximal end is continuous with the sigmoid colon. The distal end, called the *anorectal junction,* is visible on proctoscopic examination as a sawtoothlike edge, but it is not palpable. Above the anorectal junction, the rectum dilates and turns posteriorly into the hollow of the coccyx and sacrum, forming the rectal ampulla, which stores flatus and feces. The rectal wall contains three semilunar transverse folds (Houston valves), the lowest of which can be palpated by the examiner.

Physical Examination Components

1. Inspect the sacrococcygeal and perianal areas for:
   - Skin characteristics
   - Lesions
   - Pilonidal dimpling and/or tufts of hair
   - Inflammation
   - Excoriation
2. Inspect the anus for:
   - Skin characteristics and tags
   - Lesions, fissures, hemorrhoids, or polyps
   - Fistulae
   - Prolapse
3. Insert finger and assess sphincter tone.
4. Palpate the muscular ring for smoothness and evenness of pressure against examining finger.
5. Palpate the lateral, posterior, and anterior rectal walls for:
   - Nodules, masses, or polyps
   - Tenderness
   - Irregularities
6. In patients with a prostate, palpate the posterior surface of the prostate gland through the anterior rectal wall for:
   - Size
   - Contour
   - Consistency
   - Mobility
7. In patients with a uterus, palpate the cervix and uterus through the anterior rectal wall for:
   - Size
   - Shape
   - Position
   - Smoothness
   - Mobility
8. Have the patient bear down, and palpate deeper for tenderness and nodules.
9. Withdraw the finger and examine fecal material for:
   - Color
   - Consistency
   - Blood or pus
   - Occult blood by chemical test if indicated

Note: For transgender women who have had a vaginoplasty, the prostate is anterior to the vaginal wall. A digital neovaginal examination may be more effective.

The prostate gland is located at the base of the bladder and surrounds the urethra. It is composed of muscular and glandular tissue and is approximately 4 × 3 × 2 cm. The posterior surface of the prostate gland is in close contact with the anterior rectal wall and is accessible by digital examination. It is convex and divided by a shallow median sulcus into right and left lateral lobes. A third or median lobe, not palpable on examination, is composed of glandular tissue and lies between the ejaculatory duct and the urethra. It contains active secretory alveoli that contribute to ejaculatory fluid. The seminal vesicles extend outward from the prostate (Fig. 21.2).

The vagina lies in contact with the anterior rectal wall of the rectum and is separated from it by the rectovaginal septum. See Chapter 19 for a more detailed discussion.

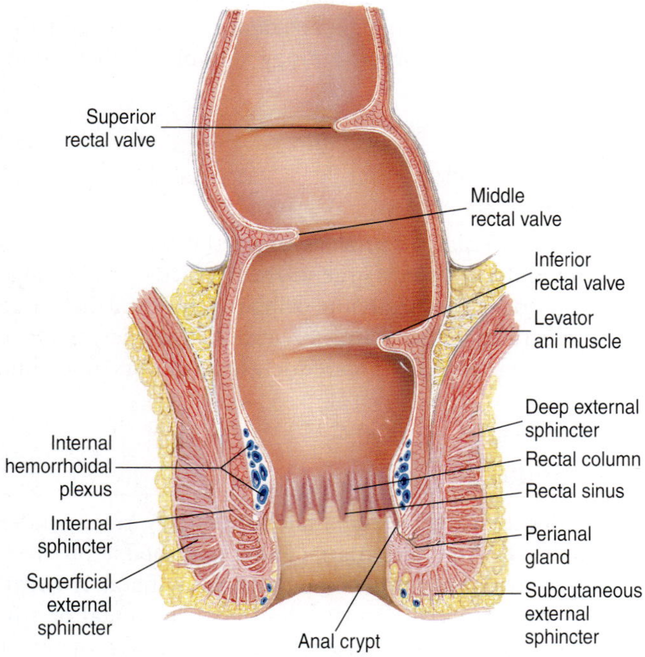

FIG. 21.1 Anatomy of the anus and rectum.

Infants and Children

At 7 weeks of gestation, a portion of the caudal hindgut is divided by an anorectal septum into a urogenital sinus and a rectum. The urogenital sinus is covered by a membrane that develops into the anal opening by 8 weeks of gestation. Most anorectal malformations result from abnormalities in this partitioning process.

The first meconium stool is ordinarily passed within the first 24 hours after birth and indicates anal patency. It is common for newborns, especially those who are breastfed, to have a stool after each feeding (the gastrocolic reflex). Both the internal and external sphincters are under involuntary reflexive control, as myelination of the spinal cord is incomplete.

By the end of the first year, the infant may have one or two bowel movements daily. Children are developmentally ready to begin toilet training between 2 and 3 years of age. Girls typically acquire bladder control before boys; bowel control typically is achieved before bladder control.

The prostate is small, inactive, and not palpable on rectal examination. The prostate remains undeveloped until puberty, at which time androgenic influences prompt its growth and maturation. The initially minimal glandular

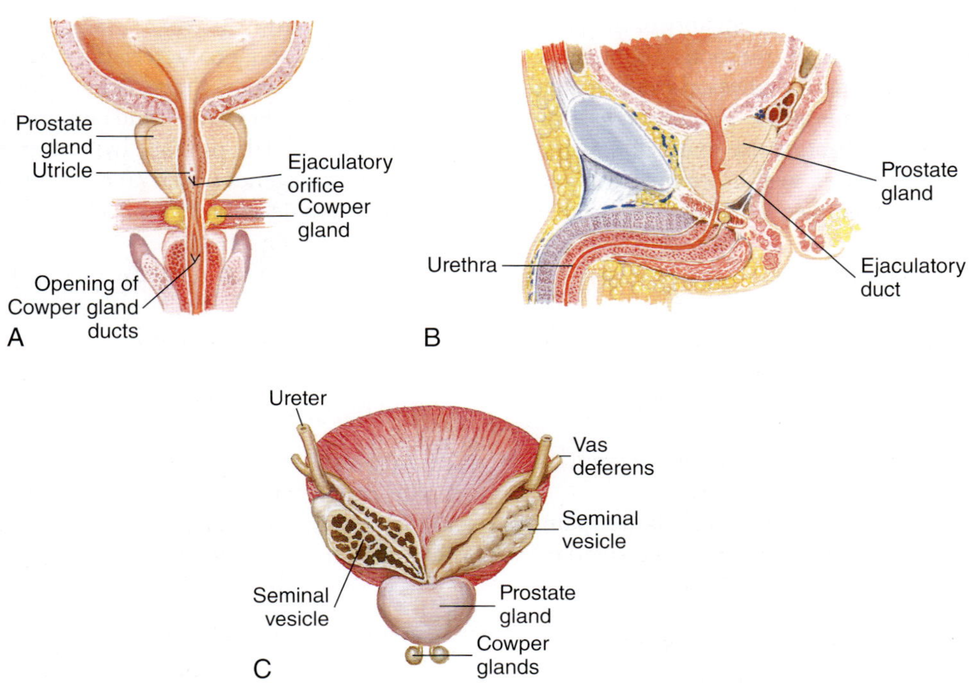

FIG. 21.2 Anatomy of the prostate gland and seminal vesicles. (A) Cross section. (B) Lateral view. (C) Posterior view.

component develops active secretory alveoli, and the prostate becomes functional.

Pregnant Patients

During pregnancy, pressure increases in the veins below the enlarged uterus. Dietary habits and hormonal changes that decrease GI tract tone and motility produce constipation. These factors predispose pregnant individuals to the development of hemorrhoids. Labor, which results in pressure on the pelvic floor by the presenting part of the fetus and expulsive efforts of the pregnant patient, may also aggravate the condition, causing protrusion and inflammation of hemorrhoids.

Older Adults

Degeneration of afferent neurons in the rectal wall interferes with the process of relaxation of the internal sphincter in response to distention of the rectum. As a result, the older adult may have a higher pressure threshold for the sensation of rectal distention with consequent retention of stool. Conversely, as the autonomically controlled internal sphincter loses tone, the external sphincter, by itself, cannot control the bowels, and the older adult may experience fecal incontinence.

The fibromuscular structures of the prostate gland atrophy, with loss of function of the secretory alveoli; however, the atrophy associated with aging is often obscured by benign hyperplasia of the glandular tissue. The muscular component of the prostate is progressively replaced by collagen.

REVIEW OF RELATED HISTORY

For each of the symptoms or conditions discussed in this section, targeted topics to include in the history of the present illness are listed. Responses to questions about these topics provide clues for focusing the physical examination and the development of an appropriate diagnostic evaluation. Questions regarding medication use (prescription and over-the-counter preparations) as well as complementary, alternative, and integrative therapies are relevant for each.

History of Present Illness

Changes in Bowel Function

- Character: number, frequency, consistency of stools; presence of mucus or blood; color (dark, bright red, black, light, or clay colored); odor
- Onset and duration: sudden or gradual, relation to dietary change, relation to stressful events
- Accompanying symptoms: incontinence, flatus, pain, fever, nausea, vomiting, cramping, abdominal distention
- Medications: iron, laxatives, stool softeners

Anal Discomfort (Itching, Pain, Stinging, Burning)

- Relation to body position and defecation
- Straining at stool
- Presence of mucus or blood
- Interference with activities of daily living or sleep
- Medications: hemorrhoid preparations

Rectal Bleeding

- Color: bright or dark red, black
- Relation to defecation
- Amount: spotting on toilet paper versus active bleeding
- Accompanying changes in stool: color, frequency, consistency, shape, odor, presence of mucus
- Associated symptoms: incontinence, flatus, rectal pain, abdominal pain or cramping, abdominal distention, weight loss
- Medications: iron, fiber additives

Changes in Urinary Function in Patients With a Prostate

- History of enlarged prostate or prostatitis
- Symptoms: hesitancy, urgency, nocturia, dysuria, change in force or caliber of stream, dribbling, urethral discharge
- Medications: antihistamines, anticholinergics, tricyclic antidepressants, 5-alpha-reductase inhibitors, hormone therapy

Past Medical History

- Gender identity: female, male, nonbinary, transgender woman, transgender man; gender assigned at birth
- Organ inventory: prostate gland; penis (natal or surgically constructed), scrotum and testicles (natal or surgically constructed), prostate gland, clitoris (natal or surgically constructed), vagina (natal or surgically constructed), cervix, uterus, fallopian tubes, ovaries
- Hemorrhoids
- Spinal cord injury
- Bowel habits and characteristics: timing, frequency, number, consistency, shape, color, odor
- Males, transgender women, and nonbinary individuals assigned male at birth: prostatic hypertrophy or carcinoma
- Females, transgender men, and nonbinary individuals assigned female at birth: episiotomy or fourth-degree laceration during delivery
- Colorectal cancer or related cancers: breast, ovarian, endometrial
- Anal, rectal, prostate surgeries

Family History

- Rectal polyps
- Colon cancer or familial cancer syndromes (see Risk Factors box in Chapter 18)
- Prostate cancer (see Risk Factors box)

Personal and Social History

- Travel history: areas with high incidence of parasitic infestation, including zones in the United States

- Diet: inclusion of fiber foods (cereals, breads, nuts, fruits, vegetables) and concentrated high-fiber foods; amount of animal fat
- Risk factors for colorectal, prostate, or anal cancer (see Risk Factors box in Chapter 18)
- Sexual practices at risk for anal human papilloma virus (HPV) infection (see Patient Safety, "Sexually Transmitted Infections" and Box 21.1)
- Vaccination status for HPV
- Use of alcohol

Risk Factors

Prostate Cancer

- Age: older than 50 years
- Race/ethnicity: more common in African Americans and in Caribbean patients of African ancestry; less common in Asian Americans and Hispanic/Latinos than in non-Hispanic White persons
- Geography: common in North America and northwestern Europe, Australia, and on Caribbean islands; less common in Asia, Africa, Central America, and South America
- Family history of prostate cancer: twice the risk with one first-degree relative; risk increases with more than one first-degree relative; the risk is higher for those who have a brother with prostate cancer than for those who have a father with it
- Inherited cancer syndromes: *BRCA1, BRCA2* mutations; hereditary nonpolyposis colorectal cancer (Lynch syndrome)
- Gonadectomy in transgender women may reduce, but does not eliminate, the risk of prostate cancer

From American Cancer Society. (2020a). *Prostate cancer risk factors.* Accessed October 8, 2020, from http://www.cancer.org/cancer/prostatecancer/detailedguide/prostate-cancer-risk-factors; Deutsch, M. B. (Ed.). (2016). *Guidelines for the primary care of transgender and gender nonbinary people* (2nd ed.). UCSF Center of Excellence for Transgender Health. http://transhealth.ucsf.edu/trans?page=guidelines-home; and Wesp, L. (2016). *Prostate and testicular cancer considerations in transgender women.* UCSF Transgender Care. https://transcare.ucsf.edu/guidelines/prostate-testicular-cancer

Risk Factors

Anal Cancer

- Infection with high-risk type of HPV
- HPV-related conditions: anal warts, cervical cancer
- Multiple sexual partners
- Receptive anal intercourse
- Cigarette smoking
- Immunosuppression: HIV infection
- Gender/ethnicity: more common in White females and Black males

From American Cancer Society. (2020b). *Risk factors for anal cancer.* Accessed October 10, 2020, from http://www.cancer.org/cancer/analcancer/detailedguide/anal-cancer-risk-factors.

Infants and Children

- Newborns: characteristics of stool
- Bowel movements accompanied by crying, straining, bleeding
- Feeding habits: types of foods, milk (formula or breast for infants), appetite

BOX 21.1 Screening for Sexually Transmitted Infections in Special Populations

The Centers for Disease Control and Prevention (CDC) has identified populations who are at risk for sexually transmitted infections based on sexual practices or, in the case of fetuses, are at risk for debilitating effects of intrauterine or perinatally transmitted infections. Adolescents, persons in correctional facilities, men who have sex with men, women who have sex with women, and transgender men and women may engage in practices that expose them to a variety of sexually transmitted diseases. The CDC has specific screening and prevention recommendations for each group, which are available at https://www.cdc.gov/sti/?CDC_AAref_Val=https://www.cdc.gov/std/tg2015/specialpops.htm

Data from U.S. Centers for Disease Control and Prevention. (2021). *Sexually transmitted infections treatment guidelines.* https://www.cdc.gov/std/treatment-guidelines/screening-recommendations

- Age at which bowel control and toilet training were achieved
- Encopresis (involuntary "fecal soiling" in children who have usually already been toilet trained)
- Associated symptoms: episodes of diarrhea or constipation; tenderness when cleaning after a stool; perianal irritations; weight loss; abdominal pain, nausea, vomiting
- Congenital anomaly: imperforate anus, myelomeningocele, aganglionic megacolon

Pregnant Patients

- Weeks of gestation and estimated date of delivery
- Exercise
- Fluid intake and dietary habits
- Medications: prenatal vitamins, iron, fiber supplements
- Use of complementary, alternative, or integrative therapies

Older Adults

- Changes in bowel habits or character: frequency, number, color, consistency, shape, odor
- Associated symptoms: weight loss, rectal or abdominal pain, incontinence, flatus, episodes of constipation or diarrhea, abdominal distention, rectal bleeding
- Dietary changes: fluid intake, intolerance for certain foods, inclusion of high-fiber foods, regularity of eating habits, appetite
- History of enlarged prostate, urinary symptoms (hesitancy, urgency, nocturia, dysuria, force and caliber of urinary stream, dribbling)

EXAMINATION AND FINDINGS

Equipment

- Gloves
- Water-soluble lubricant
- Drapes
- Penlight or other light source
- Fecal occult blood testing materials if indicated

Preparation

Although the rectal examination is generally uncomfortable and sometimes embarrassing for the patient, it provides important information that is a necessary part of a comprehensive examination. Be calm, slowly paced, and gentle in your touch. Explain what will happen step by step and let the patient know what to expect. A hurried or rough examination can cause unnecessary pain and sphincter spasm, and you can easily lose the trust and cooperation of the patient.

CLINICAL PEARL

In Pain?

The patient with an acute rectal problem will often shift uncomfortably from side to side when sitting.

Positioning

The rectal examination can be performed with the patient in any of these positions: knee-chest, lithotomy, left lateral with hips and knees flexed, or standing with the hips flexed and the upper body supported by the examining table. As a general rule, patients should be examined in the position congruent with their identified gender, taking into account also their comfort and anatomy. In patients with a prostate, the latter two positions are satisfactory and allow adequate visualization of the perianal and sacrococcygeal areas as well as acceptable positioning for the prostate examination. For transgender women who have had a vaginoplasty, the prostate is anterior to the vaginal wall. A digital neovaginal examination may provide more effective access to the prostate for palpation. In patients with vaginal cavities, the rectal examination is most often performed as part of the rectovaginal examination while the patient is in the lithotomy position (see Chapter 19).

Ask the patient to assume one of the examining positions, guiding gently with your hands when necessary. Use drapes but retain good visualization of the area. Glove both hands.

Sacrococcygeal and Perianal Areas

Inspect the sacrococcygeal (pilonidal) and perianal areas. The skin should be smooth and uninterrupted. Inspect for lumps, rashes, inflammation, excoriation, scars, pilonidal dimpling, and tufts of hair at the pilonidal area. Fungal infection and pinworm infestation can cause perianal irritation. Fungal infection is more common in adults with diabetes, and pinworms are more common in children. The best time to visualize pinworms in children is after they fall asleep. Inspection of the anus often reveals them. Palpate the area. The discovery of tenderness and inflammation should alert you to the possibility of a perianal abscess, anorectal fistula or fissure, pilonidal cyst, or pruritus ani.

Anus

Separate the patient's buttocks apart and inspect the anus. Use a penlight or lamp to assist in visualization. The skin around the anus will appear coarser and more darkly pigmented. Look for skin lesions, skin tags or warts, external hemorrhoids, fissures, and fistulae. Ask the patient to bear down. This will make fistulae, fissures, rectal prolapse, polyps, and internal hemorrhoids more readily apparent.

Sphincter

Lubricate the examining index finger of your gloved hand and press the pad of it against the anal opening (Fig. 21.3A). Ask the patient to bear down to relax the external sphincter. As relaxation occurs, slip the tip of the finger into the anal canal (see Fig. 21.3B). Warn the patient that there may be a feeling of urgency for a bowel movement and assure them that this will not happen. Ask the patient to tighten the external sphincter around your finger (Fig. 21.4A), noting its tone; it should tighten evenly with no discomfort to the patient. A lax sphincter may indicate neurologic deficit or sexual abuse. An extremely tight sphincter can result from scarring, spasticity caused by a fissure or other lesion, inflammation, or anxiety about the examination.

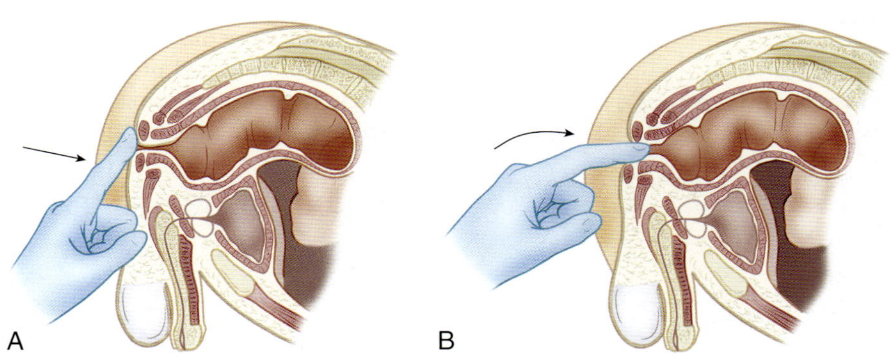

FIG. 21.3 (A) Correct procedure for introducing a finger into the rectum. Press the pad of the finger against the anal opening. (B) As the external sphincter relaxes, slip the fingertip into the anal canal. Note that the patient is in the hips-flexed position.

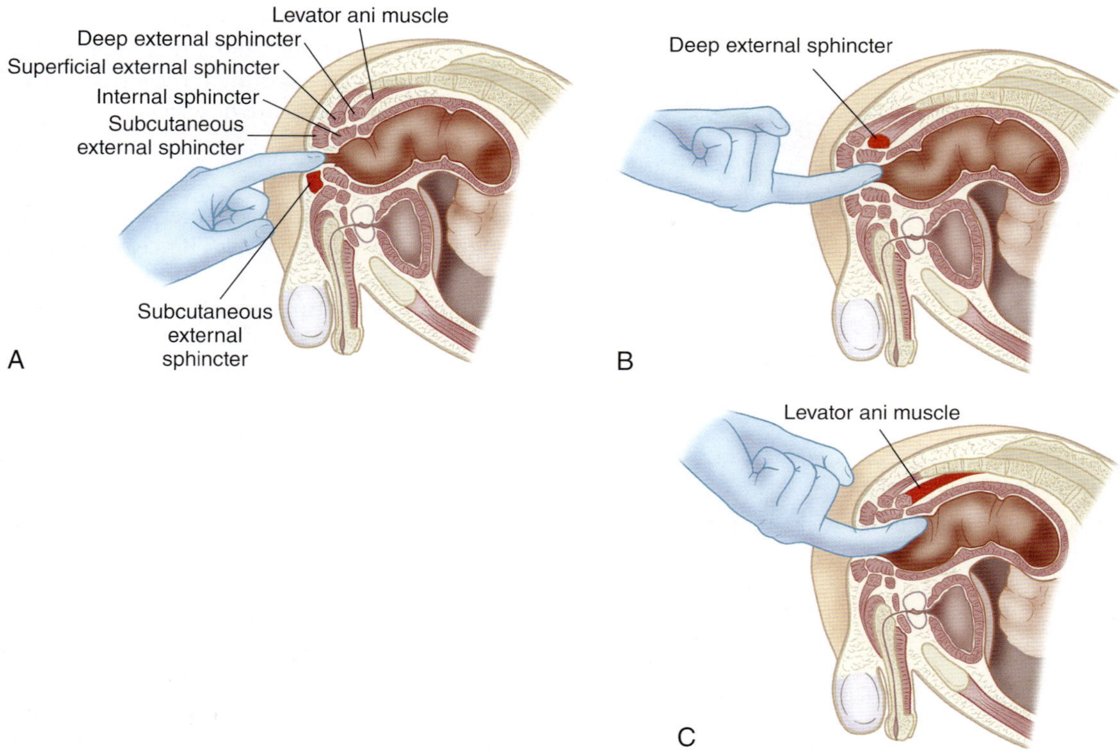

FIG. 21.4 (A) Palpation of subcutaneous external sphincter. Feel it tighten around the examining finger. (B) Palpation of deep external sphincter. (C) Palpation of the posterior rectal wall.

An anal fistula or fissure may produce such extreme tenderness that you are not able to complete the examination without local anesthesia. Rectal pain is almost always indicative of a local disease. Look for irritation, rock-hard stool in the rectum, rectal fissures, fluctuance from a perirectal abscess, or thrombosed hemorrhoids. Always inquire about previous episodes of pain.

Anal Ring

Rotate your finger to examine the muscular anal ring (see Fig. 21.4B). It should feel smooth and exert even pressure on the finger. Note any nodules or irregularities.

Lateral and Posterior Rectal Walls

Insert your finger farther and palpate in sequence the lateral and posterior rectal walls, noting any nodules, masses, irregularities, polyps, or tenderness (see Fig. 21.4C). The walls should feel smooth, even, and uninterrupted. Internal hemorrhoids are not ordinarily felt unless they are thrombosed. The examining finger can palpate a distance of about 6 to 10 cm into the rectum.

Bidigital Palpation

Bidigital palpation with the thumb and examining finger can sometimes reveal more information than palpating with the index finger alone. To perform bidigital palpation, gently press your thumb against the perianal tissue and bring your finger toward the thumb. This technique is particularly useful for detecting a perianal abscess.

Anterior Rectal Wall

Rotate the examining finger to palpate the anterior rectal wall, as noted earlier. Ask the patient to bear down. This allows you to reach a few centimeters farther into the rectum. Because the anterior rectal wall is in contact with the peritoneum, you may be able to detect the tenderness of peritoneal inflammation and the nodularity of peritoneal metastases. The nodules, called *shelf lesions,* are palpable in the peritoneal cul-de-sac. These can be felt as a hard, nodular shelf at the tip of the examining finger.

Prostate

You can palpate the posterior surface of the prostate gland (Fig. 21.5) on the anterior wall. The patient may feel the urge to urinate but offer assurance that this will not happen. Note the size, contour, consistency, and mobility of the prostate. The gland should feel like a pencil eraser—firm, smooth, and slightly movable—and it should be nontender. A healthy prostate has a diameter of about 4 cm, with less than 1 cm protrusion into the rectum. Greater protrusion denotes prostatic enlargement, which should be noted, with the amount of protrusion recorded (Box 21.2). The median sulcus may be obliterated when

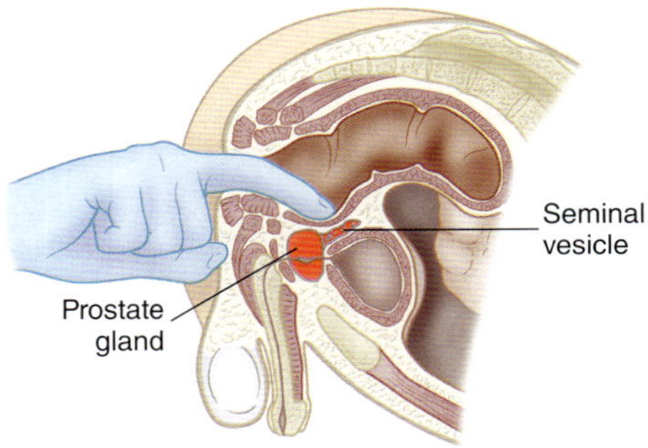

FIG. 21.5 **Palpation of the posterior surface of the prostate gland.** Feel for the lateral lobes and median sulcus.

BOX 21.2 Prostate Enlargement

Prostate enlargement is classified by the amount of protrusion into the rectum:
Grade I: 1–2 cm
Grade II: 2–3 cm
Grade III: 3–4 cm
Grade IV: more than 4 cm

the lobes are hypertrophied or neoplastic. A rubbery or boggy consistency is indicative of benign hypertrophy, whereas stony, hard nodularity may indicate carcinoma, prostatic calculi, or chronic fibrosis. A tender, fluctuant softness suggests prostatic abscess. Identify the lateral lobes and the median sulcus. The prostatic lobes should feel symmetric. The seminal vesicles are not palpable unless they are inflamed. The Evidence-Based Practice box discusses screening for prostate cancer.

Palpation of the prostate can force secretions through the urethral orifice. Secretions that appear at the meatus can be cultured and examined microscopically. Specimen preparation techniques are described in Chapter 19.

Uterus and Cervix

A retroflexed or retroverted uterus is usually palpable through rectal examination. The cervix may be palpable through the anterior rectal wall (see Chapter 19). Do not mistake these structures for a tampon or a tumor.

Stool

Slowly withdraw your finger and examine it for any fecal material, which should be soft and brown (Box 21.3). Note any blood or purulent discharge. Light tan or gray stool could indicate obstructive jaundice, whereas tarry, black stool should make you suspect upper intestinal tract bleeding. A more subtle blood loss can result in a virtually unchanged color of the stool, but even a small amount will yield a positive test for occult blood. If indicated, fecal material can be tested for blood using a chemical guaiac procedure. Common causes of rectal bleeding are identified in Box 21.4. The Evidence-Based Practice Box considers the predictive value of rectal bleeding in diagnosing colorectal cancer.

Further evaluation is indicated if there is persistent anal or rectal bleeding; any interruption in the smooth contour of the rectal wall on palpation; persistent pain with negative findings on rectal examination; or unexplained, persistent stool changes.

Evidence-Based Practice in Physical Examination

Screening for Prostate Cancer: The Controversy

The results from two large randomized clinical trials—one in the United States and one in Europe—and their updates have not settled the controversy over screening for prostate cancer. The trials had different designs, tested different populations, had different screening intervals, and had conflicting results. In the U.S. trial, the rate of death from prostate cancer was very low and did not differ significantly between the screening group and the control group (Andriole et al., 2009, 2012). In the European trial, prostate-specific antigen (PSA)–based screening reduced the relative risk of death from prostate cancer by 21% in the screening group but was associated with overdiagnosis (Schröder et al., 2009, 2012).

The Cluster Randomized Trial of PSA Testing for Prostate Cancer (CAP), reported in 2018, explored the effectiveness of a single PSA screening intervention versus standard practice without screening in 419,582 males ages 50 to 69 years in the United Kingdom. There was no significant difference in prostate cancer mortality after a median follow-up of 10 years, but the detection of low-risk prostate cancer cases increased (Martin et al., 2018).

The persistent issue is whether the benefits of prostate cancer screening are large enough to outweigh the associated harms, which include false-positive screening tests, unnecessary biopsies, and overdiagnosis. Because of the current inability to reliably distinguish tumors that will remain indolent (slow to develop) from those that will be lethal, many patients are at risk for the harms of treatment for prostate cancer that will never become symptomatic and without any improvement in health outcomes.

The U.S. Preventive Services Task Force (USPSTF) recognizes that screening offers a small potential benefit of reducing the chance of death from prostate cancer in some. They note, however, that many patients will experience the potential harms of screening, including false-positive results that require additional testing and possible prostate biopsy, overdiagnosis and overtreatment, and treatment complications. The USPSTF endorses an individual decision based on discussion with the clinician, balancing potential harms and benefits and incorporating individual values and preferences (USPSTF, 2018).

The American Cancer Society (ACS, 2023) recommends informed decision making by males with their health care provider about whether to be screened for prostate cancer or not. The decision should be made after discussion about the uncertainties, risks, and potential benefits of prostate cancer screening. The decision to perform screening for prostate cancer in transgender women should be made based on guidelines for nontransgender men (Deutsch, 2016).

BOX 21.3 Stool Characteristics in Disease

Changes in the shape, content, or consistency of stool suggest that some disease process is present. Stool characteristics can sometimes point to the type of disorder present; therefore you should be familiar with the following characteristics and associated disorders:

- Intermittent, pencil-like stools suggest a spasmodic contraction in the rectal area.
- Persistent, pencil-like stools indicate permanent stenosis from scarring or from pressure of a malignancy.
- Decreased caliber (pencil-thin stools) indicate lower rectal stricture.
- A large amount of mucus in the fecal matter is characteristic of intestinal inflammation and mucous colitis.
- Small flecks of blood-stained mucus in liquid feces are indicative of amebiasis.
- Fatty stools are seen in patients with pancreatic disorders and malabsorption syndromes, such as cystic fibrosis.
- Stools the color of aluminum (caused by a mixture of melena and fat) occur in tropical sprue, carcinoma of the hepatopancreatic ampulla, and children treated with sulfonamides for diarrhea.

BOX 21.4 Common Causes of Rectal Bleeding

There are numerous reasons that blood can appear in the feces, ranging from benign, self-limiting events to serious, life-threatening disease. Following are some common causes:

- Anal fissures
- Anaphylactoid purpura
- Aspirin-containing medications
- Bleeding disorders
- Coagulation disorders
- Colitis
- Dysentery, acute and amebic
- Esophageal varices
- Familial telangiectasia
- Foreign body trauma
- Hemorrhoids
- Hiatal hernia
- Hookworm
- Intussusception
- Iron poisoning
- Meckel diverticulum
- Neoplasms of any type
- Oral steroids
- Peptic ulcers, acute and chronic
- Polyps, single or multiple
- Regional enteritis
- Strangulated hernia
- Swallowed blood
- Thrombocytopenia
- Volvulus

Evidence-Based Practice in Physical Examination

Does Rectal Bleeding Predict Colorectal Cancer?

In a systematic review of 38 studies in 37 articles, containing 5626 colorectal cancer patients and 73,174 participants with rectal bleeding from 16 countries, the authors considered the diagnostic value of rectal bleeding in predicting colorectal cancer. The pooled sensitivity and specificity were 0.47 (95% CI: 0.45 to 0.48) and 0.96 (95% CI: 0.96 to 0.96), respectively. The overall positive predictive values ranged from 0.01 to 0.21 with a pooled value of 0.06 (95% CI: 0.05 to 0.08), meaning 6 out of 100 patients with rectal bleeding actually had colorectal cancer, which is higher than the rate of colorectal cancer in the general population. Additional findings of being over the age of 60 years, change in bowel habit, weight loss, anemia, history of colorectal cancer among first-degree relatives, and feeling of incomplete evacuation of rectum appeared to increase the predictive value of rectal bleeding. The low sensitivity points to the multiple noncancer causes of rectal bleeding. The bottom line: rectal bleeding alone is an insufficient predictor of colorectal cancer but should be considered an alarm symptom.

From Tong, G. X., Chai, J., Cheng, J., et al. (2014). Diagnostic value of rectal bleeding in predicting colorectal cancer: A systematic review. *Asian Pacific Journal of Cancer Prevention, 15*(2), 1015–1021.

TABLE 21.1 Sequence and Description of Stools in Infants

INFANTS	TYPE OF STOOL
Newborn meconium	Greenish black, viscous, contains occult blood; first stool is sterile
3–6 days old	Transitional: thin, slimy, brown to green
Breastfed	Mushy, loose, seedy, golden (mustard) yellow; frequency varies from after each feeding to every few days; nonirritating to skin
Formula-fed	Light yellow, characteristic odor, irritating to skin

Data from Lowdermilk, D. L., & Perry, S. E. (2004). *Maternity and women's health care* (8th ed.). St. Louis: Mosby.

Infants and Children

Rectal examination is generally performed on infants and children only if there is a particular problem. An examination is required when a symptom suggests an intra-abdominal or pelvic problem, a mass or tenderness, bladder distention, bleeding, or rectal or bowel abnormalities. Deviation from the expected stool pattern in infants requires investigation (Table 21.1).

It is imperative that you respect the child's modesty and always have a parent present for the examination. Careful explanation of each step in the process is necessary for the child who is old enough to understand.

Routinely inspect the anal region and perineum, examining the surrounding buttocks for redness, bruising, masses, or swelling. Inspect for swollen, tender perirectal protrusion; abscesses; and possibly rectal fistulae. Buttocks with redundant skin folds suggest chronic disease with associated malnutrition. They are also common in premature infants. Asymmetric creases may occur with developmental dysplasia of the hip. Perirectal redness and irritation are suggestive of pinworms, *Candida,* or other irritants of the diaper area. Rectal prolapse can occur as a result of constipation, diarrhea, gynecologic surgery, pelvic neuropathies, or severe coughing or straining. Hemorrhoids are rare in children, and their presence suggests a serious underlying problem such as portal hypertension. Small, flat flaps of skin around the rectum (condylomas) are typically from HPV infection, which may occur as the result of perinatal infection or sexual abuse. Sinuses, tufts of hair, and dimpling in the pilonidal area may indicate lower occult spinal deformities; the presence of these should alert the examiner for the need of diagnostic imaging to evaluate for potential spinal deformities.

Lightly touch the anal opening, which should produce anal contraction (the "anal wink"). Lack of contraction may indicate a lower spinal cord lesion or chronic abuse.

Examine the patency of the anus and its position in all newborn infants. Patency is usually confirmed by passage of meconium or initial rectal temperature. To determine patency when there is concern, insert a lubricated catheter no more than 1 cm into the rectum. Occasionally, a perianal fistula may be confused with an anal orifice. Be careful in making this judgment. Sometimes the anal orifice can seem appropriate, yet there may be atresia just inside, or a few centimeters within, the rectum. Rectal examination or insertion of a catheter does not always provide definitive assessment, and radiologic studies may be necessary. If there is no passage of stool in 24 hours in a newborn, suspect rectal atresia, Hirschsprung disease (congenital megacolon), or cystic fibrosis.

Perform the rectal examination in infants and young children with the child lying on their back. You may hold the child's feet together and flex the knees and hips on the abdomen with one hand, using the gloved index finger of your other hand for the examination (Fig. 21.6). Some health care clinicians are reluctant to use the index finger because of its size, choosing instead the fifth finger; however, even with the smallest of adult fingers, some bleeding and transient prolapse of the rectum often occurs directly after examination. Always warn the parents of this possibility.

Assess the tone of the rectal sphincter. It should feel snug but neither too tight nor too loose. A very tight sphincter can cause enough tension to produce a stenosis, which leads to stool retention and pain during a bowel movement. A lax sphincter is associated with lesions of the peripheral spinal nerves or spinal cord, *Shigella* infection, and previous fecal impactions. The presence of bruises around the anus, scars, anal tears (especially those that extend into the surrounding perianal skin), and anal dilation may be evidence of sexual abuse.

Feel for feces in the rectum. Chronic constipation in children with cognitive deficiency or emotional problems is often associated with a rectum distended with feces. A consistently empty rectum in the presence of constipation is a clue to the diagnosis of Hirschsprung disease. A fecal mass in the rectum accompanying diarrhea suggests overflow diarrhea. Stool recovered on the examining finger should be tested for occult blood, if indicated.

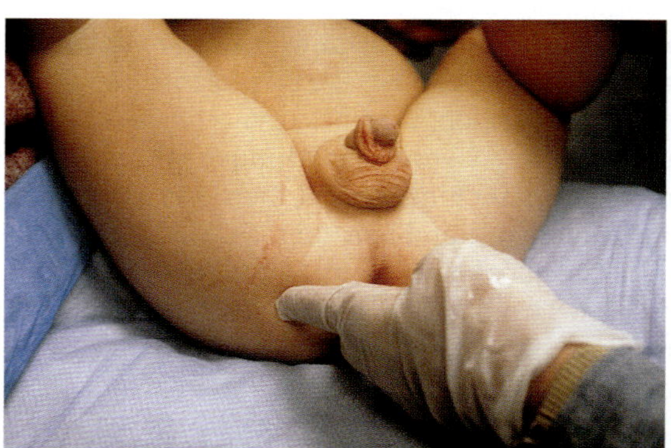

FIG. 21.6 Positioning the infant or child for rectal examination.

In young adults, a retroflexed or retroverted uterus may be palpable on rectal examination. The ovaries are not usually palpable on rectal examination.

In preadolescents, the prostate is usually not felt, and a palpable prostate suggests precocious puberty or a virilizing disease process, which should be apparent from examination of the genitalia.

Rectal examination should be part of the physical examination for adolescents who have symptoms related to the lower intestinal tract. The same procedures and guidelines that are used for adults apply to adolescents with the appropriate use of chaperones. Be especially sensitive on a first examination, and spend additional time explaining what to expect. Illustrations and models can be helpful.

Pregnant Patients

The examination of the rectum provides information about rectovaginal musculature and confirms findings about the uterus (see Chapter 19). Assessment for hemorrhoids should include both external and internal evaluation. Hemorrhoids are usually not found early in pregnancy; however, they may be an expected variation late in pregnancy. Evaluate hemorrhoids for size, extent, location (internal or external), discomfort to the patient, and signs of infection or bleeding.

> **CLINICAL PEARL**
>
> **Stool Changes in Pregnant Patients**
>
> During pregnancy, the stool color may be dark green or black if the patient is taking iron supplements. Iron may also cause diarrhea or constipation.

Older Adults

The examination procedure and findings for the older adult are much the same as those for the younger adult. The older patient may be more limited in ability to assume a position other than the left lateral. Sphincter tone may be somewhat decreased. Older adults commonly experience fecal impaction resulting from constipation. Older patients are far more likely to have an enlarged prostate, which will be felt as smooth, rubbery, and symmetric. The median sulcus may or may not be obliterated. Older adults are more likely to have polyps and are at higher risk for carcinoma, making the rectal examination particularly important in this age group.

Patient Safety

Sexually Transmitted Infections

Infected persons may spread sexually transmitted infections (STIs) through anal sex practices in which blood, semen, or other fluid is shared. STIs that affect the anus include the following:

- Herpes simplex virus (HSV) infection of the skin and mucosa, causing recurring sores and pain
- Gonorrheal infection of the mucosa, producing an infectious discharge
- HPV, causing anal warts
- Parasites that affect the entire GI tract
- Early syphilis infection, causing a painless lesion

Hepatitis and HIV are two STIs whose symptoms do not appear on the anus but can be transmitted through anal sex practices.

It is possible to acquire an STI without penetration. Oral-anal contact, whether from kissing or from oral contact with fingers that have been touching the anus, can spread bacteria and cause infection. The use of sex toys may also transmit certain infections.

Box 21.1 discusses screening recommendations for STIs in special populations.

ABNORMALITIES

ANUS, RECTUM, AND SURROUNDING SKIN

Pilonidal Cyst

Cyst or sinus near the cleft of the buttocks

PATHOPHYSIOLOGY

- Loose hairs penetrate the skin in the sacrococcygeal area
- Local inflammatory reaction causes a cyst to form around the ingrown hair
- Excessive pressure or repetitive trauma to the sacrococcygeal predisposes to development of the cyst
- Most first diagnosed in young adults, although they are usually a congenital anomaly

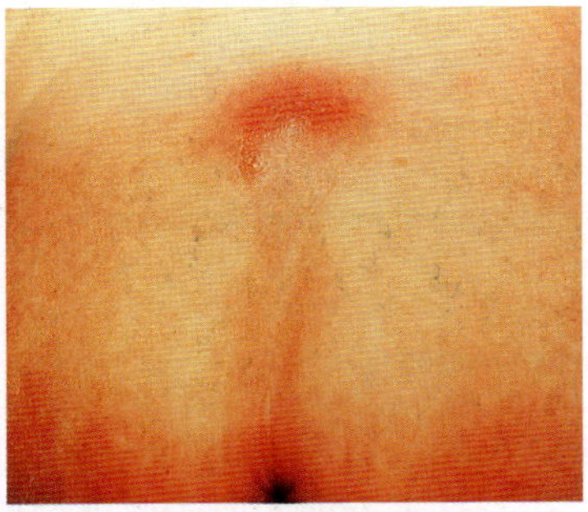

FIG. 21.7 **Pilonidal cyst.** (From Zitelli, B. J., & Davis, H. W. (2007). *Atlas of pediatric physical diagnosis* (5th ed.). St Louis: Mosby.)

PATIENT DATA

Subjective Data

- Usually asymptomatic
- May have pain with sitting and inflammation from secondary infection

Objective Data

- Cyst or sinus seen as a dimple with a sinus tract opening
- Located in the midline, superficial to the coccyx and lower sacrum (Fig. 21.7)
- Opening may contain a tuft of hair and be surrounded by erythema
- A cyst may be palpable

Anal Warts (Condyloma Acuminata)

Growths in or around the anus and genital area

PATHOPHYSIOLOGY

- Result of infection with HPV
- Virus transmitted from person to person, almost always by direct sexual contact, or through perinatal infection; considered an STI

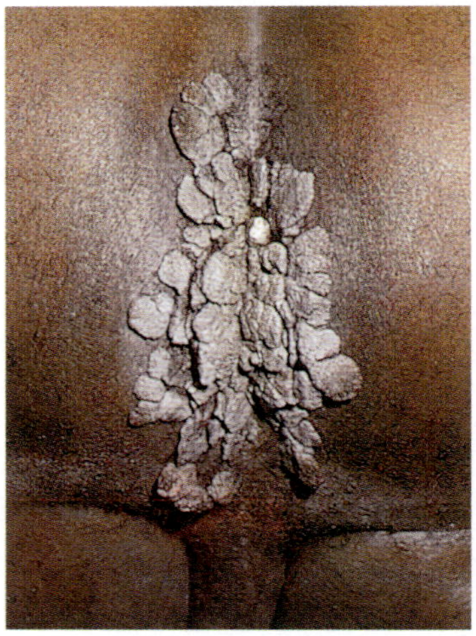

FIG. 21.8 Anal warts (condyloma acuminata). (From Morse SA, et al: *Atlas of sexually transmitted diseases and AIDS*, ed 3, St Louis, 2003, Mosby.)

OBJECTIVE DATA

Subjective Data

- Patients may be unaware that the warts are present

Objective Data

- Single or multiple papular lesions in or around the anus and genital area
- May be pearly, filiform, fungating (ulcerating and necrotic), cauliflower-like, or plaquelike (Fig. 21.8)

Perianal and Perirectal Abscesses

Infection of the anal tissue or glands

PATHOPHYSIOLOGY

- Perianal abscess: infection of the soft tissues surrounding the anal canal, with formation of a discrete abscess cavity
- Perirectal abscesses; infection of the mucus-secreting anal glands, which drain into the anal crypts; abscess formation occurs in the deeper tissues (Fig. 21.9)
- Infections caused by anaerobic organisms, usually polymicrobial

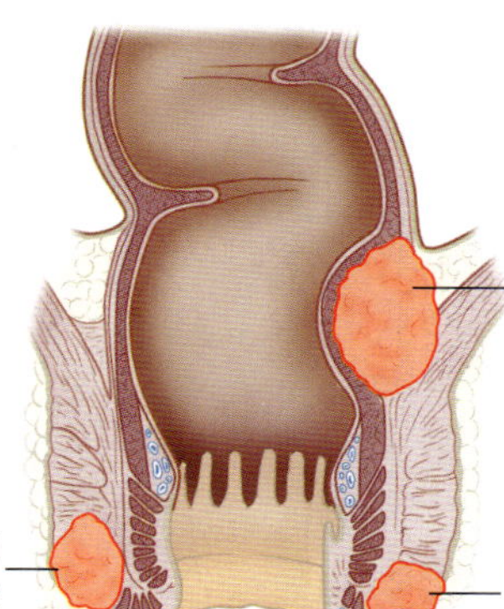

FIG. 21.9 Perianal and perirectal abscesses. Common sites of abscess formation.

PATIENT DATA

Subjective Data

- Painful and tender anal area
- Fever
- Pain on defecation or with sitting or walking
- Risk factors:
    - Crohn disease
    - Immunosuppression

Objective Data

- Perianal abscess: tender, swollen, fluctuant mass in the superficial subcutaneous tissue just adjacent to the anus
- Perirectal abscess: tender mass that may be indurated, fluctuant, or draining

Anorectal Fissure

Tear in the anal mucosa (Fig. 21.10)

PATHOPHYSIOLOGY

- Tear usually caused by traumatic passage of large, hard stools

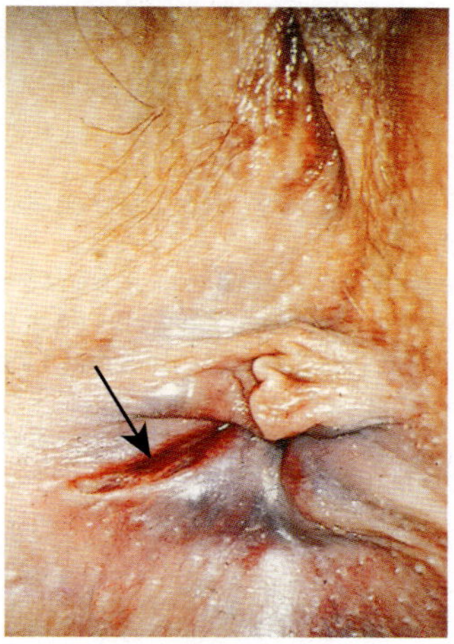

FIG. 21.10 Lateral anal fissure in adult. (Courtesy Gershon Efron, MD, Sinai Hospital of Baltimore.)

PATIENT DATA

Subjective Data

- History of hard stools
- Bleeding seen in toilet or on toilet paper
- Severe pain with passing of stool and relief after completion of bowel movement

Objective Data

- Examination is painful and may require local anesthesia
- Fissure most often in the posterior midline, although it can also occur in the anterior midline
- Sentinel skin tag may be seen at the lower edge of the fissure
- May be ulceration through which muscles of the internal sphincter are seen
- Internal sphincter is spastic

Anal Fistula

Inflammatory tract that runs from the anus or rectum and opens onto the surface of the perianal skin or other tissue

PATHOPHYSIOLOGY

- Caused by inflammation from a perianal or perirectal abscess; the abscess degrades the tissue until a tract and an opening in the skin is created

PATIENT DATA

Subjective Data

- May report chills, fever, nausea, vomiting, and malaise

Objective Data

- External opening of a fistula appears as a pink or red, elevated, granular tissue on the skin near the anus
- Palpable indurated tract may be present on digital rectal examination
- Serosanguineous or purulent drainage may appear with compression of the area

Pruritus Ani

Itching of the anal area

PATHOPHYSIOLOGY

- Commonly caused by fungal infection in adults and by parasites in children

PATIENT DATA

Subjective Data

- Anal burning or itching that may interfere with sleep

Objective Data

- Excoriation, thickening, and pigmentation of anal and perianal tissue

Hemorrhoids

Swollen veins in the lower portion of the rectum or anus

PATHOPHYSIOLOGY

- External hemorrhoids: varicose veins that originate below the anorectal line and are covered by anal skin (Fig. 21.11A)
- Internal hemorrhoids: varicose veins that originate above the anorectal junction and are covered by rectal mucosa (see Fig. 21.11B)
- Caused by pressure on the veins in the pelvic and rectal area from straining, diarrhea, constipation, prolonged sitting, or pregnancy

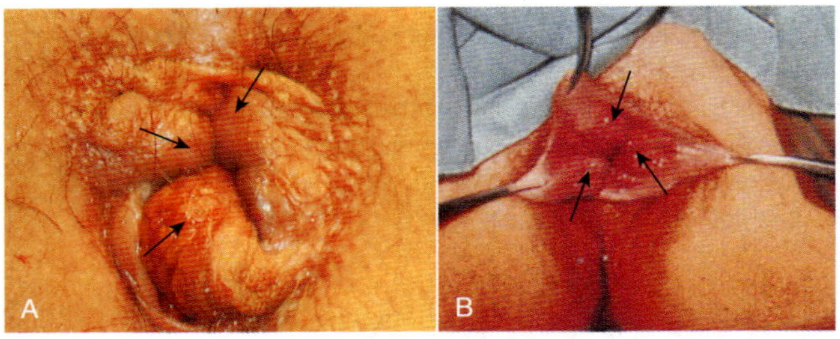

FIG. 21.11 (A) Prolapsed hemorrhoids. (B) Primary internal hemorrhoids. (Courtesy Gershon Efron, MD, Sinai Hospital of Baltimore.)

PATIENT DATA

Subjective Data

- External: may cause itching, bleeding, and discomfort
- Internal: no discomfort unless they are thrombosed, prolapsed, or infected
- Bleeding may occur with or without defecation

Objective Data

- Usually not visible at rest, they can protrude on standing and on straining at stool
- Thrombosed hemorrhoids appear as blue, shiny masses at the anus
- Internal: soft swellings that are not palpable on rectal examination and are not visible unless they prolapse through the anus; proctoscopy usually required for diagnosis
- Hemorrhoidal skin tags, which can appear at the site of resolved hemorrhoids, are fibrotic or flaccid and painless

Polyps

Abnormal growth of tissue projecting from the mucous membrane

PATHOPHYSIOLOGY

- Occur anywhere in the intestinal tract
- May be malignant or benign or have malignant potential
- Can occur singly or in profusion

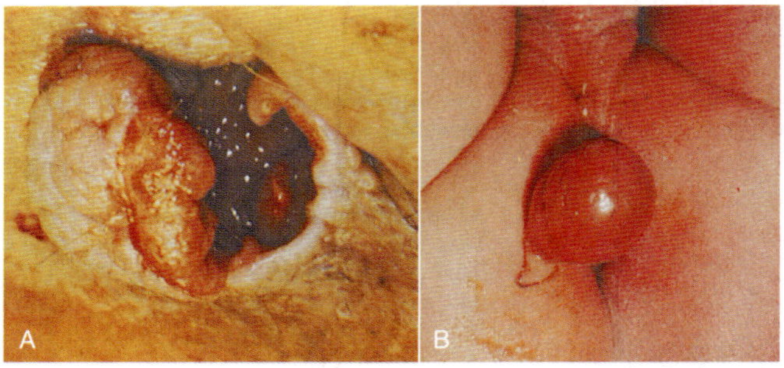

FIG. 21.12 (A) Fibroepithelial polyp of the rectum. (B) Infant with prolapsed rectal polyp. (Courtesy Gershon Efron, MD, Sinai Hospital of Baltimore.)

PATIENT DATA

Subjective Data

- Asymptomatic
- Rectal bleeding

Objective Data

- Rectal polyp may protrude through rectum (Fig. 21.12)
- Rectal polyps are sometimes palpable on rectal examination as soft nodules and can be either pedunculated (on a stalk) or sessile (closely adhering to the mucosal wall)
- Colonoscopy or proctoscopy is usually required for diagnosis, and biopsy is necessary to distinguish benign from malignant

Anal Cancer

Cancer of the anal skin, mucosa, or glands

PATHOPHYSIOLOGY

- Most are squamous cell carcinomas, which are associated with HPV infection
- About 15% are adenocarcinomas, which originate in the glands near the anus
- Remaining anal cancers are basal cell carcinoma and malignant melanoma
- Melanoma in the anus is difficult to see and is often discovered at a late stage, after the cancer has spread through layers of tissue

PATIENT DATA

Subjective Data

- May be asymptomatic
- May report:
  - Bleeding from the anus or rectum
  - Pain or pressure in the area around the anus
  - Itching or discharge from the anus
  - A lump near the anus
  - A change in bowel habits such as constipation, diarrhea, and the thinning of the stools

Objective Data

- Raised, erythematous mucosa
- White, scaling mucosa
- Pigmented mucosa
- Mucosal ulceration
- Verrucous lesion

Colorectal Cancer

Cancer of the large intestine or rectum

PATHOPHYSIOLOGY

- Adenocarcinomas comprise the large majority of colorectal cancers
- Accumulation of genetic and epigenetic alterations that affect essential cellular- and tissue-level functions
- Begins with cell proliferation with progression to adenoma and invasive carcinoma
- The *APC* tumor suppressor gene is defective in more than 80% of adenomatous polyps and colon cancers

PATIENT DATA

Subjective Data

- Bleeding is most common symptom
- Often asymptomatic
- May report:
  - Change in bowel habits or stool characteristics
  - Unexplained weight loss
  - Abdominal pain or tenderness
  - Personal or family history of colon polyps
  - Family history of colon cancer

Objective Data

- Rectal cancer may be felt as a sessile polypoid mass with nodular, raised edges and areas of ulceration; the consistency is often stony, and the contour is irregular
- Carcinoma higher in the colon not palpable
- Polyps or lesions visualized on colonoscopy or flexible sigmoidoscopy

PROSTATE

Prostatitis

Inflammation and infection of the prostate gland (Fig. 21.13)

PATHOPHYSIOLOGY

- Acute: bacterial infection including *Escherichia coli, Klebsiella,* and *Proteus*
- May be acquired as a sexually transmitted disease, from infection of an adjacent organ, or as a complication of prostate biopsy
- Chronic: may be bacterial or nonbacterial (chronic pelvic pain syndrome)

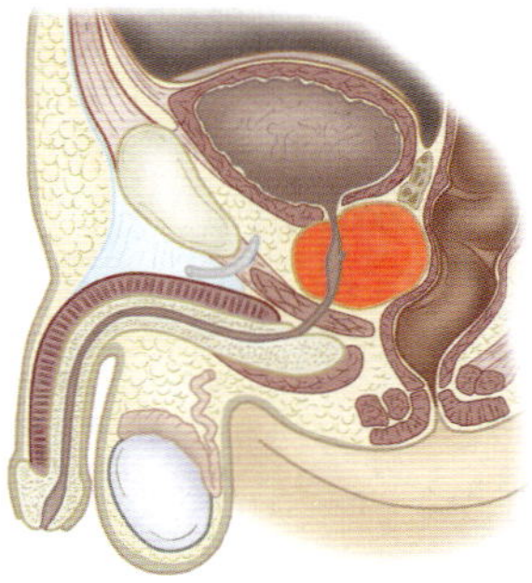

FIG. 21.13 Prostatitis.

PATIENT DATA

Subjective Data

- Acute
  - Pain
  - Urination problems
  - Sexual dysfunction
  - Fever, chills, shakes
- Chronic
  - Asymptomatic
  - Frequent bladder infections
  - Frequent urination
  - Persistent pain in the lower abdomen or back

Objective Data

- Acute
  - Gentle examination imperative; massage of the prostate can cause bacteremia
  - Prostate enlarged, acutely tender, and often asymmetric
  - Abscess may develop, felt as a fluctuant mass in the prostate
  - Seminal vesicles are often involved and may be dilated and tender on palpation; however, the prostate may feel boggy, enlarged, and tender or have palpable areas of fibrosis that simulate neoplasm
  - Bacteria in the urine
- Chronic
  - Prostate may be normal in size and consistency
  - May be enlarged and boggy
  - Prostate massage required for specimen collection

Think About It

Prostate massage is required in chronic prostatitis but contraindicated in acute prostatitis. How do you determine when to perform a prostate massage? Observation and a detailed history are essential. Patients with acute bacterial prostatitis typically appear ill and may have chills, fever, urinary frequency and urgency, perineal pain, and low back pain. They may have obstructive symptoms such as hesitancy, incomplete voiding, straining to urinate, and weak stream. They may also report painful ejaculation, hematospermia, and painful defecation. Patients with chronic prostatitis generally report recurrent urinary tract infections. Common symptoms, when present, do mirror those of acute prostatitis with urinary frequency, dysuria with or without obstructive symptoms, low back pain and perineal discomfort. However, these symptoms have been present for weeks or months. Patients with chronic prostatitis do not have the ill appearance of those with acute prostatitis and may be asymptomatic.

CLINICAL PEARL

Unexplained Fever

The search for an unexplained fever should always include the rectal examination—a rectal abscess or prostatitis may be the cause.

Benign Prostatic Hypertrophy

Nonmalignant enlargement of the prostate

PATHOPHYSIOLOGY

- Common in patients older than 50 years
- Gland begins to grow at adolescence, continuing to enlarge with advancing age (Fig. 21.14)

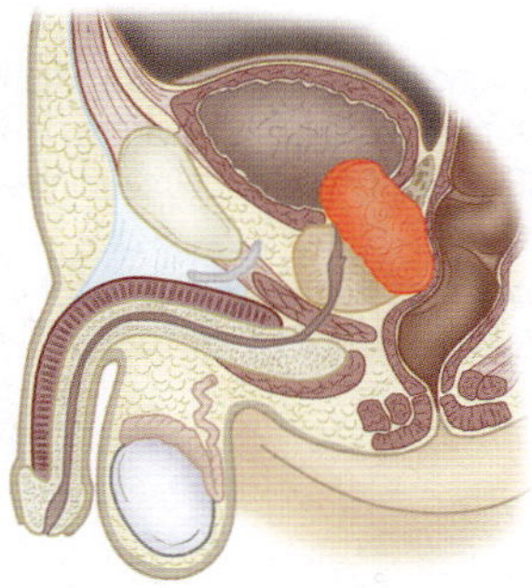

FIG. 21.14 Benign prostatic hypertrophy.

PATIENT DATA

Subjective Data

- Symptoms of urinary obstruction: hesitancy, decreased force and caliber of stream, dribbling, incomplete emptying of the bladder, frequency, urgency, nocturia, and dysuria

Objective Data

- Prostate feels smooth, rubbery, symmetric, and enlarged
- Median sulcus may or may not be obliterated

Prostate Cancer

Cancer of the prostate

PATHOPHYSIOLOGY

- More than 99% of prostate cancers are adenocarcinomas, developing from the gland cells in the prostate (Fig. 21.15)
- In most cases, prostate cancer is a relatively slow-growing cancer; a small percentage is a rapidly growing, aggressive form
- Incidence increases with age and is less frequent in patients younger than 50 years of age
- Pathogenesis poorly understood; following the initial transformation event, further mutations of a multitude of genes lead to tumor progression and metastasis

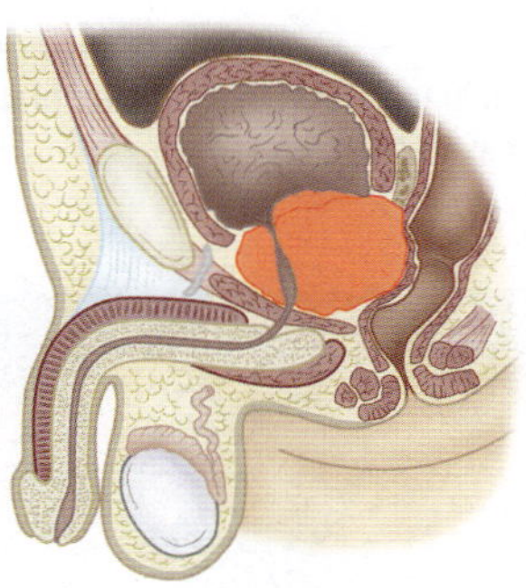

FIG. 21.15 Cancer of the prostate.

PATIENT DATA

Subjective Data

- Early carcinoma asymptomatic
- As the malignancy advances, symptoms of urinary obstruction occur (see symptoms listed for benign prostatic hyperplasia [BPH])

Objective Data

- A hard, irregular nodule may be palpable on prostate examination
- Prostate feels asymmetric, and the median sulcus may be obliterated
- Biopsy required for diagnosis

Infants and Children

Imperforate Anus

Congenital defect in which the opening to the anus is missing or blocked

PATHOPHYSIOLOGY

- A variety of anorectal malformations can occur during fetal development
- Rectum may end blindly, be stenosed, or have a fistulous connection to the perineum, urinary tract, or vagina (Fig. 21.16)

PATIENT DATA

Subjective Data

- Lack of passage of stools

Objective Data

- Condition is usually diagnosed during newborn examination on rectal examination and confirmed by lack of passage of stool within the first 48 hours of life (Figs. 21.17 and 21.18); radiographic confirmation may be necessary
- Be aware that the imperforation may be just out of the reach of the examining finger on infrequent occasions

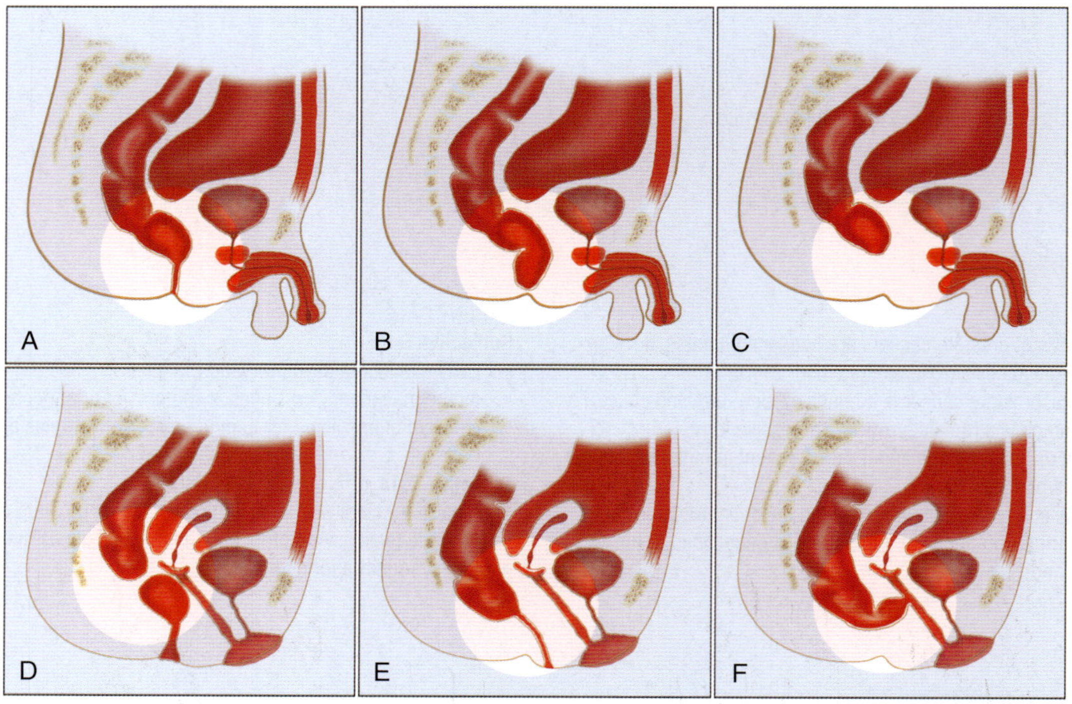

FIG. 21.16 Imperforate anus: various anorectal malformations. (A) Congenital anal stenosis. (B) Anal membrane atresia. (C) Anal agenesis. (D) Rectal atresia. (E) Rectoperineal fistula. (F) Rectovaginal fistula.

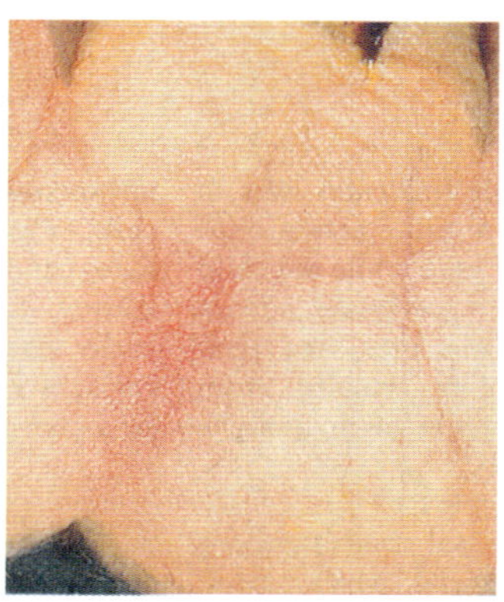

FIG. 21.17 Imperforate anus. (From Wolfe J: *400 Self-assessment picture tests in clinical medicine*, Chicago, 1984, Elsevier. From American Academy of Dermatology, 2006. By permission of Mosby International.)

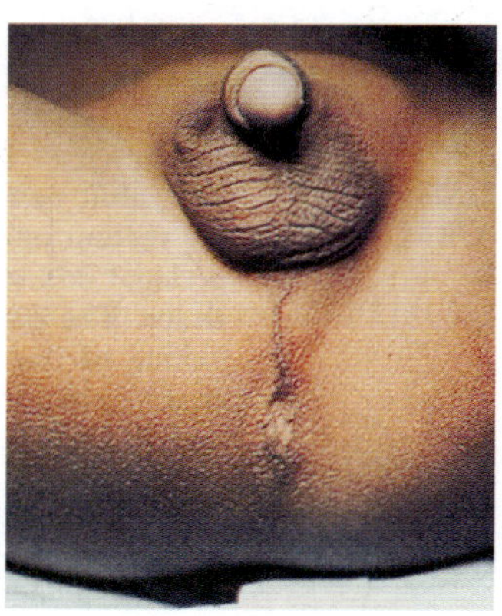

FIG. 21.18 Rectal atresia. (Courtesy Gershon Efron, MD, Sinai Hospital of Baltimore.)

Enterobiasis (Roundworm, Pinworm)

Infection caused by a small, thin, white roundworm, *Enterobius vermicularis*

PATHOPHYSIOLOGY

- Adult nematode (parasite) lives in the rectum or colon and emerges onto perianal skin to lay eggs while the child sleeps

PATIENT DATA

Subjective Data

- Intense itching of the perianal area
- Parents often describe unexplained irritability in the infant or child, especially at night

Objective Data

- Perianal irritation often results from scratching
- Can be diagnosed using Scotch tape test: press the sticky side of cellulose tape against the perianal folds, and then press the tape on a glass slide; nematodes can be seen on microscopic examination

CHAPTER

22 Musculoskeletal System

The musculoskeletal system provides the stability and mobility necessary for physical activity. Physical performance requires bones, tendons, ligaments, muscles, and joints that function smoothly and effortlessly. Because the musculoskeletal system serves as the body's main defense against external forces, injuries are common. Moreover, numerous disease processes affect the musculoskeletal system and can ultimately cause disability. The purpose of this chapter is to review a systematic approach to the evaluation of the musculoskeletal system.

Physical Examination Components

1. Inspect the skeleton and extremities and compare sides for:
   - Alignment
   - Contour and symmetry
   - Size
   - Deformity
2. Inspect the skin and subcutaneous tissues over muscles and joints for:
   - Color
   - Number of skinfolds
   - Swelling
   - Masses
3. Inspect muscles and compare sides for:
   - Size
   - Symmetry
   - Fasciculations or spasms
4. Palpate all bones, joints, and surrounding muscles for:
   - Muscle tone
   - Warmth
   - Tenderness
   - Swelling
   - Crepitus
5. Test each major joint for active and passive range of motion and compare sides.
6. Test major muscle groups for strength and compare sides.

Joints that deserve particular attention include the following:

Hands and Wrists

1. Inspect the dorsum and palm of hands for:
   - Contour
   - Position
   - Shape
   - Number and completeness of digits
2. Palpate each joint in the hand and wrist.
3. Test range of motion by the following maneuvers:
   - Metacarpophalangeal flexion (90 degrees) and hyperextension (30 degrees)
   - Thumb opposition
   - Forming a fist
   - Finger adduction and abduction
   - Wrist extension, hyperextension, and flexion
   - Radial and ulnar motion
4. Test muscle strength by the following maneuvers:
   - Wrist extension and hyperextension
   - Hand grip strength

Elbows

1. Inspect the elbows in flexed and extended positions for:
   - Contour
   - Carrying angle (5 to 15 degrees)
2. Palpate the extensor surface of the ulna, olecranon process, and medial and lateral epicondyles of the humerus.
3. Test range of motion by the following maneuvers:
   - Flexion (160 degrees)
   - Extension (180 degrees)
   - Pronation and supination (90 degrees)

Shoulders

1. Inspect shoulders and shoulder girdle for contour.
2. Palpate the joint spaces and bones of the shoulders.
3. Test range of motion by the following maneuvers:
   - Shrugging the shoulders
   - Forward flexion (180 degrees) and hyperextension (up to 50 degrees)
   - Abduction (180 degrees) and adduction (50 degrees)
   - Internal and external rotation (90 degrees)
4. Test muscle strength by the following maneuvers:
   - Shrugged shoulders
   - Abduction with forward flexion
   - Medial rotation
   - Lateral rotation

Temporomandibular Joint

1. Palpate the joint space for clicking, popping, and pain.
2. Test range of motion by having the patient perform the following:
   - Opening and closing mouth
   - Moving jaw laterally to each side
   - Protruding and retracting the jaw
3. Test strength of temporalis muscles with the patient's teeth clenched.

Physical Examination Components—cont'd

Cervical Spine

1. Inspect the neck for alignment and symmetry of skinfolds and muscles.
2. Test range of motion by the following maneuvers:
   - Forward flexion (45 degrees)
   - Hyperextension (55 degrees)
   - Lateral bending (40 degrees)
   - Rotation (70 degrees)
3. Test strength of sternocleidomastoid and trapezius muscles (cranial nerve XI, spinal accessory).

Thoracic and Lumbar Spine

1. Inspect the spine for alignment.
2. Palpate the spinal processes and paravertebral muscles.
3. Percuss for spinal tenderness.
4. Test range of motion.

Hips

1. Inspect the hips for symmetry and level of gluteal folds.
2. Palpate hips and pelvis for:
   - Instability
   - Tenderness
   - Crepitus
3. Test range of motion by the following maneuvers:
   - Flexion (120 degrees), extension (90 degrees), and hyperextension (30 degrees)
   - Adduction (30 degrees) and abduction (45 degrees)
   - Internal rotation (40 degrees)
   - External rotation (45 degrees)
4. Test muscle strength of hips with the following maneuvers:
   - Knee in flexion and extension
   - Abduction and adduction

Legs and Knees

1. Inspect the knees for natural concavities.
2. Palpate the popliteal space and joint space.
3. Test range of motion by flexion (130 degrees) and extension (0 to 15 degrees).
4. Test the strength of muscles in flexion and extension.

Feet and Ankles

1. Inspect the feet and ankles during weight bearing and non–weight bearing for:
   - Contour
   - Alignment with tibias
   - Size
   - Number of toes
2. Palpate the Achilles tendon and each metatarsal joint.
3. Test range of motion by the following maneuvers:
   - Dorsiflexion (20 degrees) and plantar flexion (45 degrees)
   - Inversion (30 degrees) and eversion (20 degrees)
   - Flexion and extension of the toes
4. Test strength of muscles in plantar flexion and dorsiflexion.

ANATOMY AND PHYSIOLOGY

The musculoskeletal system is a bony structure that provides stability to the soft tissues of the body. Its joints are held together by ligaments, attached to muscles by tendons, and cushioned by cartilage, which facilitates movement (Figs. 22.1 and 22.2). The musculoskeletal system protects vital organs; provides storage space for minerals (phosphorus, calcium, and carbonate); and produces blood cells within the bone marrow (hematopoiesis).

Most joints are synovial—freely moving articulations containing ligaments and cartilage covering the ends of the opposing bones, which are enclosed by a fibrous capsule. A synovial membrane lines the joint and secretes the serous lubricating synovial fluid. Bursae develop in the spaces of connective tissue between tendons, ligaments, and bones to promote ease of motion at points where friction would occur.

Upper Extremities

The radiocarpal joint (wrist) consists of the articulation of the radius and the carpal bones. Additional articulations occur between the proximal and distal rows of carpal bones. An articular disk separates the ulna and carpal bones, and the joint is protected by ligaments and a fibrous capsule. The wrist moves in two planes. There is flexion and extension movement as well as radial and ulnar (rotational) movement. The hand has articulations between the carpals and metacarpals, metacarpals and proximal phalanges, and middle and distal phalanges (Fig. 22.3). The forearm joints consist of the articulations between the radius and ulna at both the proximal and distal locations. These are important for pronation and supination.

The elbow consists of the articulation of the humerus, radius, and ulna. Its three contiguous surfaces are enclosed in a single synovial cavity, with the collateral ligaments of the radius and ulna securing the joint. A bursa lies between the olecranon and the skin (Fig. 22.4). The elbow is a hinge joint, permitting movement of the humerus and ulna in one plane (flexion and extension).

The glenohumeral joint (shoulder) consists of the articulation between the humerus and the glenoid fossa of the scapula. The acromion and coracoid processes and the ligament between them form the arch surrounding and protecting the joint (Fig. 22.5A). Four muscles (supraspinatus, infraspinatus, teres minor, and subscapularis) and their tendons comprise the rotator cuff, reinforcing the glenohumeral joint to stabilize the shoulder and the position of the humeral head within the joint (see Fig. 22.5B). The shoulder is a ball-and-socket joint that permits movement of the humerus in several axes.

Two additional joints adjacent to the glenohumeral joint complete the articulation of the shoulder girdle.

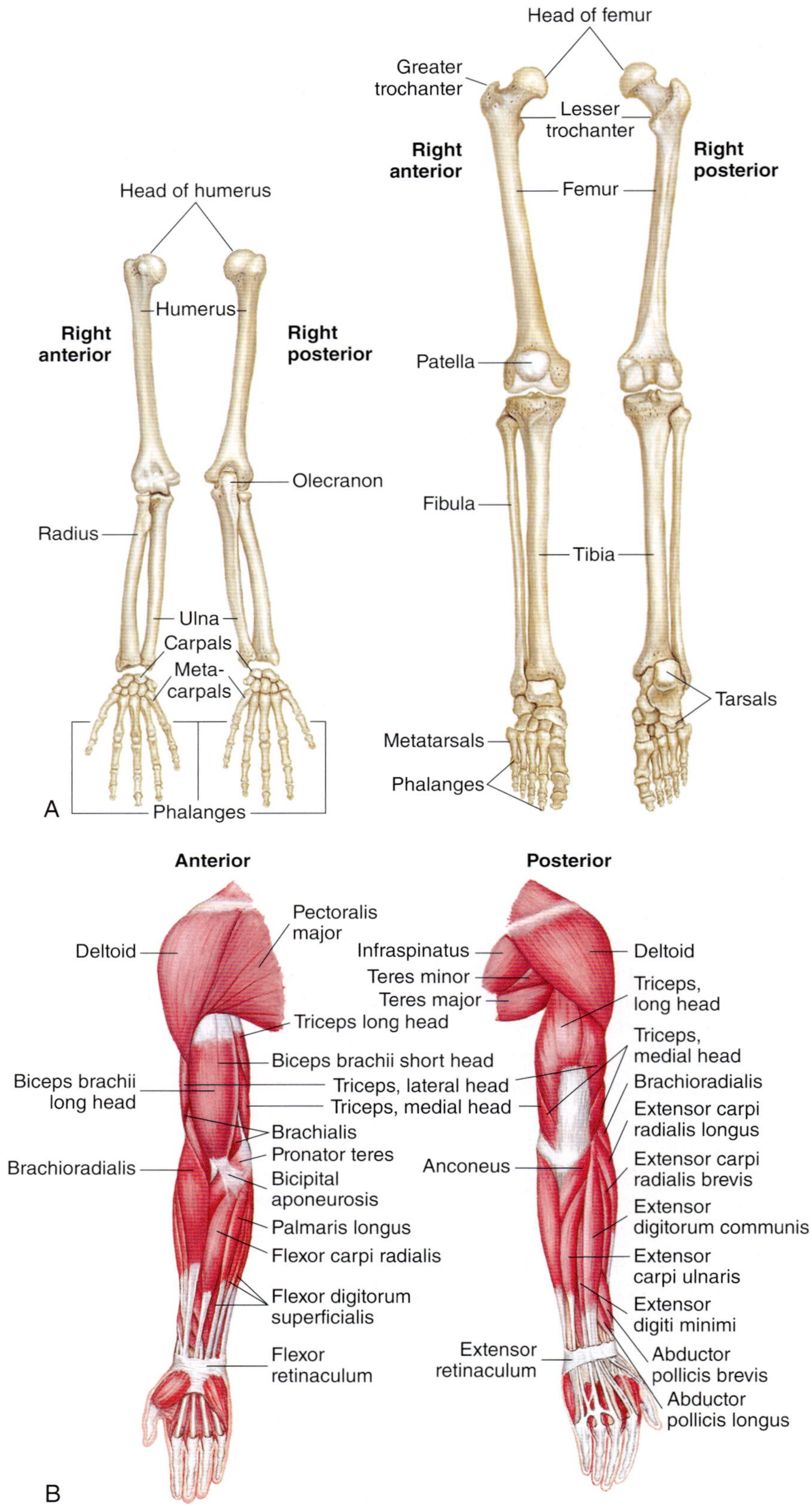

FIG. 22.1 (A) Bones of the upper and lower extremities. (B) Muscles of the upper extremities.

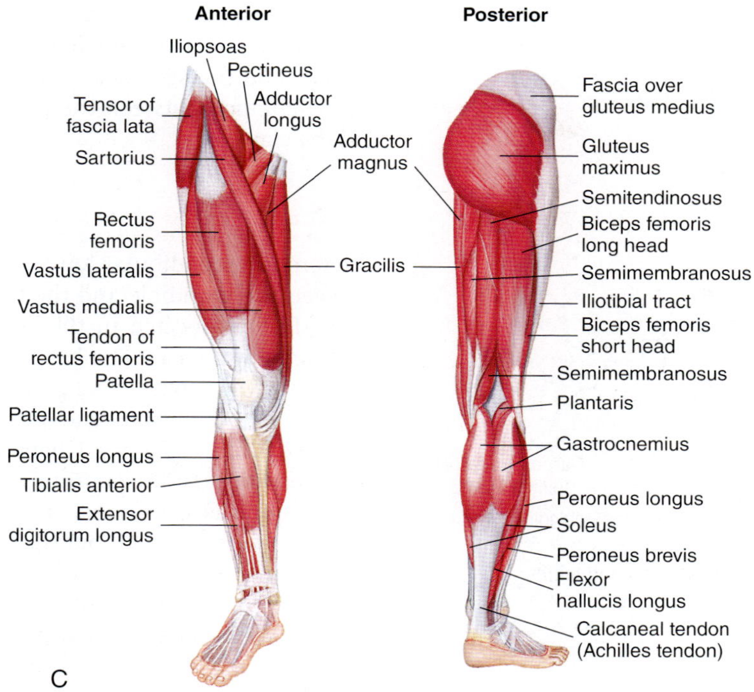

FIG. 22.1, cont'd (C) Muscles of the lower extremities.

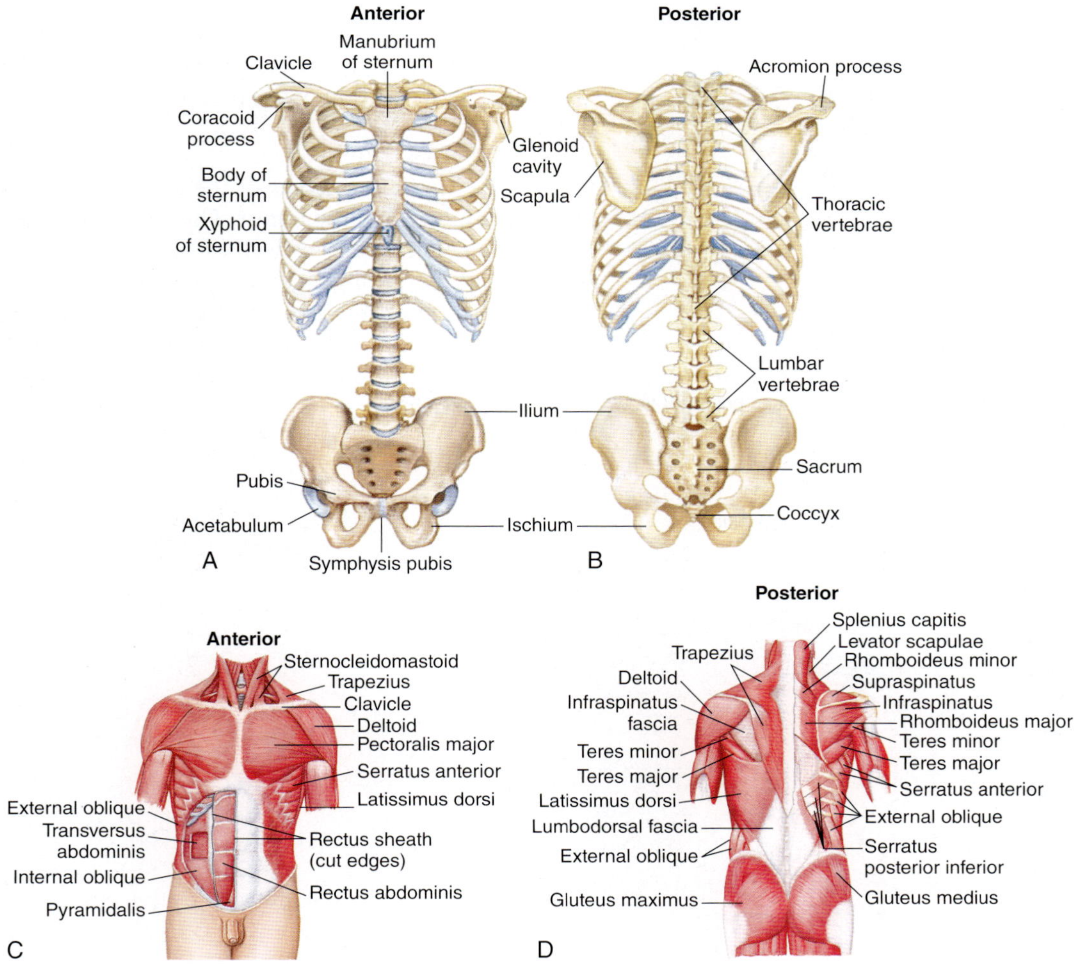

FIG. 22.2 (A) Bones of the trunk, anterior view. (B) Bones of the trunk, posterior view. (C) Superficial muscles of the trunk, anterior view. (D) Superficial muscles of the trunk, posterior view.

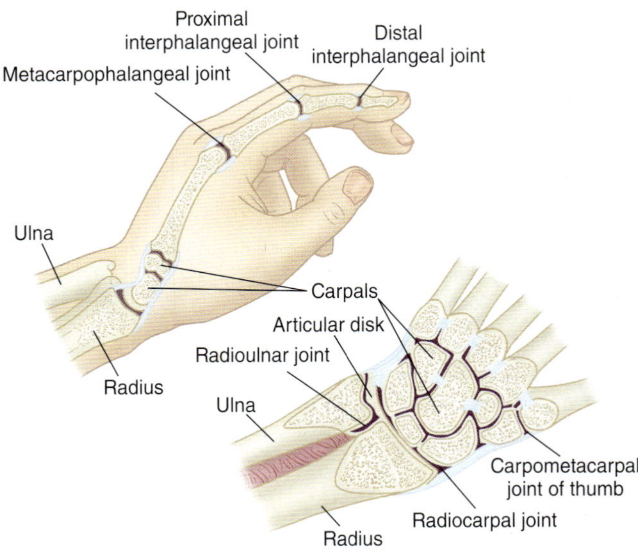

FIG. 22.3 Structures of the wrist and hand joints.

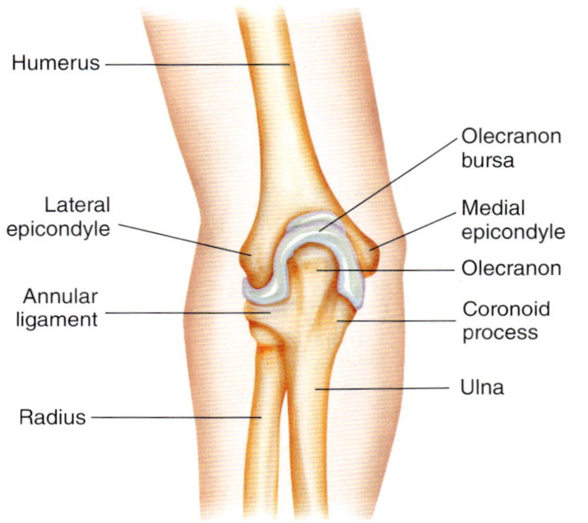

FIG. 22.4 Structures of the left elbow joint, posterior view.

These are the acromioclavicular joint, which consists of the articulation between the acromion process and the clavicle, and the sternoclavicular joint, which consists of the articulation between the manubrium of the sternum and the clavicle.

Head and Spine

The temporomandibular joint consists of the articulation between the mandible and the temporal bone in the cranium. Each is located in the depression just anterior to the tragus of the ear. The hinge action of the joint opens and closes the mouth. The gliding action permits lateral movement, protrusion, and retraction of the mandible (Figs. 22.6 and 22.7). See Chapter 11 for a description of the fused bones of the cranium.

The spine is composed of cervical, thoracic, lumbar, and sacral vertebrae. All but the sacral vertebrae are separated from each other by fibrocartilaginous disks. Each disk has a central area of fibrogelatinous material, known as the *nucleus pulposus,* that cushions the vertebral bodies (Fig. 22.8). The vertebrae form a series of joints that glide slightly over each other's surfaces, permitting movement in several axes. The cervical vertebrae are the most mobile. Flexion and extension occur between the skull and C1, whereas rotation occurs between C1 and C2. The sacral vertebrae are fused and, with the coccyx, form the posterior portion of the pelvis.

Lower Extremities

The hip joint consists of the articulation between the acetabulum and the femur. The depth of the acetabulum in the pelvic bone—as well as the joint, which is supported by three strong ligaments—helps stabilize and protect the head of the femur in the joint capsule. Multiple bursae reduce friction in the hip. The hip is a ball-and-socket joint, permitting movement of the femur on many axes (Fig. 22.9).

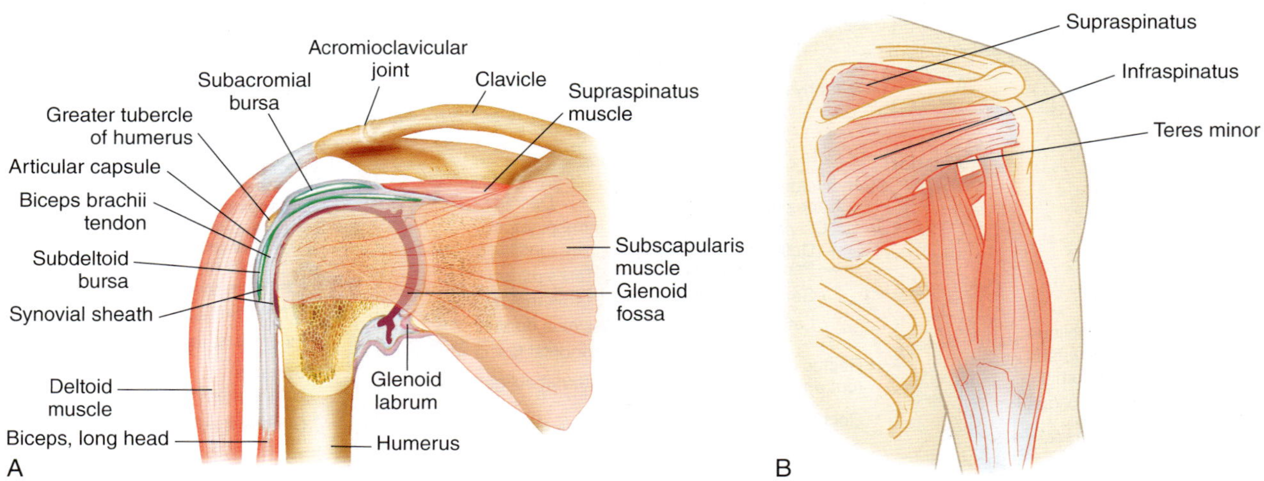

FIG. 22.5 Structures of the shoulder. (A) Structures of glenohumeral and acromioclavicular joints, anterior view. (B) Rotator cuff muscles of shoulder, posterior view.

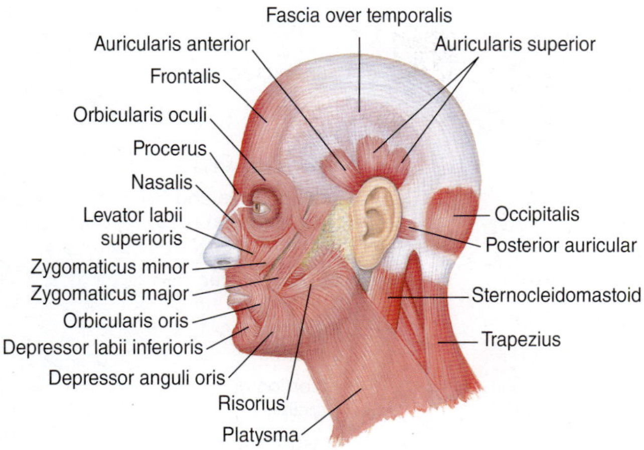

FIG. 22.6 **Muscles of the face and head, left lateral view.**

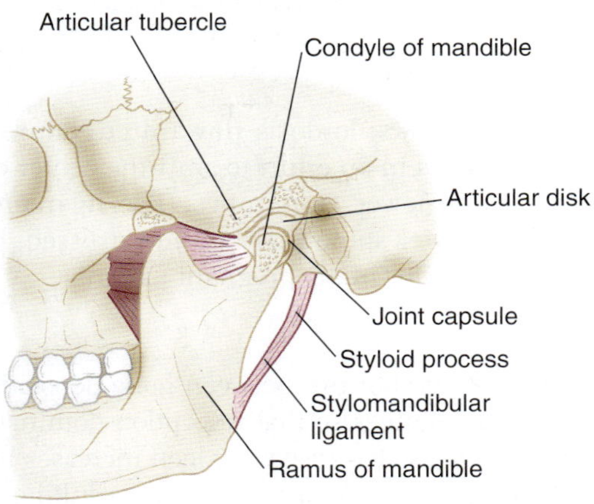

FIG. 22.7 **Structures of the temporomandibular joint.**

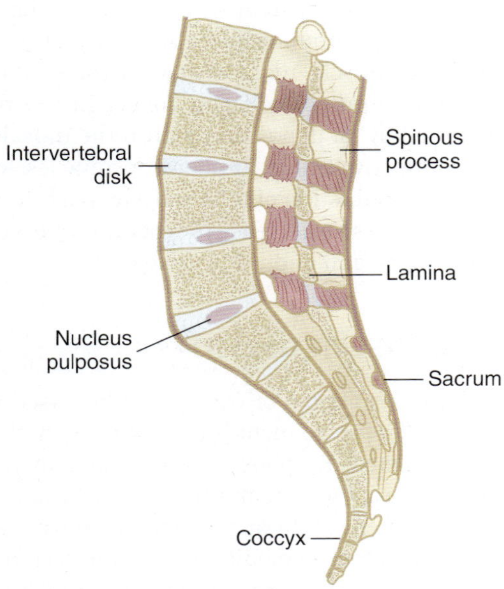

FIG. 22.8 **Structures of vertebral joints.**

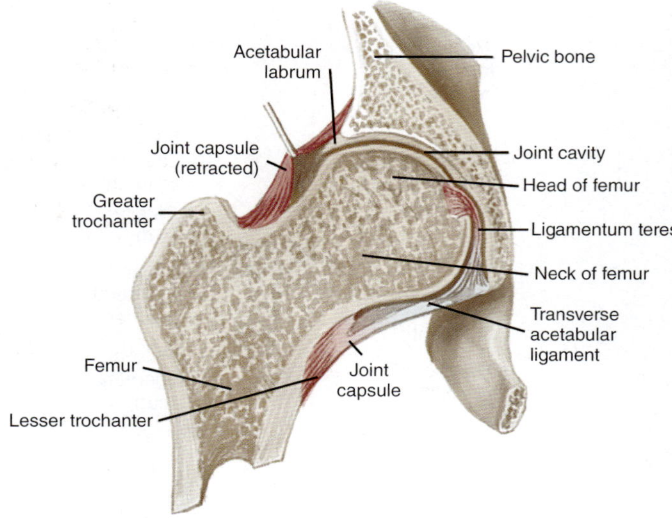

FIG. 22.9 **Structures of the hip.** (From Rothrock JC: *Alexander's care of the patient in surgery*, ed 12, St Louis, 2007, Mosby.)

The knee consists of four bones (femur, tibia, fibula, and patella), with three separate articulating compartments: the lateral tibiofemoral, the medial tibiofemoral, and the patellofemoral. Fibrocartilaginous disks (medial and lateral menisci), which cushion the tibia and femur, are attached to the tibia and the joint capsule. Collateral ligaments give medial and lateral stability to the knee. Two cruciate ligaments cross obliquely within the knee, adding anterior and posterior stability. The anterior cruciate ligament protects the knee from hyperextension. There are four separate bursae in the anterior knee that help to reduce the friction of knee movement. The knee is a hinge joint, permitting movement (flexion and extension) between the femur and tibia in one plane (Fig. 22.10).

The tibiotalar joint (ankle) consists of the articulation of the tibia, fibula, and talus. It is protected by ligaments on the medial and lateral surfaces. The tibiotalar joint is a hinge joint that permits flexion and extension (dorsiflexion and plantar flexion) in one plane. Additional joints in the ankle—the talocalcaneal joint (subtalar) and transverse tarsal joint—permit it to pivot or rotate (pronation and supination). Articulations of the foot between the tarsals and metatarsals, the metatarsals and proximal phalanges, and the middle and distal phalanges allow flexion and extension (Fig. 22.11) to occur.

Infants and Children

During fetal development, the skeletal system emerges from embryologic connective tissues to form cartilage that calcifies to become bone. Throughout infancy and childhood, long bones increase in diameter through the growth of new bone tissue around the bone shaft. Increased length of long bones results from the proliferation of cartilage at the growth plates (epiphyses). In the smaller bones, such as the carpals, ossification centers form in calcified cartilage. Ligaments are stronger than bone until

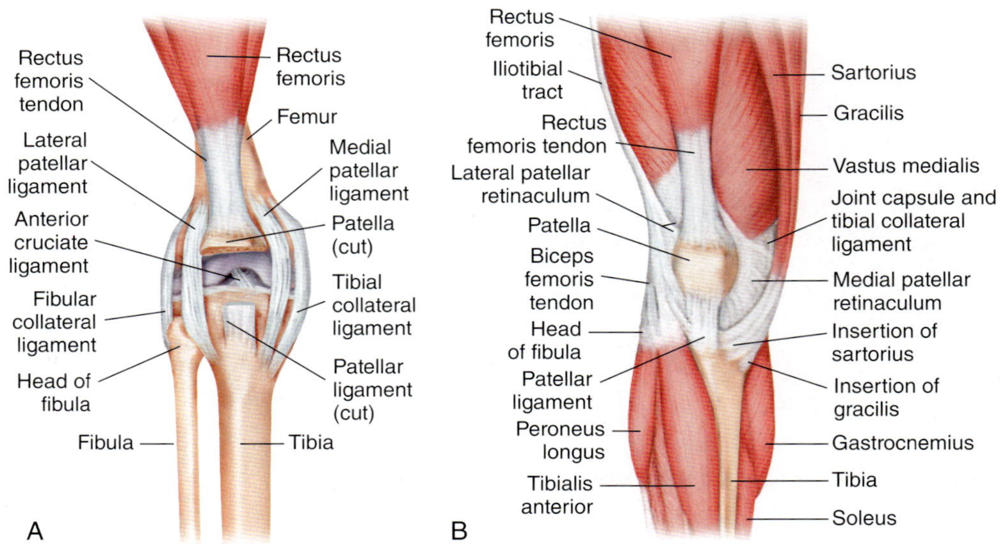

FIG. 22.10 Structures of the knee, anterior view. (A) Bones and ligaments of the joint. (B) Muscles attaching at the knee.

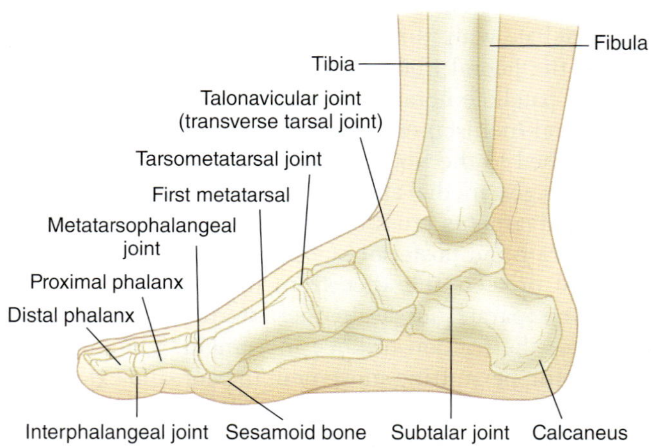

FIG. 22.11 Bones and joints of the ankle and foot.

adolescence; as such, injuries to long bones and joints are more likely to result in fractures than in sprains.

Adolescents

Rapid growth during Tanner stage 3 (see Chapter 8) results in decreased strength in the epiphyses as well as overall decreased strength and flexibility, leading to greater potential for injury. Bone growth is completed at about age 20, when the last epiphysis closes and becomes firmly fused to the shaft. Once bone growth stops, bone density and strength continue to increase. Peak bone mass is not achieved until about 35 years of age.

Pregnant Patients

Increased hormone levels contribute to the elasticity of ligaments and softening of the cartilage in the pelvis at about 12 to 20 weeks of gestation. As a result, there is increased mobility of the sacroiliac, sacrococcygeal, and symphysis pubis joints.

As the fetus grows, lordosis (inward curvature of the lower spine) occurs in an effort to shift the center of gravity back over the lower extremities. The ligaments and muscles of the lower spine may become stressed, leading to lower back pain for many pregnant patients.

Older Adults

With aging, the equilibrium between bone deposition and bone resorption changes so that resorption dominates. For menopausal females, decreased estrogen increases bone resorption and decreases calcium deposition, resulting in bone loss and decreased bone density. By 80 years of age, up to 30% of bone mass can be lost. The loss of bone density affects the entire skeleton, but the weight-bearing long bones and the vertebrae are particularly vulnerable to fractures. Bony prominences become more apparent with the loss of subcutaneous fat. The cartilage around joints also deteriorates.

Initially, the muscle mass also undergoes alteration as increased amounts of collagen collect in the tissues. This is followed by fat deposition within the muscles and fibrosis of connective tissue. Tendons become less elastic. This results in a reduction of total muscle mass, tone, and strength. A progressive decrease in reaction time, speed of movement, agility, and endurance also occurs.

REVIEW OF RELATED HISTORY

For each of the symptoms or conditions discussed in this section, targeted topics to include in the history of the present illness are listed. Responses to questions about these topics provide clues for focusing the physical examination and the development of an appropriate diagnostic evaluation. Questions regarding medication use (prescription and over-the-counter preparations) as well as complementary, alternative, and integrative therapies are relevant for each.

History of Present Illness

Joint Symptoms

- Character: stiffness or limitation of movement, change in size or contour, swelling or redness, constant pain or pain with particular motion, unilateral or bilateral involvement, interference with daily activities, joint locking or giving way
- Associated events: time of day, activity, specific movements, injury, strenuous activity, weather
- Temporal factors: change in frequency or character of episodes, better or worse as day progresses, nature of onset (sudden or gradual)
- Efforts to treat: exercise, rest, weight reduction, physical therapy, heat, ice, braces or splints
- Medications: nonsteroidal antiinflammatory drugs (NSAIDs), acetaminophen, biologic modifiers and other immunosuppressants, corticosteroids, topical analgesics, glucosamine, chondroitin, hyaluronic acid; complementary, alternative, and integrative therapies

Muscular Symptoms

- Character: limitation of movement, weakness or fatigue, paralysis, tremor, tics, spasms, clumsiness, wasting, aching, pain
- Precipitating factors: injury, strenuous activity, sudden movement, stress
- Efforts to treat: heat, ice, splints, rest, massage
- Medications: muscle relaxants, statins, NSAIDs

Skeletal Symptoms

- Character: difficulty with gait or limping; numbness, tingling, or pressure sensation; pain with movement, crepitus; deformity or change in skeletal contour
- Associated event: injury, recent fractures, strenuous activity, sudden movement, stress, postmenopause
- Efforts to treat: rest, splints, chiropractic, acupuncture
- Medications: hormone therapy, calcium, calcitonin, bisphosphonates

Injury

- Sensation at time of injury: click, pop, tearing, numbness, tingling, catching, locking, grating, snapping, warmth or coldness, ability to bear weight
- Mechanism of injury: direct trauma, overuse, sudden change of direction, forceful contraction, overstretch
- Pain: location, type, onset (sudden or gradual), aggravating or alleviating factors, position of comfort
- Swelling: location, timing (with activity or injury)
- Efforts to treat: rest, ice, heat, splints
- Medications: analgesics, NSAIDs

Back Pain

- Abrupt or gradual onset, better or worse with activity
- Character of pain and sensation: tearing, burning, or steady ache; tingling or numbness; location and distribution (unilateral or bilateral); radiation to buttocks, groin, or legs; triggered by coughing or sneezing and sudden movements
- Associated event: trauma, lifting of heavy weights, long-distance driving, sports activities, change in posture or deformity
- Efforts to treat: rest, avoid standing or sudden movements, chiropractic, acupuncture
- Medications: muscle relaxants, analgesics, NSAIDs

Past Medical History

- Trauma: nerves, soft tissue, bones, joints; residual problems; bone infection
- Surgery on joint or bone; amputation, arthroscopy
- Chronic illness: cancer, arthritis, sickle cell disease, hemophilia, osteoporosis, renal or neurologic disorder
- Skeletal deformities or congenital anomalies

Family History

- Congenital abnormalities of hip or foot
- Scoliosis or back problems
- Arthritis: rheumatoid, osteoarthritis, ankylosing spondylitis, gout
- Genetic disorders: osteogenesis imperfecta, skeletal dysplasia, rickets, hypophosphatemia, hypercalciuria

Risk Factors

Osteoarthritis

- Obesity
- Female
- Family history of osteoarthritis
- Hypermobility syndromes
- Aging (older than 40 years)
- Injury, high level of sports activities
- Peripheral neuropathy
- Occupation requiring overuse of joints

Data from Blagojevic, M., Jinks, C., Jeffery, A., & Jordan, K. P. (2010). Risk factors for onset of osteoarthritis of the knee in older adults: A systematic review and meta-analysis. *Osteoarthritis and cartilage*, *18*(1), 24–33.

Personal and Social History

- Employment: past and current, lifting and potential for unintentional injury, repetitive motions, typing/computer use, safety precautions, use of spinal support, chronic stress on joints
- Exercise: extent, type, and frequency; weight bearing; stress on specific joints; overall conditioning; sport (level of competition, type of shoes and athletic gear); warm-up and cool-down routines with exercise
- Functional abilities: personal care (eating, bathing, dressing, grooming, elimination); other activities

(housework, walking, climbing stairs, caring for pet); use of prosthesis
- Weight: recent gain, overweight or underweight for body frame
- Height: maximum height achieved, any changes
- Nutrition: amount of calcium, vitamin D, calories, and protein
- Tobacco or alcohol use

Infants and Children

- Birth history
- Presentation, large for gestational age, birth injuries (may result in fractures or nerve damage), type of delivery (vaginal vs. cesarean delivery), use of forceps
- Low birth weight, premature, resuscitation efforts, intrauterine insult or perinatal asphyxia, fetal stroke, maternal infections leading to muscle tone disorders, required ventilator support (may result in anoxia leading to muscle tone disorders)
- Fine and gross motor developmental milestones, appropriate for chronologic age
- Overweight or obese
- Quality of movement: spasticity, flaccidity
- Arm or leg pain
  - Character: localized or generalized; in muscle or joint; limitation of movement; associated with movement, trauma, or growth spurt
  - Onset: age, sudden or gradual, at night or with rest, after activity
- Participation in organized or competitive sports, weightlifting

Pregnant Patients

- Muscle cramps: nature of onset, frequency and time of occurrence, muscles involved, efforts to treat
- Back pain
- Weeks of gestation, associated with multiple pregnancies, efforts to treat
- Associated symptoms: uterine tightening, nausea, vomiting, fever, malaise (could signify musculoskeletal discomfort if not from another condition)
- Type of shoes (heels may increase lordosis)

Older Adults

- Weakness
  - Onset: sudden or gradual, localized or generalized, with activity or after sustained activity
  - Associated symptoms: stiffness of joints, muscle spasms or tension, any particular activity, dyspnea
- Increase in minor injuries: stumbling, falls, limited agility; association with poor vision
- Change in ease of movement: loss of ability to perform sudden movements, change in exercise endurance, pain, stiffness, localized to particular joints or generalized
- Nocturnal muscle spasm: frequency, associated back pain, numbness or coldness of extremities
- History of injuries or excessive use of a joint or group of joints, known joint abnormalities
- Previous fractures, bone mineral density screening
- Medications: steroids, calcium, bisphosphonates, NSAIDs

Risk Factors

Osteoporosis

- Race (White, Asian, Native American/American Indian); northwestern European descent
- Low body weight
- Increasing age
- Family history of osteoporosis, previous fractures
- Nulliparous
- Amenorrhea or menopause before 45 years of age, postmenopausal
- Sedentary lifestyle, lack of aerobic or weight-bearing exercise
- Constant dieting, inadequate calcium and vitamin D intake, excessive carbonated soft drinks per day
- Scoliosis, rheumatoid arthritis, cancer, multiple sclerosis, chronic illness
- Metabolic disorders (e.g., diabetes, hypercortisolism, malabsorption, hypogonadism, hyperthyroidism)
- Drugs that decrease bone density (e.g., thyroxine, corticosteroids, heparin, lithium, anticonvulsants, antacids with aluminum)
- Cigarette smoking or heavy alcohol use

EXAMINATION AND FINDINGS

Equipment

- Skin-marking pencil
- Goniometer
- Tape measure
- Reflex hammer

Begin your examination of the musculoskeletal system by observing the gait and posture when the patient enters the examination room. Note how the patient walks, sits, rises from sitting position, takes off a coat, and responds to other directions given during the examination. If it is your preference to shake hands with the patient when you greet them, do so gently. If they have underlying arthritis or injury involving their right hand, your firm handshake may cause them significant discomfort.

As you give specific attention to bones, joints, tendons, ligaments, and muscles, expose the body surface and view under good lighting. Position the patient to provide the greatest stability to the joints. Examine each region of the body for limb and trunk stability, muscular strength and function, and joint range of motion. Position the extremities uniformly as you examine and look for asymmetry.

Inspection

Inspect the anterior, posterior, and lateral aspects of the patient's posture (Fig. 22.12). Observe the patient's

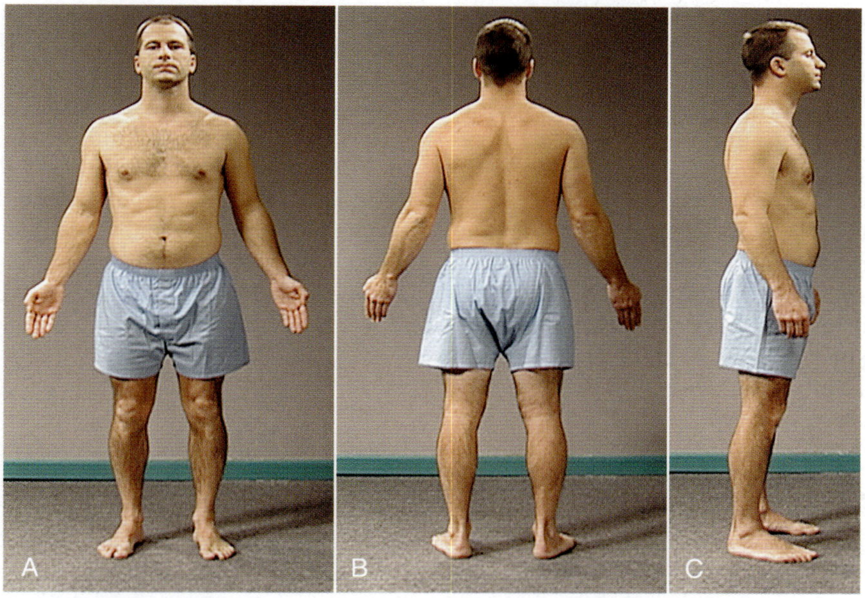

FIG. 22.12 **Inspection of overall body posture.** Note the even contour of the shoulders, level scapulae and iliac crests, alignment of the head over the gluteal folds, and symmetry and alignment of extremities. (A) Anterior view. (B) Posterior view. (C) Lateral view. The occiput, shoulders, buttocks, and heels should be able to touch the wall the patient stands against.

ability to stand erect, symmetry of body parts, and alignment of the extremities. Note any lordosis, kyphosis (overcurvature of the thoracic vertebrae), or scoliosis (curved from side to side) of the spine.

Inspect the skin and subcutaneous tissues overlying the articular structures for discoloration, swelling, and masses.

Observe the extremities for overall size, gross deformity, bony enlargement, alignment, contour, and symmetry of length and position. Expect to find bilateral symmetry in length, circumference, alignment, and the extremity position (see Clinical Pearl, "Bilateral Symmetry").

Inspect the muscles for gross hypertrophy or atrophy, fasciculations, and spasms. Muscle size should approximate symmetry bilaterally. Fasciculation (muscle twitching) occurs after injury to a muscle's motor neuron. Muscle wasting occurs after an injury as a result of pain, disease of the muscle, or damage to the motor neuron.

CLINICAL PEARL

Bilateral Symmetry

Bilateral symmetry should not be defined as absolute because there is no perfect symmetry. For example, the dominant forearm is expected to be larger in athletes who play racquet sports and in manual laborers.

Palpation

Palpate any bones, joints, tendons, and surrounding muscles if symptomatic. Palpate inflamed joints last, being aware of the patient's discomfort. Note any heat, tenderness, swelling, crepitus, pain, and resistance to movement. No discomfort should occur when you apply pressure to bones or joints. Muscle tone should be firm, not hard or doughy. Synovial thickening can sometimes be felt in joints that are close to the skin surface when the synovium is edematous or hypertrophied because of inflammation. Crepitus (a grating sound or sensation) can be felt when two irregular bony surfaces rub together as a joint moves, when two rough edges of a broken bone rub together, or with the movement of a tendon inside the tendon sheath when tenosynovitis is present.

Range of Motion and Muscle Tone

Examine both the active and passive ranges of motion for each major joint and its related muscle groups. Muscle tone is often evaluated simultaneously. Allow adequate space for the patient to move each muscle group and joint through its full range. Instruct the patient to move each joint through its range of motion as detailed in specific joint and muscle sections. Pain, limitation of motion, spastic movement, joint instability, deformity, or contracture may suggest a problem with the joint, related muscle group, or nerve supply.

Ask the patient to relax and allow you to passively move the same joints until the end of the range of motion is felt. Do not force the joint if there is pain or muscle spasm. Muscle tone may be assessed by feeling the resistance to passive stretch. During passive range of motion, the muscles should have slight tension. Passive range of motion often exceeds active range of motion by 5 degrees. The range of motion with active and passive maneuvers should be equal between contralateral joints. Discrepancies between active and passive ranges of motion may indicate true muscle weakness or a joint disorder. No crepitation or tenderness with movement should be apparent. Note the specific location of tenderness when present. Spastic muscles are harder to put through the ranges of motion. Measurements may vary if the muscle tested relaxes with gentle persistence.

When a joint appears to have an increase or a limitation in its range of motion, a goniometer (see Chapter 3) can be used to precisely measure the angle. Begin with the joint in the fully extended or neutral position and then flex the joint as far as possible. Measure the angles of greatest flexion and extension, comparing these with the expected joint flexion and extension values (Fig. 22.13).

Muscle Strength

Evaluating the strength of each muscle group is an important part of the neurologic examination. However, it is usually integrated with the examination of the associated joint for range of motion. Ask the patient first to contract the muscle you indicate by extending or flexing the joint and then to resist as you apply force against that muscle contraction (Fig. 22.14). Alternatively, tell the patient to push against your hand to feel the resistance. Compare the muscle strength bilaterally. Expect muscle strength to be bilaterally symmetric with full resistance to opposition. Full muscle strength requires a complete active range of motion.

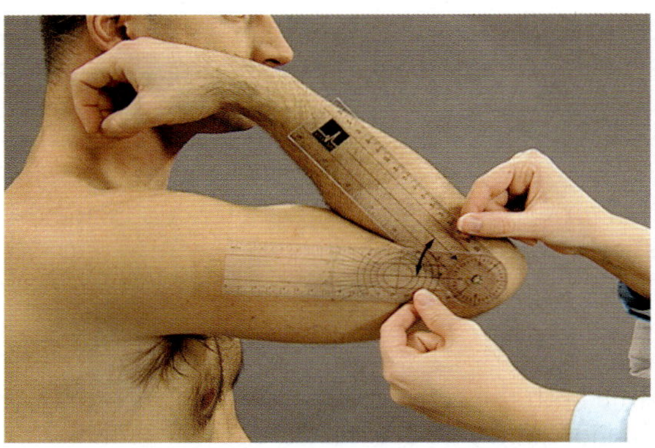

FIG. 22.13 Use of a goniometer to measure joint range of motion.

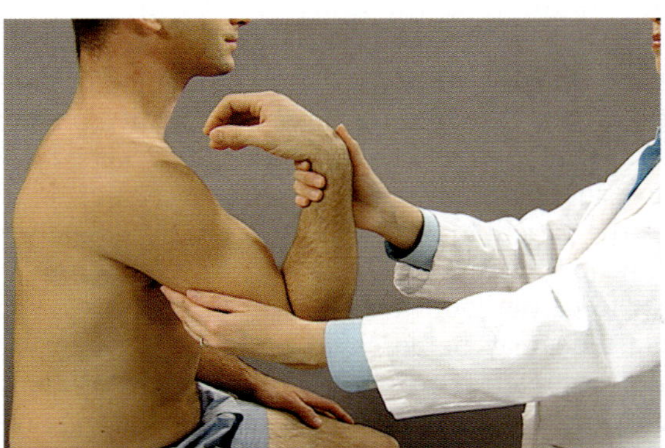

FIG. 22.14 Evaluation of muscle strength: flexion of the elbow against opposing force.

Variations in muscle strength are graded from no voluntary contraction to full muscle strength, using the scale in Table 22.1. When muscle strength is grade 3 or less, disability is present; activity cannot be accomplished in a gravity field, and external support is necessary to perform movements. Weakness may result from an underlying muscle disorder, pain, fatigue, or overstretching.

Specific Joints and Muscles

Hands and Wrists

Inspect the dorsal and palmar aspects of the hands, noting the contour, position, shape, number, and completeness of digits. Note the presence of palmar and phalangeal creases. The palmar surface of each hand should have a central depression with a prominent, rounded mound (thenar eminence) on the thumb side of the hand and a less prominent hypothenar eminence on the little finger side of the hand. Expect the fingers to fully extend when in close approximation and be aligned with the forearm. The lateral finger surfaces should gradually taper from the proximal to the distal aspects (Fig. 22.15).

Deviation of the fingers to the ulnar side and swan neck or boutonnière deformities of the fingers usually indicate rheumatoid arthritis (Fig. 22.16).

Palpate each joint in the hand and wrist. Palpate the interphalangeal joints with your thumb and index finger. The metacarpophalangeal joints are palpated with both thumbs. Palpate the wrist and radiocarpal groove with your thumbs on the dorsal surface and your fingers on the palmar aspect of the wrist (Fig. 22.17). Joint surfaces should be smooth and without nodules, swelling, bogginess, or tenderness. A firm mass over the dorsum of the wrist may be a ganglion.

Bony overgrowths in the distal interphalangeal joints, which are felt as hard, nontender nodules usually 2 to 3 mm in diameter but sometimes encompassing the entire joint, are associated with osteoarthritis. When located along the distal interphalangeal joints, they are called *Heberden*

TABLE 22.1 Assessing Muscle Strength

MUSCLE FUNCTION LEVEL	GRADE
No evidence of movement	0
Trace of movement	1
Full range of motion, but not against gravity[a]	2
Full range of motion against gravity but not against resistance	3
Full range of motion against gravity and some resistance, but weak	4
Full range of motion against gravity, full resistance	5

[a]Passive movement.

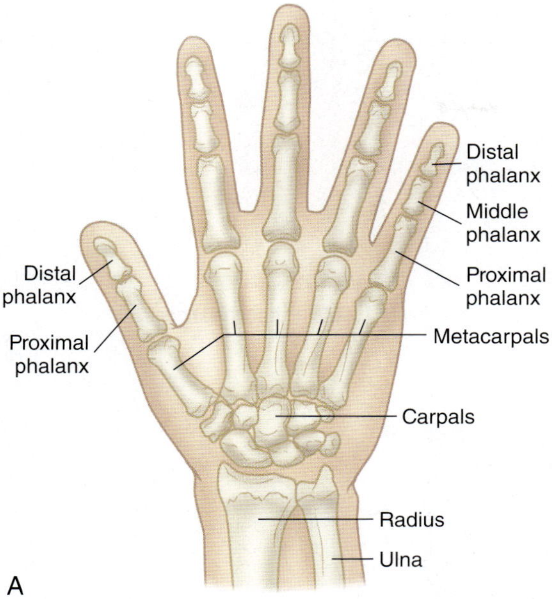

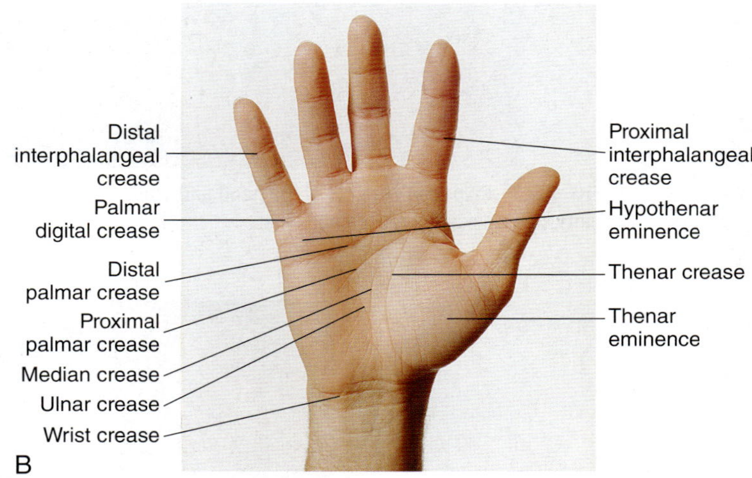

FIG. 22.15 (A) Bony structure of the right hand and wrist; note the alignment of the fingers with the radius. (B) Features of the palmar aspect of the hand; note creases, thenar eminence and hypothenar eminence, and gradual tapering of the fingers.

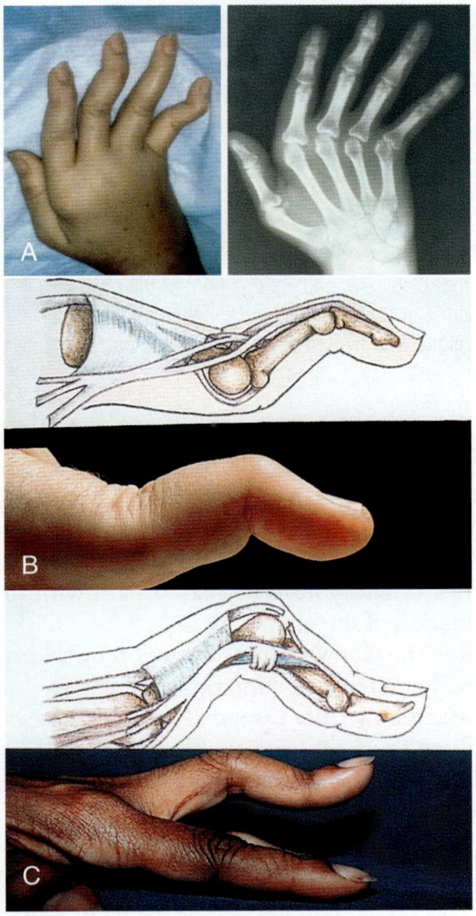

FIG. 22.16 Unexpected findings of the hand. (A) Ulnar deviation and subluxation of metacarpophalangeal joints. (B) Swan neck deformities. (C) Boutonnière deformity. (Used by permission of the American College of Rheumatology.)

nodes; those along the proximal interphalangeal joints are called *Bouchard nodes.* Painful swelling of the proximal interphalangeal joints causes spindle-shaped fingers, which are associated with the acute stage of rheumatoid arthritis (Fig. 22.18). Cystic, round, nontender swellings along tendon sheaths or joint capsules that are more prominent with flexion may indicate ganglia.

Examine the range of motion of the hand and wrist by asking the patient to perform these movements:

- Bend the fingers forward at the metacarpophalangeal joint, then stretch the fingers up and back at the knuckle. Expect metacarpophalangeal flexion of 90 degrees and hyperextension up to 30 degrees (Fig. 22.19A).
- Touch the thumb to each fingertip and to the base of the little finger; make a fist. All movements should be possible (see Fig. 22.19B and C).
- Spread the fingers apart and then touch them together. Both movements should be possible (see Fig. 22.19D).
- Bend the hand at the wrist up and down. Expect flexion of 90 degrees and hyperextension of 70 degrees (see Fig. 22.19E).
- With the palm side down, turn each hand to the right and left. Expect radial motion of 20 degrees and ulnar motion of 55 degrees (see Fig. 22.19F).

Have the patient maintain wrist flexion and hyperextension while you apply opposing force to evaluate the strength of the wrist muscles. To evaluate hand strength, have the patient tightly grip two of your fingers. To avoid painful compression from an overzealous squeeze, offer your two fingers of one hand side by side in the handshake position. Finger extension, abduction, adduction, and thumb opposition may also be used to evaluate hand strength.

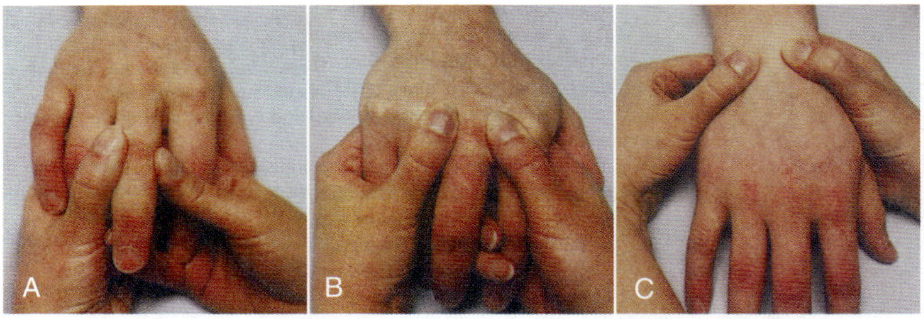

FIG. 22.17 Palpation of joints of the hand and wrist. (A) Proximal interphalangeal joints. (B) Metacarpophalangeal joints. (C) Radiocarpal groove and wrist.

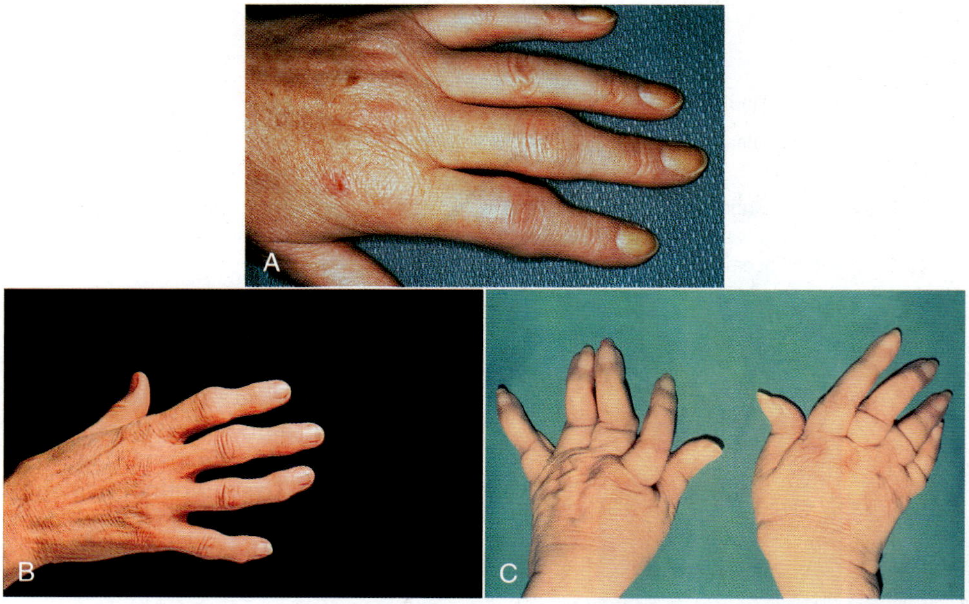

FIG. 22.18 Unexpected findings of the fingers. (A) Fusiform swelling or spindle-shaped enlargement of the proximal interphalangeal joints. (B) Degenerative joint disease; Heberden nodes at the distal interphalangeal joints and Bouchard nodes at the proximal interphalangeal joints. (C) Telescoping digits with hypermobile joints. (Used by permission of the American College of Rheumatology.)

Elbows

Inspect the contour of the patient's elbows in both flexed and extended positions. Subcutaneous nodules along pressure points of the ulnar surface may indicate a rheumatoid nodule (Fig. 22.20) or gouty tophi.

Note any deviations in the carrying angle between the humerus and radius while the arm is passively extended, palm forward. The carrying angle is usually 5 to 15 degrees laterally. Variations in carrying angle are cubitus valgus, a lateral angle exceeding 15 degrees, and cubitus varus, a medial carrying angle (Fig. 22.21).

Flex the patient's elbow 70 degrees and palpate the extensor surface of the ulna, the olecranon process, and the medial and lateral epicondyles of the humerus. Then palpate the groove on each side of the olecranon process for tenderness, swelling, and thickening of the synovial membrane (Fig. 22.22). The olecranon bursa is a fluid-filled sac that acts as a cushion between the skin and the olecranon process. Olecranon bursitis results in swelling and tenderness of the bursa. Suspect epicondylitis or tendonitis when a point tenderness exists at the lateral epicondyle or along the grooves of the olecranon process and epicondyles in addition to increased pain with pronation and supination of the elbow.

Examine the elbow's range of motion by asking the patient to perform the following movements:

- With the elbow fully extended at 0 degrees, bend and straighten the elbow. Expect flexion of 160 degrees and extension returning to 0 degrees or 180 degrees of full extension (Fig. 22.23A).
- With the elbow flexed at a right angle, rotate the hand from palm side down to palm side up. Expect pronation of 90 degrees and supination of 90 degrees (see Fig. 22.23B).
- Have the patient maintain flexion and extension while you apply opposing force to evaluate the strength of the elbow muscles.

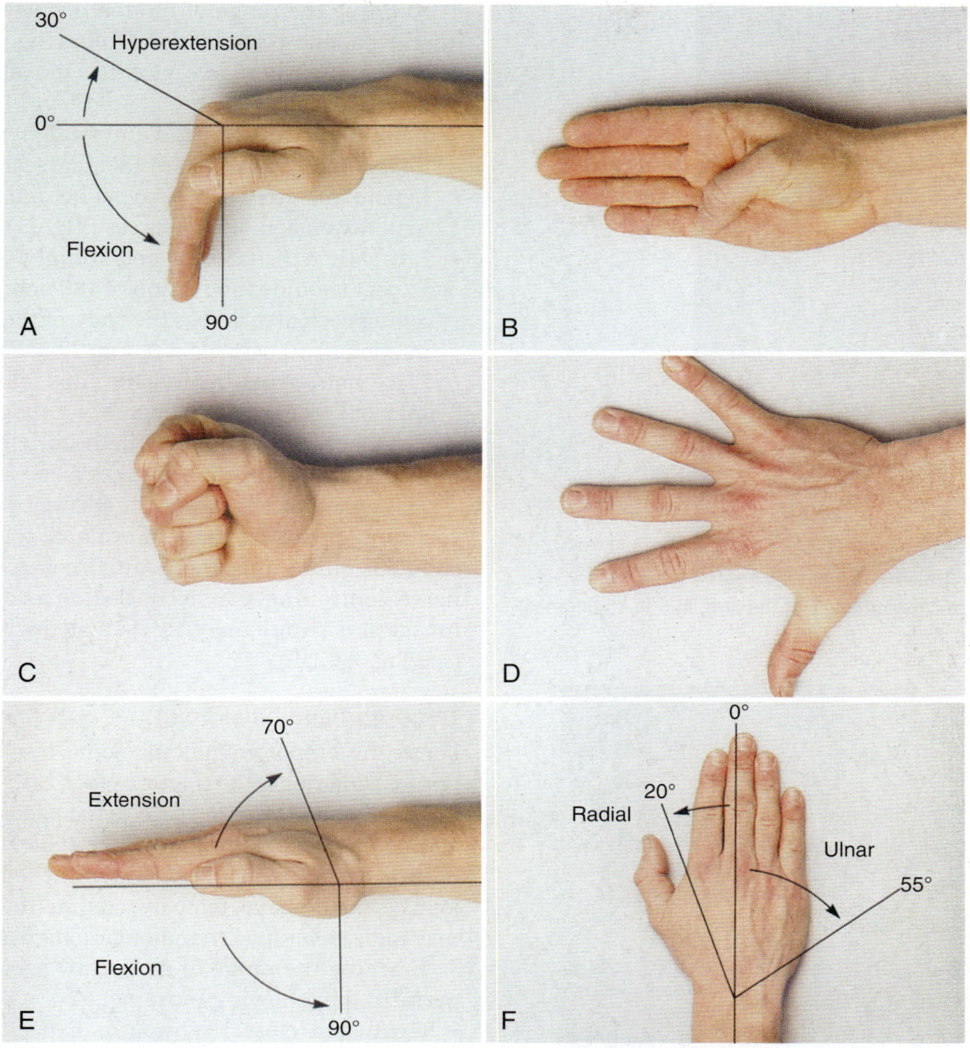

FIG. 22.19 Range of motion of the hand and wrist. (A) Metacarpophalangeal flexion and hyperextension. (B) Finger flexion: thumb to each fingertip and to the base of the little finger. (C) Finger flexion: fist formation. (D) Finger abduction. (E) Wrist flexion and hyperextension. (F) Wrist radial and ulnar movement.

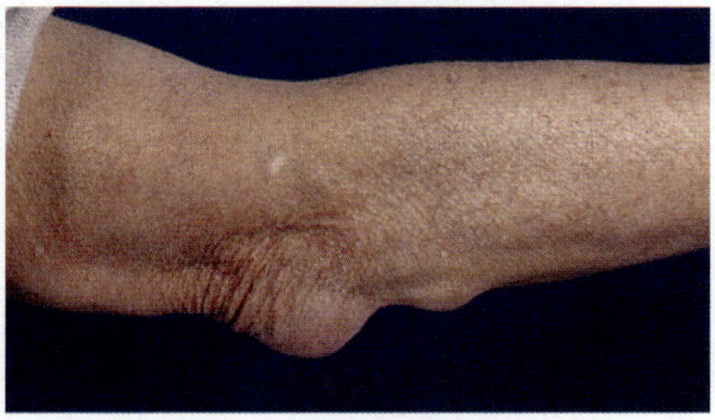

FIG. 22.20 Rheumatoid arthritis involving the elbow. Olecranon bursitis and a rheumatoid nodule are shown. (From Hochberg MC, Silman AJ, Smolen JS, et al: *Rheumatology*, ed 6, Philadelphia, 2015, Mosby.)

Shoulders

Inspect the contour of the shoulders, the shoulder girdle, the clavicles and scapulae, and the surrounding musculature. Expect symmetry of size and contour of all shoulder structures. When the shoulder contour is asymmetric and one shoulder has hollows in the rounding contour, suspect a shoulder dislocation (Fig. 22.24). Observe for a winged scapula, an outward prominence of the scapula, indicating injury to the nerve of the anterior serratus muscle (see Fig. 22.24B).

Palpate the sternoclavicular joint, clavicle, acromioclavicular joint, scapula, coracoid process, greater tubercle of the humerus, biceps groove, and area muscles. To palpate the biceps groove, rotate the arm and forearm externally. Locate the biceps muscle near the elbow and follow the muscle and its tendon into the biceps groove along the anterior aspect of the humerus. Palpate the muscle insertions of the supraspinatus, infraspinatus, and teres minor near the greater tuberosity of the humerus by lifting the elbow posteriorly to extend the shoulder. No tenderness should be noted over the muscle insertions.

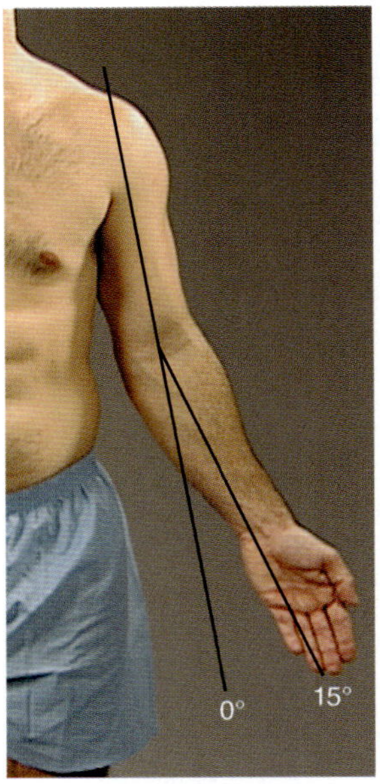

FIG. 22.21 Expected carrying angle of the arm, at 5 to 15 degrees.

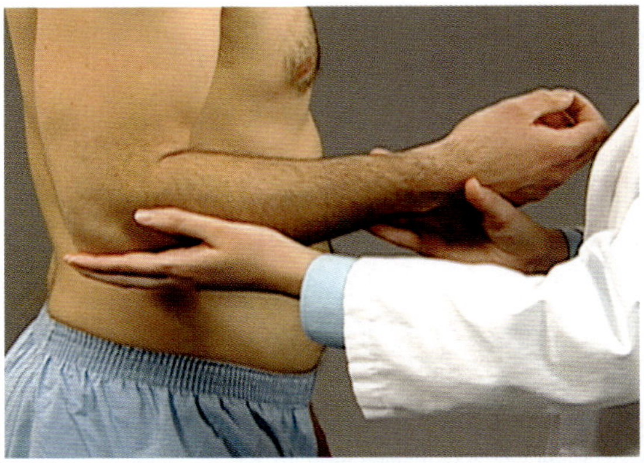

FIG. 22.22 Palpation of the olecranon process grooves.

Examine the range of motion of the shoulders by asking the patient to perform the following movements:

- Shrug the shoulders. Expect the shoulders to rise symmetrically.
- Raise both arms forward and straight up over the head. Expect forward flexion of 180 degrees.
- Extend and stretch both arms behind the back. Expect hyperextension of 50 degrees (Fig. 22.25A).
- Lift both arms laterally and straight up over the head. Expect shoulder abduction of 180 degrees.
- Swing each arm across the front of the body. Expect adduction of 50 degrees (see Fig. 22.25B).
- Place both arms behind the hips, elbows out. Expect internal rotation of 90 degrees (see Fig. 22.25C).
- Place both arms behind the head, elbows out. Expect external rotation of 90 degrees (see Fig. 22.25D).

Have the patient maintain shrugged shoulders while you apply opposing force to evaluate the strength of the shoulder girdle muscles. Cranial nerve XI (the accessory nerve controlling the sternocleidomastoid and trapezius muscles) is simultaneously evaluated with this maneuver (see Fig. 22.25E).

Temporomandibular Joint

Locate the temporomandibular joints by placing your fingertips just anterior to the tragus of each ear. Allow your fingertips to slip into the joint space as the patient's mouth opens, and gently palpate the joint space (Fig. 22.26). An audible or palpable snapping or clicking in the temporomandibular joints is not unusual, but pain, crepitus, locking, or popping may indicate temporomandibular joint dysfunction.

Examine the range of motion by asking the patient to perform the following movements:

- Open and close the mouth. Expect a space of 3 to 6 cm between the upper and lower teeth when the jaw is open.

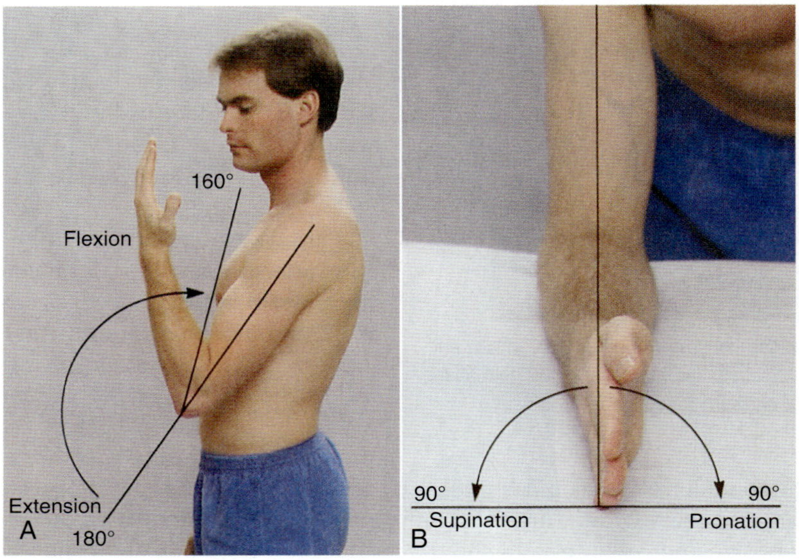

FIG. 22.23 **Range of motion of the elbow.** (A) Flexion and extension. (B) Pronation and supination.

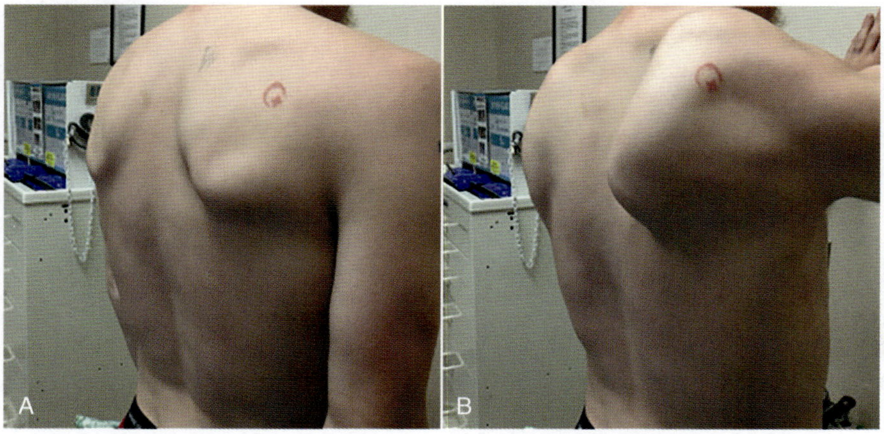

FIG. 22.24 (A) At rest, the patient has subtle prominence of the medial border of the right scapula. (B) When the patient flexes his arm forward and pushes against a wall, the medial border of the right scapula protrudes from the posterior chest wall ("winged scapula"). (From Chiu EF, et al: Ranula: *Winged scapula, Visual Journal of Emergency Medicine* 13:135–136, 2018.)

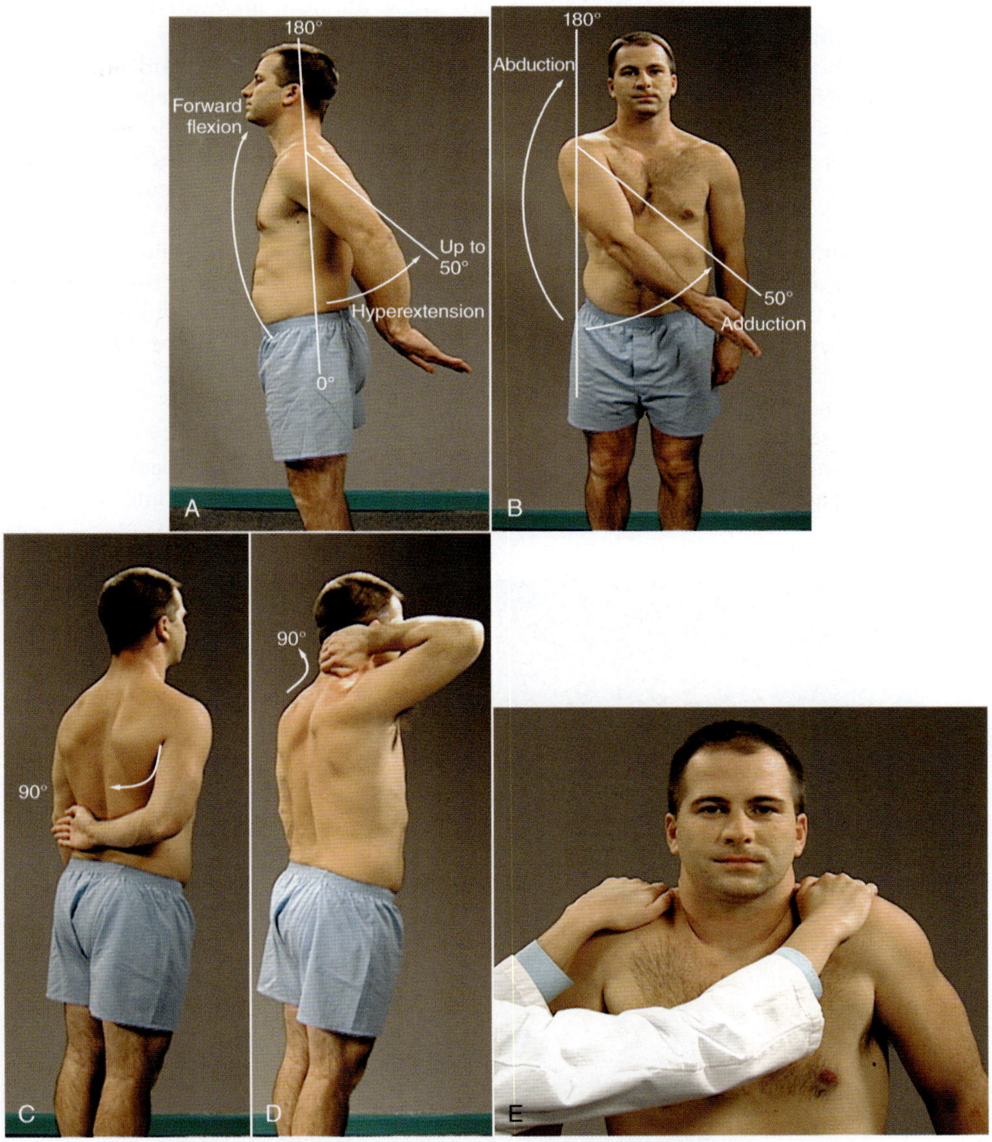

FIG. 22.25 Range of motion of the shoulder. (A) Forward flexion and hyperextension. (B) Abduction and adduction. (C) Internal rotation. (D) External rotation. (E) Shrugged shoulders.

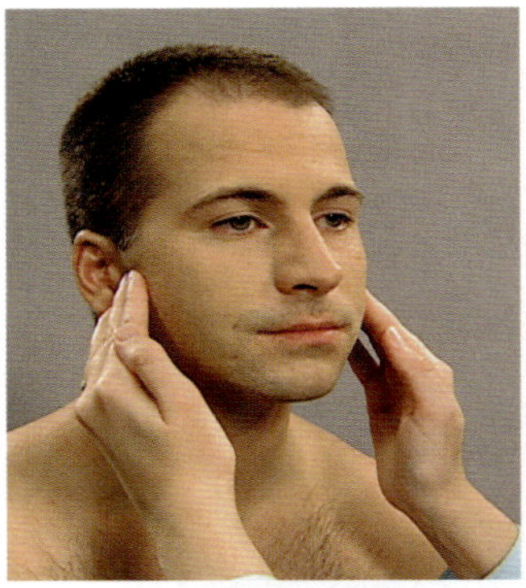

FIG. 22.26 **Palpation of the temporomandibular joint.**

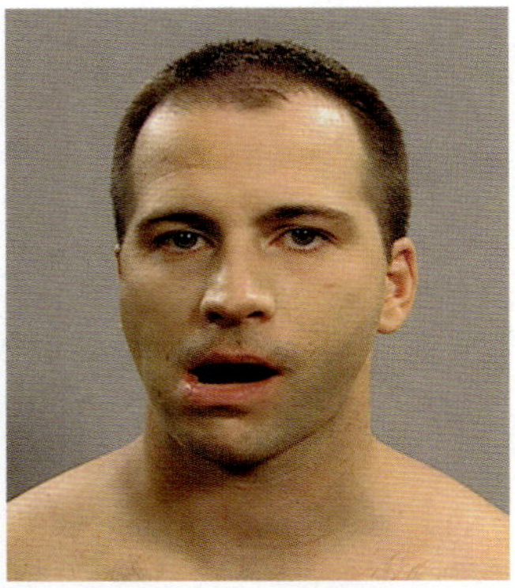

FIG. 22.27 **Lateral range of motion in the temporomandibular joint.**

- Laterally move the lower jaw to each side. The mandible should move 1 to 2 cm in each direction (Fig. 22.27).
- Protrude and retract the chin. Both movements should be possible.

The strength of the temporalis and masseter muscles may be evaluated by asking the patient to clench the teeth while you palpate the contracted muscles and apply opposing force. This maneuver simultaneously tests cranial nerve V (the trigeminal nerve).

Cervical Spine

Inspect the patient's neck from both the anterior and posterior positions, observing for alignment of the head with the shoulders and symmetry of the skinfolds and muscles. Expect the cervical spine curve to be concave with the head erect and in appropriate alignment. Palpate the posterior neck; cervical spine; and paravertebral, trapezius, and sternocleidomastoid muscles. The muscles should have good tone and appear symmetric in size, with no palpable tenderness or muscle spasm.

Evaluate the range of motion in the cervical spine by asking the patient to perform the following movements (Fig. 22.28):

- Bend the head forward, chin to the chest. Expect flexion of 45 degrees.
- Bend the head backward, chin toward the ceiling. Expect extension of 45 degrees.
- Bend the head to each side, ear to each shoulder. Expect lateral bending of 40 degrees.
- Turn the head to each side, chin to shoulder. Expect rotation of 70 degrees.

The strength of the sternocleidomastoid and trapezius muscles is evaluated with the patient maintaining each of the previous positions while you apply opposing force. With rotation, cranial nerve XI is simultaneously tested (Fig. 22.29).

Thoracic and Lumbar Spine

Major landmarks of the back include each spinal process of the vertebrae (C7 and T1 are usually the most

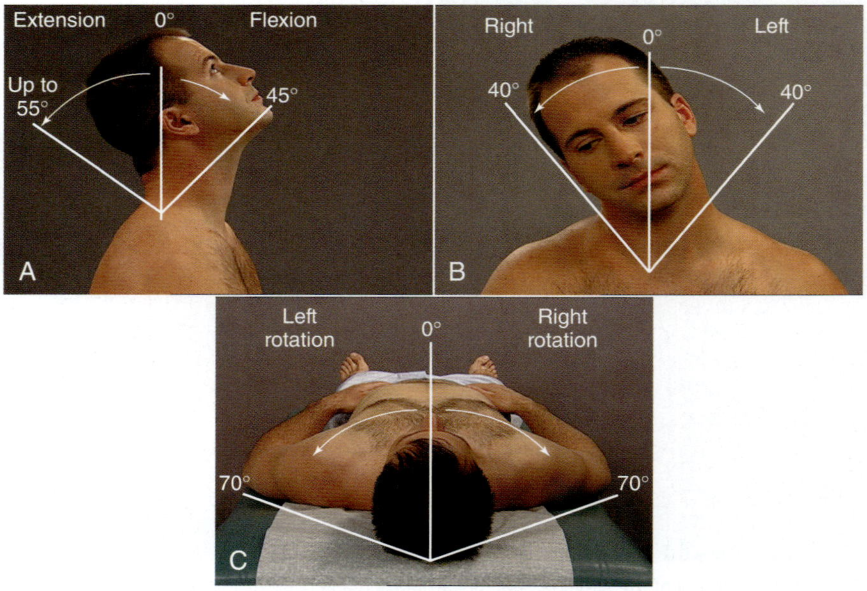

FIG. 22.28 **Range of motion of the cervical spine.** (A) Flexion and hyperextension. (B) Lateral bending. (C) Rotation.

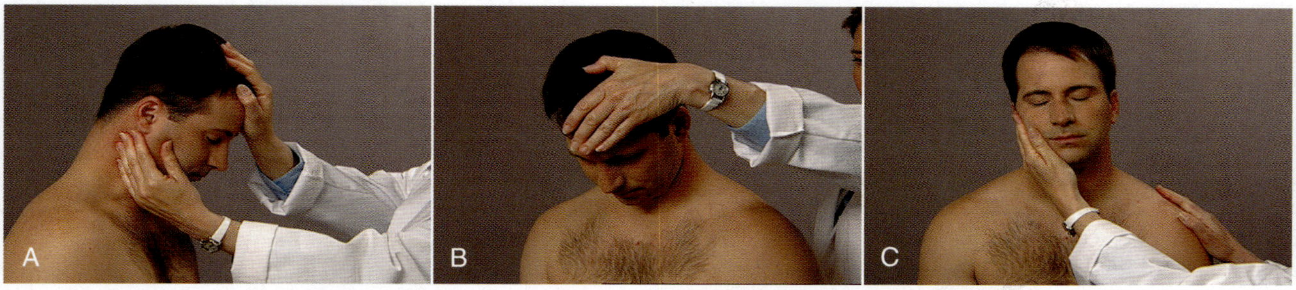

FIG. 22.29 **Examining the strength of the sternocleidomastoid and trapezius muscles.** (A) Flexion with palpation of the sternocleidomastoid muscle. (B) Extension against resistance. (C) Rotation against resistance.

prominent), scapulae, iliac crests, and paravertebral muscles (Fig. 22.30). Expect the head to be positioned directly over the gluteal cleft and the vertebrae to be straight, as indicated by symmetric shoulder, scapular, and iliac crest heights. The curve of the thoracic spine should be convex. The curve of the lumbar spine should be concave (Fig. 22.31A). The knees and feet should be in alignment with the trunk, pointing directly forward.

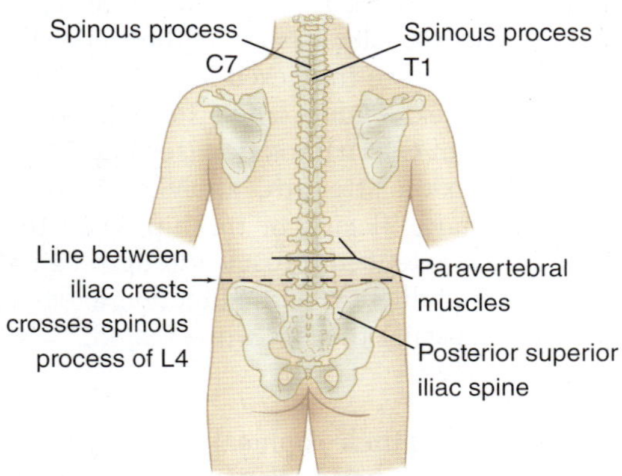

FIG. 22.30 **Landmarks of the back.**

Kyphosis may be observed in aging adults (see Fig. 22.31B). Lordosis is common in patients who are obese or pregnant (see Fig. 22.31C). A sharp angular deformity, a gibbus, is associated with a collapsed vertebra from osteoporosis (see Fig. 22.31D).

With the patient standing erect, palpate along the spinal processes and paravertebral muscles (Fig. 22.32). No muscle spasms or spinal tenderness should be present. Percuss for spinal tenderness, first by tapping each spinal process with one finger and then by percussing each side

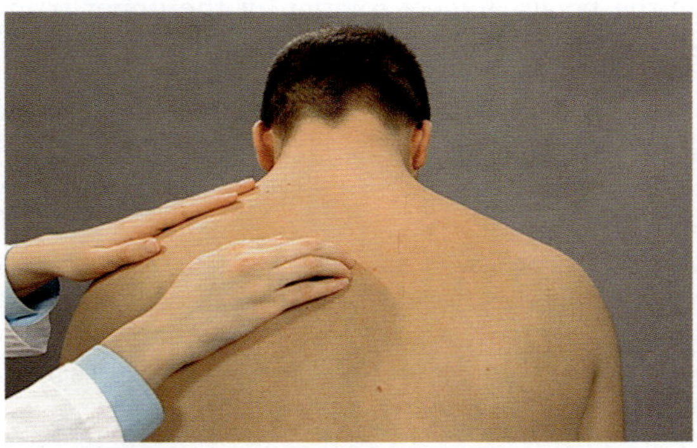

FIG. 22.32 **Palpation of the spinal processes of the vertebrae.**

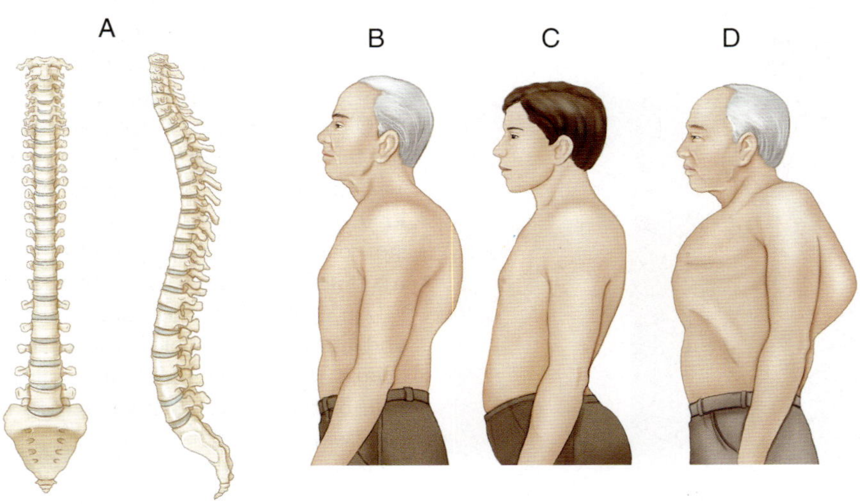

FIG. 22.31 **Deviations in spinal column curvatures.** (A) Expected spine curvatures. (B) Kyphosis. (C) Lordosis. (D) Gibbus.

of the spine along the paravertebral muscles with the ulnar aspect of your fist. No muscle spasm or spinal tenderness with palpation or percussion should be elicited.

Ask the patient to bend forward slowly and touch their toes while you observe from behind. Inspect the spine for unexpected curvature. The patient's back should remain symmetrically flat as the concave curve of the lumbar spine becomes convex with forward flexion. A lateral curvature or rib hump should make you suspect scoliosis (Fig. 22.33). Measure the degree of rotation with a scoliometer (see Chapter 3). Then have the patient rise but remain bent at the waist to fully extend the back. Reversal of the lumbar curve should be apparent.

Evaluate the range of motion by asking the patient to perform the following movements:

- Bend forward at the waist and, without bending the knees, try to touch the toes. Expect flexion of 75 to 90 degrees (Fig. 22.34A).
- Bend back at the waist as far as possible. Expect hyperextension of 30 degrees (see Fig. 22.34B).
- Bend to each side as far as possible. Expect lateral bending of 35 degrees bilaterally (see Fig. 22.34C).
- Swing the upper trunk from the waist in a circular motion from front to side to back to side while you stabilize the pelvis. Expect rotation of the upper trunk 30 degrees forward and backward (see Fig. 22.34D).

Patient Safety

Reducing the Risk for Lower Back Pain

Counsel patients on how to use appropriate techniques when lifting heavy objects to reduce the risk of lower back injury. Rather than bend over to pick up a heavy object, keep the back straight and flex the knees to get closer to the object. Keep the object close to the body and lift with the knees. Avoid twisting the back during the lift.

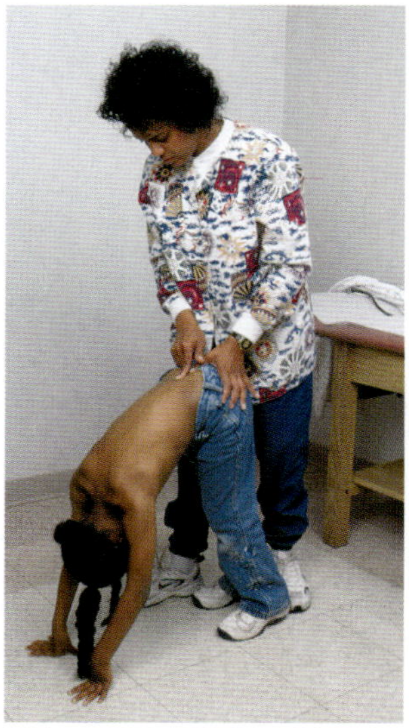

FIG. 22.33 Inspection of the spine for lateral curvature and lumbar convexity.

Hips

Inspect the hips anteriorly and posteriorly while the patient stands. Using the major landmarks of the iliac crest and the greater trochanter of the femur, note any asymmetry in the iliac crest height, the size of the buttocks, or the number and level of gluteal folds.

Examine the range of motion of the hips by asking the patient to perform the following movements:

While supine, raise the leg with the knee extended above the body. Expect up to 90 degrees of hip flexion (Fig. 22.35A).

While either standing or prone, swing the straightened leg behind the body without arching the back. Expect hip hyperextension of 30 degrees or less (see Fig. 22.35B).

While supine, raise one knee to the chest with the other leg straight. Expect hip flexion of 120 degrees (see Fig. 22.35C).

While supine, swing the leg laterally and medially with the knee straight. With the adduction movement, passively lift the opposite leg to permit the examined leg full movement. Expect up to 45 degrees of abduction and up to 30 degrees of adduction (see Fig. 22.35D).

While supine, flex the knee, keeping the foot on the table, then rotate the leg with the flexed knee toward the other leg. Expect internal rotation of 40 degrees (see Fig. 22.35E).

While supine, place the lateral aspect of the foot on the knee of the other leg; move the flexed knee toward the table (FABER test—*F*lex, *AB*duct, and *E*xternally *R*otate). Expect 45 degrees of external rotation (see Fig. 22.35F).

To test hip flexion strength, apply resistance while the patient maintains flexion of the hip when the knee is flexed and then extended. Muscle strength can also be evaluated during abduction and adduction as well as by resistance to uncrossing the legs while seated.

Legs and Knees

Inspect the knees and their popliteal spaces in both flexed and extended positions, noting the major landmarks: tibial tuberosity, medial and lateral tibial condyles, medial and lateral epicondyles of the femur, adductor tubercle of the femur, and patella (see Fig. 22.10). Inspect the extended knee for its natural concavities on the anterior aspect, on each side, and above the patella. Loss of these concavities may suggest a knee effusion.

Observe the lower leg alignment. The angle between the femur and tibia is expected to be less than 15 degrees. Variations in lower leg alignment are genu valgum (knock-knees) and genu varum (bowlegs). Excessive hyperextension of the knee with weight bearing (genu recurvatum) may indicate weakness of the quadriceps muscles.

An effusion of the knee fills the suprapatellar pouch and the concavity below the patella medially. When this occurs, the usual indentation above and on the medial side of the patella is filled out to be convex rather than concave.

Palpate the popliteal space, noting any swelling or tenderness. Fullness in the popliteal space may indicate a popliteal (Baker) cyst. Next, palpate the tibiofemoral joint space, identifying the patella, the suprapatellar pouch, and

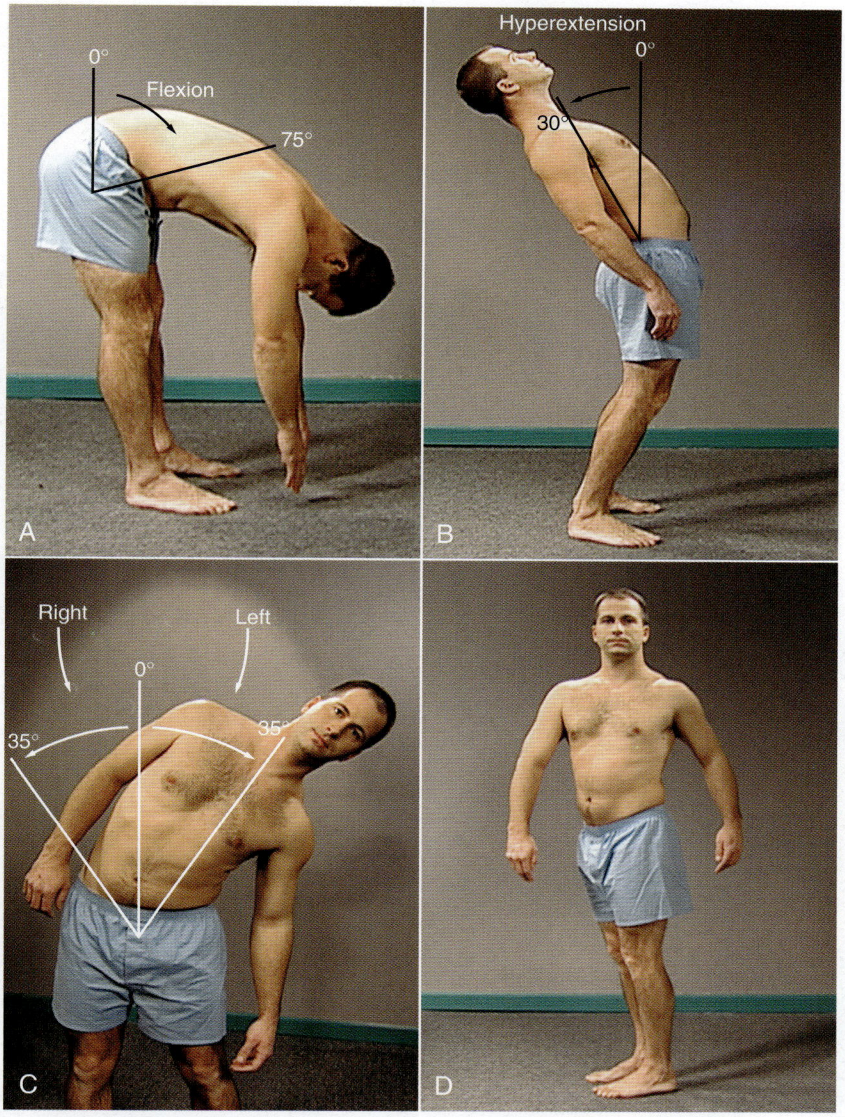

FIG. 22.34 Range of motion of the thoracic and lumbar spine. (A) Flexion. (B) Hyperextension. (C) Lateral bending. (D) Rotation of the upper trunk.

the infrapatellar fat pad. This joint should feel smooth and firm, without tenderness, swelling, bogginess, nodules, or crepitus (see "Knee Assessment" for additional assessment procedures).

Examine the knees' range of motion by asking the patient to perform the following movements (Fig. 22.36):

- Bend each knee. Expect 130 degrees of flexion.
- Straighten the leg and stretch it. Expect full extension and up to 15 degrees of hyperextension.

The strength of the knee muscles is evaluated with the patient maintaining flexion and extension while you apply opposing force. The patient may be sitting or standing for this assessment.

Feet and Ankles

Inspect the feet and ankles while the patient is bearing weight (i.e., standing and walking) and while sitting. Landmarks of the ankle include the medial malleolus, the lateral malleolus, and the Achilles tendon. Expect to observe smooth and rounded malleolar prominences, prominent heels, and prominent metatarsophalangeal joints. Calluses and corns may indicate chronic pressure or irritation.

Observe the contour of the feet and the position, size, and number of toes. The feet should be in alignment with the tibias. Common alignment variations are pes varus (in-toeing) and pes valgus (out-toeing). Weight bearing should be on the midline of the foot, on an imaginary line from the heel midline to between the second and third toes. Deviations in forefoot alignment (metatarsus varus or metatarsus valgus), heel pronation, and pain or injury often cause a shift in weight-bearing position (Fig. 22.37).

Expect the foot to have a longitudinal arch, although the foot may flatten with weight bearing (Fig. 22.38A). Common variations include pes planus (see Fig. 22.38B),

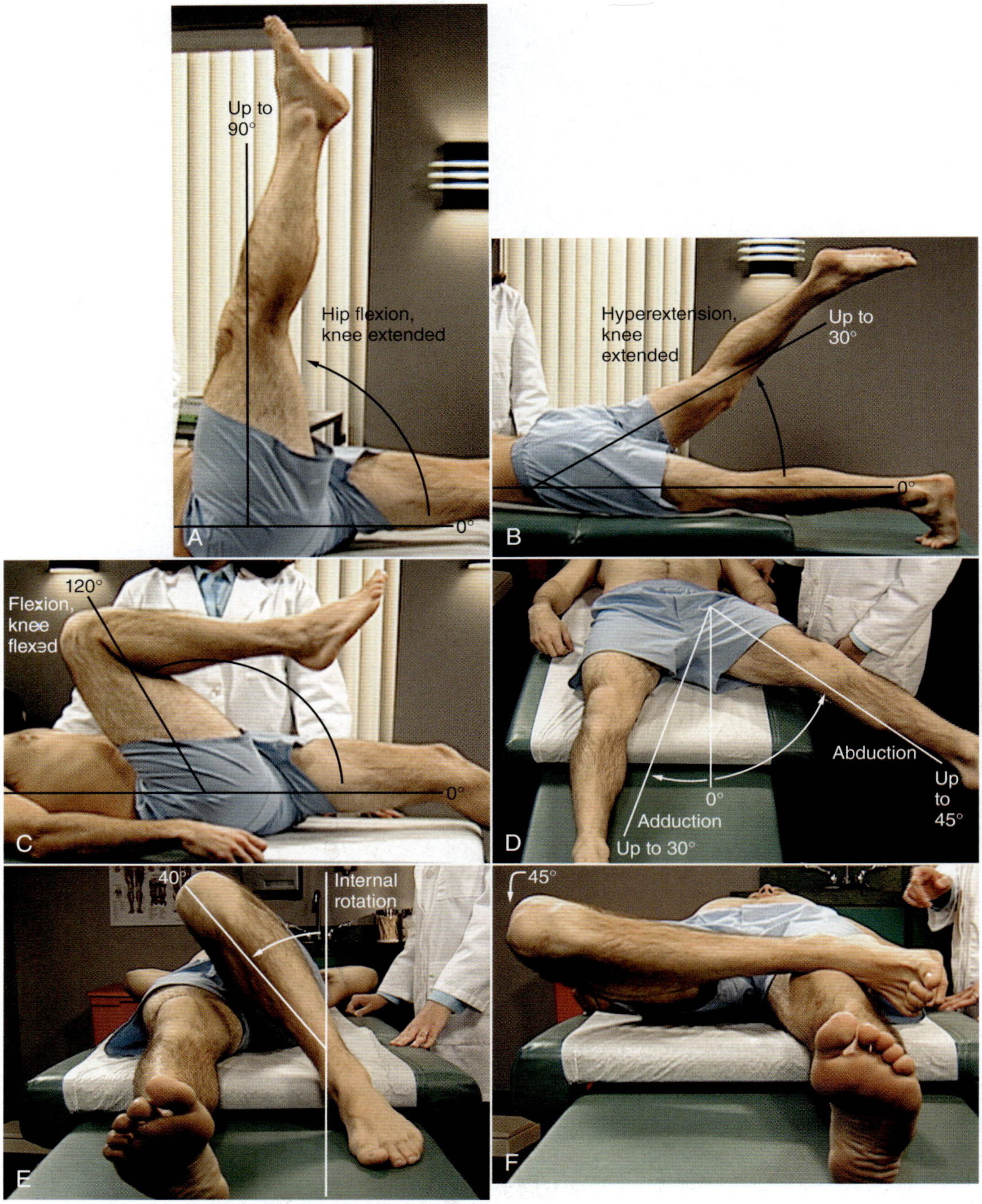

FIG. 22.35 Range of motion of the hip. (A) Hip flexion, knee extended. (B) Hip extension, knee extended. (C) Hip flexion, knee flexed. (D) Abduction. (E) Internal rotation. (F) External rotation.

a foot that remains flat even when not bearing weight, and pes cavus, a high instep (see Fig. 22.38C). Pes cavus may be associated with claw toes.

The toes should be straight forward, flat, and in alignment with each other. Several unexpected deviations of the toes can occur (Fig. 22.39). Hyperextension of the metatarsophalangeal joint with flexion of the toe's proximal joint is called *hammertoe*. A flexion deformity at the distal interphalangeal joint is called a *mallet toe*. *Claw toe* is hyperextension of the metatarsophalangeal joint with flexion of the toe's proximal and distal joints. *Hallux valgus* is lateral deviation of the great toe, which may cause overlapping with the second toe. A bursa often forms at the pressure point and, if it becomes inflamed, forms a painful bunion.

Heat, redness, swelling, and tenderness are signs of an inflamed joint, possibly caused by rheumatoid arthritis, gout, septic joint, fracture, or tendonitis. In particular, an inflamed metatarsophalangeal joint of the great toe should make you suspect gouty arthritis.

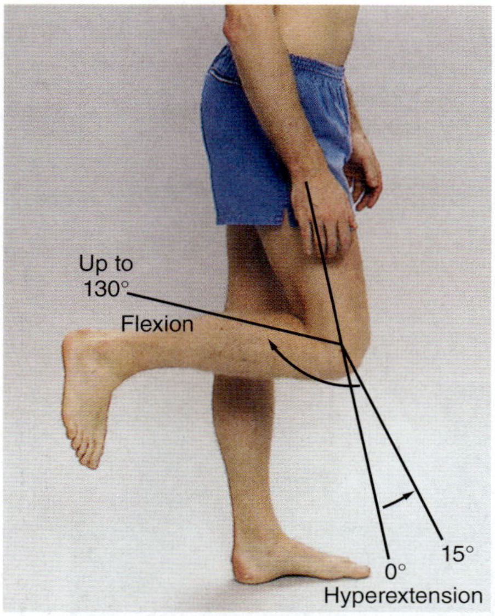

FIG. 22.36 **Range of motion of the knee: flexion and extension.**

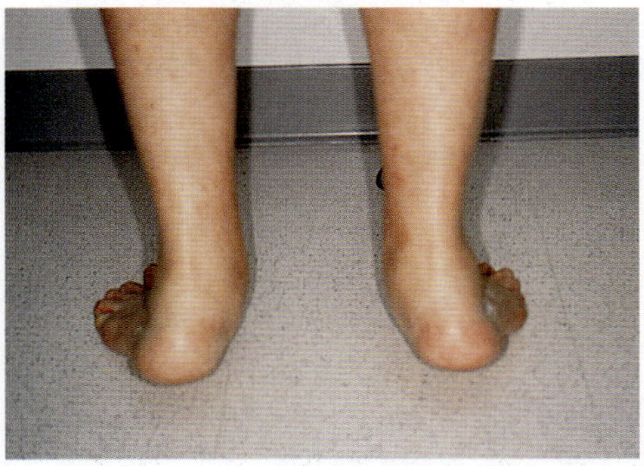

FIG. 22.37 **Pronation of the heel.** Note that weight bearing is not through the midline of the foot. (Courtesy Charles W. Bradley, DPM, MPA, and Caroline Harvey, DPM, California College of Podiatric Medicine.)

Palpate the Achilles tendon, the anterior surface of the ankle, and the medial and lateral malleoli. A persistently thickened Achilles tendon may indicate the tendonitis that can develop with spondyloarthritis or from xanthelasma of hyperlipidemia. Use the thumb and fingers of both hands to compress the forefoot and to palpate each metatarsophalangeal joint, taking note of discomfort or swelling.

Assess the range of motion of the foot and ankle by asking the patient to perform the following movements while sitting:

Point the foot toward the ceiling. Expect dorsiflexion of 20 degrees (Fig. 22.40A).

- Point the foot toward the floor. Expect plantar flexion of 45 degrees.
- Bending the foot at the ankle, turn the sole of the foot toward and then away from the other foot. Expect inversion of 30 degrees and eversion of 20 degrees (see Fig. 22.40B).
- Rotating the ankle, turn the foot away from and then toward the other foot while the examiner stabilizes the leg. Expect abduction of 10 degrees and adduction of 20 degrees (see Fig. 22.40C).
- Bend and straighten the toes. Expect flexion and extension, especially of the great toes.

Have the patient maintain dorsiflexion and plantar flexion while you apply opposing force to evaluate the strength of the ankle muscles. Abduction and adduction of the ankle and flexion, as well as extension of the great toe, may also be used to evaluate muscle strength.

For the assessment of gait, see Chapter 23.

Evidence-Based Practice in Physical Examination

Acute Ankle Injury in Adults

In cases of an acute ankle injury, the Ottawa Ankle Rules help identify the characteristics of patients needing an ankle radiograph series. There must be pain in the malleolar zone and one of the following:

- Bone tenderness along the distal 6 cm of the posterior edge of the fibula or tip of the lateral malleolus
- Bone tenderness along the distal 6 cm of the posterior edge of the tibia or tip of the medial malleolus
- Inability to bear weight for four steps both immediately after the injury and in the emergency department

Absolute exclusion criteria for an ankle radiograph series include the following: age younger than 18 years, intoxication, multiple painful (distracting) injuries, pregnancy, head injury, and neurologic deficit.

The Ottawa Ankle Rules have 95% sensitivity for detecting an ankle fracture that is present on radiography.

Data from Beckenkamp, P. R., Lin, C. C., Macaskill, P., Michaleff, Z. A., Maher, C. G., & Moseley, A. M. (2017). Diagnostic accuracy of the Ottawa ankle and midfoot rules: A systematic review with meta-analysis. *British Journal of Sports Medicine, 51*(6), 504.

ADVANCED SKILLS

Various other procedures are performed for further evaluation of specific joints of the musculoskeletal system when problems are detected with routine procedures (Table 22.2).

Hand and Wrist Assessment

Several procedures are used to evaluate the integrity of the median nerve, which innervates the palm of the hand and the palmar surface of the thumb, index and middle fingers, and half of the ring finger. Ask the patient to mark the specific locations of pain, numbness, and tingling on the Katz hand diagram (Fig. 22.41). Certain patterns of pain, numbness, and tingling are associated with carpal tunnel syndrome.

The *thumb abduction test* isolates the strength of the abductor pollicis brevis muscle, innervated only by the median nerve. Have the patient place the hand palm up and raise the thumb perpendicular to it. Apply downward pressure on the thumb to test muscle strength (Fig. 22.42A). Full resistance to this pressure is expected. Weakness is associated with carpal tunnel syndrome.

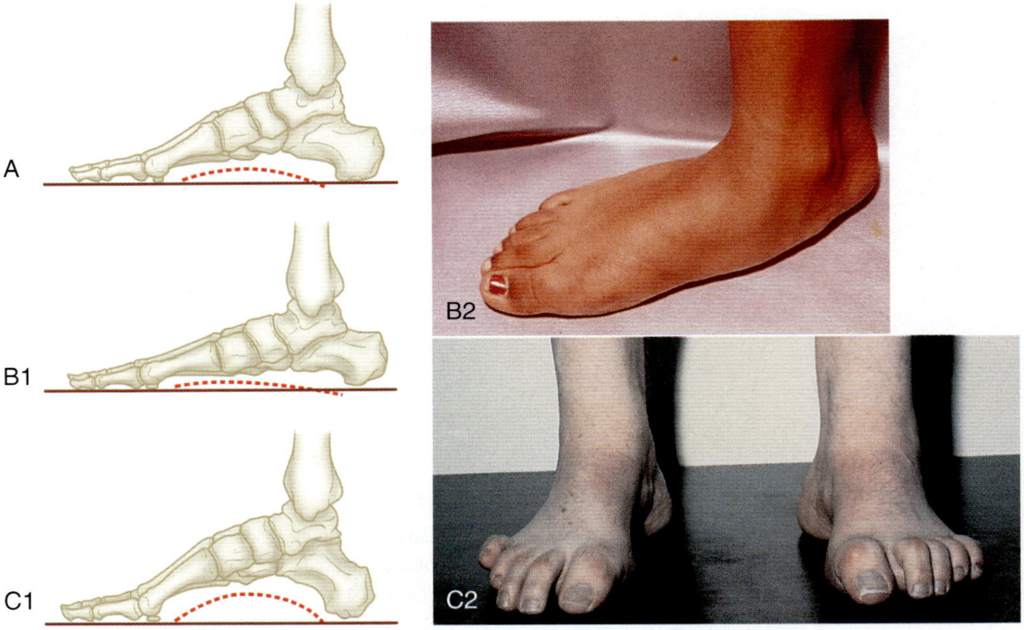

FIG. 22.38 Variations in the longitudinal arch of the foot. (A) Commonly expected arch. (B1 and B2) Pes planus (flatfoot). (C1 and C2) Pes cavus (high instep). (B2, Courtesy Charles W. Bradley, DPM, MPA, and Caroline Harvey, DPM, California College of Podiatric Medicine; C2, from Coughlin MJ, et al: *Surgery of the foot and ankle*, ed 8, 2007, Elsevier.)

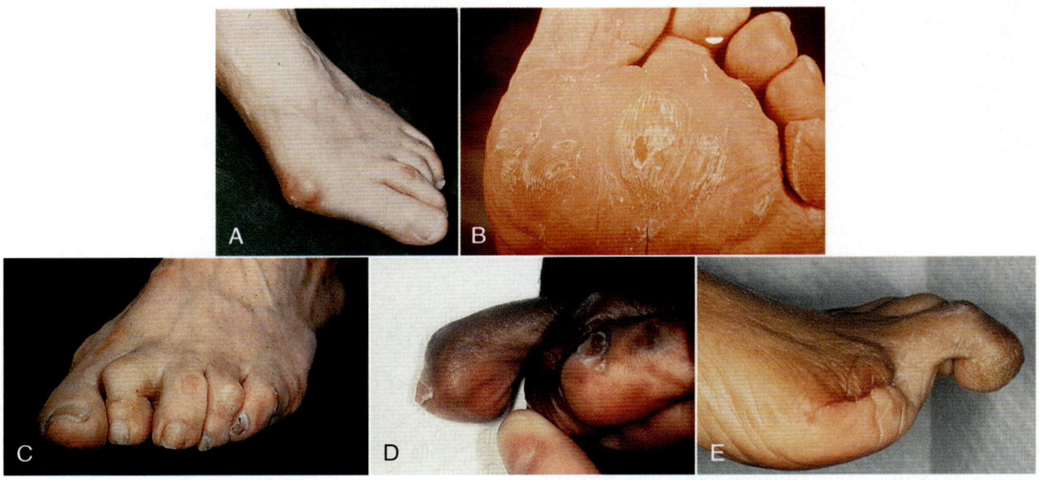

FIG. 22.39 Unexpected findings of the feet. (A) Hallux valgus with bunion. (B) Protruding metatarsal heads with callosities. (C) Hammertoes. (D) Mallet toe. (E) Claw toes. (Courtesy Charles W. Bradley, DPM, MPA, and Caroline Harvey, DPM, California College of Podiatric Medicine.)

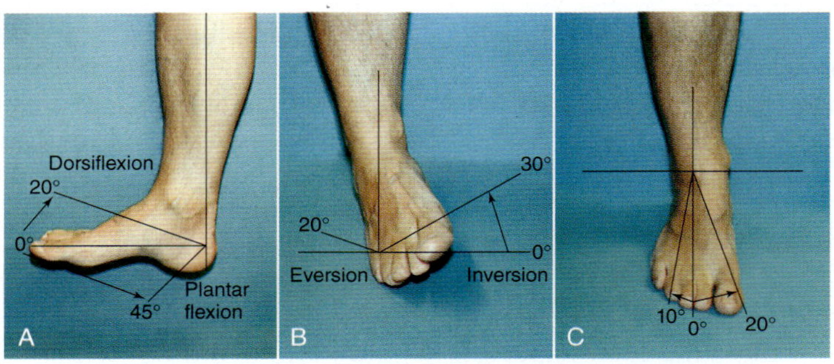

FIG. 22.40 Range of motion of the foot and ankle. (A) Dorsiflexion and plantar flexion. (B) Inversion and eversion. (C) Abduction and adduction.

TABLE 22.2 Special Procedures for Assessment of the Musculoskeletal System

PROCEDURE	CONDITION DETECTED
Limb measurement	Asymmetry in limb size
Neer test	Shoulder rotator cuff impingement or tear
Hawkins-Kennedy test	Shoulder rotator cuff impingement or tear
Katz hand diagram	Median nerve integrity
Thumb abduction test	Median nerve integrity
Tinel sign	Median nerve integrity
Phalen test	Median nerve integrity
Straight leg raising	L4, L5, S1 nerve root irritation
Femoral stretch test	L1, L2, L3, L4 nerve root irritation
Ballottement	Effusion in the knee
Bulge sign	Effusion in the knee
McMurray test	Torn meniscus in the knee
Anterior and posterior drawer test	Anterior and posterior cruciate ligament integrity
Varus-valgus stress test	Medial or lateral collateral ligament instability in knee
Lachman test	Anterior cruciate ligament integrity
Thomas test	Flexion contracture of hip
Trendelenburg sign	Weak hip abductor muscles

To perform the Phalen test, ask the patient to hold both wrists in a fully palmar-flexed position with the dorsal surfaces pressed together for 1 minute (see Fig. 22.42B). Numbness and paresthesia in the distribution of the median nerve are suggestive of carpal tunnel syndrome. The reverse Phalen test is performed by placing the palms and fingers together with full wrist extension. The Tinel sign is tested by striking the patient's wrist with your index or middle finger where the median nerve passes under the flexor retinaculum and volar carpal ligament (see Fig. 22.42C). A tingling sensation radiating from the wrist to the hand in the distribution of the median nerve is a positive Tinel sign and can indicate carpal tunnel syndrome.

Evidence-Based Practice in Physical Examination

Carpal Tunnel Syndrome

The likelihood that a patient will have a positive electrodiagnostic study for carpal tunnel syndrome is increased by the following: weakened thumb abduction, a classic or probable distribution of symptoms on the Katz hand diagram (see next page), and hypalgesia (decreased pain sensation along the thumb and median nerve distribution compared with the little finger on the same hand). The Tinel and Phelan tests are less accurate.

Data from Watson, J., Zhao, M., & Ring, D. (2010). Predictors of normal electrodiagnostic testing in the evaluation of suspected carpal tunnel syndrome. *Journal of Hand and Microsurgery, 2*(2), 47–50. http://dx.doi.org/10.1007/s12593-010-0012-9.

Shoulder Assessment

Several procedures are used to evaluate the rotator cuff for impingement (tendonitis or overuse injury from repetitive overhead activities) or a tear.

To perform the passive painful arc maneuver (Neer test), forward flex the patient's arm up to 150 degrees while depressing the scapula. This presses the greater tuberosity and supraspinatus muscle against the anteroinferior acromion. Increased shoulder pain is associated with rotator cuff inflammation or a tear (Fig. 22.43A).

The Hawkins-Kennedy test is performed by abducting the shoulder to 90 degrees, flexing the elbow to 90 degrees, and then internally rotating the arm to its limit. Increased shoulder pain is associated with rotator cuff inflammation or a possible tear (see Fig. 22.43B).

To test the strength of the rotator cuff muscles, perform the following maneuvers. A normal result is indicated by the absence of pain or weakness with these maneuvers:

To assess the supraspinatus muscle of the rotator cuff, have the patient place the arm in 90 degrees of abduction, 30 degrees of forward flexion, and internally rotated (thumbs pointing down). Apply downward pressure on the arm against patient resistance.

To assess the subscapularis muscle, have the patient hold the arm at the side, elbow flexed 90 degrees, and rotate the forearm medially against resistance.

To evaluate the infraspinatus and teres minor muscles, have the patient hold the arm at the side, elbow flexed 90 degrees, and rotate the arm laterally against resistance.

Pain and weakness with opposing force are unexpected findings and may be associated with inflammation or a tear.

Lower Spine Assessment

The straight-leg raising test is used to test for nerve root irritation or lumbar disk herniation, most commonly seen at the L4, L5, and S1 levels. Have the patient lie supine with the neck slightly flexed. Ask the patient to raise the leg, keeping the knee extended (see Fig. 22.35A). No pain should be felt below the knee with leg raising. Radicular pain below the knee may be associated with disk herniation. Flexion of the knee often eliminates the pain with leg raising. Repeat the procedure on the unaffected leg. Crossover pain in the affected leg with this maneuver is more indicative of sciatic nerve impingements.

The femoral stretch test or hip extension test is used to detect inflammation of the nerve root at the L1, L2, L3, and sometimes L4 levels. Have the patient lie prone and extend the hip. No pain is expected. Pain on extension is a positive sign of nerve root irritation (Fig. 22.44).

Hip Assessment

The Thomas test is used to detect flexion contractures of the hip that may be masked by excessive lumbar lordosis.

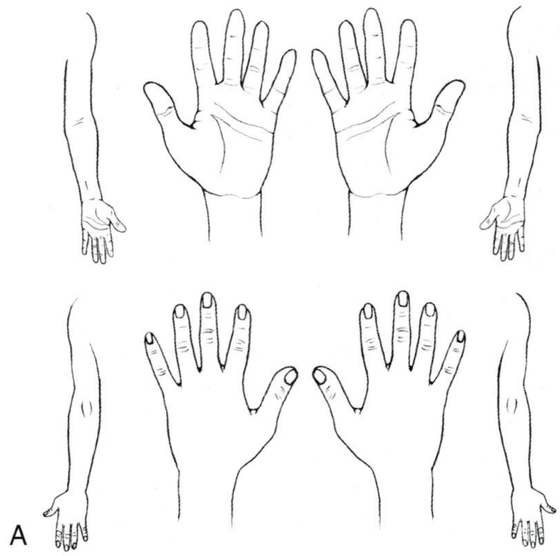

Classic pattern
Symptoms affect at least two of digits 1, 2, or 3. The classic pattern permits symptoms in the fourth and fifth digits, wrist pain, and radiation of pain proximal to the wrist, but it does not allow symptoms on the palm or dorsum of the hand.

Probable pattern
Same symptom pattern as classic, except palmar symptoms are allowed unless confined solely to the ulnar aspect. In the **possible pattern,** *not shown*, symptoms involve only one of digits 1, 2, or 3.

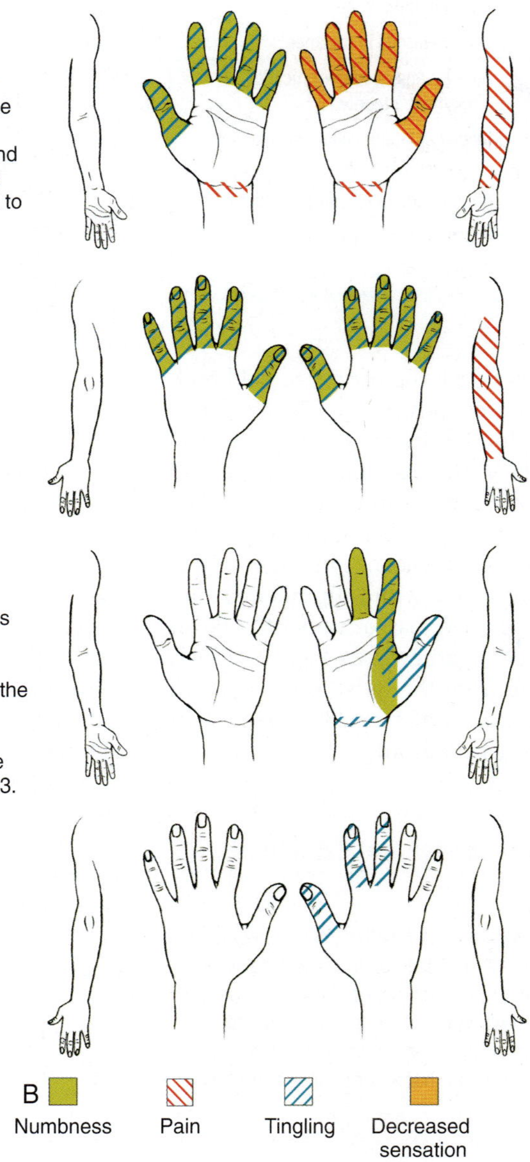

FIG. 22.41 Assessment for carpal tunnel syndrome. (A) Katz hand diagram. (B) Classic and probable patterns of pain, tingling, and numbness using the Katz hand diagram.

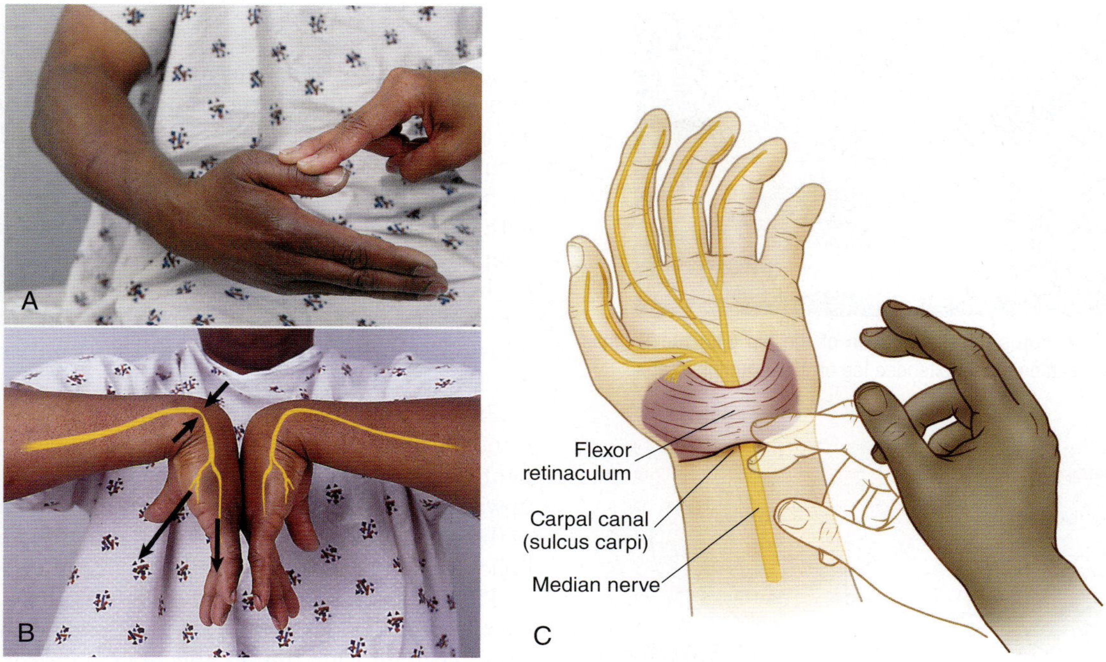

FIG. 22.42 Additional procedures for assessment of carpal tunnel syndrome. (A) Thumb abduction test. (B) Phalen maneuver. (C) Elicitation of Tinel sign.

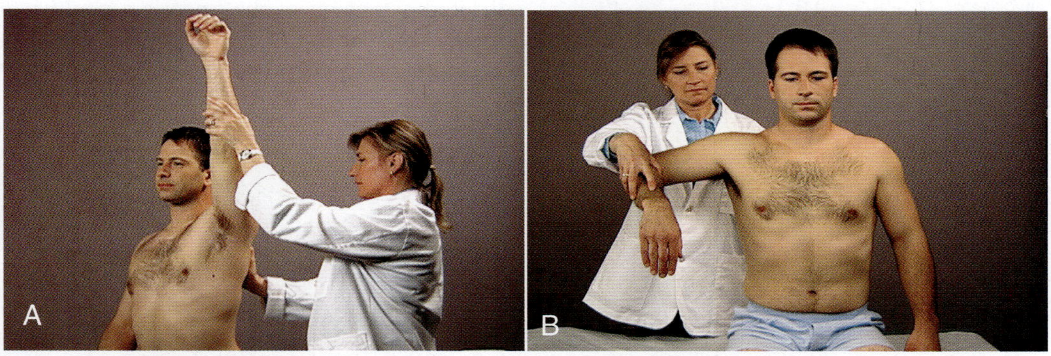

FIG. 22.43 Assessment for rotator cuff inflammation or tear. (A) Neer test. (B) Hawkins-Kennedy test.

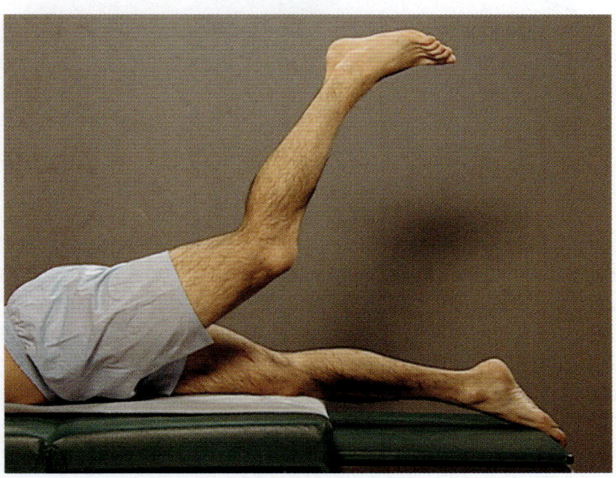

FIG. 22.44 Femoral stretch test for high lumbar nerve root irritation.

Have the patient lie supine; fully extend one leg flat on the examining table and flex the other leg with the knee to the chest. Observe the patient's ability to keep the extended leg flat on the examining table (Fig. 22.45). Lifting the extended leg off the examining table indicates a hip flexion contracture in the extended leg.

The Trendelenburg test is a maneuver to detect weak hip abductor muscles. Ask the patient to stand and balance first on one foot and then on the other. Observing from behind, note any asymmetry or change in the level of the iliac crests. When the iliac crest drops on the side of the lifted leg, this indicates the hip abductor muscles on the weight-bearing side are weak (Fig. 22.46).

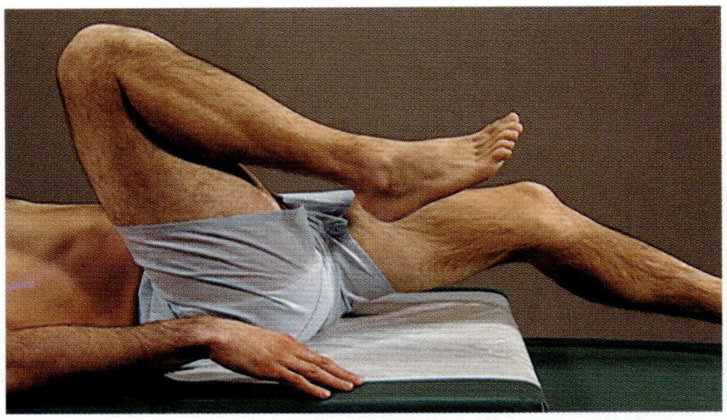

FIG. 22.45 Procedures for examination of the hip with the Thomas test. Note the elevation of the extended leg off the examining table.

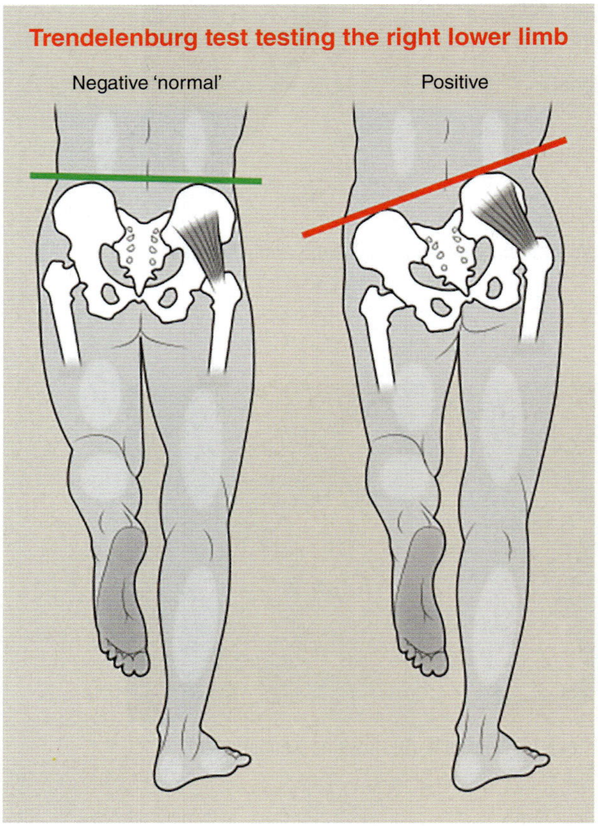

FIG. 22.46 Trendelenburg test evaluating the right lower limb. Note any asymmetry in the level of the iliac crests with weight bearing. (From Tillotson L, et al: *Examination of the hip for MRCS OSCE*, Surgery 38(2): 65–69, 2020.)

Knee Assessment

Ballottement is used to determine the presence of an effusion in the knee from excess fluid. With the knee extended, apply downward pressure on the suprapatellar pouch with the web or the thumb and forefinger of one hand and then push the patella quickly downward against the femur with a finger of your other hand. If an effusion is present, a tapping or clicking will be sensed when the patella is pushed against the femur. Release the pressure against the patella, but keep your finger lightly touching it. If an effusion is present, the patella will float out as if a fluid wave were pushing it (Fig. 22.47).

Examination for the bulge sign is also used to determine the presence of excess fluid in the knee. With the patient's knee extended, milk the medial aspect of the knee upward two or three times and then milk the lateral side of the patella. Observe for a bulge of returning fluid to the hollow area medial to the patella (Fig. 22.48).

The McMurray test is used to detect a torn medial or lateral meniscus. Have the patient lie supine and flex one knee. Position your thumb and fingers on either side of the joint space. Hold the heel with your other hand, fully flexing the knee, and rotate the foot and knee outward (valgus stress) to a lateral position. Extend and then flex the patient's knee. Any palpable or audible click, pain, or limited extension of the knee is a positive sign of a torn medial meniscus. Repeat the procedure, rotating the foot and knee inward (varus stress; Fig. 22.49). A palpable or

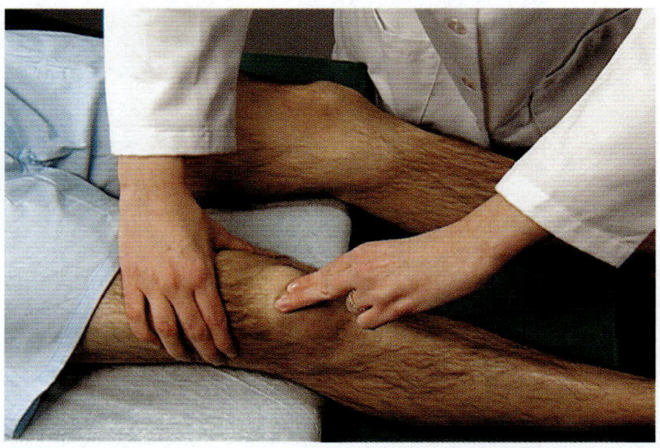

FIG. 22.47 Procedure for ballottement examination of the knee.

Evidence-Based Practice in Physical Examination

Hip Osteoarthritis

Simple tests of hip motion and observing for pain during that motion can be helpful in distinguishing patients most likely to have osteoarthritis (OA) from those who do not.

To identify patients most likely to have OA, the most useful physical findings were squat causing posterior hip pain (sensitivity, 24%; specificity, 96%); groin pain on passive abduction or adduction (sensitivity, 33%; specificity, 94%); abductor weakness (sensitivity, 44%; specificity, 90%); and decreased passive hip adduction (sensitivity, 80%; specificity, 81%). A combination of findings efficiently detects those most likely to have severe hip OA. The presence of normal passive hip adduction was most useful for suggesting the absence of OA.

Data from Metcalfe, D., Perry, D. C., Claireaux, H. A., Simel, D. L., Zogg, C. K., & Costa, M. L. (2019). Does this patient have hip osteoarthritis? The rational clinical examination systematic review. *Journal of the American Medical Association, 322*(23), 2323–2333.

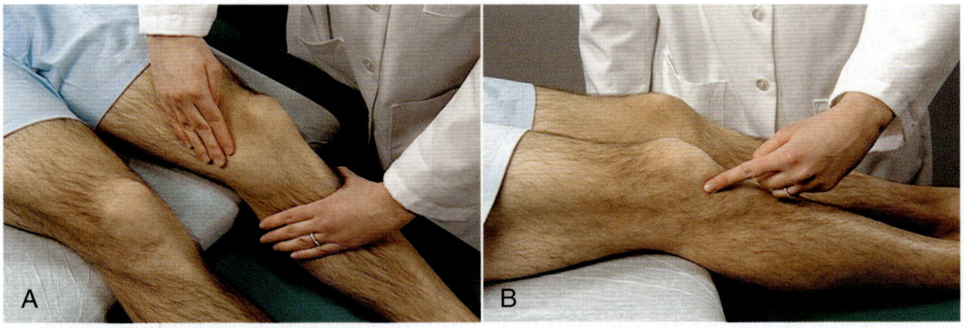

FIG. 22.48 Testing for the bulge sign in examination of the knee. (A) Milk the medial aspect of the knee two or three times. (B) Tap the lateral side of the patella.

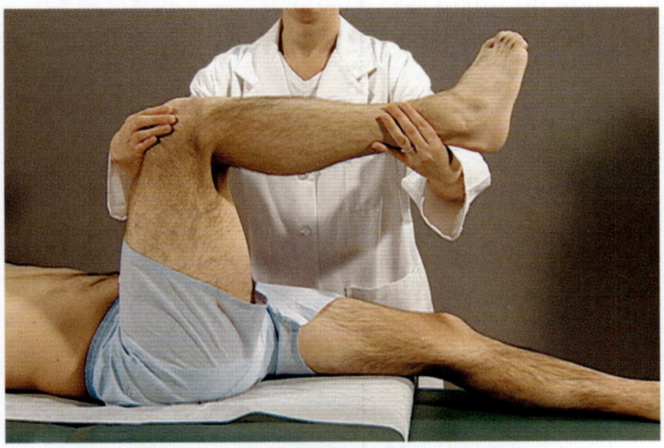

FIG. 22.49 Procedure for examination of the knee with the McMurray test. Knee is flexed after lower leg was rotated to medial position.

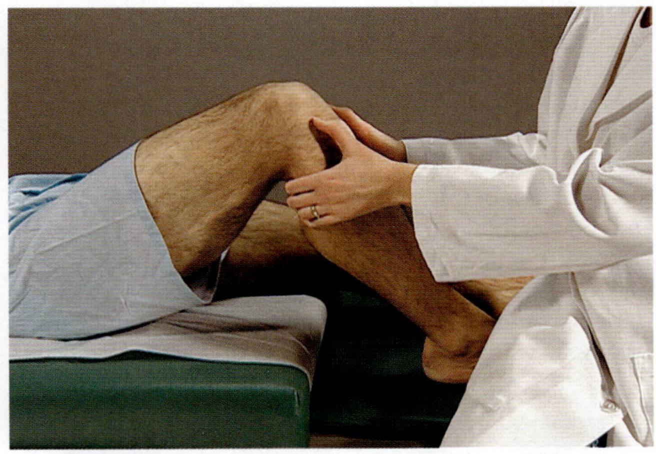

FIG. 22.50 Examination of the knee with the drawer test for anterior and posterior stability.

audible click, pain, or lack of extension is a positive sign of a torn lateral meniscus.

The anterior and posterior *drawer test* is used to identify instability of the anterior and posterior cruciate ligaments. Have the patient lie supine and flex the knee 45 to 90 degrees, placing the foot flat on the table. Place both hands on the lower leg with the thumbs on the ridge of the anterior tibia just distal to the tibial tuberosity. Draw the tibia forward, forcing the tibia to slide forward of the femur. Then push the tibia backward (Fig. 22.50). Anterior or posterior movement of the knee greater than 5 mm in either direction is an unexpected finding.

The *Lachman test* is used to evaluate anterior cruciate ligament integrity. With the patient supine, flex the knee 10 to 15 degrees with the heel on the table. Place one hand above the knee to stabilize the femur and place the other hand around the proximal tibia. While stabilizing the femur, pull the tibia anteriorly. Attempt to have the patient relax the hamstring muscles for an optimal test. Increased laxity, greater than 5 mm compared with the uninjured side, indicates injury to the ligament.

Evidence-Based Practice in Physical Examination

Acute Knee Injury

In cases of an acute knee injury, the Ottawa Knee Rules identify the characteristics of patients who should have a radiograph of the knee. The rules include any of the following findings:

- Age older than 55 years
- Tenderness at head of fibula
- Isolated tenderness of the patella
- Inability to flex the knee to 90 degrees

Data from Jalili, M., & Gharebaghi, H. (2010). Validation of the Ottawa knee rule in Iran: A prospective study. *Emergency Medicine Journal, 27*(11), 849–851, http://dx.doi.org/10.1136/emj.2009.080267

The *varus (abduction)* and *valgus (adduction) stress tests* are used to identify instability in the lateral and medial collateral ligaments. Have the patient lie supine and extend the knee. Stabilize the femur with one hand and hold the ankle with your other hand. Apply varus force against the ankle (toward the midline) and internal rotation. Excessive laxity is felt as the joint opens. Laxity in this position indicates injury to the lateral collateral ligament. Then apply valgus force against the ankle (away from the midline) and external rotation. Laxity in this position indicates injury to the medial collateral ligament (Fig. 22.51). Repeat the movements with the patient's knee flexed to 30 degrees. No excessive medial or lateral movement of the knee is expected.

Limb Measurement

When a difference in length or circumference of matching extremities is suspected, measure and compare the size of both extremities. Leg length is measured from the anterior superior iliac spine to the medial malleolus of the ankle, crossing the knee on the medial side (Fig. 22.52A). Arm length is measured from the acromion process through the olecranon process to the distal ulnar prominence. The circumference of the extremities is measured in centimeters at the same distance on each limb from a major landmark (see Fig. 22.52B). Athletes who use the dominant arm almost exclusively in their activities (e.g., pitchers and tennis players) may have some discrepancy in circumference. For most people, there should be no more than a 1-cm discrepancy in length and circumference between matching extremities.

Infants

Genetic disorders and fetal conditions can produce musculoskeletal anomalies. The fetus may experience various postural pressures leading to reduced extension of the extremities and torsions of various bones.

In a fully undressed infant, observe the posture and spontaneous generalized movements. Use a warming table when examining a newborn. No localized or generalized muscular twitching is expected. Inspect the lower back for tufts of hair, dimples, discolorations, cysts, or masses near the spine. A mass near the spine is likely to be a meningocele or myelomeningocele.

From about age 2 months, the infant should be able to lift the head and trunk from the prone position, giving you an indication of forearm strength. Assess the curvature of the spine and the strength of the paravertebral muscles with the infant in a sitting position. Kyphosis of the thoracic and lumbar spine will be apparent in the sitting position until the infant can sit without support (Fig. 22.53).

Inspect the extremities, noting symmetric flexion of arms and legs. The axillary, gluteal, femoral, and popliteal creases should be symmetric, and the limbs should move freely. No unusual proportions or asymmetry of limb length or circumference, constricted annular bands, or other deformities should be noted.

Place the newborn in a fetal position to observe how that may have contributed to any asymmetry of flexion, position, or shape of the extremities. Newborns have some resistance to full extension of the elbows, hips, and knees. Movements should be symmetric.

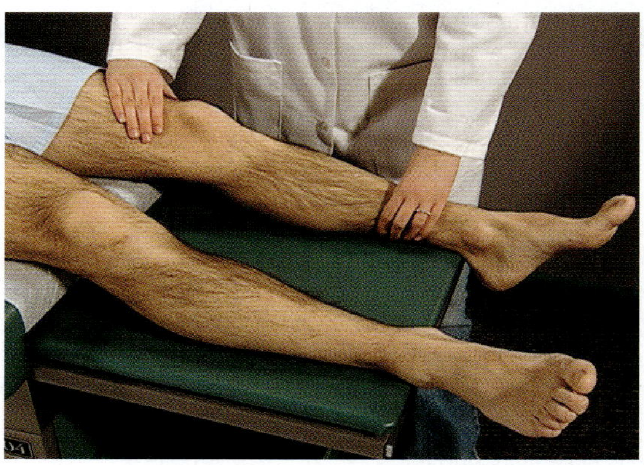

FIG. 22.51 Valgus stress test of the knee with knee extended.

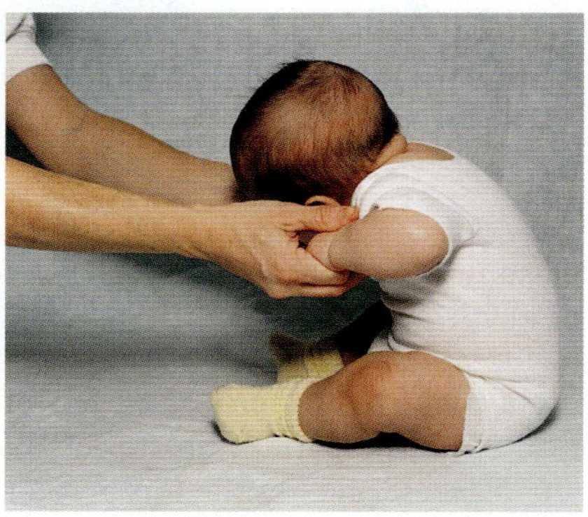

FIG. 22.53 Kyphosis, expected convex curvature of the newborn's thoracic and lumbar spine.

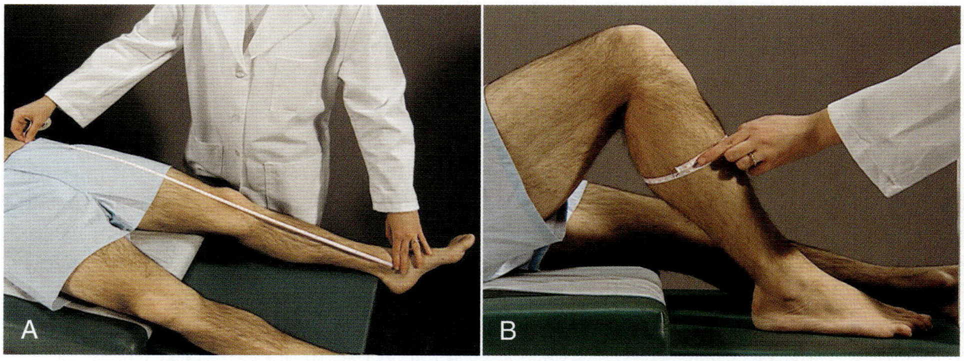

FIG. 22.52 Measuring limb length (A) and leg circumference (B).

All infants are flat footed, and many newborns have a slight varus curvature of the tibias (tibial torsion) or forefoot adduction (metatarsus adductus) from fetal positioning. The midline of the foot may bisect the third and fourth toes rather than the second and third toes. The forefoot should be flexible, straightening with abduction. It is necessary to follow tibial torsion and metatarsus adductus variations carefully, but they seldom require intervention. As growth and development take place, the expected body habitus is usually achieved.

The hands should open periodically with the fingers fully extended. Observe the palmar and phalangeal creases on each hand. A single crease extending across the entire palm is frequently associated with Down syndrome and other genetic conditions, but it may also be seen in healthy individuals. Count the fingers and toes, noting polydactyly (six or more digits on an extremity) or syndactyly (two or more digits fused together; Fig. 22.54).

Palpate the clavicles and long bones for fractures, dislocations, crepitus, masses, and tenderness. One of the most easily missed findings in the newborn is a fractured clavicle. This may be evident by a lump on the collarbone caused by the callus that forms on the healing clavicle noted in the first weeks after birth.

Position the baby with the trunk flexed and palpate each spinal process. Feel the shape of each, noting whether it is thin and well formed, as expected, or whether it is split, possibly indicating a bifid defect (Fig. 22.55).

Palpate the muscles to evaluate muscle tone, grasping the muscle to estimate its firmness. Observe for spasticity or flaccidity and, when detected, determine whether it is localized or generalized. Use passive range of motion to examine joint mobility.

The *Barlow and Ortolani maneuvers* to detect hip dislocation or subluxation should be performed each time you examine the infant during the first year of life. Using little force, test one hip at a time, stabilizing the pelvis with the other hand. With the infant supine, position yourself at the infant's feet, and flex the hip and knee to 90 degrees. For the Barlow maneuver, grasp the leg with your thumb on the inside of the thigh, the base of the thumb on the knee, and your fingers gripping the outer thigh with fingertips resting on the greater trochanter (Fig. 22.56). Adduct the thigh and gently apply downward pressure on the femur in an attempt to disengage the femoral head from the acetabulum. A positive sign is when a clunk or sensation is felt as the femoral head exits the acetabulum posteriorly. For the Ortolani maneuver, slowly abduct the thigh while maintaining axial pressure. With the fingertips on the greater trochanter, exert a lever movement in the opposite direction so that your fingertips press the head of the femur back toward the acetabulum center. If the head of the femur slips back into the acetabulum with a palpable clunk when pressure is exerted, you should suspect hip subluxation or dislocation and refer to an orthopedic surgeon for management. High-pitched clicks are common and expected. By 3 months of age, muscles and ligaments tighten, and limited abduction of the hips becomes the most reliable sign of hip subluxation or dislocation (Fig. 22.57).

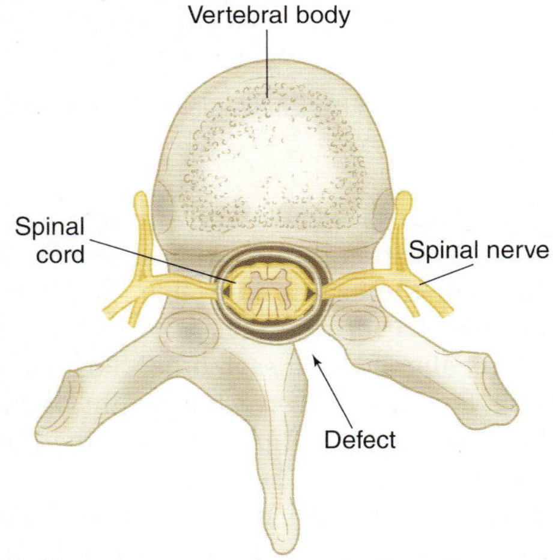

FIG. 22.55 Bifid defect of the vertebra identified by palpation.

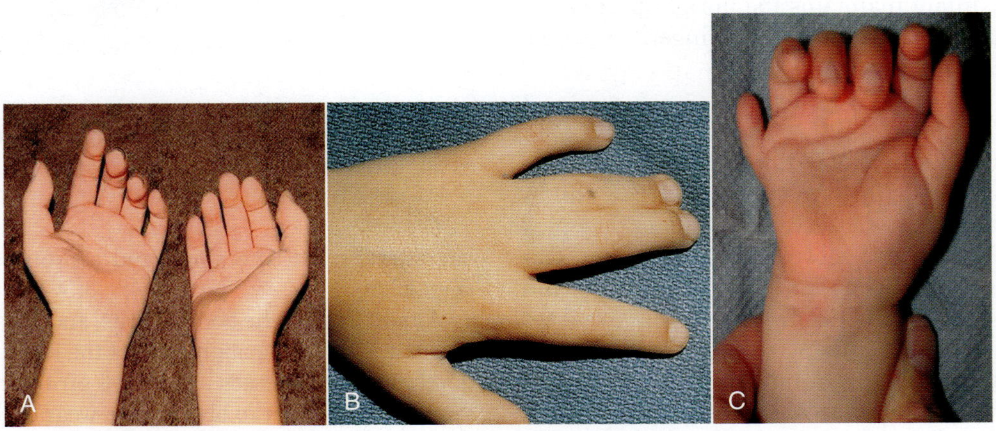

FIG. 22.54 Anomalies of the newborn's hand. (A) Simian crease. (B) Syndactyly. (C) Polydactyly. (A, from Davidson MA: developmental disabilities, part I primary care for children and adolescents with Down syndrome, *Pediatr Clin North Am* 55:1099–1111, 2008.; B, courtesy Dr. Joseph Imbriglia, Allegheny General Hospital; C, from Chung KC: Hand and upper extremity reconstruction with DVD: a volume in the procedures in reconstructive surgery series, Philadelphia, 2009, Saunders.)

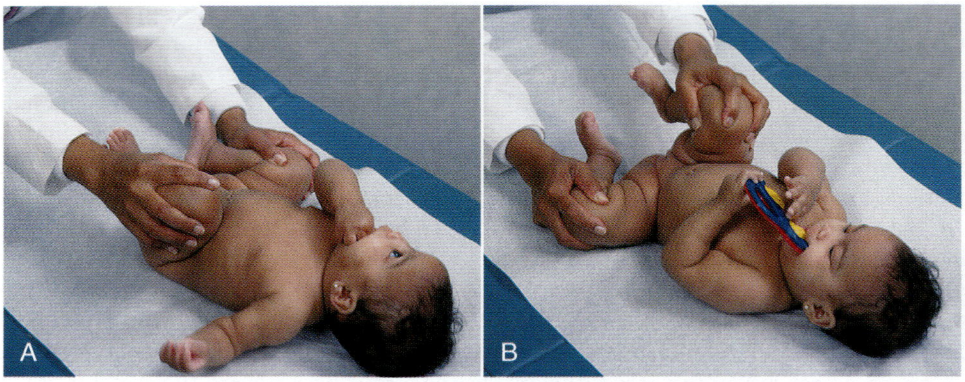

FIG. 22.56 Barlow and Ortolani maneuvers to detect hip dislocation. (A) Phase I, adduction. (B) Phase II, abduction.

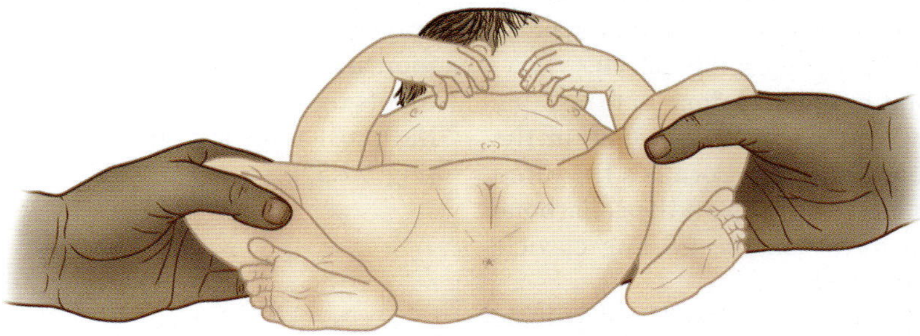

FIG. 22.57 Signs of hip dislocation: limitation of abduction and asymmetric gluteal folds.

The Galeazzi test, also called the *Allis sign,* can be used to detect hip dislocation or a shortened femur. With the infant supine on the examining table, flex both knees, keeping the feet flat on the table close to the buttocks and the femurs aligned with each other. Position yourself at the child's feet, and observe the height of the knees (Fig. 22.58). When one knee appears lower than the other, the Allis sign is positive.

General muscle strength is evaluated by holding the infant in vertical suspension with your hands under the axillae (Fig. 22.59). Adequate shoulder muscle strength is present if the infant maintains the upright position. If the infant begins to slip through your fingers, proximal muscle weakness is present.

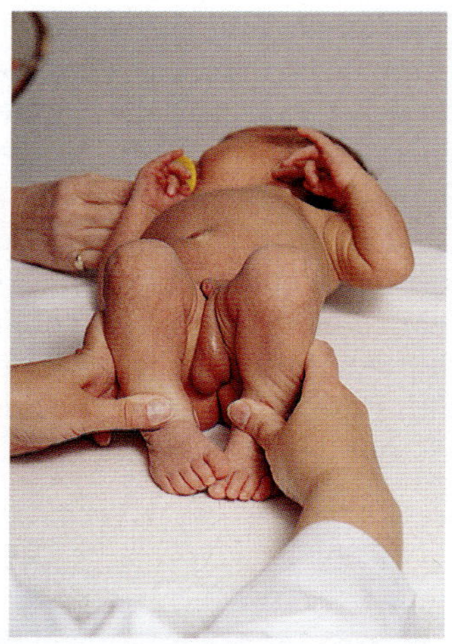

FIG. 22.58 Examination for the Allis sign. Unequal upper leg length would indicate a positive sign.

Children

Watching young children play during the history can provide a great deal of information about the child's musculoskeletal system. Observe the child as they pick up and play with toys and move around the room. Observe the toddler's ability to sit, creep, and grasp and release objects during play. Knowledge of the expected sequence of motor development will facilitate your examination. If the child shows no limitation, the musculoskeletal examination may not reveal any additional information.

Position the young child to observe motor development and musculoskeletal function. Inspect the child's spine while they are standing. Young children will have a lumbar curvature of the spine and a protuberant abdomen (Fig. 22.60).

As you inspect the bones, joints, and muscles, pay particular attention to the alignment of the legs and feet because developmental stresses are placed on the musculoskeletal system. Remember to observe the wear of the child's shoes and ask about their favorite sitting posture. The W or reverse tailor position places stress on the joints of the hips, knees, and ankles. It is commonly seen in children with in-toeing associated with femoral anteversion (Fig. 22.61).

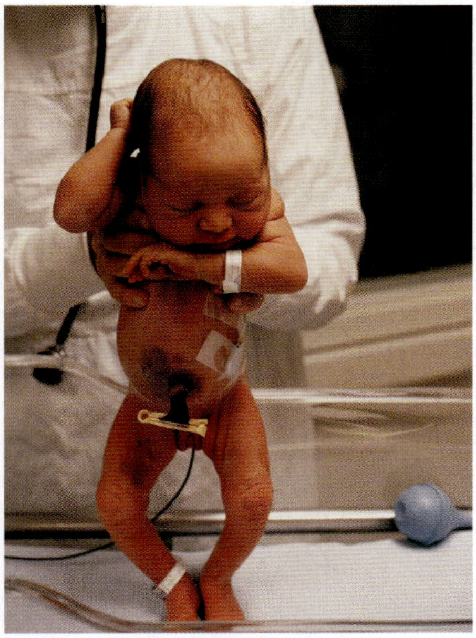

FIG. 22.59 Evaluation of shoulder muscle strength in the newborn.

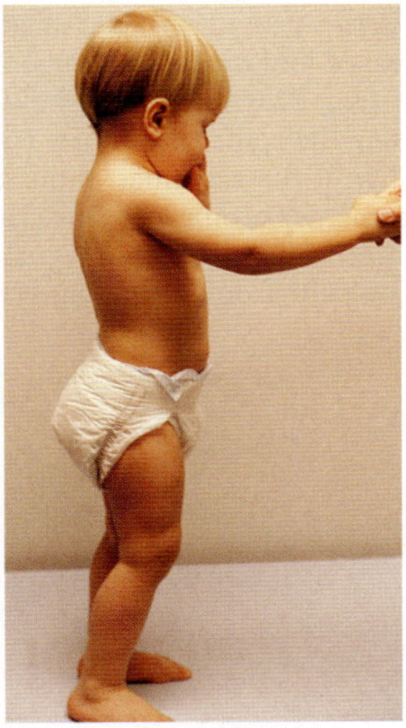

FIG. 22.60 Lumbar curvature of the toddler's spine.

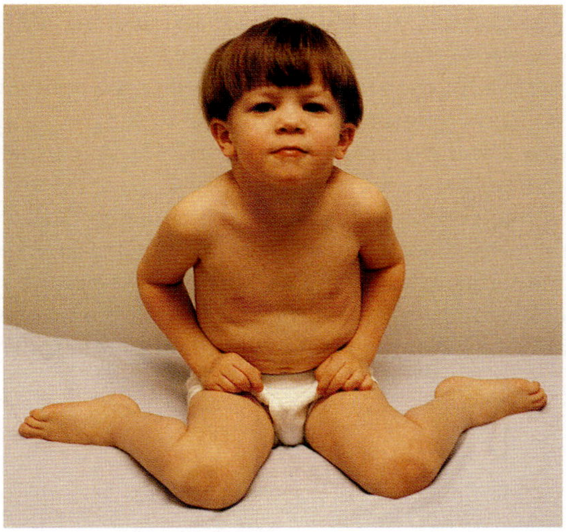

FIG. 22.61 Reverse tailor sitting position.

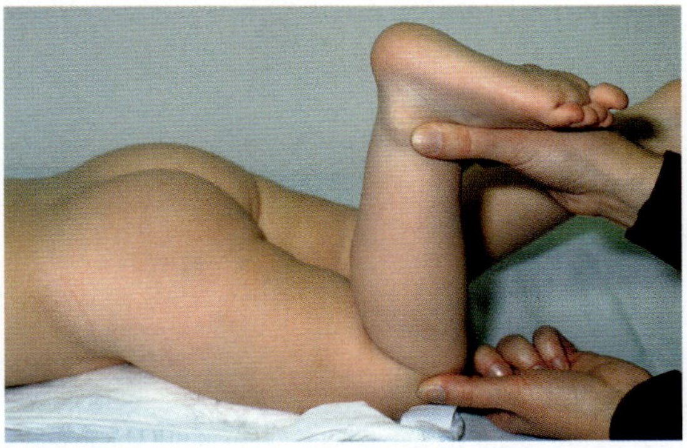

FIG. 22.62 Examination for tibial torsion.

Inspect the longitudinal arch of the foot and the position of the feet with weight bearing. A fat pad obscures the longitudinal arch of the foot until about 3 years of age; after that time, the arch should be apparent when the foot is not bearing weight. Metatarsus adductus should be resolved. The feet of the toddler will often pronate slightly inward until about 30 months of age. After that age, weight bearing should shift to the midline of the feet.

Assess for tibial torsion with the child prone on the examining table. Flex one knee 90 degrees and align the midline of the foot parallel to the femur. Using the thumb and index finger of one hand, grasp the medial and lateral malleoli of the ankle; then grasp the knee, placing your thumb and index finger on the same side of the leg (Fig. 22.62). If your thumbs are not parallel to each other, tibial torsion is present. Tibial torsion, a residual effect of fetal positioning, is expected to resolve within several years after weight bearing.

Assess for bowleg (genu varum) with the child standing, facing you, knees at your eye level. Measure the distance between the knees when the medial malleoli of the ankles are together. Genu varum is present if a space of 2.5 cm (1 inch) exists between the knees. The expected 10- to 15-degree angle at the tibiofemoral articulation increases with genu varum but remains bilaterally symmetric. On future examinations, note any increase in the angle or increased space between the knees. Genu varum is a common finding in toddlers until 18 months of age. Asymmetry of the tibiofemoral articulation angle or space between the knees should not exceed 4 cm (1.5 inches).

Evaluate for knock-knee (genu valgum) with the child standing, facing you, knees at your eye level. With the knees together, measure the distance between the medial malleoli of the ankles. Genu valgum is present if a space of 2.5 cm (1 inch) exists between the medial malleoli. As with genu varum, the tibiofemoral articulation angle will increase with genu valgum. On future examinations, note any increase in the angle or increased space between the ankles. Genu valgum is a common finding of children between 2 and 4 years of age (Fig. 22.63). Asymmetry of the tibiofemoral articulation angle or a space between the medial malleoli should not exceed 5 cm (2 inches).

Palpate the bones, muscles, and joints, paying particular attention to asymmetric body parts. Use passive range of motion to examine a joint and muscle group if some limitation of movement is noted while the child is playing.

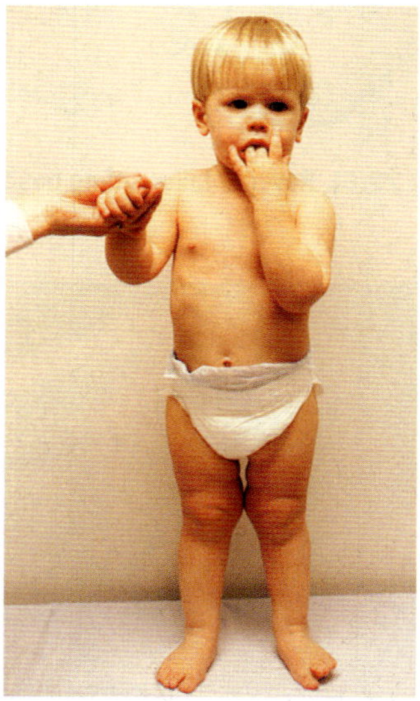

FIG. 22.63 Genu valgum (knock-knee) in the young child.

Ask the child to stand, rising from a supine position. The child with good muscle strength will rise to a standing position without using the arms for leverage. Proximal muscle weakness is indicated by the Gower sign in which the child rises from a sitting position by placing hands on the legs and pushing the trunk up (Fig. 22.64).

Adolescents

Examine older children and adolescents with the same procedures used for adults. Specific procedures for the musculoskeletal examination for sports participation are found in Chapter 25.

The spine should be smooth, with balanced concave and convex curves. No lateral curvature or rib hump with forward flexion should be apparent. The shoulders and scapulae should be level with each other within 0.5 inches, and a distance between the scapulae of 3 to 5 inches is usual (see Fig. 22.12B). Adolescents may have slight kyphosis and rounded shoulders with an interscapular space of 5 or 6 inches.

Pregnant Patients

Postural changes with pregnancy are common. The growing fetus shifts the patient's center of gravity forward, leading to increased lordosis and a compensatory forward cervical flexion (Fig. 22.65). Stooped shoulders and large breasts exaggerate the spinal curvature. Increased mobility and instability of the sacroiliac joints and symphysis pubis as the ligaments become less tense contribute to the "waddling" gait of late pregnancy. Pregnant patients can often experience pain from the pubic symphysis down

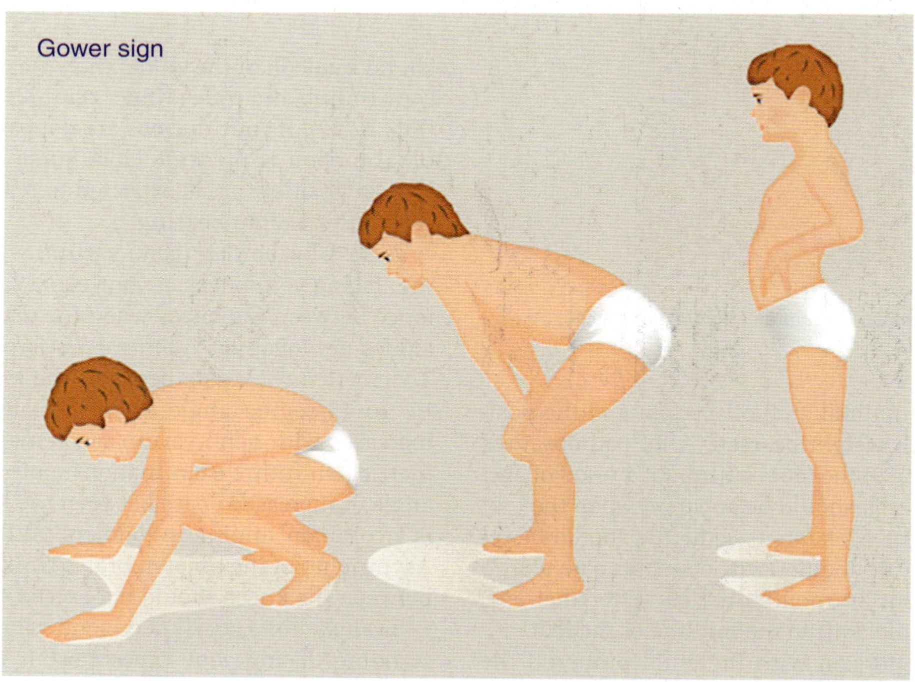

FIG. 22.64 **Gower sign.** Starting from a seated position on the floor, the child uses their hands to "climb up" their legs to achieve a standing position. This is due to weakness in the pelvis, hips, and thighs. (From Heaver C, et al: *Neuromuscular disorders: a guide for the orthopaedic surgeon*, Orthopaedics and Trauma 33(4): 239–248, 2019.)

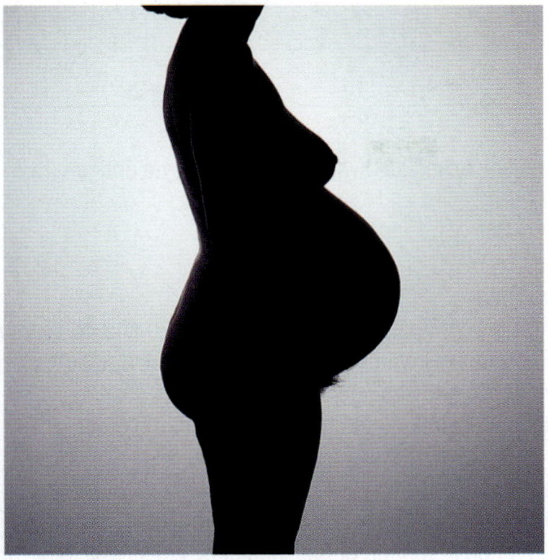

FIG. 22.65 Postural changes with pregnancy.

into the inner thigh when standing and may have a feeling that the bones are moving or snapping when walking.

During pregnancy, increases in the lumbosacral curve and anterior flexion of the head in the cervicodorsal region become apparent. To assess for lumbosacral hyperextension, ask the patient to bend forward at the waist toward the toes. Palpate the distance between the L4 and S1 spinal processes. As the patient rises to standing, from full flexion to full extension, note when the distance between L4 and S1 becomes fixed. If it becomes fixed before the spine is fully extended, the patient will be hyperextended when walking, possibly resulting in lower back pain. Most back pain resolves within 6 months after delivery.

Carpal tunnel syndrome (discussed later in the chapter) is experienced by some patients during the last trimester because of the associated fluid retention during pregnancy. Usually, the symptoms abate several weeks after delivery.

Older Adults

The older adult should be able to participate in the physical examination as described for the adult, but the response to your requests may be more slow and deliberate. Fine and gross motor skills required to perform activities of daily living such as dressing, grooming, climbing steps, and writing will provide an evaluation of the patient's joint muscle agility (see the Functional Assessment box). Joint and muscle agility have tremendous extremes among older adults.

The patient's posture may display increased dorsal kyphosis, accompanied by flexion of the hips and knees. The head may tilt backward to compensate for the increased thoracic curvature (see Fig. 22.31B). The extremities may appear to be relatively long if the trunk has diminished in length due to vertebral collapse. The base of support may be broader with the feet more widely spaced, and the patient may hold the arms away from the body to aid balancing. The reduction in total muscle mass is often related to atrophy either from disuse, as in patients with arthritis, or from loss of nerve innervation, as in patients with diabetic neuropathy.

FUNCTIONAL ASSESSMENT

Musculoskeletal Assessment

ACTIVITY TO OBSERVE	INDICATORS OF WEAKENED MUSCLE GROUPS
Rising from lying to sitting position	Rolling to one side and pushing with arms to raise to elbows; grabbing a side rail or table to pull to sitting
Rising from chair to standing	Pushing with arms to supplement weak leg muscles; upper torso thrusts forward before body rises
Walking	Lifting leg farther off floor with each step; shortened swing phase; foot may fall or slide forward; arms held out for balance or move in rowing motion
Climbing steps	Holding handrail for balance; pulling body up and forward with arms; uses stronger leg
Descending steps	Lowering weakened leg first; often descends sideways holding rail with both hands; may watch feet
Picking up item from floor	Leaning on furniture for support; bending over at waist to avoid bending knees; uses one hand on thigh to assist with lowering and raising torso
Tying shoes	Using footstool to decrease spinal flexion
Putting on and pulling up trousers or stockings	Difficulty may indicate decreased shoulder and upper arm strength; these activities are often performed in sitting position until clothing is pulled up
Putting on sweater	Putting sleeve on weaker arm or shoulder first; uses internal or external shoulder rotation to get remaining arm in sleeve
Zipping dress in back	Difficulty with this indicates weakened shoulder rotation
Combing hair	Difficulty indicates problems with grasp, wrist flexion, pronation and supination of forearm, and elbow rotation
Pushing chair away from table while seated	Standing and easing chair back with torso; difficulty indicates problems with upper arm, shoulder, lower arm strength, and wrist motion
Buttoning button or writing name	Difficulty indicates problem with manual dexterity and finger-thumb opposition

Modified from Wilson, S. F., & Giddens, J. F. (2005). *Health assessment for nursing practice* (3rd ed.). St Louis: Mosby.

ABNORMALITIES

MUSCULOSKELETAL

Ankylosing Spondylitis

A chronic inflammatory disease of the spine, ankylosing spondylitis has a genetic predisposition associated with human leukocyte antigen (HLA)–B27 and may affect the cervical, thoracic, and lumbar spine along with the sacroiliac joints (Fig. 22.66)

PATHOPHYSIOLOGY

- Inflamed intervertebral disk and longitudinal ligament ossification
- Leads to eventual fusion and severe deformity of the vertebral column

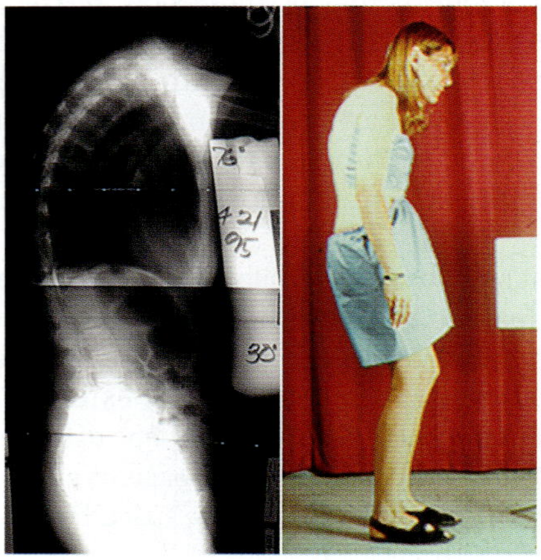

PATIENT DATA

Subjective Data

- Develops predominantly in males between 20 and 40 years of age
- Begins insidiously with inflammatory low back and buttock pain, also involving hips and shoulders
- Buttock pain can fluctuate from one side to the other

Objective Data

- Restriction in the lumbar flexion of the patient
- Limited range of motion of the shoulders, chest wall, hips, and knees may develop
- Uveitis may be present

FIG. 22.66 Gross postural changes in patient affected by ankylosing spondylitis. (From Miller RD: *Miller's anesthesia*, ed 7, Philadelphia, 2010, Churchill Livingstone.)

Lumbosacral Radiculopathy (Herniated Lumbar Disk)

Herniation of a lumbar disk that irritates the corresponding spinal nerve root

PATHOPHYSIOLOGY

- Generally caused by degenerative changes of the disk
- Most commonly occurring at the L4, L5, and S1 nerve roots
- Greatest incidence occurs between 31 and 50 years of age

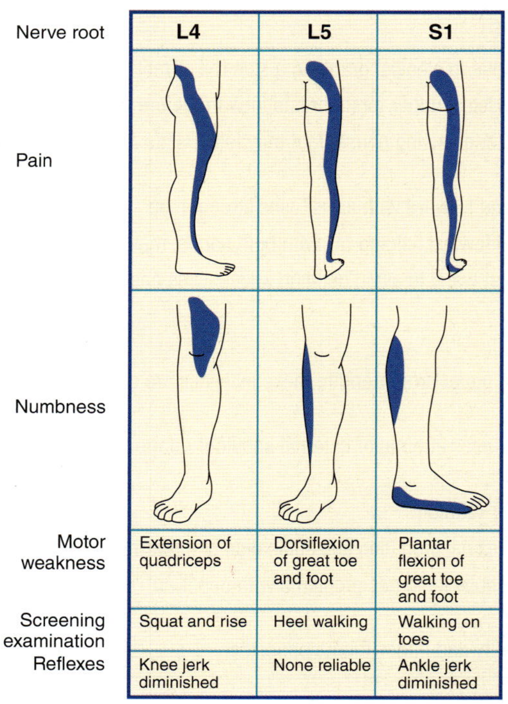

PATIENT DATA

Subjective Data

- Can be associated with lifting heavy objects
- Common symptoms include low back pain with radiation to the buttocks and posterior thigh or down the leg in the distribution of the dermatome of the nerve root
- Pain relief is often achieved by lying down

Objective Data

- Spasm and tenderness over the paraspinal musculature may be present
- Potential difficulty with heel walking (L4 and L5) or toe walking (S1)
- Numbness, tingling, or weakness in the involved extremity (Fig. 22.67)

FIG. 22.67 Distribution of paresthesia and radiating pain associated with herniated disks at the L4, L5, and S1 nerve roots. (From Thompson JM, et al: *Mosby's clinical nursing*, ed 4, St Louis, 1997, Mosby.)

Lumbar Stenosis

Narrowing of the spinal canal

PATHOPHYSIOLOGY

- Canal narrowing from bone and ligament hypertrophy may lead to entrapment of the spinal cord as it traverses the spinal canal

PATIENT DATA

Subjective Data

- Pain with walking or standing upright that often seems to originate in the buttocks and may then radiate down the legs
- Pain relief may occur with sitting or bending forward
- Pain may be worsened by prolonged standing, walking, or hyperextending the back

Objective Data

- In the early stages, the neurologic examination is frequently normal
- With progression, the examination may show lower extremity weakness and sensory loss
- A stooped forward gait may be present

Carpal Tunnel Syndrome

Compression on the median nerve (see Fig. 22.41)

PATHOPHYSIOLOGY

- Compression of the nerve within its flexor tendon sheath due to microtrauma, local edema or inflammation, repetitive motion, or vibration of the hands
- Associated with rheumatoid arthritis, gout, acromegaly, hypothyroidism, and the hormonal changes of pregnancy

PATIENT DATA

Subjective Data

- Numbness, burning, and tingling in the hands often occur at night
- Can also be elicited by flexion/extension movements of the wrist
- Pain may radiate to the arms

Objective Data

- Weakness of the thumb and flattening of the thenar eminence of the palm
- Reproduction of symptoms with provocation of the Tinel and Phalen maneuvers

Gout

A form of arthritis resulting from chronically elevated serum uric acid

PATHOPHYSIOLOGY

- Monosodium urate crystal deposition in joints and surrounding tissues results in acute inflammatory attacks

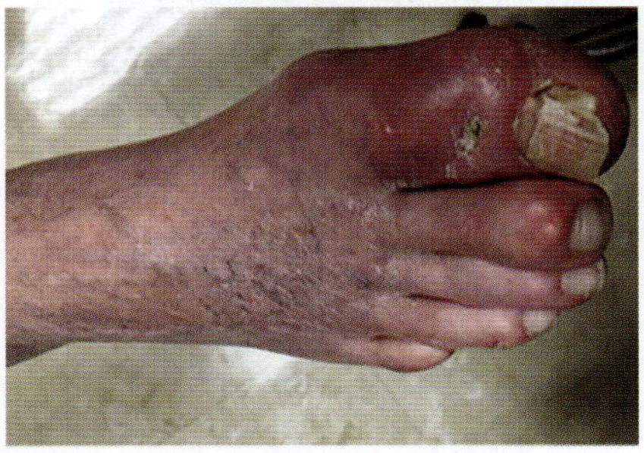

FIG. 22.68 Tophi of first and second toe with whitish material seen under the skin of the distal second toe. (From Fields TR: *The challenges of approaching and managing gout*, Rheumatic Disease Clinics of North America 45(1):145-157, 2018.)

PATIENT DATA

Subjective Data

- Sudden onset of a hot, swollen joint; exquisite pain; limited range of motion
- Primarily affects males older than 40 years and females of postmenopausal age
- Usually affects the proximal phalanx of the great toe, although the wrists, hands, ankles, and knees may be involved

Objective Data

- The skin over the swollen joint may be shiny and red or purple
- Uric acid crystals may form as tophi under the skin with chronic gout (Fig. 22.68)

Temporomandibular Joint Syndrome

Painful jaw movement

PATHOPHYSIOLOGY

- Caused by congenital anomalies, malocclusion, trauma, arthritis, and other joint diseases

PATIENT DATA

Subjective Data

- Unilateral facial pain that usually worsens with joint movement
- May be referred to any point on the face or neck

Objective Data

- Most patients have a muscle spasm, and many have clicking, popping, or crepitus in the affected joint

Osteomyelitis

An infection in the bone

PATHOPHYSIOLOGY

- Usually results from an open wound or systemic infection
- Purulent matter spreads through the cortex of the bone and into the soft tissue
- Decreased blood flow to the affected bone may lead to bone necrosis

PATIENT DATA

Subjective Data

- Dull pain develops insidiously at the involved site and progresses over days to weeks
- Limp or decreased movement in infants and children

Objective Data

- Signs of infection include edema, erythema, and warmth at the site
- Tenderness to palpation, pain with movement, and signs of inflammation such as fevers

Bursitis

Inflammation of the bursa

PATHOPHYSIOLOGY

- Due to repetitive movement and excessive pressure on the bursa
- Can also be due to infection or gout

PATIENT DATA

Subjective Data

- Common sites include the shoulder, elbow, hip, and knee, with pain and stiffness surrounding the joint around the inflamed bursa
- The pain is usually worse during activity

Objective Data

- Limitation of motion caused by swelling; pain on movement; point tenderness; and an erythematous, warm site (Fig. 22.69)
- Soreness may radiate to tendons at the site

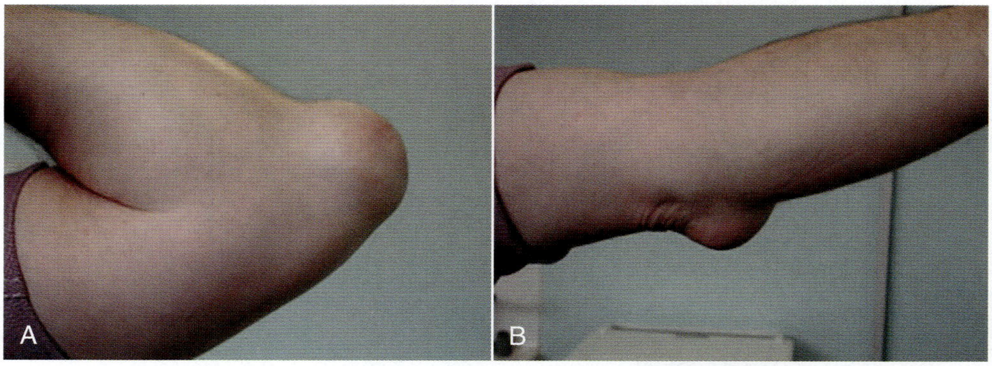

FIG. 22.69 (A) Olecranon bursitis with (B) full range of elbow extension. (From Reilly D, Kamineni S: Olecranon bursitis, *J Shoulder Elbow Surg* 25(1):158–167, 2016.)

Paget Disease of the Bone (Osteitis Deformans)

A focal metabolic disorder of the bone

PATHOPHYSIOLOGY

- Appears in persons older than 45 years
- Excessive bone resorption and bone formation produce a mosaic pattern of lamellar bone

PATIENT DATA

Subjective Data

- Vertigo and headache as a result of skull involvement
- Progressive deafness from involvement of the ossicles or neural elements may develop

Objective Data

- Bowed tibias, misshapen pelvis, or prominent skull forehead may be evident
- Frequent fractures may occur

Osteoarthritis

The deterioration of the articular cartilage covering the ends of bone in synovial joints

PATHOPHYSIOLOGY

- As a result of cartilage abrasion, pitting, and thinning, the bone surfaces are eventually exposed, with bone rubbing against bone
- Separately there can be remodeling of the bone surface and formation of bone spurs

PATIENT DATA

Subjective Data

- Pain in hands, feet, hips, knees, and cervical or lumbar spine (most commonly)
- Onset usually begins after 40 years of age and develops slowly over many years, with nearly 100% of people older than 75 years affected

Objective Data

- The joints may be enlarged due to bone growths (osteophytes; see Fig. 22.18B)
- May have crepitus and limited, painful range of motion

Rheumatoid Arthritis

A chronic systemic inflammatory disorder of the synovial tissue surrounding the joints

PATHOPHYSIOLOGY

- Cause is unknown
- Within the inflamed synovial tissue and fluid, polymorphonuclear leukocytes aggregate
- Multiple inflammatory cytokines and enzymes are released that can result in subsequent damage to bone, cartilage, and other tissues

PATIENT DATA

Subjective Data

- Joint pain and stiffness, especially in the morning or after periods of inactivity
- Constitutional symptoms of fatigue, myalgias, weight loss, and low-grade fever are common

Objective Data

- Involved joints include the hands, wrists, feet, and ankles as well as the hips, knees, and cervical spine
- Synovitis, with soft tissue swelling and effusions, is present on examination
- Nodules and characteristic deformities can develop (see Fig. 22.16)

The Differential Diagnosis table contrasts rheumatoid arthritis and osteoarthritis.

DIFFERENTIAL DIAGNOSIS

Comparison of Osteoarthritis With Rheumatoid Arthritis

SIGNS AND SYMPTOMS	OSTEOARTHRITIS	RHEUMATOID ARTHRITIS
Onset	Insidious, over many years	Gradual (typically weeks to months), although sometimes sudden (24–48 hours)
Duration of morning stiffness	Only a few minutes in the localized joints	Several hours
Pain	On motion, with prolonged activity, relieved by rest	Even at rest, may disturb sleep
Weakness	Usually localized and not severe	Often pronounced, out of proportion with muscle atrophy
Fatigue	Unusual	Often severe, with onset 4–5 hours after rising
Emotional depression and lability	Unusual	Common, coinciding with fatigue and disease activity, often relieved if in remission
Tenderness localized over afflicted joint	Common	Almost always, most sensitive indicator of inflammation
Swelling	Noninflammatory effusion common, little synovial reaction	Fusiform soft tissue enlargement, inflammatory effusion common, synovial proliferation and thickening, often symmetric, rheumatoid nodules
Heat, erythema	Unusual, minimal if present	Sometimes present
Crepitus, crackling	Coarse to medium on motion	Medium to fine
Joint enlargement	Mild with bony consistency due to osteophytes	Moderate to severe if an inflammatory effusion is present

SPORTS INJURIES

Trauma to the musculoskeletal system results in a variety of injuries to muscles, bones, and supportive joint structures. The injury may be the result of an acute incident or overuse and repetitive trauma. Often a neurovascular assessment is necessary to detect any nerve damage or circulatory impairment (Box 22.1).

BOX 22.1 Neurovascular Assessment

Assessment of circulation and nerve sensation is important when an extremity is injured. Perform the following steps to complete a neurovascular assessment distal to the injury. Use the contralateral extremity for comparison.

ASSESSMENT	UNEXPECTED FINDINGS
Color	Pallor or cyanosis
Temperature	Cool or cold
Capillary refill time	Greater than 4 seconds
Swelling	Significantly swollen
Pain	Presence of moderate to severe pain
Sensation	Numbness, tingling, pins-and-needles sensation
Movement	Decreased or no movement

Consider all the findings simultaneously to complete the neurovascular assessment. The presence of most or all of these unexpected findings indicates significantly impaired circulation and pressure or injury to the nerve, which requires emergency intervention.

Risk Factors

Sports Injury

- Poor physical conditioning
- Failure to warm up muscles adequately
- Intensity of competition
- Collision and contact sports participation
- Rapid growth
- Overuse of joints

Muscle Strain

PATHOPHYSIOLOGY

- Can be due to excessive stretching or forceful contraction beyond the muscle's functional capacity
- Often associated with improper exercise warm-up, fatigue, or previous injury

PATIENT DATA

Subjective Data

- Muscle pain
- Severity ranges from a mild intrafibrous tear to a total rupture of a single muscle

Objective Data

- Temporary muscle weakness, spasm, pain, and contusion

Dislocation

Complete separation of the contact between two bones in a joint

PATHOPHYSIOLOGY

- Often caused by pressure or force pushing the bone out of the joint; usually occurs in the setting of acute trauma

PATIENT DATA

Subjective Data

- Can occur more easily in patients with hyperextensibility conditions (e.g., Marfan, Ehlers-Danlos)

Objective Data

- Deformity and inability to use the extremity or joint as usual

Fracture

Partial or complete break in the continuity of a bone

PATHOPHYSIOLOGY

- From trauma (direct, indirect, twisting, or crushing)

PATIENT DATA

Subjective Data

- Pain, limited movement, cannot bear weight, swelling
- Felt a pop or snap with injury
- Can occur more easily in patients with bone disorders (e.g., osteogenesis imperfecta, osteoporosis, bone metastasis)

Objective Data

- Deformity, edema, pain, loss of function, color changes, and paresthesia

Tenosynovitis (Tendonitis)

Inflammation of the synovium-lined sheath around a tendon

PATHOPHYSIOLOGY

- Seen with repetitive actions associated with occupational or sports activities
- Can occur in inflammatory conditions like rheumatoid arthritis

PATIENT DATA

Subjective Data

- Pain with movement of such common sites as the shoulder, knee, heel, and wrist

Objective Data

- Point tenderness over the involved tendon
- Pain with active movement and some limitation of movement in the affected joint

Rotator Cuff Tear

Microtrauma and tearing of the rotator cuff muscles, most often the supraspinatus

PATHOPHYSIOLOGY

- Usually due to degeneration of the muscle and tendon from repeated overhead lifting and compression under the acromion
- An acute tear may also result from a fall on an outstretched arm

PATIENT DATA

Subjective Data

- Pain in the shoulder and deltoid area is common; this can awaken the patient at night

Objective Data

- Inability to maintain a lateral raised arm against resistance may develop due to pain
- Tenderness over the acromioclavicular joint
- Grating sound on movement, crepitus, and weakness in external shoulder rotation

Infants and Children

Clubfoot (Talipes Equinovarus)

Fixed congenital defect of the ankle and foot

PATHOPHYSIOLOGY

- Causes include genetic factors and external influences in the final trimester, such as intrauterine compression

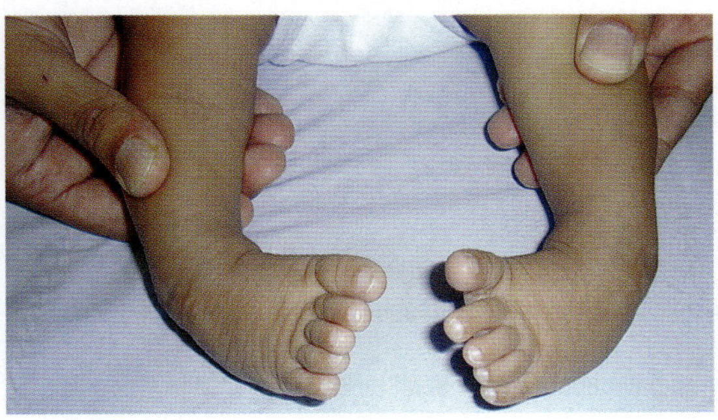

PATIENT DATA

Subjective Data

- Diagnosis is usually obvious at birth with the characteristic deformity

Objective Data

- Most common combination of position deformities includes inversion of the foot at the ankle and plantar flexion, with the toes lower than the heel (Fig. 22.70)

FIG. 22.70 Clubfoot deformity, talipes equinovarus (bilateral deviation). (From Foster A, et al: *Congenital talipes equinovarus (clubfoot)*, Surgery—Oxford international edition 25(4):171–175, 2007.)

Metatarsus Adductus (Metatarsus Varus)

The most common congenital foot deformity; can be either fixed or flexible

PATHOPHYSIOLOGY

- Defect is caused by intrauterine positioning
- Medial adduction of the toes and forefoot results from angulation at the tarsometatarsal joint

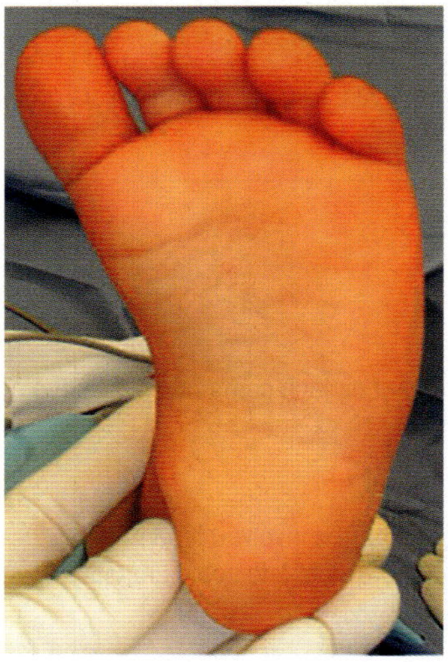

FIG. 22.71 **Metatarsus adductus.** (From Hagmann S, et al: Skewfoot, Foot and Ankle Clinics 14(3):409–434, 2009.)

PATIENT DATA

Subjective Data

- Diagnosis is usually obvious at birth with the characteristic deformity
- The heel and ankle are uninvolved (Fig. 22.71)

Objective Data

- The lateral border of the foot is convex
- A crease is sometimes apparent on the medial border of the foot

Legg-Calvé-Perthes Disease

Avascular necrosis of the femoral head

PATHOPHYSIOLOGY

- Results from a decreased blood supply to the femoral head

PATIENT DATA

Subjective Data

- Most commonly seen in young males between 3 and 11 years of age
- Pain is often referred to the medial thigh, knee, or groin
- Bilateral involvement may occur in 10% of cases

Objective Data

- Child may have a limp that is painless or antalgic (painful limp with shortened time on extremity)
- Loss of internal rotation; abduction and decreased range of motion on the affected side are seen
- Muscle weakness of the upper leg may be present if symptoms have been present for a prolonged period

Osgood-Schlatter Disease

A traction apophysitis (inflammation of a bony outgrowth) of the anterior aspect of the tibial tubercle

PATHOPHYSIOLOGY

- Inflammation of a bony outgrowth of the anterior aspect of the tibial tubercle
- Develops in association with inflammation of the anterior patellar tendon
- This self-limiting disorder is most common in young males between 9 and 15 years of age

PATIENT DATA

Subjective Data

- The child may walk with a limp
- Often describes knee pain (especially with activity)

Objective Data

- Knee swelling that is aggravated by strenuous activity
- Pain especially prominent with activity involving the quadriceps muscle
- Pain with palpation over the tibial tuberosity

Slipped Capital Femoral Epiphysis

Disorder in which the capital femoral epiphysis slips over the neck of the femur

PATHOPHYSIOLOGY

- Most common between 8 and 16 years of age, although affected females are often younger than affected males
- Majority of cases (75%) are unilateral; left side is involved more often than the right
- More common in overweight and obese patients

PATIENT DATA

Subjective Data

- The child or adolescent presents with knee pain and a limp

Objective Data

- The affected child has leg weakness and reduced internal hip rotation
- Characteristic plain radiograph shows slippage of femoral head

Muscular Dystrophy

A group of genetic disorders involving gradual degeneration of the muscle fibers

PATHOPHYSIOLOGY

- Progressive symmetric weakness and muscle atrophy or pseudohypertrophy from fatty muscle infiltrates
- Skeletal muscles and the heart may be involved
- Some forms result in only mild disability, and these patients can expect a normal life span.
- Other types produce severe disability, deformity, and death

PATIENT DATA

Subjective Data

- Early signs may include clumsiness, difficulty climbing stairs, and frequent falls

Objective Data

- Muscle atrophy and weakness with a waddling gait
- A positive Gower sign (see Fig. 22.64)
- Progressive loss of function, including ability to walk

Scoliosis

Physical deformity of the spine

PATHOPHYSIOLOGY

- A curvature of the vertebral bodies such that when viewed from the rear, the spine may look more like an "S" or a "C" rather than a straight line
- Structural scoliosis most commonly affects young females and progresses during early adolescence
- There is no known cause

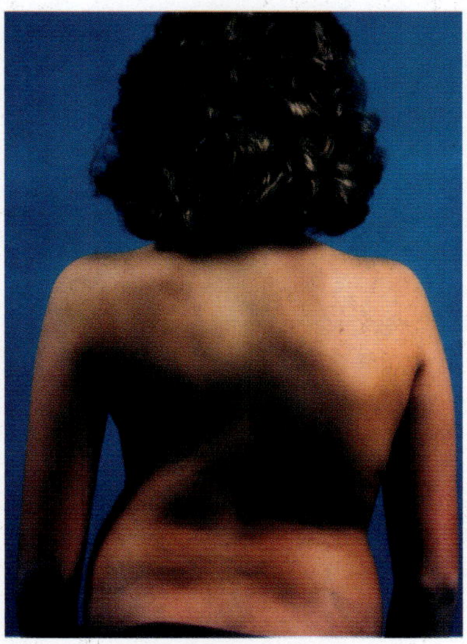

FIG. 22.72 Scoliosis, lateral curvature of the spine. Scapular asymmetry is easily discernible in the upright position. (From Herring JA: *Tachdjian's pediatric orthopaedics*, ed 5, St Louis, 2014, Elsevier.)

PATIENT DATA

Subjective Data

- May lead to back discomfort and is often associated with a leg length discrepancy

Objective Data

- Lateral curvature of the spine, rib hump as the child flexes forward to touch the toes
- Scoliometer reading of greater than or equal to 7 degrees is a positive screening test
- In severe deformities, the patient has uneven shoulder and hip levels; may have a crease on one side at the waist
- Physiologic alterations occur in the spine, chest, and pelvis (Fig. 22.72)

Radial Head Subluxation (Nursemaid's Elbow)

A dislocation injury

PATHOPHYSIOLOGY

- Caused by jerking the arm upward while the elbow is extended
- The jerking pulls apart the elbow joint and tears the margin of the annular ligament around the radial head into the joint
- Common in children 1–4 years of age

PATIENT DATA

Subjective Data

- Child complains of pain in the elbow and wrist and/or refuses to move the arm

Objective Data

- Child holds the arm slightly flexed and pronated
- Supination motion is resisted

Older Adults

Osteoporosis

A decrease in bone mass that occurs when bone resorption is more rapid than bone deposition

PATHOPHYSIOLOGY

- The bones become fragile and susceptible to spontaneous fractures
- Most commonly seen in postmenopausal females, with a female-to-male ratio of 4:1
- Glucocorticoid excess and hypogonadism are also risk factors

PATIENT DATA

Subjective Data

- Presenting symptom is usually loss of height or an acute, painful fracture
- Most common fracture sites are the hip, vertebrae, and wrist

Objective Data

- Affected persons lose height and have decreased abdominothoracic space (Fig. 22.73)
- In the spine, vertebral compression fractures lead to kyphosis or scoliosis

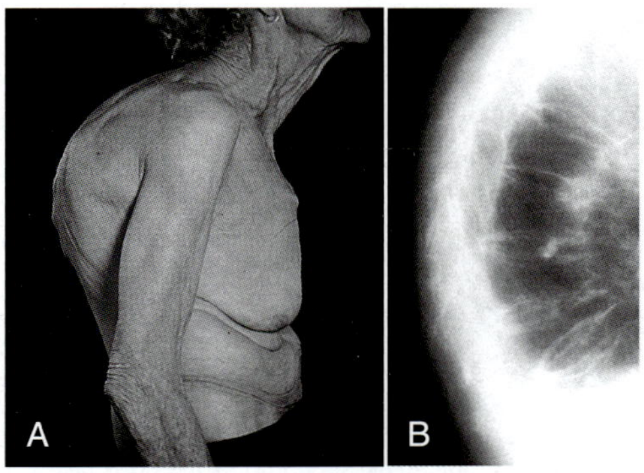

FIG. 22.73 Hallmark of osteoporosis: dowager hump. (A) Kyphosis of the upper thoracic and lower cervical spine. (B) Vertebral compression fractures. (From Hochberg MC, et al: *Rheumatology*, ed 3, St Louis, 2008, Mosby.)

Dupuytren Contracture

Contractures involving the flexor hand tendons

PATHOPHYSIOLOGY

- Cause is unknown, although there may be a hereditary component

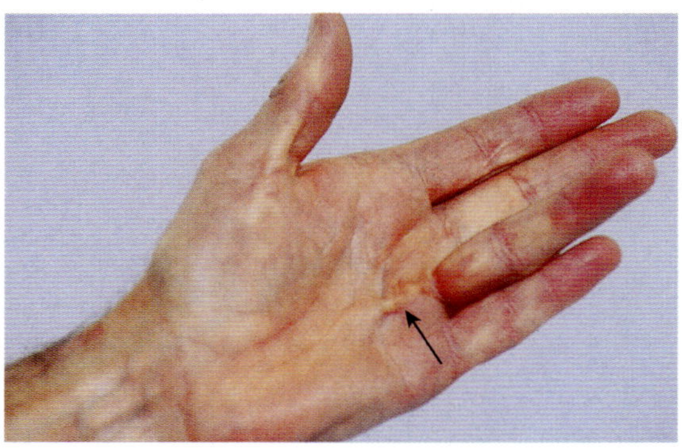

FIG. 22.74 Dupuytren contracture.

PATIENT DATA

Subjective Data

- Flexion contractures develop insidiously
- The incidence increases after age 40, occurring more frequently in males (Fig. 22.74)

Objective Data

- Flexor tendons generally of the fourth and fifth digits contract, causing the fingers to curl, with impaired extension
- These tendons are easily palpable

CHAPTER

23

Neurologic System

The nervous system, with its central and peripheral divisions, maintains and controls all body functions by its voluntary and autonomic responses. The evaluation of motor, sensory, autonomic, cognitive, and behavioral elements makes neurologic assessment one of the most complex portions of the physical examination. This chapter focuses on assessment of the cranial nerves, cerebellar function and proprioception, sensory function, and superficial and deep tendon reflexes. Assessment of mental status (cognitive function, communication, and behavior) is addressed in Chapter 7. Muscle strength assessment is addressed in Chapter 22.

Physical Examination Components

1. Test cranial nerves I through XII.
2. Evaluate coordination and fine motor skills by:
   - Rapid rhythmic alternating movements
   - Accuracy of upper and lower extremity movements
3. Evaluate balance using the Romberg test.
4. Observe the patient's gait for:
   - Posture
   - Rhythm and sequence of stride and arm movements
5. Test primary sensory responses to:
   - Superficial touch
   - Superficial pain
6. Test cortical sensory response to:
   - Vibration with a tuning fork over joints or bony prominences on upper and lower extremities
   - Position sense with movement of the great toes or a finger on each hand
   - Identification of familiar object by touch and manipulation
   - Two-point discrimination
   - Identification of letter or number "drawn" on palm of hand
   - Identification of body area when touched
7. Assess superficial and deep tendon reflexes
   - Plantar reflex
   - Abdominal reflexes
   - Cremasteric reflex in male patients
   - Biceps, brachioradialis, triceps, patellar, and Achilles deep tendon reflexes
   - Ankle clonus

ANATOMY AND PHYSIOLOGY

The central nervous system (CNS; brain and spinal cord) is the main network of coordination and control for the body. The peripheral nervous system, comprising the cranial and spinal nerves and the ascending and descending pathways, carries information to and from the CNS. The autonomic nervous system coordinates and regulates the internal organs of the body, such as cardiac muscle and smooth muscle. It has two divisions, each tending to balance the impulses of the other. The sympathetic division prods the body into action during times of physiologic and psychological stress; the parasympathetic division functions in a complementary and counterbalancing manner to conserve body resources and maintain day-to-day body functions such as digestion and elimination.

The intricate interrelationship of the nervous system divisions permits the body to perform the following:

- Receive sensory stimuli from the environment
- Identify and integrate the adaptive processes needed to maintain body functions
- Orchestrate body function changes required for adaptation and survival
- Integrate the rapid responsiveness of the CNS with the more gradual responsiveness of the endocrine system
- Control cognitive and voluntary behavioral processes (see Chapter 7)
- Control subconscious and involuntary body functions

The brain and spinal cord are protected by the skull and vertebrae, the meninges, and the cerebrospinal fluid (CSF). Three layers of meninges (pia mater, arachnoid mater, and dura mater) surround the brain and spinal cord, assisting in the production and drainage of CSF (Fig. 23.1). CSF circulates between an interconnecting system of ventricles in the brain and around the brain and spinal cord, serving as a shock absorber.

Brain

The brain receives its blood supply (approximately 20% of the total cardiac output) from the two internal carotid arteries and two vertebral arteries (Fig. 23.2). Blood drains from the brain through venous plexuses and dural sinuses

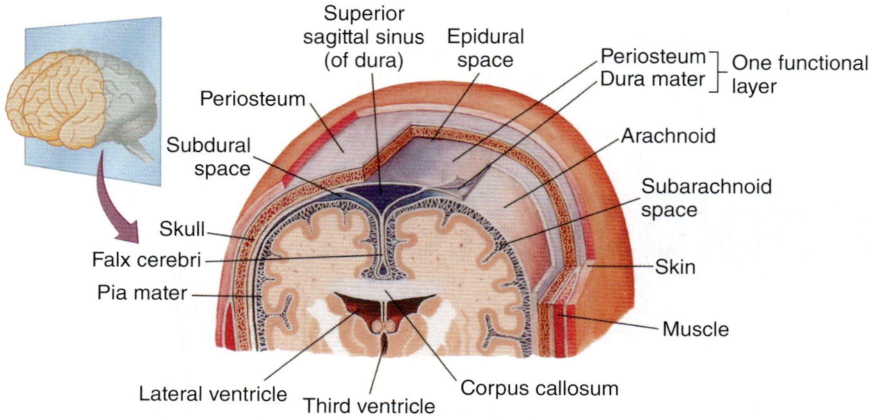

FIG. 23.1 Frontal section of the superior portion of the head as viewed from the front. Both bony and membranous coverings of the brain can be seen. (From Thibodeau, G. A., & Patton, K. T. (2003). *Anatomy and physiology* (3rd ed.). St. Louis: Mosby.)

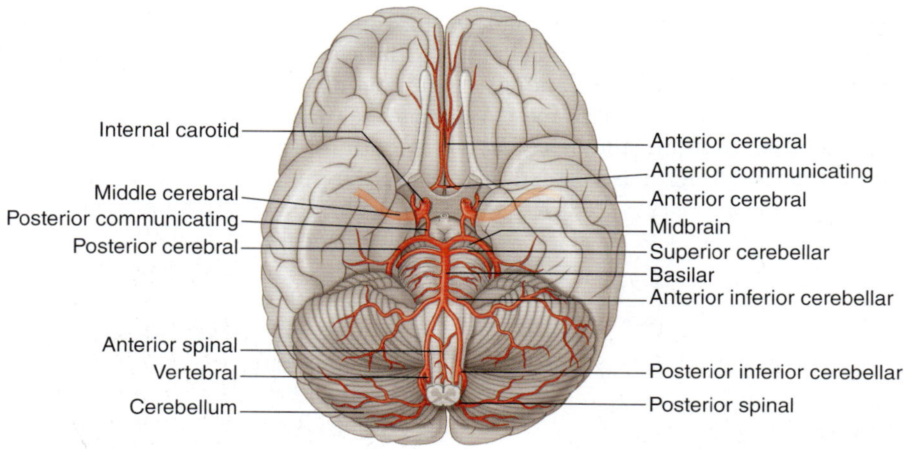

FIG. 23.2 Arterial blood supply to the brain. The internal carotid arteries supply 80%, and the vertebral basilar arteries supply 20%. (From Thibodeau, G. A., & Patton, K. T. (2007). *Anatomy and physiology* (6th ed.). St. Louis: Mosby.)

that empty into the internal jugular veins. The three major units of the brain are the cerebrum, the cerebellum, and the brainstem.

Cerebrum

Two cerebral hemispheres (right and left), each divided into lobes, form the cerebrum (Fig. 23.3; see also Fig. 7.1). The gray outer layer, the cerebral cortex, houses the higher mental functions and is responsible for general movement, visceral functions, perception, behavior, and the integration of these functions. The hemispheres control the contralateral (opposite) side of the body. The surface of the cerebrum has folds, or gyri, which are separated by sulci. When sulci are deep they are called *fissures*. Commissural fibers (corpus callosum) interconnect the counterpart areas in each hemisphere, permitting the coordination of activities between the two (see Fig. 23.1). The frontal lobe contains the motor cortex associated with voluntary skeletal movement and fine repetitive motor movements as well as the control of eye movements. Specific areas in the primary motor area

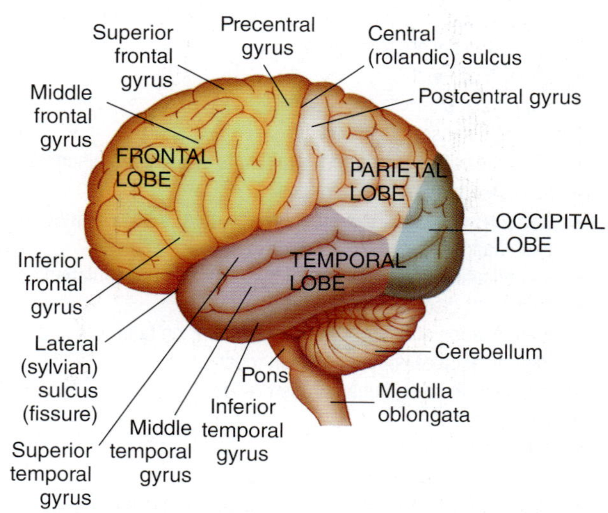

FIG. 23.3 Lobes and principal fissures of the cerebral cortex, cerebellum, and brainstem (left hemisphere, lateral view). (From McCance, K. M., & Huether, S. E. (2006). Pathophysiology: *The biologic basis for disease in adults and children* (5th ed.). St. Louis: Mosby.)

are associated with the movement of specific parts of the body. The corticospinal tracts extend from the primary motor area into the spinal cord.

The parietal lobe is primarily responsible for processing sensory data as they are received. It assists with the interpretation of tactile sensations (i.e., temperature, pressure, pain, size, shape, texture, and two-point discrimination) as well as vision, taste, smell, and hearing. Recognition of body parts and awareness of body position (proprioception) are dependent on the parietal lobe. Association fibers provide communication between the sensory and motor areas of the brain.

The occipital lobe contains the primary vision center and provides interpretation of visual data.

The temporal lobe is responsible for the perception and interpretation of sounds and determination of their source. It is also involved in the integration of taste, smell, and balance. The reception and interpretation of speech is located in the Wernicke area (see Fig 7.1). The medial temporal lobes include the hippocampi, which are essential for memory storage.

The basal ganglia system located deep within the brain functions as the extrapyramidal pathway and processing station between the cerebral motor cortex and the upper brainstem. Through its interconnections with the thalamus, motor cortex, reticular formation, and spinal cord, the basal ganglia refine motor movements.

Cerebellum

The cerebellum aids the motor cortex of the cerebrum in the integration of voluntary movement. It processes sensory information from the eyes, ears, touch receptors, and musculoskeletal system. In concert with the vestibular system, the cerebellum uses the sensory data for reflexive control of muscle tone, balance, and posture to produce steady and precise movements. As opposed to the cerebrum, the cerebellum's hemispheres have ipsilateral (same side) control of the body.

Brainstem

The brainstem is the pathway between the cerebral cortex and the spinal cord, and it controls many involuntary functions (Table 23.1). Its structures include the medulla oblongata, pons, midbrain, and diencephalon. The nuclei of the 12 cranial nerves arise from these structures. The thalamus is the major integrating center for perception and interpretation of sensations such as pain and temperature. The thalamus also relays sensory aspects of motor information between the basal ganglia and cerebellum. The pons transmits information between the brainstem and the cerebellum, where motor information from the cerebral cortex is relayed to the contralateral cerebellar hemisphere. The medulla oblongata is the site where the descending corticospinal tracts decussate (cross to the contralateral side).

Cranial Nerves

Cranial nerves are peripheral nerves that arise from the brain rather than the spinal cord. Each nerve has motor or sensory functions, and four cranial nerves have parasympathetic functions (Table 23.2).

TABLE 23.1 Structures of the Brainstem and Their Functions

STRUCTURE	FUNCTION
Medulla oblongata CN IX–XII	Respiratory, circulatory, and vasomotor activities; houses respiratory center Reflexes of swallowing, coughing, vomiting, sneezing, and hiccupping Relay center for major ascending and descending spinal tracts that decussate at the pyramid
Pons CN V–VIII	Reflexes of pupillary action and eye movement Regulates respiration; houses a portion of the respiratory center Controls voluntary muscle action with corticospinal tract pathway
Midbrain CN III and IV	Reflex center for eye and head movement Auditory relay pathway Corticospinal tract pathway
Diencephalon CN I and II Thalamus	Relays impulses between cerebrum, cerebellum, pons, and medulla (see Fig. 23.4) Conveys all sensory impulses (except olfaction) to and from cerebrum before their distribution to appropriate associative sensory areas Integrates impulses between motor cortex and cerebrum, influencing voluntary movements and motor response Controls state of consciousness, conscious perceptions of sensations, and abstract feelings Interconnected with limbic system to help manage emotions and memories
Epithalamus	Houses the pineal body that secretes melatonin and controls the sleep-wake cycle Connects limbic system to other parts of the brain
Hypothalamus and pituitary gland	Interconnects endocrine and neurologic systems to maintain temperature, water metabolism, body fluid osmolarity, feeding behavior, and neuroendocrine activity Secretes hormones for control of growth, lactation, vasoconstriction, immune response, and metabolism

Spinal Cord and Spinal Tracts

The 40- to 50-cm-long spinal cord begins at the foramen magnum, exiting the skull as a continuation of the medulla oblongata, and terminates at L1 or L2 of the vertebral column. Fibers, grouped into tracts, run through the spinal cord carrying sensory, motor, and autonomic impulses between higher centers in the brain and the body. The gray matter, arranged in a butterfly shape with anterior and posterior horns, contains the nerve cell bodies associated with sensory pathways and the autonomic nervous system. The white matter of the spinal cord contains the ascending and descending spinal tracts (Fig. 23.4).

The ascending spinal tracts (e.g., spinothalamic, spinocerebellar) mediate various sensations. These spinal tracts

TABLE 23.2 The Cranial Nerves and Their Functions

CRANIAL NERVES	FUNCTION
Olfactory (I)	Sensory: smell reception and interpretation
Optic (II)	Sensory: visual acuity and visual fields
Oculomotor (III)	Motor: raise eyelids, most extraocular movements Parasympathetic: pupillary constriction, change lens shape
Trochlear (IV)	Motor: downward, inward eye movement
Trigeminal (V)	Motor: jaw opening and clenching, chewing, and mastication Sensory: sensation to cornea, iris, lacrimal glands, conjunctiva, eyelids, forehead, nose, nasal and mouth mucosa, teeth, tongue, ear, facial skin
Abducens (VI)	Motor: lateral eye movement
Facial (VII)	Motor: movement of facial expression muscles except jaw, close eyelids, labial speech sounds (b, m, w, and rounded vowels) Sensory: taste—anterior two-thirds of tongue, sensation to pharynx Parasympathetic: secretion of saliva and tears
Acoustic (VIII)	Sensory: hearing and equilibrium
Glossopharyngeal (IX)	Motor: voluntary muscles for swallowing and phonation (guttural speech sounds) Sensory: sensation of nasopharynx, gag reflex, taste—posterior one-third of tongue Parasympathetic: secretion of salivary glands, carotid reflex
Vagus (X)	Sensory: sensation behind ear and part of external ear canal Parasympathetic: secretion of digestive enzymes; peristalsis; carotid reflex; involuntary action of heart, lungs, and digestive tract
Spinal accessory (XI)	Motor: turn head, shrug shoulders, some actions for phonation
Hypoglossal (XII)	Motor: tongue movement for speech sound articulation (l, t, d, n) and swallowing

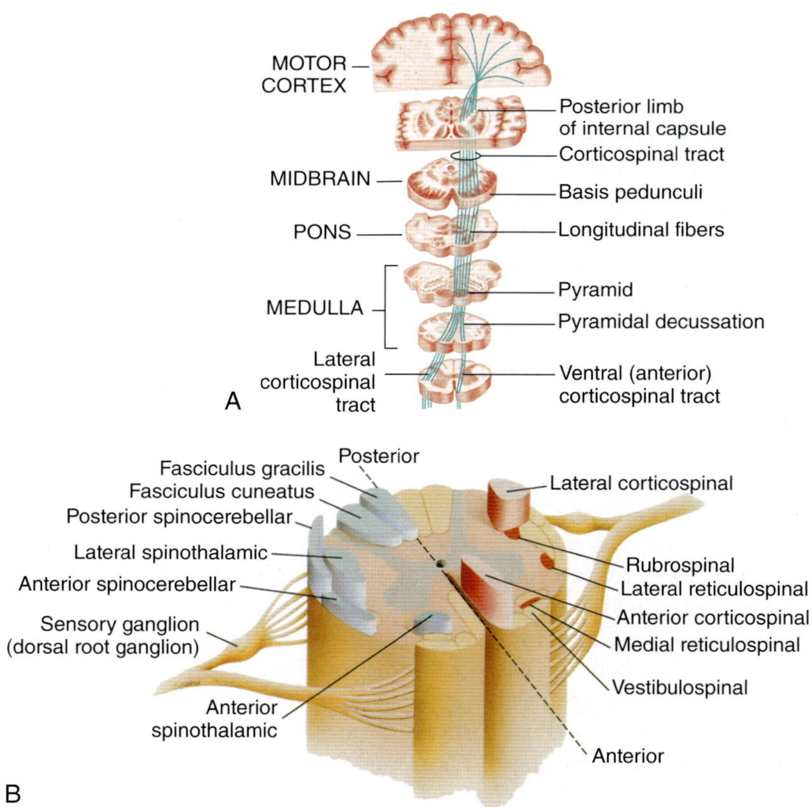

FIG. 23.4 Tracts of the spinal cord. (A) Pathway of spinal tracts from spinal cord to motor cortex. Note decussation of the pyramids at the level of the medulla. (B) Major ascending (sensory) tracts, shown here only on the left, are highlighted in *blue.* Major descending (motor) tracts, shown here only on the right, are highlighted in *red.* (A, Modified from Rudy, E. B. (1984). *Advanced neurological and neurosurgical nursing.* St. Louis: Mosby; B, from Thibodeau, G. A., & Patton, K. T. (2003). *Anatomy and physiology* (3rd ed.). St. Louis: Mosby.)

manage the sensory signals necessary to perform complex discrimination tasks. They are capable of transmitting precise information about the type of stimulus and its location. The posterior (dorsal) column spinal tract (fasciculus gracilis and fasciculus cuneatus) carries the fibers for the sensations of fine touch, two-point discrimination, and proprioception. The spinothalamic tracts carry the fibers for the sensations of light and crude touch, pressure, temperature, and pain.

The descending spinal tracts (corticospinal, reticulospinal, vestibulospinal) convey impulses from the brain to various muscle groups by inhibiting or exciting spinal activity. They also have a role in the control of muscle tone, posture, and precise motor movements. The corticospinal (pyramidal) tract permits skilled, delicate, and purposeful movements. The vestibulospinal tract causes the extensor muscles of the body to suddenly contract when a person starts to fall. The corticobulbar tract arising from the brainstem innervates the motor functions of the cranial nerves.

Upper motor neurons are nerve cell bodies for the motor pathways located within the cerebral cortex and brainstem. They comprise the descending pathways from the brain to the spinal cord. Their primary role is influencing, directing, and modifying spinal reflex arcs and circuits. The upper motor neurons can affect movement only through the lower motor neurons. The lower motor neurons, cranial and spinal motor neurons, originate in the anterior horn of the spinal cord and extend into the peripheral nervous system. They transmit neural signals directly to the muscles to permit movement. Injury to the upper motor neurons results in initial paralysis followed by partial recovery over an extended period. Injury to the lower motor neurons often results in permanent paralysis.

Spinal Nerves

Thirty-one pairs of spinal nerves arise from the spinal cord and exit at each intervertebral foramen (Fig. 23.5). The sensory and motor fibers of each spinal nerve supply and receive information in a specific body distribution of cutaneous innervation called a *dermatome* (Fig. 23.6). The anterior branches of several spinal nerves combine to form a nerve plexus (network of nerve fibers) so that a spinal nerve may lose its individuality to some extent. The spinal nerve may complement the effort of an anatomically related nerve or even help compensate for some loss of function. Numerous peripheral nerves originate from each nerve plexus.

Within the spinal cord, each spinal nerve separates into anterior and posterior roots. The motor or efferent fibers of the anterior root carry impulses from the spinal cord to the muscles and glands of the body. The sensory or afferent fibers of the posterior root carry impulses from sensory receptors of the body to the spinal cord and then on to the brain for interpretation by the cerebral sensory cortex.

A spinal afferent (sensory) neuron may initiate a reflex arc response when it receives an impulse stimulus such as a tap on a stretched muscle tendon. In this case, the response is transmitted outward by the efferent (motor) neuron in the anterior horn of the spinal cord via the spinal nerve and peripheral nerve of the skeletal muscle,

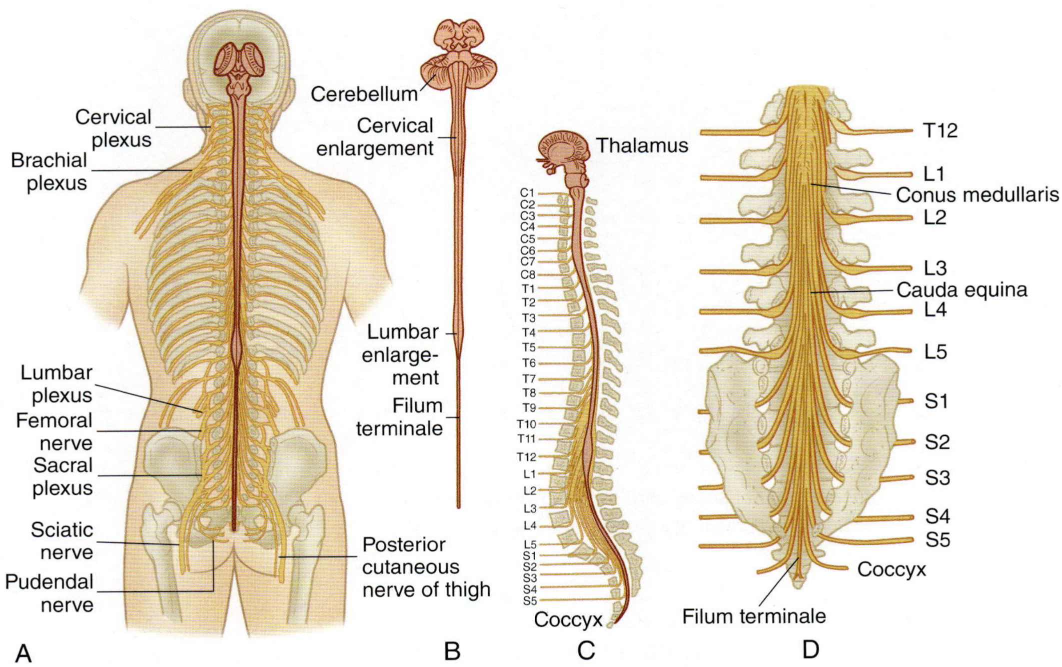

FIG. 23.5 Location of exiting spinal nerves in relation to the vertebrae. (A) Posterior view. (B) Anterior view of brainstem and spinal cord. (C) Lateral view showing relationship of spinal cord to vertebrae. (D) Enlargement of caudal area with group of nerve fibers composing the cauda equina. (Modified from Rudy, 1984.)

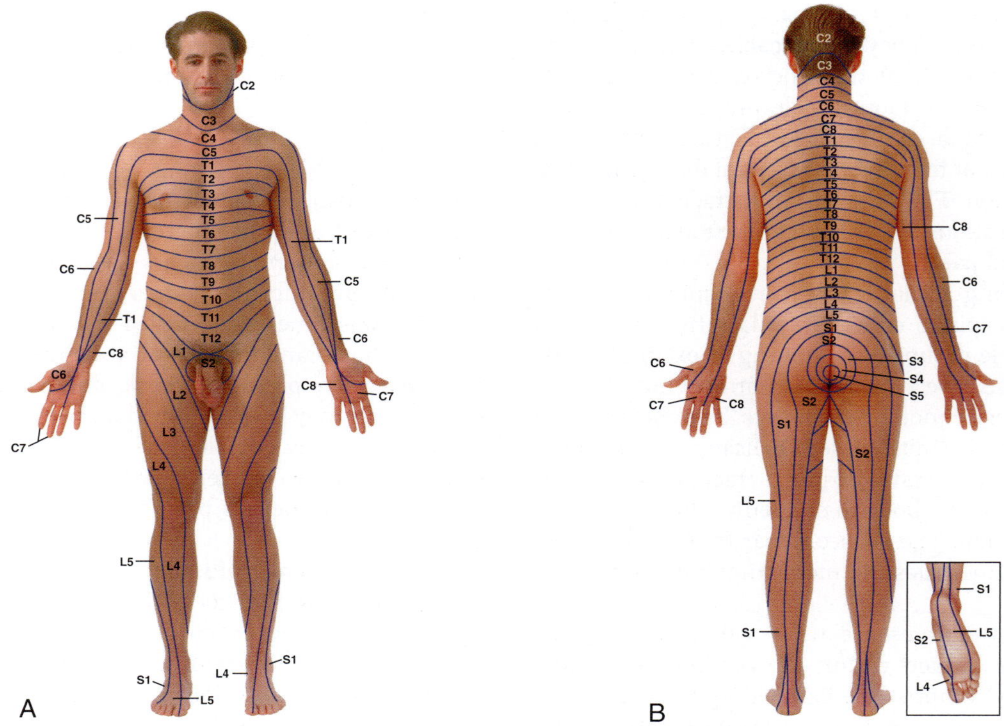

FIG. 23.6 Dermatomes of the body, the area of body surface innervated by particular spinal nerves; C1 usually has no cutaneous distribution. (A) Anterior view. (B) Posterior view. It appears that there is a distinct separation of surface area controlled by each dermatome, but there is almost always overlap between spinal nerves. *C,* Cervical; *L,* lumbar; *S,* sacral; *T,* thoracic.

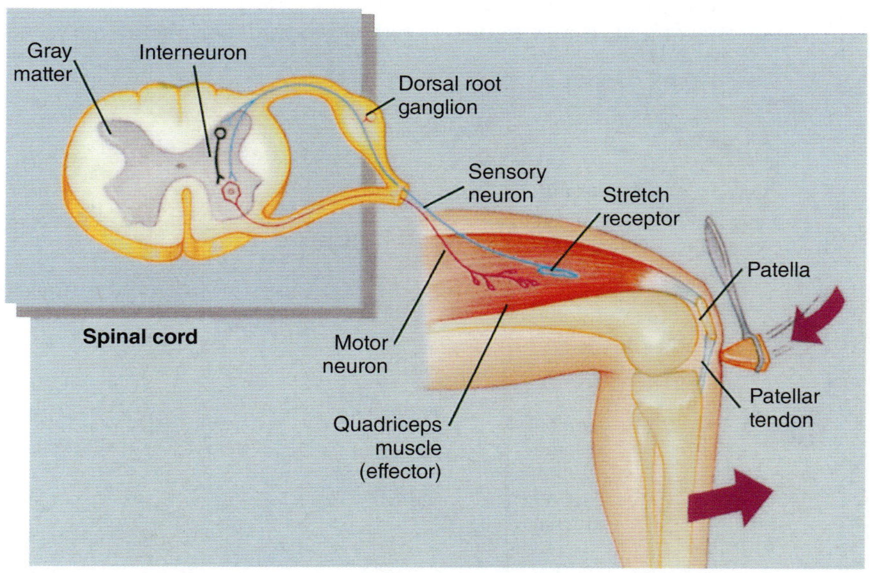

FIG. 23.7 Cross section of spinal cord showing simple reflex arc. (From Thibodeau, G. A., & Patton, K. T. (2003). *Anatomy and physiology* (3rd ed.). St. Louis: Mosby.)

stimulating a brisk contraction (Fig. 23.7). Such a reflex is dependent on intact afferent neurons, interneurons (also called *connector* or *relay neurons*), functional synapses in the spinal cord, intact efferent neurons, functional neuromuscular junctions, and competent muscle fibers.

Infants and Children

The major portion of brain growth occurs in the first year of life, along with myelinization of the brain and nervous system where axons become insulated with a myelin sheath. Any event that disrupts brain development and growth during this period (e.g., infection, poor nutrition, or trauma) can have profound effects on eventual brain function. At birth, the neurologic impulses are primarily handled by the brainstem and spinal cord, such as the following reflexes: sucking, rooting, yawning, sneezing, hiccupping, blinking at bright light, and withdrawing from painful stimuli. Some common newborn reflexes are present at birth (e.g., Moro, stepping, palmar and plantar grasp), and as the brain develops, these reflexes are inhibited as more advanced cortical functions and voluntary control take over.

Motor maturation proceeds in a cephalocaudal direction. Motor control of the head and neck develops first, followed by the trunk and extremities. Motor development progresses, enabling more complex and independent functioning. Development occurs in an orderly sequence, but the timing varies considerably among children. Many capabilities may develop simultaneously in a child.

Pregnant Patients

Hypothalamic-pituitary neurohormonal changes occur with pregnancy; however, specific alterations in the neurologic system are not well identified. During the first trimester, individuals have increased sleep needs, but they may not feel rested, even with increased sleep. Late in pregnancy, sleep can be affected due to multiple discomforts, such as back pain, frequent urination, leg cramps, and restless leg syndrome.

Older Adults

The number of cerebral neurons decreases with aging, along with decreased brain size. The vast number of neurons and neuroplasticity inhibit the appearance of clinical signs in many cases. Sensory functions such as taste, smell, hearing, and vision may be diminished. The velocity of nerve impulse conduction declines, so responses to various stimuli may be diminished, such as deep tendon reflexes. Sleep disturbances also occur. See Chapter 7 for changes in mental functioning.

REVIEW OF RELATED HISTORY

For each of the symptoms or conditions discussed in this section, particular topics to include in the history of the present illness are listed. Responses to questions about these topics provide clues for individualizing the physical examination and the development of a diagnostic evaluation appropriate for the particular patient. Questions regarding medication use (prescription and over-the-counter preparations) as well as complementary, alternative, and integrative therapies are relevant for each area.

History of Present Illness

Seizures

- Independent observer's report: fall to ground, shrill cry, motor activity, transition phase, change in color of face or lips, pupil changes or eye deviations, loss of consciousness, loss of bowel or bladder control
- Aura (perceptual sensation that may signal a seizure): irritability, tension, confusion, blurred vision, mood changes, initial focal motor seizure activity, gastrointestinal distress
- Level of consciousness: loss, impairment, duration
- Automatism: eyelid fluttering, chewing, lip smacking, swallowing
- Muscle tone: flaccid, stiff, tense, twitching; where spasm began and moved through the body; change in character of motor activity during seizure
- Postictal phase: weakness, transient paralysis, confusion, drowsiness, headaches, muscle aching, sleeping; any lateralization of signs
- Relationship of seizure to time of day, meals, fatigue, emotional stress, excitement, menses, and discontinuing or incorrect medication use; activity before episode
- Frequency of seizures; total length of seizure activity; age at first seizure
- Medications: antiepileptic; initiation of medication or complementary or alternative therapy, potential for herb or product use that interacts with prescribed antiepileptic medication

Pain

- See Chapter 6 for general pain assessment but consider "neurologic-specific" pain such as headaches associated with meningitis or encephalitis, space-occupying lesions, neck pain, sciatica, trigeminal neuralgia, or diabetic neuropathy
- Onset: sudden or progressive, associated with fever or injury
- Quality and intensity: deep or superficial; aching, boring, throbbing, sharp or stabbing, burning, pressing, stinging, cramping, gnawing, prickling, shooting; duration and constancy
- Location or path: along distribution of one or more peripheral nerves or a more general distribution; radiating from one part of the body to another
- Associated manifestations: crying, change in activity or energy level, sweating, muscle rigidity, tremor, impaired mental processes or concentration, weakness
- Efforts to treat, impact on functioning and life
- Medications: opioids or nonsteroidal antiinflammatory drugs; prescription, nonprescription, complementary or alternative therapy

Gait Coordination

- Balance: sensation of leaning when walking to doorway; unsteadiness when walking
- Vertigo: see Chapter 13 for more information
- Falling: fall in consistent direction, backward, forward; associated with looking up; legs simply giving way; stiffness of limbs
- Associated problems: arthritis of cervical spine or knees, ataxia, stroke, seizure, arrhythmias, sensory changes

- Medications: phenytoin, pyrimethamine, etoposide, vinblastine; prescription, nonprescription, complementary or alternative therapy

Weakness or Paresthesia

- Onset: sudden, with activity initiation or following sustained activity, time before symptoms begin; rapid or slow
- Character: generalized or specific body area affected (face, extremity); progressively ascending or transient; proximal or distal extremities, unilateral, bilateral, or asymmetric; difficulty walking; loss of balance or coordination; hypersensitivity to touch or burning sensation
- Associated symptoms: tingling or numbness; confusion, trouble speaking or understanding speech; severe headache; impaired vision in one or both eyes; limb feels encased in tight bandage, pain, shortness of breath, joint stiffness, spasms, muscle tension, sensory deficits; loss of urinary or bowel control; personality change
- Recent acute illness or concurrent chronic illness such as diabetes, hypertension, nutritional or vitamin deficiency
- Medications: chemotherapy, prescription, nonprescription, HIV medications, complementary or alternative therapy

Risk Factors

Stroke (Brain Attack or Cerebrovascular Accident)

- Hypertension
- Previous stroke
- Obesity
- Physical inactivity
- Smoking tobacco products
- Stress
- Sleep apnea
- Pregnancy
- Menopause
- Increased levels of serum cholesterol, lipoproteins, and triglycerides
- Use of oral contraceptives
- Sickle cell disease
- Family history of stroke, diabetes mellitus, cardiovascular disease, hypertension, and increased serum cholesterol levels
- Congenital cerebrovascular anomalies

Tremor

- Onset: sudden or gradual
- Character: worse with rest, intentional movement, or anxiety; unilateral or bilateral; body location (distal extremities, head); interference with daily activities and impact on life
- Associated problems: hyperthyroidism, familial tremor, liver or kidney disorder, alcohol use, multiple sclerosis (MS)
- Relieved by: rest, activity, alcohol
- Medications: neuroleptics, valproate, phenytoin, albuterol, pseudoephedrine, antiarrhythmics, corticosteroids, caffeine (all may cause essential tremor)

Past Medical History

- Trauma: concussion or traumatic brain injury (TBI), spinal cord injury, or localized injury; birth trauma; stroke
- Meningitis, encephalitis, lead poisoning, poliomyelitis
- Congenital anomalies, genetic syndromes
- Cardiovascular, circulatory problems: hypertension, aneurysm, peripheral vascular disease
- Neurologic disorder, brain surgery, residual effects
- Headaches (e.g., migraines)

Family History

- Hereditary disorders: neurofibromatosis, Huntington chorea, muscular dystrophy, diabetes, pernicious anemia
- Alcoholism
- Intellectual disability
- Epilepsy or seizure disorder
- Headaches
- Alzheimer disease or other dementia, Parkinson disease
- Learning disorders
- Weakness or gait disorders, cerebral palsy (CP)
- Medical or metabolic disorder: thyroid disease, hypertension, diabetes mellitus

Personal and Social History

- Environmental or occupational hazards: exposure to lead, arsenic, insecticides, organic solvents, other chemicals; operate or live on farm, handle dangerous equipment or work at heights or in water (neurologic disorder may affect employment or personal safety)
- Hand, eye, and foot dominance; family patterns of dexterity and dominance
- Ability to care for self: hygiene, activities of daily living, finances, communication, shopping; ability to fulfill work expectations
- Sleeping or eating patterns; weight loss or gain; anxiety
- Alcohol or substance use, especially mood-altering drugs

Infants

- Prenatal history: pregnant person's health, medications taken, intrauterine infections such as toxoplasmosis, Zika, syphilis, tuberculosis, rubella, cytomegalovirus, herpes, fetal movement, prior history of hypertension, preeclampsia, bleeding, history of trauma or stress, malnutrition, persistent vomiting, hypertension, drug or alcohol use
- Birth history: Apgar score, gestational age, prematurity, birth weight, presentation, use of instruments to assist in delivery, prolonged or precipitate labor, fetal distress

- Respiratory status at birth: resuscitation needed, apnea, cyanosis, need for oxygen or mechanical ventilation
- Neonatal health: jaundice (from ABO blood type incompatibility, breastfeeding, or other causes), perinatal infections, seizures, irritability, poorly coordinated suck and swallow, need for intensive care, ototoxic medication exposure
- Congenital anomalies, congenital heart disease, or other physical disabilities
- Hypotonia or hypertonia in infancy, developmental delay

Children

- Developmental milestones
  - Age attained: smiling, head control in prone position, grasping, transferring objects between hands, rolling over, sitting, crawling, independent walking, toilet trained, saying words other than "mama" and "dada" (see Chapter 24)
  - Pattern of development: similar to other children; always slower than others; loss of previously achieved function; change in the child's rate of development (progress occurred as expected until a certain age with slow progress afterward or regression)
- Performance of self-care activities: dressing, toileting, feeding
- Hyperactive or impulsive behavior; problems with schedule changes, sitting for entire meal; poor organizational skills, unable to handle more than one instruction at a time, mood change, uncontrolled anger, poor social skills; school problems
- Health problems:
  - Headaches, unexplained vomiting, lethargy, personality changes
  - Seizure activity: association with fever, frequency, duration, character of movement
  - Clumsiness, unsteady gait, progressive muscular weakness, unexplained falling, problems going up and down stairs, problems getting up after lying down on floor

Pregnant Patients

- Weeks of gestation or estimated date of delivery
- Seizure activity: past history of seizures or pregnancy-induced hypertension; frequency, duration, character of movement
- Headache: onset, character, frequency, association with hypertension; visual changes
- Nutritional status: dietary supplements such as prenatal vitamins, calcium; salt depletion

Older Adults

- Pattern of increased stumbling, falls, unsteadiness, or decreased agility; worse in the dark; safety modifications used in home
- Interference with performance of daily living tasks, social withdrawal, personality change, feelings about symptoms
- Hearing loss, vision deficit, anosmia (loss of smell)—transient or persistent
- Urinary or fecal incontinence
- Transient neurologic deficits (may indicate transient ischemic attacks)

Patient Safety

Fall Prevention for Older Adults

Ask these three screening questions to assess fall risk in adults 65 years and older:

- Have you fallen in the past year?
- Do you feel unsteady when standing or walking?
- Do you worry about falling?

A positive answer to any of the questions indicates a need for further assessment and intervention (Centers for Disease Control and Prevention, 2019b). Risk factors for falls include:

- Previous falls
- Chronic conditions such as arthritis, stroke, Parkinson disease, dementia, incontinence, and peripheral neuropathy
- Disorder of gait, balance, or vertigo
- Lower extremity muscle weakness or sensory loss
- Postural hypotension
- Impaired vision
- Improper use of an assistive device (e.g., walker or cane)
- Structural factors: lack of stair handrails or bathroom grab bars, dim lighting, slippery or uneven surfaces

EXAMINATION AND FINDINGS

Equipment

- Penlight
- Tongue blade, paper clip, cotton-tipped applicator
- Tuning forks, 200 to 400 Hz and 500 to 1000 Hz
- Familiar objects: coins, keys, paper clip
- Cotton wisp
- 5.07 monofilament (10 g force)
- Reflex hammer
- Additional items for a comprehensive diagnostic neurologic examination, typically performed by a specialist
  - Vials of aromatic substances: coffee, orange, peppermint extract, oil of cloves
  - Vials of solutions: glucose, salt, lemon or vinegar, and quinine—with applicators for taste testing
  - Test tubes of hot and cold water for temperature sensation testing

Because the neurologic examination is complex, the discussion is divided into four sections: cranial nerves, proprioception and cerebellar function, sensory function, and reflex function. Assessment of mental status is detailed in Chapter 7. Evaluation of muscle tone and strength, an integral part of the neurologic examination, is detailed in Chapter 22.

The neurologic system is assessed during the entire encounter. As you watch the patient entering the room, you gain information about the neurologic system. You can observe balance, coordination and smoothness of gait, ability to follow directions, and ability to sit and stand. The musculoskeletal examination, particularly muscle tone and strength, provides important information about the neurologic examination because the systems are interdependent. In addition to the history, a neurologic screening examination may be helpful in revealing a potential neurologic problem (Box 23.1).

Cranial Nerves

Evaluating the cranial nerves is an integral part of the neurologic examination. Ordinarily, taste and smell are not evaluated unless a problem is suspected. A patient may not recognize that some hearing, certain taste sensations, or some vision has been lost. When a sensory loss is suspected, be thoughtful about determining and documenting the extent of loss when testing the relevant cranial nerve.

Examination of some cranial nerves is described in detail in other chapters, associated with the body system in which they are most commonly evaluated. Testing of the optic (II), oculomotor (III), trochlear (IV), and abducens (VI) nerves is described in Chapter 12; the acoustic (VIII) and hypoglossal (XII) nerves in Chapter 13; and the spinal accessory nerve (XI) in Chapter 22. Table 23.3 describes a review of all cranial nerve examination procedures. Unexpected findings (focal deficits) indicate trauma or a lesion in the cerebral hemisphere or local injury to the nerve. See Clinical Pearl, "Mnemonic for Cranial Nerve Names."

BOX 23.1 Procedure for the Neurologic Screening Examination

The shorter screening examination is commonly used for health visits when no known neurologic problem is apparent.

Cranial Nerves

Cranial nerves II through XII are routinely tested; however, taste is not tested unless some aberration is found.

Proprioception and Cerebellar Function

One test is administered for each of the following: rapid rhythmic alternating movements, accuracy of movements, balance (Romberg test is given), and gait and heel-toe walking.

Sensory Function

Superficial pain and touch at a distal point in each extremity are tested; vibration and position senses are assessed by testing the great toe.

Deep Tendon Reflexes

All deep tendon reflexes are tested, excluding the plantar reflex and the test for clonus.

CLINICAL PEARL

Mnemonic for Cranial Nerve Names

One way to remember the cranial nerves is the mnemonic for the first letter of each nerve: Occasionally Old Owls Travel Through Abandoned Farm Villages Gathering Vegetables and Herbs. Classification of each cranial nerve by function—Sensory (S), Motor (M), or Both (B) can be remembered by the mnemonic: Silly Sally Makes Maple Baked Muffins But Struggles Baking Basic Muffin Mixes.

TABLE 23.3 Procedure for Cranial Nerve Examination

CRANIAL NERVE (CN)	PROCEDURE
CN I (olfactory)	Test ability to identify familiar aromatic odors, one naris at a time with eyes closed.
CN II (optic)	Test distant and near vision. Perform ophthalmoscopic examination of fundi. Test visual fields by confrontation and extinction of vision.
CN III (oculomotor), CN IV (trochlear), and CN VI (abducens)	Inspect eyelids for drooping. Inspect pupils' size for equality and their direct and consensual response to light and accommodation. Test extraocular eye movements.
CN V (trigeminal)	Inspect face for muscle atrophy and tremors. Palpate jaw muscles for tone and strength when patient clenches teeth. Test superficial pain and touch sensation in each branch (test temperature sensation if there are unexpected findings to pain or touch). Test corneal reflex.
CN VII (facial)	Inspect symmetry of facial features with various expressions (e.g., smile, frown, puffed cheeks, wrinkled forehead). Test ability to identify sweet and salty tastes on each side of the tongue.
CN VIII (acoustic)	Test sense of hearing with whisper screening tests or by audiometry. Compare bone and air conduction of sound. Test for lateralization of sound.
CN IX (glossopharyngeal), and X (vagus)	Test ability to identify sour and bitter tastes on each side of the tongue. Test gag reflex and ability to swallow. Inspect palate and uvula for symmetry with speech sounds and gag reflex. Observe for swallowing difficulty. Evaluate quality of guttural speech sounds (presence of nasal or hoarse quality to voice).
CN XI (spinal accessory)	Test trapezius muscle strength (shrug shoulders against resistance). Test sternocleidomastoid muscle strength (turn head to each side against resistance).
CN XII (hypoglossal)	Inspect tongue in mouth and while protruded for symmetry, tremors, and atrophy. Inspect tongue movement toward nose and chin. Test tongue strength with index finger when tongue is pressed against cheek. Evaluate quality of lingual speech sounds (l, t, d, n).

Olfactory (I)

The olfactory nerve is tested when a concern exists with the patient's ability to discriminate odors. Have available two or three vials of familiar aromatic odors. Use the least irritating aromatic substance (e.g., orange or peppermint extract) first so that the patient's perception of weaker odors is not impaired. Before starting the assessment, make sure the patient's nasal passages are patent. Occlude one naris at a time and ask the patient to breathe in and out.

Consider having the patient close their eyes to avoid visual cues and occlude one naris. Hold an opened vial under the open naris. Ask the patient to inspire deeply (so the odor reaches the upper nose and the olfactory mucosa) and to identify the odor (Fig. 23.8). Use a different odor to test the other side. Continue the assessment, alternating between sides with two or three odors, comparing the patient's ability to identify and discriminate between odors. Avoid offering multiple odors too quickly as this may confuse the olfactory sense.

Patients are expected to perceive an odor on each side and usually to identify it. Inflammation of the mucous membranes, allergic rhinitis, and cigarette smoking may all interfere with the ability to distinguish odors. The sense of smell may diminish with age. Anosmia, the loss of sense of smell or an inability to discriminate odors, can be caused by trauma to the cribriform plate, an olfactory tract lesion, or infection.

Optic (II)

Visual acuity and visual fields are evaluated as described in Chapter 12.

Oculomotor, Trochlear, and Abducens (III, IV, and VI)

Movement of the eyes through the six cardinal points of gaze, pupil size, shape, response to light and accommodation, and opening of the upper eyelids are described in Chapter 12.

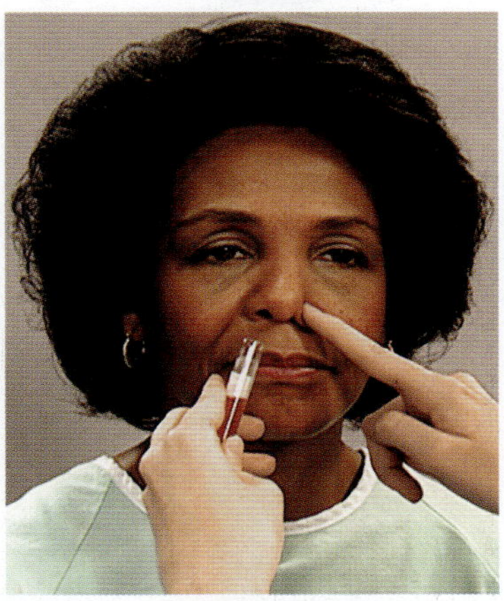

FIG. 23.8 Examination of the olfactory cranial nerve. Occlude one naris, hold the vial with aromatic substance under the nose, and ask the patient to deeply inspire. If the patient's eyes are open, make sure there are no visual cues to odors. The patient should discriminate between odors.

When assessing patients with severe headaches, the experienced examiner evaluates movement of the eyes for the presence or absence of lateral (temporal) gaze. The function of cranial nerve VI is often lost first in the presence of increased intracranial pressure.

Trigeminal (V)

Evaluate motor function by observing the face for muscle atrophy, deviation of the jaw to one side, and fasciculation (muscle twitches). Have the patient tightly clench the teeth as you palpate the muscles over the jaw, evaluating tone (Fig. 23.9). Muscle tone over the face should be symmetric without fasciculations.

The three divisions of the trigeminal nerve are evaluated for sharp, dull, and light touch sensation (Fig. 23.10). With the patient's eyes closed, touch each side of the face at the scalp, cheek, and chin areas, alternately using the sharp and smooth edges of a broken tongue blade or a paper clip. Avoid using a predictable pattern. Ask the patient

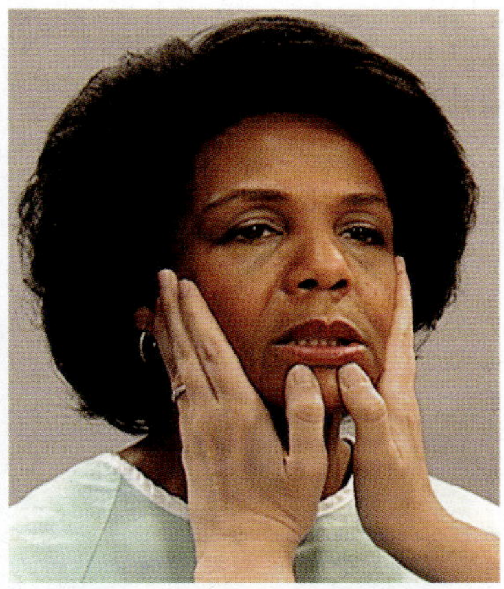

FIG. 23.9 Examination of the trigeminal cranial nerve for motor function. Have the patient tightly clench the teeth and then palpate the muscles over the jaw for tone.

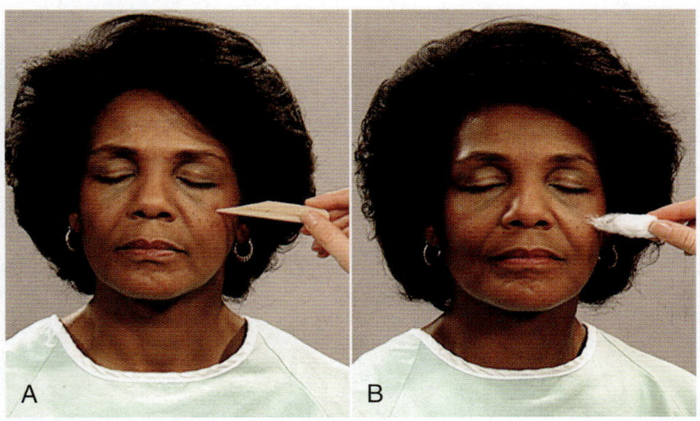

FIG. 23.10 Examination of the trigeminal cranial nerve for sensory function. Touch each side of the face at the scalp, cheek, and chin areas alternately using no predictable pattern (A) with the point and rounded edge of a paper clip or broken tongue blade and (B) with a brush or cotton wisp. Ask the patient to discriminate between sensations.

to report whether each sensation is sharp or dull. Then stroke the face in the same six areas with a cotton wisp, brush, or lightly with a finger pad, asking the patient to tell when the stimulus is felt. A wooden applicator is used to test sensation over the buccal mucosa inside the mouth. Discrimination of all stimuli is expected over all areas.

If sensation is impaired, use test tubes filled with hot and cold water to evaluate temperature sensation. Ask the patient to tell you if the tubes feel hot or cold as you touch the same six areas of the face. Contrast the discrimination of temperature with the other sensations.

When assessment of the corneal reflex is clinically indicated, have the patient look up and away from you as you approach from the side (contact lenses, if used, should be removed). Avoiding the eyelashes and the conjunctiva, lightly touch the cornea of one eye with a cotton wisp. Repeat the procedure on the other cornea. A symmetric blink reflex to corneal stimulation is expected. Patients who wear contact lenses may have a diminished or absent reflex.

Facial (VII)

Evaluate motor function by observing facial expressions after asking the patient to raise the eyebrows, squeeze the eyes shut, wrinkle the forehead, frown, smile, show the teeth, purse the lips to whistle, and puff out the cheeks (Fig. 23.11). Observe for tics, unusual facial movements, and asymmetry of expression. Listen as the patient speaks and note any difficulties with labial speech sounds (b, m, and p). Drooping of one side of the mouth, a flattened nasolabial fold, and a sagging lower eyelid are signs of muscle weakness. See the discussion of Bell palsy later in the chapter and Clinical Pearl, "Upper and Lower Neuron Disease."

> **CLINICAL PEARL**
>
> **Upper and Lower Neuron Disease**
>
> To distinguish between upper and lower neuron disease affecting the face, observe the patient's face when they are laughing or crying. When the upper motor neurons are affected, as in a stroke, voluntary movements are paralyzed, but emotional movements are preserved. In a lower motor neuron disorder, such as Bell palsy, all facial movements on the affected side are paralyzed.

To evaluate taste, a sensory function of cranial nerves VII and IX, have available the four solutions, applicators, and a card listing the tastes (bitter, sour, salty, sweet). The fifth taste, umami (savory or meaty flavor), is less commonly tested. Make sure the patient cannot see the labels on the vials. Ask the patient to keep the tongue protruded and to point out the taste perceived on the card. Apply one

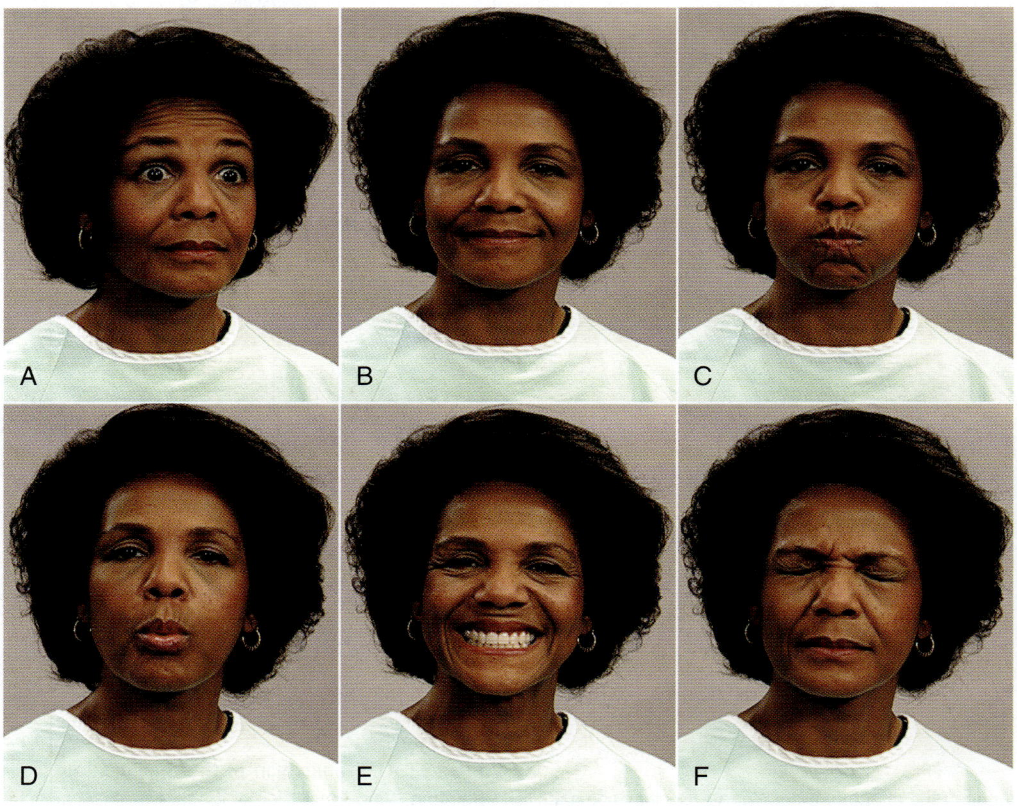

FIG. 23.11 Examination of the facial cranial nerve for motor function. Ask the patient to (A) wrinkle the forehead by raising the eyebrows, (B) smile, (C) puff out the cheeks, (D) purse the lips and blow out, (E) show the teeth, and (F) squeeze the eyes shut.

solution at a time to the lateral side of the tongue in the appropriate taste bud region (Fig. 23.12). Alternate the solutions, using a different applicator for each. Offer a sip of water after each stimulus. Each solution is used on both sides of the tongue to identify taste discrimination. The patient should identify each taste bilaterally when placed correctly on the tongue surface. Disorders of taste sensation may be related to loss of smell, traumatic brain injury, viral infection, radiation for cancer therapy, and prescription medications.

Acoustic (VIII)

Hearing is evaluated with the screening tests described in Chapter 13 or with an audiometer. Vestibular function is tested by the Romberg test (described later in this chapter). Other vestibular function tests are not routinely performed.

Glossopharyngeal (IX)

The sensory function of taste over the posterior third of the tongue may be tested during cranial nerve VII evaluation. The glossopharyngeal nerve is simultaneously tested during evaluation of the vagus nerve for nasopharyngeal sensation (gag reflex) and the motor function of swallowing.

Vagus (X)

To evaluate nasopharyngeal sensation, warn the patient you will be testing the gag reflex. Touch the posterior wall of the patient's pharynx with an applicator as you observe for upward movement of the palate and contraction of the pharyngeal muscles. Expect the uvula to remain in the midline. Drooping or absence of an arch on either side of the soft palate is unexpected.

Evaluate motor function by inspection of the soft palate for symmetry. Ask the patient to say "ah," and observe the movement of the soft palate and uvula for asymmetry. If the vagus or glossopharyngeal nerve is damaged and the palate fails to rise, the uvula will deviate from the midline.

Have the patient sip and swallow water. You can do this while examining the thyroid gland (see Chapter 11). The patient should swallow easily. No retrograde passage of water through the nose after the nasopharynx has closed off or aspiration should occur.

Listen to the patient's speech, noting any hoarseness, nasal quality, or difficulty with guttural sounds.

Spinal Accessory (XI)

Evaluation of the size, shape, and strength of the trapezius and sternocleidomastoid muscles is described in Chapter 22.

Hypoglossal (XII)

Inspect the patient's tongue while at rest on the floor of the mouth and while protruded from the mouth (Fig. 23.13). Ask the patient to move the tongue in and out of the mouth, from side to side, curled upward as if to touch the nose, and curled downward as if to lick the chin. Test the tongue's muscle strength by asking the patient to push the tongue against the cheek as you apply resistance with an index finger. When listening to the patient's

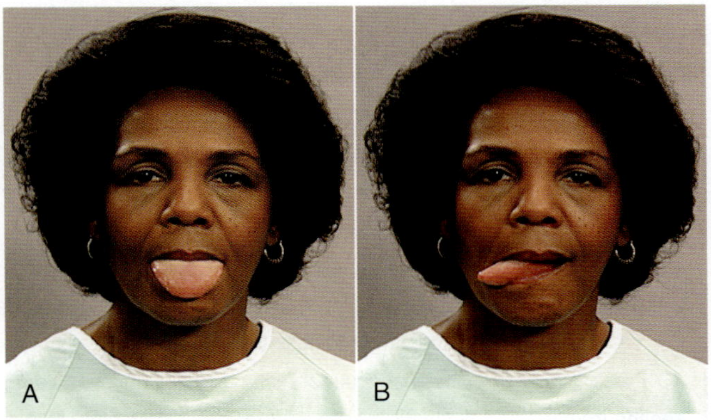

FIG. 23.13 Examination of the hypoglossal cranial nerve. (A) Inspect the protruded tongue for size, shape, symmetry, and fasciculation. (B) Observe movement of the tongue from side to side.

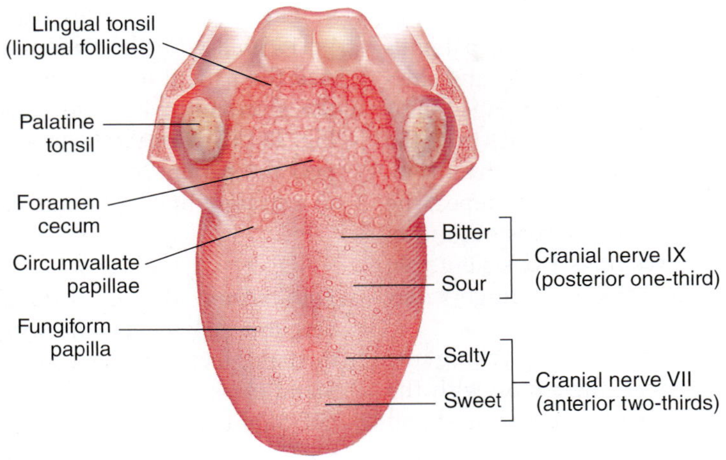

FIG. 23.12 Location of the taste bud regions tested for the sensory function of the facial and glossopharyngeal cranial nerves.

speech, expect no problems with lingual speech sounds (l, t, d, n). Any tongue fasciculations, asymmetry, atrophy, or deviation from the midline is unexpected.

Proprioception and Cerebellar Function

Coordination and Fine Motor Skills

When performing the following assessments, observe for any involuntary movements such as tremors (rhythmic oscillatory movements), tics, or fasciculations. Note the parts of the body affected, quality, rate, and rhythm (see the Differential Diagnosis table, "Tremors").

Rapid Rhythmic Alternating Movements

Ask the seated patient to pat their thighs with both hands, alternately turning up and down the palms of the hands and increasing the speed gradually (Fig. 23.14A and B). As an alternate procedure, have the patient touch the thumb to each finger on the same hand in sequence from the index finger to the little finger and back. Test one hand at a time, increasing speed gradually (see Fig. 23.14C). Expect the patient to perform movements smoothly, maintaining rhythm with increasing speed. Stiff, slowed, nonrhythmic, or jerky clonic movements are unexpected.

DIFFERENTIAL DIAGNOSIS

Tremors

TYPE OF TREMOR	CHARACTERISTICS	POTENTIAL CAUSE
Enhanced physiologic tremor	Seen with arms held extended, disappears when limb is at rest; small amplitude	Drug or alcohol withdrawal Hyperthyroidism, hypoglycemia Toxicity associated with some medications (e.g., lithium, methylxanthines, valproate, tricyclic antidepressants)
Essential tremor	Bilateral, symmetric; primarily seen in hands or outstretched arms, intention tremor May be seen in head, trunk, voice, tongue May worsen with stress or fatigue; may improve temporarily with alcohol Progressive Usually absence of other neurologic signs Lower limbs rarely affected	No consistent cerebral pathology Autosomal dominant inheritance pattern
Intention tremor	Seen during intentional movements, such as writing, pouring water in a cup, finger to nose testing Does not occur at rest	May be associated with a cerebellar disorder such as multiple sclerosis or alcohol use disorder
Resting tremor	Seen when limb is at rest Slow supination-pronation (pill-rolling) movements	Parkinson disease

Accuracy of Movements

The finger-to-nose test is performed with the patient's eyes open. Ask the patient to use an index finger and alternately touch their nose and your index finger (Fig. 23.15A and B). Position your index finger about 18 inches from the patient, allowing the patient to reach full arm extension. Move your finger several times during the test. Repeat the procedure with the other hand. Expect the patient's movements to be rapid, smooth, and accurate. Consistent past pointing (i.e., missing the examiner's index finger) may indicate cerebellar disease.

An alternate finger-to-nose test involves asking the patient to close both eyes and touch their nose with the index finger of each hand. Alternate the hands used and increase speed gradually (see Fig. 23.15C). Expect the movement to be smooth, rapid, and accurate, even with increasing speed.

The heel-to-shin test is another alternate method, performed with the patient standing, sitting, or supine. Ask the patient to run the heel of one foot up and down the shin (from knee to ankle) of the opposite leg (see Fig. 23.15D). Repeat the procedure with the other heel. Expect the patient to move the heel up and down the shin in a straight line without irregular deviations to the side.

Balance

Equilibrium Balance is initially evaluated with the Romberg test. Ask the patient (with eyes open and then closed) to stand, feet together and arms at the sides (Fig. 23.16). Stand close, prepared to catch the patient if they start to fall. Slight swaying movement of the body is expected, but not to the extent that falling is a danger. Loss of balance, a positive Romberg sign, indicates cerebellar ataxia, vestibular dysfunction, or sensory loss. If the patient staggers or

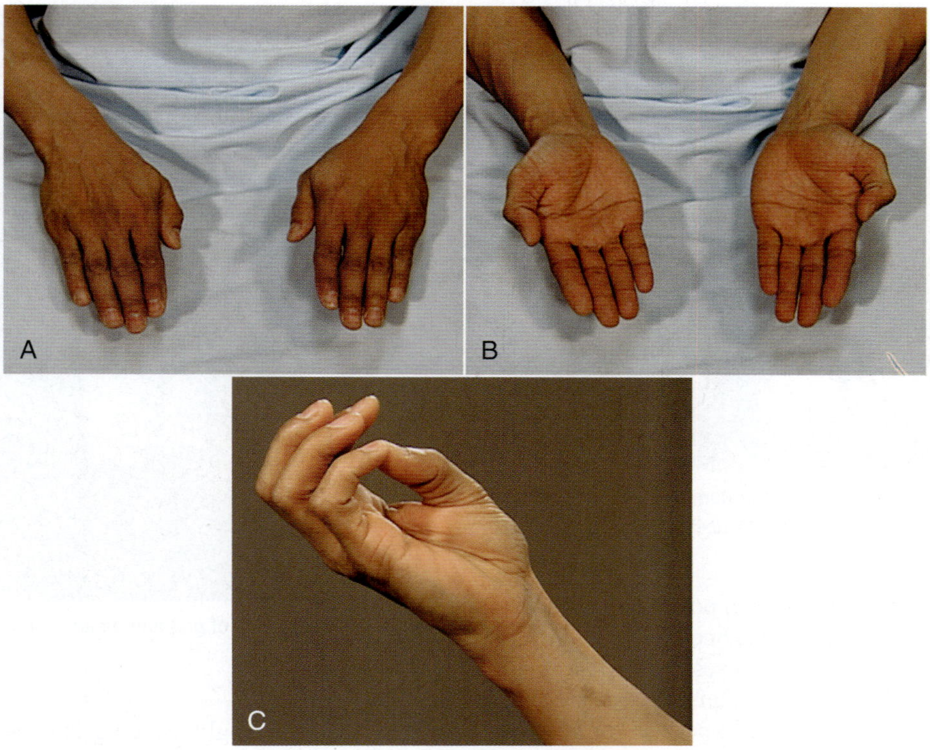

FIG. 23.14 Examination of coordination with rapid alternating movements. (A and B) Pat the knees with both hands, alternately using the palm and back of the hand. (C) Touch the thumb to each finger of the hand in sequence from index finger to small finger and back.

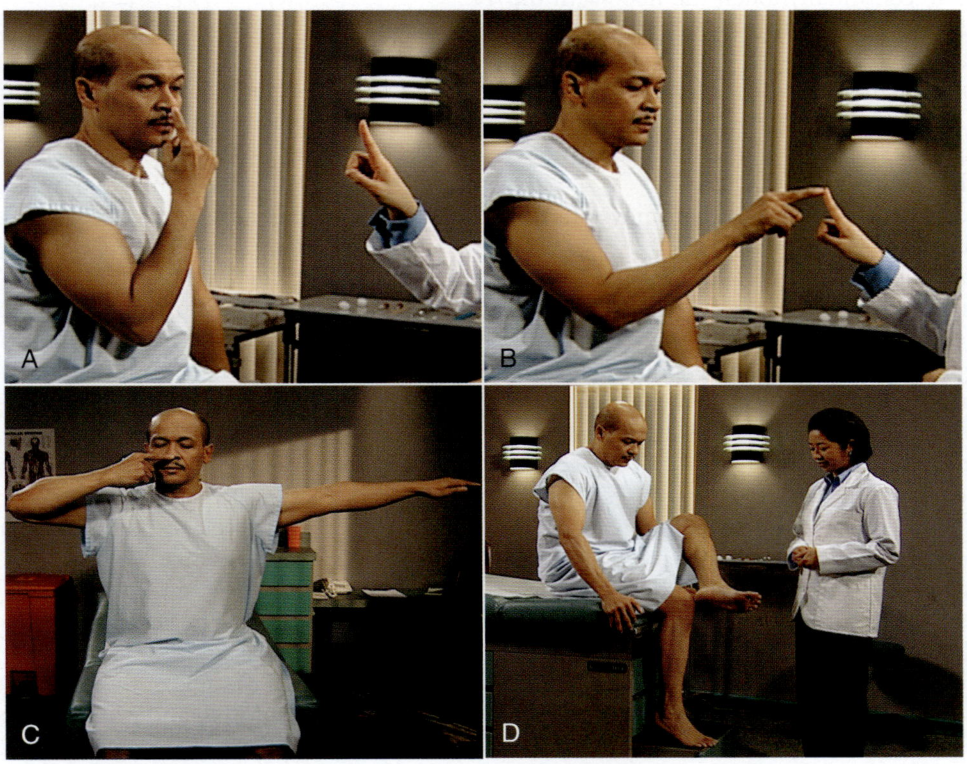

FIG. 23.15 Examination of fine motor function. (A and B) The patient alternately touches their own nose and the examiner's index finger with the index finger of one hand, (C) alternately touches their own nose with the index finger of each hand, and (D) runs the heel of one foot down the shin or tibia of the other leg.

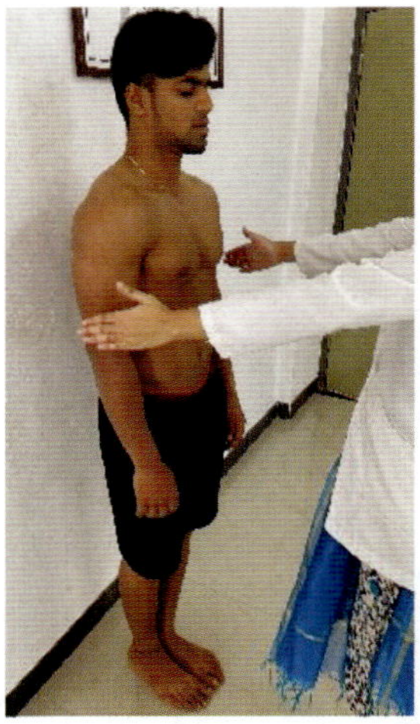

FIG. 23.16 **Evaluation of balance with the Romberg test.** (From Ramanathan, R. [2023]. *Physiology practical manual.* Elsevier.)

loses balance with the Romberg test, postpone other tests of cerebellar function requiring balance.

Ask the patient to close their eyes with their arms straight at the side of the body and stand on one foot. Repeat the test on the opposite foot. Expect slight swaying along with the ability to maintain balance on each foot for 5 seconds.

Have the patient (eyes open) hop in place first on one foot and then on the other. Expect the patient to hop on each foot for 5 seconds without loss of balance. Note any instability, a need to continually touch the floor with the opposite foot, or a tendency to fall.

Gait. Observe the patient walk without shoes around the room or down a hallway with the eyes open. Observe the expected gait sequence, noting simultaneous arm movements and upright posture:

1. The first heel strikes the floor and then moves to full contact with the floor.
2. The second heel pushes off, leaving the ground.
3. Body weight is transferred from the first heel to the ball of its foot.
4. The leg swing is accelerated as weight is removed from the second foot.
5. The second foot is lifted and travels ahead of the weight-bearing first foot, swinging through.
6. The second foot slows in preparation for heel strike.

Expect the patient to continuously sequence stance and swing, step after step. The gait should have a smooth, regular rhythm and symmetric stride length. The trunk posture should sway with the gait phase, and arm swing should be smooth and symmetric.

Heel-toe walking (tandem gait) will exaggerate any unexpected finding in gait evaluation. Direct the patient to touch the toe of one foot with the heel of the other foot (Fig. 23.17). Have the patient walk a straight line, first forward and then backward, with eyes open and arms at the sides. Consistent contact between the heel and toe should

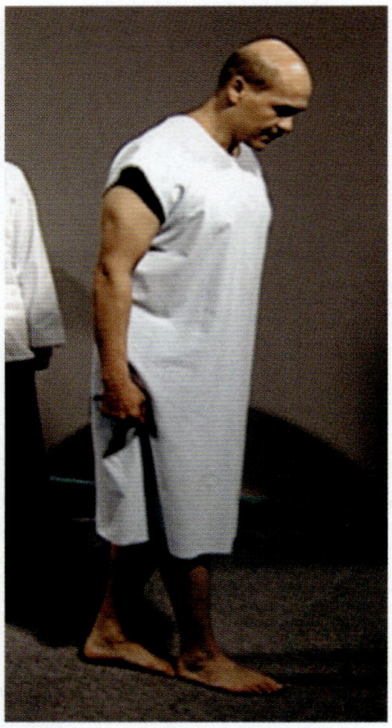

FIG. 23.17 **Evaluation of gait and balance with heel-toe walking on a straight line.**

occur, although slight swaying is expected. Note any extension of the arms for balance, instability, a tendency to fall, or lateral staggering and reeling. Note any shuffling, widely placed feet, toe walking, foot flop, leg lag, scissoring, loss of arm swing, staggering, or reeling. Fig. 23.18 and Table 23.4 describe unexpected gait patterns.

Sensory Function

Evaluate both primary and cortical discriminatory sensation by having the patient identify various sensory stimuli at the following sites: hands, lower arms, abdomen, feet, and lower legs. For the complete neurologic examination, assess each major peripheral nerve. Sensory discrimination of the face is performed when evaluating cranial nerve V as described previously.

Each sensory discrimination procedure is tested with the patient's eyes closed. Use minimal stimulation initially, increasing it gradually until the patient becomes aware of it. A stronger stimulus is needed over the back, buttocks, and heavily callused areas, where there are lower levels of sensitivity. Test contralateral areas of the body, and ask the patient to compare perceived sensations, side to side. With each type of sensory stimulus, expected findings include the following:

- Minimal differences side to side
- Correct description of sensations (e.g., hot/cold, sharp/dull)
- Recognition of the side of the body tested
- Location of sensation and whether proximal or distal to the previous stimuli

If evidence of sensory impairment is found, map the boundaries of the sensory deficit by the distribution of major peripheral nerves or dermatomes (see Fig. 23.6).

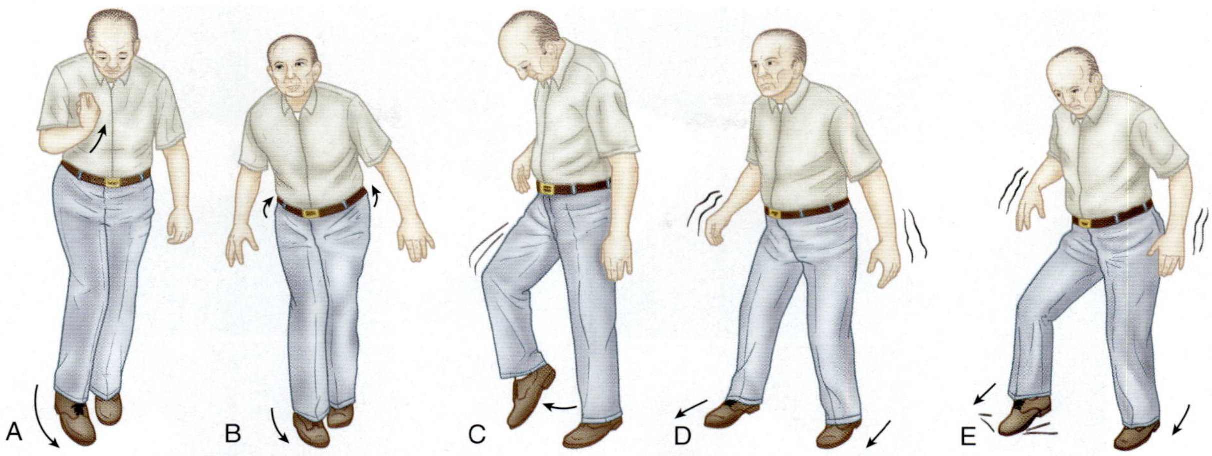

FIG. 23.18 Unexpected gait patterns. (A) Spastic hemiparesis. (B) Spastic diplegia (scissoring). (C) Steppage gait. (D) Cerebellar ataxia. (E) Sensory ataxia.

TABLE 23.4 Characteristics of Unexpected Gait Patterns

GAIT PATTERN	CHARACTERISTICS
Spastic hemiparesis	The affected leg is stiff and extended with plantar flexion of the foot; movement of the foot results from pelvic tilting upward on the involved side; the foot is dragged, often scraping the toe, or it is circled stiffly outward and forward (circumduction); the affected arm remains flexed and adducted and does not swing (see Fig. 23.18A).
Spastic diplegia (scissoring)	The patient uses short steps, dragging the ball of the foot across the floor; the legs are extended and the thighs tend to cross forward on each other at each step due to injury to the pyramidal system (see Fig. 23.18B).
Steppage	The hip and knee are elevated excessively high to lift the plantar-flexed foot off the ground; the foot is brought down to the floor with a slap; the patient is unable to walk on the heels (see Fig. 23.18C).
Dystrophic gait (waddling)	The legs are kept apart, and weight is shifted from side to side in a waddling motion due to weak hip abductor muscles; the abdomen often protrudes, and lordosis is common.
Tabetic gait	The legs are positioned far apart, lifted high, and forcibly brought down with each step; the heel stamps on the ground.
Cerebellar gait (cerebellar ataxia)	The patient's feet are wide based; staggering and lurching from side to side is often accompanied by swaying of the trunk (see Fig. 23.18D).
Sensory ataxia	The patient's gait is wide based; the feet are thrown forward and outward, bringing them down first on heels, then on toes; the patient watches the ground to guide their steps; a positive Romberg sign is present (see Fig. 23.18E).
Parkinsonian gait	The patient's posture is stooped, and the body is held rigid; steps are short and shuffling, with hesitation on starting and difficulty stopping (see Fig. 23.31C).
Dystonia	Jerky, dancing movements appear nondirectional.
Ataxia	Uncontrolled falling occurs.
Antalgic limp	The patient limits the time of weight bearing on the affected leg to limit pain.

Loss of sensation can indicate spinal tract, brainstem, or cerebral lesions.

Primary Sensory Functions

Superficial Touch. Touch the skin with a cotton wisp or with your fingertip, using light strokes. Do not depress the skin, and avoid stroking areas with hair (Fig. 23.19A). Have the patient point to the area touched or tell you when and where the sensation is felt.

Superficial Pain. Alternating the sharp and smooth edges of a broken tongue blade or paper clip, touch the skin in an unpredictable pattern. Allow 2 seconds between each stimulus to avoid a summative effect (see Fig. 23.19B). Ask the patient to identify each sensation as sharp or dull and where it is felt.

Evaluation of superficial pain and touch can be evaluated together. Alternate the use of the sharp and dull tongue blade edges with fingertip strokes to determine whether the patient can identify the change in sensation. In patients with known or suspected neuropathy, be careful with the strength of the sharp sensation used to avoid injury.

Temperature and Deep Pressure. Temperature and deep pressure sensation tests are performed only if superficial

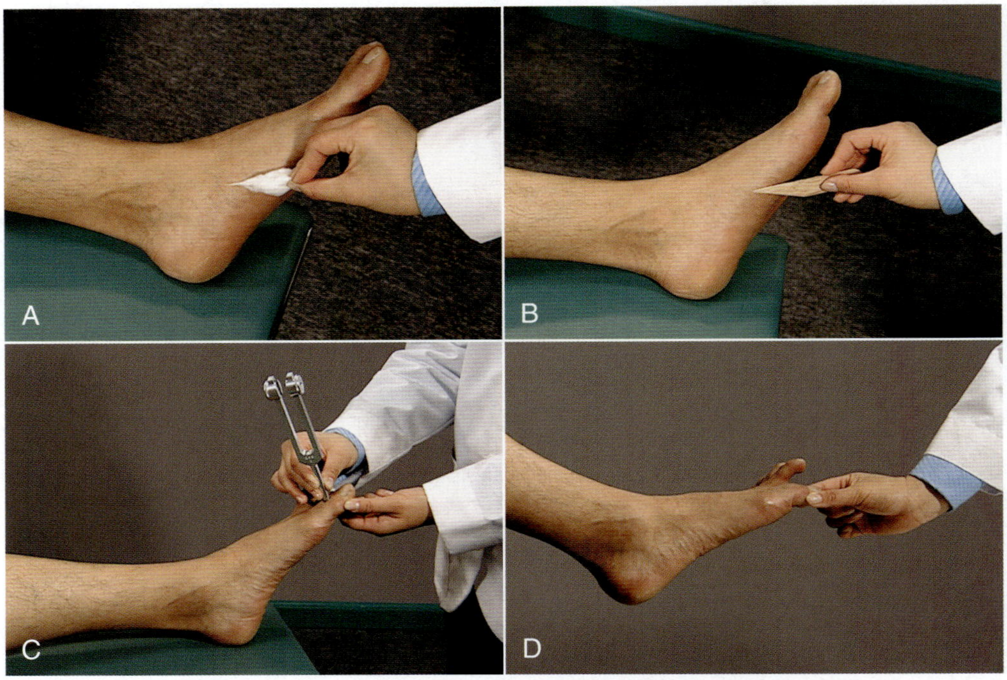

FIG. 23.19 Evaluation of primary sensory function. (A) Superficial tactile sensation; use a light stroke to touch the skin with a cotton wisp or brush. (B) Superficial pain sensation; use the sharp and rounded edge of a broken tongue blade in an unpredictable alternate pattern. (C) Vibratory sensation; place the stem of a vibrating tuning fork against several bony prominences. (D) Position sense of joints; hold the toe or finger by the lateral aspects while raising and lowering the toe.

pain sensation is not intact. To evaluate temperature sensation, roll test tubes of hot and cold water against the skin, alternating in an unpredictable pattern between the various sites. Ask the patient to indicate which temperature is perceived and where it is felt. Squeeze the trapezius, calf, or biceps muscle to evaluate deep pressure sensation. The patient should experience discomfort.

Vibration. Place the stem of a vibrating tuning fork (the tuning fork with lower Hz has slower reduction of vibration) against several bony prominences, beginning at toe and finger joints. The sternum, shoulder, elbow, wrist, shin, and ankle may also be tested (see Fig. 23.19C). Ask the patient to tell you when and where the buzzing or tingling sensation is felt. Dampen the tines on occasion before application to determine whether the patient distinguishes a difference.

Proprioception. With the patient's eyes closed, assess the great toe of each foot and a finger on each hand. Hold the joint to be tested (e.g., great toe or finger) by the lateral aspects to avoid giving a clue about the direction moved. Beginning with the joint in a neutral position, raise or lower the digit, and ask the patient which way the joint was moved (see Fig. 23.19D). Expect patients to identify the joint position.

Loss of sensory modalities may indicate peripheral neuropathy. Symmetric sensory loss indicates a polyneuropathy. See Box 23.2 for patterns of sensory loss.

Cortical Sensory Functions

Cortical or discriminatory sensory functions test cognitive ability to interpret sensations. Inability to perform these tests may indicate a lesion in the sensory cortex or the posterior columns of the spinal cord. The patient's eyes should be closed for these procedures.

Stereognosis. Hand the patient a familiar object (e.g., key, coin) to identify by touch and manipulation (Fig. 23.20A). Tactile agnosia, an inability to recognize objects by touch, suggests a parietal lobe lesion.

Two-Point Discrimination. Use two ends of a paper clip or sharp ends of a broken tongue blade and alternate touching the patient's skin with one point or both points at various locations over the body (see Fig. 23.20B). Ask the patient how many points are felt. On the fingertips and toes, two points are commonly felt when 2 to 8 mm apart. A greater distance is expected for discrimination of two points on other body parts, such as the back (40 to 70 mm) or chest and forearms (40 mm).

Extinction Phenomenon. Simultaneously touch two areas on each side of the body (e.g., cheek, hand, or other area) with the sharp edge of a broken tongue blade. Ask the patient to tell you the number of stimuli and where they are felt. Expect similar sensations to be felt bilaterally.

BOX 23.2 Patterns of Sensory Loss Injury or Defect and Description of Findings

Single Peripheral Nerve
The area of sensory loss is generally less than the anatomic distribution of the nerve. The lost sensation is greatest in the central portion of the nerve's anatomic distribution with a surrounding zone of partial loss because adjacent nerve distributions overlap. All or selected forms of sensory discrimination may be lost.

Multiple Peripheral Nerves (Polyneuropathy)
The sensory loss is most severe over legs and feet or over hands (i.e., glove-and-stocking distribution). The change from expected to impaired sensation is often gradual. All forms of sensory discrimination are usually lost.

Multiple Spinal Nerve Roots
Incomplete loss of sensation in any area of the skin usually occurs when one nerve root is affected. When two or more nerve roots are completely divided, a zone of sensory loss is surrounded by partial loss. Tendon reflexes may also be lost.

Complete Transverse Lesion of the Spinal Cord
All forms of sensation are lost below the level of the lesion. Pain, temperature, and touch sensations are lost one to two dermatomes below the lesion.

Partial Spinal Sensory Syndrome (Brown-Séquard Syndrome)
Pain and temperature sensation are lost one to two dermatomes below the lesion on the opposite side of the body from the lesion. Proprioceptive loss and motor paralysis occur on the lesion side of the body.

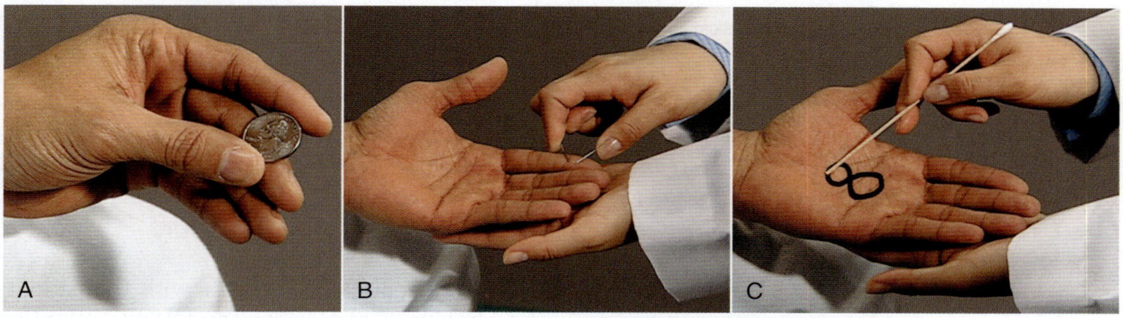

FIG. 23.20 Evaluation of cortical sensory function. (A) Stereognosis; patient identifies a familiar object by touch. (B) Two-point discrimination; using two sharp ends of a broken tongue blade or two points of a paper clip, alternately place one or two points simultaneously on the skin, and ask the patient to determine whether one or two sensations are felt. (C) Graphesthesia; draw a letter or number on the body (without actually marking skin) and ask the patient to identify it.

Graphesthesia. With a blunt pen or an applicator stick, draw a letter, number, or shape on the palm of the patient's hand (see Fig. 23.20C). Other body locations may also be used. Ask the patient to identify the figure. Repeat using a different figure on the other hand. Expect the figure to be readily recognized.

Point Location. Touch an area on the patient's skin and withdraw the stimulus. Ask the patient to point to the area touched. No difficulty localizing the stimulus should be noted. This procedure is often performed with superficial tactile sensation.

Table 23.5 provides a summary of procedures used to test the integrity of spinal tracts.

Reflexes

Both superficial and deep tendon reflexes are used to evaluate the function of specific spine segmental levels (Table 23.6).

Superficial Reflexes

The plantar reflex is routinely performed. The abdominal and cremasteric reflexes are less commonly tested, but they are important when thoracic spinal nerves need to be evaluated.

Plantar Reflex. Use the end of a reflex hammer to stroke the lateral side of the foot from the heel to the ball and then across the ball of the foot to the medial side (Fig. 23.21A). Expect plantar flexion of all toes. The Babinski sign is present when there is dorsiflexion of the great toe with or without fanning of the other toes. The Babinski sign indicates an upper motor neuron lesion or disorder affecting the corticospinal tract. It is, however, an expected finding in children younger than 2 years of age. The ticklish patient may respond with some degree of the Babinski sign, but this can be avoided with a firm touch.

Evidence-Based Practice

Babinski Sign Interpretation

A study of 107 patients with pyramidal tract disease assessed the relationship of level of pyramidal tract disease to a Babinski sign with dorsiflexion of the great toe when fanning (movement of the other toes) was or was not present. A Babinski sign with great toe dorsiflexion alone was found to occur significantly more often in patients with lesions in the brain cortex, while a Babinski sign with great toe dorsiflexion and movement of the other toes was found to occur significantly more often in patients with subcortical lesions between the cortex and spinal cord ($P < 0.001$; Deng et al., 2013).

TABLE 23.5 Procedures for Testing the Integrity of Individual Spinal Tracts for Upper and Lower Motor Neuron Disorders

SPINAL TRACTS	NEUROLOGIC TESTS
Ascending Tracts for Lower Motor Neuron Disorders	
Lateral spinothalamic	Superficial pain
	Temperature
Anterior spinothalamic	Superficial touch
	Deep pressure
Posterior column	Vibration
	Deep pressure
	Position sense
	Stereognosis
	Point location
	Two-point discrimination
Anterior and dorsal spinocerebellar	Proprioception
Descending Tracts for Upper Motor Neuron Disorders	
Lateral and anterior corticospinal	Rapid rhythmic alternating movements
	Voluntary movement
	Deep tendon reflexes
	Plantar reflex
Medial and lateral reticulospinal	Posture and Romberg
	Gait
	Instinctual motor reactions

Abdominal Reflex. With the patient supine, stroke each quadrant of the abdomen with the end of a reflex hammer or edge of a tongue blade. Elicit the upper abdominal reflexes by stroking upward and away from the umbilicus. Elicit the lower abdominal reflexes by stroking downward and away from the umbilicus (see Fig. 23.21B). Expect a slight movement of the umbilicus toward each area of stimulation to be bilaterally equal. A diminished reflex may be present in patients who are obese or whose abdominal muscles have been stretched during pregnancy. Abdominal reflexes may be absent on the side of a corticospinal tract lesion, but their presence or absence may have little clinical significance.

TABLE 23.6 Spinal Nerve Level Evaluated by Superficial and Deep Tendon Reflexes

REFLEX	SPINAL NERVE LEVEL EVALUATED
Superficial	
Upper abdominal	T8, T9, and T10
Lower abdominal	T10, T11, and T12
Cremasteric	T12, L1, and L2
Plantar	L5, S1, and S2
Deep Tendon	
Biceps	C5 and C6
Brachioradialis	C5 and C6
Triceps	C6, C7, and C8
Patellar	L2, L3, and L4
Achilles	S1 and S2

Cremasteric Reflex. Stroke the inner thigh of the male patient (proximal to distal) to elicit the cremasteric reflex. Expect the testicle and scrotum to rise on the side where a stroke occurred.

Deep Tendon Reflexes

Evaluate deep tendon reflexes with the patient either sitting or lying down. Focus the patient's attention on an alternate muscle contraction (e.g., pulling clenched hands apart) to help prevent an exaggerated or diminished response. Position the limb with slight tension on the tendon to be tapped and palpate the tendon to locate the correct point for stimulation. Hold the reflex hammer loosely between your thumb and index finger and, without striking too forcefully, briskly tap the tendon with a flick of the wrist (Fig. 23.22).

Test each reflex, comparing responses between sides. Expect symmetric visible or palpable responses. Deep tendon reflex responses are scored as shown in Table 23.7. Absent reflexes may indicate neuropathy or lower motor neuron disorder. Hyperactive reflexes suggest an upper motor neuron disorder. The characteristics of upper and lower motor neuron disorders are listed in the Differential Diagnosis table, "Characteristics of Upper and Lower Motor Neuron Disorders."

DIFFERENTIAL DIAGNOSIS

Characteristics of Upper and Lower Motor Neuron Disorders

ASSESSMENT PARAMETERS	UPPER MOTOR NEURON	LOWER MOTOR NEURON
Muscle tone	Increased tone, muscle spasticity, risk for contractures	Decreased tone, muscle flaccidity
Muscle atrophy	Little or no muscle atrophy, but decreased strength	Loss of muscle strength; muscle atrophy or wasting
Sensation	Sensation loss may affect entire limb	Sensory loss follows the distribution of dermatomes or peripheral nerves

DIFFERENTIAL DIAGNOSIS—cont'd

Characteristics of Upper and Lower Motor Neuron Disorders

ASSESSMENT PARAMETERS	UPPER MOTOR NEURON	LOWER MOTOR NEURON
Reflexes	Hyperactive deep tendon and abdominal reflexes; positive Babinski sign	Weak or absent deep tendon, plantar, and abdominal reflexes; negative plantar reflex; no pathologic reflexes
Fasciculations	No fasciculations	Fasciculations present
Motor effect	Paralysis of voluntary movements	Paralysis of muscles
Location of insult	Damage above level of brainstem affects opposite side of body; damage below brainstem affects same side of body	Damage affects muscle on same side of body

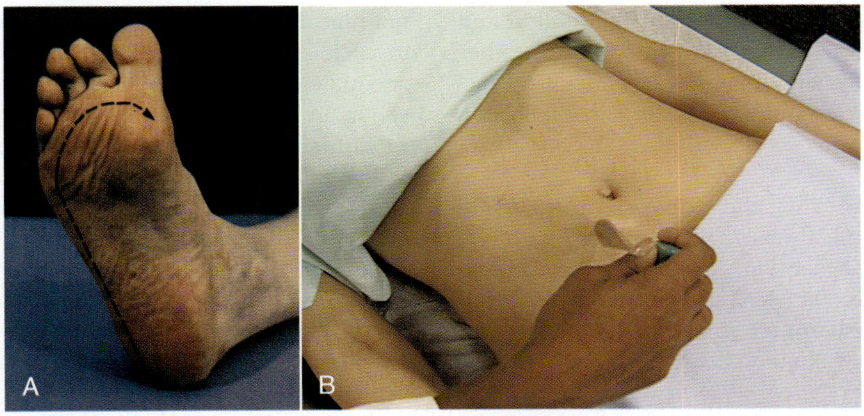

FIG. 23.21 Superficial reflexes. (A) Plantar reflex indicating the direction of the stroke and the Babinski sign—dorsiflexion of the great toe with or without fanning of the toes. (B) One of several approaches for the abdominal reflexes. Stroke the lower abdominal area downward, away from the umbilicus. Stroke the upper abdominal area upward, away from the umbilicus.

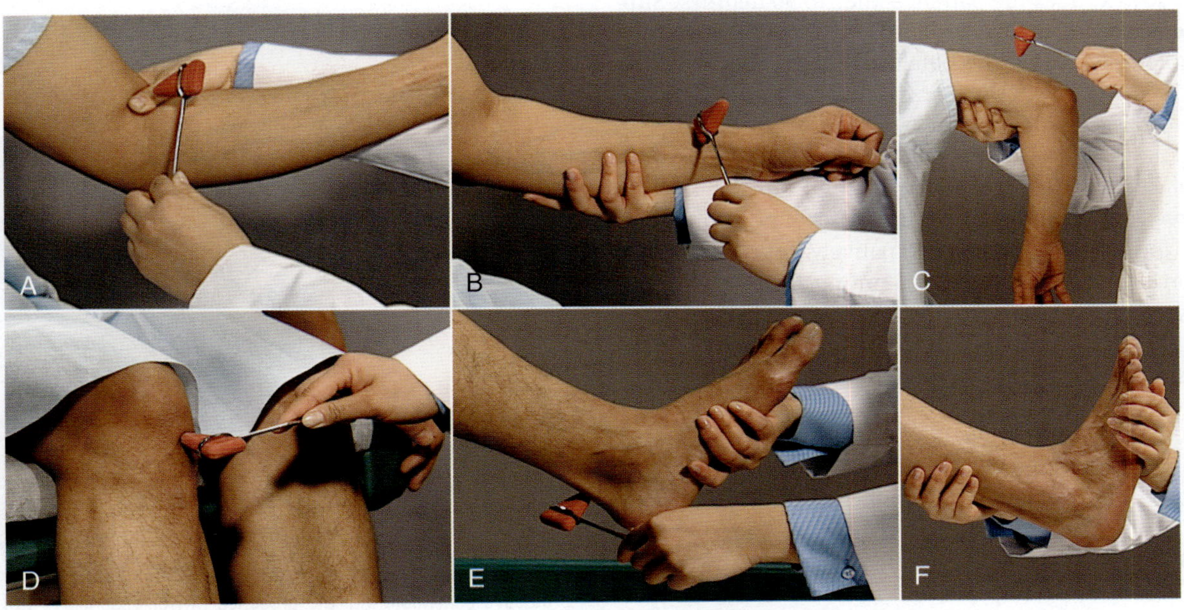

FIG. 23.22 Location of tendons for evaluation of deep tendon reflexes. (A) Biceps. (B) Brachioradialis. (C) Triceps. (D) Patellar. (E) Achilles. (F) Evaluation of ankle clonus.

TABLE 23.7 Scoring Deep Tendon Reflexes

GRADE	DEEP TENDON REFLEX RESPONSE
0	No response
1+	Sluggish or diminished
2+	Active or expected response
3+	More brisk than expected, slightly hyperactive
4+	Brisk, hyperactive, with intermittent or transient clonus

Biceps Reflex. Flex the patient's arm to 45 degrees at the elbow. Palpate the biceps tendon in the antecubital fossa (see Fig. 23.22A). Place your thumb over the tendon and your fingers under the elbow. Strike your thumb, rather than the tendon directly, with the reflex hammer. Contraction of the biceps muscle causes visible or palpable flexion of the elbow.

Brachioradialis Reflex. Flex the patient's arm up to 45 degrees and rest the forearm on your arm with the hand slightly pronated (see Fig. 23.22B). Strike the brachioradialis tendon (about 1 to 2 inches above the wrist) directly with the reflex hammer. Pronation of the forearm and flexion of the elbow should occur.

Triceps Reflex. Flex the patient's arm at the elbow up to 90 degrees, supporting the arm proximal to the antecubital fossa. Palpate the triceps tendon and strike it directly with the reflex hammer, just above the elbow (see Fig. 23.22C). Contraction of the triceps muscle causes visible or palpable extension of the elbow.

Patellar Reflex. Flex the patient's knee to 90 degrees. Support the upper leg with your hand and allow the lower leg to hang loosely. Strike the patellar tendon just below the patella (see Fig. 23.22D). Contraction of the quadriceps muscle causes extension of the lower leg.

Achilles Reflex. With the patient sitting, flex the knee to 90 degrees and keep the ankle in a neutral position, holding the foot in your hand. Alternatively, the patient may kneel on a chair with the toes pointing toward the floor. Strike the Achilles tendon at the level of the ankle malleoli (see Fig. 23.22E). Contraction of the gastrocnemius muscle causes plantar flexion of the foot.

Clonus. Test for ankle clonus, especially if the reflexes are hyperactive. Support the patient's knee in partially flexed position and briskly dorsiflex the foot with your other hand, maintaining the foot in flexion (see Fig. 23.22F). No rhythmic oscillating movements between dorsiflexion and plantar flexion should be palpated. Sustained clonus is associated with upper motor neuron disease.

ADVANCED SKILLS

Other procedures for further evaluation of the neurologic system may be performed when problems are detected with routine examination.

Protective Sensation

Use the 5.07 monofilament to test for sensation on several sites of the foot in all patients with diabetes mellitus in addition to patients with concern for peripheral neuropathy (Fig. 23.23). While the patient's eyes are closed, apply the monofilament in a random pattern to several sites on the plantar surface of the foot and on one site of the dorsal surface. Do not test over calluses or broken skin. Do not repeat a test site. The monofilament should be applied to each site for 1.5 seconds. When the filament bends, adequate pressure is applied. Patients should feel the sensation in all sites. Loss of sensation to the touch of the monofilament is an indication of peripheral neuropathy. It also indicates the loss of protective pain sensation that alerts patients to skin breakdown and injury on the foot.

Meningeal Signs

A stiff neck, or nuchal rigidity, is a sign that may be associated with meningitis and subarachnoid hemorrhage. With the patient supine, slip your hand under the head and raise it, flexing the neck. Try to make the patient's chin touch the sternum, but do not force it. Placing your hand under the shoulders when the patient is supine and raising the shoulders slightly will help relax the neck, making the determination of true stiffness more accurate. Patients generally do not resist or complain of pain. Pain and a resistance to neck motion are associated with nuchal

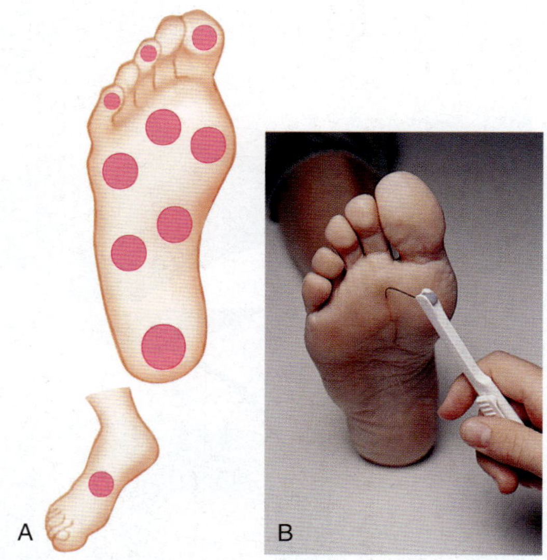

FIG. 23.23 (A) Sites for application of the 5.07 monofilament to test for protective sensation. Indicate presence (+) or absence (−) of sensory perception on a drawing of the foot. (B) Apply the monofilament to the patient's foot with just enough pressure to bend the monofilament.

rigidity. Occasionally, painful swollen lymph nodes in the neck and superficial trauma may also cause pain and resistance to neck motion.

The Brudzinski sign may also be present when neck stiffness is assessed. Involuntary flexion of the hips and knees when flexing the neck is a positive Brudzinski sign and may indicate meningeal irritation (Fig. 23.24A).

The Kernig sign is evaluated by flexing the leg at the knee and hip when the patient is supine, then attempting to straighten the leg. A positive Kernig sign is present when the patient has pain in the lower back and resistance to straightening the leg at the knee. The presence of this sign may also indicate meningeal irritation (see Fig. 23.24B).

Jolt Accentuation of Headache

For the patient presenting with fever and headache that leads to a suspected diagnosis of meningitis, jolt accentuation of headache may be performed. Ask the patient with extended feet to move the head horizontally at a rate of two to three rotations per second. A positive sign is indicated by an increased headache over the baseline. This test result may be helpful as a diagnostic sign for meningitis in emergency care settings, but supportive evidence is lacking (Iguchi et al., 2020). See Evidence-Based Practice, "Signs of Meningitis."

Evidence-Based Practice in Physical Examination

Signs of Meningitis

The classic signs of acute meningitis are fever, a stiff neck, and altered mental status, but most patients do not have all three signs. Other potential presenting symptoms include headache, rash, nausea, vomiting, chills, and myalgia. Nuchal rigidity, Brudzinski sign, Kernig sign, and jolt accentuation of headache are considered important diagnostic signs for meningitis.

Prospective studies investigating physical signs associated with meningitis in adults (e.g., nuchal rigidity, head jolt accentuation of headache, Brudzinski sign, and Kernig sign) reveal that these physical signs are seen significantly more often in patients with meningitis compared with those without meningitis, but no one sign or combination of meningeal irritation signs increases the likelihood of meningitis (Afhami et al., 2017; Akaishi et al., 2019). A lumbar puncture is needed to confirm the presence of meningitis.

Posturing

Postures that may be found in unresponsive patients are associated with a severe brain injury. Decorticate or flexor posturing is associated with injury to the corticospinal tracts above the brainstem (Fig. 23.25A). Decerebrate or extensor posturing is associated with injury to the brainstem (see Fig. 23.25B).

Infants

Neurologic problems may be suspected in infants and young children when parents report they are not doing something aligned with their developmental age or they have lost a skill previously attained. The major clues are discovered with an accurate and thorough history. Observe for dysmorphic facial features that may be suggestive of congenital conditions that include neurologic problems (e.g., low-set ears or port-wine stain).

The cranial nerves are not routinely tested as in adults, but careful observations during the physical examination provide an indirect evaluation (Table 23.8).

Observe the infant's spontaneous activity for symmetry and smoothness of movement (Fig. 23.26). Coordinated sucking and swallowing are also functions of the cerebellum. Hands are usually held in fists for the first 3 months of life, but not constantly. After 3 months the hands begin to open for longer periods. Purposeful movement (e.g., reaching and grasping for objects) begins at about 2 months of age. The infant progresses to taking objects with one hand at 6 months, transferring objects between hands at 7 months, and purposefully releasing objects by 10 months of age. No tremors or constant overshooting of movements is expected. See Clinical Pearl, "Infant Development: Rolling Over."

CLINICAL PEARL

Infant Development: Rolling Over

Infants roll over independently around 4 to 6 months of age. Since infants should sleep on their backs to reduce the risk of sudden unexpected infant death, supervised tummy time (play in prone position) when they are awake can help stimulate their gross motor development.

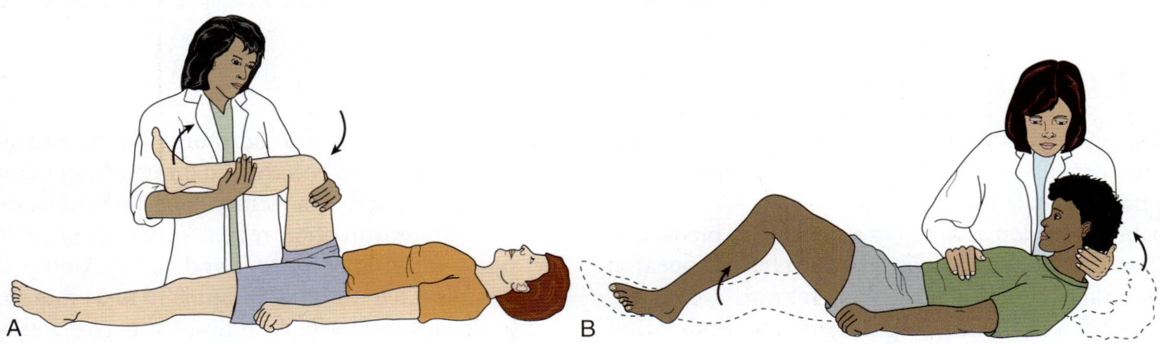

FIG. 23.24 (A) Kernig sign, flex the leg at the knee and hip when the patient is supine, and then attempt to straighten the leg. Observe for pain in the lower back and resistance to straightening the leg. (B) Brudzinski sign, flex the neck and observe for involuntary flexion of the hips and knees. (From Lewis, S. L., et al. (2007). *Medical-surgical nursing* (7th ed.). Mosby.)

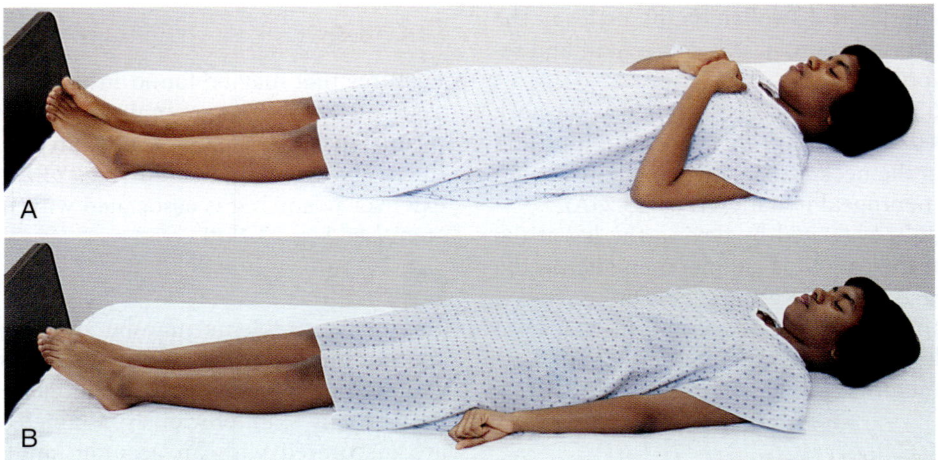

FIG. 23.25 (A) Decorticate or flexor posture. The upper arms are flexed at the elbows and held tightly toward the center of the body. The wrists and fingers are flexed, and the feet are plantar flexed. The legs are extended and internally rotated. Fine tremors or intense stiffness may be present. (B) Decerebrate or extensor posture. The arms are fully extended with forearms pronated. The wrists and fingers are flexed, and the jaw is clenched. The neck is extended, and the back may be arched. The feet are plantar flexed.

TABLE 23.8 Indirect Cranial Nerve Evaluation in Newborns and Infants

CRANIAL NERVES (CN)	PROCEDURES AND OBSERVATIONS[a]
CN II, III, IV, and VI	Optical blink reflex: shine a light at the infant's open eyes; *observe the quick closure of the eyes and dorsal flexion of the infant's head;* no response may indicate poor light perception *Gazes intensely at close object or face* *Focuses on and tracks an object with both eyes* Doll's eye maneuver (see CN VIII)
CN V	Rooting reflex: touch one corner of the infant's mouth; *the infant should open its mouth and turn its head in the direction of stimulation*; if the infant has been fed *recently,* minimal or no response is expected (see Table 23.9) Sucking reflex: place your finger in the infant's mouth, feeling the sucking action; *the tongue should push up against your finger with good strength;* note the pressure, strength, and pattern of sucking
CN VII	Observe the infant's facial expression when crying; *note the infant's ability to wrinkle the forehead and the symmetry of the smile*
CN VIII	Acoustic blink reflex: loudly clap your hands about 30 cm from the infant's head; avoid producing an air current; *note the blink in response to the sound;* no response after 2–3 days of age may indicate hearing problems; infant will habituate to repeated testing *Moves eyes in direction of sound; freezes position with high-pitched sound* Doll's eye maneuver: hold the infant under the axilla in an upright position, head held steady, facing you; rotate the infant first in one direction and then in the other; *the infant's eyes should turn in the direction of rotation and then the opposite direction when rotation stops;* if the eyes do not move in the expected direction, suspect a vestibular problem or eye muscle paralysis
CN IX and X	*Swallowing ability and gag reflex*
CN XII	*Coordinated sucking and swallowing ability* Pinch infant's nose; *mouth will open and tip of tongue will rise in a midline position*

[a]*Italics* indicate expected findings.

A withdrawal of all limbs from a painful stimulus provides a measure of sensory integrity. Other sensory functions are not routinely tested.

The patellar tendon reflexes are present at birth, and the Achilles and brachioradialis tendon reflexes appear at 6 months of age. When deep tendon reflexes are tested, the examiner can use a finger or stethoscope head, rather than the reflex hammer, to tap the tendon. In each case, expect the muscle attached to the tendon struck to contract. Interpret findings as for adults; however, one or two beats of ankle clonus are common. Infants with sustained ankle clonus should be assessed for neurologic conditions.

The plantar reflex is routinely performed as described in the adult examination reflex section. A positive Babinski sign—fanning of the toes and dorsiflexion of the great toe—is expected until the infant is 16 to 24 months of age.

The common newborn reflexes are assessed routinely to evaluate the posture and movement of the developing infant (Table 23.9). These reflexes appear and disappear in a sequence corresponding with CNS development.

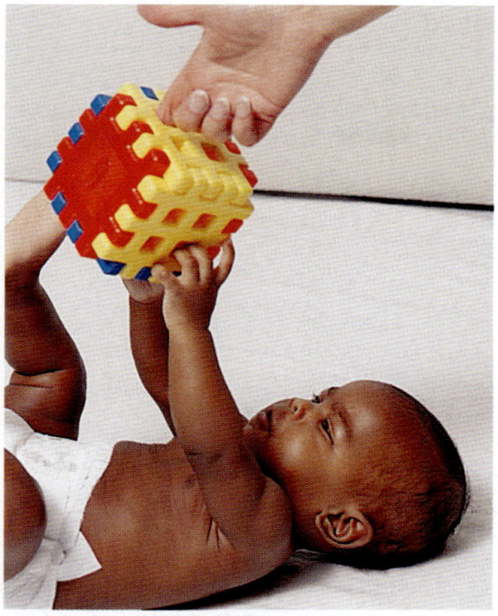

FIG. 23.26 Observe interest and purposeful movement such as reaching for the block.

Symmetry and smoothness of response are important observations. During the assessment, observe for any rhythmic twitching of the facial, extremity, and trunk musculature and for any sustained asymmetric posturing. These signs, especially in paroxysmal episodes, are associated with seizure activity.

Muscle strength and tone are especially important to evaluate in the newborn and infant (see Chapter 22). The newborn's neuromuscular development at the time of birth should be evaluated with the Ballard Clinical Assessment for gestational age (Ballard et al., 1991; see http://perinatology.com/calculators/Ballard.htm).

Children

Perform the neurologic examination of the young child by observing the neuromuscular developmental progress and skills displayed during the visit. Delay in sitting and walking may be a sign of a cerebellar disorder. Developmental screening tests (e.g., a standardized parent

TABLE 23.9 Common Newborn Reflexes Routinely Evaluated in Infants

REFLEX (APPEARANCE)	PROCEDURE AND FINDINGS[a]
Rooting reflex (birth) 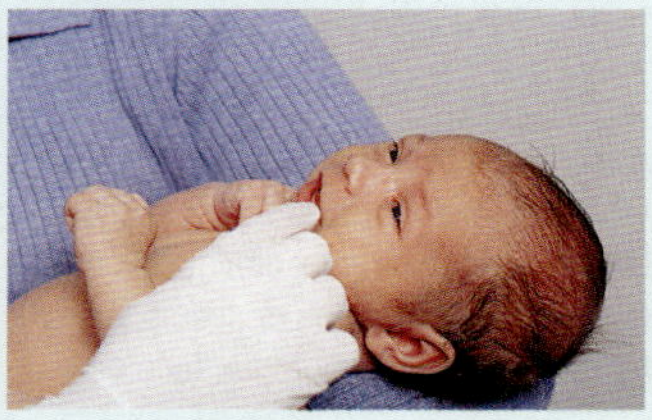	Touch the corner of the infant's mouth; *when hungry, the infant will move the head and open the mouth on the side of stimulation;* disappears by 3–4 months of age.
Palmar grasp (birth) 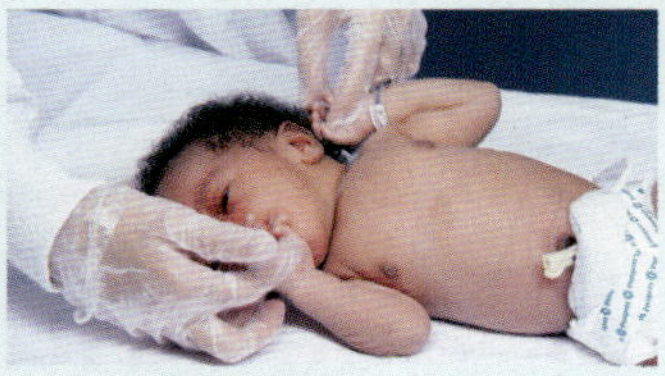	Making sure the infant's head is in midline, touch the palm of the infant's hand from the ulnar side (opposite the thumb); *note the strong grasp of your finger; sucking facilitates the grasp;* it should be strongest between 1 and 2 months of age and disappear by 3 months.
Plantar grasp (birth) 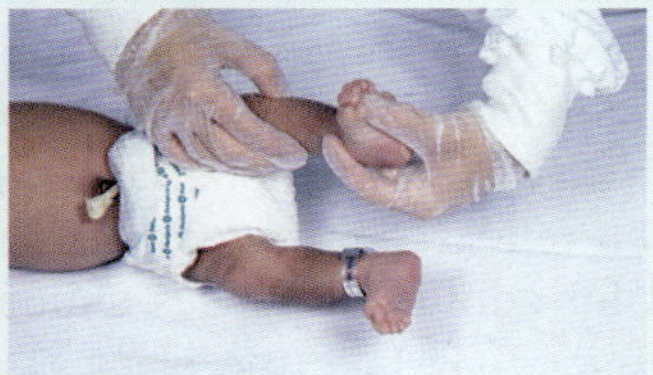	Touch the plantar surface of the infant's feet at the base of the toes; *the toes should curl downward;* the reflex should be strong up to 8 months of age.
Moro (birth) 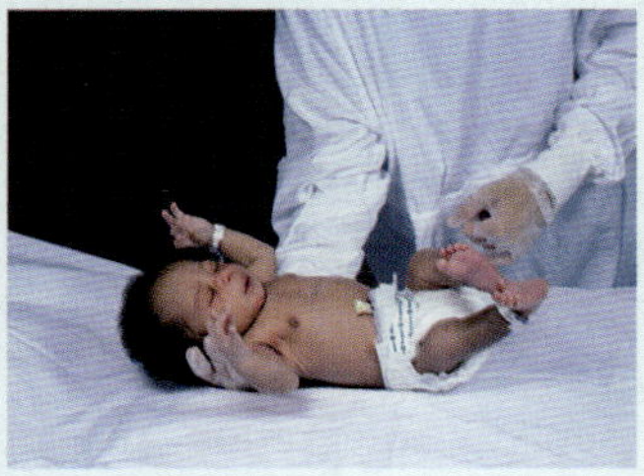	With the infant supported in a semisitting position, allow the head and trunk to drop back to a 30-degree angle; *observe symmetric abduction and extension of the arms; fingers fan out and thumb and index finger form a C; the arms then adduct in an embracing motion followed by relaxed flexion; the legs may follow a similar pattern of response;* the reflex diminishes in strength by 3–4 months and disappears by 6 months.

Continued

TABLE 23.9 Common Newborn Reflexes Routinely Evaluated in Infants—cont'd

REFLEX (APPEARANCE)	PROCEDURE AND FINDINGS[a]
Placing (4 days of age) 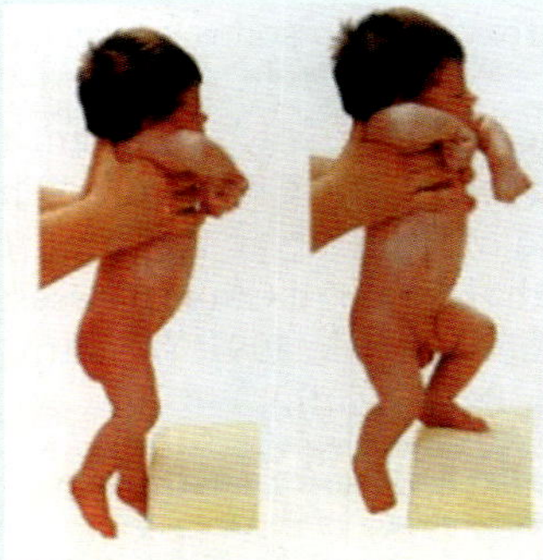 (Courtesy Zsuzsa Csontos.)	Hold the infant upright under the arms next to a table or chair; touch the dorsal side of the foot to the table or chair edge; *observe flexion of the hips and knees and lifting of the foot as if stepping up on the table;* age of disappearance varies.
Stepping (between birth and 8 weeks) 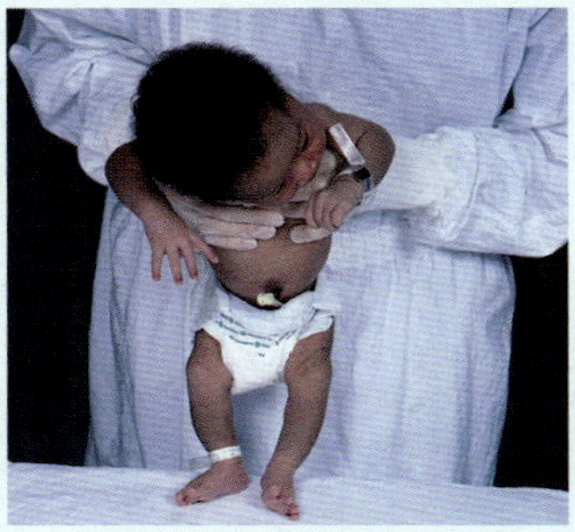	Hold the infant upright under the arms and allow the soles of the feet to touch the surface of the table; *observe for alternate flexion and extension of the legs, simulating walking;* it disappears before voluntary walking.
Asymmetric tonic neck or "fencing" (by 2–3 months) 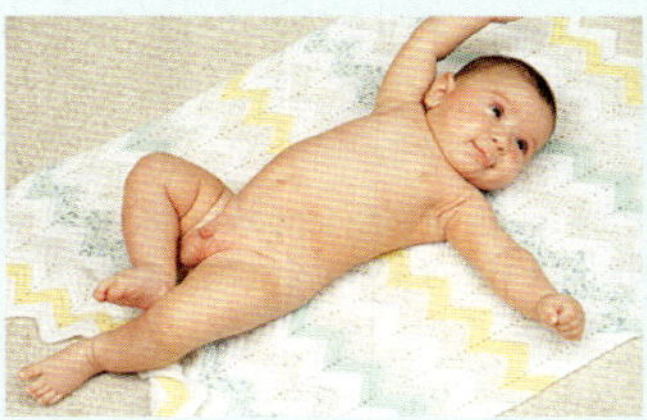	With the infant lying supine and relaxed or sleeping, turn the head to one side so the jaw is over the shoulder; observe for *extension of the arm and leg on the side to which the head is turned and for flexion of the opposite arm and leg;* turn the infant's head to the other side, observing the reversal of the extremities' posture; this reflex diminishes at 3–4 months of age and disappears by 6 months; be concerned if the infant never exhibits the reflex or seems locked in the fencing position; this reflex must disappear before the infant can roll over or bring the hands to the face.

[a]*Italics* indicate expected findings.

questionnaire) are useful tools to determine whether the child is progressing as expected with fine and gross motor skills, language, and personal-social skills.

Direct examination of cranial nerves is modified for the age of the child. Often a game is played to elicit the response. Table 23.10 describes these procedures.

Observe the young child at play, noting gait and fine motor coordination. The child beginning to walk has a wide-based gait. The older child walks with feet closer together, has better balance, and recovers more easily when unbalanced. Observe the child's skill in reaching for, grasping, and releasing toys. Expect no tremors or constant overshooting movements.

Heel-to-toe walking, hopping, and jumping are all coordination skills that develop in the young child. Ask the child to show how well they perform each skill, making this a game for the child.

Many of the techniques used in the adult neurologic examination are used for children, with some modifications for the child's level of understanding. Deep tendon reflexes are not always tested in a child who demonstrates appropriate development. When reflexes are tested, use the same techniques described for adults; responses should be the same. Your index finger may take the place of a reflex hammer and be less threatening to a child.

Evaluate light touch sensation by asking the child to close their eyes and point to where you touch. Alternatively, have the child discriminate between hard and soft textures. Use the tuning fork to evaluate vibration sensation, asking the child to point to the area where the buzzing sensation is felt. Superficial pain sensation is not routinely tested in young children to avoid causing distress.

When checking cortical sensory integration, use figures (e.g., circle, square, triangle) rather than numbers to

TABLE 23.10 Cranial Nerve Examination Procedures for Young Children

CRANIAL NERVES (CN)	PROCEDURES AND OBSERVATIONS
CN II	If the child cooperates, the Snellen letter chart, HOTV chart, or LEA symbols may be used to test vision.
	Visual fields may be tested, but the child may need the head held still.
CN III, IV, and VI	Have the child follow an object with the eyes, holding the head still if necessary. Move the object through the cardinal points of gaze to test extraocular muscle movement.
CN V	Observe the child chewing a cookie or cracker, noting bilateral jaw strength.
	With eyes closed, touch the child's forehead and cheeks with cotton or string and watch the child push it away.
CN VII	Observe the child's face when smiling, frowning, and crying.
	Ask the child to show the teeth.
	Demonstrate puffed cheeks and ask the child to imitate.
CN VIII	Observe the child turn to sounds such as a bell or whisper.
	Whisper a commonly used word behind the child's back and have them repeat the word.
	Perform audiometric testing.
CN IX and X	Elicit the gag reflex.
CN XI and XII	Instruct the older child to stick out the tongue and shrug the shoulders or raise the arms.

evaluate graphesthesia. Draw each figure twice and ask the child if the figures are the same or different. (Make sure the child understands the terms "same" and "different.") Practice once with the child's eyes open to improve response.

Pregnant Patients

Examination of pregnant patients is the same as for the adult in general. Assessment of deep tendon reflexes during the initial examination can serve as a baseline evaluation.

Older Adults

Examination of the neurologic system of the older adult is identical to that of the adult. You may need to allow more time for performing maneuvers that require coordination and movement. Assessing functional status is essential in determining the impact of any health condition on the patient.

Medications can impair CNS function and cause slowed reaction time; tremors (rhythmic, oscillating, involuntary purposeless movements); and anxiety. Problems may develop because of the dosage, number, or interaction of prescription or nonprescription medications.

Think About It

Carefully consider polypharmacy and specific categories of medications when evaluating CNS function. Medications such as benzodiazepines, CNS antidepressants, gabapentinoids, and muscle relaxants have effects that can cause sedation, orthostatic hypotension, and cognitive impairment. The potential for falls and other injuries can be higher in older adults taking these medications. A formal review by pharmacists and clinicians using the American Geriatrics Society (AGS) Beers Criteria may identify potentially inappropriate medications (American Geriatrics Society, 2023).

The older adult may have diminished smell and taste sensation. Decreased perception of all tastes (sweet, salty, bitter, sour, and umami) increases with advancing age (Barragán et al., 2018). Vision and hearing are other sensations that decline with aging. Older adults are reported to have reduced tactile and temperature sensation (warm and cold) when tested in an orofacial distribution (Heft & Robinson, 2014). Touch perception and manual dexterity (fine motor skills) also decrease with aging (Reuter et al., 2012).

In older adults, balance and strength decrease, which can affect mobility. Gait with advancing age is characterized by shorter steps with less lifting of the feet as proprioception declines. Shuffling may occur as speed, balance, and grace decrease with age. Arms are more flexed, and legs may be flexed at the hips and knees (Fig. 23.27).

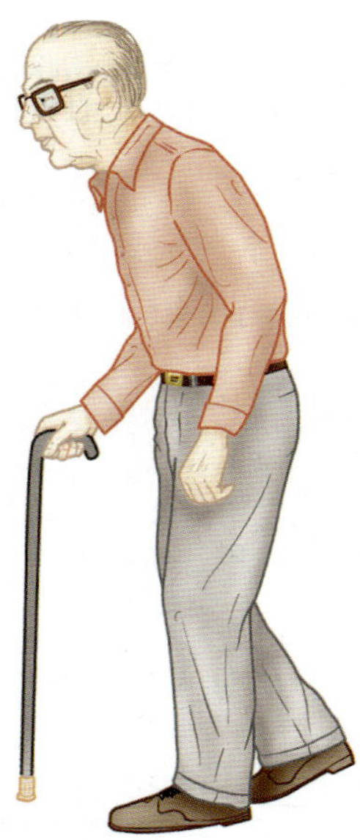

FIG. 23.27 Short, uncertain steps are characteristic of gait with advancing age.

The timed up and go (TUG) test is a simple screening test of balance, strength, and cerebellar function. Inform the patient about the actions to perform on the command "Go":

- Stand up from a chair without using the chair arms
- Walk 10 feet (3 m) to a mark on the floor
- Turn around
- Walk 10 feet (3 m) back to the chair
- Sit down without using chair arms

Walking assistive devices can be used, but no assistance from the examiner is provided. Ask the patient to do this quickly and safely. Begin timing the patient's performance when you say, "Go." Most healthy older adults can perform the test within 10 seconds. Performance of 12 seconds or longer indicates a higher risk for falls (Centers for Disease Control and Prevention, 2017). The TUG performance measures functional mobility, gait speed, and falls in older adults (Knobe et al., 2016).

See the Functional Assessment box for the Performance Oriented Mobility Assessment (POMA) Tool, also known as the Tinetti Balance and Gait Assessment Tool, which can be used for older adults who are at risk for falls, for people who have difficulty performing daily activities requiring mobility, or for those performing a task that involves unsupported standing. This tool is useful to monitor changes in gait and balance over time, such as for individuals with MS.

FUNCTIONAL ASSESSMENT

Performance-Oriented Mobility Assessment Tool

Balance Tests

Nine positions and position changes are evaluated.

Instructions: The patient is seated in a hard, armless chair. The following maneuvers are tested.

Maneuver	Response	Score
1. Sitting balance	Leans or slides in chair	= 0
	Steady, safe	= 1 ______
2. Rises (ask patient to rise without using arms)	Unable without help	= 0
	Able, uses arms to help	= 1
	Able without using arms	= 2 ______
3. Attempts to rise	Unable without help	= 0
	Able, requires more than one attempt	= 1
	Able to arise, one attempt	= 2 ______
4. Immediate standing balance (first 5 seconds)	Unsteady (swaggers, moves feet, trunk sways)	= 0
	Steady but uses walker or other support	= 1
	Steady without walker or other support	= 2 ______
5. Standing balance (once stance balances)	Unsteady	= 0
	Steady but wide stance (medial heels more than 4 inches apart) or uses cane or other support	= 1
	Narrow stance without support	= 2 ______
6. Nudged (subject at maximum position with feet as close together as possible, examiner pushes lightly on subject's sternum with palm of hand three times)	Begins to fall	= 0
	Staggers, grabs, catches self	= 1
	Steady	= 2 ______
7. Eyes closed (at maximum position, as in 6)	Unsteady	= 0
	Steady	= 1 ______
8. Turning 360 degrees	Discontinuous steps	= 0
	Continuous steps	= 1 ______
	Unsteady (grabs, staggers)	= 0
	Steady	= 1 ______
9. Sitting down	Unsafe (misjudges distance, falls into chair)	= 0
	Uses arm or not a smooth motion	= 1
	Safe, smooth motion	= 2 ______

Balance Score: __________ of 16

FUNCTIONAL ASSESSMENT—cont'd

Gait Tests

Initial instructions: The patient stands with examiner, walks down the hallway or across the room for at least 10 feet, first at "usual" pace, then back at "rapid but safe" pace (using usual walking aids).

Item	Observation	Score
1. Initiation of gait (immediately after being told "Go")	Any hesitancy or multiple attempts to start	= 0
	No hesitancy	= 1 ______
2. Step length and height	Right swing foot does not pass left foot with stance	= 0
	Passes left stance foot	= 1 ______
	Right foot does not clear floor completely with step	= 0
	Right foot completely clears floor	= 1 ______
	Left swing foot does not pass right stance foot with step	= 0
	Passes right stance foot	= 1 ______
	Left foot does not clear floor completely with step	= 0
	Left foot completely clears floor	= 1 ______
3. Step symmetry	Right and left step lengths not equal (estimate)	= 0
	Right and left step lengths appear equal	= 1 ______
4. Step continuity	Stopping or discontinuity between steps	= 0
	Steps appear continuous	= 1 ______
5. Path (estimated in relation to floor tiles, 12 inches square; observe excursion of one of the subject's feet over about 10 feet of the course)	Marked deviation	= 0
	Mild/moderate deviation or uses walking aid	= 1
	Straight without walking aid	= 2 ______
6. Trunk	Marked sway or uses walking aid	= 0
	No sway, but flexion of knees or back, or spreads arms out	= 1 while walking
	No sway, no flexion, no use of arms, and no use of walking aid	= 2 ______
7. Walking stance	Heels apart	= 0
	Heels almost touching while walking	= 1 ______

Gait Score: ________ of 12

Balance and Gait Score: ________ of 28

A score lower than 21 indicates a high risk for recurrent falls (Knobe, M., Giesen, M., Plate, S., Gradl-Dietsch, G., Buecking, B., Eschbach, D., van Laack, W., & Pape, H. C. (2016). The Aachen Mobility and Balance Index to measure physiological falls risk: A comparison with the Tinetti POMA Scale. *European Journal of Trauma and Emergency Surgery, 42*(5), 537–545.).

From Tinetti, M. E. (1986). Performance-oriented assessment of mobility problems in elderly patients. *Journal of the American Geriatrics Society, 34*(2), 119–126.

Check for fine motor abilities by observing the patient put on a sweater or button a jacket without assistance. Tactile and vibratory sensation, as well as position sense, may be reduced in the older adult. These patients may need stronger stimuli to detect sensation.

Changes in deep tendon reflexes occur with aging. The older adult usually has less brisk or even absent reflexes, with response diminishing in the lower extremities before the upper extremities are affected. The Achilles and plantar reflexes may be absent or difficult to elicit in some older adults. The superficial reflexes (e.g., abdominal and cremasteric) may also disappear. There is typically an increase in benign essential tremor with aging. Fine motor coordination and agility may be impaired.

ABNORMALITIES

Disorders of the central and peripheral nervous systems occur in different ways. A static disorder may develop at any age and not get better or worse, even though the clinical manifestation may change with time (e.g., CP). An individual may have been well until function is lost with a degenerative condition (e.g., MS) and it progressively worsens. Some problems are intermittent (e.g., seizures), and others are genetic (e.g., Huntington disease) or related to a metabolic disorder (e.g., vitamin B_{12} deficiency).

Disorders of the Central Nervous System

MULTIPLE SCLEROSIS

A progressive autoimmune disorder characterized by a combination of inflammation and degeneration of the myelin of the brain's white matter, leading to decreased brain mass and obstructed transmission of nerve impulses

PATHOPHYSIOLOGY

- Etiology is unknown; risk factors may include smoking, vitamin D deficiency, and Epstein-Barr virus infection
- Lesions occur in both white and gray matter; irreversible CNS tissue damage results
- Gradual, but unpredictable, progression, with or without remissions; symptom onset between 20 and 40 years of age, females affected twice as often as males

PATIENT DATA

Subjective Data

- Fatigue, weakness
- Urinary frequency, urgency, or hesitancy
- Sexual dysfunction
- Vertigo, numbness
- Blurred vision, diplopia, loss of vision
- Emotional changes
- Relapse symptoms develop rapidly over hours or days, and symptoms take weeks to recede

Objective Data

- Muscle weakness, ataxia
- Hyperactive deep tendon reflexes
- Paresthesia, sensory loss, such as loss of vibration sense
- Intention tremor
- Optic neuritis
- Cognitive changes
- Magnetic resonance imaging (MRI) reveals demyelinated plaques, macrophage infiltration, and abnormal iron deposition

Seizure Disorder (Epilepsy)

A chronic disorder characterized by recurrent, unprovoked bursts of electrical brain activity

PATHOPHYSIOLOGY

- Episodic abnormal electrical discharges (excessive concurrent firing) of cerebral neurons may be caused by a CNS disorder, a CNS structural defect, or a disorder that affects functioning of the CNS; examples include brain injury, infection, toxins, stroke, brain tumor, biochemical disorder, congenital malformations, and hypoxic syndromes

PATIENT DATA

Subjective Data

- History of prior seizure
- Premonition or aura (headache, mood change, anxiety, irritability, lethargy, changes in appetite, dizziness, and lightheadedness)
- Body is stiff and rigid, followed by rhythmic jerking movements
- Eyes roll upward
- Drooling
- Loss of bladder or bowel control

Objective Data

- Tonic phase: brief flexion and characteristic cry with contraction of abdominal muscles, followed by generalized extension for 10–15 min; loss of consciousness for 1–2 min, eyes deviated upward, and dilated pupils
- Clonic phase: contractions alternate with muscle relaxation
- Postictal state: coma followed by confusion and lethargy
- Common electroencephalographic findings of spikes and waves

Encephalitis

Acute inflammation of the brain and spinal cord involving the meninges, often due to a virus

PATHOPHYSIOLOGY

- Virus may be transmitted by the bite of an arthropod or a mosquito, such as with West Nile virus, Eastern equine encephalitis, and Japanese encephalitis; herpes simplex virus (HSV) may be another cause
- Nerve cell degeneration occurs leading to edema, increased intracranial pressure, and areas of necrosis

PATIENT DATA

Subjective Data

- Mild viral illness with fever
- Recovery and quiet stage followed by onset of lethargy, restlessness, and mental confusion

Objective Data

- Altered mental status, confusion, stupor, coma
- Photophobia
- Stiff neck
- Muscle weakness, paralysis, ataxia

Meningitis

Inflammation of the meninges of the brain or spinal cord

PATHOPHYSIOLOGY

- Bacterial, viral, or fungal pathogens colonize in the upper respiratory tract, invade the bloodstream, and cross the blood-brain barrier to infect the CSF and meninges

PATIENT DATA

Subjective Data

- Fever, chills
- Headache, stiff neck
- Lethargy, malaise
- Vomiting
- Irritability
- Seizures

Objective Data

- Altered mental status, confusion
- Nuchal rigidity
- Fever
- Brudzinski and Kernig signs may be positive
- Jolt accentuation of headache may be seen
- Petechiae and purpura may be seen with meningococcal meningitis
- See the Evidence-Based Practice box on signs of meningitis earlier in chapter
- Lumbar puncture and CSF culture confirm the diagnosis

Intracranial Tumor

An abnormal growth within the cranial cavity that may be a primary or metastatic cancer

PATHOPHYSIOLOGY

- Mass causes displacement of tissue and pressure, affecting CSF circulation; function is threatened through compression and destruction of tissues
- Incidence of primary brain tumors increases until about 70 years old and then decreases (Boss & Huether, 2019)

PATIENT DATA

Subjective Data

- Persistent headache, may awaken patient from sleep
- Nausea, early morning vomiting
- Unsteady gait, impaired coordination
- Memory loss and confusion
- Reduced visual acuity, visual loss, diplopia
- Behavior or personality change
- Seizure

Objective Data

- Signs may vary by location of tumor
- Altered consciousness, confusion
- Papilledema
- Cranial nerve impairment
- Aphasia, language disorder
- Vision loss—hemianopia, nystagmus
- Gait disturbances, ataxia
- Brain imaging by computed tomography (CT) scan or MRI confirms the diagnosis

Pseudotumor Cerebri (Idiopathic Intracranial Hypertension)

A clinical syndrome of elevated cerebrospinal fluid (CSF) pressure that mimics brain tumors

PATHOPHYSIOLOGY

- Etiology is unknown, but proposed causes are excess CSF production or malabsorption; obstructed venous drainage of CSF is also a potential cause
- Obesity is considered a contributing factor (Burkett et al., 2018)
- Most common in women of childbearing age with obesity (Burkett et al., 2018)

PATIENT DATA

Subjective Data

- Severe daily headache
- Transient episodes of visual acuity or visual field loss, unilateral or bilateral
- Tinnitus or whooshing sound in ears
- Back pain

Objective Data

- Papilledema
- Inferior nasal visual field defect
- Decreased visual acuity
- Abducens nerve palsy
- Alert, unimpaired consciousness
- Absence of focal neurologic signs
- CT scan or MRI reveals no cause of increased intracranial pressure

Stroke (Brain Attack or Cerebrovascular Accident)

Sudden interruption of blood supply to a part of the brain or the rupture of a blood vessel, spilling blood into spaces around brain cells

PATHOPHYSIOLOGY

- Ischemic strokes (most common cause) occur when a thrombus or embolism interrupts the blood supply, oxygen, and nutrients to the brain, and brain cells die (Fig. 23.28)
- Intracerebral or subarachnoid bleeding causes about 13% of hemorrhagic strokes, often within the distribution of the anterior circulation of the brain (Boss & Huether, 2019); brain cells die due to the bleeding into or around the brain

PATIENT DATA

Subjective Data

Sudden onset of:

- Numbness or weakness, especially on one side of the body
- Confusion, trouble speaking, or speech not understood
- Vision disturbance in one or both eyes
- Dizziness, weakness, or loss of balance or coordination
- Severe headache with no known cause

Objective Data

- Signs vary by part of the brain affected; see the accompanying Differential Diagnosis table
- Elevated blood pressure
- Altered level of consciousness
- Difficulty managing secretions
- Weakness or paralysis of extremities or facial muscles, unilateral or bilateral
- Aphasia, receptive or expressive
- Articulation impairment
- Impaired horizontal gaze or hemianopia
- Brain imaging with CT and MRI diagnose the type of stroke

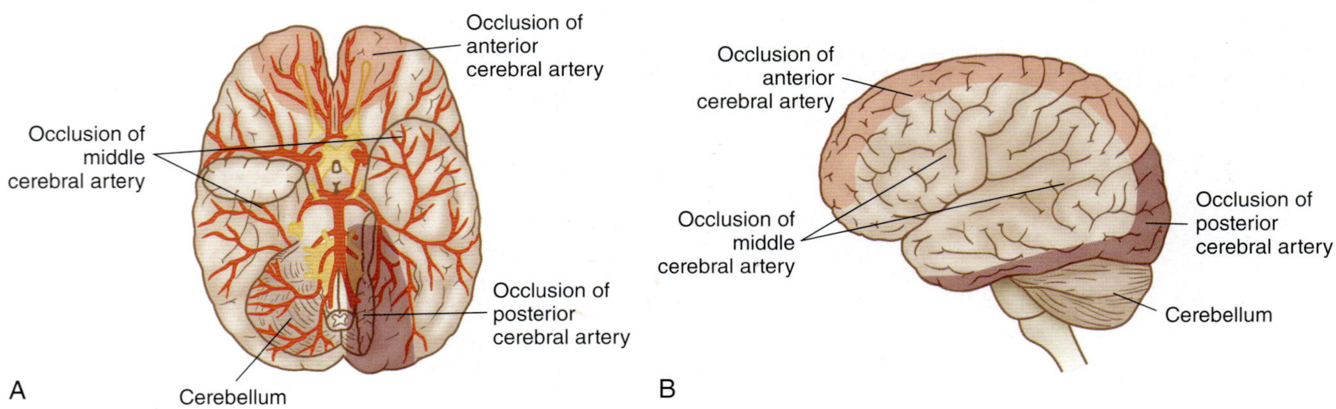

FIG. 23.28 Areas of the brain affected by occlusion of the anterior, middle, and posterior cerebral artery branches. (A) Inferior view. (B) Lateral view. (Modified from Rudy, E. B. (1984). *Advanced neurological and neurosurgical nursing.* St. Louis: Mosby.)

DIFFERENTIAL DIAGNOSIS

Neurologic Signs Associated With Stroke by Artery Affected

ARTERY AFFECTED	NEUROLOGIC SIGNS
Internal Carotid Artery Supplies the cerebral hemispheres and diencephalon by the ophthalmic and ipsilateral hemisphere arteries	Unilateral blindness Severe contralateral hemiplegia and hemianesthesia Profound aphasia
Middle Cerebral Artery Supplies frontal lobe, parietal lobe, cortical surfaces of temporal lobe (affecting structures of higher cerebral processes of communication; language interpretation; perception and interpretation of space, sensation, form, and voluntary movement)	Alterations in communication, cognition, mobility, and sensation Contralateral homonymous hemianopia (see Chapter 12) Contralateral hemiplegia or hemiparesis, motor and sensory loss, greater in face and arm than the leg
Anterior Cerebral Artery Supplies superior surfaces of frontal and parietal lobes and medial surface of cerebral hemispheres (includes motor and somesthetic cortex serving the legs), basal ganglia, corpus callosum	Emotional lability Confusion, amnesia, personality changes Urinary incontinence Contralateral hemiplegia or hemiparesis, greater in lower than upper extremities
Posterior Cerebral Artery Supplies medial and inferior temporal lobes, medial occipital lobe, thalamus, posterior hypothalamus, and visual receptive area	Hemianesthesia Contralateral hemiplegia, greater in face and upper extremities than in lower extremities, cerebellar ataxia, tremor Visual loss—homonymous hemianopia, cortical blindness Receptive aphasia Memory deficits
Vertebral or Basilar Arteries Supply the brainstem and cerebellum	Transient ischemic attacks
Incomplete occlusion	Unilateral and bilateral weakness of extremities; upper motor neuron weakness involving face, tongue, and throat; loss of vibratory sense, two-point discrimination, and position sense Diplopia, homonymous hemianopia Nausea, vertigo, tinnitus, and syncope Dysphagia Dysarthria Sometimes confusion and drowsiness
Anterior portion of pons	"Locked-in" syndrome—no movement except eyelids; sensation and consciousness preserved
Complete occlusion or hemorrhage	Coma Miotic pupils Decerebrate rigidity Respiratory and circulatory abnormalities Death
Posterior Inferior Cerebellar Artery Supplies the lateral and posterior portions of the medulla	Wallenberg syndrome (swallowing difficulty, hoarseness, dizziness, nausea and vomiting, nystagmus, and problems with balance and gait coordination) Ipsilateral anesthesia of face and cornea for pain and temperature (touch preserved) Ipsilateral Horner syndrome (see Chapter 12) Contralateral loss of pain and temperature sensation in trunk and extremities Ipsilateral decompensation of movement
Anterior Inferior and Superior Cerebellar Arteries Supply the cerebellum	Difficulty in articulation, swallowing, gross movements of limbs; nystagmus

Continued

DIFFERENTIAL DIAGNOSIS—cont'd

Neurologic Signs Associated With Stroke by Artery Affected

ARTERY AFFECTED	NEUROLOGIC SIGNS
Anterior Spinal Artery Supplies the anterior spinal cord	Flaccid paralysis, below level of lesion Loss of pain, touch, temperature sensation (proprioception preserved)
Posterior Spinal Artery Supplies the posterior spinal cord	Sensory loss, particularly proprioception, vibration, touch, and pressure (movement preserved)

Disorders of the Peripheral Nervous System

Adults

Myasthenia Gravis

Autoimmune disorder of neuromuscular junction involved with muscle activation

PATHOPHYSIOLOGY

- Etiology is unknown, but some genetic forms exist along with several subtypes
- Autoantibodies against the acetylcholine receptor sites cause their destruction and block the transmission of nerve impulses across the neuromuscular junction to direct muscle contraction; inflammatory changes in the postsynaptic membranes lead to muscle dysfunction
- Peak incidence occurs in young adults at 30 years of age, and incidence increases until 50 years of age (Gilhus et al., 2015)

PATIENT DATA

Subjective Data

- Drooping eyelids
- Double vision
- Difficulty swallowing or speaking
- Fluctuating fatigue or weakness (worse with exercise, improves with rest)
- Inability to work with arms raised above head
- Difficulty walking
- Symptoms worsen later in the day and improve with rest

Objective Data

- Ptosis that develops within 2 min of upward gaze
- Facial weakness when puffing out cheeks
- Hypophonia
- Difficulty managing secretions
- Respiratory compromise or failure
- Weakness of skeletal muscles without reflex, sensory, or coordination abnormalities

Guillain-Barré Syndrome

Postinfectious disorder following a nonspecific gastrointestinal or respiratory infection that causes an acute neuromuscular paralysis

PATHOPHYSIOLOGY

- Autoimmune disorder triggered by a bacterial or viral infection (including the Zika virus) or other immune stimulant that causes an autoimmune response that damages the peripheral nerves and associated spinal roots, leading to denervation and atrophy

PATIENT DATA

Subjective Data

- History of recent illness and recovery
- Rapidly progressive weakness in more than two extremities
- Paresthesia
- Muscle or back pain
- Double vision

Objective Data

- Distal ascending weakness, usually bilateral and symmetric
- Diminished tendon reflexes
- Ataxia, progressing to flaccid paralysis
- Facial nerve weakness (Bell palsy), diplopia
- Dysphagia, difficulty handling secretions
- Respiratory distress
- Lumbar puncture reveals increased protein in CSF

Trigeminal Neuralgia (Tic Douloureux)

Recurrent paroxysmal sharp pain that radiates into one or more branches of the fifth cranial nerve

PATHOPHYSIOLOGY

- Often caused by a small artery that chronically compresses the fifth cranial nerve causing demyelination; may also be caused by venous compression
- Rare before age 40 years, average age of onset is 60 years; females are more commonly affected than males

PATIENT DATA

Subjective Data

- Sharp pain episodes on one side of the face that last seconds to minutes; pain is rarely bilateral
- Potential pain triggers are chewing, swallowing, talking, washing the face, brushing the teeth, exposure to cold, and even a breeze across the face
- Episodes may occur several times a day to several times a month followed by a pain-free period

Objective Data

- May be normal neurologic findings
- May have slight sensory impairment in the regions of pain
- Pain occurs in the distribution of one or more divisions of the facial nerve

Bell Palsy

Acute paralysis or weakness of one side of the face that may have partial or complete resolution

PATHOPHYSIOLOGY

- Etiology is unknown; may be an inflammatory reaction that compresses the facial nerve (cranial nerve VII), such as a herpes simplex or herpes zoster viral infection reactivation
- Facial nerve swelling and compression against the temporal bone occurs, followed by demyelination (De Ru et al., 2015)

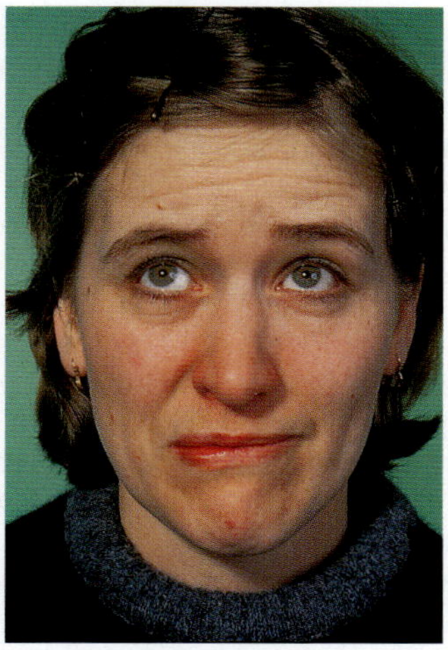

FIG. 23.29 Characteristic features of Bell palsy. (From Forbes, C. D., & Jackson, W. F. (2003). *Color atlas and text of clinical medicine* (3rd ed.). London: Mosby Ltd.)

PATIENT DATA

Subjective Data

- Rapidly progressive muscle weakness on one side of face (over 2–3 days)
- Feeling of facial numbness

Objective Data

- Facial creases and nasolabial fold disappear on affected side (Fig. 23.29)
- Eyelid will not close on affected side and lower lid sags; leads to eye irritation; eye may tear excessively
- Food and saliva may pool in affected side of mouth
- Facial sensation is intact

Peripheral Neuropathy

Disorder of the peripheral nervous system that results in motor and sensory loss in the distribution of one or more nerves

PATHOPHYSIOLOGY

- Common causes are diabetes mellitus or alcohol use disorder; other causes include nerve compression (compartment syndrome), HIV infection, nutritional disorders, and neurotoxic chemotherapy
- Inflammatory processes from biochemical exposures (hyperglycemia, lipoproteins, neurotoxins) damage axons and nerve fibers and may lead to sensory deficits
- Present in 8% of the general population by 55 years of age, but present in up to 66% of patients with diabetes (Watson et al., 2015)

PATIENT DATA

Subjective Data

- Gradual onset of numbness, tingling, burning, and cramping, most commonly in the hands and feet
- Night pain in one or both feet
- Early signs may be unusual sensations of walking on cotton, floors feeling strange, or inability to distinguish between coins by feel
- Tripping over feet, falling
- Sensation of burning accompanied by hyperalgesia and allodynia (all sensation is painful)

Objective Data

- Reduced sensation in the foot with the monofilament; reduced pain or touch sensation
- Distal pulses may be diminished
- Diminished or absent ankle and knee reflexes
- Decreased or no vibratory sensation below the knees; temperature sensation may be less impaired
- Distal muscle weakness, inability to stand on toes or heels
- Skin ulceration or injuries to extremities the patient does not feel

Children

Cerebral Palsy

Group of permanent disorders of movement and posture development associated with nonprogressive (static) disturbances that occurred in the developing fetal or infant brain

PATHOPHYSIOLOGY

- Major contributing lesions include infection, trauma, and anoxia in the perinatal period; intracerebral hemorrhage or subarachnoid hemorrhage injures the immature periventricular white matter in the fetus or premature infant; kernicterus and genetic factors may also contribute to its development
- Prevalence is 1 per 323 children in the United States (Butterfield & Huether, 2019)

PATIENT DATA

Subjective Data

- Delays in gross motor development that become more obvious as the infant ages
- Activity limitation, stiff joints and positioning
- May have hearing, speech, and language disorders
- Feeding difficulties, poor sucking and swallowing coordination
- Seizures

Objective Data

- Cognitive impairment or learning disabilities may be present
- Spastic CP: hypertonicity, tremors, scissor gait, toe walking
- Persistent primitive reflexes, exaggerated deep tendon reflexes
- Dyskinetic CP: involuntary, slow, writhing movements of the extremities; tremors may be present
- Exaggerated posturing, inconsistent muscle tone that varies during the day
- Ataxic: abnormalities of movement involving balance and position of trunk and extremities
- Intention tremors, past pointing
- Increased or decreased muscle tone, may have hypotonia as infant
- Instability, wide-based gait

Myelomeningocele (Spina Bifida)

Congenital vertebral defect (commonly at the lumbar or sacral level) that allows spinal cord contents to protrude

PATHOPHYSIOLOGY

- Cause is unknown but associated with excessive use of alcohol, medications used for seizures and acne, genetic factors, and pregnant person's health conditions (folic acid deficiency, diabetes mellitus, and maternal obesity)
- An estimated 1645 infants are born with the condition each year in the United States, with a higher incidence in Hispanic compared with non-Hispanic White and Black infants (Centers for Disease Control and Prevention, 2019)

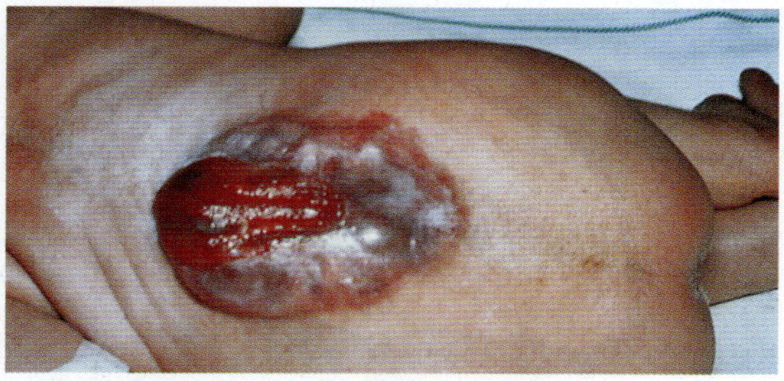

FIG. 23.30 **Myelomeningocele.** (From Zitelli, B. J., & Davis, H. W. (1997). *Atlas of pediatric physical diagnosis* (3rd ed.). St. Louis: Mosby.)

PATIENT DATA

Subjective Data

- May have loss of bowel control or constipation
- May have loss of bladder control (incontinence or urinary retention)
- Mobility problems

Objective Data

- Exposed meningeal sac filled with fluid and nerves is apparent at birth (Fig. 23.30)
- Extent of sensory deficit and paralysis or weakness depend on spinal cord level of defect (the higher the defect, the greater the neurologic dysfunction); may not be symmetric
- Rapidly increasing head circumference (hydrocephalus)
- May have hip or foot abnormalities
- Learning disabilities and perceptual motor skills

Abusive Head Trauma

Inflicted head injury in young children, including "shaken baby syndrome" resulting from biomechanical forces like shaking

PATHOPHYSIOLOGY

- Inflicted rotational and contact forces as occurs with shaking can result in brain injury, spinal hemorrhage, intracranial hemorrhage, and retinal hemorrhage
- 32 to 38 cases per 100,000 children each year in under 1-year-olds; fatal in about one-quarter of cases (Narang et al., 2020)

PATIENT DATA

Subjective Data

- Irritability or lethargy
- Decreased food intake
- Breathing difficulty or apnea
- Seizure
- Loss of consciousness

Objective Data

- Reported history of present illness may not match the nature and severity of findings
- Altered level of consciousness
- Seizures
- Bilateral retinal hemorrhages with retinal detachments or folds (see Fig. 12.53)
- Absence of visible trauma to the head; fingerprint bruises may be seen on infant's upper arms and body
- Bruising, bite marks, or burns may also be seen in some infants
- CT scan reveals subdural or subarachnoid hemorrhage
- Signs of old and new fractures of long bones and ribs may be seen on radiographs

Older Adults

Parkinson Disease

Slowly progressive, degenerative neurologic disorder in which motor function is primarily affected along with behavioral and cognitive problems

PATHOPHYSIOLOGY

- Destruction of neurons that transmit dopamine results in systemic neurologic and nonmotor symptoms leading to abnormal movement
- About 10% of cases are familial, with the majority being idiopathic
- Secondary parkinsonism may be caused by other neurologic disorders or certain drugs
- Onset after 40 years of age, with increasing incidence after 60 years of age; incidence is higher in males than in females (Boss & Huether, 2019).

PATIENT DATA

Subjective Data

- Tremors (sometimes unilateral) occur initially at rest and with fatigue, disappearing with intended movement and sleep; progresses to pill-rolling movement of fingers bilaterally and head tremor
- Slowing of voluntary and automatic movements, "feel wooden," freezing or unable to continue movements
- Numbness, aching, tingling, and muscle soreness occur in many patients (Fig. 23.31)
- Difficulty swallowing, drooling

Objective Data

- Tremors
- Muscular rigidity, cogwheel rigidity with jerks
- Stooped posture, balance and postural instability
- Short steps, shuffling, freezing gait; gait may accelerate to maintain upright posture
- Slow, slurred, monotonous speech; voice softening
- Impaired cognition, dementia

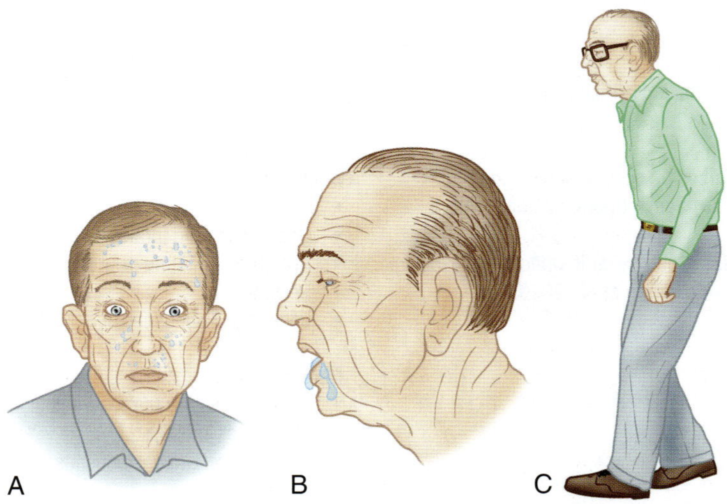

FIG. 23.31 Characteristic features of Parkinson disease. (A) Excessive sweating. (B) Drooling with excess saliva. (C) Gait with rapid, short, shuffling steps and reduced arm swinging. (Modified Rudy, E. B. (1984). *Advanced neurological and neurosurgical nursing.* St. Louis: Mosby.)

Normal Pressure Hydrocephalus

Syndrome simulating degenerative diseases that is caused by noncommunicating hydrocephalus (dilated ventricles with intracranial pressure within expected ranges)

PATHOPHYSIOLOGY

- Etiology is unknown, but it is associated with aging, and may be related to brain trauma, subarachnoid hemorrhage, brain tumor, or an infection such as meningitis
- Increased CSF enlarges the ventricles
- Present in 2%–6% of persons with dementia (Piscascia et al., 2015)

PATIENT DATA

Subjective Data

- Gait impairment is the first symptom
- Unsteadiness and difficulty turning
- Forgetfulness, cognitive impairment
- Urinary frequency that progresses to urgency and incontinence over time

Objective Data

Triad of findings include:

- Gait impairment (wide-based stance; short, small steps; and reduced floor clearance)
- Cognitive impairment, attention, and executive function impaired, impaired memory
- Urinary incontinence
- Brain CT and MRI reveal enlarged ventricles not attributable to brain atrophy or a congenital problem

Postpolio Syndrome (Progressive Postpoliomyelitis Muscular Atrophy)

Reappearance of neurologic signs 10 or more years after an acute poliomyelitis infection

PATHOPHYSIOLOGY

- During recovery from the initial polio infection, damaged neurons sent out axonal links to activate muscle fibers that had neurons killed by the poliovirus; surviving motor neurons activate many more muscle fibers, and with aging, the overloaded neurons die, causing symptoms

PATIENT DATA

Subjective Data

- History of paralytic or nonparalytic polio
- New-onset muscle weakness, muscle cramps
- Increased pain sensitivity
- Fatigue, reduced endurance
- Cold intolerance
- Difficulty swallowing or speaking
- Shortness of breath
- Difficulty sleeping

Objective Data

- Focal and asymmetric muscle weakness and atrophy
- Fasciculations
- Dysphagia, dysarthria
- Sleep apnea, hypoventilation

CHAPTER

24 Head-to-Toe Examination

This chapter provides you with the opportunity to integrate your knowledge regarding obtaining an interview and health history and performing the physical examination. It offers a suggested approach and sequence for performing all steps of the physical examination. However, each patient presents with unique circumstances, and flexibility in your approach and examination sequence is encouraged. With experience, you will adapt easily while being attentive to the patient and ensuring their active participation in their own care.

The relationship with the patient begins with respect and good manners. The relationship becomes well established through the powerful therapeutic effect of carefully listening to what the patient says, exploring concerns, and explaining information without patronizing or judging. These actions communicate to the patient that you care and that they are your full partner (Box 24.1).

Building the history and performing the physical examination vary based on your style and comfort. Be flexible in your history-taking routine so that the patient's unique story is revealed. Consider starting the interview with "Tell me about yourself," and then listen to their response.

The physical examination, the "laying on of hands," is integral to the history, making it possible to understand the objective findings—the disease—but also the great variety of subjective findings that modify the patient's experience with the disease. Technological expertise is a complement to, rather than a substitute for, the skillful physical examination.

Beginning the Examination Process

At the Start

At the initial visit, explain your level of training and experience. The pressure and uncertainty you feel about your ability will lessen as time, experience, and appropriate supervision help build your self-confidence.

The history and physical examination do not have to be completed in a special sequence or in the same sequence in which you will record them. They can be integrated to meet the needs of the patient or the demands of the moment. For example, if deviations from the expected physical findings are found, ask additional questions during the physical examination to expand or clarify historical information heard earlier. If a patient has a concern about their skin, it is often helpful to examine the skin concern before proceeding with gathering a history. In young children, it is helpful to assess the child's appearance prior to conducting the examination and base the sequence of the physical examination on their activity level. If the child is quiet, assessing the cardiovascular and respiratory system first is less threatening and may provide a more accurate assessment of their condition. In this case, you are adapting to circumstances by using clinical judgment. This varies with the nature of the patient's concern; age, gender, and cultural background of the patient; and even findings during the physical examination.

The patient with a concern and a probable vulnerability may be uneasy, anxious, or even fearful (Box 24.2). Patients evaluate you during the examination and gauge their anxiety by your manner, hesitations in speech, changes in facial expression, and time spent examining a part of their body. Some patients equate the gravity of the situation with the length of time you spend, but others equate length of time with thoroughness. One approach is to consistently provide an explanation about which part of the examination comes next and to be honest about any potential discomfort or pain and how long it will last. Check with your clinical supervisor before sharing your opinion about unexpected examination findings. This is especially true for areas the patient or parent cannot visually observe such as cardiac, lung, or ear examination. Avoid inappropriate reassurance, and do not offer premature assumptions about unexpected findings.

Once you have obtained the basic history, assess the urgency, the nature of the concerns, and the body systems involved. Then perform the physical examination, paying particular attention to the body systems of potential concern. You may need to ask more questions or even return to the physical examination to gather all of the needed information. Occasionally a patient or parent will share a photo of a finding that has resolved, such as urticaria, or a stool in a diaper they fear is abnormal. They may share an audio recording of a croupy cough. Be open to other methods to identify abnormal physical findings.

Do not assume that your initial list of differential diagnoses is accurate. The patient may have an unusual presentation of a common problem, a common presentation of a rare condition, more than one disease process, a

BOX 24.1 A Few Reminders for Developing an Effective Relationship With Patients

- Ensure good communication with courtesy and provision of comfort, connection, and confirmation (see Box 2.2, Chapter 2).
- Dress neatly and be well groomed.
- Patients are culturally diverse, so use the patient's language if possible. It is important for you to be understood, so use colloquialisms if needed. Do not use complex medical terminology.
- Avoid distraction and interruption, except for an emergency.
- Adapt to the patient's circumstances. An older adult in a wheelchair is a different challenge than the infant on the parent's lap.
- Be flexible, but be certain at the end that all the necessary observations were made.
- Make sure the examining table is positioned so you can access the patient from every side.
- Have the patient comfortably draped, paying attention to modesty at every age. Adequately expose the part of the body to be examined, or you may lose the vital finding.
- Always consider the need for a chaperone.
- Keep your hands and stethoscope warm.
- Do not probe too vigorously when examining tender areas.
- Explain what you are doing and anticipate the patient's concern about what comes next. State the reasons for examining an area and warn of any potential discomfort.
- Ask the patient to do things; never order. Say "please" and "thank you." Occasionally ask if the patient is comfortable or has any questions.
- Observe the patient's demeanor and body language. Apathy, disinterest, or inability to offer a social smile are equally worrisome in adults, infants, and children.
- Be objective as you assess the patient. Make no premature assumptions about what you find.
- Describe first without diagnosing. Do not voice impressions prematurely. For example, a lump in the neck may be a swollen node and not a cyst. Diagnosis can usually wait until all the data are in.
- Remember that physical findings have meanings that vary according to age.
- Be reassuring only when you honestly can. Do not make promises you cannot keep.
- Pace the assessment according to the circumstances, the sense of urgency, and the recognition of fatigue and frailty. It is not necessary to do it all at once. Allow for rest and return later to finish up.

co-occurring emotional or social problem, a new illness superimposed on an existing one, or a combination of any of these factors. Do not ignore any fact or finding that does not fit your initial hypothesis or assume that a single diagnosis exists when two or more may be present. Do not misidentify findings to fit your initial hypothesis regarding the patient's symptoms and fall prey to premature closure (see Clinical Pearl, "Respecting Your Instincts"). With all pathophysiologic and psychosocial possibilities in mind and with probabilities and urgency dominant, constantly challenge yourself and resist being tightly bound by your initial impressions. See Chapter 4 for more information on clinical reasoning.

BOX 24.2 The Patient We Define as Difficult

Sometimes we find ourselves reacting negatively when patients do the following:

- Seem insatiable in their demands, wanting and feeling entitled to preferential treatment, seeming always on the edge of a lawsuit, and often impressed with their self-determined status in society (the VIP) but are really quite dependent
- Deny conditions or seem self-destructive—for example, being inattentive to instructions or not following treatment regimens
- Reject, distrust, always test your competency and reliability, and express pessimism about the efficacy of your effort

Try to understand the patient's needs and insecurities. Remember that patients often bring fears and worries to the encounter that are unrelated to their health (e.g., recent argument with partner, financial stress). Show respect and use all available supportive resources. Strategies that may help include the following: be clear and precise, keep all promises, set firm limits on what you can do, and try to maintain a compassionate approach. This may enable your partnership to mature, even if it is painful at times.

Despite patients' vulnerabilities, they often are inclined to give the health care provider a chance to gain their trust and respect.

CLINICAL PEARL

Respecting Your Instincts

Respect your instincts whenever you come across the unexpected, whenever your sense of what you might call normal has been violated. Pay attention when that happens, even if it does not seem to make sense or you cannot explain it easily.

Accuracy

You and the patient have responsibility for the reliability of findings and observations, but yours is greater. Take the time with open-ended questions to ensure that the patient has the opportunity to report fully and accurately. Ask follow-up questions as needed. Several things can limit the patient's ability to observe well and to report accurately:

- *Sensory deprivation.* A partial or total loss of any sense (e.g., vision, hearing, touch, taste, or smell) is clearly constraining. Do not expect the unaffected senses to be heightened. This may occur with some persons, but not all.
- *Emotional constraints, apparent and unapparent.* Patients who are psychotic, delirious, depressed, or otherwise seriously emotionally affected may confuse you. When you suspect this, carefully and objectively assess mental status during the history and physical examination.
- *Language barriers.* Patients may speak a language different from yours. Translation can be difficult in the best of circumstances, even when using a professional interpreter. Passing messages among three persons could potentially change the meaning and interpretation of important information, and confusion may be the result. Even using the same language may be a problem if the patient has a limited vocabulary,

HEAD-TO-TOE EXAMINATION

speaks English as a second language, or cannot read it very well.

- *Cultural barriers.* Consider the probable differences between you and the patient with candor and compassionate inquiry (see Chapter 1). Gender, race, and ethnicity may be obvious differences. Consider other barriers, such as the life experiences among persons who are overweight versus underweight, those with hearing impairment versus normal hearing, gravely ill versus well, transgender versus cisgender, and older versus younger. Display respectful curiosity by encouraging conversation about such differences. Uniformity is not part of the human condition.

Identify limitations that may affect accuracy, and take steps to enhance reliability. For example, the patient with a hearing impairment may need a response that facilitates communication such as use of a telephonic device for the hearing impaired, loud language, written questions, sign language, or lip reading enhanced with good lighting, speaking slowly, and/or keeping your lips visible to the patient. Remember that a person with hearing impairment cannot read lips through a mask, and those with severe vision impairment cannot see your gestures.

Family, friends, or an emergency medical technician are a frequent resource for collateral information. If possible, make the patient aware that others are providing information. When possible, the patient should set the limits regarding information that can be shared. Autonomy and confidentiality are factors to consider.

At times a patient may be considered a "poor historian" because of life situations, disease state, limited cognition, indifference, or apathy. Other situations may involve patients with emotional or psychological disorders that lead to distortions such as overstatements or understatements of reality. Each of these possibilities requires skill and sensitivity to obtain the most accurate information possible. Often collateral information or supporting information from previous health records is needed. Avoid using the descriptor "unreliable" in the health record because of its negative connotation.

The Potential for Error

We are all susceptible to error. A practitioner may palpate the same abdomen at different times on the same day and conclude that the liver span is somewhat different each time. Multiple health care providers may palpate the same abdomen on the same day and report different liver spans. This demonstrates the potential for error in each of us, and the same error may occur with many of the diagnostic tests ordered for our patients (Box 24.3). Every observation has a certain sensitivity (i.e., the assurance that if a patient has an abnormal examination finding that it will be found) and specificity (e.g., the assurance that a healthy patient will not have the abnormal finding). No observation or test has 100% sensitivity and specificity. Candidly question yourself and seek confirmation from others when necessary to minimize your errors.

BOX 24.3 Humans and Machines

Your perceptions of the patient from looking, listening, touching, and smelling are better than any machine. Mechanical imaging cannot capture vitality, apathy, or cognitive awareness, but technology can expand our insights. Just like our observations, technological procedures do not always result in highly sensitive or specific findings. Other potential limitations include needle anxiety and pain, use of irradiation, potentially toxic contrast agents, and, in the case of magnetic resonance imaging, intimidating sound and confinement. Remember that all technological procedures, as well as all that we do, have a potential cost to the human body, to emotion, and to finances.

Uncertainty

The potential for error increases uncertainty and the health care provider's discomfort. It is more comforting to think in a deterministic or mechanistic fashion, seeking certain and fixed knowledge and avoiding subjective impressions. We cannot always express our findings in numbers, and probabilities cannot be avoided, but we attempt to do so. For example, we use scales (assessment tools) that have several variables requiring a subjective judgment and the assignment of a fixed number to quantify each variable leading to a total score (consider the Glasgow Coma Scale and the Apgar score). That fixed number is really a pseudoquantification or proxy indicator of severity. Such scales may provide a false comfort in the apparent certainty of numbers. The mature clinician is one who is comfortable with probabilities and making decisions with a degree of uncertainty.

Examination Sequence

Adults and Adolescents

No one right way exists to perform the physical examination so that the process flows smoothly, minimizes the number of times the patient has to change positions, and conserves patient energy (e.g., when the patient is ill or frail). You need to adapt to the particular setting *and* patient condition *or* abilities. Box 24.4 gives a list of supplies you should have on hand. Be sure to wash your hands and don the appropriate personal protective equipment (PPE) prior to the examination.

Modesty matters, but do not let it deter examinations essential for appropriate care. Have comfortable patient gowns and appropriate drapes available. Close doors and curtains. It is also best to leave the room when the patient undresses and prepares for the examination. Do not assume that the patient has the same comfort with the situation that you do.

Always consider the need for a chaperone for the patient, especially for age, gender, specific examinations (e.g., genitourinary, breast, and rectal examinations), or with psychologically unstable patients. Consider a patient's sensibilities or the "difficult" patient when making a chaperone decision (see Box 24.2). The chaperone may also be valuable in assisting with patient positioning.

BOX 24.4 Equipment Supplies for Physical Examination

Basic Materials

Cotton balls
Cotton-tipped applicator sticks
Drapes
Examining gloves
Gauze squares
Lubricant
Marking pen
Measuring tape
Monofilament 5.07 (optional)
Nasal speculum
Odor-testing substances (optional)
Ophthalmoscope
Otoscope with pneumatic bulb
Penlight
Percussion hammer
Pulse oximeter
Ruler
Sharp and dull testing implements
Sphygmomanometer
Stethoscope with diaphragm and bell
Taste-testing substances (optional)
Thermometer
Tongue blades
Tuning forks
Vaginal speculum
Visual acuity screening charts for near and far vision

Materials for Gathering Specimens

Culture media
Glass slides
KOH (potassium hydroxide)
Occult blood–testing materials
Pap smear spatula/brush/broom, fixative, and container
Saline
Sterile cotton-tipped applicators

Become familiar with your health care facility's policy regarding chaperones to provide assurance to patients that the examination will be performed in a professional manner and to protect the health care provider should the patient make a false accusation.

General Inspection

Begin the inspection as you greet the patient, looking for problematic signs. You can perform parts of your physical examination any time the patient is in your view, during the history, or even in the waiting room (Fig. 24.1). If you go to the waiting room to invite the patient into your examining room, take a moment to observe the appropriateness of dress and grooming, manner of sitting, degree of relaxation, relationship with others in the room, and their degree of situational awareness. On this first greeting, you can take note of the manner with which you are met and the palm's moistness when you shake hands. Remember not to squeeze too hard when the patient is unknown to you

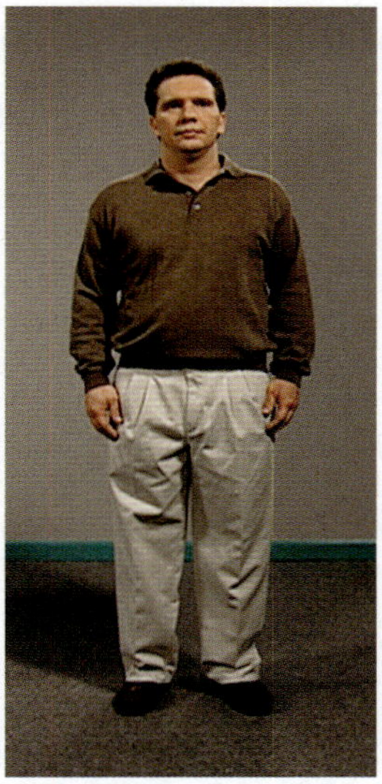

FIG. 24.1 Observe the patient while entering the examining room for manner, dress, interest or apprehension, and mobility.

and may have arthritic, painful hands. Observe the gait as the patient walks with you, the luster of the eyes, and the expression of emotion. All of this contributes to your examination, along with the initial assessments of the following:

- Skin color
- Facial expression
- Mobility
  - Use of assistive devices
  - Gait
  - Sitting, rising from chair
  - Taking off coat
- Dress and posture
- Speech pattern, disorders, preferred language
- Difficulty hearing, assistive devices
- Stature and build
- Musculoskeletal deformities
- Vision problems, assistive devices
- Eye contact with examiner
- Orientation, mental alertness
- Nutritional state
- Respiratory problems
- Individuals accompanying patient
- Developmental milestones in children

Preparation

After completing the interview, you or an assistant can instruct the patient to empty their bladder, remove as much clothing as is necessary, and put on a gown. Ask for a chaperone when appropriate. Modifications in the suggested sequence that follows are often necessary when the patient has disabilities (Box 24.5).

Measurements

Patient measurements (e.g., height, weight, and temperature) may be taken by an assistant in advance. In some

BOX 24.5 Examining People With Physical Disabilities

Variations in the approach to physical examination may be required for the patient with disabilities. What body systems are affected? What is the degree of impairment? What specific assistance does the patient require? Be flexible. For example, for an episodic visit, it may not be necessary for the patient to undress fully, using up energy and time. Removing or rearranging the examination room furnishings will provide the space needed to maneuver a wheelchair. Some patient examination positions can be varied without compromising the quality of the examination (e.g., alternative positions for the genitourinary examination; see Chapter 19). Some patients may need just a bit more than usual assistance from a family member or an assistant in getting set for the maneuvers of the examination. Patience and a gentle approach pay off.

cases you as the examiner will obtain all measurements or repeat certain ones (e.g., blood pressure if the initial measurement was elevated). Height and weight are often measured on the way to the examining room, and body mass index (BMI) is calculated. Vital signs (temperature, pulse, respirations, blood pressure, pain assessment, and sometimes oxygen saturation) may be obtained at the start of the physical examination or during the body system assessment. Assessment of distance vision and hearing may be performed by an assistant or at a convenient time during the physical examination.

Patient Seated, Wearing Gown

Patient is seated on examining table; examiner stands in front of patient (Fig. 24.2).

Head and Face

- Inspect skin characteristics.
- Inspect symmetry and external characteristics of eyes and ears.

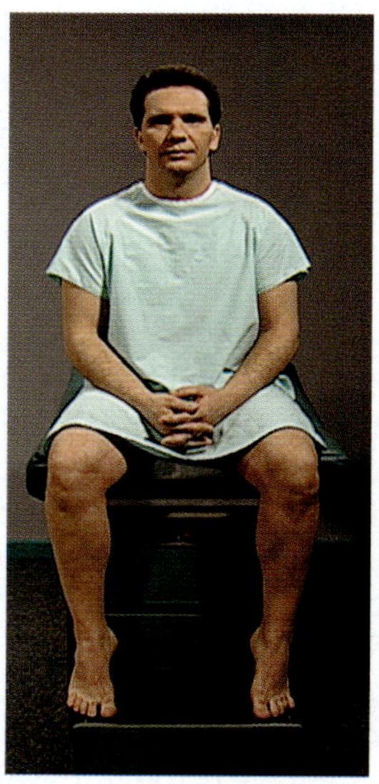

FIG. 24.2 Face the patient who is seated on the examining table.

- Inspect configuration of skull.
- Inspect and palpate scalp and hair for texture, distribution, and quantity.
- Palpate facial bones.
- Palpate temporomandibular joint while patient opens and closes mouth.
- Palpate and percuss sinus regions.
- Inspect ability to clench teeth, squeeze eyes tightly shut, wrinkle forehead, smile, stick out tongue, and puff out cheeks (cranial nerve [CN] V, VII).
- Test light-touch sensation of forehead, cheeks, and chin (CN V).

Eyes

- External examination:
  - Inspect eyelids, eyelashes, and palpebral folds.
  - Determine alignment of eyebrows.
  - Inspect sclera, conjunctiva, and iris.
  - Palpate lacrimal apparatus.
  - Near vision screening: Rosenbaum chart (CN II)
- Eye function:
  - Test pupillary response to light and accommodation.
  - Perform cover-uncover test and corneal light reflex.
  - Test extraocular eye movements (CN III, IV, VI).
  - Assess visual fields (CN II).
  - Test corneal reflexes (CN V), if indicated.
- Ophthalmoscopic examination:
  - Assess red reflex.
  - Inspect lens.
  - Inspect disc, cup margins, vessels, and retinal surface.

Ears

- External ear
  - Inspect surface characteristics, alignment, and placement.
  - Palpate auricle.
- Screen hearing with whisper test (CN VIII).
- Perform otoscopic examination.
  - Inspect canals.
  - Inspect tympanic membranes for landmarks, effusion, redness, bulging, and deformities.
- Perform Rinne and Weber tests.

Nose

- Inspect structure and position of septum.
- Determine patency of each nostril.
- Inspect mucosa, septum, and turbinates with nasal speculum.
- Assess olfactory function: Test sense of smell (CN I) when clinically necessary.

Mouth and Pharynx

- Inspect lips, buccal mucosa, gums, hard and soft palates, and floor of mouth for color, surface characteristics, and any other apparent abnormalities.
- Inspect oropharynx. Note anteroposterior pillars, uvula, tonsils, posterior pharynx, and mouth odor.

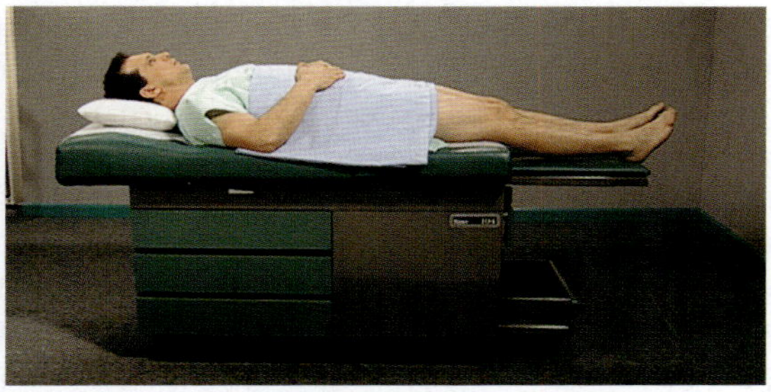

FIG. 24.7 Examine the patient in supine position with legs exposed.

Hips

- Palpate hips for stability.
- Assess range of motion and strength of hips.

Patient Sitting, Lap Draped

Assist the patient to a sitting position. The patient should have the gown on with a drape across the lap (Fig. 24.8).

Musculoskeletal

- Observe patient moving from lying to sitting position.
- Note coordination, use of muscles, and ease of movement.

Neurologic

- Test sensory function.
  - Assess dull and sharp sensation of forehead, paranasal sinus area, lower arms, hands, lower legs, and feet.
  - Test vibratory sensation of wrists and ankles.
  - Test position sense of upper and lower extremities (e.g., great toe and finger).
  - Test two-point discrimination of palms, thighs, and back.
  - Test stereognosis and graphesthesia.
- Assess upper extremity fine motor function and coordination. Ask the patient to perform the following tasks:
  - Touch the nose with alternating index fingers.
  - Rapidly alternate fingers to thumb.
  - Rapidly move index finger between the patient's nose and the examiner's finger.

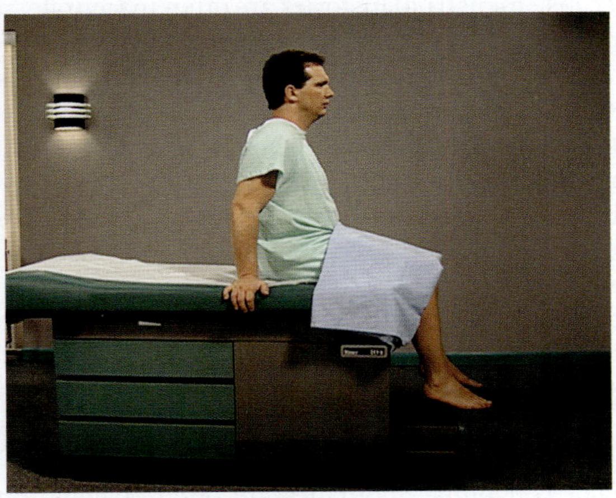

FIG. 24.8 Examine the patient seated with a drape across the lap.

- Assess lower extremity fine motor function and coordination, asking the patient to do the following:
  - Run heel down tibia of opposite leg.
  - Cross leg over opposite knee rapidly, and alternate legs.
- Test deep tendon reflexes and compare bilaterally: biceps, triceps, brachioradial, patellar, and Achilles.
- Test plantar reflex bilaterally.

Patient Standing

Assist patient to a standing position (Fig. 24.9). Examiner stands next to patient.

Spine

- Inspect and palpate spine as patient bends over at waist.
- Assess range of motion: flexion, hyperextension, lateral bending, rotation of upper trunk.

Neurologic

- Observe gait.
- Assess proprioception and cerebellar function.
- Perform the Romberg test.
- Ask the patient to walk heel to toe.
- Ask the patient to stand on one foot, then the other, with eyes closed.
- Ask the patient to hop in place on one foot, then the other.

Abdominal/Genital

- Assess for inguinal and femoral hernias.

Patient With Female Genitalia, Lithotomy Position

Assist patients into lithotomy position and drape appropriately (Fig. 24.10). Examiner is seated.

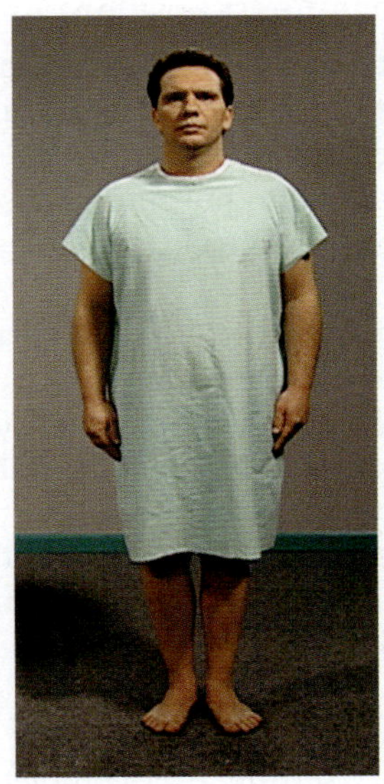

FIG. 24.9 Examine the patient while standing.

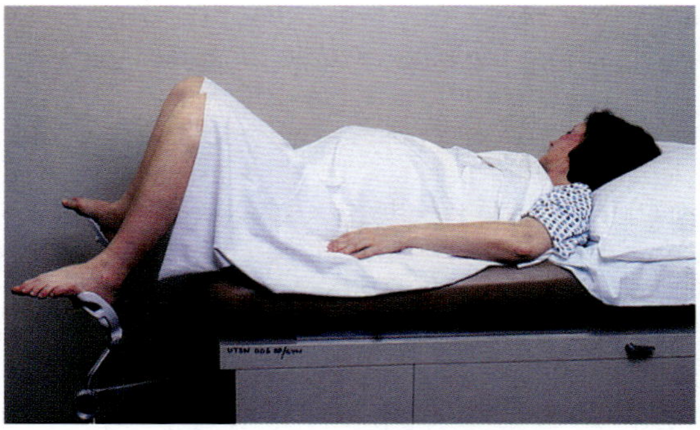

FIG. 24.10 Examining the patient in lithotomy position, appropriately draped.

External Genitalia

- Inspect pubic hair, labia, clitoris, urethral opening, vaginal opening, perineal and perianal areas, and anus.
- Palpate labia and Bartholin glands; milk Skene glands.

Internal Genitalia

- Perform speculum examination:
  - Inspect vagina and cervix.
  - Collect Pap smear/human papillomavirus (HPV) and other necessary specimens.
- Perform bimanual palpation to assess for characteristics of vagina, cervix, uterus, and adnexa. Examiner is standing.
- Perform rectovaginal examination to assess rectovaginal septum and broad ligaments.
- Perform rectal examination:
  - Assess anal sphincter tone and surface characteristics; palpate circumferentially for rectal mass.
  - Obtain rectal culture if needed.
  - Note characteristics of stool when gloved finger is removed.

Patients With a Prostate, Bending Forward (Lateral Decubitus or Knee-Chest Positions Are Also Possible)

Assist patients to lean over the examining table (or into knee-chest position or lateral decubitus position if preferred). Examiner is behind the patient. Ask the patient to point toes inward and to put their arms and chest on the table to help relax the buttocks and make the examination easier.

- Inspect sacrococcygeal and perianal areas.
- Perform rectal examination:
  - Palpate sphincter tone and surface characteristics; palpate circumferentially for rectal mass.
  - Obtain rectal culture if needed.
  - Palpate prostate gland and seminal vesicles.
  - Note characteristics of stool when gloved finger is removed. Test for occult blood.

Concluding the Examination

In the ambulatory setting after completing the examination and time allows, excuse yourself to allow the patient to get dressed. Take the time to organize your thoughts regarding the history, physical findings, and proposed plan of care. Add initial notes to the health record, especially for abnormalities found. When you return, discuss these thoughts to the extent that you can, and ask any needed additional questions. This is a final time during the visit for review, reflection, and an opportunity to address questions, concerns, or stressful matters. Discuss the plan of care that may include laboratory and other diagnostic tests as well as medications and treatments. Make sure the patient's accompanying family member is included in this discussion, if appropriate. You must be sure that the patient has a clear understanding of the situation or plan going forward. To be assured of this, you may request the patient to "teach back" what you have just instructed (Caplin & Saunders, 2015). This is also the ideal time to ask your patient, "Do you have any other thoughts or questions before we end our visit?"

If the patient is examined in a hospital bed, remember to put everything back in order when you are finished. Make sure the patient is comfortably settled in an appropriate manner, with the bed lowered and the side rails up if the clinical condition warrants and nursing call buttons within easy reach.

Physical Examination of Infants

Newborns

The newborn has a greater risk and better potential for health than patients of other ages. The Apgar score (see Chapter 14), taken at 1 and 5 minutes of age, provides insight into the newborn's in utero, intrapartum, and immediate postnatal experience. A low score for several of the variables—color, heart rate, respirations, muscle tone, and reflex irritability—is evidence of difficulty of transition. Further investigation of the reason for cyanosis, increased irritability, tachypnea, tachycardia, or loss of muscle tone is needed. The Apgar score is not an actual quantitative measure. It is an assessment of combined objective and subjective observations that allows for comparison over time and communication between observers.

Because menstrual histories are often inaccurate, more objective means of estimating the newborn's gestational age are required. The Ballard Gestational Age Assessment Tool contains six physical and six neuromuscular newborn characteristics that should be evaluated within 36 hours of birth to establish or confirm the preterm newborn's gestational age (see Chapter 8). The full-term newborn (40 weeks' gestation) commonly has the following physical characteristics: many creases on the sole of the foot, breast nodule of 4-mm diameter, cartilage present in the helix of the ear, and testes descended into the scrotum covered with rugae. Increasing muscle tone with a posture of predominantly flexed extremities is another sign of increased maturity.

Major congenital anomalies are often obvious during inspection, but exceptions occur, such as a life-threatening diaphragmatic hernia. Maintain a high index of suspicion. Search for clues about potential health conditions from information about the newborn's intrauterine life, the mother's labor and delivery experience, and the family history. For example, the newborn may be at risk if the mother has a fever during or after delivery or if herpetic lesions are present around the mother's mouth or genitalia. The mother's use of drugs—prescribed, over the counter, or illicit—may have an impact. Some drugs may have teratogenic effects. The mother's frequent use of sedatives or opioids may cause irritability, jitteriness, poor sucking, and other problems as the newborn goes through withdrawal (neonatal abstinence syndrome). Problems with earlier pregnancies may be relevant to the newborn's intrauterine life. The fate of siblings may suggest the fate of your present patient.

Carefully inspect the unclothed newborn, being careful to prevent hypothermia. If the newborn is full-term with an Apgar score of 8 or higher, the newborn may be skin to skin with the mother following birth. An abbreviated examination can be performed during this period, and a more thorough examination can be performed after the initial skin-to-skin period of 1 to 2 hours. You can learn a lot before touching, handling, or using an instrument. Note the baby's degree of awareness or apathy, the posture (e.g., unusual flaccidity, tension, spasticity), skin color, unexpected gross deformities, or unusual facies. The responsive, eager infant with a strong suck is reassuring. Note the presence or absence of spontaneity in the baby's behavior.

Observe a feeding. Often the baby demonstrates interest in life by latching on to the breast or bottle eagerly and with strength. Always observe the interaction between parents and between parent and infant.

When you begin the physical examination, examine the anterior and posterior chest if the newborn is quiet first, then palpate the head and fontanels (best done with baby upright), followed by the extremities and abdomen, and finally examine the rest of the baby. Use a gentle touch that will not obscure unusual findings. Chest percussion is generally of little value because of the relatively small chest and the examiner's relatively large hands and fingers. Abdominal percussion may have value, especially when the abdomen is distended.

Older Infants

No best sequence exists for the infant physical examination. Vary the sequence as appropriate for the infant's age and whether awake or asleep at the start, taking advantage of opportunities presented throughout the examination. Aim for infant cooperation for as long as possible. The sleeping infant offers a wonderful chance to auscultate the heart, lungs, and abdomen and to observe the infant's position at rest. Observe as much as you can before touching (e.g., the quality and rate of respiration, flaring of the alae nasi, skin color, even the visible apical thrust). Defer to the end anything invasive (e.g., examination of the ears, throat, and eyes).

If the infant is crying, all is not lost. Evaluate the quality or lustiness of the cry, lung excursion, and facial symmetry. Assess the mouth and pharynx for integrity of the soft palate and cranial nerves IX, X, and XII. Is stridor or hoarseness present? Examine the posterior tongue for the length and thickness of the lingual frenulum to identify a tongue-tie (ankyloglossia), which can interfere with deep latch and successful breastfeeding. The crying infant needs to take a breath, so be ready to listen to the heart and lungs each time a breath is taken. Over several intervals of breathing, you can hear enough of the heart and lung sounds. A crying baby may keep the eyes tightly shut, but the parent can stand and hold the infant over the shoulder while you stand behind the parent. At this point, the child will often stop crying for a moment and open the eyes. If you are poised with an ophthalmoscope, you can quickly assess the red reflex, corneal light reflex, and pupillary response to light.

Observe the infant during feeding to evaluate sucking and swallowing coordination, CN XII, and alertness and responsiveness. Seizing these advantages often requires a change in the examination sequence to suit the moment. Give the older infant less than a year of age something to hold in each hand. You may be able gauge the infant's interest in the objects and also have some freedom to use the stethoscope without having it grabbed.

Examination Sequence for Infants

The following is a suggested examination sequence of the newborn or young infant. The infant's temperature, weight (unclothed), length (lying), and head circumference are usually measured first. Weight, length, and head circumference are plotted on a growth curve for the infant's age and gender and then compared with prior measurements to assess growth (see Chapter 8).

General Inspection

Inspect the undressed, supine newborn on a warming table; inspect the older infant preferably on a parent's lap (Fig. 24.11).

- Assess positioning or posture at rest: symmetry and size of extremities, the newborn's assumption of in

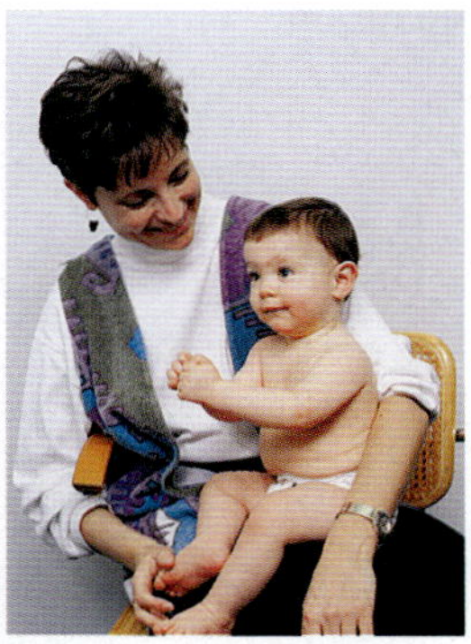

FIG. 24.11 Infants are often more comfortable when examined on a parent's lap.

utero position (flexion of extremities, unusual flaccidity or spasticity), and any difference in positioning between upper and lower extremities.

- Lift the infant's upper body a couple of inches, and with a sudden dropping motion assess the Moro newborn reflex response.
- Note voluntary movement of extremities.
- Inspect the skin for color and for meconium staining and vernix in a newborn.
- Note the presence of tremors.
- Assess for any apparent anomalies.
- Inspect the face for symmetry of features and spacing and position of features (e.g., intercanthal distance, presence and characteristics of the philtrum).

Chest, Lungs, and Heart

- Inspect the following: chest structure, symmetry of expansion with respiration; presence of retractions, heaves, or lifts (Fig. 24.12).
- Note the quality of respirations and count the rate.
- Inspect the breasts for nipple and tissue development.
- Palpate the chest and precordium.
- Locate the apical impulse (point of maximal impulse); note any thrills.
- Auscultate the entire anterior and lateral chest for breath sounds; note any bowel sounds.
- Auscultate each cardiac listening area for S_1 and S_2, splitting, and murmurs.
- Count the apical pulse rate.

Abdomen

- Inspect shape, configuration, and movement with respirations. Note a scaphoid or distended appearance.
- Inspect the umbilicus.
    - Inspect the newborn cord stump, count the vessels, note oozing of blood.
    - If the stump has fallen off, inspect the area for lesions, erythema, drainage, and foul odor.
- Auscultate each quadrant for bowel sounds.
- Lightly palpate all areas. Note size of liver, muscle tone, bladder, and spleen tip (Fig. 24.13).
- Palpate more deeply for kidneys, any masses; note any muscle rigidity or tenseness.
- Percuss each quadrant.

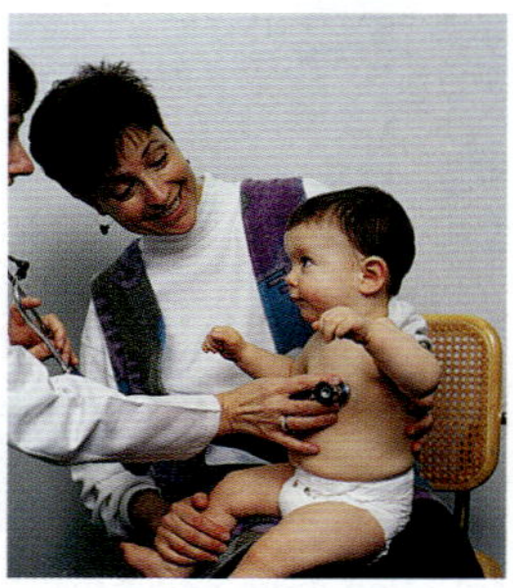

FIG. 24.12 Examining the chest of an infant on the parent's lap.

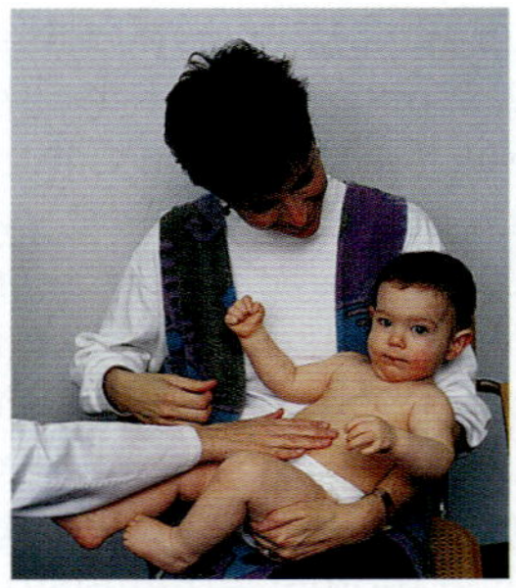

FIG. 24.13 Examining the infant's abdomen while reclining on the parent's lap.

- Check skin turgor.
- Palpate the inguinal area for femoral pulses and lymph nodes.

Head and Neck. Inspection and palpation can be done before or simultaneously with use of invasive instruments (Fig. 24.14).

- Inspect head shape: molding, swelling, scalp electrode site, and hairline.
- Palpate the head: anterior and posterior fontanels, sutures, areas of swelling or asymmetry. Measure fontanels in two dimensions.
- Perform ultrasound or transilluminate the newborn's skull if clinically necessary.
- Inspect the ears: shape, position, and alignment of auricles, pits, and sinuses.
- Perform the otoscopic examination assessing the patency of the auditory canals and characteristics of the tympanic membranes.
- Evaluate hearing.
- Inspect the eyes:
    - Assess the swelling of eyelids, discharge, size, shape, position, epicanthal folds, and conjunctivae.
    - Examine the pupils and their response to light.
    - Assess the corneal light reflex.
    - Examine the red reflex using the ophthalmoscope. Perform an ophthalmoscopic examination when age and cooperation permit.
    - Inspect eye movement when tracking a light or following a moving picture or face; note nystagmus.
    - Evaluate vision.

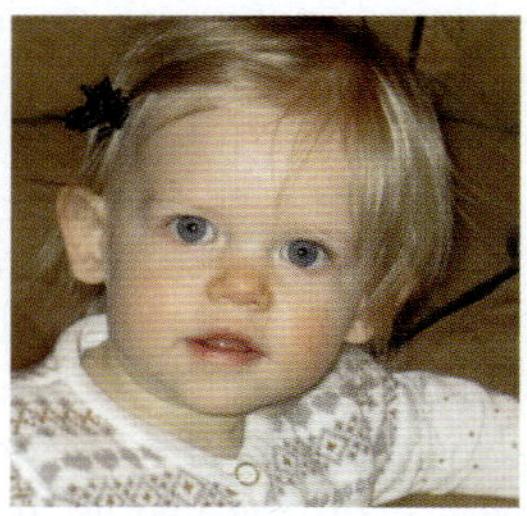

FIG. 24.14 Inspect and palpate the infant's face. (Courtesy Jennifer Hermes.)

- Inspect the nose:
  - Note flaring, discharge, size, and shape.
  - Inspect the nasal mucosa and alignment of the septum.
- Check patency of choanae (observe respiratory effort while alternately occluding each naris when mouth is closed).
- Inspect the mouth: lips, gums, hard and soft palates; size of tongue; excessive secretions in the newborn, drooling in the infant; presence of teeth, lesions.
- Palpate the mouth. Insert gloved small finger into the mouth to palpate hard and soft palates with finger pad and to evaluate suck.
- Stimulate gag reflex.
- Stroke each side of mouth to evaluate the rooting reflex.
- Lift infant's trunk, allowing head to fall back and rest against the table, slightly hyperextended. Inspect and palpate the position of the trachea.
- Inspect for alignment of head with neck.
- Inspect the neck for webbing, excess skinfolds.
- Palpate neck for masses, thyroid, muscle tone.
- Palpate lymph nodes: anterior and posterior cervical, preauricular, postauricular, submental, sublingual, tonsillar, supraclavicular.
- Palpate the clavicles for integrity. Note crepitus.
- Rotate the head to each side to assess passive range of motion.
- Observe the asymmetric tonic neck reflex response.

Upper Extremities

- Inspect and palpate arms.
- Move arms through the expected range of motion.
- Palpate the brachial or radial pulses; compare quality and timing with femoral pulses.
- Open the hands: Inspect nails and palmar and phalangeal creases, webbing of fingers; count fingers.
- Place a finger in infant's palms to evaluate palmar grasp newborn reflex.
- Keeping fingers in infant's hands, pull the infant slowly to sitting position, evaluate grasp and arm strength; evaluate head control.

Lower Extremities

- Inspect the legs and feet for alignment and symmetry of skinfolds (Fig. 24.15).
- Palpate the bones and muscles of each leg.
- Move legs through the expected range of motion; adduct and abduct the hips.
- Palpate the femoral and dorsalis pedis pulses.
- Count the toes.
- Elicit the plantar, patellar, and Achilles reflexes.
- Measure the blood pressure in the lower extremity when the femoral pulse is diminished, absent, or if clinically indicated.

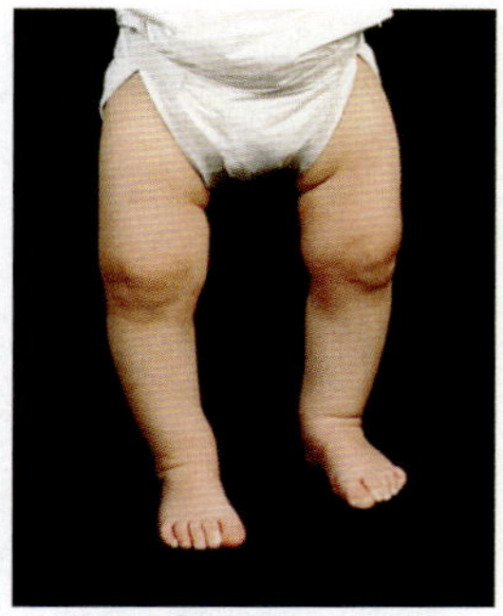

FIG. 24.15 Examine the infant's lower extremities. (From Atlas of Pediatric Physical Diagnosis, 7th edition, 2018, Zitelli, B., McIntire, S. & Nowalk, A. Elsevier, ISBN: 978-0-323-39303-4, page 809, Figure 22.93A.)

Genitals and Rectum

- Female genitalia:
  - Inspect external genitalia, noting size of clitoris, any discharge, hymenal opening, and any ambiguity of structures.
- Male genitalia:
  - Inspect placement of urethral opening without fully retracting the foreskin.
  - Inspect scrotum for rugae and presence of contents; note any ambiguity of structures.
  - Palpate scrotum for the testes, presence of hernia or hydrocele.
  - Transilluminate the scrotum when a mass other than testes is noted.
  - Observe voiding for strength of stream.
- Inspect rectum and assess sphincter tone. If the newborn does not pass meconium within 24 hours of birth, evaluate rectal patency with a soft catheter.

Neurologic

- Hold the infant in vertical suspension, facing you with your hands under the axillae to assess general body strength and tone. Without gripping the infant's chest, keep your hands under the infant's axillae, and note whether the baby begins to slip through your hands or maintains its position.
- Observe infant's open eyes for the sunsetting sign (portion of iris and pupil lying below lower eyelid).
- Hold the infant in horizontal suspension, with hands around the chest. Note the infant's ability to maintain a straight back, lift the head upright, and flex the extremities—all signs of good muscle tone.
- Perform the doll's eyes maneuver.
- Elicit the stepping and placing newborn reflexes.

Back. Position the newborn prone on the warming table or have the parent hold the infant upright over the shoulder (Fig. 24.16).

- Inspect spine. Observe for alignment, symmetry of muscle development, any masses, tufts of hair, dimples, skin pigmentation or discoloration, or defects over lower spine.

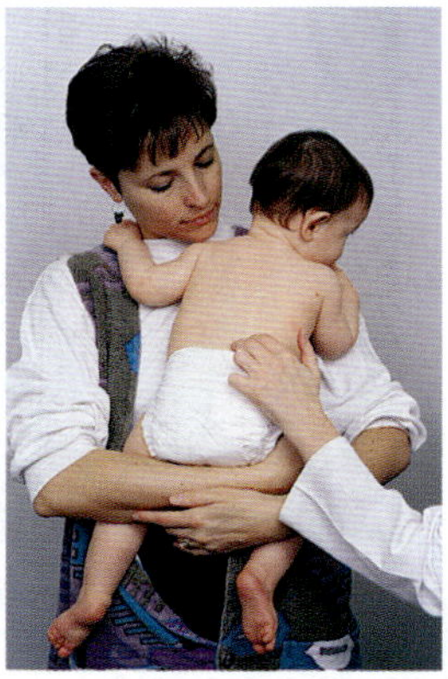

FIG. 24.16 Examining the infant's back while held by the parent.

- Palpate each spinal process for defects.
- Auscultate posterior chest for breath sounds, any heart sounds.
- Inspect symmetry of gluteal folds.

Behavior. Throughout examination of the newborn, note the alertness, ability to be quieted or consoled, and the response to handling. With an older infant, note alertness, responsiveness to the parent or other adult caregivers, and the ability of the parent to sense and respond to the infant's need for consolation. The child's ability at any age to react socially offers clues to physical and emotional well-being. The classic example is the "social smile"—the smile meant for you that we learn to expect from infants by the time they are 2 to 3 months old. Consider each of the following as you evaluate the infant's behavior:

- Is that smile real and meant for you?
- Is the infant playful, alert, and responsive or are dullness and apparent apathy present?
- If the infant is fearful, does your soothing effort help ease the fear?
- Does the infant move freely, show interest in the immediate environment, and reach for toys?
- Note the response to voices or noise: quieting, stopping movement, turning toward sounds indicating hearing.

Newborn hearing screening and congenital heart disease screening should be conducted prior to newborn discharge from the hospital.

Examination Sequence of Children

For children small enough, the parent's lap is a splendid examining table. It is helpful during the interview to keep the child and parent together and to observe their interaction. How they feel about each other is conveyed through touch, soothing and reassuring gestures, and the child's response. Take note of the obvious and subtle ways in which children and parents communicate with each other. If interaction is minimal and the child does not look to the parent for help, the family dynamics may be devoid of warmth and affection. Ask the parent to be present if you need to perform procedures (e.g., venipuncture) because this will be reassuring to the child. Most parents accept the request to be present, and the reaction to your request gives you more information about family dynamics and emotional resources.

With the young child, as you build the history you can help prepare the child for the physical examination at the same time by establishing some reassuring contact. For example, playing with the child (providing a ball, blocks, or an age-appropriate book) may reveal developmental progress and help win cooperation. A few pleasant words, relaxed moments, and patience can break the ice. Children do not know your routine. Often you are a stranger, and the environment may be frightening. Not every child will be smiling and happy about an examination.

Flexibility is important when examining young children. Avoid rushing, and do not persist if the child is anxious. Be thorough, but unless there is urgency, you may defer some aspects of the examination for when the child is more relaxed and less afraid of you. Children may be fearful because they have had procedures that hurt (e.g., immunizations), or they do not want to be separated from a trusted, familiar figure. In some cases, children have been victims of abuse or have witnessed violence in their homes and communities. It is important to recognize that anxiety or fear in a child may be a manifestation of trauma. It is important to respect the child's fear; to explain what is going to happen; and to be honest, firm, unapologetic, and gently expeditious. You also need to develop comfort in working in the presence of a parent who is sharply observant, sometimes tentative, or sometimes hostile. Do not separate the child from the parent for the sole purpose of improving your personal comfort.

General Inspection

General inspection may begin in the waiting room or as the child enters the examining room. The temperature, weight, length or height, and head circumference (up to age 2 years) are usually obtained earlier. Offer toys or paper and crayons to entertain the child, to develop rapport, and to evaluate development and neurologic status. For well-child visits, the parent should have already completed a developmental screening questionnaire to provide information about the child's language, motor coordination, and social skills. Evaluate mental status as the child interacts with you and with the parent. Take seriously and investigate any sense of possible stress in the parent-child relationship and any parental report of a developmental concern.

The following sequence is a guideline. Take advantage of opportunities the child presents during the examination to make your observations. The sequence of examination may vary with each child (Box 24.6).

Child Playing

The child playing in the examination room offers an opportunity to evaluate both the musculoskeletal and

BOX 24.6 Some Tips for Examining a Young Child

- Tell a story or ask about the child's experience (e.g., toys, school, games, or friends) to help attract attention or, at times, to distract.
- Avoid restraining the child or having adults looming over the examining table as this increases the child's apprehension and decreases cooperation. If the child's arms and head must be kept still (e.g., to look at the ears), the child is often less distressed if seated on the parent's lap and held by the parent's arms.
- Use the tongue blade only at the end of the examination if it must be used. Ease the tendency to gag by moistening it first with warm water.
- Ask a child to "blow out" your flashlight as a way to introduce your instruments. Offer them as toys (they will not break), or draw a doll's face on a tongue blade. You might even get down on the floor with the child, or use your own lap as an examining table. Anything goes (within bounds of propriety) to get the information you need.
- Enlist the help of the ticklish child. Place your hand on top of the child's to gently probe the abdomen or the axilla. The diaphragm of your stethoscope can also serve as a probe.
- Hold babies; feed them. You will know each other better.
- Be patient with discomfort or resistance. If the situation allows, come back to that portion of the examination later when calm may be restored.
- Use brief, specific, polite directions. Do not ask the child's permission for each step. It is better to say, "Please open your mouth" rather than "Do you want to open your mouth?" After all, what will you do next if the answer is "no"?
- Offer choices when possible, such as "Which ear should I check first?"

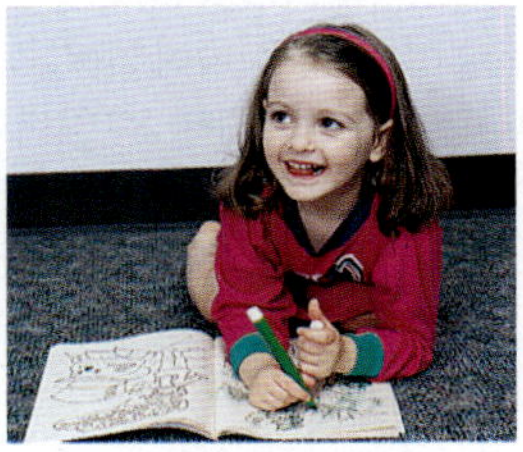

FIG. 24.17 Provide toys or other items to observe the child's development.

neurologic systems while developing a rapport with the child (Fig. 24.17).

- Observe the child's spontaneous activities.
- Ask the child to demonstrate some skills: turning pages in a book, building block towers, drawing geometric figures, or coloring.
- Evaluate gait, jumping, hopping, and range of motion.
- Muscle strength: Observe the child rise from sitting on the floor, climbing on the parent's lap, stooping, and recovering.

Child on Parent's Lap

The parent's lap is a fine and helpful examining table. Begin with the child sitting and undressed except for the diaper or underpants (Fig. 24.18).

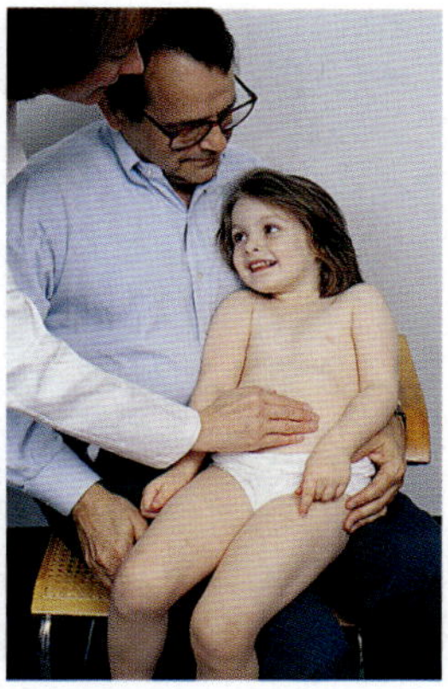

FIG. 24.18 Young children can also be examined on the parent's lap.

Upper Extremities

- Inspect arms for movement, size, shape, and skin lesions.
- Observe use of the hands; inspect hands for number and configuration of fingers and palmar creases.
- Palpate radial pulses.
- Elicit biceps and triceps reflexes when the child cooperates.
- Take the blood pressure at a time when the child is comfortable with you. The child should be seated on a chair with the back supported and feet on the floor if possible.

Lower Extremities (May Stand for Part of the Examination)

- Inspect the legs for movement, size, shape, alignment, and lesions.
- Inspect the feet for alignment, longitudinal arch, and number of toes.
- Palpate the dorsalis pedis pulse.
- Elicit the plantar reflex and, if cooperative, the Achilles and patellar reflexes.

Head and Neck

- Inspect head and face (Fig. 24.19):
  - Inspect shape, hairline, and hair.
  - Inspect eyelids, palpebral folds, conjunctivae, sclerae, and irides.
  - Inspect position of auricles.
  - Inspect for facial symmetry.
- Palpate the skull for irregularities and depressions; hair for texture.
- Inspect neck for alignment, webbing, and voluntary movement.
- Palpate neck, noting the trachea and its position, thyroid, muscle tone, and lymph nodes.

Chest, Heart, and Lungs

- Inspect the chest for respiratory movement, size, shape, precordial movement, deformity, and nipple and breast development.

HEAD-TO-TOE EXAMINATION

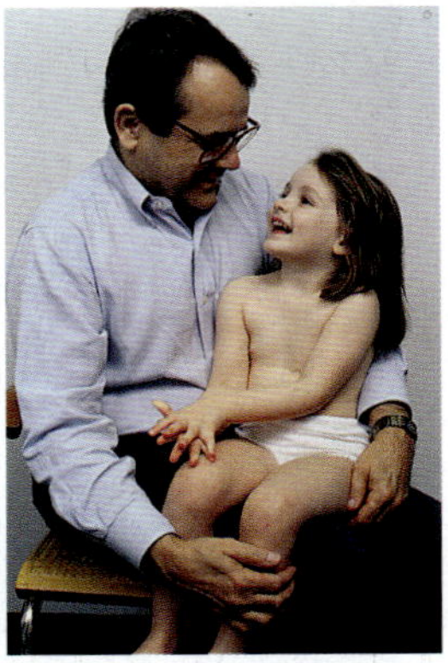

FIG. 24.19 Inspect and palpate the child's head and neck.

- Palpate the anterior chest, locate the point of maximal impulse; note tactile fremitus in the talking or crying child.
- Auscultate the anterior, lateral, and posterior chest for breath sounds; count respirations.
- Auscultate all cardiac listening areas for S_1 and S_2, splitting, and murmurs; count the apical pulse.

Child Relatively Supine, Still on Lap, Diaper Loosened

- Inspect the abdomen.
- Auscultate for bowel sounds.
- Palpate the abdomen. Identify the size of the liver and any other palpable organs or masses.
- Percuss the abdomen.
- Palpate the femoral pulses, compare with radial pulses.
- Palpate for inguinal lymph nodes.
- Inspect the external genitalia.
- Male genitalia. Palpate scrotum for descent of testes and other masses.

Child Standing

- Inspect spinal alignment as the child bends slowly forward to touch toes (Fig. 24.20).
- Observe posture from anterior, posterior, and lateral views.
- Observe gait.

Child Returns to Parent's Lap

Reduce the child's fear of the funduscopic, otoscopic, and oropharyngeal examinations by permitting the child to

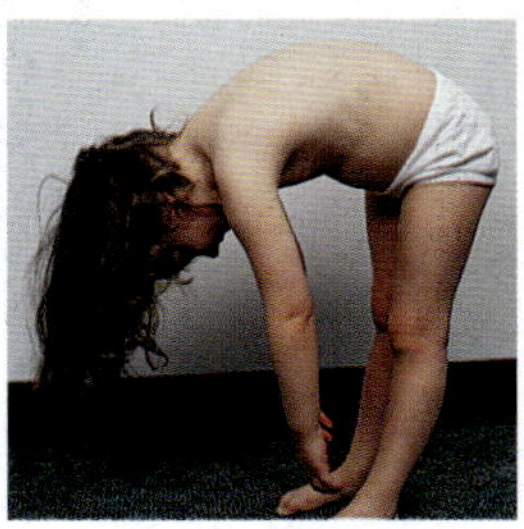

FIG. 24.20 Examine the child while standing and bending to touch the toes.

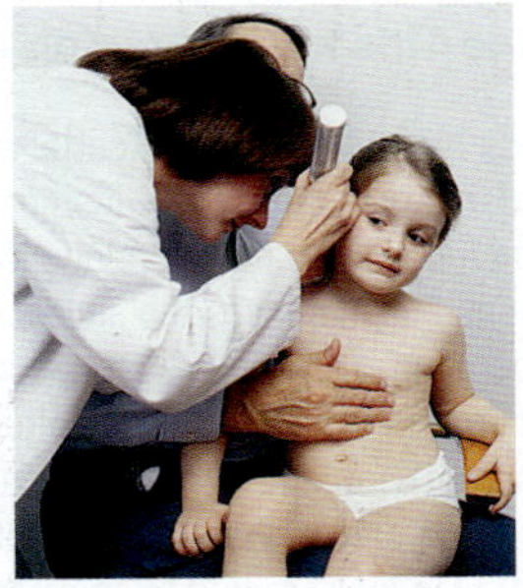

FIG. 24.21 With some children, it is better to postpone the use of instruments until the end of the examination.

handle the instruments, "blow out" the light, or use them on a doll or the parent. Attempt to gain the child's cooperation, even if it takes more time (Fig. 24.21). If successful in gaining cooperation, future visits will be more pleasant for the child and for you. Only as a last resort restrain the child for these examinations. After finishing these preliminary maneuvers, perform the following:

- Perform vision screening with the Snellen chart, HOTV chart, or LEA symbols beginning at about age 3 years (see Chapter 12).
- Inspect the eyes: pupillary light reflex, red reflex, corneal light reflex, and extraocular movements.
- Perform the funduscopic examination.
- Perform the otoscopic examination.
- Evaluate hearing.
- Inspect the nasal mucosa.
- Inspect the mouth and pharynx.

By the time the child is school age, it is usually possible to use an examination sequence similar to that for adults.

Physical Examination in Pregnant Patients and Older Adults

Pregnant Patients

Pregnancy requires frequent abdominal and pelvic evaluations to assess the patient's status and fetal well-being. Late in pregnancy, the patient may find it difficult to assume the supine position without experiencing hypotension. Ask for this position only when necessary, and provide alternatives by elevating the backrest or by supplying pillows to allow the side-lying position. Abdominal assessment is more comfortable for the patient and more accurate if the bladder is empty. Urinary urgency and frequency are common during pregnancy.

The baseline physical examination is important. A healthy patient may not have had a recent examination before becoming pregnant. Baseline vital signs, height, current weight, and prepregnancy weight should be recorded. The examination may be performed in the same sequence used for other adults with special attention paid to the abdomen and pelvic examination. All physical findings that may be significant later in pregnancy or that may potentially affect the fetus should be addressed and documented (e.g., cervical abnormalities, hyperthyroidism, cardiac problems, hypertension, and infections).

Older Adults

Physical examination of the older adult may require some changes from the usual adult process. Patients who are older and/or frail have difficulty assuming the lithotomy and knee-chest positions. Sometimes an alternative position is required or patients need additional assistance (see Chapter 19). The quality of assessment data is not compromised with these changes. Your skill and patience are far more important in ensuring accuracy. A hurried pace or impatience may fluster or confuse an older adult patient. Neurologic testing reaction time may be longer or may require more intense stimuli.

Functional assessment (see Chapter 1) is an essential examination of every older adult, regardless of how well they are coping in the community environment. Consider how the patient walks, follows instructions, undresses, and maneuvers to the examining table. This tells you about mobility, balance, fine motor skills (e.g., unbuttoning clothes), and range of motion as well as some clues about perceptual abilities and cognition. Some older adults have more than one condition that suggests poor health.

For many, the bottom line is not a physical defect but something else that gets in the way of successful daily living. Perceptions of ill health may be associated with physical disease or another problem, such as the loss or impairment of a significant relationship (e.g., illness, death, divorce), changed living arrangements, inadequate understanding about one's problems, poor self-image, or substance abuse. Secondary gains from complaining (e.g., indulgent family response by providing extra comforts or attention or distraction from other problems) may also be involved.

Functional assessment is the determination of how well the patient can deal with the consistent demands of life. This includes self-care and daily living activities such as the ability to drive a car, use public transportation, prepare a meal, manage finances, and use a telephone. It includes a comprehensive history, physical examination, and social assessment. In particular:

- Obtain a listing of all medications (e.g., prescribed and over-the-counter drugs, especially hypnotics, sedatives, and laxatives). Ask the patient to bring in all medications prescribed by all health care providers and all nonprescribed medications, including herbs, vitamins, and other complementary and alternative therapies.
- Review function, including activities of daily living (ADLs), evaluating the degree of independence versus need for caretaker assistance:
  - *Basic ADLs:* bathing, dressing, toileting, ambulation, feeding
  - *Instrumental ADLs:* housekeeping, grocery shopping, meal preparation, medication adherence, communication skills, financial management
  - Use of assistive devices for ambulation and function: cane, walker, commode chair, hospital bed
- Systems review, particularly common geriatric problems:
  - Nutritional status, evidence of malnutrition
  - Urinary incontinence
  - Memory changes, signs of cognitive impairment
  - Depression
  - Medication-induced delirium
  - Prior falls or fear of falling
- Social situation:
  - Identification of caretakers and probable caretakers, including those who maintain the home environment
  - Assessment of caretaker abilities
  - Assessment of financial resources, housing status, food security, and health insurance, with particular attention to long-term services not ordinarily covered by insurance: personal grooming, home care, medication supervision
  - Existence of advance directives and an assigned health care agent (durable power of attorney for health care decisions by a family member or trusted person)
- Physical examination with particular focus on the following:
  - Mental status with specific attention to cognition, memory, and mood
  - Respiratory examination for dyspnea on exertion
  - Blood pressure for orthostatic hypotension
  - Musculoskeletal evaluation of strength with special attention on ability to independently rise from the bed and a chair
  - Neurologic examination of balance, coordination, gait
  - Skin for signs of decubitus ulcers or venous stasis ulcers

The Closing Discussion

Each interaction with a patient is unique. You will at times be worried, rushed, and tired. Because you are human, you may respond differently to people who are dying, to children, to older adults, to persons of different sexual orientation or gender identity, and to persons of different cultural groups. Be aware of your biases, learn about your patients with genuine curiosity, and demonstrate respect (Box 24.7).

You are at the point of organizing the information you have assembled into a usable whole, ready for providing care, caring, and problem solving. Be disciplined enough to pursue complete information, even when the solution seems obvious (because sometimes the obvious is wrong), and be courageous enough to make the decision for urgency when the data are incomplete.

Following analysis of all findings and initial impressions from the history and physical examination, clinical reasoning is used to guide the identification of the diagnosis or need for additional diagnostic testing (see

BOX 24.7 How Are You Doing?

As a health care professional you should constantly assess how you communicated while building the history and doing the physical examination:

- Were you courteous and demonstrating respect?
- Did you provide comfort?
- Did you connect with the patient?
- Did you confirm your understanding and the patient's understanding of what happened?

Did You, at the Start?

- Say "hello" and appropriately greet the patient and others present. Use the patient's preferred name and pronouns.
- Introduce yourself and ask others present how they are related to the patient.
- Give attention to everyone's comfort.
- Position yourself to foster communication with the patient seated closest to you and without the barrier of a computer.
- Minimize noise as much as possible.
- Explain your approach to the history and physical examination.
- Assess the patient's approach and understanding.
- Begin with a comfortable, open-ended question, such as, "How can I be of help?" or "What concerns do you have?"

Did You, as You Talked With the Patient?

- Make it easy for the patient to talk.
- Move appropriately from open-ended questions to specific questions.
- Clarify what was unclear as well as you could.
- Steer the course of the interview unobtrusively.
- Ask one question at a time, leaving time for the answer.
- Offer occasional repetition of what you have heard to let the patient know you are really listening.

Did You, Throughout?

- Maintain appropriate eye contact.
- Sit comfortably.
- Pace the conversation, allowing enough time for the patient's comments, expressions, thoughts, and feelings.
- Empathize when appropriate.
- Restate your willingness to help when appropriate.
- Confirm that you and the patient are allies, working together to find appropriate outcomes.
- Ensure the necessary understandings between you and the patient.

Did You, at the Finish?

- Summarize and recheck for accuracy.
- Ask if any other questions or concerns need to be addressed.
- Appropriately indicate next steps.
- Say "thank you" with appreciation and with an appropriate "good-bye."

Chapter 4). Make sure that information is well-documented to ensure competent care to the patient and for protection should there ever be a legal challenge to your care (see Chapter 5).

Summary information is shared with the patient in this health care visit. Follow guidelines for effective communication and partnership with the patient when having this discussion. When bad news must be shared, plan how to do this effectively (Box 24.8).

Serving the whole patient—their physical, emotional, and social needs—demands discipline and flexibility within that discipline. Contrary to the view of some, the building of a history and the performance of a physical examination are still and will remain the heart, soul, and mind of an alliance with the patient.

BOX 24.8 The Stressful Moment

For patients of any age and those who support them, certain principles are guides when disturbing or bad news must be communicated. First, turn off your mobile devices and arrange a quiet setting, as free as possible of ambient noise and distraction.

- If you do not know the patient well, try to involve family members or other trusted persons who are essential for emotional and practical support. Consider their base of knowledge, experience, and understanding of the situation.
- Be specific in all details, providing information in a deliberate flow adjusted to the needs of the patient, allowing time for questions and for frequent repetition whenever necessary.
- Use jargon-free language adapted to the patient's understanding.
- Inform the patient immediately unless, for example, the sensorium is clouded. Otherwise, there is seldom, if any, justification for delay in offering information.

Sports Participation Evaluation

CHAPTER 25

Overview of Preparticipation Physical Evaluation

Each year, about 60 million U.S. children, youth, and young adults participate in organized sports and are required by state and local school districts to have a preparticipation physical evaluation (PPE). Cases of death and serious injury on the playing field, usually among college and professional athletes, keep concerns about the risks of sports participation in the public eye.

The overall goals of the PPE are to determine the general physical and psychological health of an athlete, ensure safe participation in appropriate physical activity, and not restrict participation unnecessarily. Whether athletes receive the PPE in the context of an ongoing primary care relationship or as a focused preseason checkup, the following objectives of the evaluation are universal:

- To identify conditions that may interfere with a person's ability to participate in a sport
- To identify existing health conditions for a person that may increase the risk of injury or death during sports participation
- To help select an appropriate sport for a person's particular abilities and physical status

Sports and disciplined physical effort enhance fitness and coordination, increase self-esteem, and provide positive social experiences for participants, including individuals with physical and intellectual disabilities (Box 25.1). Few children and youth have conditions that should limit participation, and most of these conditions are known before the PPE takes place (see Clinical Pearls, "Atlantoaxial Instability," and "Hypertension in the Pediatric and Adolescent Athlete").

Approaches to Preparticipation Physical Evaluations

Ideally, the PPE occurs in the primary care setting by a clinician with whom the individual has a longitudinal relationship and knows the patient's medical, behavioral, social, and family history. The American Academy of Pediatrics (AAP) recommends the PPE occur during the annual well-child visit (American Academy of Pediatrics, 2021). The PPE is individualized and tailored to the specific needs of the particular patient. The PPE may be the only opportunity to assess an athlete's health and safety, including mental health, substance use, and concerns unrelated to sports participation.

Another approach to the PPE is the group-based station method in which a large number of patients are evaluated in a single session by multiple clinicians. Each clinician takes responsibility for a specific aspect of the evaluation at a station dedicated to that purpose. The station method can involve clinicians from a variety of disciplines such as medicine, nursing, athletic training, and physical therapy. Athletes move from one station to the next, with historical and objective information documented throughout on a standard form.

CLINICAL PEARL

Atlantoaxial Instability

Individuals with Down syndrome are at a slightly increased risk of atlantoaxial subluxation. Because cervical spine radiographs do not accurately predict risk of spine problems in asymptomatic children and adolescents, the AAP no longer supports routine radiologic screening. However, it is important to discuss spinal cord injury risk with parents of children with Down syndrome who will be participating in sports (especially football, soccer, and gymnastics). Of note, trampoline use should be avoided by all children with or without Down syndrome, unless participation is part of a structured program with safety measures and supervision in place. For children with Down syndrome, inform parents to remind clinical staff about maintaining a neutral cervical spine position during anesthetic, surgical, and radiologic procedures. During visits, inquire about neck or radicular pain, weakness, change in gait, and bowel or bladder function and perform a careful neurologic examination. If a child has physical examination findings of myelopathy, including increased deep tendon reflexes; a positive Babinski sign; ankle clonus or a change in tone, strength, or gait, immediately refer them to a neurosurgeon with expertise in atlantoaxial instability (Bull & Committee on Genetics, 2022).

Think About It

As you perform a PPE on a pediatric patient for middle school soccer, you notice mild thoracic scoliosis. His mother tells you he has always had flat feet and his chest wall seems to be caved more inward than when he was younger. As he shows you how far he can bend his fingers back, you recognize he has pectus excavatum. Your patient has a number of features consistent with Marfan syndrome, and you refer him to cardiology for an echocardiogram to assess his aortic root for dilatation and ophthalmology to check for lens dislocation (Fig. 25.1).

BOX 25.1 Special Olympics: Promoting Sports Participation in Individuals With Disabilities

The Special Olympics offers an opportunity for year-round sports training and athletic competition to approximately 2.5 million individuals with intellectual disabilities (www.specialolympics.org). The official sports include aquatics, track and field, basketball, golf, gymnastics, softball, tennis, and volleyball, among others. Participants must be at least 8 years old. A PPE is required for admission to the program.

The clinician should not restrict participation based on a patient's intellectual disability alone. The thorough PPE outlined in this chapter should guide decisions about sports participation clearance, as it does for nondisabled patients. A supplemental history form is publicly available on the AAP website (https://www.aap.org/en/patient-care/preparticipation-physical-evaluation/), and athlete medical forms can be found on the AAP and Special Olympics websites. Past experience indicates there is some risk of eye injury in badminton, basketball, floor hockey, handball, soccer, softball, and tennis. An increased risk for those with atlantoaxial instability is associated with alpine skiing, diving, equestrian sports, gymnastics, high jump, soccer, and swimming.

The same care is due for persons seeking to join in the Paralympic Games, an opportunity offered by a different organizing group for athletes with a physical disability of a serious nature, such as amputation, cerebral palsy, spinal cord impairment, or visual impairment. These athletes, however, need not have an intellectual disability.

Compared with nonparticipants, Special Olympics participants have demonstrated higher self-esteem and greater perceived physical competence and peer acceptance. Considering the physical, emotional, and social benefits of sports participation and physical activity, the AAP Council on Children with Disabilities urges pediatric clinicians to promote the participation of children with disabilities. Clinicians should help individuals and families overcome barriers to participation and become aware of resources like the Special Olympics and the National Center on Physical Activity and Disability (Carbone et al., 2021).

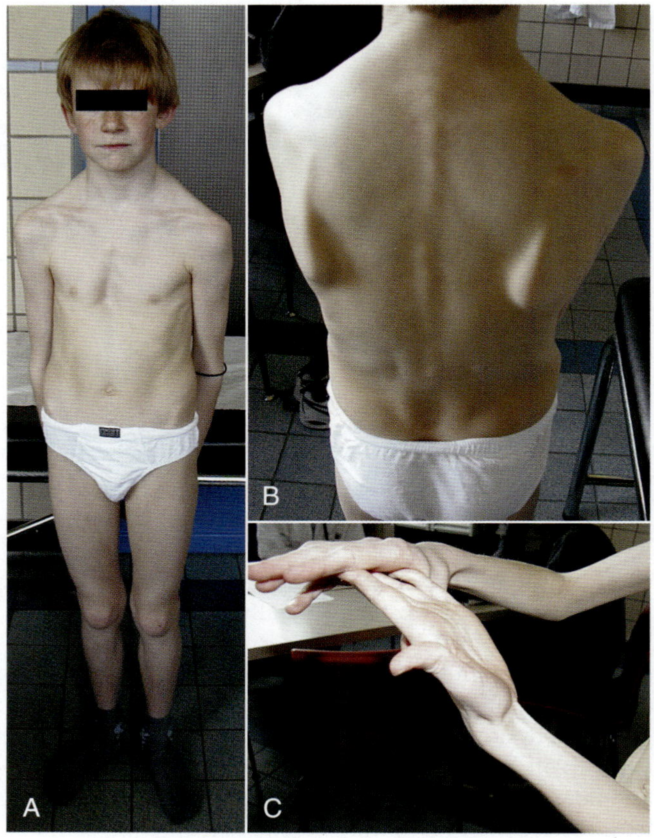

FIG. 25.1 Marfan syndrome clinical features in a 12-year-old. (A) Pectus excavatum and long bone overgrowth. (B) Beginning scoliosis at the onset of growth acceleration. (C) Arachnodactyly and hypermobility of the small joints. (From Callewaert B, Malfait F, Loeys B, De Paepe A. (2008). Ehlers-Danlos syndromes and Marfan syndrome. *Best Pract Res Clin Rheumatol. 22*(1):165-189.)

A checkout station is critical to the success of this approach. The person in charge of this station reviews the data collected during the evaluation and coordinates any necessary follow-up testing or referrals, communicating directly with the athlete (and parents, if appropriate) and generating a written report. The PPE station format is not a comprehensive service for addressing issues unrelated to sports participation and does not typically provide privacy for the disclosure of health-risk behaviors or other concerns. The PPE may also be provided by urgent care centers and retail clinics. When a PPE occurs outside of the primary care setting, the report should be sent to the patient's primary care provider, and the need for patients to concurrently receive routine health maintenance care should be emphasized. Since it is best to receive care from a consistent clinician who knows the patient's health, family, and social history, the AAP does not recommend the use of these alternative settings (American Academy of Pediatrics, 2021).

Focus of Preparticipation Physical Evaluations

The PPE should be completed at least 6 to 8 weeks in advance of the planned sports activity so that any needed specialist evaluations, rehabilitation, or therapy can be completed before participation begins. Primary care providers are often asked to complete a sports participation form based on a prior visit. Because the overall goal of the PPE is to ensure safe participation in a specific sport, clinicians should emphasize the importance of scheduling a complete PPE visit. Once an initial, thorough PPE has been completed, subsequent PPEs may be shorter and should focus on interim problems and concerns. Collegiate athletes should have a PPE and a comprehensive health assessment upon entry into the athletic program with annual or more frequent follow-up evaluations based on injury or illness since the initial PPE. For middle school and high school athletes in the United States, the required frequency for having a PPE is determined by each state as recommended by the National Federation of State High School Associations (nfhs.org).

CLINICAL PEARL

Hypertension in the Pediatric and Adolescent Athlete

Hypertension is the most common cardiovascular condition seen in competitive athletes. Blood pressure measurement is particularly important during the PPE for young athletes. In the pediatric population, the diagnosis of hypertension is made when blood pressure measurements on three or more occasions are above cutoffs based on the child's sex, age, and height percentile. Patients should be assessed for substances known to increase blood pressure (e.g., over-the-counter supplements, alcohol, tobacco, and highly caffeinated beverages). For children under 13 years of age, stage 1 hypertension is defined as blood pressure measurements >95th to <95th percentile + 12 mmHg or 130/80 to 139/89 mmHg (whichever is lower). Stage 2 hypertension is defined as blood pressure measurements ≥95th percentile + 12 mmHg or ≥140/90 mmHg (whichever is lower). Similar to adults, for youth 13 years of age and older, stage 1 hypertension is defined as repeated measurements 130/80 to 139/89 mmHg, and stage 2 hypertension is diagnosed when measurements are ≥140/90 mmHg. Like adults, if the patient has stage 1 hypertension and is asymptomatic, recommend lifestyle modification and recheck the blood pressure in 1 to 2 weeks. If the blood pressure remains at the stage 2 level, upper and lower extremity blood pressures should be measured to rule out coarctation of the aorta, nutrition and/or weight management guidance should be considered, and follow-up should occur in 3 months. If stage 1 hypertension persists, evaluation for an etiology, comorbid conditions, and assessment is warranted. Subspecialist referral and pharmacotherapy may be indicated. Similar guidance should be followed for patients with stage 2 hypertension, but follow-up and referral to a subspecialist should occur sooner (within 1 week). Symptomatic patients with stage 2 hypertension should be referred immediately to a pediatric emergency care setting. Since physical activity can reduce blood pressure over time, sports participation should be encouraged in youth with hypertension after evaluation by a medical subspecialist (e.g., cardiologist and/or nephrologist). All youth athletes with hypertension should be assessed for left ventricular hypertrophy (LVH) by echocardiogram prior to sports participation. The AAP recommends restriction from high-static sports for youth with stage 2 hypertension until their blood pressure is in the normal range after making lifestyle changes and/or initiating pharmacotherapy (AAP, 2017).

The physical examination component of the PPE should center on high-yield areas, particularly those related to sports participation and issues identified by the history. Items such as auscultation of the lung fields and otoscopy are low yield unless the patient is symptomatic at the time of the evaluation. Such findings can distract clinicians from the more important PPE cardiac and orthopedic examinations.

The recommended PPE history and physical examination forms are shown in Box 25.2 and were developed by the American Academy of Family Physicians, AAP, American College of Sports Medicine, American Medical Society for Sports Medicine, American Orthopedic Society for Sports Medicine, and American Osteopathic Academy of Sports Medicine. The PPE history form is available in English and Spanish. Many clinicians may be less comfortable with the orthopedic component of the physical examination. Garrick developed a "2-minute" screening orthopedic examination to be used in conjunction with a thorough history. This 14-step musculoskeletal examination consists of observing the athlete in a variety of positions and postures that highlight asymmetries in range of motion, strength, and muscle bulk (Fig. 25.2; Miller, 2019). These asymmetries serve to identify acute or old, poorly rehabilitated injuries. The steps pictured in Fig. 25.2 help in assessing most of the following:

- Posture and general muscle contour bilaterally
- Patient's "duck walk," four steps with knees completely bent
- Spine for curvature and lumbar extension, fingers touching toes with knees straight
- Shoulder and clavicle for dislocation
- Neck, shoulders, elbows, forearms, hands, fingers, and hips for range of motion
- Knee ligaments for drawer sign

Evidence-Based Practice in Physical Examination

The Particular Value of a Careful History

The only proven benefit of the PPE is the recognition of athletes at risk for later orthopedic injury. With a careful history, recent or poorly rehabilitated injuries that can become worse with sports participation can be detected. The history can identify up to 88% of general conditions and 67% to 75% of musculoskeletal conditions relevant for sports participation (MacDonald et al., 2021). Asthma is a good example. Unless a patient is in respiratory distress when evaluated, asthma will not be detected during the physical examination. The incidence of sudden cardiac death is estimated to be 1 in 50,000 to 1 in 80,000 athletes (Sweeting et al., 2018). To identify patients with structural and arrhythmogenic heart conditions, patients should be assessed for personal history of exertional symptoms (e.g., chest pain, dyspnea), prior detection of a heart murmur, unexplained syncope or near-syncope, physical findings consistent with Marfan syndrome, and family history of premature serious heart conditions (before age 50) or sudden unexplained death (McDonald et al., 2021).

Although rare, sudden and unexpected deaths in athletes usually occur off the field or court and are most often caused by unintentional injury, suicide, homicide, and drug overdose (Sweeting et al., 2018). In an epidemiologic study examining U.S. data between 2007 and 2015, 45 deaths were reported in youth 6 to 17 years of age who were participating in organized sports (middle school, youth league, and recreational). The majority of deaths (80%) were in males, most (76%) were cardiac related, and many (71%) occurred during practice (Endres et al., 2019). Conditions leading to these uncommon events are rarely associated with detectable physical findings. They may, however, be associated with symptoms revealed by a careful medical and family history during the PPE. For adolescent-age patients, it is important to obtain the health history from both the adolescent and the parents or caregivers. The expert consensus recommendation history form includes medical, mental health, and family heart health questions and remains an essential component of the PPE (Box 25.2). A thorough history can detect up to 90% of medical conditions and 70% of musculoskeletal conditions identified during a PPE (Miller & Peterson, 2019).

BOX 25.2

This form should be placed into the athlete's medical file and should not be shared with schools or sports organizations. The Medical Eligibility Form is the only form that should be submitted to a school or sports organization.
Disclaimer: Athletes who have a current Preparticipation Physical Evaluation (per state and local guidance) on file should not need to complete another History Form.

■ PREPARTICIPATION PHYSICAL EVALUATION (Interim Guidance)

HISTORY FORM

Note: Complete and sign this form (with your parents if younger than 18) before your appointment.

Name: ______________________ Date of birth: ______________

Date of examination: ______________ Sport(s): ______________________

Sex assigned at birth (F, M, or intersex): ________ How do you identify your gender? (F, M, non-binary, or another gender): ________

Have you had COVID-19? (check one): ☐ Y ☐ N

Have you been immunized for COVID-19? (check one): ☐ Y ☐ N If yes, have you had: ☐ One shot ☐ Two shots ☐ Three shots ☐ Booster date(s) ______________

List past and current medical conditions. ______________________

Have you ever had surgery? If yes, list all past surgical procedures. ______________________

Medicines and supplements: List all current prescriptions, over-the-counter medicines, and supplements (herbal and nutritional).

Do you have any allergies? If yes, please list all your allergies (ie, medicines, pollens, food, stinging insects).

Patient Health Questionnaire Version 4 (PHQ-4)

Over the last 2 weeks, how often have you been bothered by any of the following problems? (Circle response.)

	Not at all	Several days	Over half the days	Nearly every day
Feeling nervous, anxious, or on edge	0	1	2	3
Not being able to stop or control worrying	0	1	2	3
Little interest or pleasure in doing things	0	1	2	3
Feeling down, depressed, or hopeless	0	1	2	3

(A sum of ≥3 is considered positive on either subscale [questions 1 and 2, or questions 3 and 4] for screening purposes.)

GENERAL QUESTIONS (Explain "Yes" answers at the end of this form. Circle questions if you don't know the answer.)	Yes	No
1. Do you have any concerns that you would like to discuss with your provider?		
2. Has a provider ever denied or restricted your participation in sports for any reason?		
3. Do you have any ongoing medical issues or recent illness?		
HEART HEALTH QUESTIONS ABOUT YOU	**Yes**	**No**
4. Have you ever passed out or nearly passed out during or after exercise?		
5. Have you ever had discomfort, pain, tightness, or pressure in your chest during exercise?		
6. Does your heart ever race, flutter in your chest, or skip beats (irregular beats) during exercise?		
7. Has a doctor ever told you that you have any heart problems?		
8. Has a doctor ever requested a test for your heart? For example, electrocardiography (ECG) or echocardiography.		

HEART HEALTH QUESTIONS ABOUT YOU (*CONTINUED*)		Yes	No
9. Do you get light-headed or feel shorter of breath than your friends during exercise?			
10. Have you ever had a seizure?			
HEART HEALTH QUESTIONS ABOUT YOUR FAMILY	**Unsure**	**Yes**	**No**
11. Has any family member or relative died of heart problems or had an unexpected or unexplained sudden death before age 35 years (including drowning or unexplained car crash)?			
12. Does anyone in your family have a genetic heart problem such as hypertrophic cardie myopathy (HCM), Marfan syndrome, arrhyth -mogenic right ventricular cardiomyopathy (ARVC), long QT syndrome (LQTS), short QTsyndrome (SQTS), Brugada syndrome, or catecholaminergic polymorphic ventricular tachycardia (CPVT)?			
13. Has anyone in your family had a pacemaker or an implanted defibrillator before age 35?			

BOX 25.2—cont'd

BONE AND JOINT QUESTIONS		Yes	No
14. Have you ever had a stress fracture or an injury to a bone, muscle, ligament, joint, or tendon that caused you to miss a practice or game?			
15. Do you have a bone, muscle, ligament, or joint injury that bothers you?			
MEDICAL QUESTIONS		**Yes**	**No**
16. Do you cough, wheeze, or have difficulty breathing during or after exercise?			
17. Are you missing a kidney, an eye, a testicle, your spleen, or any other organ?			
18. Do you have groin or testicle pain or a painful bulge or hernia in the groin area?			
19. Do you have any recurring skin rashes or rashes that come and go, including herpes or methicillin-resistant Staphylococcus aureus (MRSA)?			
20. Have you had a concussion or head injury that caused confusion, a prolonged headache, or memory problems?			
21. Have you ever had numbness, had tingling, had weakness in your arms or legs, or been unable to move your arms or legs after being hit or falling?			
22. Have you ever become ill while exercising in the heat?			
23. Do you or does someone in your family have sickle cell trait or disease?	Unsure		
24. Have you ever had or do you have any problems with your eyes or vision?			

MEDICAL QUESTIONS (*CONTINUED)*		Yes	No
25. Do you worry about your weight?			
26. Are you trying to or has anyone recommended that you gain or lose weight?			
27. Are you on a special diet or do you avoid certain types of foods or food groups?			
28. Have you ever had an eating disorder?			
MENSTRUAL QUESTIONS	**N/A**	**Yes**	**No**
29. Have you ever had a menstrual period?			
30. How old were you when you had your first menstrual period?			
31. When was your most recent menstrual period?			
32. How many periods have you had in the past 12 months?			

Explain "Yes" answers here.

____

____

____

____

____

____

____

____

____

____

____

____

I hereby state that, to the best of my knowledge, my answers to the questions on this form are complete and correct.

Signature of athlete: ____

Signature of parent or guardian: ____

Date: ______________________________

Continued

BOX 25.2—cont'd

This form should be placed into the athlete's medical file and should *not* be shared with schools or sports organizations.

PREPARTICIPATION PHYSICAL EVALUATION

PHYSICAL EXAMINATION FORM

Name: ______________________________ Date of birth: ______________

PHYSICIAN REMINDERS

1. Consider additional questions on more-sensitive issues.
   - Do you feel stressed out or under a lot of pressure?
   - Do you ever feel sad, hopeless, depressed, or anxious?
   - Do you feel safe at your home or residence?
   - Have you ever tried cigarettes, e-cigarettes, chewing tobacco, snuff, or dip?
   - During the past 30 days, did you use chewing tobacco, snuff, or dip?
   - Do you drink alcohol or use any other drugs?
   - Have you ever taken anabolic steroids or used any other performance-enhancing supplement?
   - Have you ever taken any supplements to help you gain or lose weight or improve your performance?
   - Do you wear a seat belt, use a helmet, and use condoms?
2. Consider reviewing questions on cardiovascular symptoms (Q4–Q13 of history form).

EXAMINATION		
Height: Weight:		
BP: / (/) Pulse: Vision: R 20/ L 20/ Corrected: ☐ Y ☐ N		
MEDICAL	**NORMAL**	**ABNORMAL FINDINGS**
Appearance • Marfan stigmata (kyphoscoliosis, high-arched palate, pectus excavatum, arachnodactyly, hyperlaxity, myopia, mitral valve prolapse [MVP], and aortic insufficiency)		
Eyes, ears, nose, and throat • Pupils equal • Hearing		
Lymph nodes		
Heart[a] • Murmurs (auscultation standing, auscultation supine, and ± Valsalva maneuver)		
Lungs		
Abdomen		
Skin • Herpes simplex virus (HSV), lesions suggestive of methicillin-resistant Staphylococcus aureus (MRSA), or tinea corporis		
Neurological		
MUSCULOSKELETAL	**NORMAL**	**ABNORMAL FINDINGS**
Neck		
Back		
Shoulder and arm		
Elbow and forearm		
Wrist, hand, and fingers		
Hip and thigh		
Knee		
Leg and ankle		
Foot and toes		
Functional • Double-leg squat test, single-leg squat test, and box drop or step drop test		

[a]Consider electrocardiography (ECG), echocardiography, referral to a cardiologist for abnormal cardiac history or examination findings, or a combination of those.

Name of health care professional (print or type): ______________________ Date: __________

Address: ______________________________ Phone: __________

Signature of health care professional: ______________________ , MD, DO, NP, or PA

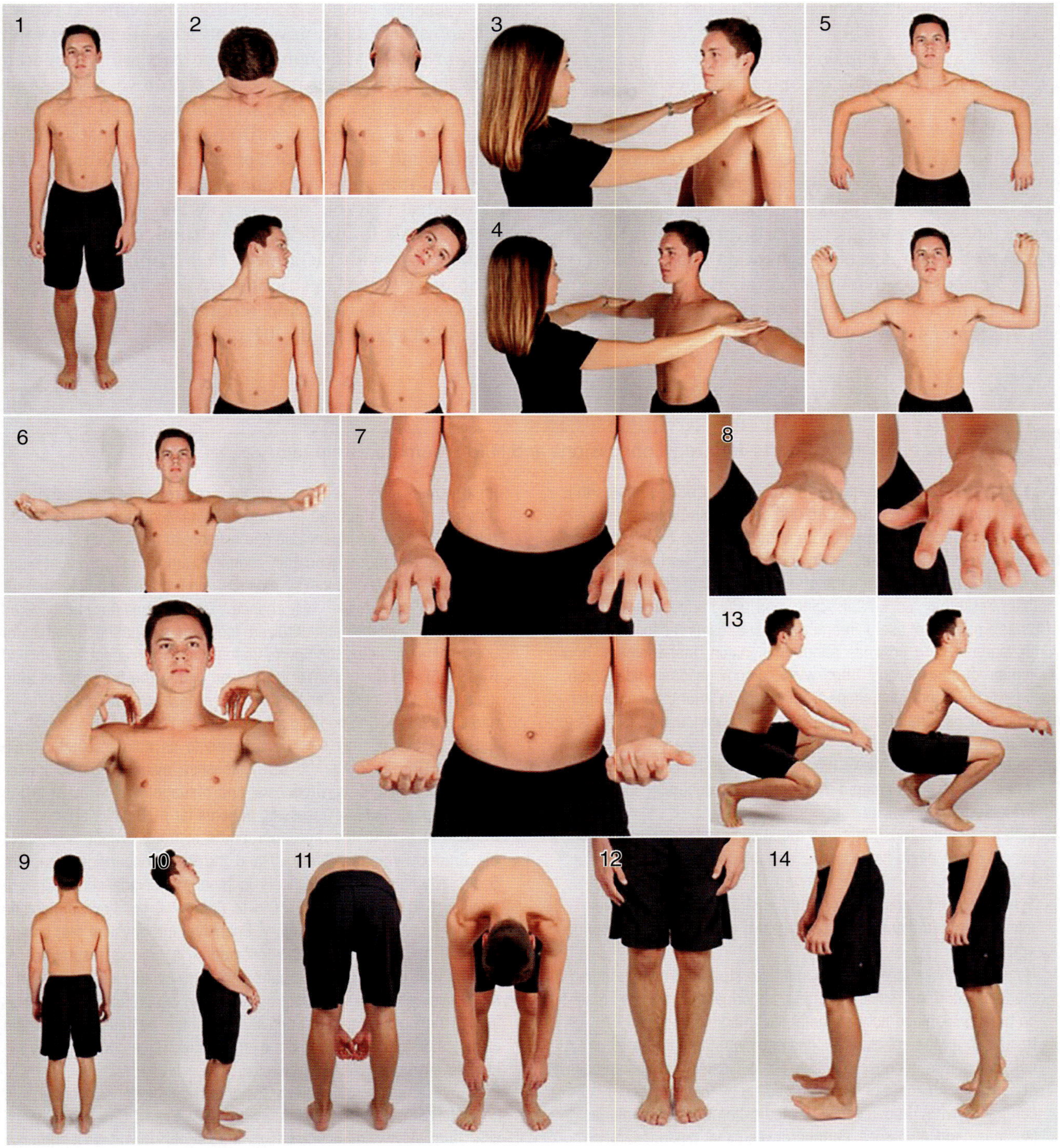

FIG. 25.2 Musculoskeletal screening examination. The general musculoskeletal screening examination consists of the following: (1) inspection, athlete standing, facing toward examiner (symmetry of trunk, upper extremities); (2) forward flexion, extension, rotation, lateral flexion of neck (range of motion, cervical spine); (3) resisted shoulder shrug (strength, trapezius); (4) resisted shoulder abduction (strength, deltoid); (5) internal and external rotation of shoulder (range of motion, glenohumeral joint); (6) extension and flexion of elbow (range of motion, elbow and wrist); (7) pronation and supination of the elbow (range of motion, elbow and wrist); (8) clench fist, then spread fingers (range of motion, hand and fingers); (9) inspection, athlete facing away from examiner (symmetry of trunk, upper extremities); (10) back extension, knees straight (spondylolysis/spondylolisthesis); (11) back flexion with knees straight, facing toward and away from the examiner (range of motion, thoracic and lumbosacral spine; spine curvature; hamstring flexibility); (12) inspection of the lower extremities, contraction of quadriceps muscles (alignment, symmetry); (13) "duck walk" four steps (motion of hip, knee, and ankle; strength; balance); and (14) standing on toes, then on heels (symmetry, calf; strength; balance). (From Miller, S. M., & Peterson, A. R. (2019). The sports preparticipation evaluation. *Pediatrics in Review*, *40*(3), 108–128.)

The clinician should also assess the following:

- Gait
- Patient's ability to hop on each foot
- Patient's ability to walk on tiptoes and heels

Guidance After Preparticipation Physical Evaluations

Patients with findings from the PPE may require evaluation by clinicians with appropriate knowledge and experience to assess the safety of a given sport for the athlete. This may include professionals in sports medicine, orthopedic surgery, cardiology, neurology, physical therapy, and others. Box 25.3 discusses guidelines for patients who have experienced a concussion. Two conditions considered absolute contraindications to sports participation are myocarditis and fever. Myocarditis is the third most common cause of sudden cardiac death in young athletes after hypertrophic cardiomyopathy and anomalous coronary artery (Spencer & Quraishi, 2023). Fever may occur with myocarditis, and it is independently associated with an increased risk of heat-related illness. A good rule: Do not suggest that an athlete "play through" an injury or a problem. If a condition is identified that may restrict a patient's participation, referral to a specialist may be necessary. When it is determined there is risk to participation, shared decision making should occur with the athlete, their family, and an interdisciplinary team. Restricting participation may lead to psychological distress, and emotional support should be offered (McDonald et al., 2021)

BOX 25.3 Patient Safety: Sports-Related Concussions and Mild Traumatic Brain Injury

The Centers for Disease Control and Prevention (CDC) estimates that in the United States more than 280,000 children and adolescents are treated each year in emergency departments (EDs) for sports- and recreation-related traumatic brain injuries (TBIs; Sarmiento et al., 2019). Sports associated with the greatest number of ED visits include football, basketball, soccer, bicycling, and playground activities. The CDC has a number of useful interactive online resources for clinicians, youth, parents, and coaches about recognition, management, and prevention of concussions (http://www.cdc.gov/headsup/index.html). Based on the recommendations from the Sixth International Conference on Concussion in Sport, "a sports-related concussion (SRC) is a traumatic brain injury:

1. Caused by a direct blow to the head, neck, or body, resulting in an impulsive force transmitted to the brain that occurs in sports and exercise-related activities.
2. Initiates a neurotransmitter and metabolic cascade, with possible axonal injury, blood flow change, and inflammation affecting the brain.
3. Symptoms and signs may present immediately, or evolve over minutes or hours, and commonly resolve within days, but may be prolonged.
4. No abnormalities [are] seen on standard structural neuroimaging studies, but in the research setting, abnormalities may be present on functional, blood flow, or metabolic imaging studies.
5. Results in a range of clinical signs and symptoms that may or may not involve loss of consciousness. The clinical symptoms and signs of concussion cannot be explained solely by (but may occur concomitantly with) drug, alcohol, or medication use, other injuries (such as cervical injuries, peripheral vestibular dysfunction), or other comorbidities (such as psychological factors or coexisting medical conditions)" (Patricios et al., 2023).

Evaluation should involve a comprehensive history and complete neurologic examination, determination of clinical status (i.e., improvement or worsening since the occurrence of the injury), and determination of the need for head imaging. A diagnosis of a sports-related concussion can include one or more of the following features: co-clinical symptoms (somatic, cognitive, emotional), physical signs (e.g., loss of consciousness), balance impairment, cognitive impairment, and sleep/wake disturbance. These domains are covered in publicly available standardized tools for evaluating athletes for concussion, including the Sports Concussion Assessment Tool version 6 (SCAT6) and Child SCAT6 to be used within the first 7 days after injury and the Sports Concussion Office Assessment Tool (SCOAT6) and Child SCOAT6 to be used after the initial 72 hours.

A concussion may also be referred to as mild traumatic brain injury (mTBI). In 2018, the CDC published evidence-based guidelines on the diagnosis, prognosis, and management of mTBI in the pediatric population. In assessing patients for mTBI, they recommend the use of a validated, age-appropriate symptom rating scale, like the Graded Symptom Checklist and the Post Concussion Symptom Scale. When an mTBI diagnosis is made, clinicians should inform families that most children (70% to 80%) will not have difficulties beyond 1 to 3 months postinjury. Cognitive and physical rest should occur in the first several days followed by a gradual resumption of activity that does not exacerbate symptoms, with close monitoring. An active rehabilitation program with the progressive reintroduction of noncontact aerobic activity may then be introduced, again closely monitoring for symptom exacerbation. Once children have remained asymptomatic with increasing their level of physical activity, they can return to full activity. Social and emotional support should be routinely assessed in children with mTBI. The CDC Heads Up website (http://www.cdc.gov/headsup/index.html) includes a number of resources for resuming physical activity and returning to school. For children who have prolonged symptoms or academic challenges, health care providers should refer families to a TBI specialist (Lumba-Brown et al., 2018).

Patient Safety

Female Athlete Triad and Relative Energy Deficiency in Sport

A trio of conditions—low energy availability with or without disordered eating, menstrual dysfunction, and low bone mineral density—define the female athlete triad. In a study of 323 collegiate female athletes, 25% were found to be at moderate to high risk for suffering a bone stress injury. Young females at greater risk were more likely to participate in sports that stress the need to be lean (cross-country running, gymnastics, and lacrosse). Of 16 sports, cross-country runners experienced the highest proportion of injuries (Tenforde et al., 2017). In 2014, the International Olympic Committee (IOC) renamed the triad to relative energy deficiency in sport (RED-S) that occurs in both males and females as the result of insufficient caloric intake and/or excessive energy expenditure. In addition to bone health and menstrual function, RED-S can negatively affect an individual's metabolism, immunity, protein synthesis, cardiovascular system, and mental well-being (Statuta et al., 2017). While there is ongoing debate, experts believe the female athletic triad and RED-S should be considered separate entities (De Souza et al., 2022). Early recognition of both is essential, and the PPE is an ideal time for assessing risk factors. A review of prior injuries, diet, weight loss, exercise, menstrual history, and mood changes should be routine.

Identify an energy deficit, in which calorie expenditure exceeds calorie intake. This may sometimes occur unintentionally, but at other times intentionally (e.g., binging and purging; using laxatives, diuretics, and diet pills). The body may adapt at first so that the problem may have a subtle onset. In studies using screening questionnaires, the prevalence of eating disorders in elite athletes ranged from 0% to 13.6% for males and 7.4% to 50% for females (Fatt et al., 2024). Clinicians should review responses on the PPE history form, which includes questions about weight perception, plans to gain or lose weight, special diets, and history of an eating disorder (see Box 25.2).

Primary amenorrhea (no onset of menses by 16 years of age), secondary amenorrhea (no periods for three cycles in a row or 6 months), or oligomenorrhea (intervals between periods longer than 35 days) are all possibilities in female patients with these conditions. These findings are not a normal response to exercise. Secondary amenorrhea occurs in approximately 2% to 5% of the general female population. In a 5-year retrospective study of female college athletes, 20% reported menstrual disturbances (Ackerman & Misra, 2018). More than half of adult bone calcium is deposited during the teenage years, making this a particularly vulnerable time. A too-thin body encourages a low estrogen state and the possibility of menstrual dysfunction and a resultant osteopenia or osteoporosis. The risk of stress fracture increases. A multidisciplinary team is often needed to support athletes with the goal of correcting and maintaining energy balance. Questions about menses are also included on the PPE history form.

CHAPTER

26 Emergency or Life-Threatening Situations

An emergency situation, whether it is unresponsiveness, an acute medical condition, drug overdose, or trauma, requires a change in the usual sequence of history taking and examination. Life-threatening conditions, such as airway obstruction, cardiac arrest, hypovolemic shock, and respiratory failure, must be identified rapidly and managed. The steps to complete the assessment for life-threatening conditions take seconds, not minutes. The rapid sequential assessment process focuses on patient physiology to identify priority lifesaving interventions.

In an emergency, the patient is assessed and treatment priorities are established based on the presenting physiologic findings, with a goal of physiologic stability rather than making a diagnosis. National organizations such as the American College of Surgeons Committee on Trauma and the American Heart Association have defined an approach for the emergency assessment of patients with trauma and cardiac arrest. Using this approach, the patient's vital functions are determined quickly through a rapid primary assessment with resuscitation of vital functions as necessary (Box 26.1 presents the basic life support assessment sequence). During the emergency, the responding examiners need to protect themselves with appropriate personal protective equipment (PPE).

Emergency Assessment of the Injured Patient

The Primary Survey

The primary survey or initial assessment is rapidly completed. With a stable patient, it may only take 30 seconds, but it may take several minutes when a mechanism of injury or the patient's physiologic responses make you suspect a potential critical condition. The patient history, obtained during the primary survey, is often limited to the chief concern (e.g., the mechanism of injury or primary symptom). The primary survey (initial assessment) includes addressing basic life support and integrates rapid assessment for life-threatening injuries.

Hemorrhage. Perform a rapid inspection for excessive bleeding. Control visible bleeding with manual pressure while continuing the primary survey, and estimate the amount of blood loss from visible blood on dressings or pooled around the patient. A tourniquet around an extremity proximal to the injury may be needed in cases of uncontrolled bleeding.

Airway and Cervical Spine. The patency of the upper airway and responsiveness are assessed by asking the patient a question. If the patient answers, the patient is responsive, and the airway is open at this time (Box 26.2). Keep the patient talking so that you know the airway is being maintained. Have suction equipment readily available to prevent aspiration in case the patient vomits.

If the patient does not respond, place your ear close to the patient's nose and mouth to detect any air movement (Fig. 26.1), while simultaneously looking for chest movement. Look for any blood, vomitus, teeth, or foreign bodies that may be obstructing the airway. Determine whether any fractures of the mandible, face, or larynx could be obstructing the airway.

If the airway is obstructed and the patient is supine, use a chin lift or jaw thrust (if any potential injury to the cervical spine has occurred) to raise the tongue (the most common cause of airway obstruction) out of the oropharynx (Fig. 26.2). Do not hyperextend, hyperflex, or rotate the patient's head and neck to establish or maintain the airway. Remove blood, vomitus, or foreign bodies from the airway by suction. Endotracheal intubation is frequently performed to control and protect the airway, especially when the patient is unresponsive.

The cervical spine must be stabilized when performing any airway maneuvers or moving the patient in cases of multisystem injury or trauma above the clavicles. Excessive movement of the cervical spine can convert a fracture or dislocation without neurologic damage to one with neurologic injury. Stabilize the cervical spine by manually maintaining the neck in a neutral position, in alignment with the body (Fig. 26.3) until a cervical collar can be applied. Once the patient's vital functions are more stable, radiologic imaging of all seven cervical vertebrae is often obtained to diagnose the presence or absence of cervical spine injury.

Breathing. Expose the patient's chest to assess breathing effort and to observe bilateral chest movement synchronized with breathing. Identify paradoxical chest movement (the entire chest does not rise and fall in synchrony), open chest wounds, and bruising. Note the rate and depth

BOX 26.1 Basic Life Support Survey for an Unconscious Patient

First: Check for responsiveness and for abnormal (gasping) or absent breathing (no chest movement).
Second: Call for emergency responders and get a defibrillator if one is available, or send someone to do this.
Third: Check for the carotid pulse for 10 seconds.
- If no pulse, begin cardiopulmonary resuscitation. Perform chest compressions at a rate of 100 per minute, interrupting after 30 compressions to give 2 breaths. Repeat cycles of 30 compressions and 2 breaths.
- If a pulse is present, begin rescue breathing at 10 to 12 breaths per minute.

Fourth: If no pulse, use the defibrillator when it arrives to check for a shockable rhythm.
- Provide shocks as indicated.
- Resume cardiopulmonary resuscitation immediately after each shock.

Modified from Kleinman, M. E., Brennan, E. E., Goldberger, Z. D., et al. (2015). Part 5: Adult basic life support and cardiopulmonary resuscitation quality. *Circulation, 132*(Suppl. 2), S414–S435.

BOX 26.2 Assessment of Airway Patency

Signs of Obstruction
- Hoarse voice and/or cough, sometimes characterized as a "bark"
- Apprehension: tense, deeply worried facial expression
- Stridor: severity related to extent of obstruction and the patient's respiratory effort
  - Inspiratory: obstruction at the glottis, epiglottis
  - Expiratory: obstruction below the glottis (wheezing)
- Retraction
  - Suprasternal notch: obstruction at or above trachea
  - Intercostal and subcostal, below suprasternal notch: obstruction in bronchial tree or below
- Altered mental status
- Drooling (difficulty swallowing): obstruction at glottis or above
- Bleeding from mouth or nose
- Subcutaneous emphysema, particularly with trauma
- Facial or mandible fracture, often palpable

Symptoms of Obstruction
- Respiratory distress: dyspnea, tachypnea
- Difficulty swallowing
- Pain, such as a sore throat
- Cough and associated strain or change in voice
- Behavior change: restlessness or lethargy

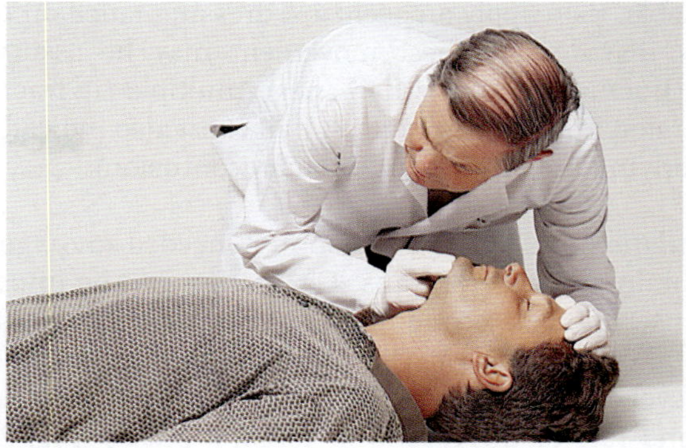

FIG. 26.1 Look, listen, and feel for adequate breathing to assess patency of the upper airway.

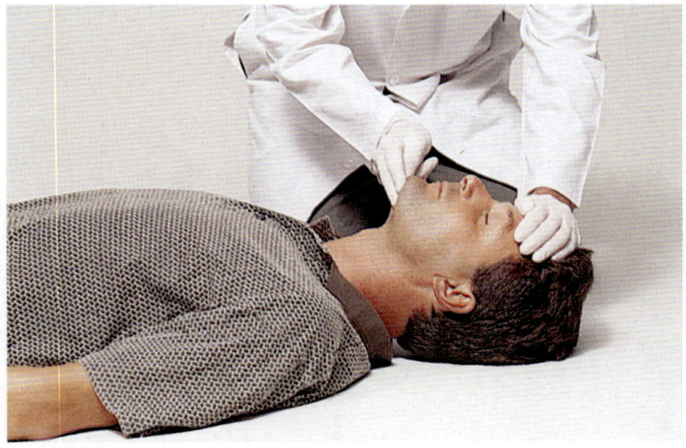

FIG. 26.2 Use a chin lift to lift the tongue out of the oropharynx and ensure an open airway.

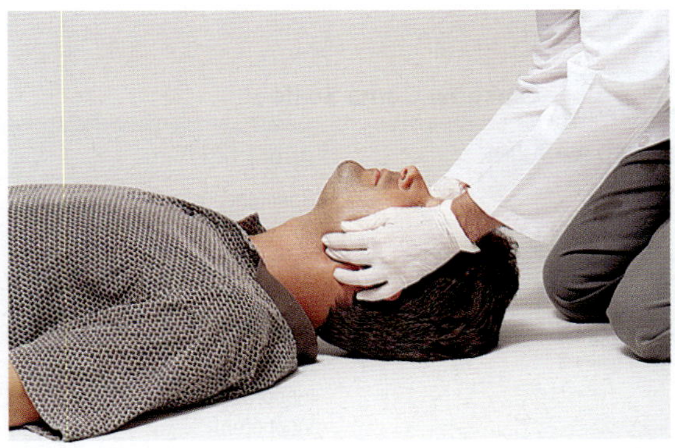

FIG. 26.3 Properly position both hands to stabilize and maintain the head and neck in a neutral position in alignment with the body.

of respirations. Use the stethoscope to auscultate for the presence of bilateral breath sounds. Note any signs of respiratory distress such as retractions, tachypnea, and cyanosis. Apply a pulse oximeter if available.

Palpate the upper chest and neck for crepitation, a sign of air leakage into soft tissue. Bruising should alert you to the possibility of a pulmonary contusion (bruising of the lung tissue caused by the energy of an external impact transmitted through the chest wall). This injury may result in a pneumothorax (air leakage into the pleural space causing lung collapse).

Provide high concentration oxygen and ventilatory assistance with a bag-valve-mask, when needed, as the primary survey assessment continues. Cover open chest wounds immediately with a hand to minimize the entry of atmospheric air into the chest until definitive treatment is available, then apply an occlusive dressing taped on three sides. Paradoxical chest movement may be associated with fractured ribs or a flail chest (multiple rib fractures separated from the rib cage). A flail chest also indicates an underlying lung injury (pulmonary contusion).

Circulation. Adequate circulation is needed to oxygenate the brain and other organs. Circulation can be impaired because of cardiac conditions, hemorrhage, dehydration, and other medical conditions. To assess circulation, note the level of responsiveness; skin color; and presence, quality, and rate of the carotid or femoral pulses (Fig. 26.4). Use the capillary refill time to assess the adequacy of tissue perfusion. Press firmly over a nail bed or bony prominence (e.g., chin, forehead, or sternum) until the skin blanches. Remove the pressure and count the seconds it takes for color to return. A capillary refill time in excess of 2 seconds in a central location (e.g., sternum or chin) indicates poor perfusion.

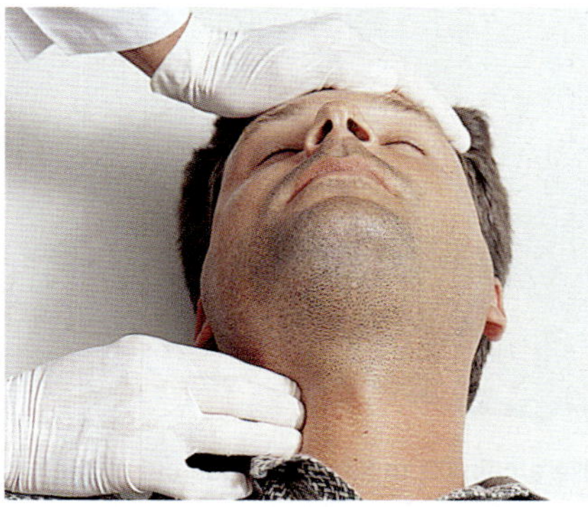

FIG. 26.4 Check the carotid pulse to confirm circulation, one side at a time.

Perform a quick total body appraisal for additional bleeding sites, being especially careful to look and feel for dampness in dark clothing that may hide hemorrhage. Consider the possibility of internal hemorrhage with some mechanisms of injury. Hypovolemic shock can occur with significant blood loss from external bleeding or from internal bleeding into the thoracic and abdominal cavities (see "Shock State" in "Abnormalities"). Replacement of intravascular volume is initiated with warmed intravenous fluids and then blood products for hemorrhage.

Disability. A brief neurologic evaluation is performed to identify significant disability. Assess the patient's responsiveness with AVPU or level of consciousness with the Glasgow Coma Scale (Table 26.1). (See Clinical Pearl, *Mnemonic AVPU*.) This tool allows numeric scoring of the patient's verbal, motor, and eye-opening responses to specific stimuli to assess the cerebral cortex and brainstem function. Different versions are available for the adult and young child. The Glasgow Coma Scale score should be repeated at intervals to detect changes. A decreased or decreasing level of consciousness may indicate severe brain injury as well as hypoxemia or hypovolemic shock, necessitating a reevaluation of the patient's airway, breathing, and circulation. See Table 7.1 in Chapter 7 for common causes of unresponsiveness. Additional neurologic assessments to be performed include the pupillary size and reactivity, lateralizing signs, or spinal cord injury level.

TABLE 26.1 Glasgow Coma Scale

ASSESSED BEHAVIOR	ADULT CRITERIA	INFANT AND YOUNG CHILD CRITERIA	SCORE
Eye opening	Spontaneous opening	Spontaneous opening	4
	To verbal stimuli	To loud noise or voice	3
	To pain	To pain	2
	No response	No response	1
Verbal response	Oriented to appropriate stimulation	Smiles, coos, cries	5
	Confused	Irritable, cries	4
	Inappropriate words	Inappropriate crying	3
	Incoherent	Grunts, moans	2
	None	No response	1
Motor response	Obeys commands	Spontaneous movement	6
	Localizes pain	Withdraws from touch	5
	Withdraws from pain	Withdraws from pain	4
	Flexion to pain (decorticate)	Abnormal flexion (decorticate)	3
	Extension to pain (decerebrate)	Abnormal extension (decerebrate)	2
	None	No response	1

The patient's best response in each category is matched to the criteria for scoring. Appropriate verbal stimuli are questions eliciting the patient's level of orientation to person, place, and time. Painful stimuli are used when necessary to obtain eye opening and motor responses. Begin with less painful stimuli (e.g., pinching the skin) and progress to squeezing muscle mass or tendons if there is no response. Three scores are summed for the total Glasgow Coma Scale score. A maximum score of 15 indicates the optimal level of consciousness, and a minimal score of 3 indicates deepest coma.

Modified from Bethel, J. (2012). Emergency care of children and adults with head injury. *Nursing Standard (Royal College of Nursing (Great Britain): 1987), 26*(43), 49–58; James, H. E. (1986). Neurologic evaluation and support of the child with acute brain insult. *Pediatric Annals, 15*(1), 16; Teasdale, G., & Jennett, B. (1974). Assessment of coma and impaired consciousness: A practical scale. *Lancet, 2*, 81–84; and Teasdale, G., Maas, A., Lecky, F., et al. (2014). The Glasgow Coma Scale at 40 years: Standing the test of time. *Lancet Neurology, 13*, 844–854.

CLINICAL PEARL

Mnemonic AVPU

A quick way to initially assess a patient's level of responsiveness is with the *mnemonic AVPU*:
A Alert: no stimuli needed
V Verbal stimuli: responsive to
P Painful stimuli: responsive to
U Unresponsive to verbal and pain stimuli

Exposure and Environmental Control. In cases of trauma, undress the patient as completely as possible to facilitate a brief body search for major injuries that may have been missed during the prior steps of the primary survey. Hypothermia is a concern, so use warm blankets, warmed intravenous fluids, and a warm environment to maintain the patient's body temperature. See Clinical Pearl, "Delay Secondary Assessment to Resuscitate."

CLINICAL PEARL

Delay Secondary Assessment to Resuscitate

Lifesaving measures—hemorrhage control, chest compressions, airway management, defibrillation, oxygen, assisted ventilation, intravenous fluids, and medications—are initiated first, rather than after completion of the assessment. Once the life-threatening problem is stabilized, the initial assessment is continued or repeated. Only when all vital functions have been assessed and treated is an effort made to identify the cause or diagnose the emergency condition through a more detailed head-to-toe assessment and history.

Secondary Assessment of the Injured Patient

Assess the vital signs (heart and respiratory rates, blood pressure, oxygen saturation) before beginning the head-to-toe survey of the body to identify additional injuries. Compare the patient's vital sign values to expected values for age and condition. Recognize that vital sign values above or below those expected for the person's age may indicate physiologic derangement or preexisting health conditions.

History. Usually someone other than the examiner obtains an abbreviated history from the patient, family, emergency medical technicians, or scene bystanders. Pertinent information is then shared with the examiner during the assessment process. See Clinical Pearl, "AMPLE Abbreviated History."

CLINICAL PEARL

AMPLE Abbreviated History

This history focuses on information relevant to the emergency condition. Use the *mnemonic AMPLE* to remember the key categories of this history.
A Allergies
M Medications or drugs of any type currently being used by the patient
P Past illnesses (e.g., diabetes, epilepsy, hypertension); Pregnancy
L Last meal
E Events preceding the precipitating event; Environment related to the injury

Identify the mechanism of injury that describes the nature and force of the energy transmitted to the body. Because the mechanism of injury is associated with patterns of injury, it provides important clues about physiologic responses and interventions needed (see "Blunt Trauma" and "Penetrating Trauma" sections). It is also important to identify potential exposure to hazardous materials (e.g., chemicals or toxins).

Head and Neck. Inspect and palpate the face, head, and scalp, looking for any depressions, bone instability, crepitus, lacerations, contusions, penetrating injuries, or drainage from the ears or nose. Clear or amber-colored drainage from the nose or ears may indicate a basilar skull fracture with a cerebrospinal fluid leak. Use an otoscope to inspect the tympanic membranes for blood in the middle ear. Note any bruising around the eyes (raccoon eyes) or behind the ears (Battle sign), indicating a basilar skull fracture (Fig. 26.5). Assess facial structures for any fractures.

Examine the eyes for pupillary size and responsiveness to light. Examine the retinas and conjunctivae for hemorrhage and the lens for dislocation. A quick visual examination of both eyes is performed by asking a conscious patient to read the words on the side of any container. Extraocular movements are also examined.

Inspect the neck for unexpected findings such as penetrating injury, bruising (e.g., seatbelt mark), and tracheal deviation from the midline. Palpate for deformity and crepitus. Auscultate the carotid arteries for bruits. Be certain that the neck is manually maintained in neutral position until radiographic studies confirm the absence of cervical injury when cervical injury is suspected. See Clinical Pearl, "Identifying Risk for Cervical Spine Injury."

CLINICAL PEARL

Identifying Risk for Cervical Spine Injury

Factors that place an injured patient at higher risk for cervical spine injury include a history of a fall from a height greater than 3 feet or five stairs, high-speed motor vehicle crash with rollover or ejection, all-terrain vehicle crash, or bicycle collision with a fixed object. Injured patients 65 years or older are at greater risk. Cervical spine fractures and dislocations can result from severe trauma caused by events including falls, motor vehicle accidents, and sports injuries. Common symptoms of cervical spine injury often include neck pain, which can move to other areas, such as the head, jaw, and shoulders. Additionally, individuals with such injuries may experience sensations of numbness and weakness in various parts of the body.

Chest. Inspect the anterior and posterior chest for bruising and obvious signs of deformity. Palpate the sternum, each rib, and clavicle. Note pain and dyspnea. Blunt sternal pressure will be painful if any attached ribs are fractured. Patterns of bruising may indicate the mechanism of injury, such as a steering wheel or tire track, and may signal a possible pulmonary contusion.

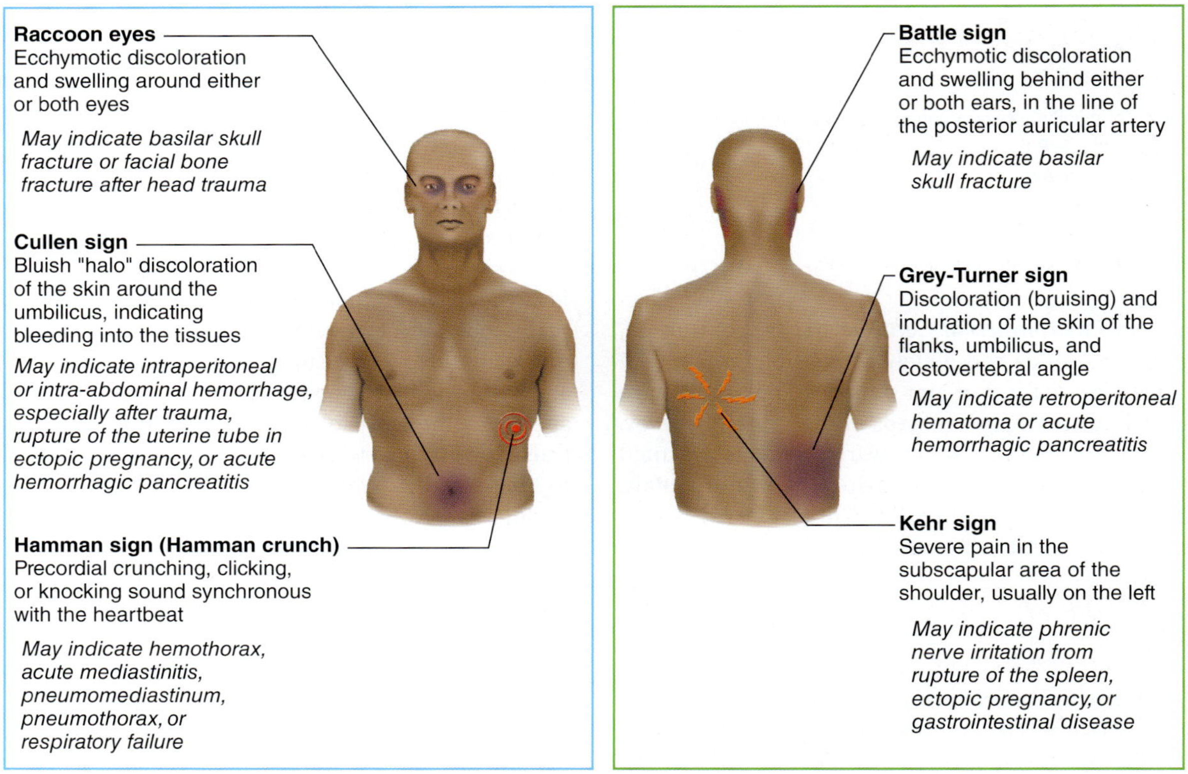

FIG. 26.5 Signs that indicate serious injury associated with trauma.

Auscultate breath sounds at the apex, base, and midaxillary areas. Note any diminished or absent breath sounds, which may indicate a pneumothorax or hemothorax (bleeding into the pleural space). Auscultate the heart for clarity of heart sounds. Distant, muffled heart sounds may indicate cardiac tamponade, a life-threatening condition where blood fills the pericardial space; however, heart sounds may be difficult to hear in a noisy environment. Distended neck veins (increased jugular venous pressure) may indicate cardiac tamponade, pneumothorax, or any problem that causes obstruction of the cardiovascular system. However, hypovolemia may prevent distention of neck veins. A tension pneumothorax may manifest with decreased breath sounds, hyperresonance to percussion, and shock. Chest imaging is used to confirm examination findings when time permits.

Abdomen. Inspect the abdomen for bruising and distention. Gently palpate the abdomen, noting guarding and pain. Solid and hollow organs (e.g., intestines) in the abdomen may be ruptured as a result of blunt trauma and result in occult hemorrhage; pain and distention may indicate an underlying hemorrhage (see Fig. 26.5). Diagnostic imaging may be performed.

Extremities and Back. Inspect and palpate all extremities for signs of fractures or deformities, crepitus, pain, and lack of spontaneous movement. Palpation of the bones with rotational or three-point pressure along the shaft helps identify fractures where alignment has been maintained. Note any wounds over the site of a suspected fracture, the possible indication of an open fracture. Palpate all peripheral pulses. It is particularly important to document skin temperature, capillary refill time, and the presence of distal pulses in extremities with a suspected fracture.

Maintain cervical spine stabilization and alignment of the thoracic and lumbar spine when inspecting the back. Use three people to log-roll the patient.

Suspect pelvic fractures if bruising is seen over the iliac wings, pubis, labia, or scrotum and by pain on palpation. If the patient is unconscious, an experienced examiner should test for mobility of the pelvic ring by placing gentle anterior and posterior pressure against the iliac wings and symphysis pubis with the heels of the hands. The maneuver is not repeated as it can cause additional bleeding. Pelvic fractures are associated with occult hemorrhage, which may become a life-threatening condition.

Rectum and Perineum. Inspect the peritoneum for bruising, lacerations, or urethral bleeding. Perform a rectal examination to detect blood within the bowel lumen, a high-riding prostate (associated with genitourinary injury), pelvic fractures, the integrity of the abdominal wall, and the quality of sphincter tone. A vaginal examination is sometimes performed to assess for bleeding and lacerations.

Neurologic Examination. Perform a more complete neurologic evaluation once the patient's condition has been stabilized. Reassess the patient's Glasgow Coma Scale score (see Table 26.1) as well as pupillary size and reactivity. Then perform a more detailed motor and sensory evaluation (see Chapter 23). Note any paralysis or paresis, which suggests major injury to the spinal column or peripheral nervous system. Record the location of pain and its intensity.

Reevaluate the Patient. Reevaluate the patient frequently so that any new signs and symptoms are not overlooked. Perform the primary survey every 5 minutes and compare the results with those obtained in previous assessments to detect if deterioration in the patient's condition is occurring. Monitor vital signs continuously. Frequently monitor the patient's level of consciousness to detect deterioration in neurologic functioning. As life-threatening conditions are managed, other equally life-threatening problems may develop and less severe conditions may become evident. A high index of suspicion and constant alertness during the examination may lead to earlier recognition of conditions and their needed management.

Injury Mechanisms

When the patient has been injured, a history of the injury and identification of the injury mechanism (blunt or penetrating) will help to determine the severity of the injury.

Blunt Trauma

Blunt trauma mechanisms include motor vehicle crashes, falls, being struck by an object, and various recreational or sports activities. The force, surface the body struck, direction of impact, and body part affected determine the severity and pattern of injuries. For example, motor vehicle crashes account for the majority of severe blunt trauma cases. Emergency personnel at the scene should describe the appearance of the vehicle, the damage sustained to the passenger compartment, and passenger restraint. From that information the emergency trauma team can identify the areas of the body that absorbed the greatest transfer of energy and suspect specific injuries. The following are some examples (American College of Surgeons, 2018):

- A bent steering wheel may be associated with an anterior flail chest, pneumothorax, aortic disruption, myocardial contusion, and fractured spleen or liver.
- A bull's-eye fracture of the windshield may be associated with a cervical spine injury and brain injury. The delta V (change in force) associated with deceleration of the brain's movement within the skull has a relationship with the severity of the brain injury. The initial impact (coup injury) is that closest to the point of impact. The brain then moves in the skull and is again injured as it strikes the opposite side of the skull (contrecoup) during deceleration.
- Side impact may be associated with contralateral neck sprain or cervical fracture; lateral flail chest; pneumothorax; aortic disruption; ruptured diaphragm; fractured spleen, kidney, or liver (depending on the side of impact); and fractured pelvis or acetabulum.
- Rear impact collision can result in cervical spine injury or soft tissue injury of the neck.
- Persons ejected from a vehicle are at high risk for multiple severe injuries.

Penetrating Trauma

Penetrating trauma mechanisms include firearm injuries, stabbings, and impalement. Two factors help determine the type of injury and subsequent management:

- The region of the body and organs in the path of the penetrating object
- The transfer of energy is determined by the force of impact by the penetrating object, such as the velocity of the missile, caliber, and distance from the source. Energy transfer is also determined by the rate or change in speed once the missile is inside the patient's body.

Burns

Burns should alert the examiner to the possibility of airway inflammation from smoke, heat, and toxic chemical inhalation and carbon monoxide poisoning. Anticipate airway obstruction in all cases of burns to the face, inhalation injury, hoarseness, and carbon deposits in the mouth or nose. Suspect and assess for additional injuries if the patient was injured in an explosion or might have fallen while attempting to escape a fire. The body surface area and burn depth are determined (Fig. 26.6).

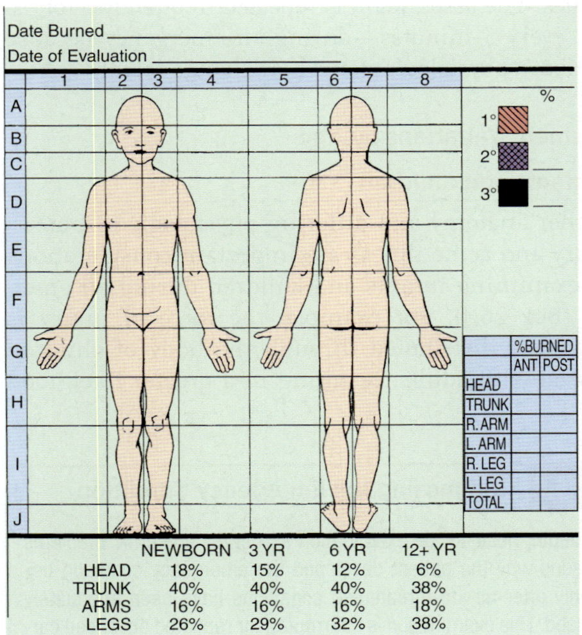

FIG. 26.6 To estimate the total body surface area burned, mark the areas of the patient's burns on the chart. Then estimate the area of each body part burned, using the percentage of body surface area for each body part according to the age of the patient. Insert the percentages into the chart, and sum to obtain the total body surface area burned. *ANT*, Anterior; *POST*, posterior.

Assessment of an Acute Medical Emergency

Advanced Cardiac Life Support Survey

Once the basic life support survey has been completed and the patient is conscious, additional assessment is needed. Perform a systematic rapid examination of the patient's vital functions and physiologic status in a sequence known as the CABs (Circulation, *A*irway, *B*reathing). This rapid assessment process is also known as the *primary survey* or *initial assessment*. The immediate goal is to identify life-threatening conditions such as no pulse, airway obstruction, or impaired ventilation and hypoxemia—the physiologic responses to an acute medical emergency.

- **Circulation:** Identify the presence of the carotid pulse. If there is no pulse after 15 seconds, begin chest compressions. When available, attach a cardiac monitor or defibrillator to identify the cardiac rhythm and potential need for defibrillation.
- **Airway:** Identify an obstructed airway or need for an airway management device (e.g., endotracheal tube).
- **Breathing:** Identify the adequacy of ventilation and oxygenation, including oxygen saturation.
- **Differential diagnosis:** This is the beginning of the physical examination to find and treat reversible causes of the emergency (Box 26.3).

As with serious injuries, the advanced cardiac life support survey is interrupted to manage a life-threatening physiologic condition as soon as it is detected. For example, if a patient is not breathing, rescue breaths, oxygen, and assisted ventilation must be provided before the assessment continues. The assessment is repeated frequently—for example, every 5 minutes—during an emergency because the patient's physiologic status may change rapidly.

Assessment Variations by Age

Infants and Children

A smaller anatomy and differing physiologic responses to injury and acute illness are important considerations when examining infants and children during an emergency (Box 26.4). For example, the force of injury is more widely distributed through the body of children compared with adults, resulting in a greater likelihood of multiple injuries. Additionally, cardiac arrest is rarely a primary event in children as it is in adults; however, some children do experience ventricular fibrillation and cardiac arrest. The child more commonly experiences respiratory and ventilatory failure or shock that progresses to respiratory arrest and subsequent cardiac arrest (American Heart Association, 2016). For this reason, repeated primary assessment of the child with respiratory distress is essential so that deterioration to respiratory failure is prevented.

The assessment sequence and assessment priorities for the infant and child are the same for adults. The child's size, blood volume, and fluid requirements may be smaller, and the disease or the mechanism of injury may be different, but the airway, breathing, and circulation must be ensured. Keep the infant or child warm to prevent hypothermia, which makes all conditions more difficult to manage. Involve the parents as much as possible every step of the way.

During respiratory failure, carbon dioxide is not effectively exhaled, resulting in hypoxia. In the event of hypovolemic shock (poor tissue perfusion), blood is shunted to the vital organs, allowing the child a short period of physiologic compensation. Progression to hypoxemia, acidosis (low blood pH), and tissue acidosis occurs if hypoxia and poor tissue perfusion are not reversed. Early intervention usually prevents progression to cardiac arrest.

Considerations in the emergency assessment of the infant and child include the following:

- A crying or talking child has, at that moment, a patent airway.
- Assessment with AVPU level of responsiveness (see Clinical Pearl, *Mnemonic AVPU*, earlier in the chapter) is as helpful with children as with adults.
- If the child is responsive, attempt to establish rapport with the child consistent with the situation. Try to get as much information as possible when the child will communicate, such as "Please use one finger to show me where it hurts."
- The approximate expected systolic blood pressure for a child older than 1 year: 80 + (2 × child's age in years). This estimated value can be used until the child is stabilized, when a comparison can be made with the actual norms for the child's age, gender, and height percentile.
- Capillary refill time longer than 2 seconds is a marker of poor tissue perfusion, just as for adults.
- Because of the young child's large body surface area, exposure of the body for assessment causes significant heat loss. Try to keep an infant or child warm with heat lamps or a warming blanket during assessment and treatment.
- The mnemonic AMPLE (see Clinical Pearl, "AMPLE Abbreviated History," earlier in the chapter) is also useful for remembering the key elements of the child's history of the emergency. If an infant is only a few weeks old, add questions about the gestational age,

BOX 26.3 Diagnosing the Emergency Condition

An in-depth, head-to-toe examination to identify anatomic problems or reasons why the patient developed the emergency condition begins only after all life-threatening conditions have been adequately addressed. This examination is interrupted for repeated advanced cardiac life support surveys or if any life-threatening condition develops.

Special procedures required for patient assessment, such as imaging and laboratory studies, are usually conducted during the differential diagnosis assessment. Sometimes the reason for a medical emergency may not be readily evident. Table 26.2 defines eight primary symptoms that may be associated with a life-threatening condition.

TABLE 26.2 Symptoms and Risks of Serious and Life-Threatening Conditions

PRIMARY SYMPTOMS	POSSIBLE ACCOMPANYING SYMPTOMS	POSSIBLE DIAGNOSIS	RISK
Vomiting blood or black or dark brown material that resembles coffee grounds	Recurrent bouts of gnawing pain in the upper part of the abdomen Black or tarlike stool Weakness Pallor Progressive fatigue Increased awareness of a rapid heartbeat (palpitations)	Bleeding ulcer of the stomach or duodenum, bleeding from esophageal varices	Possibly fatal hemorrhage
Crushing pain in the center of the chest	Radiation of the pain to the left arm, neck, jaw, shoulder Sweating Nausea and vomiting Unrelenting indigestion Shortness of breath Cool, clammy skin Fainting Feeling of impending doom	Myocardial infarction	Many deaths occur within minutes or hours of the attack, so the speed of treatment is crucial.
Severe throbbing pain in and around one bloodshot eye	Blurred or acute loss of vision in the affected eye Pain, headache Eyeball is both tender and firm to the touch Abnormal sensitivity to light (photosensitivity) Fixed and dilated pupil	Acute glaucoma	Delay in treatment can result in permanent blindness in affected eye. In many cases vision loss occurs very quickly.
Flashes of light in the field of vision of one eye	Absence of pain in the affected eye Black cobweblike floating spots Partial loss of vision spreading as a curtainlike shadow from the top or one side of the eye	Retinal detachment	Extension of detachment with delayed treatment leading to permanent loss of peripheral or central vision depending on area of detachment
Sudden and progressively more severe abdominal pain	Nausea and vomiting Swollen or tender abdomen Severe constipation Temperature greater than 100°F (38°C)	Acute abdomen (e.g., appendicitis, intestinal obstruction)	Delayed treatment can result in rupture or ischemic destruction of the involved organ and peritonitis.
Sudden feeling of weakness and unsteadiness that may result in momentary loss of consciousness	Weakness or paralysis of arm(s) or leg(s) Numbness and/or tingling in any part of the body Excruciating headache Confusion Difficulty speaking Blurred or double vision or loss of vision in one eye	Transient ischemic attack (TIA) or stroke (brain attack)	TIA: Signs last 24 hours, but it may signal an impending stroke. Stroke: The outcome depends on the location and extent of brain deprived of blood supply (see Fig. 23.28). Some are fatal, some cause permanent disability, and some have no long-lasting effect.
Sudden onset of difficulty breathing (often in the middle of the night) and worsens rapidly	Restlessness, anxiety, and sense of doom Increased distress when lying down Swollen ankles Cough producing frothy pink or brownish, blood-flecked sputum Audible bubbling sound when breathing Crackles on auscultation Bluish lips and nail beds Profuse sweating	Pulmonary edema, related to sudden left-sided heart failure	Delayed treatment can be fatal.

any problems during pregnancy and delivery, and any health problems.

- Evaluate the meaning of signs and symptoms with deliberate speed (Table 26.3).
- The child's weight in kilograms is essential for calculating resuscitation medication dosages and intravenous fluid volumes. Parents usually know the child's weight in pounds. The conversion factor is 2.2 lb. = 1 kg. If the weight is not known, a length-based resuscitation tape provides a reasonably close estimate of weight and can guide decisions about the size of equipment, fluid volume, and drug dosages appropriate for the child.

Older Adults

The impaired neurologic and motor function consequent to aging leads to decreased alertness and response to external stimuli; these changes associated with a more active lifestyle conducted by older people expose them to a higher risk of being victims of traumatic events and serious injuries. Trauma is actually the fifth leading cause of

BOX 26.4 Ways in Which Children Differ Physically From Adults

Although children differ physically from adults, the closer they are in age to an adult, the more like an adult they become.

Characteristics of Young Children

Skin

- The skin is thinner, with less subcutaneous fat, and is less protective against burns and more likely to develop hypothermia.

Head

- Until about age 4 years, the head is larger and heavier relative to the rest of the body.
- The bones of the skull are softer and are separated by fibrous tissue and cartilage until about age 5 years; this is somewhat protective against increased intracranial pressure, at least for a short time.
- The developing brain, particularly to age 5 years, is more vulnerable to injury, infection, and poisons. The dura, very firmly attached to the skull, has bridging veins to the brain, which are apt to tear and bleed with inflicted injury, such as with abusive shaking.

Airway

- Nasal passages are relatively smaller and more easily obstructed with discharge or foreign bodies. Because newborns and young infants are obligate nose breathers, they are particularly vulnerable.
- The tongue is relatively larger and more easily able to obstruct the upper airway.
- The trachea is narrower and its cartilage more elastic and collapsible, and is therefore more vulnerable to edema, pressure, and inflammation; hyperextension or flexion can crimp and obstruct.
- The epiglottis is higher and more anterior and is therefore more "available" for aspiration.

Chest and Lungs

- The rib cage is more elastic and flexible, less vulnerable to fracture, and more apt to allow retraction during increased respiratory distress.
- The mediastinum is more mobile and more vulnerable to tension pneumothorax.
- Chest muscles are not well developed. Their use, in addition to the expected diaphragmatic effort, suggests respiratory distress; they tire more easily with prolonged effort.
- The higher metabolic rate and greater oxygen requirement increase vulnerability to hypoxemia.

Heart and Circulation

- Infants and children have a smaller total circulating blood volume but will lose as much blood as an adult from a similar laceration.
- When a significant blood or fluid volume is lost, children compensate and maintain their blood pressure longer than adults do, even to the point of cardiac arrest.
- Bradycardia, usually the initial response to hypoxemia in neonates, may herald cardiac arrest.

Abdomen

- The liver and spleen are relatively larger and more vascular and are less protected by the ribs and abdominal muscles, making them more susceptible to injury.

Extremities

- Bones are not fully calcified and are softer than bones of adults until puberty; more vulnerable to fracture.

Nervous System

- An infant is able to feel pain anywhere in the body but cannot always localize or isolate it; older infants and toddlers can push your hand away from a painful location.
- Children who appear passive in stressful situations and do not seek comforting reassurance from parents may have an altered, depressed level of consciousness or, if alert, may be providing a clue to child abuse.

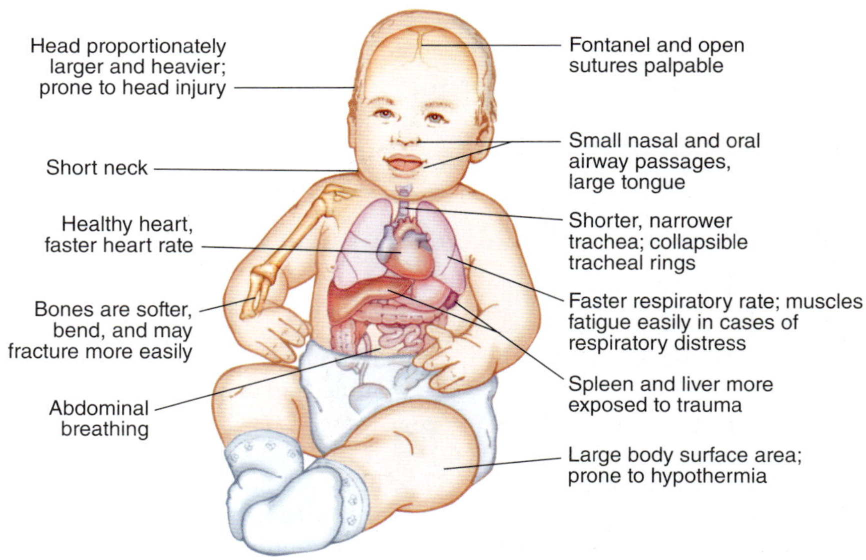

From Child Health Nursing, 3rd Edition, Ball, J., Bindler, R., Cowen, K., & Shaw, M. ISBN: 978-0134624723 Pearson. 2013.

TABLE 26.3 Assessment Findings That Indicate a Sense of Urgency in Infants and Children

PHYSIOLOGY AFFECTED	SIGNS AND SYMPTOMS OF CONCERN
Responsiveness	• Combative or inconsolable • Decreased responsiveness, lethargy • Poor muscle tone • Weak or high-pitched cry, moaning • Personality change, failure to make eye contact, glassy-eyed stare, lack of interest in play or interaction • Does not recognize parents
Airway and breathing	• Respiratory rate greater than 60 breaths per minute, sustained, especially with oxygen administration • Respiratory rate less than 20 breaths per minute, especially in the presence of acute illness or with injury to the chest or abdomen • Respiratory distress, nasal flaring, retractions (intercostal, supraclavicular, and sternal) • Airway sounds: stridor, muffled speech, grunting, signs of obstruction • Head bobbing with each breath: impending respiratory failure • Position: tripod, refusing to lie down • Asymmetric chest movements or see-saw respirations (chest rises as abdomen falls and vice versa)
Circulation	• Pale, cool skin—mottling, pallor, and peripheral cyanosis are indicators of poor tissue perfusion or respiratory distress • Pulses—absence of peripheral pulses indicates poor tissue perfusion; absent central pulse is an ominous sign • Capillary refill time—greater than 2 seconds indicates poor tissue perfusion, hypothermia, constricted blood flow (e.g., tight cast) • Sunken fontanel, doughy skin texture, dry mucous membrane may indicate hypovolemia due to dehydration • Heart rate—greater than 160 or less than 80 per minute in child under age 5 years; greater than 140 per minute in child 5 years and older • Bradycardia—sign of impending cardiac arrest • Sustained sinus tachycardia—indicates hypovolemia • Blood pressure—hypotension is a late sign of hypovolemia, indicates cardiovascular decompensation (a decrease of 10 mm Hg is significant) • Oliguria

death in all age groups and the eighth cause of death in the older population.

Organ system changes with aging affect physiologic reserves during an emergency:

- Arthritic changes may limit mobility of the neck and temporomandibular joint and make it more difficult to open the mouth and obtain an airway. Dentures or teeth that easily break may also interfere with obtaining an airway.
- Older adults may have a spine injury even with ground-level falls.
- The muscles in the upper airway weaken with age, leading to less effective cough and gag reflexes. The older adult has a higher potential for aspiration and obstruction.
- Increased stiffness of the rib cage may lead to an increased rate of rib fractures and pulmonary contusion in cases of chest wall injuries.
- Older adults have a decreased energy reserve, and the increased work of breathing may lead to respiratory failure more quickly than in younger adults.
- Hypoxia is not well tolerated by older adults.
- Cardiovascular changes include coronary artery stenosis, changes in the conduction system, dysrhythmias, and decreased ventricular filling associated with a lower cardiac output.
- Hypotension and hypovolemia increase the risk for myocardial ischemia. The older adult is less able to compensate quickly for low perfusion states. Knowledge of the older adult's usual blood pressure reading is important when assessing for a falling blood pressure and shock.
- Hypovolemia may be present with a heart rate and blood pressure that are considered within adult normal limits because older adults may have hypertension. Patients taking beta-blocker medications are unable to compensate and increase their heart rate in cases of shock or dehydration.
- Patients on anticoagulation therapy will have increased bleeding.
- Nerve endings deteriorate, and perception of pain may be reduced.
- Chronic mental status changes may be present in an older adult, making assessment of responsiveness and cognition difficult.
- The skin has thinner subcutaneous fat and is injured more easily. Hypothermia is also a greater risk in older adults.

Legal Considerations

Records

Medical issues may arise during emergency situations, and precise records of your sequential observations, evaluation, and interventions prescribed and performed are essential. Pertinent negatives are as important as pertinent positives. Flow sheets (in the electronic health record [EHR] or on paper for transfer to the EHR) that enable chronologic recording of emergency assessments and care provided are commonly used.

Consent for Treatment

Written informed consent for procedures and health care is usually obtained before treatment. In life-threatening emergencies, when the patient is unconscious or incapacitated, the needed emergency assessment and treatment are provided. Implied consent for treatment is based on the principle that a reasonably competent person would have consented for treatment, and delay in care could cause death or irreparable harm to the patient.

Trauma Due to Violence

If the patient's injury could be associated with physical violence or sexual assault, health care providers must preserve evidence. Any such injuries must be reported to legal authorities. All items, such as bullets and clothing, must be retained for law enforcement personnel, with a documented chain of possession by health professionals.

Medical Orders for Life-Sustaining Treatment

Make a conscientious effort to learn whether a patient has made an advance directive—a formal statement of desired medical care in the event of a catastrophic injury or illness. Such a document states conditions under which a patient wants specific medical interventions to be used, limited, or forbidden when unable to make health care decisions. Each state has a name for an advance directive, such as "durable or medical power of attorney" or "designated health care agent." A close relative or other trusted person is designated to make health care decisions when the patient is unable to do so. Both documents are especially important if the illness or injury results in a cognitive impairment that prevents participation in medical decision making. A central concern is the extent to which life-sustaining measures should be instituted.

Summary

In contrast to most health care situations, in an emergency situation, diagnosis is not made before the initiation of treatment. Rather, the life-threatening physiologic signs of disease or trauma are identified rapidly and treated immediately. The diagnosis causing the physiologic signs is investigated after the patient's physiologic condition is stabilized, and a thorough examination can then be performed.

ABNORMALITIES

Upper Airway Obstruction

Compromise of the airway space, resulting in impaired respiratory exchange

PATHOPHYSIOLOGY

Potential causes include the following:

- Aspirated foreign body or chemicals
- Inflammation of the airway due to smoke or other chemical inhalation
- Infection such as laryngotracheitis (croup) or retropharyngeal abscess
- Trauma to the neck or face
- Tumor or goiter

PATIENT DATA

Subjective Data

- History of a choking episode or exposure to chemicals or smoke
- History of infection with fever
- Fatigue
- Shortness of breath
- Sore throat

Objective Data

- Patient may grasp neck with inability to speak
- Apnea
- Severe dyspnea and tachypnea
- Stridor or hoarseness
- Dysphagia, drooling
- Extreme anxiety progressing to altered mental status (lethargy to coma)
- Tripod positioning

Hypoxemia

Severely reduced blood oxygen levels in major organs

PATHOPHYSIOLOGY

- Results from conditions (e.g., upper airway obstruction, asthma, and hypovolemic shock) that cause respiratory distress, poor tissue perfusion, or ventilatory failure
- May result from severe lung injury (e.g., pulmonary contusion) with increased permeability of alveoli

PATIENT DATA

Subjective Data

- History of choking episode, reactive airway disease (asthma), or chronic respiratory condition
- Thoracic injury
- Shortness of breath
- Fatigue

Objective Data

- Severe dyspnea and tachypnea
- Pallor, mottling, or cyanosis
- Altered mental status (lethargy to coma; anxiety and combativeness may precede lethargy)
- Tachycardia

Shock State

An abnormality of the circulatory system that results in inadequate organ perfusion and tissue oxygenation

PATHOPHYSIOLOGY

- Hypovolemic shock results from hemorrhage associated with injury or gastrointestinal bleeding, dehydration, or fluid loss associated with burn injury
- Septic shock is caused by several different organisms, leading to a systemic inflammatory response syndrome that impairs circulatory functioning and clotting functioning
- Obstructive shock may result from an injury above the diaphragm causing poor cardiac functioning (e.g., myocardial contusion or tension pneumothorax)
- Distributive shock may result from septic shock or an injury to the spinal cord when loss of sympathetic nervous system tone causes blood to pool in the extremities

PATIENT DATA

Subjective Data

- Anxiety
- History and mechanism of injury with potential for hypovolemia or circulatory system impairment or of overwhelming infection
- Vomiting and diarrhea
- Black, tarry stools
- Abdominal pain
- Rapid heart rate
- Shortness of breath
- Fatigue
- Feels cold
- Fever

Objective Data

- Pallor, cold extremities
- Diaphoresis
- Coma (or altered mental status)
- Tachycardia
- Decreasing systolic blood pressure or hypotension
- Delayed capillary refill time
- Tachypnea, respiratory distress
- Oliguria
- Circulatory collapse
- In adults with septic shock, the systolic blood pressure is less than 90 mm Hg or 40 mm or more below the usual systolic reading (Dellinger et al., 2019)

Ventilatory Failure

Compromised exhalation of carbon dioxide because of alveolar hypoventilation

PATHOPHYSIOLOGY

- Numerous disorders can cause or progress to ventilatory failure if not proactively managed, including upper airway obstruction, central nervous system disorder, increased intracranial pressure, Guillain-Barré syndrome, drug overdose, pulmonary contusion, flail chest, or severe kyphoscoliosis

PATIENT DATA

Subjective Data

- History or mechanism of injury placing individual at risk
- Headache
- Respiratory distress
- Apprehension

Objective Data

- Altered mental status—confusion or lethargy progressing to coma (may be subtle if the process is chronic)
- Slowed respiratory rate
- Paradoxical respirations
- Blood gases reveal hypoxemia and hypercapnia

Increased Intracranial Pressure

An increase in volume of brain tissue, blood, or cerebrospinal fluid (CSF) within the closed space of the skull that results in elevated pressure

PATHOPHYSIOLOGY

- Intracranial causes include brain trauma (cerebral edema, hematoma), tumor, ischemic stroke, brain abscess, or hydrocephalus
- Extracranial causes include anoxic insult (hypoxia or hypercarbia), seizure, significant hypoglycemia or hyperglycemia, other metabolic disorders, or hyperpyrexia

PATIENT DATA

Subjective Data

- History of brain injury, seizure, stroke, or other condition
- Headache
- Nausea and vomiting

Objective Data

- Changes in mental status, lethargy, irritability, slowed responsiveness; may progress to stupor or coma
- Seizures or syncope
- Papilledema
- Cranial nerve palsy, particularly VI (abducens paralysis)
- Cushing triad: bradycardia, rising blood pressure, and irregular respirations
- Also in infants: bulging fontanel, irritable or high-pitched cry, inconsolable, change in vital signs
- Radiographic studies may reveal a mass, generalized edema, or excessive CSF

Pulmonary Embolism

Migration of a blood clot from the deep veins of the legs or pelvis to the lung vasculature

PATHOPHYSIOLOGY

- Venous stasis and endothelial injury can lead to adhesion of platelets and clot formation
- Certain individuals may be predisposed due to hematologic disease, such as those with clotting abnormalities
- Family history of deep vein thrombosis

PATIENT DATA

Subjective Data

- History of reduced mobility or bed bound, surgery in past month, long airplane trip
- Shortness of breath
- Stabbing and sharp chest pain that worsens with breathing or coughing
- Cough, coughing up blood
- Palpitations
- Anxiety
- Leg pain and swelling
- Use of oral contraceptives

Objective Data

- Tachycardia
- Diaphoresis
- Tachypnea
- Pain with deep leg vein palpation, unilateral swelling
- Syncope
- Cough, hemoptysis
- A ventilation/perfusion lung scan may diagnose the condition

Status Asthmaticus

An acute severe asthma exacerbation that does not respond to usual treatment in the emergency department

PATHOPHYSIOLOGY

- Chronic inflammation of the airway is present in asthma, and a variety of physical, chemical, and pharmacologic stimuli trigger bronchospasm and mucus obstruction of the intrapulmonary airways

PATIENT DATA

Subjective Data

- History of dyspnea and increasing use of medication over a period of many days or sudden onset of symptoms
- Shortness of breath
- Wheezing
- Coughing
- Fatigue

Objective Data

- Ability to say only a few words between breaths
- Tachycardia (often more than 130 beats/min in adults)
- Tachypnea (may be variable)
- Hypertension
- Dyspnea
- Hypoxemia
- Wheezing (unless airflow is so diminished that it obscures wheezing)
- Pulsus paradoxus greater than 20 mm Hg
- Altered mental status may be present

Status Epilepticus

A prolonged seizure or series of seizures that occur without recovery of consciousness

PATHOPHYSIOLOGY

- May occur in patients with various seizure disorders, including generalized and partial seizures
- May occur in association with an acute illness, a febrile illness, trauma, or stroke (Hocker et al., 2014)

PATIENT DATA

Subjective Data

- History of seizures, neurologic disorder, or injury
- Shaking movements
- Loss of consciousness and unresponsive for longer than usual

Objective Data

- Tonic-clonic movements with unresponsiveness for longer than 5 minutes or two or more seizures without return to baseline, despite appropriate emergency antiepileptic medications, may be prolonged as much as 30–60 minutes (movements may be diminished by drugs used to manage the seizures)
- Hypotension
- Cardiac dysrhythmias
- Fever
- Pallor to cyanosis
- Hypoxemia may result from impaired respirations during tonic stage
- Hypoglycemia due to increased metabolic rate

References

Chapter 1

Bertakis, K. D., & Azari, R. (2012). Patient-centered care: The influence of patient and resident physician gender and gender concordance in primary care. *Journal of Women's Health, 21,* 326–333.

Borkan, J. M., Culhane-Pera, K. A., & Goldman, R. E. (2008). Towards cultural humility in healthcare for a culturally diverse Rhode Island. *Medicine and Health, Rhode Island, 91*(12), 361–364.

Bukutu, C., Deol, J., & Vohra, S. (2008). Complementary, holistic, and integrative medicine: Therapies for acute otitis media. *Pediatrics in* Review, *29*(6), 193–199.

Calzone, K. A., Jenkins, J., Nicol, N., Skirton, H., Feero, W. G., & Green, E. D. (2013). Relevance of genomics to healthcare and nursing practice. *Journal of Nursing Scholarship, 45*(1), 1–2.

Campinha-Bacote, J. (2011). Delivering patient-centered care in the midst of a cultural conflict: The role of cultural competence. *Online Journal of Issues in Nursing,* 16(2), 5.

Center for Excellence for Transgender Health. (2016). *Department of family and community medicine, University of California San Francisco: Guidelines for the primary and gender-affirming care of transgender and gender nonbinary people* (2nd ed.). www.transhealth.ucsf.edu/guidelines

DeCamp, L. R., Kuo, D. Z., Flores, G., O'Connor, K., & Minkovitz, C. S. (2013). Changes in language services use by U.S. pediatricians. *Pediatrics, 132*(2), e396–e406.

Demmer, L. A., & Waggoner, D. J. (2014). Professional medical education and genomics. *Annual Review of Genomics and Human* Genetics, *15,* 507–516.

Dittus, P. J., Michael, S. L., Becasen, J. S., Gloppen, K. M., McCarthy, K., & Guilamo-Ramos, V. (2015). Parental monitoring and its associations with adolescent sexual risk behavior: A meta-analysis. *Pediatrics, 136*(6), e1587–e1599.

Duello, T. M., Rivedal, S., Wickland, C., & Weller, A. (2021). Race and genetics versus 'race' in genetics: A systematic review of the use of African ancestry in genetic studies. *Evolution, Medicine, and Public Health, 9*(1), 232–245. https://doi.org/10.1093/emph/eoab018

Fahlberg, B., Foronda, C., & Baptiste, D. (2016). Cultural humility: The key to patient/family partnerships for making difficult decisions. *Nursing, 46*(9), 14–16.

Fashner, J., Ericson, K., & Werner, S. (2012). Treatment of the common cold in children and adults. *American Family Physician, 86,* 153–159.

FitzGerald, C., & Hurst, S. (2017). Implicit bias in healthcare professionals: A systematic review. *BMC Medical Ethics, 18*(1), 19.

Flores, G. (2010). Committee on Pediatric Research: Technical report—racial and ethnic disparities in the health and health care of children. *Pediatrics, 125,* e979–e1020.

Foronda, C., MacWilliams, B., & McArthur, E. (2016). Interprofessional communication in healthcare: An integrative review. *Nurse Education in Practice, 19,* 36–40.

Garrido, P., Aldaz, A., Vera, R., Calleja, M. A., de Álava, E., Martín, M., Matías-Guiu, X., & Palacios, J. (2018). Proposal for the creation of a national strategy for precision medicine in cancer: A position statement of SEOM, SEAP, and SEFH. *Clinical & Translational Oncology, 20*(4), 443–447.

Ginsburg, G. S., & Phillips, K. A. (2018). Precision medicine: From science to value. *Health* Affairs, *37*(5), 694–701.

Kota, K. K., Salazar, L. F., Culbreth, R. E., Crosby, R. A., & Jones, J. (2020). Psychosocial mediators of perceived stigma and suicidal ideation among transgender women. *BMC Public Health, 20,* 125. https://doi.org/10.1186/s12889-020-8177-z

Manuel, J. K., Satre, D. D., Tsoh, J., Moreno-John, G., Ramos, J. S., McCance-Katz, E. F., & Satterfield, J. M. (2015). Adapting screening, brief intervention, and referral to treatment for alcohol and drugs to culturally diverse clinical populations. *Journal of Addiction Medicine, 9*(5), 343–351.

Office of Disease Prevention and Health Promotion. *Health people 2020: Lesbian, gay, bisexual and transgender health.* 2010. https://www.healthypeople.gov/2020/topics-objectives/topic/lesbian-gay-bisexual-and-transgender-health

Pesola, F., Shelton, K. H., Heron, J., Munafò, M., Hickman, M., & van den Bree, M. B. (2015). The developmental relationship between depressive symptoms in adolescence and harmful drinking in emerging adulthood: The role of peers and parents. *Journal of Youth and Adolescence, 44*(9), 1752–1766.

Pickett-Blakely, O., Bleich, S. N., & Cooper, L. A. (2011). Patient-physician gender concordance and weight-related counseling of obese patients. *American Journal of Preventive Medicine, 40*(6), 616–619.

Posadzki, P., Watson, L. K., & Ernst, E. (2013). Adverse effects of herbal medicines: An overview of systematic reviews. *Clinical Medicine (London, England), 13*(1), 7–12.

Purnell, L. D. (Ed.). (2013). *Transcultural health care: A culturally competent approach* (4th ed.). Philadelphia: F. A. Davis.

Richeson, J. A., & Sommers, S. R. (2016). Toward a social psychology of race and race relations for the twenty-first century. *Annual Review of Psychology, 67,* 439–463.

Saha, S., Beach, M. C., & Cooper, L. A. (2008). Patient centeredness, cultural competence and healthcare quality. *Journal of the National Medical Association, 100*(11), 1275–1285.

Schwartz, S. J., Weisskirch, R. S., Zamboanga, B. L., Castillo, L. G., Ham, L. S., Huynh, Q. L., Park, I. J., Donovan, R., Kim, S. Y., Vernon, M., Davis, M. J., & Cano, M. A. (2011). Dimensions of acculturation: Associations with health risk behaviors among college students from immigrant families. *Journal of Counseling Psychology, 58*(1), 27–41.

Shao, Z., Richie, W. D., & Bailey, R. K. (2016). Racial and ethnic disparity in major depressive disorder. *Journal of Racial and Ethnic Health Disparities, 3*(4), 692–705.

Stubbe, D. E. (2020). Practicing cultural competence and cultural humility in the care of diverse patients. *Focus, 18*(1), 49–51.

Stulc, D. M. (1991). The family as a bearer of culture. In J. M. Cookfair (Ed.), *Nursing process and practice in the community.* St. Louis: Mosby.

Trent, M., Dooley, D. G., Dougé, J., Section on Adolescent Health, Council on community Pediatrics, & Committee on Adolescence. (2019). The impact of racism on child and adolescent health. *Pediatrics, 144*(2), e20191765.

Tsugawa, Y., Jena, A. B., Figueroa, J. F., Orav, E. J., Blumenthal, D. M., & Jha, A. K. (2017). Comparison of hospital mortality and readmission rates for Medicare patients treated by male vs female physicians. *JAMA Internal Medicine, 177*(2), 206–213.

University of California—San Francisco (UCSF). *Transition roadmap*. 2019. https://transcare.ucsf.edu/transition-roadmap

Van Berckelaer, A. C., Mitra, N., & Pati, S. (2011). Predictors of well child care adherence over time in a cohort of urban Medicaid-eligible infants. *BMC Pediatrics, 11*(1), 36.

Visscher, P. M., Wray, N. R., Zhang, Q., Sklar, P., McCarthy, M. I., Brown, M. A., & Yang, J. (2017). 10 Years of GWAS discovery: Biology, function, and translation. *American Journal of Human Genetics, 101*(1), 5–22.

White, A. A. 3rd, & Stubblefield-Tave, B. Some advice for physicians and other clinicians treating minorities, women, and other patients at risk of receiving health care disparities. *Journal of Racial and Ethnic Health Disparities, 4*(3), 472–479.

Williams, D. R., Lawrence, J. A., & Davis, B. A. (2019). Racism and health: Evidence and needed research. *Annual Review of Public Health, 40*, 105–125. https://doi.org/10.1146/annurev-publhealth-040218-043750

World Health Organization. (2010). *Framework for action on interprofessional education and collaborative practice*. Geneva: Author. http://www.who.int/hrh/resources/framework_action/en/

Chapter 2

Appelbaum, P. S. (2007). Clinical practice. Assessment of patients' competence to consent to treatment. *The New England Journal of Medicine, 357*(18), 1834–1840.

Artandi, M. K., & Stewart, R. W. (2018). The outpatient physical examination. *The Medical Clinics of North America, 102*(3), 465–473.

Augustyn, M., Parker, S., Groves, B. M., & Zuckerman, B. (1995). Silent victims: Children who witness violence. *Contemporary Pediatrics, 12*, 35.

Auster, S. (January 6, 2004). Spirituality and medicine. Personal communication (from the Uniformed services University of the Heath Sciences).

Bandeen-Roche, K., Seplaki, C. L., Huang, J., Buta, B., Kalyani, R. R., Varadhan, R., Xue, Q. L., Walston, J. D., & Kasper, J. D. (2015). Frailty in older adults: A nationally representative profile in the United States. *The Journals of Gerontology. Series A, Biological Sciences and Medical Sciences, 70*(11), 1427–1434. http://dx.doi.org/10.1093/gerona/glv133

BLUE CAMPAIGN. *What is human trafficking?* https://www.dhs.gov/blue-campaign/what-human-trafficking

Bradley, K. A., Bush, K. R., Epler, A. J., Dobie, D. J., Davis, T. M., Sporleder, J. L., Maynard, C., Burman, M. L., & Kivlahan, D. R. (2003). Two brief alcohol-screening tests From the Alcohol Use Disorders Identification Test (AUDIT): Validation in a female Veterans Affairs patient population. *Archives of Internal Medicine, 163*(7), 821–829.

Brown, R. L., & Rounds, L. A. (1995). Conjoint screening questionnaires for alcohol and other drug abuse: Criterion validity in a primary care practice. *Wisconsin Medical Journal, 94*(3), 135–140.

Bush, K., Kivlahan, D. R., McDonell, M. B., Fihn, S. D., & Bradley, K. A. (1998). For the ambulatory care quality improvement Project (ACQUIP): The AUDIT alcohol Consumption questions (AUDIT-C): An effective brief screening test for problem drinking. *Archives of Internal Medicine, 158*(16), 1789–1795. http://dx.doi.org/10.1001/archinte.158.16.1789

Cahill, S., Singal, R., Grasso, C., King, D., Mayer, K., Baker, K., & Makadon, H. (2014). Do ask, do tell: High levels of acceptability by patients of routine collection of sexual orientation and gender identity data in four diverse American community health centers. *PLoS One, 9*(9), e107104.

Chen, P. H., Rovi, S., Vega, M., Jacobs, A., & Johnson, M. S. (2005). Screening for domestic violence in a predominantly Hispanic clinical setting. *Family Practice, 22*(6), 617–623. http://dx.doi.org/10.1093/fampra/cmi075

Curlin, F. A., Lawrence, R. E., Chin, M. H., & Lantos, J. D. (2007). Religion, conscience, and controversial clinical practices. *The New England Journal of Medicine, 356*(6), 593–600. http://dx.doi.org/10.1056/NEJMsa065316

Dank, M., Yu, L., Vasquez-Noriega, C., Gelatt, J., & Pergamit, M. (2017). *Pretesting a human trafficking screening tool in the child welfare and runaway and homeless youth systems*. https://www.urban.org/research/publication/pretesting-human-trafficking-screening-tool-child-welfare-and-runaway-and-homeless-youth-systems

Disease. Merriam-Webster.com.

Fosarelli, P. (2003). Children and the development of faith: Implications for pediatric practice. *Contemporary Pediatrics, 20*, 85.

George, A., Shamim, S., Johnson, M., Ajwani, S., Bhole, S., Blinkhorn, A., Ellis, S., & Andrews, K. (2011). Periodontal treatment during pregnancy and birth outcomes: A meta-analysis of randomised trials. *International Journal of Evidence-Based Healthcare, 9*(2), 122–147. http://dx.doi.org/10.1111/j.1744-1609.2011.00210.x

Ginsburg, K. R. (2021). The SSHADESS screening: A strength-based psychosocial assessment. In K. R. Ginsburg & Z. B. R. McClain (Eds.), *Reaching teens: Strength-based, trauma-sensitive, resilience-building communication strategies rooted in positive youth development* (2nd ed., pp. 225–228). American Academy of Pediatrics.

Gold, A. (2010). Physicians' "right of conscience"- beyond politics. *The Journal of Law, Medicine & Ethics, 38*, 134–142. http://dx.doi.org/10.1111/j.1748-720X.2010.00473.x

Goldenring, J. M., & Rosen, D. S. (2004). Getting into adolescent heads: An essential update. *Contemporary Pediatrics, 21*(1), 64–90.

Goroll, A. H. (2015). Toward trusting therapeutic relationships—in favor of the annual physical. *The New England Journal of Medicine, 373*(16), 1487–1489. doi:10.1056/NEJMp1508270

Greenwald, A. G., & Banaji, M. R. (1995). Implicit social cognition: Attitudes, self-esteem, and stereotypes. *Psychological Review, 102*(1), 4–27.

Henry, S. G., Fuhrel-Forbis, A., Rogers, M. A., & Eggly, S. (2012). Association between nonverbal communication during clinical interactions and outcomes: A systematic review and meta-analysis. *Patient Education and Counseling, 86*(3), 297–315. http://dx.doi.org/10.1016/j.pec.2011.07.006

Houry, D., Feldhaus, K., Peery, B., Abbott, J., Lowenstein, S. R., al-Bataa-de-Montero, S., & Levine, S. (2004). A positive domestic violence screen predicts future domestic violence. *Journal of Interpersonal Violence, 19*(9), 955–966. https://doi.org/10.1177/0886260504267999

Institute of Medicine. (2001). *Crossing the quality chasm: A new health system for the 21st century*. Washington DC: National Academies Press.

Kliegman, R., Stanton, B., & Geme, J. W. S., (Eds.). (2016). *Nelson textbook of pediatrics* (20th ed.). Philadelphia: Elsevier.

Knight, J. R., Sherritt, L., Shrier, L. A., Harris, S. K., & Chang, G. (2002). Validity of the CRAFFT substance abuse screening test among adolescent clinic patients. *Archives of Pediatrics & Adolescent Medicine, 156*(6), 607–614.

Kroenke, K., Spitzer, R. L., & Williams, J. B. (2001). The PHQ-9: Validity of a brief depression severity measure. *Journal of General Internal Medicine, 16*(9), 606–613. doi:10.1046/j.1525-1497.2001.016009606.x

MacMillan, H. L., Wathen, C. N., Jamieson, E., Boyle, M., McNutt, L. A., Worster, A., Lent, B., Webb, M., & McMaster Violence Against Women Research Group. (2006). Approaches to screening for intimate partner violence in health care settings: A randomized trial. *JAMA, 296*(5), 530–536. http://dx.doi.org/10.1001/jama.296.5.530

Magauran, B. G., Jr. (2009). Risk management for the emergency physician: Competency and decision-making capacity, informed consent, and refusal of care against medical advice. *Emergency Medicine Clinics of North America, 27*(4), 605–614.Narayan, M. C. (2019). Addressing implicit bias in nursing: A review. *The American Journal of Nursing, 119*(7), 36–43. http://dx.doi.org/10.1097/01.NAJ.0000569340.27659.5a

Nelson, H. D., Bougatsos, C., & Blazina, I. (2012). *Screening women for intimate partner violence and elderly and vulnerable adults for abuse: Systematic review to update the 2004 U.S. Preventive Services Task Force Recommendation, Evidence syntheses, No 92.* Rockville, MD: Agency for Healthcare Research and Quality (US). http://www.ncbi.nlm.nih.gov/books/NBK97297

Nelson, H. D., Nygren, P., McInerney, Y., Klein, J., & U. S. Preventive Services Task Force (2004). Screening women and elderly adults for family and intimate partner violence: A review of the evidence for the U. S. Preventive Services Task Force. *Annals of Internal Medicine, 140*(5), 387–396.

O'Connor, E., Rossom, R. C., Henninger, M., Groom, H. C., & Burda, B. U. (2016). primary care screening for and treatment of depression in pregnant and postpartum women: Evidence report and systematic review for the US Preventive Services Task Force. *JAMA, 315*(4), 388–406. http://dx.doi.org/10.1001/jama.2015.18948

O'Hara, M. W., & McCabe, J. E. (2013). Postpartum depression: Current status and future directions. *Annual Review of Clinical Psychology, 9,* 379–407. http://dx.doi.org/10.1146/annurev-clinpsy-050212-185612

Olson, L. M., Radecki, L., Frintner, M. P., Weiss, K. B., Korfmacher, J., & Siegel, R. M. (2007). At what age can children report dependably on their asthma health status? *Pediatrics, 119*(1), e93–e102. http://dx.doi.org/10.1542/peds.2005-3211

Pitts, M., Mitchell, A., Smith, A., & Patel, S. (2006). *Private lives: A report on the health and wellbeing of GLBTI Australians.* Australian Research Centre in Sex, Health and Society, La Trobe University. https://www.livingwell.org.au/wp-content/uploads/2012/11/private_lives_report_1_0.pdf

Pritlove, C., Juando-Prats, C., Ala-Leppilampi, K., & Parsons, J. A. (2019). The good, the bad, and the ugly of implicit bias. *Lancet (London, England), 393*(10171), 502–504. http://dx.doi.org/10.1016/s0140-6736(18)32267-0

Puchalski, C., & Romer, A. L. (2000). Taking a spiritual history allows clinicians to understand patients more fully. *Journal of Palliative Medicine, 3*(1), 129–137.

Roberts, S. J., Chandler, G. E., & Kalmakis, K. (2019). A model for trauma-informed primary care. *Journal of the American Association of Nurse Practitioners, 31*(2), 139–144. http://dx.doi.org/10.1097/JXX.0000000000000116

Sokol, R. J., Martier, S. S., & Ager, J. W. (1989). The T-ACE questions: Practical prenatal detection of risk-drinking. *American Journal of Obstetrics and Gynecology, 160*(4), 863–870.

Stead, L. F., Buitrago, D., Preciado, N., Sanchez, G., Hartmann-Boyce, J., & Lancaster, T. (2013). Physician advice for smoking cessation. *The Cochrane Database of Systematic Reviews, 2013*(5), CD000165. http://dx.doi.org/10.1002/14651858.CD000165.pub4

Substance Abuse and Mental Health Services Administration. (2014). *Trauma-informed care in behavioral health services* (TIP Series 57; HHS Publication No. SMA 13-4801). Rockville, MD: U.S. Department of Health and Human Services.

United States. (1982). President's Commission for the study of ethical problems in medicine and biomedical and behavioral research. *United States Code Annotated. United States,* Title 42 Sect. 300v as added 1978.

Weiss-Laxer, N. S., Platt, R., Osborne, L. M., Kimmel, M., Solomon, B. S., Mendelson, T., Webb, L., & Riley, A. W. (2016). Beyond screening: A review of pediatric primary care models to address maternal depression. *Pediatric Research, 79*(1-2), 197–204. http://dx.doi.org/10.1038/pr.2015.214

Whitton, S. W., Dyar, C., Mustanski, B., & Newcomb, M. E. (2019) Intimate partner violence experiences of sexual and gender minority adolescents and young adults assigned female at birth. *Psychology of Women Quarterly, 43*(2), 232–249. http://dx.doi.org/10.1177/0361684319838972

Whitton, S. W., Newcomb, M. E., Messinger, A. M., Byck, G., & Mustanski, B. (2016). A longitudinal study of IPV victimization among sexual minority youth. *Journal of Interpersonal Violence, 34*(5), 912–945. doi:10.1177/0886260516646093

Williams, D. R., & Wyatt, R. (2015). Racial bias in health care and health: Challenges and opportunities. *JAMA, 314*(6), 555–556. doi:10.1001/jama.2015.9260

Yang, Q., Liu, T., Valdez, R., Moonesinghe, R., & Khoury, M. J. (2010). Improvements in ability to detect undiagnosed diabetes by using information on family history among adults in the United States. *American Journal of Epidemiology, 171*(10), 1079–1089. http://dx.doi.org/10.1093/aje/kwq026

Chapter 3

American Academy of Pediatrics, Committee on Practice and Ambulatory Medicine, & Section on Ophthalmology. (2016). Procedures for the evaluation of the visual system by pediatricians. *Pediatrics, 137*(1), e20153597. http://pediatrics.aappublications.org/content/pediatrics/early/2015/12/07/peds.2015-3597.full.pdf. Accessed June 15, 2024.

Centers for Disease Control and Prevention. (2016). *Guide to* infection *prevention for outpatient setting: Minimum expectations for safe care, Version 2.3.* https://www.cdc.gov/infection-control/media/pdfs/outpatient-guide-508.pdf?CDC_AAref_Val=https://www.cdc.gov/infectioncontrol/pdf/outpatient/guide.pdf accessed June 15, 2024.

Centers for Disease Control and Prevention. (2024). *Infection control guidelines and guidance library.* https://www.cdc.gov/infectioncontrol/guidelines/index.html. Accessed June 15, 2024.

Kippenberger, S., Havlíček, J., Bernd, A., Thaçi, D., Kaufmann, R., & Meissner, M. (2012). 'Nosing around' the human skin: What information is concealed in skin odour? *Experimental Dermatology, 21*(9), 655–659. https://doi.org/10.1111/j.1600-0625.2012.01545.x

McGee, S. R. (1995). Percussion and physical diagnosis: Separating myth from science. *Disease-a-Month, 41*(10), 641–692.

National Institute for Occupational Safety and Health (NIOSH). (2023, August 10). *Latex allergy: A prevention guide, Publication Number 98-213, 1998.* http://www.cdc.gov/niosh/docs/98-113/. Accessed June 15, 2024.

Pecoraro, V., Petri, D., Costantino, G., Squizzato, A., Moja, L., Virgili, G, & Lucenteforte, E. (2021). The diagnostic accuracy of digital, infrared and mercury-in-glass thermometers in measuring body temperature: A systematic review and network meta-analysis. *Internal and Emergency Medicine, 16,* 1071–1083. https://link.springer.com/article/10.1007/s11739-020-02556-0

Ravindra, K., Gandhi, S., & Sivuni, A. (2018). Olfactory diagnosis in skin. *Clinical Dermatology Review, 2*(1), 38-40.

Seah, J. J., Zhao, J., Wang, Y., & Lee, H. P. (2023). Review on the advancements of stethoscope types in chest auscultation. *Diagnostics (Basel), 13*(9), 1545–2023.

Shi, D., Zhang, L. Y., & Li, H. X. (2020). Diagnostic test accuracy of new generation tympanic thermometry in children under different cutoffs: A systematic review and meta-analysis. *BMC Pediatrics, 20,* 210.

Siegel, J. D., Rhinehart, E., Jackson, M., & Chiarello, L. (2023). *2007 Guideline for isolation precautions: Preventing transmission of infectious agents in healthcare settings, June 2007.* https://www.cdc.gov/infection-control/hcp/isolation-precautions/index.html. Accessed June 15, 2024.

Sollai, S., Dani, C., Berti, E., Fancelli, C., Galli, L., de Martino, M., & Chiappini, E. (2016). Performance of a non-contact infrared thermometer in healthy newborns. *BMJ Open, 6*(3), e008695. https://pubmed.ncbi.nlm.nih.gov/26983944/

Sonthalia, S., Yumeen, S., & Kaliyadan, F. (2024). Dermoscopy overview and extradiagnostic applications. [Updated 2023 Aug 8]. In *StatPearls* [Internet]. Treasure Island, FL: StatPearls Publishing. https://www.ncbi.nlm.nih.gov/books/NBK537131/

Chapter 4

DiClemente, C., & Prochaska, J. (1998). Toward a comprehensive transtheoretical model of change. In W. R. Miller & N. Healther (Eds.), *Treating addictive behaviors.* New York: Plenum Press.

Hilliard, A. A., Weinberg, S. E., Tierney, L. M., Midthun, D. E., & Saint, S. (2004). Occam's razor versus Saint's triad. *New England Journal of Medicine, 350,* 599–603.

Thorburn, W. M. (1918). The myth of Occam's razor. *Mind, 27*(107), 345–353.

Chapter 5

Altman, R. L., Lin, C. T., & Earnest, M. (2023). Problem-oriented documentation: Design and widespread adoption of a novel toolkit in a commercial electronic health record. *JAMIA Open, 6*(1), ooad005.

Barth, O., Anderson, B., Jones, K., Nickles, A., Dawkins, K., Burnett, A., & Quartermus, K. (2024). An innovative approach to using electronic health records through health information exchange to build a Chronic Disease Registry in Michigan. *Preventing Chronic Disease, 21,* E41. doi:10.5888/pcd21.230413

Camacho, E. M., Gavan, S., Keers, R. N., Chuter, A., & Elliott, R. A. (2024). Estimating the impact on patient safety of enabling the digital transfer of patients' prescription information in the English NHS. *BMJ Quality & Safety, 33*(11), 726–737. https://doi.org/10.1136/bmjqs-2023-016675

Cheng, C. G., Wu, D. C., Lu, J. C., Yu, C. P., Lin, H. L., Wang, M. C., & Cheng, C. A. (2022). Restricted use of copy and paste in electronic health records potentially improves healthcare quality. *Medicine, 101*(4), e28644. https://doi.org/10.1097/MD.0000000000028644

Dahmke, H., Cabrera-Diaz, F., Heizmann, M., Stoop, S., Schuetz, P., Fiumefreddo, R., & Zaugg, C. (2024). Development and validation of a clinical decision support system to prevent anticoagulant duplications. *International Journal of Medical Informatics, 187,* 105446. https://doi.org/10.1016/j.ijmedinf.2024.105446

Duckie, C. L., Boston, K. A., Champagne, B., Thompson, J., Halpern, D. J., & Granger, B. B. (2024). Improving hypertension control in the black patient population: A quality improvement study of workflow redesign using the electronic health record to integrate self-monitoring, education, and reporting. *Journal of Nursing Care Quality, 39*(2), 175–182.

Ichiuji, M., Asakura, L., Cain, C., Aye, N., Kolevska, T., Chen, D., Brasfield, F. M., & Kotak, D. (2024). Improving routine use of clinical pathway decision support through integration of an EHR with a clinical library resource designed to provide evidence-based guidance within oncology workflows. *BMC Health Services Research, 24*(1), 560. https://doi.org/10.1186/s12913-024-11018-8

Tillman, B. F., Domenico, H. J., Moore, R. P., Byrne, D. W., Morton, C. T., Mixon, A. S., & French, B. (2024). A real-time prognostic model for venous thromboembolic events among hospitalized adults. *Research and Practice in Thrombosis and Haemostasis, 8*(4), 102433. https://doi.org/10.1016/j.rpth.2024.102433

Ye, J., Woods, D., Jordan, N., & Starren, J. (2024). The role of artificial intelligence for the application of integrating electronic health records and patient-generated data in clinical decision support. *AMIA Joint Summits on Translational Science proceedings. AMIA Joint Summits on Translational Science, 2024,* 459–467.

Chapter 6

American Academy of Pediatrics. (2016). Committee on Fetus and newborn and Section on Anesthesiology and pain medicine: Prevention and management of procedural pain in the neonate: An update. *Pediatrics, 137*(2), e20154271.

Antony, K. M., Racusin, D. A., & Aagaard, K. (2017). Maternal physiology. In S. G. Gabbe, J. R. Niebyl, J. L. Simpson, M. B. Landon, H. L. Galan, E. R. M. Jauniaux, D. A. Driscoll, V. Berghella, & W. A. Grobman (Eds.), *Obstetrics: Normal and problem pregnancies* (7th ed., pp. 38–63). Philadelphia: Elsevier.

Cohen, S. P., Caterina, M. J., Yang, S. Y., Socolovsky, M., & Sommer, C. (2024). Pain in the context of sensory deafferentation. *Anesthesiology, 140*(4), 824–848. https://doi.org/10.1097/ALN.0000000000004881

Flynn, J. T., Kaelber, D. C., Baker-Smith, C. M., Blowey, D., Carroll, A. E., Daniels, S. R., de Ferranti, S. D., Dionne, J. M., Falkner, B., Flinn, S. K., Gidding, S. S., Goodwin, C., Leu, M G., Powers, M. E., Rea, C., Samuels, J., Simasek, M., Thaker, V. V., Urbina, E. M., & Subcommittee on screening and management of high blood pressure in children. (2017). Clinical practice guideline for screening and management of high blood pressure in children and adolescents. *Pediatrics, 140*(3), e20171904. http://dx.doi.org/10.1542/peds.2017-1904

Foo, L., Tay, J., Lees, C. C., McEniery, C. M., & Wilkinson, I. B. (2015). Hypertension in pregnancy: Natural history and treatment options. *Current Hypertension Reports, 17*(5), 36. http://dx.doi.org/10.1007/s11906-015-0545-1

Gidding, S. S., Baker-Smith, C. M., Brady, T. M., Flynn, J. T., Malle, L. M., South, A. M., Tran, A. M., Urbina, E. M., &

Bonita, F. (2023). Pediatric primary hypertension: An underrecognized condition: A scientific statement from the American Heart Association. *Hypertension, 80*(1), e1–e15. https://doi.org/10.1161/HYP.0000000000000228; https://doi.org/10.1161/crossmarkpolicy

Huether, S. E., & Rodway, G. W. (2019). Pain, temperature regulation, sleep, and sensory function. In K. L. McCance, S. E. Huether, V. L. Brashers, & N. S. Rote (Eds.), *Pathophysiology: The biologic basis for disease in adults and children* (8th ed., pp. 468–503). St Louis: Elsevier

Lawson, S. L., Hogg, M. M., Moore, C. G., Anderson, W. E., Osipoff, P. S., Runyon, M. S., & Reynolds, S. L. (2021). Pediatric pain assessment in the emergency department: Patient and caregiver agreement using the wong-baker FACES and the faces pain scale-revised. *Pediatric Emergency Care, 37*(12), e950–e954. doi:10.1097/PEC.0000000000001837

Llerena, A., Tran, K., Choudhary, D., Hausmann, J., Goldgof, D., Sun, Y., & Prescott, S. M. (2023). Neonatal pain assessment: Do we have the right tools? *Frontiers in Pediatrics, 10,* 1022751. doi:10.3389/fped.2022.1022751

Luger, R. K., & Kight, B. P. (204). Hypertension in pregnancy. [Updated 2022 Oct 3]. In *StatPearls* [Internet]. Treasure Island, FL: StatPearls Publishing. https://www.ncbi.nlm.nih.gov/books/NBK430839

Merkel, S. I., Voepel-Lewis, T., Shayevitz, J. R., & Malviya, S. (1997). The FLACC: A behavioral scale for scoring postoperative pain in young children. *Pediatric Nursing, 23*(3), 293–297.

Mullins, S., Hosseini, F., Gibson, W., & Thake, M. (2022). Physiological changes from ageing regarding pain perception and its impact on pain management for older adults. *Clinical Medicine (London, England), 22*(4), 307–310. doi:10.7861/clinmed.22.4.phys

Osilla, E. V., Marsidi, J. L., Shumway, K. R., & Sharma, S. (2024). Physiology, temperature regulation. [Updated 2023 Jul 30]. In *StatPearls* [Internet]. Treasure Island, FL: StatPearls Publishing. https://www.ncbi.nlm.nih.gov/books/NBK507838/

Rantala, A., Hakala, M., & Pölkki, T. (2022). Women's perceptions of the pain assessment and non-pharmacological pain relief methods used during labor: A cross-sectional survey. *European Journal of Midwifery, 6,* 21. https://doi.org/10.18332/ejm/146136

Ringer, M., & Lappin, S. L. (2024). Orthostatic hypotension. [Updated 2023 May 16]. In *StatPearls* [Internet]. Treasure Island, FL: StatPearls Publishing. https://www.ncbi.nlm.nih.gov/books/NBK448192/

Sansone, L., Gentile, C., Grasso, E. A., Di Ludovico, A., La Bella, S., Chiarelli, F., & Breda, L. (2023). Pain evaluation and treatment in children: A practical approach. *Children (Basel, Switzerland), 10*(7), 1212. doi:10.3390/children10071212

Shen, M., Tan, H., Zhou, S., Smith, G. N., Walker, M. C., & Wen, S. W. (2017). Trajectory of blood pressure change during pregnancy and the role of pre-gravid blood pressure: A functional data analysis approach. *Scientific Reports, 7*(1), 6227. doi:10.1038/s41598-017-06606-0

Su, Y. C., Chien, C. Y., Chaou, C. H., Hsu, K. H., Gao, S. Y., & Ng, C. J. (2022). Revising vital signs criteria for accurate triage of older adults in the emergency department. *International Journal of General Medicine, 15,* 6227–6235. https://doi.org/10.2147/IJGM.S373396

Vemu, P. L., Yang, E., & Ebinger, J. (2024, February 5). *2023 ESH hypertension guideline update: Bringing us closer together across the pond.* American College of Cardiology. http://www.acc.org/Membership/Person?id=1a73e76d-81a9-4773-a843-77392d3d58f4

Warden, V., Hurley, A. C., & Volicer, L. (2003). Development and psychometric evaluation of the Pain Assessment in Advanced Dementia (PAINAD) scale. *Journal of the American Medical Directors Association, 4*(1), 9–15.

Whelton, P. K., Carey, R. M., Aronow, W. S., Casey, D. E., Jr, Collins, K. J., Dennison Himmelfarb, C., DePalma, S. M., Gidding, S., Jamerson, K. A., Jones, D. W., MacLaughlin, E. J., Muntner, P., Ovbiagele, B., Smith, S. C., Jr, Spencer, C. C., Stafford, R. S., Taler, S. J., Thomas, R. J., Williams, K. A., Sr, Williamson, J. D., ... Wright, J. T., Jr. (2018). 2017 ACC/AHA/AAPA/ABC/ACPM/AGS/APhA/ASH/ASPC/NMA/PCNA guideline for the prevention, detection, evaluation, and management of high blood pressure in adults: A report of the American College of Cardiology/American Heart Association Task Force on Clinical Practice Guidelines. *Journal of the American College of Cardiology, 71*(19), e127–e248.

Chapter 7

Abayomi, S. N., Sritharan, P., Yan, E., Saripella, A., Alhamdah, Y., Englesakis, M., Tartaglia, M. C., He, D., & Chung, F. (2024). The diagnostic accuracy of the Mini-Cog screening tool for the detection of cognitive impairment-A systematic review and meta-analysis. *PLoS One, 19*(3), e0298686. doi:10.1371/journal.pone.0298686

Bennett, C. (2019). Caring for patients with delirium. *Nursing, 49*(9), 17–20.

Boss, B. J., & Huether, S. E. (2019). Alterations in cognitive systems, cerebral hemodynamics, and motor function. In K. L. McCance, S. E. Huether, V. L. Brashers, & N. S. Rote (Eds.), *Pathophysiology: The biologic basis for disease in adults and children* (8th ed., pp. 504–549). St. Louis: Elsevier.

Centers for Disease Control and Prevention. *Data and statistics on ADHD.* https://www.cdc.gov/adhd/data/index.html. Accessed August 13, 2024.

Edemekong, P. F., Bomgaars, D. L., Sukumaran, S., & Schoo, C. (2024). Activities of daily living. [Updated 2023 Jun 26]. In: *StatPearls [Internet].* Treasure Island, FL: StatPearls Publishing. https://www.ncbi.nlm.nih.gov/books/NBK470404/

Folstein, M. F., & Folstein, S. B. (2020). *Mini-mental State Examination* (2nd ed.). https://www.parinc.com/Products/Pkey/238

Hodges, H., Fealko, C., & Soares, N. (2020). Autism spectrum disorder: Definition, epidemiology, causes, and clinical evaluation. *Translational Pediatrics, 9*(Suppl. 1), S55–S65. doi:10.21037/tp.2019.09.09

Hudomiet, P., Hurd, M. D., & Rohwedder, S. (2022). Trends in inequalities in the prevalence of dementia in the United States. *Proceedings of the National Academy of Sciences of the United States of America, 119*(46), e2212205119. doi:10.1073/pnas.2212205119

Hwang, A. B., Boes, S., Nyffeler, T., & Schuepfer, G. (2019). Validity of screening instruments for the detection of dementia and mild cognitive impairment in hospital inpatients: A systematic review of diagnostic accuracy studies. *PLoS One, 14*(7), e0219569. http://dx.doi.org/10.1371/journal.pone.0219569

Islam, N., Hashem, R., Gad, M., Brown, A., Levis, B., Renoux, C., Thombs, B. D., & McInnes, M. D. (2023). Accuracy of the Montreal Cognitive Assessment tool for detecting mild cognitive impairment: A systematic review and meta-analysis. *Alzheimer's & Dementia, 19*(7), 3235–3243. doi:10.1002/alz.13040

Kwan, M. (2018). Development, behavior, and mental health. In B. Engorn & J. Flerlage (Eds.), *The Harriet Lane handbook* (21st ed., pp. 195–214). Philadelphia: Elsevier/Mosby.

Nandakumar, A. L., Vande Voort, J. L., Nakonezny, P. A., Orth, S. S., Romanowicz, M., Sonmez, A. I., Ward, J. A., Rackley, S. J., Huxsahl, J. E., & Croarkin, P. E. (2019). Psychometric properties of the Patient Health Questionnaire-9 modified for major depressive disorder in adolescents. *Journal of Child and Adolescent Psychopharmacology, 29*(1), 34–40, http://dx.doi.org/10.1089/cap.2018.0112

National Institute of Mental Health. (2024, August). *Suicide prevention health topic*. https://www.nimh.nih.gov/health/topics/suicide-prevention#part_2474. Accessed August 7, 2024.

National Institutes of Health. (2017). National Institute on Deafness and other Communication disorders: Speech and language developmental milestones. https://www.nidcd.nih.gov/health/speech-and-language#1

Nguyen, B. L., Lyons, B. H., Forsberg, K., Wilson, R. F., Liu, G. S., Betz, C. J., & Blair, J. M. (2024). Surveillance for violent deaths - National Violent Death Reporting System, 48 states, the District of Columbia, and Puerto Rico, 2021. *Morbidity and Mortality Weekly Report. Surveillance Summaries (Washington, D.C.: 2002), 73*(5), 1–44. doi:10.15585/mmwr.ss7305a1

Pinto, T. C. C., Machado, L., Bulgacov, T. M., Rodrigues-Júnior, A. L., Costa, M. L. G., Ximenes, R. C. C., & Sougey, E. B. (2019). Is the Montreal Cognitive Assessment (MoCA) screening superior to the Mini-Mental State Examination (MMSE) in the detection of mild cognitive impairment (MCI) and Alzheimer's Disease (AD) in the elderly? *International Psychogeriatrics, 31*(4), 491–504. doi:10.1017/S1041610218001370

Posner, J., Polanczyk, G. V., & Sonuga-Barke, E. (2020). Attention-deficit hyperactivity disorder. *Lancet (London, England), 395*(10222), 450–462. doi:10.1016/S0140-6736(19)33004-1

Posner, K., Brent, D., Lucas, C., Gould, M., Stanley, B., Brown, G., Fisher, P., Zelazny, J., Burke, A., Oquendo, M., & Mann, J. (2016). *Columbia- Suicide Severity Rating Scale (C-SSRS)*. Research Foundation for Mental Hygiene, Inc. http://cssrs.columbia.edu/wp-content/uploads/C-SSRS_Pediatric-SLC_11.14.16.pdf

Substance Abuse and Mental Health Services Administration. (2016). An introduction to bipolar disorder and co-occurring substance use disorders. *Advisory. 15*(2).

Takahashi, L. K. (2019). Neurobiology of schizophrenia, mood disorders, anxiety disorders, and obsessive-compulsive disorder. In K. L. McCance, S. E. Huether, V. L. Brashers, & N. S. Rote (Eds.), *Pathophysiology: The biologic basis for disease in adults and children* (8th ed., pp. 600–618). St. Louis: Elsevier.

Ulep, M. G., Saraon, S. K., & McLea, S. (2019). Alzheimer disease. *Journal of the American Association of Nurse Practitioners, 14*(3), 129–135.

US Preventive Services Task Force, Barry, M. J., Nicholson, W. K., Silverstein, M., Chelmow, D., Coker, T. R., Davidson, K. W., Davis, E. M., Donahue, K. E., Jaén, C. R., Li, L., Ogedegbe, G., Pbert, L., Rao, G., Ruiz, J. M., Stevermer, J. J., Tsevat, J., Underwood, S. M., & Wong, J. B. (2023). Screening for depression and suicide risk in adults: US Preventive Services Task Force recommendation statement. *JAMA, 329*(23), 2057–2067.

Wilkinson, A., Anderson, S., & Wheeler, S. B. (2017). Screening for and treating postpartum depression and psychosis: A cost-effective analysis. *Maternal and Child Health Journal, 21*(4), 903–914. http://dx.doi.org/10.1007/s10995-016-2192-9

Wischenka, D. M., Marquez, C., & Felsted, K. F. (2016). Benefits of physical activity on cognitive functioning in older adults. *Annual Review of Gerontology and Geriatrics, 36*(1), 103–122. http://dx.doi.org/10.1891/0198-8794.103

Chapter 8

Abacı, A., & Besci, Ö. (2024). A Current perspective on delayed puberty and its management. *Journal of Clinical Research in Pediatric Endocrinology, 16*(4), 379–400.

Alonso, G. F. (2024). Precocious puberty, pandemic and beyond. *Pituitary, 27*, 916–924. https://doi.org/10.1007/s11102-024-01434-8

Alves, F. C. R., Moreira, A., & Moutinho, O. (2024). Maternal and long-term offspring outcomes of obesity during pregnancy. *Archives of Gynecology and Obstetrics, 309*, 2315–2321. https://doi.org/10.1007/s00404-023-07349-2

Amati, F., McCann, L., Castañeda-Gutiérrez, E., Prior, E., van Loo-Bouwman, C. A., Abrahamse-Berkeveld, M., Oliveros, E., Ozanne, S., Symonds, M. E., Chang, C. Y., & Modi, N. (2024). Infant fat mass and later child and adolescent health outcomes: A systematic review. *Archives of Disease in Childhood, 109*(2), 125–129. doi:10.1136/archdischild-2023-325798

Arab, L., Wesseling-Perry, K., Jardack, P., Henry, J., & Winter, A. (2010). Eight self-administered 24-hour dietary recalls using the Internet are feasible in African Americans and Whites: The Energetics study. *Journal of the American Dietetic Association, 110*(6), 857–864.

Ashwell, M., & Gibson, S. (2016). Waist-to-height ratio as an indicator of 'early health risk': Simpler and more predictive than using a 'matrix' based on BMI and waist circumference. *BMJ Open, 6*(3), e010159.

Barlow, S. E. (2007). Expert committee recommendations regarding the prevention, assessment, and treatment of child and adolescent overweight and obesity: Summary report. *Pediatrics, 120*(Suppl. 4), S164–S192.

Barton, A. W., Yu, T., Gong, Q., Chen, E., Miller, G. E., & Brody, G. H. (2024). . Skin-deep resilience and early adolescence: Neighborhood disadvantage, executive functioning, and pubertal development in minority youth. *Journal of Youth and Adolescence, 53*, 284–293. https://doi.org/10.1007/s10964-023-01911-6

Bennett, J. P., Wong, M. C., Liu, Y. E., Quon, B. K., Kelly, N. N., Garber, A. K., Heymsfield, S. B., & Shepherd, J. A. (2024). Trunk-to-leg volume and appendicular lean mass from a commercial 3-dimensional optical body scanner for disease risk identification. *Clinical Nutrition, 43*(10), 2430–2437. https://doi.org/10.1016/j.clnu.2024.09.028

Bioletto, F., Varaldo, E., Gasco, V., Maccario, M., Arvat, E., Ghigo, E., & Grottoli, S. (2025). Central and peripheral regulation of the GH/IGF-1 axis: GHRH and beyond. *Reviews in Endocrine & Metabolic Disorders, 26*(3), 321–342. https://doi.org/10.1007/s11154-024-09933-6

Boyd, M., Brown, C. C., & Goudie, A. (2024). Association between prepregnancy body mass index and newborn breastfeeding initiation. *Breastfeeding Medicine, 19*(4), 275–283.

Centers for Disease Control and Prevention. (2000). *Growth charts*. National Center for Health Statistics. http://www.cdc.gov/growthcharts

Centers for Disease Control and Prevention. (2009). *World Health Organization growth standards*. National Center for Health Statistics.

Centers for Disease Control and Prevention. (2013). *Skin cancer risk factors*. http://www.cdc.gov/cancer/skin/basic_info/risk_factors.htm

Chan, V., Cao, L., Wong, M. M. H., Lo, K., & Tam, W. (2024). Diagnostic accuracy of waist-to-height ratio, waist circumference, and body mass index in identifying metabolic syndrome and its components in older adults: A systematic review and meta-analysis. *Current Developments in Nutrition, 8*(1), 102061.

Cromer, B. (2011). Adolescent physical and social development. In R. M. Kliegman, B. F. Stanton, J. W. St. Geme III, N. F. Schor, & R. E. Behrman (Eds.), *Nelson textbook of pediatrics* (19th ed.). Elsevier/Saunders.

Emmerich, S. D., Fryar, C. D., Stierman, B., & Ogden, C. L. (2024, September). *Obesity and severe obesity prevalence in adults: United States, August 2021–August 2023* (*NCHS Data Brief No. 508*). National Center for Health Statistics. https://www.cdc.gov/nchs/products/index.htm

Fiegelman, S. (2011). The first year. In R. M. Kliegman, B. F. Stanton, J. W. St. Geme III, N. F. Schor, & R. E. Behrman (Eds.), *Nelson textbook of pediatrics* (19th ed.). Philadelphia: Elsevier/Saunders.

Food and Nutrition Board. (2003). *Prenatal weight gain curve by weeks of gestation*. Washington, DC: National Academies Press.

Grummer-Strawn, L. M., Reinold, C., & Krebs, N. F. (2010). Use of World Health Organization and CDC growth charts for children aged 0–59 months in the United States. *MMWR Recommendations and Reports, 59*(RR-9), 1–15.

Hales, C. M., Carroll, M. D., Fryar, C. D., & Ogden, C. L. (2020). *Prevalence of obesity and severe obesity among adults: United States, 2017–2018 (NCHS Data Brief No. 360)*. Hyattsville, MD: National Center for Health Statistics.

Harris, J. A., Jackson, C. M., Paterson, D. J., & Scammon, R. E. (1930). *The measurement of man*. Minneapolis: University of Minnesota Press.

Hawkes, C. P., Mostoufi-Moab, S., McCormack, S. E., Grimberg, A., & Zemel, B. S. (2020). Sitting height to standing height ratio reference charts for children in the United States. *The Journal of Pediatrics, 226*, 221–227.e15. doi:10.1016/j.jpeds.2020.06.051

Hockenberry, M. H., & Wilson, D. (2017). *Wong's essentials of pediatric nursing* (10th ed.). St Louis: Elsevier.

Howe, L. D., Chaturvedi, N., Lawlor, D. A., Ferreira, D. L., Fraser, A., Davey Smith, G., Tilling, K., & Hughes, A. D. (2014). Rapid increases in infant adiposity and overweight/obesity in childhood are associated with higher central and brachial blood pressure in early adulthood. *Journal of Hypertension, 32*(9), 1789–1796.

Institute of Medicine and National Research Council. (2009). *Weight gain during pregnancy: Reexamining the guidelines*. Washington, DC: National Academies Press. http://www.nap.edu/catalog.php?record_id=12584

Kalyani, R. R., Corriere, M., & Ferrucci, L. (2014). Age-related and disease-related muscle loss: The effect of diabetes, obesity, and other diseases. *The Lancet. Diabetes & Endocrinology, 2*(10), 819–829.

Keane, V. (2011). Assessment of growth. In R. M. Kliegman, B. F. Stanton, J. W. St. Geme, N. F. Schor, & R. E. Behrman (Eds.), *Nelson textbook of pediatrics* (19th ed.). Philadelphia, PA: Elsevier/Saunders.

Leung, A. K. C., Lam, J. M., & Hon, K. L. (2024). Premature thelarche: An updated review. *Current Pediatric Reviews, 20*(4), 500–509.

Liu, G. T., Volpe, N. J., & Galetta, S. L. (2010). *Neuro-ophthalmology: Diagnosis and management* (2nd ed.). London, UK: Saunders.

Low, M. J. (2011). Neuroendocrinology. In S. Melmed, K. S. Polonsky, P. R. Larsen, & H. M. Kronenberg (Eds.), *Williams textbook of endocrinology* (12th ed.). Philadelphia, PA: Elsevier/Saunders.

Marković, S., Cerovac, A., Cerovac, E., Marković, D., Bogdanović, G., & Kunosić, S. (2020). Antenatal care and weight gain in adolescent compared to adult pregnancy. *International Journal of Preventive Medicine, 11*, 115. https://doi.org/10.4103/ijpvm.IJPVM_374_19

Martinez, G. M. (2020). *Trends and patterns in menarche in the United States, 1995 through 2013–2017* (National Health Statistics Report No. 146). Hyattsville, MD: National Center for Health Statistics.

McCance, K. L., Huether, S. E., Brashers, V. L., & Rote, C. L. (2015). *Pathophysiology: The biologic basis for disease in adults and children* (7th ed.). St. Louis, MO: Elsevier Mosby.

Muth, N. D., Bolling, C., Hannon, T., Sharifi, M., Section on Obesity, & Committee on Nutrition (2024). The role of the pediatrician in the promotion of healthy, active living. *Pediatrics, 153*(3), e2023065480.

Nguyen, J. C., Patel, V., Jaramillo, D., & Caine, D. (2024). The growing skeleton. In D. Caine, J. C. Nguyen, & M. Grady (Eds.), *Physeal stress injuries in young athletes. Contemporary pediatric and adolescent sports medicine*. Cham: Springer. https://doi.org/10.1007/978-3-031-70455-0_1

Pabla, P., Jones, E. J., Piasecki, M., & Phillips, B. E. (2024). Skeletal muscle dysfunction with advancing age. *Clinical Science (London), 138*(14), 863–882. https://doi.org/10.1042/CS20231197

Patton, K. T., & Thibodeau, G. (2016). *Anatomy & physiology* (9th ed.). St Louis: Elsevier.

Reiter, E. O., & Rosenfield, R. G. (2008). Endocrine regulation of growth. In H. M. Kronenberg, S. Melmed, K. S. Polonsky, & P. R. Larsen (Eds.), *Williams textbook of endocrinology* (11th ed., pp. 857–879). Philadelphia, PA: Saunders Elsevier.

Roddick, C., Harris, M., & Hofman, P. L. (2025). The metabolic programming of pubertal onset. *Clinical Endocrinology, 102*(5), 526–538. https://doi.org/10.1111/cen.15138

Rogol, A. D. (2010). Sex steroids, growth hormone, leptin and the pubertal growth spurt. *Endocrine Development, 17*, 77–85.

Sakata, I., & Sakai, T. (2010). Ghrelin cells in the gastrointestinal tract. *International Journal of Peptides, 2010*, 945056. http://dx.doi.org/10.1155/2010/945056

Teede, H. J., Bailey, C., Moran, L. J., Bahri Khomami, M., Enticott, J., Ranasinha, S., Rogozińska, E., Skouteris, H., Boyle, J. A., Thangaratinam, S., & Harrison, C. L. (2022). Gestational weight gain and pregnancy outcomes: A systematic review and meta-analysis. *JAMA Internal Medicine, 182*(2), 106–114. doi:10.1001/jamainternmed.2021.6373

U.S. Department of Agriculture, U.S. Department of Health and Human Services. (2020). *Dietary guidelines for Americans, 2020-2025* (9th ed.). U.S. Department of Agriculture. DietaryGuidelines.gov.

U.S. Department of Agriculture. (n.d.). *ChooseMyPlate.gov*. U.S. Department of Agriculture.

U.S. Department of Health and Human Services. (2018). *Physical activity guidelines for Americans* (2nd ed.). Washington, DC: U.S. Department of Health and Human Services.

Van Wieringen, J. C., Wafelbakker, F., Verbrugge, H. P., & de Haas, J. H. (1971). *Growth diagrams 1965 Netherlands: Second national survey on 0-24 year olds*. Groningen, Netherlands: Wolters-Noordhoff Publishing.

Vasiloglou, M. F., Marcano, I., Lizama, S., Papathanail, I., Spanakis, E. K., & Mougiakakou, S. (2023). Multimedia data-based mobile applications for dietary assessment. *Journal of Diabetes Science and Technology, 17*(4), 1056–1065.

Wen, J., Tian, Y. E., Skampardoni, I., Yang, Z., Cui, Y., Anagnostakis, F., Mamourian, E., Zhao, B., Toga, A. W., Zalesky, A., & Davatzikos, C. (2024). The genetic architecture of biological age in nine human organ systems. *Nature Aging, 4*(9), 1290–1307. https://doi.org/10.1038/s43587-024-00662-8

Werner, H., Weinstein, D., & Bentov, I. (2008). Similarities and differences between insulin and IGF-I: Structures, receptors, and signalling pathways. *Archives of Physiology and Biochemistry, 114*(1), 17–22.

Zitelli, B. J., McIntire, S. C., & Nowalk, A. J. (2012). *Zitelli and Davis' atlas of pediatric physical diagnosis* (6th ed.). Philadelphia: Saunders.

Zonuzirad, M. (2024). Cellular and molecular biology of neurodevelopment. In R Kelishadi (Ed.), *Nature, nurture, and neurodevelopment.* Singapore: Springer. https://doi.org/10.1007/978-981-97-7433-3_3

Chapter 9

Baran, R., Dawber, P. R., & Levene, G. M. (1991). *Color atlas of the hair, scalp, and nails.* St Louis: Mosby.

Baren, J. M., Rothrock, S. G., Brennan, J. A., & Brown, L. (2008). *Pediatric emergency medicine.* Philadelphia: Saunders.

Brzoza, Z. (2007). Pruritic urticarial papules and plaques of pregnancy. *Journal of Midwifery & Women's Health, 52*(1), 44–48.

Buchanan, K., Fletcher, H. M., & Reid, M. (2010). Prevention of striae gravidarum with cocoa butter cream. *International Journal of Gynaecology and Obstetrics, 108*(1), 65–68.

Busam, K. J. (2016). Dermatopathology: A volume in the series: Foundations in diagnostic pathology (2nd ed.). Philadelphia: Saunders.

Callen, J. P., Greer, K. E., Paller, A. S., & Swinyer, L. J. (2000). *Color atlas of dermatology* (2nd ed.). Philadelphia: Saunders.

Carey, W. D. (2010). *Current clinical medicine* (2nd ed.). Philadelphia: Saunders.

Centers for Disease Control and Prevention. (2013). *Skin cancer risk factors.* http://www.cdc.gov/cancer/skin/basic_info/risk_factors.htm

Champagne, C., & Farrant, P. (2015). Hair loss in infancy and childhood. *Pediatric Child Health, 25*(2), 66–71.

Cordoro, K. M., & Ganz, J. E. (2005). Training room management of medical conditions: Sports dermatology. *Clinical Sports Medicine, 24*(3), 565–598.

Cuppett, M., & Walsh, K. (2012). *General medical conditions in the athlete* (2nd ed.). St Louis: Mosby.

Di Chiacchio, N., & Di Chiacchio, N. G. (2015). Best way to treat an ingrown toenail. *Dermatologic Clinics, 33*(2), 277–282.

Drago, F., Broccolo, F., Ciccarese, G., Rebora, A., & Parodi, A. (2015). Persistent pityriasis rosea: An unusual form of pityriasis rosea with persistent active HHV-6 and HHV-7 infection. *Dermatology, 230*(1), 23–26.

Ferri, F. F. (2009). Ferri's color atlas and text of clinical medicine. Philadelphia: Saunders.

Gawkrodger, D., & Ardern-Jones, M. R. (2017). *Dermatology: An illustrated color text* (6th ed.). Edinburgh: Elsevier.

Glynn, M., & Drake, W. M. (2012). Hutchison's clinical methods: An integrated approach to clinical practice (23rd ed.). Edinburgh: Saunders.

Goldman, L., & Schafer, A. I. (2016). *Goldman-Cecil medicine* (25th ed.). Philadelphia: Saunders.

Goldman, M. P., & Fitzpatrick, R. E. (1994). Cutaneous laser surgery: The art and science of selective photothermolysis. St Louis: Mosby.

Hochberg, M. C., Silman, A. J., Smolen, J. S., Weinblatt, M. E., & Weisman, M. H. (2015). *Rheumatology* (6th ed.). Philadelphia: Mosby.

Hoffbrand, A. V., Pettit, J. E., & Vyas, P. (2010). *Color atlas of clinical hematology* (4th ed.). Philadelphia: Mosby.

Ignatavicius, D. D., & Workman, M. L. (2016). *Medical-surgical nursing: Patient-centered collaborative care.* St Louis: Elsevier.

James, W. D., Berger, T. G., & Elston, D. M. (2016). *Andrews' diseases of the skin: Clinical dermatology* (12th ed.). Philadelphia: Elsevier.

Keimig, E. L. (2015). Granuloma annulare. *Dermatologic Clinics, 33*(3), 315–329.

Kliegman, R. M., & Stanton, B. M. D. (2016). *Nelson textbook of pediatrics* (20th ed.). Philadelphia: Elsevier.

Kremer, J. R., & Muller, C. P. (2009). Measles in Europe—There is room for improvement. *Lancet, 373*, 356–358.

Kumar, P., & Clark, M. L. (2017). *Kumar and Clark's clinical medicine* (9th ed.). Edinburgh: Elsevier.

Lawrence, C. M., & Cox, N. H. (1993). *Physical signs in dermatology: Color atlas and text.* St Louis: Mosby.

Lemmi, F. O., & Lemmi, C. A. E. (2000). *Physical assessment findings [CD-ROM].* Philadelphia: Saunders.

Morison, M., & Moffatt, C. (1994). *A colour guide to the assessment and management of leg ulcers* (2nd ed.). St Louis: Mosby.

National. *Pressure Ulcer Advisory Panel.* (2014). http://www.npuap.org/wp-content/uploads/2014/08/Quick-Reference-Guide-DIGITAL-NPUAP-EPUAP-PPPIA-Jan2016.pdf

Neville, B. W., Damm, D. D., Allen, C. M., & Chi, A. C. (2016). *Oral and maxillofacial pathology* (4th ed.). St Louis: Elsevier.

Paller, A. S., & Mancini, A. J. (2016). Hurwitz clinical pediatric dermatology: A textbook of skin disorders of childhood and adolescence (5th ed.). Edinburgh: Elsevier.

Salvo, S. (2014). *Mosby's pathology for massage therapists* (3rd ed.). St Louis: Mosby.

Scheinfeld, N. S. (2004). Obesity and dermatology. *Clinical Dermatology, 22*(4), 303–309.

Scher, R. K., & Daniel, C. R. (2005). *Nails: Diagnosis, therapy, surgery* (3rd ed.). Philadelphia: Saunders.

Spicknall, K. E., Zirwas, M. J., & English, J. C. (2005). Clubbing: An update on diagnosis, differential diagnosis, pathophysiology, and clinical relevance. *Journal of the American Academy of Dermatology, 52*(6), 1020–1028.

Swartz, M. H. (2014). *Textbook of physical diagnosis* (7th ed.). Philadelphia: Saunders.

Taïeb, A., & Boralevi, F. (2007). Hypermelanoses of the newborn and of the infant. *Dermatologic Clinics, 25*(3), 327–336.

Thompson, J. M., McFarland, G. K., Hirsch, J. E., & Baird, K. (2002). *Mosby's clinical nursing* (5th ed.). St Louis: Mosby.

Tunzi, M., & Gray, G. R. (2007). Common skin conditions during pregnancy. *American Family Physician, 75*(2), 211–218.

Tüzün, Y., Wolf, R., Kutlubay, Z., & Engin, B. (2014). Rosacea and rhinophyma. *Clinics in Dermatology, 32*(1), 35–46.

Weston, W. L., Lane, A. T., & Morelli, J. G. (2007). *Color textbook of pediatric dermatology* (4th ed.). St Louis: Mosby.

White, G. M. (1994). *Color atlas of regional dermatology.* St Louis: Mosby.

Wollina, U. (2011). Rosacea and rhinophyma in the elderly. *Clinics in Dermatology, 29*(1), 61–68.

Zaoutis, L. B., & Chiang, V. W. (2007). *Comprehensive pediatric hospital medicine*. Philadelphia: Mosby.

Zitelli, B. J., McIntire, S. C., & Nowalk, A. J. (2012). *Zitelli and Davis' atlas of pediatric physical diagnosis* (6th ed.). Philadelphia: Saunders.

Chapter 10

Armitage, J. (2023). Approach to the patient with lymphadenopathy and splenomegaly. In L. Goldman & A. I. Safer (Eds.), *Goldman's Cecil medicine* (27th ed.). Philadelphia: Elsevier.

Bamji, M., Stone, R. K., Kaul, A., Usmani, G., Schachter, F. F., & Wasserman, E. (1986). Palpable lymph nodes in healthy newborns and infants. *Pediatrics, 78*(4), 573–575.

Coates, E. E., Costner, P. J., Nason, M. C., Herrin, D. M., Conant, S., Herscovitch, P., Sarwar, U. N., Holman, L., Mitchell, J., Yamshchikov, G., Koup, R. A., Graham, B. S., Millo, C. M., Ledgerwood, J. E., & VRC 900 Study Team. (2017). Lymph node activation by PET/CT following vaccination with licensed vaccines for human papillomaviruses. *Clinical Nuclear Medicine, 42*(5), 329–334.

Dains, J. E., et al. (2024). Advanced health assessment and clinical diagnosis in primary care (7th ed.). St. Louis: Elsevier.

Executive Committee of the International Society of Lymphology. (2020). The diagnosis and treatment of peripheral lymphedema: 2020 Consensus Document of the International Society of Lymphology. *Lymphology, 53*(1), 3-19. https://journals.librarypublishing.arizona.edu/lymph/article/id/4649/

Gabbe, S. G., et al. (2020). *Obstetrics: Normal and problem pregnancies* (8th ed.). Philadelphia: Elsevier.

Ho, T. C., Shen, D. H., Chang, C. C., Chan, H. P., Chuang, K. P., Yuan, C. H., Chen, C. N., Yang, M. H., & Tyan, Y. C. (2023). Immune response related to lymphadenopathy post COVID-19 vaccination. *Vaccines, 11*(3), 696.

Pereira, M. P., Flores, P., & Neto, A. S. (2019). Neck and supraclavicular lymphadenopathy secondary to 9-valent human papillomavirus vaccination. *BMJ Case Reports, 12*(11), e231582.

Studdiford, J., Lamb, K., Horvath, K., Altshuler, M., & Stonehouse, A. (2008). Development of unilateral cervical and supraclavicular lymphadenopathy after human papilloma virus vaccination. *Pharmacotherapy, 28*(9), 1194–1197.

Chapter 11

No references for this chapter.

Chapter 12

American Academy of Ophthalmology Pediatric Ophthalmology/Strabismus Panel. (2012). *Preferred practice pattern guidelines: Pediatric eye evaluations.* San Francisco, CA: American Academy of Ophthalmology. www.aao.org/ppp

American Academy of Pediatrics Section on Ophthalmology. (2012). Committee on practice and ambulatory medicine, American Academy of Ophthalmology, American Association for pediatric Ophthalmology and Strabismus, American Association of Certified Orthoptists: Instrument-based pediatric vision screening policy statement. *Pediatrics, 130*(5), 983–986, http://dx.doi.org/10.1542/peds.2012-2548

Courage, M. L., & Adams, R. J. (1990). Visual acuity assessment from birth to three years using the acuity card procedure: Cross-sectional and longitudinal samples. *Optometry and Vision Science, 67*(9), 713–718.

Donahue, S. P., Baker, C. N., Committee on practice and ambulatory medicine, Section on Ophthalmology, American Association of Certified Orthoptists, American Association for pediatric Ophthalmology and Strabismus, & American Academy of Ophthalmology. (2015). Procedures for the evaluation of the visual system by pediatricians. *Pediatrics, 3597,* 2015, http://dx.doi.org/10.1542/peds.2015-3597

Fierson, W. M., American Academy of Pediatrics Section on Ophthalmology, American Academy of Ophthalmology, American Association for Pediatric Ophthalmology and Strabismus, & American Association of Certified Orthoptists. (2018). Screening examination of premature infants for retinopathy of prematurity. *Pediatrics, 142*(6), e20183061.

Harjasouliha, A., Raiji, V., & Garcia Gonzalez, J. M. (2017). *Review of hypertensive retinopathy. Disease-a-Month,* 63(3), 63–69. http://www.sciencedirect.com/science/article/pii/S0011502916300839

Loh, A. R., & Chiang, M. F. (2018). Pediatric vision screening. *Pediatrics in Review, 39*(5), 225–234.

Sokol, S. (1978). Measurement of infant visual acuity from pattern reversal evoked potentials. *Vision Research, 18*(1), 33–39.

U.S. Preventive Services Task Force. (2011). Vision screening for children 1 to 5 years of age: U.S. Preventive Services Task Force recommendation statement. *Pediatrics, 127,* 340–346.

Chapter 13

American Cancer Society. (2021). *Risk factors for oral cavity and oropharyngeal cancers.* https://www.cancer.org/cancer/types/oral-cavity-and-oropharyngeal-cancer/causes-risks-prevention/risk-factors.html

American Speech-Language-Hearing Association. (2024). *Communication milestones: Birth to 1 Year (asha.org).* https://www.asha.org/public/developmental-milestones/communication-milestones-birth-to-1-year/

Bhattacharyya, I., & Chehal, H. K. (2011). White lesions. *Otolaryngologic Clinics of North America, 44,* 109–131.

Bochner, R. E., Gangar, M., & Belamarich, P. F. (2017). A clinical approach to tonsillitis, tonsillar hypertrophy, and peritonsillar and retropharyngeal abscesses. *Pediatrics in Review, 38*(2), 81–82.

Bower, C., Reilly, B. K., Richerson, J., Hecht, J. L., American Academy of Pediatrics Committee on Practice & Ambulatory Medicine, & Section on Otolaryngology-Head and Neck Surgery. (2023). Hearing Assessment in Infants, Children, and Adolescents: Recommendations Beyond Neonatal Screening. *Pediatrics, 152*(3), e2023063288.

DeMuri, G. P., & Wald, E. R. (2010). Acute sinusitis: Clinical manifestations and treatment options. *Pediatric Annals, 39*(1), 34–40.

Feltner, C., Wallace, I. F., Kistler, C. E., Coker-Schwimmer, M., & Jonas, D. E. (2021). Screening for hearing loss in older adults: Updated evidence report and systematic review for the US Preventive Services Task Force. *JAMA, 325*(12), 1202–1215.

Fine, A. M., Nizet, V., & Mandl, K. D. (2012). Large-scale validation of the Centor and McIsaac scores to predict group A streptococcal pharyngitis. *Archives of Internal Medicine, 172*(11), 847–852.

Iwata, J. (2021). Gene-environment interplay and MicroRNAs in cleft lip and cleft palate. *Oral Science International, 18*(1), 3–13.

Kraft, C. T., Malhotra, S., Boerst, A., & Thorne, M. C. (2014). Risk indicators for congenital and delayed-onset hearing loss. *Otology & Neurotology, 35*(10), 1839–1843.

Marur, S., & Forastiere, A. A. (2016). Head and neck squamous cell carcinoma: Update on epidemiology, diagnosis, and treatment. *Mayo Clinic Proceedings, 91*(3), 386–396.

McShefferty, D., Whitmer, W. M., Swan, I. R. C., & Akeroyd, M. A. (2013). The effect of experience on the sensitivity and specificity of the whispered voice test: A diagnostic accuracy study. *BMJ Open, 3*(4), e002394.

National Institute for Deafness and Communication Disorders (NIDCD). (2023, March). *Age-related hearing loss (Presbycusis), Publication Number 23-DC-4235.*

Powell, E. L., Powell, J., Samuel, J. R., & Wilson, J. A. (2013). A review of the pathogenesis of adult peritonsillar abscess: Time for a re-evaluation. *Journal of Antimicrobial Chemotherapy, 68*(9), 1941–1950.

Silk, H. (2014). Diseases of the mouth. *Primary Care, 41*(1), 75–90.

Swartz, M. H. (2020). The ear and nose. In M. H. Swartz (Ed.), *Textbook of physical diagnosis: History and examination* (8th ed., pp. 228–248). Elsevier.

Tan, H. L., Kheirandish-Gozal, L., Abel, F., & Gozal, D. (2016). Craniofacial syndromes and sleep-related breathing disorders. *Sleep Medicine Reviews, 27,* 74–88.

Van Laer, L., Dietz, H., & Loeys, B. (2014). Loeys-Dietz syndrome. *Advances in Experimental Medicine and Biology, 802,* 95–105.

Chapter 14

Hochberg, M. C., et al. (2015). *Rheumatology* (6th ed.). Philadelphia: Elsevier.

Hockenberry, M. J. (2009). *Wong's essentials of pediatric nursing* (8th ed.). St. Louis Mosby/Elsevier.

Wilson, S. F., & Giddens, J. F. (2017). *Health assessment for nursing practice* (6th ed.). St. Louis: Elsevier.

Chapter 15

Abellan van Kan, G., Rolland, Y. M., Morley, J. E., & Vellas, B. (2008). Frailty: Toward a clinical definition. *Journal of the American Medical Directors Association, 2,* 71–72.

American Heart Association. (2024). *American Heart Association recommendations for physical activity in adults and kids.* https://www.heart.org/en/healthy-living/fitness/fitness-basics/aha-recs-for-physical-activity-in-adults

Arnett, D. K., Blumenthal, R. S., Albert, M. A., Buroker, A. B., Goldberger, Z. D., Hahn, E. J., Himmelfarb, C. D., Khera, A., Lloyd-Jones, D., McEvoy, J. W., Michos, E. D., Miedema, M. D., Muñoz, D., Smith, S. C. Jr., Virani, S. S., Williams, K. A. Sr., Yeboah, J., & Ziaeian B. (2019). 2019 ACC/AHA guideline on the primary prevention of cardiovascular disease: A report of the American College of Cardiology/American Heart Association Task Force on Clinical Practice Guidelines. *Circulation, 140,* e596–e646. doi:10.1161/CIR.0000000000000678

Department of Health and Human Services. (2008). *Physical activity guidelines for Americans.* http://www.health.gov/paguidelines/default.aspx

Gewitz, M. H., Baltimore, R. S., Tani, L. Y., Sable, C. A., Shulman, S. T., Carapetis, J., Remenyi, B., Taubert, K. A., Bolger, A. F., Beerman, L., Mayosi, B. M., Beaton, A., Pandian, N. G., Kaplan, E. L., & American Heart Association Committee on Rheumatic Fever, Endocarditis, and Kawasaki Disease of the Council on Cardiovascular Disease in the Young. (2015). Revision of the Jones criteria for the diagnosis of acute rheumatic fever in the era of Doppler echocardiography: A scientific statement from the American heart Association. *Circulation, 131,* 1806–1818.

Kelder, J. C., Cramer, M. J., van Wijngaarden, J., van Tooren, R., Mosterd, A., Moons, K. G., Lammers, J. W., Cowie, M. R., Grobbee, D. E., & Hoes, A. W. (2011). The diagnostic value of physical examination and additional testing in primary care patients with suspected heart failure. *Circulation, 124*(25), 2865–2873. doi:10.1161/CIRCULATIONAHA.111.019216

Lahiri, S., & Sanyahumbi, A. (2021). Acute rheumatic fever. *Pediatrics in Review, 42*(5), 221–232. https://doi.org/10.1542/pir.2019-0288

Mikrou, P., & Ramesh, P. (2017). General paediatric evaluation of heart murmurs. *Paediatrics & Child Health, 27*(2), 90–92. http://dx.doi.org/10.1016/j.paed.2016.09.004

Stone, N. J., Robinson, J. G., Lichtenstein, A. H., Bairey Merz, C. N., Blum, C. B., Eckel, R. H., Goldberg, A. C., Gordon, D., Levy, D., Lloyd-Jones, D. M., McBride, P., Schwartz, J. S., Shero, S. T., Smith, S. C., Jr, Watson, K., Wilson, P. W., & American College of Cardiology/American Heart Association Task Force on Practice Guidelines (2014). 2013 ACC/AHA guideline on the treatment of blood cholesterol to reduce atherosclerotic cardiovascular risk in adults: A report of the American College of Cardiology/American Heart Association Task Force on Practice Guidelines. *Journal of the American College of Cardiology, 63*(25 Pt B), 2889–2934. http://dx.doi.org/10.1016/j.jacc.2013.11.002

Walsh, B., Fogg, C., Harris, S., Roderick, P., de Lusignan, S., England, T., Clegg, A., Brailsford, S., & Fraser, S. D. S. (2023). Frailty transitions and prevalence in an ageing population: Longitudinal analysis of primary care data from an open cohort of adults aged 50 and over in England, 2006-2017. *Age and Ageing, 52*(5), afad058. doi:10.1093/ageing/afad058

Chapter 16

Anuforo, A., Evbayekha, E., Agwuegbo, C., Okafor, T. L., Antia, A., Adabale, O., Ugoala, O. S., Okorare, O., Phagoora, J., Alagbo, H. O., Shamaki, G. R., & Disreal Bob-Manuel, T. (2024). Superficial venous disease-an updated review. *Annals of Vascular Surgery, 105,* 106–124. https://doi.org/10.1016/j.avsg.2024.01.009

Herrick, A. L., & Wigley, F. M. (2020). Raynaud's phenomenon. *Best Practice & Research. Clinical Rheumatology, 34*(1), 101474. doi:10.1016/j.berh.2019.101474

Ives, C. W., Sinkey, R., Rajapreyar, I., Tita, A. T. N., & Oparil, S. (2020). Preeclampsia-pathophysiology and clinical presentations: JACC State-of-the-art review. *Journal of the American College of Cardiology, 76*(14), 1690–1702. https://doi.org/10.1016/j.jacc.2020.08.014

Omar, H. R., & Guglin, M. (2018). Extent of jugular venous distension and lower extremity edema are the best tools from history and physical examination to identify heart failure exacerbation. *Herz, 43*(8), 752–758. English.

Rife, E., & Gedalia, A. (2020). Kawasaki disease: An update. *Current Rheumatology Reports, 22*(10), 75. doi:10.1007/s11926-020-00941-4

Thomas, D. C., Thomas, P., Pillai, D. P., Joseph, D., Lingaiah, U., Mathai, B. C., Ravi, A., Chhabra, S., & Pitchumani, P. K. (2022). Giant cell arteritis: A case-based narrative review of the literature. *Current Pain and Headache Reports, 26*(10), 725–740. doi:10.1007/s11916-022-01075-1

Chapter 17

American Cancer Society. (2022). *Breast cancer risk and prevention.* https://www.cancer.org/cancer/types/breast-cancer/risk-and-prevention.html. Accessed March 15, 2025.

American Cancer Society. (2023, December 19). American Cancer Society recommendations for the early detection of breast cancer.

REFERENCES

Barton, M., Harris, R., & Fletcher, S. W. (1999). Does this patient have breast cancer? The screening clinical breast examination: Should it be done? How? *Journal of the American Medical Association, 282*(13), 1270–1280.

Dains, J. E., Baumannet, L. C., & Scheibel, P. (2024). *Advanced health assessment and clinical diagnosis in primary care* (7th ed.). St Louis: Elsevier.

Deutsch, M. B. (Ed.). *Guidelines for the primary care of transgender and gender nonbinary people* (2nd ed.). UCSF Center of Excellence for Transgender Health; 2016. https://transcare.ucsf.edu/guidelines

Henderson, J. T., Webber, E. M., Weyrich, M. S., Miller, M., & Melnikow, J. (2024). Screening for breast cancer: Evidence report and systematic review for the US Preventive Services Task Force. *JAMA, 331*(22), 1931–1946.

https://www.cancer.org/cancer/types/breast-cancer/screening-tests-and-early-detection/american-cancer-society-recommendations-for-the-early-detection-of-breast-cancer.html. Accessed March 15, 2025.

Laufer, S., Cohen, E. R., Kwan, C., D'Angelo, A. L., Yudkowsky, R., Boulet, J. R., McGaghie, W. C., & Pugh, C. M. (2015). Sensor technology in assessments of clinical skill. *The New England Journal of Medicine, 372*(8), 784–786.

Laufer, S., D'Angelo, A. D., Kwan, C., Ray, R. D., Yudkowsky, R., Boulet, J. R., McGaghie, W. C., & Pugh, C. M. (2017). Rescuing the clinical breast examination: Advances in classifying technique and assessing physician competency. *Annals of Surgery, 266*(6), 1069–1074.

McDonald, S., Saslow, D., & Alciati, M. H. (2004). Performance and reporting of clinical breast examination: A review of the literature. *CA: A Cancer Journal for Clinicians, 54*, 345–361.

Myers, E. R., Moorman, P., Gierisch, J. M., Havrilesky, L. J., Grimm, L. J., Ghate, S., Davidson, B., Mongtomery, R. C., Crowley, M. J., McCrory, D. C., Kendrick, A., & Sanders, G. D. (2015). Benefits and Harms of Breast Cancer Screening: A Systematic Review. *JAMA, 314*(15), 1615–1634.

National Cancer Institute. (2024, April 24). *Genetics of breast and ovarian cancer (PDQ®)*. https://www.cancer.gov/types/breast/hp/breast-ovarian-genetics-pdq#section/all. Accessed March 15, 2025.

National Cancer Institute. (2024, March 15). *Breast cancer prevention (PDQ®)–health professional version*. https://www.cancer.gov/types/breast/hp/breast-prevention-pdq#_558. Accessed March 15, 2025.

Saslow, D., Hannan, J., Osuch, J., Alciati, M. H., Baines, C., Barton, M., Bobo, J. K., Coleman, C., Dolan, M., Gaumer, G., Kopans, D., Kutner, S., Lane, D. S., Lawson, H., Meissner, H., Moorman, C., Pennypacker, H., Pierce, P., Sciandra, E., Smith, R., ... Coates, R. (2004). Clinical breast examination: Practical recommendations for optimizing performance and reporting. *CA: A Cancer Journal for Clinicians, 54*(6), 327–344.

Saunders, K. J., Pilgrim, C. A., & Pennypacker, H. S. (1986). Increased proficiency of search in breast self-examination. *Cancer, 58*, 2531–2537.

U.S. Preventive Services Task Force. (2024). *Breast cancer: Screening*. https://www.uspreventiveservicestaskforce.org/uspstf/recommendation/breast-cancer-screening. Accessed October 10, 2024.

Uçar, A., Saka, N., Baş, F., Bundak, R., Günöz, H., & Darendeliler, F. (2012). Is premature thelarche in the first two years of life transient? *Journal of Clinical Research in Pediatric Endocrinology, 4*(3), 140–145.

Chapter 18

Abdella Bahta, N. N., Zeinert, P., Rosenberg, J., & Fonnes, S. (2023). The Alvarado score is the most impactful diagnostic tool for appendicitis: A bibliometric analysis. *The Journal of Surgical Research, 291*, 557–566.

Aldulaimi, S., & Mendez, A. M. (2021). Splenomegaly: Diagnosis and management in adults. *American Family Physician, 104*(3), 271–276.

Amatya, P., Shah, D., Gupta, N., & Bhatta, N. K. (2014). Clinical and ultrasonographic measurement of liver size in normal children. *Indian Journal of Pediatrics, 81*(5), 441–445.

American Cancer Society. (2024). *Colorectal cancer risk factors*. https://www.cancer.org/cancer/types/colon-rectal-cancer/causes-risks-prevention/risk-factors.html

Bartlett, A., Williams, R., & Hilton, M. (2016). Splenic rupture in infectious mononucleosis: A systematic review of published case reports. *Injury, 47*(3), 531–538.

Ben Kridis, W., Boudawara, T., & Khanfir, A. (2023). Sister Mary Joseph's nodule revealing cholangiocarcinoma. *Frontline Gastroenterology, 14*(6), 530–531.

Centers for Disease Control and Prevention. (2020). *The ABCs of hepatitis—for health professionals*. https://www.cdc.gov/hepatitis/resources/professionals/pdfs/abctable.pdf. Accessed November 21, 2024.

Dains, J. E., Baumann, L. C., & Scheibel, P. (2024). *Advanced health assessment & clinical diagnosis in primary care* (7th ed.). St Louis: Elsevier.

Drossman, D. A. (2016). Functional gastrointestinal disorders: History, pathophysiology, clinical features and Rome IV. *Gastroenterology, 150*(6), 1262–1279.

Felman, M., Friedman, L. S., & Brandt, L. J. (2006). *Sleisenger and Fordtran's gastrointestinal and liver disease* (8th ed.). Elsevier.

Harris, S., & Naina, H. V. (2008). Cullen's sign revisited. *The American Journal of Medicine, 121*(8), 682–683.

Harvey, S., Matthai, S., & King, D. A. (2023). How to use the Bristol Stool Chart in childhood constipation. *Archives of Disease in Childhood – Education and Practice Edition, 108*(5), 335–339.

Kularatna, M., Lauti, M., Haran, C., MacFater, W., Sheikh, L., Huang, Y., McCall, J., & MacCormick, A. D.. (2017). Clinical prediction rules for appendicitis in adults: Which is best? *World Journal of Surgery, 41*(7), 1769–1781.

Kulik, D. M., Uleryk, E. M., & Maguire, J. L. (2013). Does this child have appendicitis? A systematic review of clinical prediction rules for children with acute abdominal pain. *Journal of Clinical Epidemiology, 66*(1), 95–104.

Le, M. H., Le, D. M., Baez, T. C., Wu, Y., Ito, T., Lee, E. Y., Lee, K., Stave, C. D., Henry, L., Barnett, S. D., Cheung, R., & Nguyen, M. H. (2023). Global incidence of non-alcoholic fatty liver disease: A systematic review and meta-analysis of 63 studies and 1,201,807 persons. *Journal of Hepatology, 79*(2), 287–295.

Lederle, F. A., & Simel, D. L. (1999). The rational clinical examination: Does this patient have abdominal aortic aneurysm? *JAMA, 281*(1), 77–82.

LeFevre, M. L., U.S. Preventive Services Task Force. (2014). Screening for abdominal aortic aneurysm: U.S. Preventive services task force recommendation statement. *Annals of Internal Medicine, 161*(4), 281–290.

Lissauer, T., & Will, C. (2017). *Illustrated textbook of paediatrics* (5th ed.). Elsevier.

Loloi, J., Patel, N., McDevitt, P., Bruno, M. A., & Riley, T. (2019). How strongly do physical examination estimates and ultrasound measurements of liver size correlate? A prospective study. *The American Journal of Medicine, 132*(1), 103–108. http://dx.doi.org/10.1016/j.amjmed.2018.09.012

Marin, J. R., & Alpern, E. R. (2011). Abdominal pain in children. *Emergency Medicine Clinics of North America, 29*(2), 401–428, ix–x.

Marinis, A., Yiallourou, A., Samanides, L., Dafnios, N., Anastasopoulos, G., Vassiliou, I., & Theodosopoulos, T. (2009). Intussusception of the bowel in adults: A review. *World Journal of Gastroenterology, 15*(4), 407.

Petrick, J. L., Kelly, S. P., Altekruse, S. F., McGlynn, K. A., & Rosenberg, P. S. (2016). Future of hepatocellular carcinoma incidence in the United States forecast through 2030. *Journal of Clinical Oncology, 34*(15), 1787–1794.

Rossi, B. V., Ference, E. H., Zurakowski, D., Scholz, S., Feins, N. R., Chow, J. S., & Laufer, M. R. (2012). The clinical presentation and surgical management of adnexal torsion in the pediatric and adolescent population. *Journal of Pediatric and Adolescent Gynecology, 25*(2), 109–113.

Simel, D. L. (2009). Update: Ascites. In D. L. Simel & D. Rennie (Eds.), *The rational clinical examination evidence-based clinical diagnosis*. New York: McGraw Hill.

U.S. Preventive Services Task Force, Davidson, K. W., Barry, M. J., Mangione, C. M., Cabana, M., Caughey, A. B., Davis, E. M., Donahue, K. E., Doubeni, C. A., Krist, A. H., Kubik, M., Li, L., Ogedegbe, G., Owens, D. K., Pbert, L., Silverstein, M., Stevermer, J., Tseng, C. W., & Wong, J. B. (2021). Screening for colorectal cancer: US Preventive Services Task Force recommendation statement. *JAMA, 325*(19), 1965–1977.

U.S. Preventive Services Task Force. (2019). *Final recommendation statement: Abdominal aortic aneurysm screening.* Rockville, MD: U.S. Department of Health and Human Services, Agency for Healthcare Research and Quality. http://www.uspreventiveservicestaskforce.org/Page/Document/UpdateSummaryFinal/abdominal-aortic-aneurysm-screening

Veloso, F. T. (2016). Clinical predictors of Crohn's disease course. *European Journal of Gastroenterology & Hepatology, 28*(10), 1122–1125.

Wilson, S. F., & Giddens, J. F. (2009). *Health assessment for nursing practice* (4th ed.). St Louis: Mosby.

Zitelli, B. J., McIntire, S. C., Nowalk, A. J., Zitelli, B. J., & Davis, H. W. (2018). *Zitelli and Davis' atlas of pediatric physical diagnosis* (7th ed.). Philadelphia: Elsevier.

Chapter 19

American Academy of Pediatrics. (2023). *HPV.* https://www.aap.org/en/news-room/campaigns-and-toolkits/human-papillomavirus-hpv/?srsltid=AfmBOoojENM_hTDlAuj3tIghh4Du6L511Gd3nw-gdiYeyPpXByZcEYxt. Accessed September 24, 2024.

American Cancer Society. (2019). *Endometrial cancer risk factors.* https://www.cancer.org/cancer/endometrial-cancer/causes-risks-prevention/risk-factors.html. Accessed September 24, 2024.

American Cancer Society. (2020). *Risk factors for cervical cancer.* https://www.cancer.org/cancer/types/cervical-cancer/causes-risks-prevention/risk-factors.html. Accessed September 24, 2024.

American Cancer Society. (2021). *Ovarian cancer risk factors.* https://www.cancer.org/cancer/types/ovarian-cancer/causes-risks-prevention/risk-factors.html. Accessed September 24, 2024.

American Cancer Society. (2021). *The American Cancer Society guidelines for the prevention and early detection of cervical cancer.* https://www.cancer.org/cancer/types/cervical-cancer/detection-diagnosis-staging/cervical-cancer-screening-guidelines.html. Accessed September 24, 2024.

American Congress of Obstetricians and Gynecologists statement on HPV vaccination. (2019). https://www.acog.org/news/news-releases/2019/06/acog-statement-on-hpv-vaccination. Accessed September 24, 2024.

Borg, K., Snowdon, C., & Hodes, D. (2014). Child sexual abuse: Recognition and response when there is a suspicion or allegation. *Paediatrics and Child Health, 24*(12), 536–543.

Centers for Disease Control and Prevention. (2024). *Human papillomavirus (HPV).* http://www.cdc.gov/hpv/index.html. Accessed September 25, 2024.

Charoenkwan, K., Ninunanahaeminda, K., Khunamornpong, S., Srisomboon, J., & Thorner, P. S. (2008). Effects of gel lubricant on cervical cytology. *Acta Cytologica, 52*(6), 654–658.

Dains, J. E., Baumann, L. C., & Scheibel, P. (2024). *Advanced health assessment and clinical diagnosis in primary care* (7th ed.). St. Louis: Elsevier.

Deutsch, M. B. (Ed.). *Guidelines for the primary care of transgender and gender nonbinary people* (2nd ed.). UCSF Center of Excellence for Transgender Health; 2016. https://prevention.ucsf.edu/transhealth

Fox, G. N. (1985). Teaching first trimester uterine sizing. *Journal of Family Practice, 21*(5), 400–401.

Gilson, M., Desai, A., Cardoza-Favarato, G., Vroman, P., & Thornton, J. A. (2006). Does gel affect cytology or comfort in the screening papanicolaou smear? *Journal of the American Board of Family Medicine, 19*(4), 340–344.

Griffith, W. F., Stuart, G. S., Gluck, K. L., & Heartwell, S. F. (2005). Vaginal speculum lubrication and its effects on cervical cytology and microbiology. *Contraception, 72*(1), 60–64.

Haka-Ikse, K., & Mian, M. (1993). Sexuality in children. *Pediatrics in Review, 14*(10), 401–407.

Harer, W. B. J., Valenzuela, G., & Lebo, D. (2003). Lubrication of the vaginal introitus and external speculum had no effect on Papanicolaou smear interpretation [Commentary]. *Evidence-Based Medicine, 8*(3), 79.

Hornor, G. (2004). Sexual behavior in children. Normal or not? *Journal of Pediatric Health Care, 18*(2), 57–64.

Jenny, C., Crawford-Jakubiak, J. E., Committee on Child Abuse and Neglect, & American Academy of Pediatrics. (2013). The evaluation of children in the primary care setting when sexual abuse is suspected. *Pediatrics, 132*(2), e558–e567. http://dx.doi.org/10.1542/peds.2013-1741; http://pediatrics.aappublications.org/content/pediatrics/132/2/e558.full.pdf

Kellogg, N. D. (2010). Sexual behaviors in children: Evaluation and management. *American Family Physician, 82*(10), 1233–1238.

Koop, C. E. (1988). *The Surgeon General's letter on child sexual abuse.* Rockville, MD: Department of Health and Human Services, Public Health Service.

Köşüş, A., Köşüş, N., Duran, M., Haltaş, H., Hızlı, D., & Kafalı, H. (2012). Effect of liquid-based gel application during speculum examination on satisfactory level of smear examination. *Archives of Gynecology and Obstetrics, 285*(6), 1599–1602.

Lin, S. N., Taylor, J., Alperstein, S., Hoda, R., & Holcomb, K. (2014). Does speculum lubricant affect liquid-based Papanicolaou test adequacy? *Cancer Cytopathology, 122*(3), 221–226. http://dx.doi.org/10.1002/cncy.21369.

Mallants, C., & Casteels, K. (2008). Practical approach to childhood masturbation—a review. *European Journal of Pediatrics, 167*(10), 1111–1117.

McClain, N., Girardet, R., Lahoti, S., Cheung, K., Berger, K., & McNeese, M. (2000). Evaluation of sexual abuse in the pediatric patient. *Journal of Pediatric Health Care, 14*(3), 93–102.
Munro, M. G., Critchley, H. O. D., Fraser, I. S., & FIGO Menstrual Disorders Committee (2018). The two FIGO systems for normal and abnormal uterine bleeding symptoms and classification of causes of abnormal uterine bleeding in the reproductive years: 2018 revisions. *International Journal of Gynaecology and Obstetrics, 143*(3), 393–408. https://doi.org/10.1002/ijgo.12666
Thompson, J. M., McFarland, G. K., Tucker, S. M., Hirsch, J. E. (1997). *Clinical nursing* (4th ed.). St. Louis: Mosby.
U.S. Preventive Services Task Force. (2018). *Final recommendation statement cervical cancer: Screening.* https://www.uspreventiveservicestaskforce.org/Page/Document/RecommendationStatementFinal/cervical-cancer-screening#rationale. Accessed September 26, 2024.
Wang, Z., Asokan, G., Onnela, J. P., Baird, D. D., Jukic, A. M. Z., Wilcox, A. J., Curry, C. L., Fischer-Colbrie, T., Williams, M. A., Hauser, R., Coull, B. A., & Mahalingaiah, S. (2024). Menarche and time to cycle regularity among individuals born between 1950 and 2005 in the US. *JAMA Network Open, 7*(5), e2412854. doi:10.1001/jamanetworkopen.2024.12854
Zardawi, I. M., Catterall, N., Duncan, J., Sullivan, J., & Warwick, L. (2003). Effects of lubricant gel on conventional and liquid-based cervical smears [letter]. *Acta Cytologica, 47*(4), 704–705.

Chapter 20

American Academy of Pediatrics. (2023). *HPV.* https://www.aap.org/en/news-room/campaigns-and-toolkits/human-papillomavirus-hpv/?srsltid=AfmBOoojENM_hTDlAuj3tIghh4Du6L511Gd3nw-gdiYeyPpXByZcEYxt. Accessed September 30, 2024.
American Cancer Society. (2018). *Risk factors for penile cancer.* https://www.cancer.org/cancer/types/penile-cancer/causes-risks-prevention/risk-factors.html. Accessed September 30, 2024.
American Cancer Society. (2024). *Risk factors for testicular cancer.* https://www.cancer.org/cancer/types/testicular-cancer/causes-risks-prevention/risk-factors.html. Accessed September 30, 2024.
Centers for Disease Control and Prevention. (2024). *Human papillomavirus (HPV).* http://www.cdc.gov/hpv/index.html. Accessed September 30, 2024.
Choudhury, P., Saroya, K. K., Anand, S., Agarwal, P., Jain, V., Dhua, A. K., Yadav, D. K., Agarwala, S., Bajpai, M., Mawar, S., Afroz, M., Verma, V., Singh, H., & Goel, P. (2023). Unjumbling the TWIST score for testicular torsion: Systematic review and meta-analysis. *Pediatric Surgery International, 39*(1), 137.
Dains, J. E., Baumann, L. C., & Scheibel, P. (2024). *Advanced health assessment and clinical diagnosis in primary care* (7th ed.). St. Louis: Elsevier.
Deutsch, M. B. (Ed.). *Guidelines for the primary care of transgender and gender nonbinary people* (2nd ed.). UCSF Center of Excellence for Transgender Health; 2016. http://transhealth.ucsf.edu/trans?page=guidelines-home
Kim, A. G., & Jarboe, M. D. (2020). Inguinal and other hernias. *Advances in Pediatrics, 67,* 131–143.
Kryger, J. V., et al. (2022). Acute and chronic scrotal swelling. In R. Kleigman, et al. (Eds.). *Nelson Symptom Based Diagnosis* (2nd ed., pp. 409–420.e2). Elsevier.
Lacy, A., Smith, A., Koyfman, A., & Long, B. (2023). High risk and low prevalence diseases: Testicular torsion. *American Journal of Emergency Medicine, 66,* 98–104.
Offenbacher, J., & Barbera, A. (2019). Penile emergencies. *Emergency Medicine Clinics of North America, 37*(4), 583–592.
Shakil, A., Aparicio, K., Barta, E., & Munez, K. (2020). Inguinal hernias: Diagnosis and management. *American Family Physician, 102*(8), 487–492.

Chapter 21

Andriole, G. L., Crawford, E. D., Grubb, R. L., 3rd, Buys, S. S., Chia, D., Church, T. R., Fouad, M. N., Gelmann, E. P., Kvale, P. A., Reding, D. J., Weissfeld, J. L., Yokochi, L. A., O'Brien, B., Clapp, J. D., Rathmell, J. M., Riley, T. L., Hayes, R. B., Kramer, B. S., Izmirlian, G., Miller, A. B., ... PLCO Project Team. (2009). Mortality results from a randomized prostate-cancer screening trial. *New England Journal of Medicine, 360,* 1310–1319.
Andriole, G. L., Crawford, E. D., Grubb, R. L. III, Buys, S. S., Chia, D., Church, T. R., Fouad, M. N., Isaacs, C., Kvale, P. A., Reding, D. J., Weissfeld, J. L., Yokochi, L. A., O'Brien, B., Ragard, L. R., Clapp, J. D., Rathmell, J. M., Riley, T. L., Hsing, A. W., Izmirlian, G., Pinsky, P. F., ... PLCO Project Team. (2012). Prostate cancer screening in the randomized prostate, Lung, colorectal, and Ovarian cancer screening trial: Mortality results after 13 years of follow-up. *Journal of the National Cancer Institute, 104*(2), 125–132.
Centers for Disease Control and Prevention. *Sexually transmitted treatment guidelines 2015: Special populations.* http://www.cdc.gov/std/tg2015/specialpops.htm. Accessed October 10, 2019.
Dains, J. E., Baumann, L. C., & Scheibel, P. (2024). *Advanced health assessment and clinical diagnosis in primary care* (7th ed.). St. Louis: Elsevier.
Deutsch, M. B. (Ed.). (2016). *Guidelines for the primary care of transgender and gender nonbinary people* (2nd ed.). UCSF Center of Excellence for Transgender Health. http://transhealth.ucsf.edu/trans?page=guidelines-home
Lowdermilk, D. L., & Perry, S. E. (2004). *Maternity and women's health care* (8th ed.). St. Louis: Mosby.
Martin, R. M., Donovan, J. L., Turner, E. L., Metcalfe, C., Young, G. J., Walsh, E. I., Lane, J. A., Noble, S., Oliver, S. E., Evans, S., Sterne, J. A. C., Holding, P., Ben-Shlomo, Y., Brindle, P., Williams, N. J., Hill, E. M., Ng, S. Y., Toole, J., Tazewell, M. K., Hughes, L. J., ... CAP Trial Group. (2018). Effect of a low-intensity PSA-based screening intervention on prostate cancer mortality: The CAP Randomized Clinical Trial. *JAMA, 319*(9), 883–895.
Schröder, F. H., Hugosson, J., Roobol, M. J., Tammela, T. L., Ciatto, S., Nelen, V., Kwiatkowski, M., Lujan, M., Lilja, H., Zappa, M., Denis, L. J., Recker, F., Berenguer, A., Määttänen, L., Bangma, C. H., Aus, G., Villers, A., Rebillard, X., van der Kwast, T., Blijenberg, B. G., ... ERSPC Investigators. (2009). Screening and prostate-cancer mortality in a randomized European study. *New England Journal of Medicine, 360,* 1320–1328.
Schröder, F. H., Hugosson, J., Roobol, M. J., Tammela, T. L., Ciatto, S., Nelen, V., Kwiatkowski, M., Lujan, M., Lilja, H., Zappa, M., Denis, L. J., Recker, F., Páez, A., Määttänen, L., Bangma, C. H., Aus, G., Carlsson, S., Villers, A., Rebillard, X., van der Kwast, T., ... ERSPC Investigators. (2012). Prostate-cancer mortality at 11 years of follow-up. *New England Journal of Medicine, 366,* 981–990.

Tong, G. X., Chai, J., Cheng, J., Xia, Y., Feng, R., Zhang, L., & Wang, D. B. (2014). Diagnostic value of rectal bleeding in predicting colorectal cancer: A systematic review. *Asian Pacific Journal of Cancer Prevention, 15*(2), 1015–1021.

Wesp, L. (2016). *Prostate and testicular cancer considerations in transgender women.* UCSF Transgender Care. https://transcare.ucsf.edu/guidelines/prostate-testicular-cancer

U.S. Preventive Services Task Force. (2018, May). *Prostate cancer: Screening: Final recommendation statement.* https://www.uspreventiveservicestaskforce.org/Page/Document/RecommendationStatementFinal/prostate-cancer-screening

American Cancer Society. (2023, November 20). *American Cancer Society recommendations for prostate cancer early detection.* http://www.cancer.org/cancer/prostate-cancer/detection-diagnosis-staging/acs-recommendations.html

American Cancer Society. (2020a, June 9). *Prostate cancer risk factors.* http://www.cancer.org/cancer/prostatecancer/detailedguide/prostate-cancer-risk-factors. Accessed October 8, 2020.

American Cancer Society. (2020b, July 8,). *Risk factors for anal cancer.* http://www.cancer.org/cancer/analcancer/detailedguide/anal-cancer-risk-factors. Accessed October 10, 2020.

Chapter 22

Beckenkamp, P. R., Lin, C. C., Macaskill, P., Michaleff, Z. A., Maher, C. G., & Moseley, A. M. (2017). Diagnostic accuracy of the Ottawa ankle and midfoot rules: A systematic review with meta-analysis. *British Journal of Sports Medicine, 51*(6), 504.

Blagojevic, M., Jinks, C., Jeffery, A., & Jordan, K. P. (2010). Risk factors for onset of osteoarthritis of the knee in older adults: A systematic review and meta-analysis. *Osteoarthritis and Cartilage, 18*(1), 24–33.

Jalili, M., & Gharebaghi, H. (2010). Validation of the Ottawa knee rule in Iran: A prospective study. *Emergency Medicine Journal, 27*(11), 849–851. http://dx.doi.org/10.1136/emj.2009.080267

Metcalfe, D., Perry, D. C., Claireaux, H. A., Simel, D. L., Zogg, C. K., & Costa, M. L. (2019). Does this patient have hip osteoarthritis? The rational clinical examination systematic review. *Journal of the American Medical Association, 322*(23), 2323–2333.

Watson, J., Zhao, M., & Ring D. (2010). Predictors of normal electrodiagnostic testing in the evaluation of suspected carpal tunnel syndrome. *Journal of Hand and Microsurgery, 2*(2), 47–50. http://dx.doi.org/10.1007/s12593-010-0012-9

Wilson, S. F., & Giddens, J. F. (2005). *Health assessment for nursing practice* (3rd ed.). St. Louis: Mosby.

Chapter 23

Afhami, S., Dehghan Manshadi, S. A., & Rezahosseini, O. (2017). Jolt accentuation of headache: Can this maneuver rule out acute meningitis? *BMC Research Notes, 10,* 540. http://dx.doi.org/10.1186/s13104-017-2877-1

Akaishi, T., Kobayashi, J., Abe, M., Ishizawa, K., Nakashima, I., Aoki, M., & Ishii, T. (2019). Sensitivity and specificity of meningeal signs in patients with meningitis. *Journal of General and Family Medicine, 20*(5), 193–198. https://doi.org/10.1002/jgf2.268

Ballard, J. L., Khoury, J. C., Wedig, K., Wang, L., Eilers-Walsman, B. L., & Lipp, R. (1991). New Ballard Score, expanded to include extremely premature infants. *The Journal of Pediatrics, 119*(3), 417–423.

Barragán, R., Coltell, O., Portolés, O., Asensio, E. M., Sorlí, J. V., Ortega-Azorín, C., González, J. I., Sáiz, C., Fernández-Carrión, R., Ordovas, J. M., & Corella, D. (2018). Bitter, sweet, salty, sour and umami taste perception decreases with age: Sex-specific analysis, modulation by genetic variants and taste-preference associations in 18 to 80 year-old subjects. *Nutrients, 10*(10), 1539. http://dx.doi.org/10.3390/nu10101539.

Boss, B. J., & Huether, S. E. (2019). Disorders of the central and peripheral nervous systems and the neuromuscular junction. In K. L. McCance, S. E. Huether, V. L. Brashers, & N. S. Rote (Eds.), *Pathophysiology: The biologic basis for disease in adults and children* (8th ed., pp. 550–599). St. Louis: Elsevier.

Burkett, J. G., & Ailani, J. (2018). An up to date review of pseudotumor cerebri syndrome. *Current Neurology and Neuroscience Reports, 18,* 33 http://dx.doi.org/10.1007/s11910-018-0839-1

Butterfield, R. J., & Huether, S. E. (2019). Alterations in neurologic function in children. In K. L. McCance, S. E. Huether, V. L. Brashers, & N. S. Rote (Eds.), *Pathophysiology: The biologic basis for disease in adults and children* (8th ed., pp 619–643). St. Louis: Elsevier.

By the 2023 American Geriatrics Society Beers Criteria® Update Expert Panel. (2023). American Geriatrics Society 2023 updated AGS Beers Criteria® for potentially inappropriate medication use in older adults. *Journal of the American Geriatrics Society, 71*(7), 2052–2081. doi:10.1111/jgs.18372

Centers for Disease Control and Prevention. (2017). *Assessment: Timed get up and go.* https://www.cdc.gov/steadi/pdf/TUG_test-print.pdf

Centers for Disease Control and Prevention. (2019). *Data and statistics on spina bifida.* https://www.cdc.gov/ncbddd/spinabifida/data.html

Centers for Disease Control and Prevention. (2019). *STEADI: Stopping elderly accidents, deaths, and injuries.* http://cdc.gov/steadi

De Ru, J. A., Brennan, P. A., & Martens, E. (2015). Antiviral agents convey added benefit over steroids alone in Bell's palsy; decompression should be considered in patients who are not recovering. *Journal of Laryngology and Otology, 129*(4), 300–306.

Deng, T., Jia, J. P., Zhang, T., Guo, D., & Yang, L. (2013). Cortical versus non-cortical lesions affect expression of Babinski sign. *Neurological Sciences, 34*(6), 855–859.

Gilhus, N. E., & Verschuuren, J. J. (2015). Myasthenia gravis: Subgroup classification and therapeutic strategies. *The Lancet. Neurology, 14*(10), 1023–1036.

Heft, M. W., & Robinson, M. E. (2014). Age differences in suprathreshold sensory function. *Age (Dordrecht, Netherlands),* 36(1), 1–8.

Iguchi, M., Noguchi, Y., Yamamoto, S., Tanaka, Y., & Tsujimoto, H. (2020). Diagnostic test accuracy of jolt accentuation for headache in acute meningitis in the emergency setting. *Cochrane Database of Systematic Reviews,* 6(6), CD012824. doi:10.1002/14651858.CD012824

Knobe, M., Giesen, M., Plate, S., Gradl-Dietsch, G., Buecking, B., Eschbach, D., van Laack, W., & Pape, H. C. (2016). The Aachen mobility and Balance index to measure physiological falls risk: A comparison with the Tinetti POMA scale. *European Journal of Trauma and Emergency Surgery, 42,* 537–545. http://dx.doi.org/10.1007/s00068-016-0693-2

Narang, S. K., Fingarson, A., Lukefahr, J., & COUNCIL ON CHILD ABUSE AND NEGLECT. (2020). Abusive head trauma in infants and children. *Pediatrics, 145*(4), e20200203. doi:10.1542/peds.2020-0203

Picascia, M., Zangaglia, R., Bernini, S., Minafra, B., Sinforiani, E., & Pacchetti, C. (2015). A review of cognitive impairment and differential diagnosis in idiopathic normal pressure hydrocephalus. *Functional Neurology, 30*(4), 217–228.

Reuter, E. M., Voelcker-Rehage, C., Vieluf, S., & Godde, B. (2012). Touch perception throughout working life: Effects of age and expertise. *Experimental Brain Research, 216*(2), 287–297.

Tinetti, M. E. (1986). Performance-oriented assessment of mobility problems in elderly patients. *Journal of the American Geriatrics Society, 34*(2), 119–126.

Watson, J. C., & Dyck, J. B. (2015). Peripheral neuropathy: A practical guide for diagnosis and symptom management. *Mayo Clinic Proceedings, 90*(7), 940–951.

Chapter 24

Caplin, M., & Saunders, T. (2015). Utilizing teach-back to reinforce patient education: A step-by-step approach. *Orthopedic Nursing, 34*(6), 365–368.

Chapter 25

Ackerman, K. E., & Misra, M. (2018). Amenorrhoea in adolescent female athletes. *The Lancet. Child & Adolescent Health, 2*(9), 677–688.

2019 Preparticipation physical evaluation medical history and physical examination forms, endorsed by the American Academy of Family Physicians, American Academy of Pediatrics, American College of Sports Medicine, American Medical Society for Sports Medicine, American Orthopedic Society for Sports Medicine, and American Osteopathic Academy of Sports Medicine. Forms updated 2023 and publicly. https://www.aap.org/en/patient-care/preparticipation-physical-evaluation/. Accessed November 25, 2024.

American Academy of Pediatrics. (2021). *Sports physical: When, where, who should do it?* https://www.healthychildren.org/English/healthy-living/sports/Pages/Sports-Physical-PPE.aspx

Berry, S. A., Geleske, T. A., Holm, I., Hopkin, R. J., Introne, W. J., Lyons, M. J., Monteil, D. C., Scheuerle, A., Stoler, J. M., Vergano, S. A., Chen, E., Hamid, R., Downs, S. M., ... Spire, P. (2022). Health supervision for children and adolescents with Down syndrome. *Pediatrics, 149*(5), e2022057010.

Carbone, P. S., Smith, P. J., Lewis, C., & LeBlanc, C. (2021). Promoting the participation of children and adolescents with disabilities in sports, recreation, and physical activity. *Pediatrics, 148*(6), e2021054664.

De Souza, M. J., Strock, N. C. A., Ricker, E. A., Koltun, K. J., Barrack, M., Joy, E., Nattiv, A., Hutchinson, M., Misra, M., & Williams, N. I. (2022). The path towards progress: A critical review to advance the science of the female and male athlete triad and relative energy deficiency in sport. *Sports Medicine (Auckland, N.Z.), 52*(1), 13–23.

Endres, B. D., Kerr, Z. Y., Stearns, R. L., Adams, W. M., Hosokawa, Y., Huggins, R. A., Kucera, K. L., & Casa, D. J. (2019). Epidemiology of Sudden Death in Organized Youth Sports in the United States, 2007-2015. *Journal of Athletic Training, 54*(4), 349–355.

Fatt, S. J., George, E., Hay, P., Jeacocke, N., Gotkiewicz, E., & Mitchison, D. (2024). An umbrella review of body image concerns, disordered eating, and eating disorders in elite athletes. *Journal of Clinical Medicine, 13*(14), 4171.

Flynn, J. T., Kaelber, D. C., Baker-Smith, C. M., et al. (2017). Subcommittee on screening and management of high blood pressure in children: Clinical practice guideline for screening and management of high blood pressure in children and adolescents. *Pediatrics, 140*(3), e2017190.

Lumba-Brown, A., Yeates, K. O., Sarmiento, K., Breiding, M. J., Haegerich, T. M., Gioia, G. A., Turner, M., Benzel, E. C., Suskauer, S. J., Giza, C. C., Joseph, M., Broomand, C., Weissman, B., Gordon, W., Wright, D. W., Moser, R. S., McAvoy, K., Ewing-Cobbs, L., Duhaime, A. C., Putukian, M., ... Timmons, S. D. (2018). Diagnosis and Management of Mild Traumatic Brain Injury in Children: A Systematic Review. *JAMA Pediatrics, 172*(11), e182847.

MacDonald, J., Schaefer, M., & Stumph, J. (2021). The preparticipation physical evaluation. *American Family Physician, 103*(9), 539–546.

Miller, S. M., & Peterson, A. R. (2019). The sports preparticipation evaluation. *Pediatrics in Review, 40*(3), 108–128.

Patricios, J. S., Schneider, K. J., Dvorak, J., Ahmed, O. H., Blauwet, C., Cantu, R. C., Davis, G. A., Echemendia, R. J., Makdissi, M., McNamee, M., Broglio, S., Emery, C. A., Feddermann-Demont, N., Fuller, G. W., Giza, C. C., Guskiewicz, K. M., Hainline, B., Iverson, G. L., Kutcher, J. S., Leddy, J. J., ... Meeuwisse, W. (2023). Consensus statement on concussion in sport: The 6th International conference on concussion in sport-Amsterdam, October 2022. *British Journal of Sports Medicine, 57*(11), 695–711.

Sarmiento, K., Thomas, K. E., Daugherty, J., Waltzman, D., Haarbauer-Krupa, J. K., Peterson, A. B., Haileyesus, T., & Breiding, M. J. (2019). Emergency department visits for sports- and recreation-related traumatic brain injuries among children - United States, 2010-2016. *MMWR. Morbidity and Mortality Weekly Report, 68*(10), 237–242.

Spencer, R., & Quraishi, S. (2023). Athlete Screening and sudden cardiac death. *Pediatrics in Review, 44*(12), 669–681.

Statuta, S. M., Asif, I. M., & Drezner, J. A. (2017). Relative energy deficiency in sport (RED-S). *British Journal of Sports Medicine, 51*(21), 1570–1571.

Sweeting, J., & Semsarian, C. (2018). Sudden Cardiac death in athletes. *Heart, Lung & Circulation, 27*(9), 1072–1077.

Tenforde, A. S., Carlson, J. L., Chang, A., Sainani, K. L., Shultz, R., Kim, J. H., Cutti, P., Golden, N. H., & Fredericson, M. (2017). Association of the female athlete triad risk assessment stratification to the development of bone stress injuries in collegiate athletes. *American Journal of Sports Medicine, 45*(2), 302–310.

Chapter 26

Ali, A., Vahdata, S. S., Ghaffarzad, A., Mousavi, H., & Mirza-Aghazadeh-Attari, M. (2018). National emergency x-radiography utilization study guidelines versus Canadian C-spine guidelines on trauma patients: A prospective analytical study. *PLoS One, 13*(11), e0206283, http://dx.doi.org/10.1371/journal.pone.0206283

American College of Surgeons Committee on Trauma. (2018). *ATLS: Advanced trauma life support* (10th ed.). Chicago, IL: Author.

American Heart Association. (2016). *Pediatric advanced life support: Provider manual.* Dallas, TX: Author.

Bethel, J. (2012). Emergency care of children and adults with head injury. *Nursing Standard, 26*(43), 49–58.

Bhimani, A. D., Macrinici, V., Ghelani, S., Huang, E. Y., Khan, N. I., Saw, T. A., & Mejia, A. (2018). Delving deeper into informed consent: Legal and ethical dilemmas of emergency consent, surrogate consent, and intraoperative consultation. *Orthopedics, 41*(6), e741–e746. http://dx.doi.org/10.3928/01477447-20180912-10

Ciottone, G. (2024). *Ciottone's disaster medicine* (3rd ed.). Elsevier.

Cremonini, C., et al. (2024). Geriatric trauma. In V. Boccardi & L. Marano (Eds.), *The frail surgical patient. Practical issues in geriatrics.* Springer, Cham. https://doi.org/10.1007/978-3-031-77707-3_17

Dellinger, R. P., Roy, A., & Parillo, J. E. (2019). Severe sepsis and septic shock. In J. E. Parillo & R. P. Dellinger (Eds.), *Critical care medicine: Principles of diagnosis and management in the adult* (5th ed., pp. 323–345). Philadelphia, PA: Elsevier.

Hocker, S., Tatum, W. O., LaRoche, S., & Freeman, W. D. (2014). Refractory and super-refractory status epilepticus—an update. *Current Neurology and Neuroscience Reports, 14*(6), 452.

James, H. E. (1986). Neurologic evaluation and support of the child with acute brain insult. *Pediatric Annals, 15*(1), 17.

Kleinman, M. E., Brennan, E. E., Goldberger, Z. D., Swor, R. A., Terry, M., Bobrow, B. J., Gazmuri, R. J., Travers, A. H., & Rea, T. (2015). Part 5: Adult basic life support and cardiopulmonary resuscitation quality: 2015 American Heart Association Guidelines Update for Cardiopulmonary Resuscitation and Emergency Cardiovascular Care. *Circulation, 132*(Suppl. 2), S414–S435.

Maconochie, I. K., et al. (2021). Pediatric Life Support 2020 International Consensus on cardiopulmonary resuscitation and emergency cardiovascular care science with treatment recommendations. *Pediatrics, 147*(Suppl. 1), e2020038505B. doi:10.1542/peds.2020-038505B

Schur, J. D. (2014). Geriatric trauma. In J. A. Marx, R. S. Hockberger, R. M. Walls, et al. *Rosen's emergency medicine* (8th ed., pp. 324–329.e2). Philadelphia: Elsevier.

Teasdale, G., & Jennett, B. (1974). Assessment of coma and impaired consciousness: A practical scale. *Lancet, 2*:81–84.

Teasdale, G., Maas, A., Lecky, F., Manley, G., Stocchetti, N., & Murray, G. (2014). The Glasgow Coma Scale at 40 years: Standing the test of time. *The Lancet. Neurology, 13,* 844–854.

Yaseen, M., Ali, M., Ali, S., Hussain, A., Joo, M. I., & Kim, H. C. (2024). Cervical spine fracture detection and classification using two-stage deep learning methodology. In *IEEE Access* (Vol. 12, pp. 72131-72142).

Index

Note: Page numbers followed by "f" indicate figures, "t" indicate tables, and "b" indicate boxes.

INDEX

INDEX

P

INDEX

Q

R

X

Z

Features Box

CLINICAL PEARLS

DIFFERENTIAL DIAGNOSIS

Evidence-Based Practice in Physical Examination

FUNCTIONAL ASSESSMENT

Patient Safety

Physical Examination Components